CARE OF THE CARDIAC SURGICAL PATIENT

Robert S. Litwak, M.D.

Professor of Surgery
Mount Sinai School of Medicine
Attending Surgeon and Chief
Division of Cardiothoracic Surgery
The Mount Sinai Hospital
New York, New York

Roy A. Jurado, M.D.

Associate Professor of Surgery
Mount Sinai School of Medicine
Associate Attending Surgeon
Division of Cardiothoracic Surgery
The Mount Sinai Hospital
New York, New York

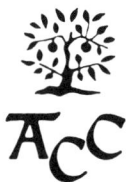

APPLETON-CENTURY-CROFTS / Norwalk, Connecticut

Copyright © 1982 by APPLETON-CENTURY-CROFTS
A Publishing Division of Prentice-Hall, Inc.

All rights reserved. This book, or any parts thereof, may not be used or reproduced in any manner without written permission. For information, address Appleton-Century-Crofts, 25 Van Zant Street, East Norwalk, CT 06855.

82 83 84 85 86 / 10 9 8 7 6 5 4 3 2 1

Prentice-Hall International, Inc., London
Prentice-Hall of Australia, Pty. Ltd., Sydney
Prentice-Hall of India Private Limited, New Delhi
Prentice-Hall of Japan, Inc., Tokyo
Prentice-Hall of Southeast Asia (Pte.) Ltd., Singapore
Whitehall Books Ltd., Wellington, New Zealand

NOTICE: The authors and publisher of this book have made every effort to ensure that drug dosages cited herein are accurate and in accord with standards accepted at the time of publication. The user is advised, however, to consult product information accompanying any drug they intend to administer to ascertain that the recommended dosage or contraindications for its use have not been changed.

Library of Congress Cataloging in Publication Data
  Main entry under title:

  Care of the cardiac surgical patient.

    Includes bibliographies and index.
    1. Heart—Surgery. 2. Heart—Surgery—Complications and sequelae. 3. Therapeutics, Surgical. I. *Litwak*, Robert S.   II. Jurado, Roy A. [DNLM: 1. Heart surgery. 2. Intraoperative care.   WG 169 L782c]
  RD598.C356 1982   617'.412   82-8779
    ISBN 0-8385-1062-0   AACR2

Text design: Gloria J. Moyer
Cover design: Lynn M. Luchetti

PRINTED IN THE UNITED STATES OF AMERICA

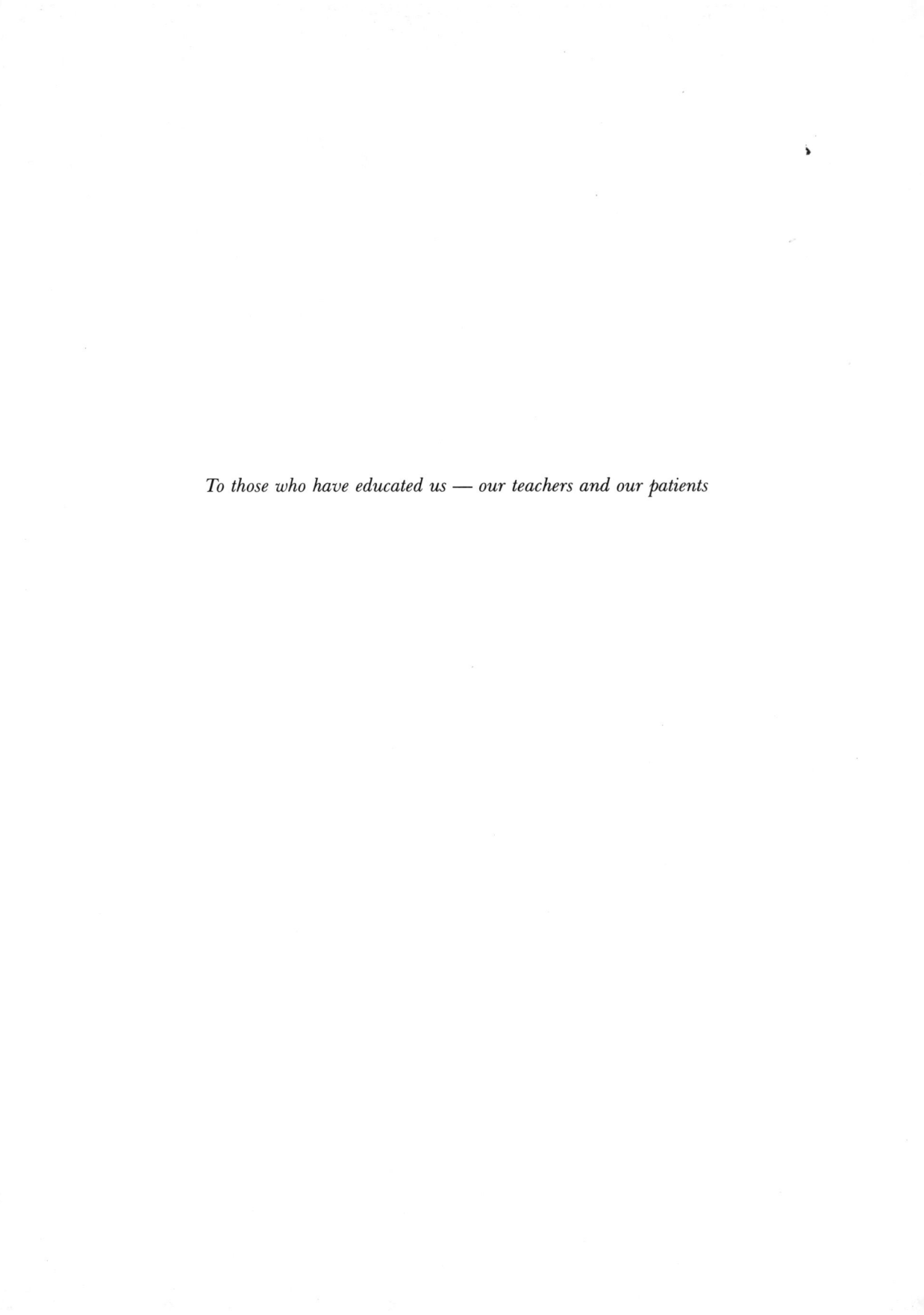

To those who have educated us — our teachers and our patients

Contributors

Stuart H. Bartle, M.D.
Assistant Clinical Professor Psychiatry
Mount Sinai School of Medicine
Assistant Attending in Psychiatry
Mount Sinai Hospital
New York, New York

John H. L. Bland, M.B., B.Chir. (Deceased)
Assistant Professor of Anesthesia
Harvard Medical School
Associate Anesthetist,
 Massachusetts General Hospital
Boston, Massachusetts

Edwin G. Brown, M.D.
Associate Professor of Pediatrics
Mount Sinai School of Medicine
Associate Attending Pediatrician and
Director, Newborn Services
The Mount Sinai Hospital
New York, New York

Murray Budabin, M.D.
Assistant Clinical Professor of Neurology
Mount Sinai School of Medicine
Assistant Attending in Neurology
The Mount Sinai Hospital
New York, New York

Simon Dack, M.D.
Clinical Professor of Medicine (Emeritus)
Mount Sinai School of Medicine
Consultant Cardiologist
The Mount Sinai Hospital
New York, New York

Manuel R. Estioko, M.D.
Assistant Professor of Surgery
Mount Sinai School of Medicine
Assistant Attending Surgeon
Division of Cardiothoracic Surgery
The Mount Sinai Hospital
New York, New York

Stanley Giannelli, M.D.
Professor of Surgery
New York Medical College
Attending Cardiothoracic Surgeon
St. Vincent's Hospital & Medical Center
New York, New York

Sheldon Glabman, M.D.
Associate Professor of Medicine
Mount Sinai School of Medicine
Director, Robert W. Johnson, Jr. Renal
 Treatment Center
The Mount Sinai Hospital
New York, New York

Frank Gollan, M.D.
Assistant Chief of Nuclear Medicine
Veteran's Administration Hospital
Miami, Florida
Professor of Surgery in Anesthesiology
University of Miami School of Medicine
Miami, Florida

Alvin J. Gordon, M.D.
Clinical Professor of Medicine
Mount Sinai Medical School
Attending Physician for Cardiology
The Mount Sinai Hospital
New York, New York

J. Donald Hill, M.D.
Chairman, Department of Cardiovascular
　Surgery
Presbyterian Hospital
Pacific Medical Center
San Francisco, California

Joseph Jagust, M.D.
Assistant Clinical Professor of
　Anesthesiology
Mount Sinai School of Medicine
Associate Attending in Anesthesiology
The Mount Sinai Hospital
New York, New York

Roy A. Jurado, M.D.
Associate Professor of Surgery
Mount Sinai School of Medicine
Associate Attending Surgeon
Division of Cardiothoracic Surgery
The Mount Sinai Hospital
New York, New York

Gerard A. Kaiser, M.D.
DeWitt and Lucille Daughtry Professor
Chief of Thoracic and Cardiovascular
　Surgery
University of Miami School of Medicine
Jackson Memorial Hospital
Miami, Florida

Arnold M. Katz, M.D.
Professor of Medicine
School of Medicine
Head, Division of Cardiology
University of Connecticut Health Center
Farmington, Connecticut

Demetrios G. Lappas, M.D.
Associate Professor of Anesthesia
Harvard Medical School
Associate Anesthetist
Massachusetts General Hospital
Boston, Massachusetts

Myron B. Laver, M.D.
Professor and Chairman
Department of Anesthesia
University of Basel
Basel, Switzerland

Robert S. Litwak, M.D.
Professor of Surgery
Mount Sinai School of Medicine
Attending Surgeon and Chief
Division of Cardiothoracic Surgery
The Mount Sinai Hospital
New York, New York

C. Harold Mielke, Jr., M.D.
Associate Professor of Medicine
University of California San Francisco
Chief of Hematology Research
Presbyterian Hospital of
　Pacific Medical Center
San Francisco, California

Burt R. Meyers, M.D.
Professor of Medicine, Division of Infectious
　Diseases
Mount Sinai School of Medicine
Attending Physician
The Mount Sinai Hospital
New York, New York

John J. Osborn, M.D.
Associate Professor of Pediatrics
Stanford University
Stanford, California
Director of the Institute of Biomedical
　Engineering Sciences
Pacific Medical Center
San Francisco, California

CONTRIBUTORS

Sidney Owitz, M.D.
Assistant Clinical Professor of
  Anesthesiology
Mount Sinai School of Medicine
Associate Attending in Anesthesiology
The Mount Sinai Hospital
New York, New York

E. Converse Peirce, II, M.D.
The Henry Kaufmann Professor of
  Hyperbaric Surgery
Mount Sinai School of Medicine,
  New York, New York
Section Chief in Surgery
Veteran's Administration Medical Center
Bronx, New York

Robert Rodvien, M.D.
Senior Scientist
Institute of Medical Sciences
San Francisco, California
Chief of Hematology
Presbyterian Hospital of
  Pacific Medical Center
San Francisco, California

Beat von Albertini, M.D.
Clinical Assistant Professor of Medicine
Stanford Hemodialysis Center
Stanford University School of Medicine
Stanford, California

Albert L. Waldo, M.D.
Professor of Medicine
Director Cardiac Arrhythmia Service
The School of Medicine
University of Alabama in Birmingham
Birmingham, Alabama

Contents

Preface xiii

1. Optimal Body Perfusion 1
   Frank Gollan, M.D.

2. Concepts of Patient Care 17
   Robert S. Litwak, M.D.; Simon Dack, M.D.

3. Preoperative Evaluation and Care 25
   Roy A. Jurado, M.D.

4. Anesthesia for Cardiac Surgery 43
   John H. L. Bland, M.B., B.Chir.; Demetrios G. Lappas, M.D.

5. Open Intracardiac Operation Employing Extracorporeal
   Circulation 65
   Robert S. Litwak, M.D.; Stanley Giannelli, M.D.

6. Patient Surveillance and General Care 119
   Roy A. Jurado, M.D.; John J. Osborn, M.D.

7. Concepts of Acid-Base Balance 161
   E. Converse Peirce II, M.D.

8. Myocardial Energetics 183
   Arnold M. Katz, M.D.

9. Analysis, Maintenance, and Support of Cardiac Function
   After Cardiac Surgery 199
   Robert S. Litwak, M.D.

10. Electrophysiologic Considerations for the Cardiac Surgical
    Patient 241
    Albert L. Waldo, M.D.; Gerard A. Kaiser, M.D.

11. Lung Function Following Open Heart Surgery 281
    Myron B. Laver, M.D.

12. Concepts of Ventilatory and Respiratory Care 309
    *Roy A. Jurado, M.D.; Joseph Jagust, M.D.;
    Sidney Owitz, M.D.*

13. Management of Ventilatory and Respiratory Complications 337
    Roy A. Jurado, M.D.; Sidney Owitz, M.D.;
    Joseph Jagust, M.D.

14. Renal Failure in Cardiac Surgery 355
    Sheldon Glabman, M.D.; Beat von Albertini, M.D.;
    Robert S. Litwak, M.D.

15. Bleeding and Hemorrhagic Complications 367
    J. Donald Hill, M.D.; Robert Rodvien, M.D.;
    C. Harold Mielke, Jr., M.D.

16. Neurologic Complications of Cardiac Surgery 387
    Murray Budabin, M.D.

17. Psychiatric Complications of Cardiac Surgery 395
    Stuart H. Bartle, M.D.

18. Infections Associated with Open Heart Surgery 403
    Burt R. Meyers, M.D.; Roy A. Jurado, M.D.

19. Operative and Postoperative Care of the Neonate and
    Pediatric Cardiac Surgical Patient 433
    Robert S. Litwak, M.D.; Edwin G. Brown, M.D.

20. Permanent Cardiac Pacemakers: Management and Problems 455
    Alvin J. Gordon, M.D.; Manuel R. Estioko, M.D.

21. Special Techniques of Care Employed in the Cardiac Surgical
    Intensive Care Unit 489
    Roy A. Jurado, M.D.

22. Cardiac Surgical Pharmacology 541
    Roy A. Jurado, M.D.

    Index 599

Preface

THIS TEXT IS the outgrowth of a brief compendium which dealt with perioperative care of cardiac surgical patients and was written some years ago primarily for our cardiothoracic surgical residents. We were pleasantly surprised to learn that the notes were being requested by medical residents and cardiology fellows as well. Encouraged by our colleagues, we expanded the material into this book. In preparing this text the editors and authors constantly have been mindful of the many basic science and clinical investigators—both known and unknown—whose contributions have been seminal to the genesis and maturation of cardiac surgery. One recalls Claude Bernard's observation: "The names of the prime movers of science disappear gradually in a general fusion, and the more science advances, the more impersonal and detached it becomes."

Books such as this are useful only if they bring together information in a fashion that does not result in a superannuated effort as a consequence of the necessary temporal delay between textual development and publication. Toward this end, and recognizing that specific methods and techniques will change, this text seeks to emphasize understanding of well documented and relatively unchanging *concepts* of normal and abnormal subsystem performance associated with cardiac disease as well as those additional distortions imposed by contemporary cardiac surgical management.

Multiple authorship has necessitated that the editors take occasional editorial liberties in attempting to adhere to the central theme of the text and to avoid unnecessary repetition. However, the reader will discern some occasional overlap which was permitted whenever it was deemed to be helpful in the development of a concept. The editors express their profound thanks to our colleagues who have contributed their special expertise to this text and we pray that they will indulge us in the editorial traumata to which their efforts occasionally have been subjected.

We also wish to express our appreciation to Doctor Howard Shiang for his editorial and photographic guidance and Maureen Jones and Ellen Felten for their medical artistry. The secretarial staff, in particular Dagmar Martinez, Doris Toback, Marion Carter, Victoria Afanador and Marian Wezmar, labored mightily and without complaint in this endeavor and we are most grateful. Finally, our sincere appreciation is extended to Mr. Robert E. McGrath and John Morgan of Appleton-Century-Crofts whose meticulous attention to detail and their insistence on maintenance of high publication standards will hopefully allow this book to make a useful contribution to the field.

CARE OF THE CARDIAC SURGICAL PATIENT

1. Optimal Body Perfusion

Frank Gollan

Upon this gifted age, in its dark hour
Rains from the sky a meteoric shower
Of facts . . . they lie unquestioned, uncombined,
Wisdom enough to teach us of our ills
Is daily spun, but there exists no loom
To weave it into fabric.

Edna St. Vincent Millay

There is little doubt that in the middle of the twentieth century the dramatic advent of open heart surgery heralded the opening of the last frontier of surgery. For the first time in the history of medicine and of civilization, people were able to free themselves temporarily from the reliance on their own heart and lungs, and to control the flow, composition, and temperature of blood at their own will. The ability to operate without haste on an empty, quiescent, and viable heart is an achievement to be recorded in the ascent of humankind. The development of body perfusion physiology has made it possible to snatch a quarter of a million patients a year all over the world from untimely death. In this chapter I will try to bring this new field into the broad context of comparative physiology, and then consider the possible applicability of these concepts to acute myocardial infarction in particular.

Even before John Gibbon, Jr. bypassed the heart and lungs of a patient in 1953, some physiologists realized that with pump-oxygenators they could extend controlled perfusion of an isolated organ to an isolated organism. At that time a most unusual thing happened. The closer they adhered to the normal physiologic conditions the worse were the results, and the more they deviated from the accepted rules, the more experimental dogs survived. This occurred because the artificial heart and lung machines—except for their names—were able to meet only the demands of the core of the human body, not those of the periphery. They were able to supply the 71 percent of total blood flow to 7 percent of body weight comprising the internal organs, but left 93 percent of body weight, consisting of skin, muscle, and residual tissue, underperfused (Fig. 1–1).

After one hour of cardiopulmonary bypass a severe oxygen debt developed in the peripheral muscle mass, and experimental animals died in prolonged shock. Only those surgeons who did not trust the brainless dinosaur machines and continued to operate with lightning speed became pioneers in open heart surgery. For short periods of time the peripheral tissues with their low oxygen consumption were able to withstand the induced ischemia, but in longer operations the accumulated oxygen debt could not be paid off by the patient, only by the next of kin. There are no exceptions to Haldane's stern rule: "Anoxia does not stop the machine, it wrecks it." This experience does not hold out much hope for an artificial heart inside the chest to prolong the span or improve the quality of life,

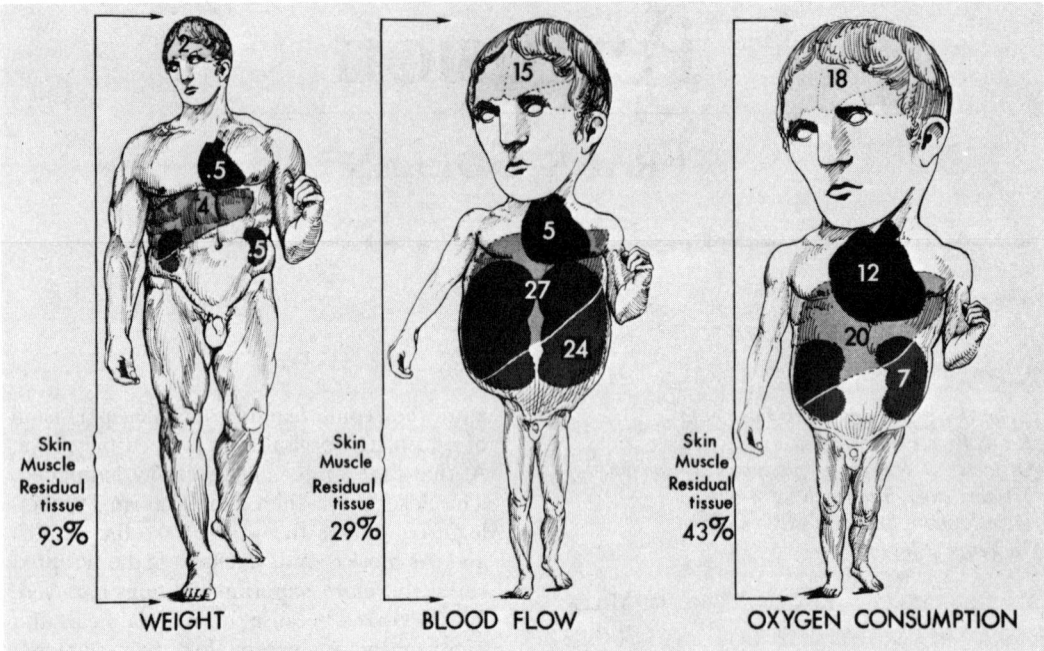

Figure 1–1. The differences between weight, blood flow, and oxygen consumption of human organs can be visualized by the metamorphosis of people who have grown or shrunk accordingly.

which requires an automatic increase of muscle blood flow the moment a patient feels strong enough to get out of bed.

However, by the powerful tool of strictly controlled experimentation on total body perfusion, the following prerequisites for optimal perfusion emerged.

REQUIREMENTS OF OPTIMAL TISSUE PERFUSION

Procedure	Mechanism
• High Flow Rate	• Low Viscosity
• Hemodilution	• Low Oxygen Consumption
• Blood Cooling	
• Hypercarbia	• Preferential Core Perfusion
• Slight Hypoxemia	
• Capillary Perfusion	• Vasolidation

At present, the first three requirements have found widespread clinical applications. The need for the highest blood flow obtainable is self-evident.

At first thought, it appears illogical to dilute the blood, because practically all of the oxygen is bound to the hemoglobin of red cells and only a negligible amount is physically dissolved in the water of the blood plasma and of the red cells. Still, a creature on this earth has evolved without any blood pigment to combine with oxygen (Fig. 1–2). The transparent, glasslike icefish sustains its sluggish life in the cold Antarctic Ocean by physically dissolved oxygen only. Without any red cells, the icefish is the world champion of low blood viscosity. It is possible to maintain the life of dogs without hemoglobin by using a pump-oxygenator for a rapid blood exchange with a cold plasma expander. This physiologic metamorphosis of a dog into an icefish has actually been applied clinically in poisoning with carbon monoxide and short-acting barbiturates, severe transfusion reactions, Reye's Syndrome, and some cases of postnecrotic hepatic coma.

Whenever the oxygen content of the blood is reduced, adrenalin is released and

OPTIMAL BODY PERFUSION

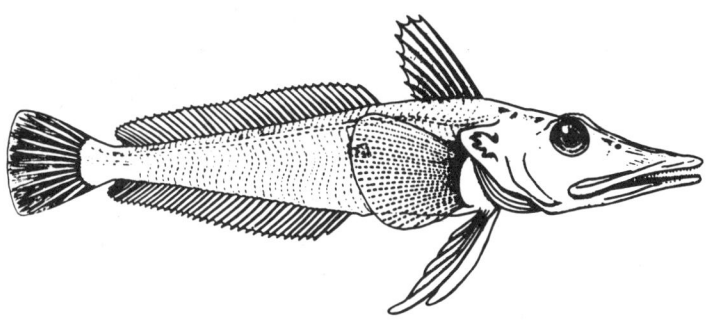

Figure 1–2. *Chaenocephalus*, which the Eskimos call icefish or crocodile fish, lives without the benefits or drawbacks of red blood cells.

the cardiac output goes up; or, whatever the blood lacks in oxygen, the heart makes up by speed. Since the product of the cardiac output and the arterial oxygen content results in the total oxygen delivery to the body, the question arises as to the optimal conditions to deliver the greatest amount of oxygen to the tissues (Fig. 1–3). Against all expectations this does not happen at a normal hematocrit; but at a hematocrit of 30 percent, the increased cardiac output supplies the greatest amount of oxygen (Messmer et al., 1972). Normally, the tremendous surplus of red cells is held as a reserve in functionally inactive capillaries, to be mobilized for active fight or flight duty. Since our patients are not training for the Olympic Games, they will be better off with a lower blood viscosity and a higher cardiac output.

The regional distribution of blood flow is proportionately increased during anemia or induced hemodilution, except for the heart, which in a retrograde fashion helps itself to the first and bigger piece of the pie before dividing the rest to all the other organs (Fig. 1–4). This preferential treatment for the never-resting heart is fully justified because it has the highest consumption of oxygen per gram of tissue and its meals are constantly interrupted by its systolic work. The second heart sound tolls the bell to start the diastolic lunch break and the first heart sound ends it abruptly. Fortunately, the coronary flow is excessive during hemodilution and particularly after a period of ischemia (Bassenge et al., 1972).

The third prerequisite to improve the oxygen balance of the peripheral tissues during total body perfusion is the induction of hypothermia. The natural masters of self-induced hypothermia are the hibernating animals, whose winterized biologic clock, identified as a neuropolypeptide, reduces first their heart rate and then their temperature to just a few degrees above the freezing point of water (Swan, 1974). They can live off their brown fat deposits for many months because, in spite of the increase of blood viscosity due to low

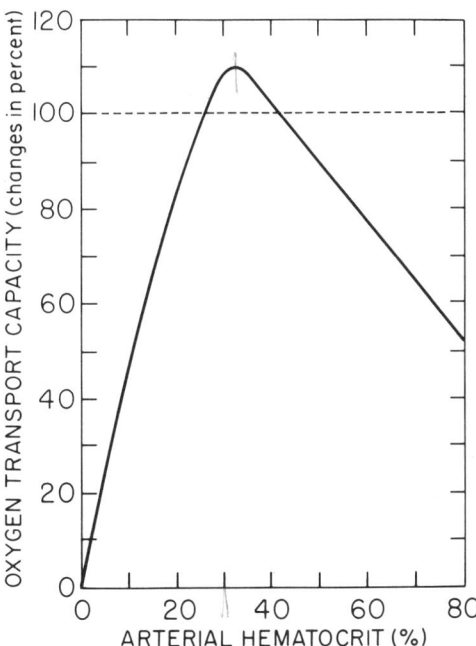

Figure 1–3. Under normal conditions the highest oxygen delivery to the tissues occurs at the abnormally low hematocrit of 30 percent.

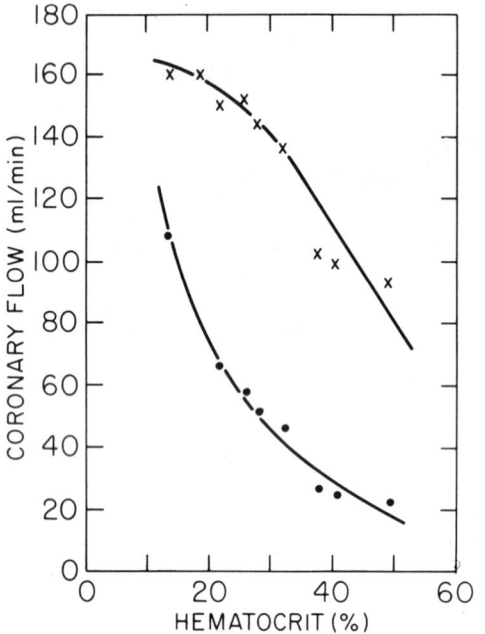

Figure 1-4. During hemodilution the coronary circulation is favored, particularly after ischemia (● at rest; x reactive hyperemia).

temperature, enough water is liberated by fat metabolism to prevent hemoconcentration. Although their total cardiac output is reduced by the slow heart rate to only a fraction of the awake state, the distribution again favors the heart (Fig. 1-5) (Bullard and Funkhausen, 1962).

Perfusion hypothermia, in contradistinction to peripheral cooling, imitates the inimitable hibernators because the much faster temperature changes of the internal organs prove that much more cooled or rewarmed blood is reaching the core than the periphery of the body (Fig. 1-6) (Gollan, 1959).

The fourth prerequisite for optimal body perfusion is mild hypercarbia. Since CO_2 is an end product of mammalian combustion and is retained in chronic obstructive pulmonary disease, we have become conditioned to consider it as a bad waste product and, like the good guys in the western movies, we are honor bound to drive it out of the body. However, even in asphyxia we can blame CO_2 only for guilt by association for having found it in the compromising company of anoxia. In fact, CO_2 protects humans from lack of oxygen, as Antonio Mosso discovered in his cou-

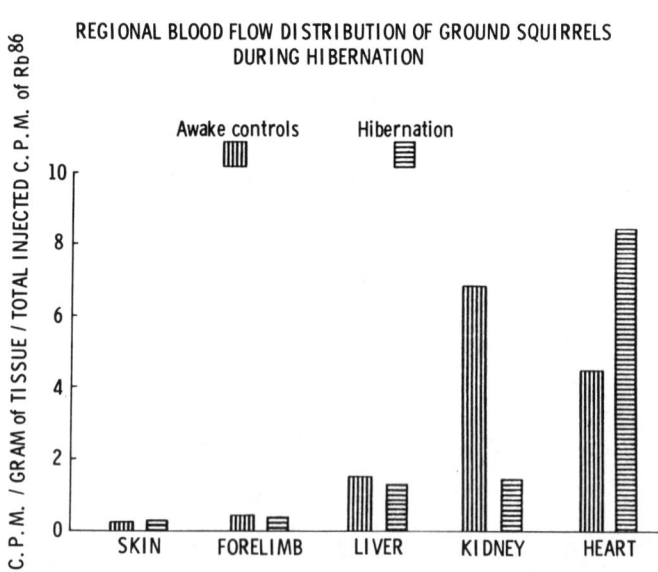

Figure 1-5. Hibernating animals divert blood flow from all organs to their hearts.

OPTIMAL BODY PERFUSION

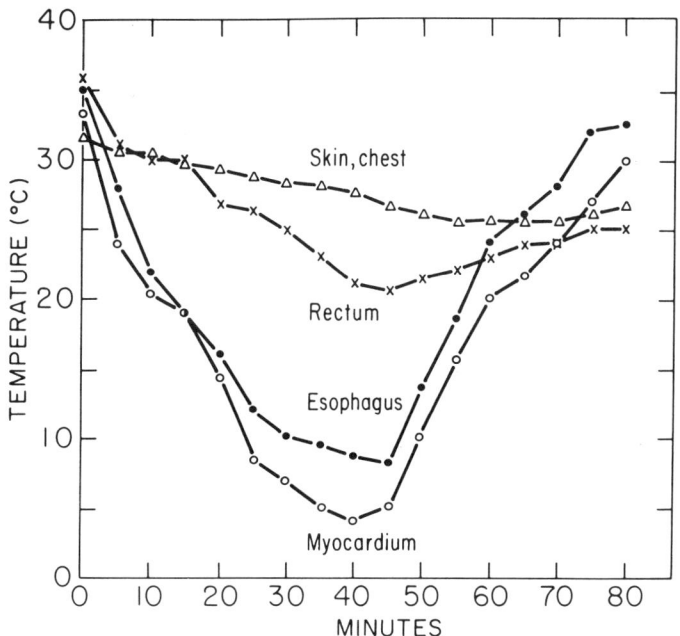

Figure 1-6. The rapid cooling rate of the heart during bloodstream cooling expresses the higher flow rate as measured by this continuous thermodilution method.

rageous experiments on mountain sickness at the end of the last century.

The well-known CO_2 effect on the cerebral circulation can be tested easily in a self-experiment by rebreathing oxygen and monitoring the electrical impedance pulses (rheoencephalogram, or REG) by electrodes on the forehead (Fig. 1-7). When the expiratory Pco_2 increases to about 65 torr, the cerebral blood flow doubles.

There is little appreciation that CO_2 has a similar, though not as marked, effect on the coronary circulation (Fig. 1-8) (Eberlein, 1966).

One cineangiographic picture (Fig. 1-9) showing the coronary vasodilatation caused by hypoxemia and to hypercarbia (West and Guzman, 1959) is worth a thousand-word printout.

Figuratively speaking, the vasoactive effect of oxygen and carbon dioxide transforms the functional shape of humans (Fig. 1-10). The higher the Po_2, the more systemic vasoconstriction; the higher the Pco_2, the more regional vasodilatation.

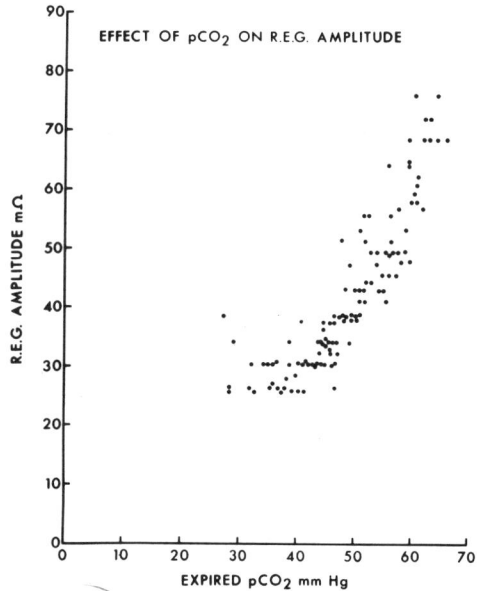

Figure 1-7. The dependence of cerebral blood flow on arterial Pco_2 can be demonstrated by the higher amplitudes of the electrical impedance pulse on the forehead.

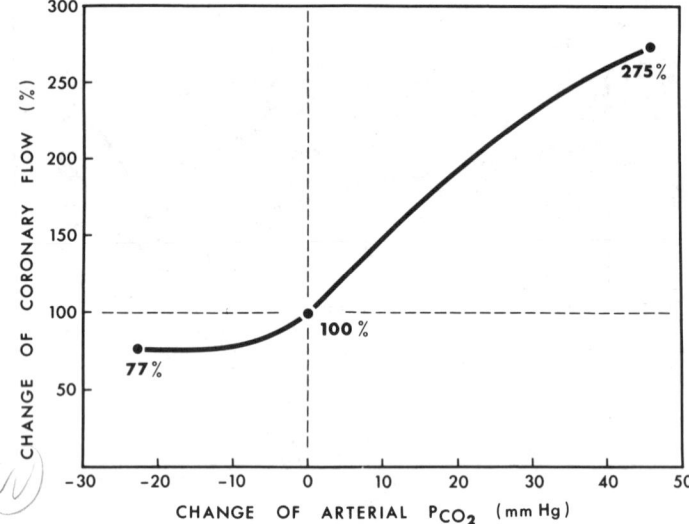

Figure 1–8. The direct relationship between coronary blood flow and arterial P_{CO_2} suggests that P_{CO_2} may be the metabolic factor regulating blood flow.

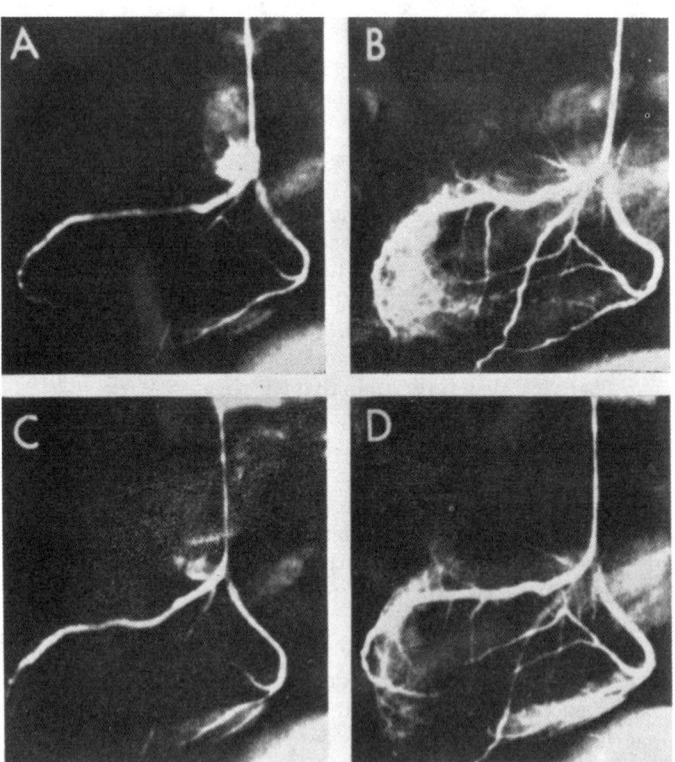

Figure 1–9. Coronary angiograms during control periods (**A** and **C**), during hypoxemia (**B**:5 percent O_2) and hypercarbia (**D**:21 percent O_2, 15 percent CO_2).

OPTIMAL BODY PERFUSION

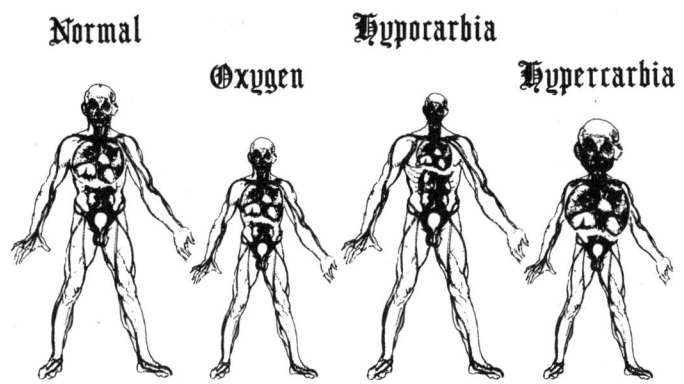

Figure 1–10. The pharmacologic effect of gas tensions on the distribution of blood flow in our body.

The last of the prerequisites for optimal body perfusion is hypoxemia, or at least the prevention of hyperoxemia. In the coronary cineangiogram we have seen that the greatest vasodilatation occurred when the subject inhaled 5 percent oxygen in nitrogen for 30 seconds. The world literature on the effects of hypoxia on the body is vast. It strikes home when, as illustrated in Figure 1–11, we realize that all of us have lived for about 280 days of

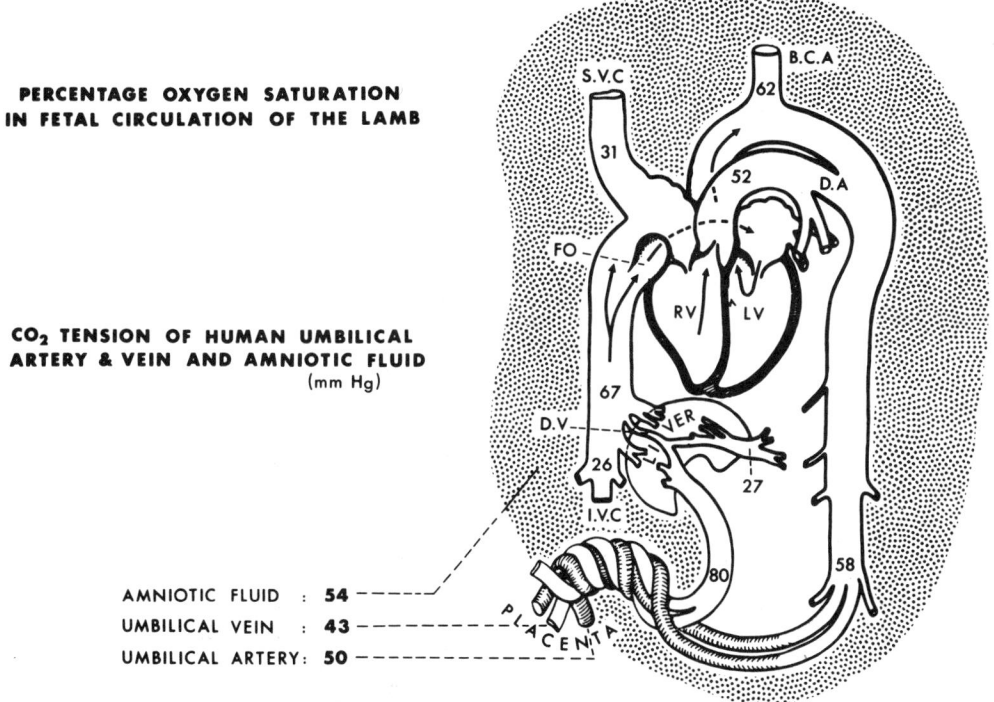

Figure 1–11. The chronic hypoxemia and hypercarbia during fetal life.

fetal life with an arterial oxygen saturation of about 60 percent (Born et al., 1954) and a P_{CO_2} of about 50 torr (Räiha and Kauraniemi, 1962).

This leads to a redistribution of blood flow to the brain and to the other internal organs that show the greatest vascularity and rate of growth. One of the most powerful stimuli of growth is a decreased tissue P_{O_2}, which we can see not only in the fetus but also in the secondary polycythemia of high altitude and chronic pulmonary disease, as well as in the anaerobic metabolism of malignancies. In fact, the first living forms developed on earth without oxygen.

Instead of the traditional classification of anoxia into static, anoxic, anemic, and toxic categories, it may be more practical for the clinician to think of two categories only: anoxia with increased flow, as in anemia and hypoxemia; and anoxia with decreased flow, as in ischemia (Fig. 1–12).

This binary classification of anoxia has prognostic value because it tells us something about the anoxic tolerance. Anoxic tolerance in anemia and hypoxemia is very high because the increased rate of blood flow washes away the acid products of anaerobic metabolism (Fig. 1–13). Such patients suffer from lack of exercise tolerance, but not from acute tissue damage. In ischemia, however, the anoxic tolerance is exceedingly short because the reduced or lacking blood flow permits the intracellular accumulation of lactic acid. Be it the obstruction of a major artery, as in coronary occlusion, or the embolization of capillaries, as in disseminated intravascular clotting, the excessively high hydrogen ion concentration damages the membranes, the organelles, and the ground substance of the cells. This is true not only for intact organisms, but for every single cell defending its intracellular individuality against the onrushing extracellular seawater. As long as there is enough phosphorus-bound energy available to man all the pumps, the dikes will hold. During an illness there may be considerable intrusions and the cells may swell. Given enough energy and time, the seawater can be

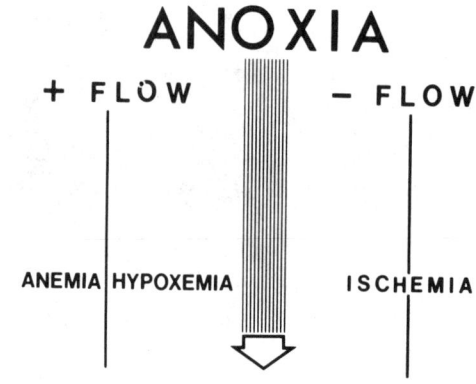

Figure 1–12. The classification of anoxia into high flow and low flow states.

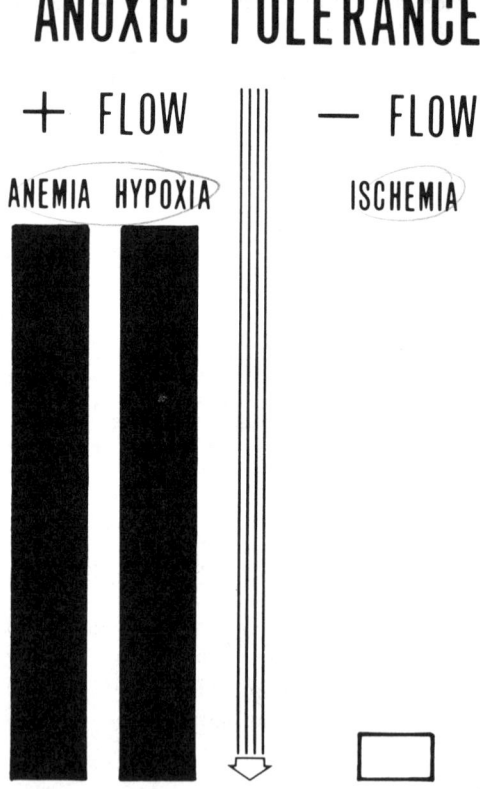

Figure 1–13. The anoxic tolerance of high flow and low flow states.

bailed out and the dikes can be repaired. However, a sudden crash by an excessively high hydrogen ion wave can overwhelm the cellular defenses, and water, sodium, and calcium will establish themselves inside the walls, while potassium is forced to escape to the outside (Fig. 1–14). When the seawater has inundated the cellular territory, life's journey comes to an end.

Specific membrane pumps have been accused of being the lone criminals who release the suicidal packages of lethal enzymes from the lysozymes. Considering the indiscriminate destruction of the most delicate structures within the cell, the proposition that ischemia may affect intracellular water itself has gained support. Intracellular water forms a liquid crystalline structure at the huge interface area of the nonpolar proteins. This lattice stabilizes the spatial configuration of all high molecular compounds in contact with intracellular water (Fig. 1–15).

If the protein surface is polarized by the free, radical hydrogen assailants, the stabilization of water is lost, and the spatial dislocation and anarchy do not permit the normal chemical linkages to take place (Drost-Hansen, 1965).

Although we consider ischemia a life-threatening event in clinical medicine, many animals have adopted ischemia as a way of life in their evolutionary drive for the survival of the fittest. The champions of self-induced ischemia are the diving animals (Scholander, 1963). Breathing air, the seal has a cardiac output of about 8 liters per minute (Fig. 1–16), but only 1.8 percent goes to the brain and only 2.2 percent to the heart. However, the moment the seal sticks its nose under water, it accomplishes spontaneously a much greater feat than its trained act of balancing a ball on it. In a split second, a reflex via the carotid sinus slows down its heart rate and its cardiac output drops from about 8 liters to about 0.6 liters per minute. But of that trickle of blood, 34 percent now goes to the brain and about 15 percent to the heart. The diving seal has changed into a heart-lung preparation.

This miraculous redistribution of blood from the periphery to the core has been called the master switch of life. When the seal comes up for air, normal blood flow is restored and all the accumulated lactic acid in the muscle cells is washed away. The seal can dive for as long as 20 minutes, which happens to be the

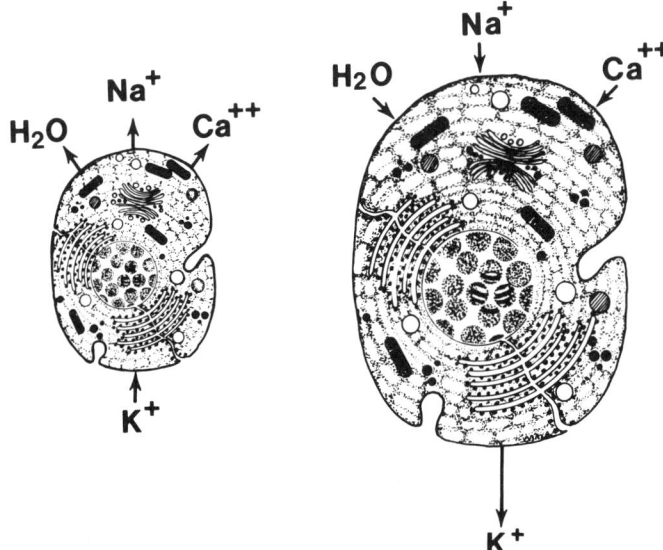

Figure 1–14. Intracellular water and electrolyte shifts caused by ischemia (on the right). Sodium and calcium enter while potassium is lost from the swollen cell. A normal cell is on the left.

Figure 1-15. Normally structured intracellular water at a protein boundary (**A**) and "atypical, malignant" appearance of intracellular water at an abnormally polarized surface (**B**).

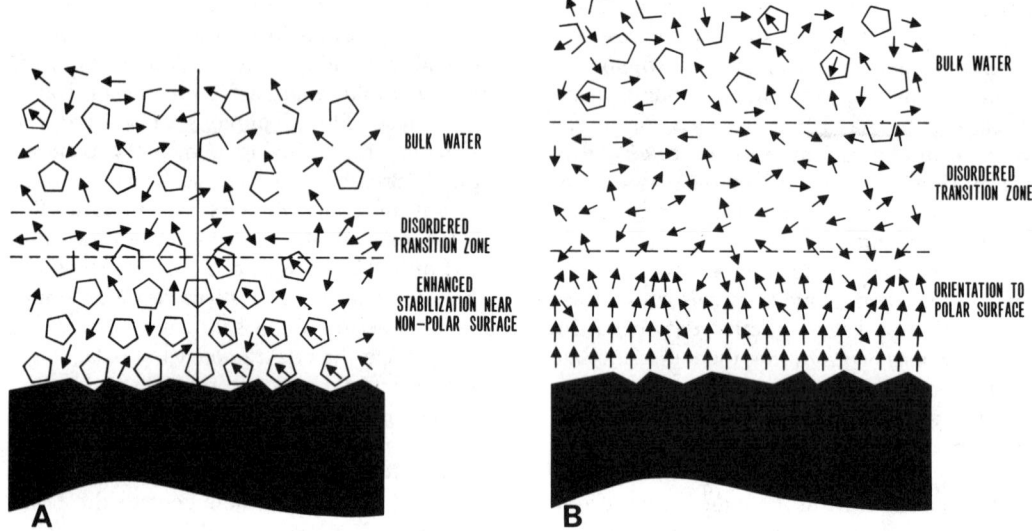

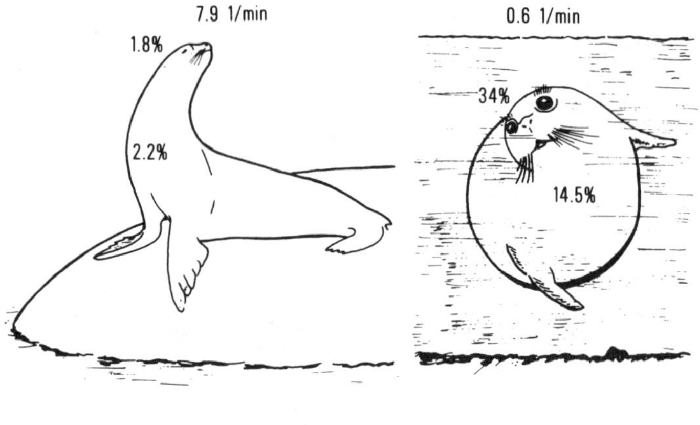

Figure 1-16. The master switch of life in diving animals. Distribution of cardiac output on land (left) and under water (right).

ischemic tolerance time of muscle at normal body temperature.

The human fetus can stay under water for nine months, and when it takes its first breath of atmospheric air, the much higher P_{O_2} inhibits a prostaglandin-induced dilatation and finally closes the ductus arteriosus. The newborn baby also eliminates lactic acid, and the excreted amount reflects the ischemia suffered during an easy or a difficult delivery (Fig. 1-17) (Scholander, 1963).

While under water in utero the baby never suffered from ischemia the way a diving animal does. After all, the baby did not get there by diving. While weightless in the amniotic fluid it was always tethered to its mother, like astronauts to their life support systems during a space walk. Nevertheless, when the

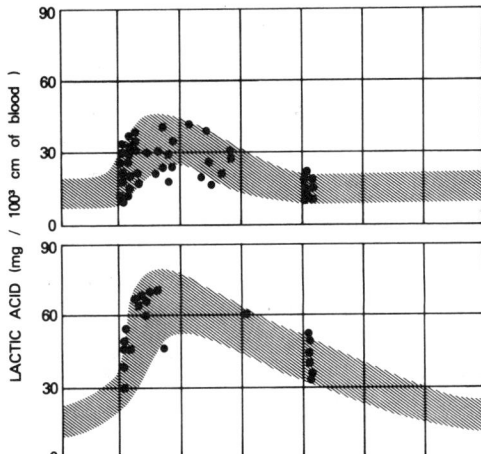

Figure 1–17. Neonatal excretion of lactic acid after a normal (upper curve) and a difficult delivery (lower curve).

baby is born the capillary bed in the periphery is still so sparse that a roentgenogram of the vascular tree (Fig. 1–18) resembles the blood distribution of the diving seal (Eckstein, 1933).

The pulling of the master switch of life in intentional or accidental submersion must be a deeply rooted reflex in all living creatures, because even the sloth possesses it, although it never thinks of going close to water. Unfortunately, this wisdom of the diving animal's body to cope with prolonged ischemia of all peripheral tissues does not apply to ischemia of the heart. No instant redistribution of blood flow within the myocardium can take place, since the only available distributor has been damaged. There is no other pump to receive a reflex message to send more blood to the heart, lungs, and brain, and the wisdom of the body fails. After the acute occlusion of a coronary artery there is no immediate dilatation of the remaining arteries—as a homeostatic imperative would demand—and vasoconstriction adds insult to injury.

In the hours and days following a coronary occlusion, myocardial edema, round cell infiltration, and necrosis may further weaken the pumping action. Even though the heart is

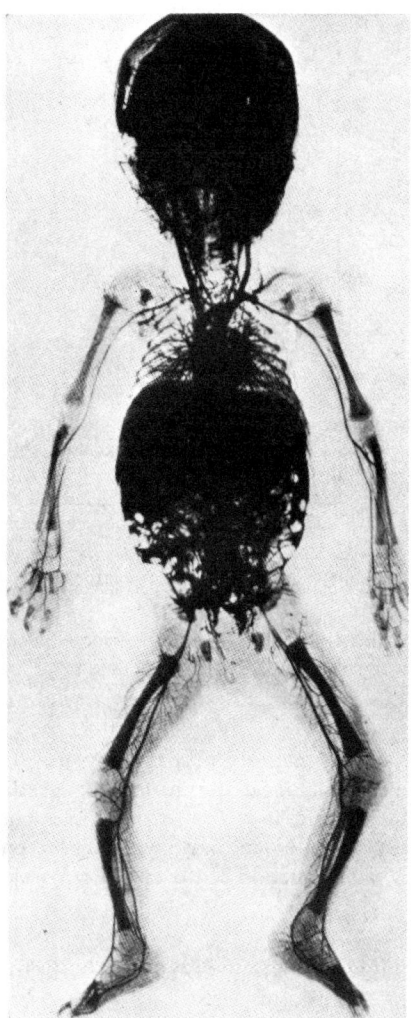

Figure 1–18. Angiogram of newborn infant, showing a vascular tree that is predominantly visceral.

less than 0.5 percent of the body weight, failure of the vital circulation throws the rest of the body into a vicious cycle. In what way are the criteria of adequate total body perfusion affected?

On the first day of an acute myocardial infarction the hematocrit is increased, and an increased viscosity of blood causes reduced capillary blood flow (Fig. 1–19) (Kung-ming et al., 1975).

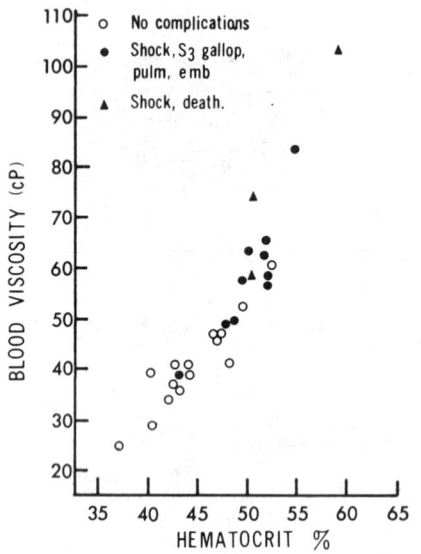

BLOOD VISCOSITY AFTER ACUTE MYOCARDIAL INFARCTION

Figure 1-19. The severity of myocardial infarction is directly related to hematocrit and blood viscosity.

of the blood. Because of the justified fear of increased irritability of the heart by hypothermia, no clinical report on the use of reduced body temperature is available. However, in dog experiments it has been shown that peripheral cooling to 30C, or cutting the oxygen consumption in half, is not followed by a higher frequency of arrhythmias or a lower survival rate.

Most patients with acute myocardial infarction hyperventilate, which may be due to fever, anxiety, or hypoxemia. There is a marked difference in mortality (Fig. 1-20) if one takes the variables of Pco_2 and pH out of their clinical complexity and compares patients who hyperventilated with those who did not (Mokhtar and Weil, 1976). No information is available on the possibility of a further reduction of the 30 percent mortality of the patients with normal Pco_2 and arterial pH if a moderate degree of hypercarbia had been induced.

Without the aid of any laboratory, a Puerto Rican country doctor by the name of Jose A. Amadeo (1944) observed that in the same rural population only his anemic patients with parasitic infestations had a low incidence of myocardial infarction. Stimulated by this well-documented and imaginatively written report, Zoll et al. (1951) injected the coronary

The majority of patients with an acute myocardial infarction have a low-grade fever during the first few days. This causes an increased demand for oxygen and a tendency for agglutination of the corpuscular elements

MORTALITY OF ACUTE MYOCARDIAL INFARCTION AND RESPIRATORY ALKALOSIS

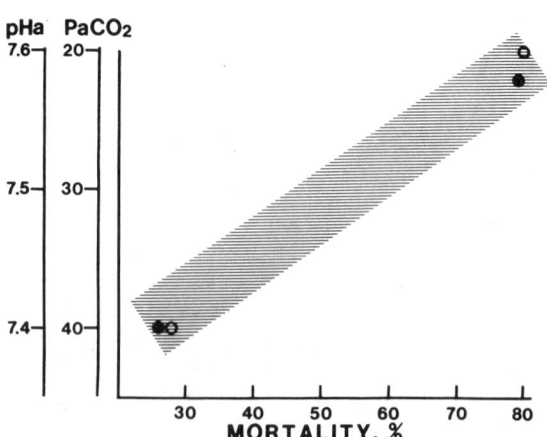

Figure 1-20. The mortality of acute myocardial infarction is also directly related to respiratory alkalosis.

blood vessels of 1,050 cadavers with an organosilicone fluid that hardened at room temperature. A large percentage of the hearts from patients who died with accompanying anemia had an increased collateral circulation (Fig. 1–21). In patients who died with marked coronary artery disease, about 90 percent of those with anemia had an increased collateral circulation, compared with about 50 percent of those with normal hematocrit.

Finally, let us look at the effects of hypoxemia on myocardial infarction. For obvious reasons this condition has never been intentionally induced in humans, but animal experiments on uncomplicated hypoxemia and coronary flow after acute coronary occlusion are available. They show that the mass of the infarcted area in the hypoxemic animals is only about one third the size of that in the animals with normal arterial oxygen content (Fig. 1–22) (Bishop and Bloor, 1974). Thus, in chronic hypoxemia there is a greater blood flow to the infarcted tissue, resulting in smaller infarct size.

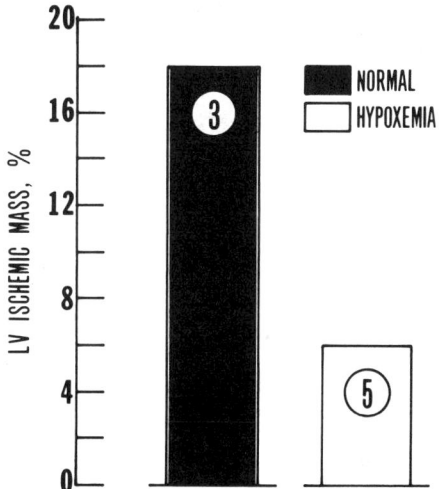

Figure 1–22. The size of experimental myocardial infarcts is markedly decreased by hypoxemia.

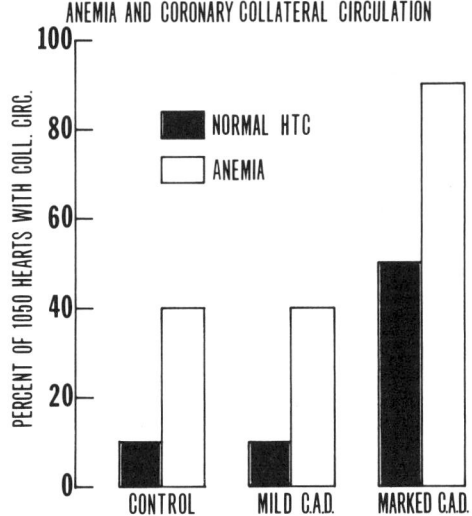

Figure 1–21. Anemia increased the degree of collateral circulation in subjects without and with mild coronary artery disease, but particularly in patients with marked coronary artery disease.

At present only a legalistic case based on circumstantial evidence can be made for the proposition that hemodilution, hypothermia, hypercarbia, and hypoxemia be even considered in the treatment of acute myocardial infarction. Only controlled animal experimentation on these single and combined modalities can supply the incontrovertible evidence needed.

We have tested the effect of hemodilution and hypothermia in greyhounds in whom congestive failure had been induced by an overdose of sodium pentobarbital (Fig. 1–23). Racing greyhounds lend themselves ideally to such experiments because they have a cardiac output of human proportion and a hematocrit of about 55 percent.

The extent of congestive failure can be estimated from the high heart rate, low stroke volume, and high left ventricular end-diastolic pressure. Hemodilution to a hematocrit of 30 percent "watered down" all values, but particularly arterial blood pressure, left ventricular end-diastolic pressure, and stroke work. When the body temperature was then lowered to 30C, a marked improvement of cardiac function was produced. This was manifest-

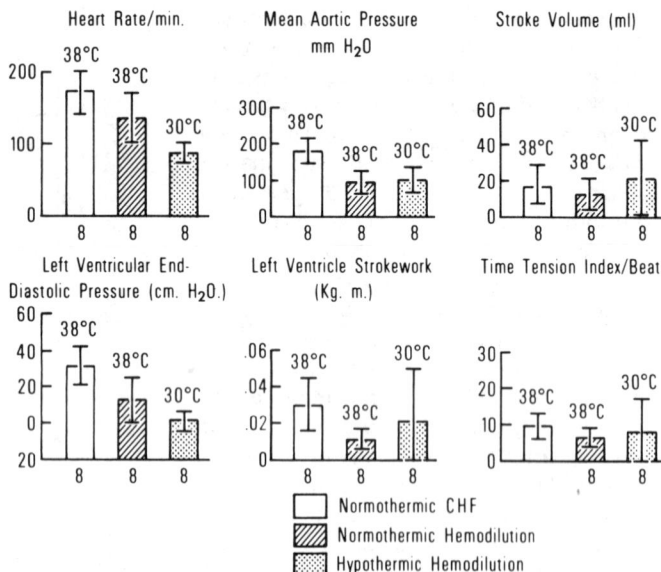

Figure 1–23. Left ventricular function in experimental congestive heart failure can be improved by hemodilution and mild hypothermia.

ed in a reduction of heart rate and left ventricular end-diastolic pressure, and an increase in stroke volume, stroke work, and the time-tension index. The improved myocardial contractility in the hypothermic heart at 30C has been known for a long time and may be due to the relatively prolonged isometric relaxation time as compared to the systolic activity phase. The hypothermic increase in blood viscosity with its capillary perfusion deficits had been prevented by previous blood dilution. More evidence that the combined principles of extracorporeal circulation are also valid in pump failure of the intracorporeal circulation is needed. If successful, such physiologic measures may be more efficient, noninvasive, and cost-containing than the mechanical assist devices.

Hemodilution, hypothermia, hypercarbia, and hypoxemia are not physiologic in humans and deviate from the constancy of their internal environment. Still, these are not unnatural conditions, and many animals, such as the icefish, the hibernator, the diving animals, and fetuses, make successful use of them in their survival. In healthy young people most of the energy consumed is converted into the maintenance of Claude Bernard's constant internal environment. However, we do not honor his name by adhering rigidly to his concept, when the energy requirements for normalcy are not available anymore. We rather honor his spirit by taking the principles of optimal extracorporeal circulation and weaving them into a concept of a controlled change of the internal environment. This artificial change in the internal environment may have to be maintained until human beings are able again to generate enough energy to return to their customary place in nature.

"This is an art which does mend nature,—change it rather: But the art itself is nature."

SHAKESPEARE

REFERENCES

Amadeo J A: A suggestion for improving the structure of the coronary circulatory system without surgical intervention. Am Heart J 28:699–713, 1944.

Bassenge E, Schmid-Schönbein H, Von Restorff W, Volger E: Effect of hemodilution on coronary hemodynamics in conscious dogs. In Hemodilution, Theoretical Basis and Clinical Application, Int Symp Rottach-Egern, 1971. Basel, Karger, 1972, pp 174–183.

Bishop S P, Bloor C M: Regional myocardial blood flow following coronary occlusion in unanesthetized normal and hypoxemic dogs. Am J Cardiol 33:127, 1974.

Born G V R, Dawes G S, Mott J C, Widdicombe J G: Changes in the heart and lungs at birth. Cold Springs Harbor Symp Quant Biol 19:102–108, 1954.

Bullard R W, Funkhausen G F: Estimated regional blood flow by rubidium-86 distribution during arousal from hibernation. Am J Physiol 204:266–270, 1962.

Drost-Hansen W: The effects of biologic systems of higher-order phase transitions in water. Ann NY Acad Sci 125:471–501, 1965.

Eberlein H J: Koronardurchblutung and Sauerstoffversorgung des Herzens unter verschiedenen CO_2 Spannungen und Anesthetica. Arch Kreislaufforschung 50:18–87, 1966.

Eckstein A: Über den peripheren Kreislauf bei Frühgeborenen. Z Kinderheilkunde 54:317, 1933.

Gollan F: Physiology of Cardiac Surgery. Hypothermia, Extracorporeal Circulation, and Extracorporeal Cooling. Springfield, Ill, Thomas, 1959.

Kung-ming F, Shu C, Bigger J T: Observations on blood viscosity changes after acute myocardial infarction. Circulation 51:1079–1084, 1975.

Messmer K, Sunder-Plassman L, Klovekorn WP, Holper K: Circulatory significance of hemodilution: rheological changes and limitations. Basel, Karger, Adv Microcirc 41:1–77, 1972.

Mokhtar S, Weil M H: Increased mortality of acute myocardial infarction in patients with alkalosis. Fed Proc 35:349, 1976.

Räiha N R, Kauraniemi T V: Carbon dioxide tension and acid-base balance of human amniotic fluid at the end of gestation. Biol Neonate 4:25–31, 1962.

Scholander P F: The master switch of life. Sci Am 209:92–107, 1963.

Swan H: Thermoregulation and Bioenergetics. New York, Elsevier, 1974.

West J W, Guzman S W: Coronary dilatation and constriction visualized by selective arteriography. Circ Res 7:527–536, 1959.

Zoll P M, Wessler S, Schlesinger M J: Interarterial coronary anastomoses in the human heart, with particular reference to anemia and relative cardiac anoxia. Circulation 4:797–815, 1951.

2. Concepts of Patient Care

ROBERT S. LITWAK   SIMON DACK

THE GOAL OF PATIENT CARE

Fundamental to survival of the patient undergoing cardiac surgery or any traumatic event is the continued adequate operation of those physical systems that permit maintenance of intracellular functional integrity. The nature of intracellular reaction processes and the integrative mechanisms that are constantly operative to maintain them are still incompletely understood.

It is a common observation that patients with significant heart disease not only survive but are able to function reasonably well for many years. If the patient as a whole is considered to be a complex *system* composed of numerous interrelated *subsystems* (Kirklin, 1971), the survival of cardiac patients is testimony to the capacity of the body's multiple subsystem compensatory mechanisms to sustain satisfactory levels of cellular metabolic activity. In large measure, this reflects the capability of the cardiovascular subsystem in general and the heart in particular to modify and maintain its operational capacity to sustain sufficient levels of blood flow so that the voracious demands of the cells are satisfied.

The diseased heart frequently makes this accommodation by invoking functional mechanisms that characteristically are less efficient. Should therapeutic interventions not improve the ratio between the work that the heart performs and the total energy expended in accomplishing that work, i.e., efficiency, a stage of myocardial deterioration ultimately is reached where, despite all possible functional compensation, intracellular oxidative metabolism and the necessary transmembrane molecular exchanges cannot be sustained and the patient dies. Thus, it follows that the principle underlying preoperative and postoperative management of the patient subjected to a cardiac operation is the *implementation of therapeutic intervention that permits movement toward or maintenance of optimal steady-state conditions within the cell.*

TRANSPORT, EXCHANGE, AND CELLULAR FUNCTION

Since present knowledge does not permit facile manipulation of intracellular events, our efforts must largely be confined to support of subserving systems that participate in the uptake and transport of oxygen, substrates, and metabolic end products to and from the proximate vicinity of the cells. If one were to attempt to define the two processes central to life support, it is apparent that they would be *diffusion* and *bulk transport (blood flow).*

Diffusion

Diffusional processes in the body function effectively because of the extraordinarily close anatomic relationships between individual capillaries and each cell. It has been estimated that almost every cell of the body is no further than 25 to 50 microns from a capillary, an arrangement allowing vast extracellular-intracellular exchanges within a fraction of a second in the normal subject. Over relatively large distances diffusion would be a slow process, but over the short distance between capillary and cell, diffusion of a molecule capable of traversing a cell membrane (such as oxygen or carbon dioxide) takes place with great rapidity, provided that there is a marked concentration difference of such a molecular species existing within the cell from that in the surrounding milieu.

Rushmer (1961, 1965) has picturesquely described these concepts by a hypothetical consideration of the comparative speeds of diffusion of 100 percent oxygen into a tissue cylinder (devoid of oxygen) 10 mm in diameter and a similar cylinder with a diameter of 0.7 mm. Although the relative difference between the diameters is approximately 14 to 1, it would take the larger tissue cylinder virtually three hours (11,100 seconds) to become 90 percent saturated, whereas the smaller cylinder would achieve a similar saturation level in only 54 seconds, more than a 200-fold time difference. Hill (1928) has calculated that a single cell 7 microns in diameter would be saturated in 0.0054 second (Fig. 2–1).

The physical factors affecting the rate of diffusion of substances are expressed in the equation originally formulated by Adolph

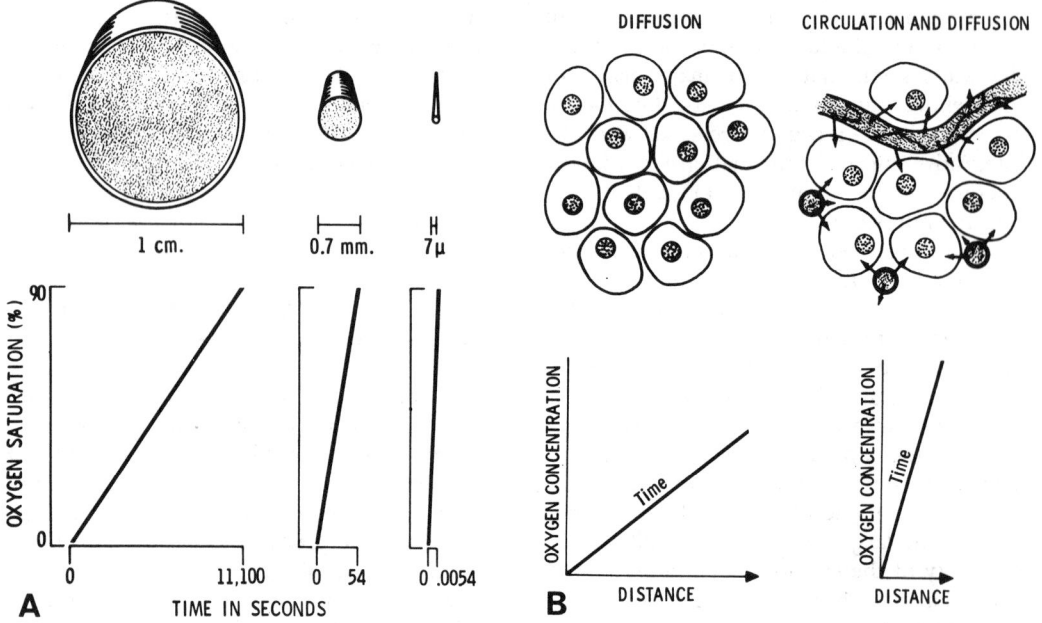

Figure 2–1. Characteristics of diffusion. Molecular species such as oxygen diffuse through protoplasm relatively slowly over long distances but quite rapidly over short distances. In the latter circumstance the concentration gradients are steep and diffusion takes place rapidly. **A.** Diffusion of pure oxygen through protoplasmic tubes of varying diameters. A cylinder 1 cm in diameter would require over 3 hours (11,100 seconds) to become 90 percent saturated. In comparison, a cylinder only 7 μ in diameter would achieve a similar level of saturation in only 0.0054 second because of the steep concentration gradient. **B.** Similar to the large protoplasmic tube in **A**, packed cell masses not immediately adjacent to capillaries have flattened concentration gradients so that diffusion is slow. On the other hand, contiguity of capillaries and cells permits high concentration gradients to exist if blood flow is adequate, thereby facilitating molecular exchanges. *(Redrawn with permission from Rushmer, RF, General characteristics of the cardiovascular system. In Ruch, TC, and Patton, HD, eds, Physiology and Biophysics. Philadelphia: Saunders, 1965.)*

Fick in 1855 and summarized by Guyton (1971) in descriptive terms:

$$R_d \propto \frac{D_c \times A_{cs} \times T}{MW \times D}, \text{ where}$$

R_d = diffusion rate
D_c = concentration difference
A_{cs} = cross-sectional area
T = temperature
MW = molecular weight
D = distance

The equation emphasizes a point made earlier that the greater the concentration difference (gradient) of a substance the greater will be the rate of diffusion from one area to another. Similarly, the greater the cross-sectional area of the chamber in which diffusion is taking place and the higher the temperature (which increases molecular motion) the greater the rate of diffusion. It can also be seen that increasing both the molecular weight and the distance to be traversed will have the effect of reducing diffusion rate.

Blood Flow

Molecules such as oxygen and carbon dioxide are lipid-soluble and pass across capillary and cell membranes virtually unimpeded simply by becoming dissolved in the lipid structure of the membranes and diffusing through them just as random diffusion of a substance would occur in water. Hence it can be appreciated that the prime factor limiting the exchange of oxygen, carbon dioxide, and similar molecular species between the blood and cells cannot be diffusion but *blood flow* at the capillary level. Only with adequate blood flow can steep concentration gradients be maintained across the cell membrane so that adequate diffusional exchanges can take place.

Normal levels of cardiac output result in movement of the subject's total blood volume around the circulation about once every 60 seconds. During that one minute, bidirectional diffusion across the capillary membranes occurs at a volume approximately 45 times that of the cardiac output, thereby facilitating virtually instantaneous transcapillary exchange.

Despite the reduction in blood flow that frequently results from heart disease, patients survive because transport of adequate quantities of metabolic substrates and end products is still possible. Thus, a built-in safety factor permits maintenance of an acceptable steady state despite suboptimal circulatory conditions. The safety factor varies for different molecular species. For example, at normal conditions, oxygen can be transported to the cells up to three times the usual amount by the simple expedient of increased oxygen extraction from the hemoglobin, a threefold level of safety. Calculation of safety factor multiples for other substances reveals the following comparisons: a 25-fold safety factor for carbon dioxide, glucose 30-fold, and nitrogenous wastes 480-fold (Guyton et al., 1973).

It is apparent that oxygen is the most flow-limited of all known life-sustaining molecules. It follows that when cardiac output falls and remains below one-third normal, cellular death becomes a virtual certainty, since oxygen delivery will be insufficient even though there is adequate transport of other substances.

The nature and rate of compartmental exchanges can be adversely influenced by structural and functional mechanisms that accompany aging and organ dysfunction, the latter due to either intrinsic disease, acute trauma, or a combination of both. In patients with heart disease requiring surgery who have major reductions of systemic and pulmonary blood flow and pressures, the consequences of altered exchange rates between the capillaries and cells can be life-threatening. Therefore, a concept of the mechanisms and magnitude of the interrelated patterns of diffusion and flow in both health and disease is fundamental to proper care of patients undergoing intracardiac surgery. Further consideration of these matters will be found in subsequent chapters. Comprehensive discussions about transport and exchange kinetics will be found in the contributions of Landis and Pappenheimer (1963) and Reeve and Guyton (1967).

HOMEOSTASIS

How relatively simple it would be to understand body function and apply this information to patient care if only each organ subsystem performed compatibly but completely separately from all the others. Indeed, the understandable tendency to concentrate one's attention on problems affecting a single organ such as the heart or lungs tends to be momentarily persuasive that performance analysis and therapy based on such considerations might have a rational basis.

But it is elemental that multicellular organisms survive solely because there is precise functional integration of all subsystems, which operate at levels in accordance with changing body requirements. This necessitates a means of sensing the changing state and an ordering of a measured response by exquisitely sensitive balancing mechanisms. The response is expressed by a change in the performance characteristics of at least one but generally a number of subsystems so that an optimal level of stability is approached or achieved.

These concepts lead us to an appreciation of the central role played by physiologic control and regulatory mechanisms in maintaining the body economy, ideas brilliantly anticipated by Claude Bernard (1878), who wrote: "It is the fixity of the *milieu interieur* which is the condition of free and independent life. . . . All the vital mechanisms, however varied they may be, have only one object, that of preserving constant the conditions of life in the internal environment." This autoregulatory system was recognized by Richet (1900), who commented that "the living being is stable. . . . By an apparent contradiction it maintains its stability only if it is excitable and capable of modifying itself according to external stimuli and adjusting its responses to the stimulation. In a sense it is stable because it is able to be modified—the slight instability is the necessary condition for the true stability of the organism." Cannon (1929), searching for a descriptive means of characterizing these processes, wrote, "The coordinated physiological reactions which maintain most of the steady states in the body are so complex and are so peculiar to the living organism, that it has been suggested that a specific designation for these states be employed—*homeostasis*."

Biologic Feedback Systems

More recently, the application of control system theory has conceptually defined homeostasis as an error-signal system (Yamamoto, 1965) in which the organism achieves stability by feedback responses to error (the disparity between the actual and optimal state). Characteristic of biologic feedback systems that attempt to maintain stability are: (1) the ability to detect an error by means of a sensor; (2) determination of the magnitude of the error by comparison with an optimal reference value; (3) generation of an error signal (the difference between the reference value and sensed value); (4) feedback of error signal to an effector mechanism; and (5) a proportioned response that tends to reduce the error (Fig. 2–2). These functions are components of *negative feedback systems,* control mechanisms performing in closed loops to make physiologic adjustments so that an optimal steady state level is approached (Fig. 2–3). For example, a sudden rise in systemic arterial pressure will excite a regulatory mechanism that will cause a series of reactions, all of which tend to lower the pressure toward normal levels. Conversely, a sudden fall in blood pressure will prompt reactions that tend to increase the pressure. In both situations the negative feedback mechanism functions in a fashion that tends to reduce the deviation (error) from the body's established normal set point for systemic arterial pressure.

On the other hand, a *positive feedback system* is one in which the output response tends to increase the error and in so doing produces more instability of the system, which may lead to death. These positive feedback systems are more commonly termed vicious cycles. The magnitude of the error often determines whether the feedback response will be negative or positive.

A readily understood example is a comparison of the cardiac output responses to

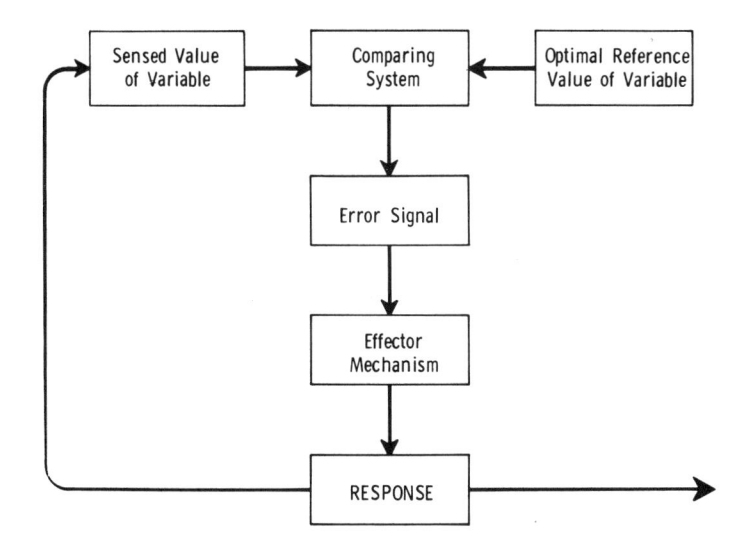

Figure 2-2. Diagram of the functional components of a negative feedback control system. A sensed value for any variable is compared with an optimal value for that variable and the difference between those values, the error, signals an effector mechanism, which effects a response. The response characteristically tends to reduce the error.

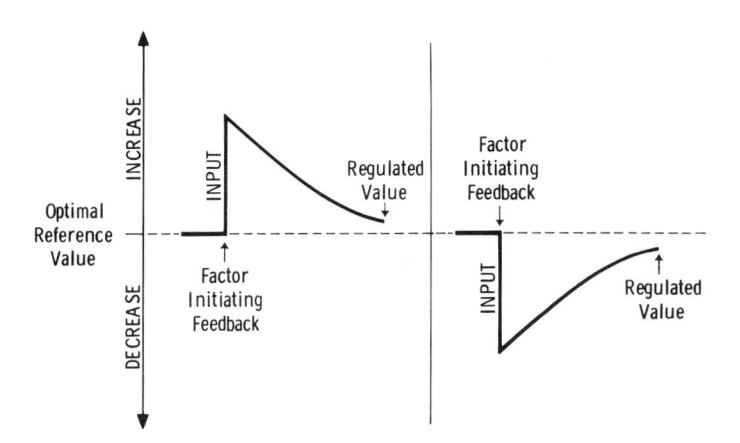

Figure 2-3. Diagram of the characteristic tendency of a negative feedback loop to reduce a detected error in a compensatory fashion so that the regulated value approaches an optimal reference value. The illustration depicts an optimally controlled mean value (identical to the reference value), which is altered suddenly. The deviation from the mean is detected and an error signal generated (input). The effector mechanism is then actuated, producing a response that returns the value toward the optimal reference value. (Adapted with permission from Guyton and Crowell, 1961.)

moderate and severe hemorrhage. Figure 2-4 depicts a hypothetic illustration of the pumping effectiveness of the heart when 1 and 2 liters of blood are suddenly removed from the subject, whose cardiac output is 5 liters per minute. It is apparent that moderate hemorrhage (1 liter) is well-tolerated and cardiac output returns to normal in several hours. A negative feedback system has come into play, involving reduction of the peripheral vascular bed, cardiac rate, and stroke volume accommodation to the altered state, and a plasma refill mechanism that operates until the blood volume is again normalized in that subject. The totality of these factors tends to reduce the error and return the cardiac output toward normal.

However, sudden severe hemorrhage (2 liters) gives rise to a positive feedback mechanism. A sharp drop in cardiac output accompanies the hemorrhage, followed by a further fall over the course of the next few hours. The

Figure 2-4. The effect of moderate and severe hemorrhage on cardiac output. The magnitude of the deviation (error) from the optimal reference value is the critical determinant of the response. Moderate hemorrhage (one liter) invokes negative feedback with restoration of cardiac output to normal within hours whereas severe hemorrhage is followed by positive feedback and ultimate failure of the system. (Adapted with permission from Guyton, A C, *Textbook of Medical Physiology.* 4th ed. Philadelphia: Saunders, 1971, p 7.)

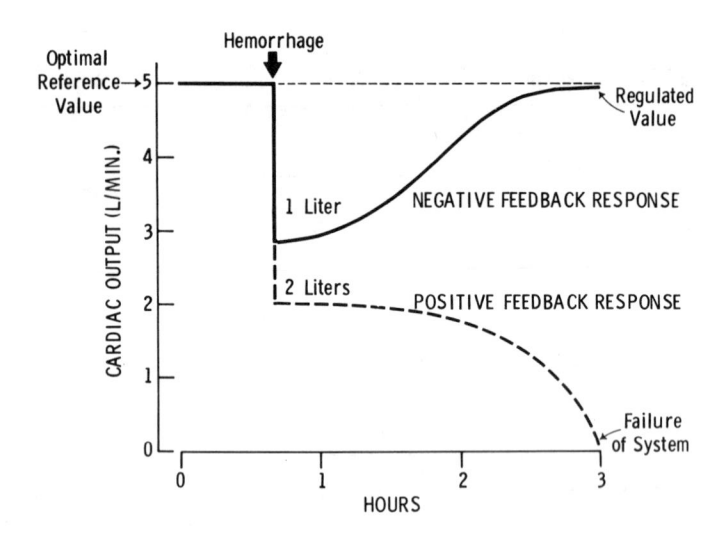

marked hypovolemic low output state worsens as acidemia, reduced coronary blood flow, and hypotension contribute to a further decrement in cardiac performance, which, in turn, contributes to more hypotension, acidemia, and additional reduction in systemic and coronary blood flow until function of the body cell mass ceases. In this situation each cycle in the feedback system has increased the magnitude of the error.

In summary, homeostatic integration of body subsystems is possible because of thousands of negative feedback mechanisms that both control and regulate function. However, there are discrete limits within which homeostatic mechanisms can operate. As we have seen, marked deviations from the normal functional set point tend to provoke positive feedback responses, with their tendency to further aggravate an already compromised situation. Where reduced or altered function has been imposed by the single or combined effects of the extremes of age, disease, and surgical trauma, the capacity of negative feedback systems to restore satisfactory stability characteristically is reduced and the propensity for appearance of destructive positive feedback is accentuated.

These considerations lead us to a painful awareness that current knowledge of normal body performance, derangements of function, and the effects of therapy are still largely qualitative. In the past decade the use of systems analysis techniques increasingly has allowed a more quantitative assessment of physiologic events (Guyton et al., 1973). Expanded application of this powerful tool may be expected to be of major importance in developing further understanding of physiologic events and ultimately improving clinical practice.

THE SCOPE OF PATIENT CARE

Safe conduct of a patient through cardiac surgery involves design and implementation of a logical plan that concerns itself with the details of (1) making a complete preoperative diagnosis, (2) thoughtful preoperative care, (3) performance of a physiologically sound and technically precise operation, and (4) meticulous and appropriate postoperative care. Failure to fulfill the requirements of any of these four precepts introduces an additional risk factor that is largely avoidable. Implicit in these rules is that the ideal way to manage complications is to avoid them, which is best accomplished with a carefully conducted care plan.

Preoperative Diagnosis

Selection of appropriate surgical candidates and proper operative design requires precise delineation of cardiovascular anatomic arrangements, quantitative determination of cardiac performance abnormalities, and assessment of the altered physiologic state imposed by the heart disease on other subsystems. It is of equal importance that a comprehensive search be made for unrelated disease processes that might influence both the advisability of operation and the outcome.

Preoperative Management

In nonemergency circumstances, preoperative management should attempt to bring the patient to an optimal state of improvement before surgery. Design and implementation of *appropriate* therapy require an integrated knowledge of the altered physiologic state imposed by the combined elements of (1) the patient's cardiac dysfunction, (2) the effects of anesthesia, extracorporeal circulation, and intracardiac surgery on organ function, and (3) constitutional factors that modify the response to trauma; i.e., age, nutritional state, and coexisting disease. These considerations, which will be amplified in Chapter 3, are of particular importance in patients who have been in chronic heart failure, since overly aggressive preoperative therapy may readily set the stage for serious intraoperative and postoperative problems.

Intraoperative Management

Survival after cardiac surgery and the level of sustained clinical improvement are both primarily influenced by intraoperative events; i.e., conduct of the operation and completeness of the repair. The most common cause of death after cardiac operations is low cardiac output. Therefore, the varyingly traumatic measures of anesthesia, extracorporeal circulation, and intracardiac manipulation must be favorably counterbalanced by prompt improvement in cardiac performance and the general physiologic state. A minimally traumatic, technically precise correction in a patient coming to the operating room with adequate myocardial contractility provides the basis for a favorable outcome.

Postoperative Care

Appropriate supportive therapy in the postoperative period is the fourth element that allows uncomplicated convalescence following cardiac surgery to be anticipated with a high degree of certainty. Proper therapy can make the difference between survival and death in patients coming to operations with significant cardiorespiratory, renal, and hepatic dysfunction. However, excellent postoperative care almost never can compensate for a poorly designed or inadequately executed operation, although it is entirely possible for a patient who has had a satisfactory surgical procedure to succumb if postoperative care is inadequate.

It seems appropriate to stress that the concept of postoperative care must be extended beyond the period of hospitalization, since a substantial challenge to the patient will present itself when he or she returns home and resumes daily activities. Residual myocardial or pulmonary problems and anticipation of possible late complications of either the operation or special therapy (such as warfarin administration) make it mandatory that a plan of posthospital management be constructed in collaboration with the patient's local physician so that optimal care and surveillance can be continued.

This discussion is intended to suggest an *interdependency* of the four elements that together contribute to the successful response of a patient undergoing an intracardiac operation. This interdependency requires knowledgeable medical and surgical teamwork, since a poorly selected candidate is likely to have an unhappy outcome regardless of the excellent quality of the operative or postoperative care, just as a properly selected patient will come to an equally bad end if the surgery or subsequent care is unsatisfactory.

REFERENCES

Bernard C: Lecons sur les Phénomènes de la Vie Communs aux Animaux et aux Végétaux. Paris, Ballier, 1878, Tom I, p 113.

Cannon W B: Organization for physiological homeostasis. Physiol Rev 9:399, 1929.

Guyton A C: Textbook of Medical Physiology, 4th ed. Philadelphia, Saunders, 1971, p 40.

———, Crowell J W: Dynamics of the heart in shock (Part III). Fed Proc 20:51, 1961.

———, Jones C E, Coleman T G: Circulatory Physiology: Cardiac Output and Its Regulation. Philadelphia, Saunders, 1973, p 4.

Hill A V: The diffusion of oxygen and lactic acid through the tissues. Proc R Soc Lond [Biol] 104B:39, 1928.

Kirklin J W: Circulation and cardiac failure. In Kinney J M, Egdahl R H, Zuidema G D (eds): American College of Surgeons Manual of Preoperative and Postoperative Care, 2nd ed. Philadelphia, Saunders, 1971. pp 195–210.

Landis E M, Pappenheimer J R: Exchange of substances through the capillary walls. In Handbook of Physiology. Section 2. Circulation, Vol II. Washington, DC, American Physiological Society, 1963, pp 961–1034.

Reeve E B, Guyton A C (eds): Physical Bases of Circulatory Transport: Regulation and Exchange. Philadelphia, Saunders, 1967.

Richet C: Dictionnaire de Physiologie. Paris, 1900, Vol 4, p 721. Cited by Cannon W B, in Organization for Physiological Homeostasis. Physiol Rev 9:399, 1929.

Rushmer R F: General characteristics of the cardiovascular system. In Ruch T C, Patton H D (eds): Physiology and Biophysics. Philadelphia, Saunders, 1965, pp 543–549.

———: Cardiovascular Dynamics, 2nd ed. Philadelphia, Saunders, 1961, p 1.

Yamamoto W S: Homeostasis, continuity, and feedback. In Yamamoto W S, Brobeck J R (eds): Physiologic Controls and Regulations. Philadelphia, Saunders, 1965, pp 14–31.

RECOMMENDED READING

Behrendt D M, Austen W G: Patient Care in Cardiac Surgery (2nd ed). Boston, Little, Brown, 1976.

Braimbridge M V: Postoperative Cardiac Intensive Care, 2nd ed. Oxford, London, Edinburgh, Blackwell Scientific, 1972.

Roe B B: Perioperative Management in Cardiothoracic Surgery. Boston, Little, Brown, 1981.

3. Preoperative Evaluation and Care

Roy A. Jurado

While the overall mortality from cardiac operations has steadily declined through the years, the operative risk remains high for patients who come to surgery with complex cardiovascular lesions requiring complicated repair and for those with significant preoperative physiologic handicaps and derangements, which may or may not be directly related to the primary cardiovascular disease. The essentials of preoperative care of patients admitted for cardiac surgery involve application of the same rules of precise medical care one would apply to noncardiac patients. The ultimate aim is to reduce operative and postoperative risks by optimizing conditions under which physiologic homeostasis might be achieved, thereby improving the patient's ability to react to and counteract derangements caused by operative trauma, stress, and infection. Successful attainment of this objective requires, among other things, intimate knowledge of the patient's general condition, the extent and severity of the primary cardiovascular disease, and the accompanying physiologic derangements. This chapter will confine itself to discussions of special management programs believed essential to the attainment of this goal. For a comprehensive discussion of surgical indications—another aspect of preoperative evaluation—the reader is referred to standard textbooks on cardiology and cardiac surgery.

The importance of a well-planned and precise hemodynamic investigation cannot be overemphasized. A clear-cut definition in the preoperative phase of the nature of the anatomic and hemodynamic defect, as well as the accompanying physiologic derangements, is one of the basic elements of a succesful outcome of cardiac surgery. With very few exceptions, patients referred for surgery have had thorough clinical evaluation, including both noninvasive and invasive studies. Most patients will have had hemodynamic studies carried out with or without angiography, prior to their admission or transfer to the surgical service. Thus, very frequently, the *surgical work-up* serves a supplemental function.

PREOPERATIVE EVALUATION: THE SURGICAL WORK-UP

Admission History

It is important for the surgical staff to obtain a careful history, which may elucidate pertinent facts not previously recalled by the patient. This should include a detailed list of all recent medications and the patient's response to them. Particular attention should be paid to recent use of cardiotonic, diuretic, and myocardial depressant drugs (e.g., antiarrhythmics and β-adrenergic blockers) and to previous antibiotic, antihypertensive, and corticosteroid therapy. It is vital that a history be elicited of any drug toxicity, sensitivity, or allergy. Review of the medical history should particularly seek any clues to bleeding tendency or other subsystem disease.

The physical examination must not neglect what may be considered "nonessentials," such as rectal and pelvic examinations. It is important to eliminate potential sources of postoperative infection before elective cardiac surgery. Toward this end, sites of chronic infection (tonsils, sinuses, or carious teeth) should be identified and, if possible, treated before proceeding with surgery.

Laboratory Studies

Table 3-1 lists certain basic laboratory studies that should be conducted in all patients requiring open intracardiac operations. For patients who have lesions that will not require the use of cardiopulmonary bypass, the schedule of tests should be modified accordingly. Thus, in the absence of a bleeding history, the coagulation screen can usually be eliminated with relative safety.

Chest Roentgenography. A chest x-ray should be obtained routinely on admission despite previous studies in the recent past. Examination of the heart and the aorta provides valuable information about the overall cardiac size, size of cardiac chambers and thoracic aorta, and calcification in valves, pericardium, coronary arteries, and aorta. Examination of the lung fields and pulmonary vessels yields similar information, including enlargement of the pulmonary artery and pulmonary vascular patterns that reflect normal or abnormal physiologic states. Inspection of the chest roentgenogram allows recognition and estimation of the severity of changes secondary to pulmonary venous hypertension, pulmonary arterial hypertension, and increased or decreased pulmonary blood flow. Primary and secondary pulmonary parenchymal changes and the presence or absence of pleural or pericardial effusions can also be discerned. Thus, the chest roentgenogram provides valuable gross anatomic and pathologic data.

Electrocardiography. An electrocardiogram should also be obtained on admission. The electrocardiogram reflects the electrophysiologic state of the heart. Disturbances of rate and rhythm, disorders of cardiac muscle, chamber enlargement, ischemic changes, and recent or previous myocardial damage can be discerned by electrocardiography. It may like-

TABLE 3-1 A SUGGESTED LIST OF BASIC PREOPERATIVE LABORATORY STUDIES IN PATIENTS REQUIRING OPEN INTRACARDIAC OPERATIONS

*Cardiopulmonary Evaluation**
  Chest fluoro-roentgenography
  Electrocardiography
  Serum enzymes (SGOT, LDH, CK, MB-CK), if indicated
  Pulmonary function tests, if indicated
  Arterial blood gases, if indicated

Hematologic Evaluation
  Erythrocyte count, hemoglobin, hematrocrit determinations [including mean corpuscular volume (MCV) and hemoglobin concentration (MCH)]
  Leukocyte count (total and differential)
  Thrombocyte (platelet) count
  Clotting time
  Bleeding time
  Rumpel-Leeds test
  Prothrombin time (one stage)
  Partial thromboplastin time
  Prothrombin consumption
  Fibrinogen
  Clot retraction or lysis

Renal-Metabolic Screen
  Urinalysis
  Blood urea nitrogen, creatinine
  Serum electrolytes
  Fasting blood sugar
  Serum lipids and cholesterol

Hepatic Screen
  Serum bilirubin
  Serum proteins, albumin/globulin ratio
  Prothrombin time (one stage)
  Alkaline phosphatase
  Serum glutamic pyruvic transaminase (SGPT)
  Serum glutamic oxalacetic transaminase (SGOT)
  Lactic acid dehydrogenase (LDH)

*Presupposes prior noninvasive and invasive cardiologic evaluation.

wise uncover evidence of digitalis and other cardiac drug toxicity or further myocardial deterioration by the presence of atrial or ventricular arrhythmias or varying degrees of block. Finally, postoperative comparison with these studies frequently is helpful.

Hematologic Tests. Admission laboratory studies should include an assessment of formed-element function and the oxygen-carrying capacity of the circulating blood. A detailed coagulation profile is obtained if the patient gives a familial or personal history of a hemorrhagic disorder. In the absence of such a positive history the following simple screening tests will suffice. (1) A platelet count should be obtained, since thrombocytopenic states may exist without a definite bleeding history. (2) The bleeding time is measured from a standard wound. This is frequently abnormal when either platelet or vascular pathology exists. (3) The partial thromboplastin time (PTT) is checked. The test determines the recalcification time of platelet-poor plasma to which cephalin (a platelet substitute) has been added. Variability of tests results due to numerical variation of platelets is thereby eliminated. The PTT test is prolonged if there is a deficiency of any coagulation factor except Factor VII and platelets. (4) The one-stage "prothrombin" time test is administered. This measures the time required for recalcified oxalated or citrated plasma to clot in the presence of tissue thromboplastin. Deficiencies of Factor I (fibrinogen), Factor II (prothrombin), Factor V (Ac-globulin), Factor VII (serum prothrombin conversion accelerator), and Factor X (Stuart-Prower factor) result in prolongation of the test time. Actually, the test is poorly named because it does not specifically measure prothrombin activity per se but rather the combined effect of the factors enumerated above. This by no means detracts from the importance of the test, for it is a reliable and simple method of studying the extrinsic coagulation system. The possibility of overlooking a clinically significant coagulation defect is remote if all four screening studies outlined above are carefully performed and interpreted.

The patient's blood type is determined and the appropriate blood order is placed with the blood bank.

Liver and Kidney Function Tests. Initial laboratory studies should include liver and renal function screening. Thus measurements of total serum protein, albumin and globulin, one-stage prothrombin time, serum bilirubin, alkaline phosphatase, and serum enzyme studies are obtained as well as a clean catch urinalysis, blood urea nitrogen, creatinine, and serum electrolytes. Should any of these initial studies prove abnormal, a complete evaluation of the suspected organ system is advisable. Frequently, patients who have been in chronic congestive heart failure may have measurable hepatic and renal dysfunction primarily related to congestive phenomena in the former and reduced blood flow in the latter. A general pattern of improved organ function can be anticipated with adequate medical therapy of the cardiac failure. Similarly, successful cardiac surgery, with its attendant reduction in congestive hepatomegaly and increased cardiac output, is generally accompanied by a progressive improvement in hepatic and renal function.

Ancillary Laboratory Examinations
Certain patients may require additional laboratory studies preoperatively.

Enzyme Markers of Myocardial Damage. In patients admitted for myocardial revascularization surgery who manifest angina persisting into the immediate preoperative period, it is important to ascertain that acute myocardial necrosis has not developed before carrying out coronary artery bypass grafting. When the electrocardiogram is equivocal, as in cases of nontransmural infarcts, other diagnostic tests are necessary.

Irreversibly injured myocardial cells release a number of enzymes into the circulation, where they can be measured by specific clinical reactions (Sobel and Shell, 1972). Patients with acute myocardial infarction show increased serum or plasma activity of many enzymes. In experimental myocardial infarction, a small but significant myocardial venoarterial difference in enzyme activity has been demonstrated (Pasyk et al., 1971) and elevated levels of plasma enzymes have been shown to correlate with corresponding depletion of these same enzymes from infarcted tissue (Jennings et al., 1957; Shell et al., 1971). Thus, determinations of serum activity of creatine-kinase (CK), glutamic oxaloacetic transferase (SGOT), and lactic dehydrogenase (LDH) have become standard tests in the laboratory diagnosis of acute myocardial infarction.

At present, elevation of serum CK activity is the most sensitive biochemical indicator of acute myocardial infarction (Smith, 1967; Goldberg and Windfield, 1972; Sobel and Shell, 1972; Vasudevan et al., 1978). In the interpretation of serum CK values, it is important to remember that there is a 15 percent incidence of false-positive results occurring primarily in patients with muscle disease, skeletal muscle trauma, intramuscular injections, vigorous exercise, alcohol intoxication, diabetes mellitus, and pulmonary embolism (Sobel and Shell, 1972). One should also remember that serum CK values in women are normally two thirds of those in men. Following the onset of acute myocardial infarction, serum CK activity rises above the normal range within six to eight hours, peaks at about 24 hours, and slowly returns to normal within three to four days after the onset of chest pains (Sobel and Shell, 1972).

Electrophoretic studies have identified three isoenzymes of CK—BB, MM, and MB. The BB isoenzyme appears to be found mainly in extracts of brain and kidney, while the MM isoenzyme predominates in skeletal muscle. Both MM and MB isoenzymes are found in cardiac muscle. The small intestine, tongue, and diaphragm also may contain minor quantities of the MB isoenzyme (Smith, 1972; Roberts and Sobel, 1973). However, for practical purposes, elevated serum MB CK activity may be considered to be the result of acute myocardial necrosis despite the presence of small amounts of MB CK isoenzyme in noncardiac tissue (Roberts et al., 1975). The development of the radioimmunoassay method of measurement of serum MB CK activity has helped improve the accuracy, sensitivity, and specificity of the test and has established it as the most reliable biochemical test for acute myocardial infarction (Roberts et al., 1975). Elevations of MB CK activity also can occur in other forms of injury to cardiac muscle, such as those resulting from cardiac surgery, trauma, and myocarditis (Alderman et al., 1973; Tonkins et al., 1975), and the differentiation can only be made by correlating the enzyme activity changes with the clinical picture.

Elevations of SGOT and LDH activity are useful but less specific biochemical tests for acute myocardial necrosis. The guidelines for their interpretation have been reviewed comprehensively elsewhere (Agress and Kin, 1960; Sobel and Shell, 1972).

Pulmonary Function Tests. Pulmonary function is frequently impaired to some degree after cardiac surgery, particularly following operations requiring use of extracorporeal circulation. These problems take on grave significance particularly if they are superimposed on lungs and preexisting pathology. When borderline respiratory function is suspected, quantitative evaluation of the pulmonary defect is essential. This requires a careful assessment of ventilation, respiration, and pulmonary circulation. Refer to standard texts on applied respiratory physiology for a comprehensive discussion of the subject.

FACTORS AFFECTING SURGICAL RISK

The decision to operate is based on a careful analysis of information obtained from the clinical history, physical examination, laboratory studies, and special diagnostic tests. Frequently, the available information also allows a reasonable estimate of the risks involved to be made and the optimal timing of the operation to be determined. In this section, consideration will be given to those factors that are believed to influence surgical morbidity and mortality.

General Factors

Age. The extremes of age impose certain physiologic handicaps on the patient. Senescence brings a decline of vitality, progressive lowering of biologic efficiency, and diminution of the capacity of the organism to maintain itself as an efficient machine. Certain changes in structure and function occur at the cellular level. While the homeostatic mechanisms may appear intact in the resting state, there is a sharply limited capability to maintain body economy under conditions of stress and trauma. Between the ages of 30 and 75, maximum oxygen uptake during exercise decreases 60 percent and maximum ventilation volume 47 percent (Shock, 1962). Vital capacity decreases 44 percent, and cardiac output at rest, 30 percent. Exercise tests performed on elderly patients focus attention on their uneven mixing, poor diffusion, reduced perfusion efficiency, rigidity of chest walls, and diminished compliance (Norris and Shock, 1960). In addition to defective alveolar ventilation there is interference with bronchial elimination of secretions containing particulate matter (Prindle, 1961).

Because of these mechanical and functional deficiencies, carbon dioxide elimination may be interfered with, setting the stage for the ready development of respiratory acidosis. It has been reported that patients over 60 years of age are two to three times more likely to develop postoperative respiratory complications (Dripps and Deming, 1946; Thoren, 1954; Klug and McPherson, 1959; Nunn, 1965; Modell and Moya, 1966; Davis and Spence, 1972). Renal plasma flow is reduced 50 percent, glomerular filtration rate 31 percent, the number of renal glomeruli, 44 percent, and renal tubular function, 44 percent. These alterations in renal function result in impairment in the ability to handle inappropriate sodium and water loads and a reduction in the capacity to secrete hydrogen ions. Consequently, there is a greater tendency to retain excess water, and with the occurrence of an extra physiologic or pathologic load on the mechanism of maintaining the hydrogen ion concentration, there is rapid decompensation. Both adrenal and gonadal activity decrease, basal metabolic rate is reduced 16 percent, and the blood water content, 18 percent, but the speed of return of blood acidity to equilibrium after exercise declines 33 percent. Brain weight decreases 10 percent and the blood flow to the brain, 20 percent. Table 3–2 summarizes the physiologic handicaps imposed by aging.

TABLE 3–2 SOME PHYSIOLOGIC HANDICAPS IMPOSED BY AGING

Cardiovascular
- Reduction of resting cardiac output
- Hazards imposed by coronary arteriosclerosis (conduction abnormalities, myocardial fibrosis, etc.)
- Reduced plasma volume

Respiratory
- Reduction of resting maximum ventilation volume
- Reduction of resting vital capacity
- Reduction of oxygen uptake postexercise
- Increased chest wall rigidity
- Diminution of lung compliance
- Increased ventilation/perfusion abnormalities
- Defective alveolar ventilation
- Decreased efficiency to eliminate tracheobronchial secretions

Renal
- Reduction in number of functional glomeruli
- Reduced glomerular filtration rate
- Reduced renal plasma flow
- Impaired ability to handle inappropriate sodium and water loads
- Reduced capacity to secrete hydrogen ions

Others
- Reduced cerebral blood flow
- Reduced basal metabolic rate
- Decreased adrenal and gonadal activity
- Sharply limited capability to maintain body economy under stress conditions

At the other end of the spectrum are the very young, whose response to disease is quite different from that of adults (Cooke and Levin, 1968; Rickham, 1969; Haller and Talbert, 1972). One important difference is the much greater lability of infants and neonates, especially the prematures. Infants have a higher metabolic rate, higher oxygen consumption, and a more rapid turnover of water and metabolites. They are much more susceptible to changes in ambient temperature because their temperature control mechanisms are not yet fully developed; furthermore, they tend to lose heat much more rapidly than adults because of their greater body surface area compared to mass. If the infant's body temperature is significantly above or below normal, there is a corresponding marked increase in oxygen consumption.

Respiratory problems after surgery are much more common in infants for a number of reasons. First, they mobilize secretions poorly because of inadequate cough reflexes. Second, because the ribs are soft and horizontal and the accessory respiratory msucles are not yet well developed, intercostal action contributes much less to ventilation than the diaphragm. Third, the narrow infant airway is much more readily compromised by edema, retained secretions, or a poorly chosen endotracheal tube. Fourth, compared to adults, infants and neonates do not tolerate cardiopulmonary bypass well.

Renal function in the newborn also is immature, reflected in an inability to concentrate and conserve fluid and electrolytes. The glomerular filtration rate is decreased and tubular reabsorptive capacity likewise diminished. It is apparent that congestive failure may rapidly ensue when overhydration occurs, since the decreased glomerular filtration rate limits renal excretion. Furthermore, the newborn's ability to ward off infection is diminished because of immature immune response mechanisms. Table 3-3 summarizes some physiologic peculiarities in the very young that alter their response to disease, operative trauma, and stress.

TABLE 3-3 SOME PHYSIOLOGIC PECULIARITIES IN NEONATES AND INFANTS THAT ALTER THEIR RESPONSE TO STRESS AND DISEASE

Cardiovascular

Circulating blood volume per kg body weight relatively greater

Total circulating blood volume small

Proportion of total body water to lean body mass greater compared to adults (82 percent vs. 73 percent)

Extracellular fluid compartment increased

Respiratory

Oxygen consumption higher

Obligatory nose-breather

Inadequate cough reflexes and weak thoracic musculature

Pliable, horizontal ribs contribute less to ventilation

Narrow, short airway more easily obstructed

Renal and Metabolic

Glomerular filtration rate decreased

Tubular reabsorption of fluid and electrolytes (concentrating ability) diminished

Others

Basal metabolic rate higher

Immature temperature-regulating mechanism

Greater surface area relative to body mass

Decreased phagocytic capacity of leukocytes

Diminished capability for immunoglobulin synthesis

These physiologic handicaps inherent in the elderly and the very young pose serious problems of management, since the permissible margins of error are small. The organ systems of both groups are sharply limited in their ability to successfully cope with potential operative and postoperative problems such as sudden blood loss, hypoxia, anemia, inappropriate fluid and electrolyte loads, and fever. In the evaluation of the patient's condition, it is important to discriminate between the effects of age and the primary disease and the effects of concomitant pathologic conditions, although these frequently are additive.

Nutritional Status. Proper assessment of the nutritional status of the patient is an equally important aspect of preoperative care. The potential dangers of both inadequate nutrition and obesity are well-known. Malnutrition, with its accompanying hypoproteinemia and hypoalbuminemia, can have many adverse effects. Hypoproteinemia appears to impair wound healing (Thompson et al., 1938) and antibody production (Cannon et al., 1944) while possibly decreasing resistance to infection (Wohl et al., 1949; Rhoads, 1953). Moreover, the hypoproteinemic patient appears to be more sensitive to large quantities of intravenously administered saline (Jones and Eaton, 1933) and has a greater tendency to develop interstitial edema from loss of plasma oncotic pressure. In addition, experimental evidence shows that hypoproteinemic animals are more susceptible to hemorrhagic shock (Radvin et al., 1944), the clinical counterpart of which has been seen frequently in humans.

Chronic loss of protein, when severe, is frequently accompanied by skeletal muscle wasting, as seen in advanced malnutrition and cardiac cachexia. This may bring about a loss of strength and function of the abdominal, intercostal, shoulder, and diaphragmatic muscles. As a result of muscle weakness, full ventilatory excursions may no longer be possible and the patient's ability to expel mucus from his or her tracheobronchial tree may be seriously impaired, thus setting the stage for respiratory complications. Chronically debilitated and cachectic patients are twice as likely to develop postoperative respiratory complications (Golebiowski, 1971).

Obesity, on the other hand, is associated with a higher incidence of degenerative diseases such as atherosclerosis and diabetes; moreover, obesity reduces ventilatory reserve and increases the risk of postoperative respiratory failure. Obese patients frequently show a reduction in functional residual capacity without a change in residual volume; the expiratory reserve volume is reduced (Tucker and Sieker, 1960) and the maximum breathing capacity is low (Cullen and Formel, 1962). The dead weight of the subcutaneous fat in the abdomen and chest wall restricts the freedom of motion of the thoracic cage, increases the resistance to expansion of the thorax, and reduces the total compliance of the respiratory system. This decrease in compliance correlates with the decrease in lung volumes observed in obese patients (Naimark and Cherniack, 1960), so that at any lung volume the respiratory compliance in the obese person is frequently half the normal value (Waltemath and Bergman, 1974).

Hypoxemia also is encountered frequently and usually is the result of abnormal relationships between ventilation and perfusion (Said, 1960). Many obese people show elevations in arterial-alveolar oxygen tension gradients, reflecting an increase in venous admixture. The latter is most commonly caused by low ventilation-perfusion ratios. In obese people, perfusion to dependent areas of the lungs is normal but is accomplished by little or no ventilation in those areas (Holley et al., 1967; Barrera et al., 1969). This decrease in ventilation is believed to be secondary to closure of small airways (Couture et al., 1970), which is a tendency often found in obese patients with low expiratory reserve volumes and aggravated by recumbency. Closure of the small airways in the dependent portions of the lungs combined with the normal increase in blood flow to these areas brought about by the influence of gravity produces marked abnormalities in ventilation-perfusion and hypoxemia (Barrera et al., 1967; Douglas and Chong, 1972).

With the superimposition of acute lung disease, obese patients are much more likely to develop hypercarbia from alveolar hypoventilation because, very often, they are functioning at already low lung volumes and reduced total respiratory compliance. These factors increase the likelihood of acute respiratory failure developing postoperatively. It has been reported that obese patients (body weight at least 30 percent greater than ideal) are two times more likely to develop postoperative respiratory complications (Thoren, 1954; Gould, 1962; Latimer et al., 1971).

It is apparent from the foregoing discussion that, whenever feasible, the patient's nutritional status should be restored to as near normal as possible before surgery. The nutritional program should be coordinated with the overall therapeutic plan and timetable for clinical care. Thus, complete replenishment of protein deficits may not be feasible in a patient with chronic congestive heart failure from rheumatic mitral and tricuspid valve disease before surgical correction of the underlying hemodynamic defects. On the other hand, an obese cardiac who is in no immediate danger of dying should, whenever practicable, promptly be placed on a weight-reducing program to shed excess adipose tissue prior to elective cardiac surgery.

Physiologic Derangements Secondary to Cardiac Disease. Of prime importance is the degree of cardiac dysfunction and the secondary functional alterations the heart disease imposes on other vital organs, such as the lungs, liver, kidneys, and brain. Frequently, abnormalities in pulmonary function accompany left-heart dysfunction. For instance, left-sided failure results in pulmonary venous hypertension with engorgement of the lungs, rigidity, and loss of parenchymal elasticity, diminution of pulmonary compliance, reduction in vital capacity, and impairment of gaseous exchange across the alveolocapillary membrane. On the other hand, right-sided failure results primarily in elevation of the systemic venous and capillary pressures, and in sodium and water retention. The organs predominantly involved are the liver, kidneys, spleen, and gastrointestinal tract, where alterations in function almost invariably occur as a result of chronic passive congestion. Aberrations in cerebral function sometimes may be attributable to congestive changes, but more frequently are caused by either concomitant cerebral arteriosclerosis or infarcts and encephalomalacia from cerebral embolization of cardiac origin.

The presence of associated pulmonary, hepatic, renal, or cerebral dysfunction, or any combination thereof, increases the risks of surgical therapy. Therefore, it is mandatory that the nature and magnitude of the functional alterations be carefully assessed preoperatively.

Intercurrent Conditions. A number of metabolic disorders are of surgical interest. Perhaps the most common condition is diabetes mellitus; disorders involving other endocrine systems (i.e., adrenal insufficiency, thyrotoxicosis, hypothyroidism) are less frequently encountered. Because each of these disorders may adversely affect the patient's response to operative trauma and stress, their recognition and control prior to surgery are of utmost importance.

Hypertensive disease, when superimposed on surgical cardiac disease, is of serious therapeutic import because of the high incidence of coronary atherosclerosis and cardiac hypertrophy associated with it. In addition, the increased peripheral vascular resistance (afterload) seen in hypertensives, especially those with chronically elevated diastolic pressures, may set the stage for a low cardiac output state postoperatively. Finally, many hypertensive patients may have been treated with drugs such as reserpine, promethazine, or chlorpromazine. These drugs may abolish reflexes controlling vasomotor tone (Eckenhoff, 1956), an effect that may last as long as two weeks after the drug has been discontinued. As a result, induction of anesthesia may initiate sudden or severe hypotension, which may not be well-tolerated by a patient with a significantly reduced cardiac output. Treatment of the hypotension consists of the prompt administration of α-adrenergic agents, such as metaraminol or levarterenol. It is good practice to stop antihypertensive agents, which have as their primary action depletion of adrenergic mediators, two weeks before the projected operation date to prevent such accidents.

The adverse effects of associated chronic bronchopulmonary disease are well known. These patients are more likely to develop postoperative respiratory complications from increased tracheobronchial secretions, bronchospasm, or atelectasis. Maximal improvement of pulmonary function is one of the important goals of preoperative preparation. This will be discussed in more detail in Chapters 6 and 12.

The detection of abnormal function of any vital organ system clearly complicates postoperative care and may compromise survival. These findings do not constitute absolute contraindications, but the additional risk must be weighed against the sum of natural history of the nonoperated lesion and the coexisting disease.

Specific Determinants of Surgical Risk

The progressive decline in hospital mortality following open intracardiac operations observed in recent years has, in large measure, been due to improvements in surgical, perfusion, and myocardial protection techniques. In spite of these advances, however, hospital mortality continues to be adversely affected by the nature and complexity of the cardiac lesion(s) and by the severity of the cardiac dysfunction present before repair. It is clearly beyond the scope of this chapter to discuss each condition from the standpoint of surgical indications, patient selection, and specific factors affecting surgical risk. Suffice it to say here that each specific cardiac lesion or combination of lesions affects hospital mortality in its own unique way.

PREOPERATIVE CARE

Preoperative Hospitalization Period and Psychologic Preparation

The period of preoperative hospitalization is governed by the time required to bring the patient to an optimally stable condition. Patients who have no history of antecedent heart failure can be admitted two to four days before the projected surgical date. On the other hand, patients who have been in chronic congestive heart failure may require several weeks or even months of hospital therapy before surgery can be carried out.

Frequently, during the course of prolonged hospital care, preoperative cardiac patients become markedly depressed and, as time wears on, they may evince increasing fear over the outcome of their surgery. It should be remembered that any patient admitted for cardiac surgery enters the hospital with varying degrees of apprehension because of the very nature of the operation to be performed. The problem becomes markedly worse if the period of preoperative hospitalization is necessarily prolonged.

Management of these emotional problems demands, above all, the expenditure of time by both the physician and nursing staff in understanding the basis for and the magnitude of the patient's anxiety. Patients often are reassured to know that their fears are not unique; that, indeed, virtually all patients experience some measure of them. Further, it is helpful to point out to patients who have been hospitalized for a considerable period that the consequence of such meticulous care will be clearly apparent to them in the postoperative period. Such a casual statement distinctly implies that the medical staff fully expects to see the patient in the latter period and goes a long way in helping the patient to develop a positive viewpoint at a most difficult time. The medical staff's inability to comprehend the intensity of these fears frequently results in denegration of their importance. However, Kennedy and Bakst (1966) have shown that the emotional state of the patient has a direct influence on the morbidity and mortality of cardiac surgery.

Shortly before surgery patients are informed of what they will experience in the immediate postoperative period. In particular, they are told that they must anticipate some discomfort at the operative site and drainage catheters. If prolonged endotracheal intubation or a tracheostomy is anticipated, this too is discussed, with particular emphasis on the rationale and on the temporary inability to speak. In general, the more the patient is aware of what to expect, the smoother will be the emotional response to surgery.

Management of Patients in Cardiac Failure

The principle underlying all cardiac therapy is the favorable alteration of the balance of factors influencing cardiac performance to improve the heart's mechanical efficiency. The therapeutic elements are: (1) limitation of physical activities, which proportionately reduces the load imposed on the heart; (2) improvement in cardiac function by pharmacologic agents, primarily digitalis glycosides; and (3) control of fluid retention by limitation of sodium intake and the use of diuretics, which improves renal excretion of sodium and water.

Rest. Rest in bed or chair is designed to reduce metabolic expenditure to a minimum, thereby requiring proportionally less cardiac work. Patients are placed on graded rest routines as dictated by the presence and severity of cardiac failure; those in severe congestive failure are placed on complete bed rest and those with milder incapacitation are permitted out of bed except at specified rest intervals. Significant clinical improvement has been observed in severely ill patients after several months of bed rest even though they were initially refractory to all therapy. Reduction in dyspnea, orthopnea, hepatomegaly, and a gradual diuresis can be seen, and the patients describe a general feeling of relative well-being. Proper timing of surgery is of vital importance in this latter group, for even the most dramatic improvement represents a short period of equilibrium in which the patient's cardiac reserve is still sufficient to satisfy his or her basal metabolic requirements. Waiting for "further improvement" may invite disaster should the patient's cardiac performance suddenly deteriorate. On the other hand, premature surgery will be equally hazardous and probably disastrous unless maximal improvement has been accomplished. At best, the timing of corrective cardiac surgery in these people is difficult.

Digitalis Glycosides. Digitalis has been the therapeutic keystone in the treatment of cardiac failure since William Withering (1785) first described its use in dropsy and a variety of other conditions. The two clinical effects of digitalis are: (1) improved myocardial contractility; and (2) slowing and control of the cardiac rate by increasing the refractory period of the atrioventricular node and bundle (His) and by increasing the vagal response of the sinoatrial node and conduction system. The precise nature of the cellular action of digitalis glycosides in improving myocardial contractility is still controversial (Olsen, 1961; Luchi and Conn, 1965; Lee and Klaus, 1971), although their positive inotropic effect was clearly established more than forty years ago in the classic experiment of Cattell and Gold (1938).

Most patients admitted for surgery of valvular heart disease have previously been in failure and are already on digitalis. They require only maintenance therapy. If they have been on one of the long-acting glycosides, such as digitalis leaf or digitoxin, they are switched to digoxin, a preparation with a shorter duration of action, so that potential postsurgical problems of drug toxicity are minimized. The medication is stopped one day before surgery, since there is a tendency toward enhancement of digitalis effect following use of extracorporeal circulation, especially when dilute perfusates not containing potassium are employed.

Sodium Restriction and Diuretics. Sodium and water retention due to congestive heart failure can be effectively managed by reduced sodium intake (Schroeder, 1941) and supplemental diuretic therapy. The reader is referred to Friedberg (1966), who has detailed a variety of sodium restrictive regimens. Patients admitted with a history of cardiac failure are placed on a diet permitting one to two grams of sodium daily; those patients with overt signs of congestive failure may require even more stringent restriction. From a practical standpoint, it is difficult to maintain patients on highly restrictive sodium diets; the menus are unappetizing and the food is frequently protein deficient. Children or adults who have no history or clinical evidence of failure are permitted a regular diet.

The majority of patients in failure who are admitted for cardiac surgery have previously been treated with diuretics. Therapy with either one of the benzothiadiazide or loop diuretics is continued as necessary to control fluid retention. Oral potassium supplements should be given. Continued diuretic therapy may readily lead to serious hyponatremia and combined hypokalemic-hypochloremic metabolic alkalosis. Moreover, the ability of diuretics to provoke severe plasma volume depletion cannot be overemphasized. Thus, overly vigorous diuretic administration can set the stage for serious intraoperative or postoperative problems related either to arrhythmias or low cardiac output. These difficulties may be particularly aggravated if extracorporeal circulation has been employed, since measurements made after bypass suggest movement of water out of the plasma and possibly the cells (Cleland et al., 1966). Further, use of dilute perfusate is generally associated with reduced serum potassium and chloride levels in the postoperative period (Deiter et al., 1970; Vasko et al., 1973). Ebert et al. (1965) have called particular attention to the relationships between postperfusion hypokalemia and life-threatening arrhythmias in patients who have undergone lengthy diuretic treatment. Thus, for all these reasons, diuretic therapy should be discontinued about five days before elective surgery.

Antiarrhythmic Drugs. Antifibrillatory drugs such as quinidine and procaine amide sometimes are employed preoperatively, especially where there has been recent onset of atrial fibrillation in patients with mitral valve disease. Although the theoretical advantage of having a patient enter the operating room in normal sinus rhythm is apparent, the practical problem of avoiding an arrhythmic "breakthrough" requires administration of drug increments that can significantly depress myocardial contractility. It is therefore advisable to accept the presence of atrial fibrillation, control the ventricular rate with digitalis, and discontinue all antifibrillatory medications at least one week before the projected surgical date. Pharmacologic or electrical cardioversion can then be attempted at an appropriate time in the postoperative period.

Management of Patients with Coronary Artery Disease

Most patients admitted for myocardial revascularization surgery are on chronic propranolol therapy. In view of the negative inotropic properties of propranolol, some concern has been expressed about the advisability of continuing drug administration into the immediate postoperative period (Viljoen et al., 1972). However, more recent studies have shown that therapeutic doses of propranolol can be administered to within 24 hours or less before surgery without profound hemodynamic depression (Caralps et al., 1974; Jones et al., 1976; Kopriva et al., 1978a; Kopriva et al., 1978b; Slogoff et al., 1978). Indeed, it has been shown that withdrawal of beta blockade may be harmful, especially if the drug is discontinued abruptly (Miller et al., 1975; Jones et al., 1976; Boudoulas et al., 1977). While the underlying pathogenetic mechanism remains uncertain, there seems little doubt that the syndrome of propranolol withdrawal does exist (summarized by Shand and Wood, 1978).

Thus, on the basis of presently available information, certain guidelines for propranolol use in patients undergoing myocardial revascularization can be laid down. (1) It seems prudent to continue propranolol therapy into the eve of surgery to prevent the emergence of acute ischemic events. (2) If the clinical situation requires discontinuance of the drug a few days before surgery, the propranolol dose should be tapered gradually, avoiding abrupt withdrawal of beta blockade.

(3) Propranolol can be administered without serious consequences up to just before anesthetic induction; thus, there should be no hesitation in maintaining maximal beta blockade into the preanesthetic period if the clinical situation demands (e.g., severe preinfarction angina).

Some patients with coronary artery disease may require intraaortic balloon counterpulsation support preoperatively. The general principles of management of such patients are discussed in Chapter 21.

Management of Patients with Congenital Heart Disease

Patients with cyanotic heart disease deserve special mention. In the presence of marked polycythemia (hematocrit >60 vol%; hemoglobin >20 gm per 100 ml), preoperative phlebotomy may be useful. The excess red cell volume is removed and replaced with fresh frozen plasma. Such treatments have been shown to improve cardiac output by reducing blood viscosity (Rosenthal et al., 1970), correct certain coagulation abnormalities (Wedemeyer et al., 1973; Ekert and Shears, 1974), and reduce postoperative bleeding (von Kaulla et al., 1967). Red cell volume reduction is achieved over the course of a few phlebotomy treatments during the week before the operation. However, such procedures may not be practical in infants. Extremely cyanotic children awaiting surgery should be given intravenous fluids while oral intake is withheld to reduce the likelihood of intravascular thrombosis.

General Measures

Preventive Respiratory Care. The hallmark of the management program is the prevention of operative and postoperative respiratory complications. In this regard, meticulous preoperative preparation and anticipatory care are of paramount importance. When indicated, a careful quantitative assessment is made of the patient's total pulmonary reserve. The presence of significant pulmonary disease does not necessarily contraindicate surgery, but does alert the staff to potential postoperative complications, including the need for postoperative ventilatory assistance.

Following identification of those conditions known to predispose to the development of postoperative pulmonary complications, appropriate corrective measures are initiated whenever applicable. For instance, smoking should be forbidden starting at least two to three weeks preoperatively. It has been reported that cigarette smokers (ten cigarettes per day) are two to seven times more likely to develop postoperative respiratory complications (Morton 1944; Collins et al., 1968; Latimer et al., 1971; Laszlo et al., 1973). Respiratory infections should be eliminated by appropriate antibiotic therapy. It has been shown that a combination of cessation of smoking and preoperative eradication of respiratory infection results in a 50 percent reduction in complications (Collins et al., 1968).

Proper physical and psychologic preparation are extremely important (Roe, 1960; Rogers et al., 1972). Patients should be properly trained to carry out the various essential respiratory maneuvers (deep breathing, coughing, wound splinting) and oriented to the chest physiotherapy techniques that are going to be employed in the postoperative period. As pointed out in a previous section, patients should be forewarned of what they can expect in the way of postoperative discomfort, pain, drainage tubes, and the like. The patient's perceptions and responses to pain can be altered by proper preoperative instruction and reassurance, resulting in reduction of postoperative analgesic requirements.

In the presence of chronic productive bronchitis, accompanied by copious and purulent secretions, an intensive management program should be instituted three to five days preoperatively. This includes the use of high humidity aerosols, chest physiotherapy, and postural drainage. In some cases, the use of bronchodilators, mucolytics, or appropriate antibiotics also may be helpful, but the emphasis should be on physical measures to evacuate secretions. Therapy is continued until the bronchial secretions are reduced to a stable minimum and bronchospasm has been controlled.

It has been our experience that patients who are made aware of the hazards of pulmonary complications will cooperate more actively in their prevention. Thus, an orderly program of preoperative instruction has proved to be of great value, particularly in the elderly or chronically ill. Specifically, patients are taught the proper techniques for achieving optimal ventilation and effective coughing and proper use of respiratory therapy apparatus (e.g., blow bottles or incentive spirometers). Professional chest physiotherapists can be extremely helpful in this regard, although other trained personnel can be relied on to carry out this task.

Antibiotic Therapy. Prophylactic antibiotic therapy is a widely accepted practice in cardiac surgery even though its efficacy has never been conclusively demonstrated by a carefully designed, prospective randomized study involving a large number of patients. This approach is based on a number of clinical and experimental observations that suggest increased vulnerability of the cardiac surgical patient to postoperative infection. The rationale for prophylactic antibiotic therapy is discussed in greater detail in Chapter 18.

A variety of antibiotic regimens have been employed with equal success. We have found the following simple regimen for prophylaxis to be effective. Cefazolin has been used in adults and children, while a combination of penicillin and gentamycin has been employed in infants. In cases of penicillin or cephalosporin hypersensitivity, a combination of vancomycin and gentamycin is preferred. Antibiotic administration is begun the night before surgery, continued the morning of the operation and immediately after it, and maintained postoperatively for five days.

Question of Preoperative "Prophylactic" Digitalization. There is disagreement as to the advisability of "prophylactically" digitalizing patients before surgery without evidence of cardiac failure or atrial fibrillation (Lyons et al., 1960; Kloster et al., 1966; Bristow and Griswold, 1965; Selzer et al., 1966; Burman, 1972). The arguments advanced for such a course are based on the belief that the inotropic action of the drug can effectively counter the deleterious effects of anesthesia, hypothermia, myocardial hypoxia, and the physical traumata of ventriculotomy, retraction, and suturing. This attitude has been reinforced by recent observations that have refuted the previously held concept that digitalis exerted a toxic effect on normal myocardium and thereby reduced the cardiac output (Harrison and Leonard, 1926; Burwell et al., 1927; Dock and Tainter, 1930). More recent observations have indicated that the cardiac output is not significantly altered in normal subjects when digitalis is administered (Williams et al., 1958; Dresdale et al., 1959; Selzer et al., 1959). Further, it has been shown that digitalis exerts a positive inotropic action in normal human subjects (Mason and Braunwald, 1963) and reduces the postexercise oxygen debt in cardiac patients without heart failure (Kahler et al., 1963).

Despite the theoretical advantages, there are several reasons why routine preoperative digitalization of all patients subjected to cardiac surgery is not advisable. First, in patients undergoing open intracardiac operations employing extracorporeal circulation, the postperfusion digitalization state is uncertain (Beall et al., 1963; Ebert et al., 1963). Second, there is some evidence that patients may be more sensitive to digitalis after open intracardiac operations (Morrison and Killip, 1973; Krasula et al., 1974). Third, the evidence that prophylactic digitalization helps reduce the incidence of postoperative arrhythmias is not firm. In a prospective randomized study of patients undergoing coronary artery bypass, Johnson et al. (1976) demonstrated a significant decrease in postoperative supraventricular tachyarrhythmias. These results are at variance with those of another study. Tyras et al. (1979) demonstrated that prophylactic digitalization was of no benefit in the prevention of supraventricular arrhythmias; indeed, such therapy may have predisposed to the development of these arrhythmias in their patients.

Fourth, we have not been impressed that preoperative prophylactic digitalization of patients not in failure has demonstrably altered the clinical results. The postoperative cardiac performance in these patients is generally satisfactory, and they usually go through surgery without need of any supportive therapy unless the surgical repair requires an anatomic and hemodynamic compromise, such as certain cases of tetralogy of Fallot where extensive reconstruction of the right ventricular outflow tract and pulmonary artery trunk may be necessary. Under these circumstances, digitalization may be safely deferred until discontinuance of extracorporeal circulation.

In the great majority of cases, there seems to be little need to confuse the postoperative picture with such prophylaxis; in particular, the diagnosis and therapy of arrhythmias are made substantially easier if the possibility of digitalis toxicity can be eliminated. An important exception is the patient with mitral stenosis and normal sinus rhythm who requires surgery. In this situation, preoperative digitalization is carried out because of the frequency of atrial fibrillation or flutter and their related and undesirable rapid ventricular responses in the postoperative period (Bailey, 1955). Should an atrial arrhythmia develop, the ventricular rate will be more readily controlled if prior digitalization has been effected. If preoperative prophylactic digitalization is elected in such a case, there is no true therapeutic end point, and maximal dosage schedules should not be employed (Bristow and Griswold, 1965). Similar therapeutic principles govern digitalis administration in infants and children. Digitalization is carried out preoperatively only if the classical indications of failure or supraventricular arrhythmias are apparent (Neill, 1965).

Patients undergoing coronary artery bypass merit special consideration. At this institution, such patients are placed in a program of prophylactic digitalization in the immediate *postoperative* period. This practice is based on our experience, corroborated by others (O'Kane et al., 1972), that postoperative digitalization reduces both the frequency and severity of supraventricular tachyarrhythmias.

Preparation for Surgery

As pointed out previously, the patient's general condition determines the length of the preoperative hospitalization period. Once an optimally stable condition has been achieved, an orderly program of care is initiated to ensure a smooth transition into the intraoperative period.

Preoperative Skin Preparation. The goal of this regimen is the reduction of the bacterial content of the patient's skin, particularly in the vicinity of the planned surgical incision(s). This is achieved through a program of mechanical scrubbing that is started two days before the operation (conceivably this program could be started before the patient enters the hospital). Ideally, this should be done twice a day using a soft, nontraumatic, iodophor-impregnated sponge, brush, or cloth. In this manner, grease, dirt, desquamated epithelium, and loose resident bacteria are removed. Iodophor seems ideally suited for this purpose because of its bactericidal and penetrating properties.

Other Preparations. Preoperative visits are made by members of the surgical, medical, anesthesiology, and nursing staff on the day before surgery. The responsible surgeon will have taken the time to review with the patient in clear and simple terms the proposed surgical procedure and its rationale. Candid discussions of inherent risks and potential complications should be conducted in a way that will not make the patient unduly fearful and apprehensive.

The patient is made familiar with the cardiac surgical intensive care unit (or recovery room), the postoperative nursing care procedures, the monitoring apparatus, and other equipment that will be used in the postoperative period. Patients have found it particularly reassuring to be visited by a nurse from the intensive care unit or postoperative recovery area, who gives a general description of the surgical care unit and its surroundings and eliminates the anonymity of the personnel who will be intimately involved in the patient's postoperative recovery. The same visiting nurse becomes acquainted with the patient's condition and formulates a postoperative nursing care plan based on his or her own evaluation of the patient.

Similarly, the physician staff makes a final general assessment of the patient's condition. This normally includes analysis of the latest results of pertinent laboratory tests, including radiographs, and a final review of the hemodynamic data and pertinent angiograms. In addition, it is good practice to review the overall operative plan with the members of the operating team, the perfusionists, and the scrub nurse, especially if the case turns out to be anything but "routine."

Preoperative Orders. Table 3–4 outlines a set of typical preoperative orders for a patient scheduled for an open intracardiac operation. All patients are shaven from chin to feet, including the axillary areas, back, both arms and forearms, pubic area, and frequently the perineal area as well. They are required to continue the iodophor scrub previously prescribed and to take a shower or bath. Antibiotic therapy is started the evening before surgery. Digitalis preparations are held on the morning of surgery, while diuretics and antiarrhythmic drugs will have been discontinued by then. A quick check is made with the blood bank on the availability of required blood and blood products. The patient is given a good sedative the evening before surgery.

TABLE 3–4 TYPICAL SET OF PREOPERATIVE ORDERS FOR ADULT OPEN HEART SURGERY

1. NPO after midnight
2. Consent for operation and photography
3. Continue iodophor skin scrub
4. Continue chest physiotherapy training
5. Skin preparation: shave from chin to feet including back, both axillae, forearms and arms, pubic area
6. Type and crossmatch for 4 units of CPD blood. Order 2 units of fresh frozen plasma
7. Hold digitalis morning of surgery
8. Antibiotics: Cefazolin 2 gm IM or IV, night before and morning of operation (Use vancomycin and gentamycin if patient is allergic to cephalosporin and congeners)
9. Calculation of heparin and protamine dose on chart: Heparin—200 IU/kg Protamine sulfate—3 mg/kg
10. Chest x-ray and angiograms to OR

REFERENCES

Agress C M, Kin J H C: Evaluation of enzyme tests in the diagnosis of heart disease. Am J Cardiol 6:641, 1960.

Alderman E L, Matlof H J, Shumway N E, Harrison D C: Evaluation of enzyme testing for the detection of myocardial infarction following direct coronary surgery. Circulation 48:135, 1973.

Bailey C P: Surgery of the Heart. Philadelphia, Lea and Febiger, 1955, p 543.

Barrera F, Reidenberg M M, Winters W L: Pulmonary function in the obese patient. Am J Med Sci 254:785, 1967.

———, ———, ———, Hungspreugs S: Ventilation-perfusion relationships in the obese patient. J Appl Physiol 26:420, 1969.

Beall A C Jr, Johnson P C, Driscoll T, Alexander J K, Dennis E, McNamara D, Cooley D, DeBakey M E: Effect of total cardiopulmonary bypass on myocardial and blood digoxin concentration in man. Am J Cardiol 11:194, 1963.

Boudoulas H, Lewis R P, Kates R E, Dalamangas G: Hypersensitivity to adrenergic stimulation after propranolol withdrawal in normal subjects. Ann Intern Med 87:433, 1977.

Bristow J D, Griswold H E: The use of digitalis in cardiovascular surgery. Prog Cardiovasc Dis 7:387, 1965.

Burman S: The prophylactic use of digitalis before thoracotomy. Ann Thorac Surg 14:359, 1972.

Burwell C S, Neighbors De W, Regen E M: The effect of digitalis upon the output of the heart in normal man. J Clin Invest 5: 125, 1927.

Cannon P R, Wissler R W, Woolridge R L, Benditt E P: Relationship of protein deficiency to surgical infection. Ann Surg 120:514, 1944.

Caralps J M, Mulet J, Wienke H R, Moran J M, Pifarre R: Results of coronary artery surgery in patients receiving propranolol. J Thorac Cardiovasc Surg 67:526, 1974.

Cattell M, Gold H: Influence of digitalis glycosides on the force of contraction of mammalian cardiac muscle. J Pharmacol Exp Ther 62:116, 1938.

Cleland J, Pluth J R, Tauxe W N, Kirklin J W: Blood volume and body fluid compartment changes soon after closed and open intracardiac surgery. J Thorac Cardiovasc Surg 52:698, 1966.

Collins C D, Drake C S, Knowelden J: Chest complications following upper abdominal surgery: their anticipation and prevention. Br Med J 1:401, 1968.

Cooke R E, Levin S: The Biologic Basis of Pediatric Practice. New York, McGraw-Hill, 1968.

Couture J, Picken J, Trop D, Ruff F, Lousada N, Houseley E, Bates D V: Airway closure in normal obese and anesthetized supine subjects. Fed Proc 29:269, 1970.

Cullen J H, Formel P F: The respiratory defects in extreme obesity. Am J Med 32:525, 1962.

Davis A G, Spence A A: Postoperative hypoxemia and age. Anesthesiology 37:663, 1972.

Deiter R A, Neville W E, Pifarre R: Hypokalemia following hemodilution cardiopulmonary bypass. Ann Surg 171:17, 1970.

Dock W, Tainter M L: Circulatory changes after full therapeutic doses of digitalis with critical discussion of views on cardiac output. J Clin Invest 8:467, 1930.

Douglas F G, Chong P Y: Influence of obesity on peripheral airways patency. J Appl Physiol 33:559, 1972.

Dresdale D T, Yuceoglue Y Z, Michtom R J, Schultz M, Lunger M: Effects of lanatoside C on cardiovascular hemodynamics. Acute digitalizing doses in subjects with normal hearts and with heart disease without failure. Am J Cardiol 4:88, 1959.

Dripps R D, Deming M V N: Postoperative atelectasis and pneumonia. Diagnosis, etiology and management based upon 1,240 cases of upper abdominal surgery. Ann Surg 124:94, 1946.

Ebert P A, Jude J R, Gaertner R A: Persistent hypokalemia following open heart surgery. Circulation 31(Suppl):137, 1965.

———, Morrow A G, Austen W G: Clinical studies of the effect of extracorporeal circulation on myocardial digoxin concentration. Am J Cardiol 11:201, 1963.

Eckenhoff J E: Some preoperative warnings of potential operating room deaths. N Eng J Med 255:1075, 1956.

Ekert H, Shears M: Preoperative and postoperative platelet function in cyanotic congenital heart disease. J Thorac Cardiovasc Surg 67:184, 1974.

Friedberg C K: Diseases of the Heart, 3rd ed. Philadelphia, London, Saunders, 1966, p 346.

Goldberg D M, Windfield D A: Diagnostic accuracy of serum enzyme assays for myocardial infarction in a general hospital population. Br Heart J 34:597, 1972.

Golebiowski A: Pulmonary resection in patients over 70 years of age. J Thor Cardiovasc Surg, 1971.

Gould A B Jr: Effect of obesity on respiratory complications following general anesthesia. Anesth Analg (Cleve) 41:448, 1962.

Haller J A Jr, Talbert J L: Surgical Emergencies in the Newborn. Philadelphia, Lea & Febiger, 1972, p 1.

Harrison T R, Leonard B W: The effect of digitalis upon the output of the heart of dogs and its bearing on the action of the drug in heart disease. J Clin Invest 3:1, 1926.

Holley H S, Milic-Emili J, Becklake M R, Bates D V: Regional distribution of pulmonary ventilation and perfusion in obesity. J Clin Invest 46:475, 1967.

Johnson L W, Dickstein R A, Fruehan C T, Kane P, Potts J L, Smuylan H, Webb W R, Eich R H: Prophylactic digitalization for coronary artery bypass surgery. Circulation 53:819, 1976.

Jennings R B, Kaltenbach J P, Smetters G W: Enzymatic changes in acute myocardial ischemic injury. Arch Pathol 64:10, 1957.

Jones C M, Eaton F B: Postoperative nutritional edema. Arch Surg 27:159, 1933.

Jones E, Kaplan J A, Dorney E R, King S B III, Douglas J S Jr, Hatcher C R Jr: Propranolol therapy in patients undergoing myocardial revascularization. Am J Cardiol 38:697, 1976.

Kahler R L, Thompson R H, Buskirk E R, Frye R L, Braunwald E: Studies on digitalis. VI. Reduction of the oxygen debt after exercise with digoxin in cardiac patients without heart failure. Circulation 27:397, 1963.

Kennedy J A, Bakst A: The influence of emotions on the outcome of surgery: a predictive study. Bull N Y Acad Med 42:811, 1966.

Kloster F E, Bristow J D, Starr A, McCord C W, Griswold H E: Serial cardiac output and blood volume studies following cardiac valve replacement. Circulation 33:528, 1966.

Klug T J, McPherson R C: Postoperative complications in the elderly surgical patient. Am J Surg 97:713, 1959.

Kopriva C J, Brown A C D, Pappas G: Hemodynamics during general anesthesia in patients receiving propranolol. Anesthesiology 48:78, 1978a.

———, Guinazu, A, Barash P G: Massive propranolol therapy and uncomplicated cardiac surgery. J A M A 239:1157, 1978b.

Krasula R W, Hastreiter A R, Levitsky S, Yanagi R, Soyka L F: Serum, atrial and urinary digoxin levels during cardiopulmonary bypass. Circulation 49:1047, 1974.

Laszlo G, Archer G G, Darrell J H, Dawson J M, Fletcher C M: The diagnosis and prophylaxis of pulmonary complications of surgical operation. Br J Surg 60:129, 1973.

Latimer R G, Dickman M, Day W C, Gunn M L, Schmidt C duW: Ventilatory patterns and pulmonary complications after upper abdominal surgery determined by preoperative and postoperative computerized spirometry and blood gas analysis. Am J Surg 122:622, 1971.

Lee K S, Klaus W: The subcellular basis for the mechanism of inotropic action of cardiac glycosides. Pharmacol Rev 23:193, 1971.

Luchi R J, Conn H L Jr: Digitalis action on the cells: fable, fact and fancy. Prog Cardiovasc Dis 7:336, 1965.

Lyons W S, DuShane J W, Kirklin J W: Postoperative care after whole-body perfusion and open intracardiac operations. JAMA 173:625, 1960.

Mason D T, Braunwald E: Studies on digitalis. IX. Effects of ouabain on the nonfailing human heart. J Clin Invest 42:1105, 1963.

Miller R R, Olson H G, Amsterdam E A, Mason D T: Propranolol withdrawal rebound phenomenon. N Engl J Med 292:416, 1975.

Modell J H, Moya F: Postoperative pulmonary complications. Incidence and management. Anesth Analg (Cleve) 45:432, 1966.

Morrison J, Killip T: Serum digitalis and arrhythmias in patients undergoing cardiopulmonary bypass. Circulation 47:341, 1973.

Morton H J V: Tobacco smoking and pulmonary complications after operation. Lancet 1:368, 1944.

Naimark A, Cherniack R M: Compliance of the respiratory system and its components in health and obesity. J Appl Physiol 15:377, 1960.

Neill C A: The use of digitalis in infants and children. Prog Cardiovasc Dis 7:399, 1965.

Norris A H, Shock N W: Exercise in adult years—with special reference to the advanced years. In Johnson W R (ed): Science of Medicine of Exercise and Sports. New York, Harper & Row, 1960, p 466.

Nunn J F: Influence of age and other factors on hypoxaemia in the postoperative period. Lancet 2:466, 1965.

O'Kane H, Geha A, Baue A, Kleiger R, Krone R, Oliver G C: Prophylactic digitalization in aortocoronary bypass patients. Circulation 45, 46 (Suppl II):II–199, 1972.

Olsen R E: The contractile proteins of heart muscle. Am J Med 30:692, 1961.

Pasyk S, Bloor C M, Khouri E M, Gregg D E: Systemic and coronary effects of coronary artery occlusion in the unanesthetized dog. Am J Physiol 220:646, 1971.

Prindle R A: The disaster potential of community air pollution. In Farber S M, Wilson R H L (eds): The Air We Breathe. Springfield, Ill, Thomas, 1961, p 177.

Radvin I S, McNamer H G, Kamholz J H, Rhoads J E: Effect of hypoproteinemia on susceptibility to shock resulting from hemorrhage. Arch Surg 48:491, 1944.

Rhoads J E: Supranormal dietary requirements of acutely ill patients. J Am Diet Assoc 29:897, 1953.

Rickham P P: Neonatal physiology and its effect on pre- and postoperative management. In Rickham P P, Johnston J H (eds): Neonatal Surgery. New York, Appleton-Century-Crofts, 1969, p 33.

Roberts R, Gowda K S, Ludbrook P A, Sobel B E: Specificity of elevated serum MB creatine phosphokinase activity in the diagnosis of acute myocardial infarction. Am J Cardiol 36:433, 1975.

———, Sobel B E: Isoenzymes of creatine phosphokinase and diagnosis of acute myocardial infarction. Ann Intern Med 79:741, 1973.

Roe B B: Prevention and treatment of respiratory complications in surgery. N Engl J Med 263:547, 1960.

Rogers R M, Weiler C, Ruppenthal B: Impact of the respiratory intensive care unit on survival of patients with acute respiratory failure. Chest 62:94, 1972.

Rosenthal A, Nathan D G, Marty A T, Button L N, Miettinen O S, Nadas A S: Acute hemodynamic effects of red cell volume reduction in polycythemia of cyanotic congenital heart disease. Circulation 42:297, 1970.

Said S I: Abnormalities of pulmonary gas exchange in obesity. Ann Intern Med 53:1121, 1960.

Schroeder H A: The importance of restriction of salt as compared to water. Am Heart J 22:141, 1941.

Selzer A, Hultgren H N, Ebnother C L, Bradley H W, Stone A O: Effect of digoxin on the circulation in normal man. Br Heart J 21:335, 1959.

———, Kelley J J Jr, Gerbode F, Kerth W J, Osborn J J, Popper R W: Case against routine use of digitalis in patients undergoing cardiac surgery. JAMA 195:141, 1966.

Shand P G, Wood A J J: Propranolol withdrawal syndrome—why? (Editorial). Circulation 58:202, 1978.

Shell W E, Kiekshus J K, Sobel B E: Quantitative assessment of the extent of myocardial infarction in the conscious dog by means of analysis of serial changes in serum creatine phosphokinase activity. J Clin Invest 50:2614, 1971.

Shock N W: The physiology of aging. Sci Am 206:100, 1962.

Slogoff S, Keats A S, Ott E: Preoperative propranolol therapy and aorto-coronary bypass operation. J A M A 240:1487, 1978.

Sobel B E, Shell W E: Serum enzyme determinations in the diagnosis and assessment of myocardial infarction. Circulation 45:471, 1972.

Smith A F: Separation of tissue and serum creatine kinase isoenzymes on polyacrylamide gel slabs. Clin Chim Acta 39:351, 1972.

———: Diagnostic value of serum creatine kinase in a coronary care unit. Lancet 2:178, 1967.

Thompson W D, Radvin I S, Frank I L: Effect of hypoproteinemia on wound disruption. Arch Surg 36:500, 1938.

Thoren L: Postoperative pulmonary complications. Observations on their prevention by means of physiotherapy. Acta Chir Scand 107:193, 1954.

Tonkins A M, Lester R M, Gunthrow C E, Roe C R, Dackel D B, Wagner G S: Persistence of MB isoenzyme of creatine phosphokinase in the serum after minor iatrogenic cardiac trauma. Absence of postmortem evidence of myocardial infarction. Circulation 51:627, 1975.

Tucker D H, Sieker H O: The effect of change in body position on lung volumes and intrapulmonary gas mixing in patients with obesity, heart failure and emphysema. Am Rev Respir Dis 82:787, 1960.

Tyras D H, Stothert J C Jr, Kaiser G C, Barner H B, Codd J E, Willman V L: Supraventricular tachyarrhythmias after myocardial revascularization: a randomized trial of prophylactic digitalization. J Thorac Cardiovasc Surg 77:310, 1979.

Vasko K A, DeWall R A, Riley A M: Hypokalemia, physiological abnormalities during cardiopulmonary bypass. Ann Thorac Surg 15:347, 1973.

Vasudevan G, Mercer D W, Varat M A: Lactic dehydrogenase isoenzyme determination in the diagnosis of acute myocardial infarction. Circulation 57:1055, 1978.

Viljoen J F, Estafanous F G, Kellner G A: Propranolol and cardiac surgery. J Thorac Cardiovasc Surg 64:876, 1972.

Von Kaulla K N, Paton B C, Rosenkrantz J G, von Kaulla E, Wasantapniek S: Preoperative correction of coagulation in tetralogy of Fallot. Arch Surg 94:107, 1967.

Waltemath C L, Bergman N A: Respiratory compliance in obese patients. Anesthesiology 41:84, 1974.

Wedemeyer A L, Castaneda A R, Edson J R, Krivit W: Serial coagulation studies in patients undergoing Mustard's procedure. Ann Thorac Surg 15:120, 1973.

Williams M H Jr, Zohman L R, Ratner A C: Hemodynamic effects of cardiac glycosides on normal human subjects during rest and exercise. J Appl Physiol 13:417, 1958.

Withering W: An Account of the Foxglove and Some of its Medical Uses: With Practical Remarks on Dropsy and Other Diseases. Birmingham, M Swinney, 1785.

Wohl M D, Reinholt J G, Rose S B: Antibody response in patients with hypoproteinemia. Arch Intern Med, 83:402, 1949.

4. Anesthesia for Cardiac Surgery

JOHN H.L. BLAND[†]   DEMETRIOS G. LAPPAS

Anesthesia for cardiac surgery has evolved as a highly specialized activity following the rapid increase in the number of operations performed on the heart and great vessels. Initially, adequate intraoperative support required a better understanding of pathophysiology as it applied to acquired valvular and congenital heart disease. The challenge has intensified with the enormous success reported in surgery for severe coronary artery disease and the need to steer a safe intraoperative course for the patient whose myocardial blood flow is barely adequate for survival.

The cardiac anesthetist should participate in the total care of the patient. Proper management of the patient in need of open heart surgery depends primarily on an understanding of the pathophysiology of the principal lesion, the problems of surgery and cardiopulmonary bypass, as well as the physiology of the respiratory, renal, and hepatic systems, and depends proportionately less on the choice of the anesthetic drug. Successful management with the least intraoperative damage can be achieved only by careful attention to all these factors.

PREOPERATIVE CARE

Preanesthetic Visit

The cardiac patient brings to the operation a remarkable complexity of biochemical, pharmacologic, and physiologic abnormalities. A preoperative evaluation of the patient's status is performed to determine the degree and severity of cardiovascular disease and the associated organ involvement. In addition to the routine review of the patient's history for previous hospitalization and associated disease, a careful search for the onset of symptoms should be conducted. A history of chest pain, dyspnea, syncope, palpitation, peripheral edema, hemoptysis, pulmonary congestion and edema should be carefully evaluated. Exercise tolerance, in particular, is an excellent means of classifying severity of impairment. In patients with coronary artery disease, the characteristics of angina pectoris should be carefully assessed. The patient who develops severe angina on minimal exertion is very susceptible to perturbations that alter the balance between the demand for and availability of myocardial oxygen.

The physical examination often may provide additional information about the severity of heart disease and complications one may encounter. Special diagnostic procedures, such as cardiac catheterization and angiography, exercise tests, cardiac imaging studies, and preoperative pulmonary function tests provide useful objective data.

The anesthetist must be aware of the drugs these cardiac patients receive preoperatively, since previous chronic drug therapy may interact with anesthetics. Preoperative digitalization or continuation of digitalis ther-

---

[†]Deceased

apy up to the time of operation has been recommended as a measure to minimize the incidence of intraoperative or postoperative supraventricular tachyarrhythmias (Deutch and Dalen, 1969; Johnson et al., 1976). The evidence to support this practice is equivocal. The incidence of arrhythmias, particularly atrial arrhythmias, may vary between 13 and 61 percent during general anesthesia (Katz and Bigger, 1970). Several factors may be responsible for this high frequency, including muscle relaxants (i.e., succinylcholine), light anesthesia, unrecognized myocardial ischemia, fluctuation in serum electrolyte concentrations, or respiratory alkalosis. The most common cause of arrhythmias in digitalized patients is intraoperative hypokalemia. The combination of chronic heart disease, overzealous digitalis and diuretic therapy, and sympathetic stimulation are likely to result in arrhythmias in the perioperative period. Differentiation between digitalis and perioperative stimuli as causative factors for arrhythmias is difficult, if not impossible.

The decision whether to discontinue digitalis before the operation, as is ordinarily done, must rest on the combined experience of the anesthesiologist, cardiologist, and surgeon. In general, preoperative digitalization is to be discontinued if it is intended solely to counteract perioperative physiologic alterations. Digitalis therapy is best continued until the evening before the operation in patients with chronic atrial fibrillation when control of heart rate may be a problem (i.e., ventricular rate in excess of 80 heartbeats/min), unless digitalis intoxication is suspected. Acute digitalization is warranted in the patient who has heart failure before the operation.

In patients on chronic diuretic therapy, intravascular volume and total body potassium content probably are reduced, and the relative hypovolemia can result in prerenal azotemia. This reduced intravascular blood volume can render induction of anesthesia more difficult; therefore, diuretics should be omitted for five days prior to surgery. Generally, it is safer to anesthetize a patient with mild residual congestive heart failure than attempt induction when a tight cardiac regimen has resulted in excellent compensation but runs a high risk of severe hypotension because of the markedly contracted blood volume. Chronic diuretic therapy invariably leads to potassium and chloride depletion, with a resulting metabolic alkalosis (Lockey et al., 1966). The degree of the alkalosis may reflect the extent of potassium depletion.

Administration of potassium chloride must be anticipated during the intra- and postoperative period to correct for severe fluctuation in serum K^+ concentrations. Intraoperative disturbances of heart rate and conduction are commonly the result of such changes. The presence of normal potassium values preoperatively is no guarantee against profound intraoperative hypokalemias. Induction of anesthesia and the use of muscle relaxants such as succinylcholine may result in marked aberrations in potassium concentrations, with the appearance of severe arrhythmias.

β-Adrenergic blocking drugs commonly are administered chronically, to control refractory or frequent angina pectoris, arrhythmias of ventricular origin, and, occasionally, essential hypertension. Early reports have supported the discontinuation of propranolol use at least two days before the operation to avoid profound hemodynamic depression during anesthesia (Faulkner et al., 1973). Withdrawal of beta-blocker therapy may make little difference to the course of the operation in some patients with controlled heart rate and no angina at rest; however, the absence of beta blockade in others may prove detrimental (Boudoulas et al., 1977; Myers and Wisenberg, 1977).

The relationships among chronic beta blockade, the myocardial depressant effects of anesthetic drugs, and the patient's reaction to intraoperative sympathetic stimuli must be considered when the question of withdrawal is raised (Robinson, 1967; Myers and Wisenberg, 1977). Discontinuation of propranolol may be hazardous if a patient is having attacks of angina that persist even with bed rest and sedation. Beta blockade should be continued in patients with unstable or crescendo angina, hypertension, ventricular arrhythmias, and tachycardia, until the day of the operation. Occasionally, a reduction in propranolol dosage before the operation is in order, if concern is aroused by depressed myocardial contractility and an elevated left-sided filling pressure. The potential for difficulty with general anesthesia during beta blockade cannot be ignored; yet the problems are rare, and a safe course is likely if the anesthetic is delivered judiciously and under the guidance of proper monitoring of arterial blood pressure, pulmonary capillary pressure, and electrocardiogram. An individualized approach demands understanding of the clinical pharmacology of beta blockers (Nies and Shand, 1975).

Finally, nitrates should not be discontinued, as well as insulin, anticonvulsive therapy, and inotropic therapy (catecholamines, vasopressors, etc.).

Patients awaiting cardiac surgery may, understandably, be terrified by their forthcoming ordeal. Judicious sedation in addition to the immediate preoperative medication is invariably necessary. Reliance on sedation alone is insufficient. A simple but direct explanation of the procedures contemplated by various members of the team often reassures the patient that care is administered by a team whose integrated efforts are likely to result in success. It is important that the patient be informed of such preoperative procedures as cannulation of arteries and veins, and the methods for induction of anesthesia. The patient should also be informed of what to expect on emergence from anesthesia. A careful, sympathetic, unhurried, informative preoperative visit will relieve the patient's anxiety. (Egbert et al., 1964).

Preoperative Assessment of the Respiratory System

Lung function tests such as vital capacity (VC), forced expired volume during first second (FEV_1), maximal breathing capacity (MBC), and maximal midexpiratory flow rate (MEFR) may be impaired either by primary lung disease or lung dysfunction secondary to heart disease. In the latter instance, improvement in the cardiac status postoperatively is usually associated with marked improvement in pulmonary function. Thus, in the patient with chronic heart disease and abnormal pulmonary hemodynamics, detailed preoperative evaluation of lung function is of limited predictive value when translated to the postoperative period, because it is often difficult to decide how much impairment is secondary to cardiac disease and therefore potentially rapidly reversible consequent to a successful operation.

The vital capacity may be reduced by a decrease in lung compliance caused by pulmonary venous congestion (McFadden and Ingram, 1980), pleural effusion, or simply an enormously dilated heart that prevents appropriate expansion of dependent lobes. Small airway obstruction, manifested by "wheezing," a reduced FEV_1, or MEFR, is commonly secondary to severe pulmonary venous congestion or pulmonary edema and may be mistakenly considered a result of primary bronchial asthma. The MBC is commonly impaired in the cardiac patient because, in addition to reflecting both restrictive as well as obstructive deficits, it is in essence an exercise tolerance test.

Cessation of smoking must be encouraged—better still, insisted on—by the cardiologist at the time of the patient's initial referral. Unfortunately, cessation often is not accomplished until a few days preoperatively, and the contribution of this factor to the development of postoperative ventilatory difficulties must not be overlooked.

If the patient has a chronic productive cough, culture of the sputum and an appropriate course of antibiotics must be combined with intense preoperative physiotherapy and regular postural drainage.

All patients should be seen preoperatively by a chest physiotherapist for instruction in the deep breathing and effective coughing that will be required postoperatively.

A thoracotomy incision is now rarely used for operations that require extracorporeal circulatory support. The median sternotomy incision is of particular benefit over the thoracotomy incision to the patient with lung disease. Less postoperative pain and interference with mechanics of the chest wall facilitate deep breathing and effective coughing. The avoidance of a pleurotomy may lessen postoperative impairment of lung function (Ghia and Andersen, 1970).

Premedication

It is imperative that a cardiac patient be well premedicated for proper placement of intravascular cannulae and induction of anesthesia. Several combinations of drugs have been proposed, all of which probably are satisfactory, provided their effect is evaluated according to requirements set by local and personal circumstances. In our experience, based on the method we use for induction and maintenance of anesthesia, a combination of morphine, scopolamine, and diazepam has been most satisfactory (Katz et al., 1974). Adult patients with heart valve disease receive 0.1 mg/kg morphine (but not more than a total of 7 mg morphine) and 0.05 mg/kg scopolamine, injected intramuscularly. This dose should be reduced to half that amount in patients with cachexia, critical valve stenosis, and congestive heart failure.

Premedication should be omitted in patients in cardiogenic shock, in emergency cardiac cases, and in patients with severe cardiorespiratory abnormalities until proper hemodynamic monitoring and ventilatory support are available. Patients with coronary artery disease and normal ventricular function tend to be more apprehensive and require heavier premedication. To these patients, 5 to 10 mg diazepam should be administered orally with a minimal amount of water two hours prior to anesthesia. The amnestic properties of both diazepam and scopolamine are particularly desirable. Since premedication occasionally may suppress respiration and cause a decrease in arterial Po_2, oxygen supplementation with a face mask should be given after premedication in patients with low Po_2, and respiratory problems. Finally, sublingual tablets of nitroglycerin should be available for use at any time.

ANESTHETIC MANAGEMENT

Monitoring

In most patients scheduled for cardiac operation, monitoring of the electrocardiogram, central venous, and direct intraarterial blood pressures is adequate. In addition, a Swan-Ganz catheter, i.e., balloon-tipped, is inserted to obtain pulmonary arterial and pulmonary capillary wedge pressures and to measure cardiac output, as necessary.

All cannulations are performed percutaneously before induction of anesthesia, under local anesthesia with 1 percent lidocaine. We generally cannulate the radial artery with a No. 18 or 20 plastic cannula. The insertion of the cannula should always be preceded by the Allen test to appraise the adequacy of the ulnar collateral circulation to the hand. If both radial arteries are not suitable for cannulation, a cannula can be inserted percutaneously into the femoral artery. A central venous catheter for pressure recording or drug administration is inserted via an antecubital, jugular, or subclavian vein. The Swan–Ganz catheter is inserted when clinically indicated (Lappas and Gayes, 1979). The procedure is not time-consuming and can be performed with little discomfort to the patient.

Insertion of the Swan-Ganz pulmonary artery catheter is indicated for patients with pulmonary hypertension, left or right ventricular failure, unstable angina, left main coronary artery disease, recent myocardial infarction, left ventricular aneurysm, and for patients in whom an intraaortic mechanical assist device has been placed preoperatively. Evaluation of the advantages and disadvantages of placement of the catheter will determine the contraindications on an individual basis. Lack of proper monitoring facilities and lack of experienced personnel are important factors against the placement of the catheter.

Pulmonary and tricuspid stenosis and the presence of cardiac dysrrhythmias are among the considerations in deciding against placement of the catheter. Although passage of the catheter into the pulmonary artery is relatively innocuous, the potential hazards and complications, such as arrhythmias, thrombus formation, and rupture of pulmonary artery branch should not be disregarded.

During cannulation the patient should be allowed to breathe oxygen by face mask, and small quantities of intravenous diazepam (e.g., 2.5 mg/dose) should be administered as indicated, to relieve apprehension and discomfort.

Continuous ECG display is essential, both to provide basic information about rate and type of conduction and to permit early detection of ominous cardiac arrhythmias and myocardial ischemic changes. The ECG is obtained routinely by using traditional limb leads. Lead II is most often used, especially for evaluation of atrial activity. Simultaneous recording of the precordial V lead, particularly in patients with coronary artery disease, should also be used as an indicator of S-T segment changes and myocardial ischemia, which may be absent in the standard limb lead (Fig. 4–1).

Arterial blood gases, hematocrit, and serum electrolytes are measured at regular intervals throughout the operation. As with the continuous recording of hemodynamic performance, regular measurement of blood gases, urine output, and other values allows for the early recognition of trends and frequently is helpful in the avoidance of disasters.

Anesthetics

The earlier days of cardiac surgery required a light level of anesthesia with appropriate reliance on an intact autonomic nervous system to sustain myocardial function in the patient with a failing heart but competent coronary arteries (Chidsey et al., 1965). The ideal anesthetic for this group would have been one with no depressant effect on the myocardium and little or no effect on peripheral vascular tone. These requirements have been modified to suit the particular needs of patients who are candidates for myocardial revascularization. Their needs are different from those of patients with chronic congestive heart failure, because they require sufficient depth of anesthesia to abolish an excessive intraoperative sympathetic response, which may result in tachycardia and hypertension.

All anesthetics used during cardiac operations must be nonflammable, and except for nitrous oxide, sufficiently potent to allow for the administration of high concentrations of oxygen (Dowdy and Kaya, 1968; Stoelting et al., 1972; Lappas et al., 1975b; Lappas et al., 1976).

Anesthetic practice for cardiac surgery in the United States has been collated by Dalton

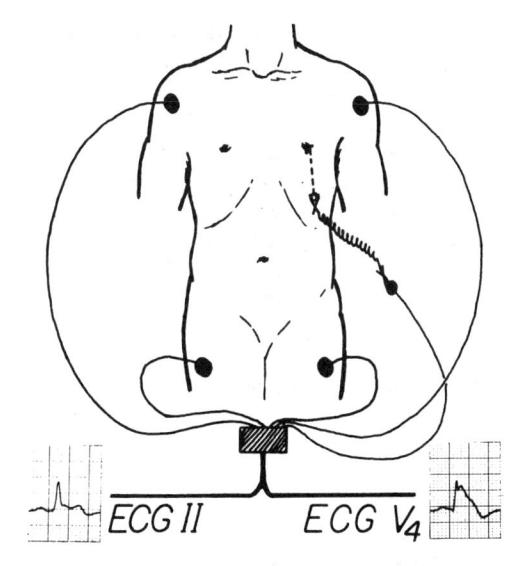

Figure 4–1. Schematic representation of placement of V_4 needle electrodes allowing continuous recording of both the V_4 lead and any chosen limb lead. A sterile needle is inserted by the surgeon after the chest has been prepared. The needle is then attached to a sterile wire and passed to the head of the table before being covered with adhesive drapes. Note the difference in ischemic changes observed in lead II and lead V_4 in a patient with severe coronary artery disease. *(Reproduced with the kind permission of Dr. B. Dalton.)*

(1972). Morphine and halothane were used as principal drugs with equal frequency and constituted 60 percent of the total anesthetics administered; the remainder included a combination of nitrous oxide with muscle relaxants, methoxyflurane, enflurane, or so-called neuroleptanalgesia (i.e., combination of a synthetic narcotic and butyrophenone derivative). We have little evidence that particular anesthetic drugs or techniques offer special advantages to the patient with cardiovascular disease.

Although anesthesia requirements to suit the particular needs of the cardiac surgical patient vary, certain principles should be observed to minimize surgical risks. The selection of the anesthetic drugs should be appropriate to ensure adequate physiologic conditions, thus preserving myocardial performance and blood flow to satisfy whole-body metabolic requirements. Furthermore, an imbalance between myocardial oxygen demand and supply should be prevented by attenuating the sympathetic response of endotracheal intubation and surgical incision (Fig. 4–2). Patients with abnormal heart function resulting from valvular or coronary artery disease have an increased sympathetic tone needed to maintain hemodynamic homeostasis (Cohn, 1973). Anesthetic drugs may either modify or accentuate vascular tone in these patients. In this case, induction of anesthesia should be performed with patience, drugs should be administered slowly, and cardiovascular function must be protected at all costs, including prophylactic infusion of alpha or beta agonists, occasionally in combination with vasodilator drugs.

The need to establish appropriate intraoperative conditions in patients with brittle hemodynamic function, accompanied by the need for a smooth transition from the operative to the postoperative phase, resulted in the use of morphine in large quantities (2 to 3 mg/kg intravenously) as the principal anesthetic drug (Lowenstein et al., 1969). The advantages provided by this drug are many. Morphine has no depressant effect on the myocardium and no effect on cardiac rhyth-

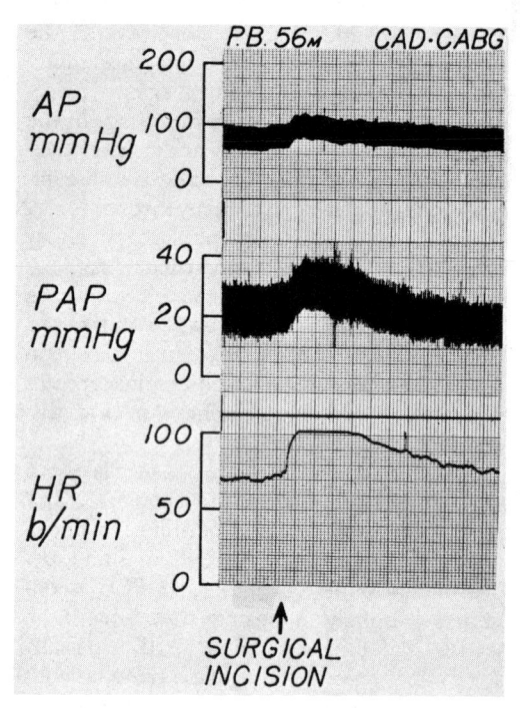

Figure 4–2. Effect of surgical incision on hemodynamics in a 56-year-old male patient with severe coronary artery disease (CAD) undergoing coronary artery bypass grafting (CABG). Note the increase in heart rate (HR) and arterial pressure (AP) with incision. The concomitant increase in HR and AP must have increased the myocardial oxygen requirements, leading to left ventricular dysfunction as indicated by the increased pulmonary arterial pressure, reflecting an increase in LV filling pressure.

micity. It also allows for ventilation with high concentrations of inspired oxygen, and there is no risk of sudden awakening and acute perception of pain if hemodynamic deterioration requires discontinuation of an inhalation anesthetic. In addition, because of its long duration of action, large quantities of morphine given at the beginning of the operation provide significant postoperative analgesia. Although large doses of morphine result in satisfactory analgesia, the hypnotic effect is inconsistent, and occasional intraoperative awareness of the environment has been observed. Therefore, the amnesic properties of diazepam are particularly desirable. We have been administering incremental doses of diazepam (2.5 mg intravenously) during induction of anesthesia, for a total of 0.5 mg/kg. In our experience, diazepam administered intravenously in small doses is tolerated well and hemodynamics are maintained.

Morphine, used in large quantities, may sustain hemodynamic function, but carries the risk of an unabated response to sympathetic stimulation. In addition, the disadvantage associated with all potent narcotics is their prolonged duration of action, with a requirement for extended postoperative mechanical ventilation, an argument not necessarily valid if the patient is hemodynamically unstable. Another undesirable side effect that accompanies the administration of large quantities of morphine is the increased requirement for intravascular component therapy, in which there is a risk of hypervolemia as venomotor tone begins to increase (Stanley et al., 1973; Stanley et al., 1974).

Administration of morphine may result in a significant decrease in arterial blood pressure, depending on the characteristics of the resistance and capacitance vessels, the level of sympathetic tone and circulating catecholamine concentration, the available intravascular constituents, and the ability of the heart to increase stroke volume as systemic vascular resistance decreases. In patients with heart failure, resistance vessel tone is consistently increased and infusion of narcotics may profoundly influence arterial blood pressure, a change not necessarily apparent in the patient with normal ventricular function. Lowenstein et al. (1969) reported that in patients with aortic valve disease the intravenous administration of morphine (1.0 mg/kg) caused a consistent reduction in systemic vascular resistance associated with a modest increase in cardiac output (Fig. 4–3). This response was less apparent in the absence of heart disease.

The effects of large doses of intravenous morphine in patients with coronary artery disease, but without left or right ventricular failure, have been studied recently by Lappas et al. (1975b). Morphine administered at a rate of 5 mg/min to a total of 2 mg/kg BW caused no change in left and right heart filling pressures (RHFP and LHFP) until a dose of 1.5 mg/kg had been reached. At 2 mg/kg, LHFP and RHFP rose significantly from approximately 7 to 10.5 mm Hg on the left ($p <0.01$) and 3 to 5 mm Hg on the right ($p <0.05$). Systemic arterial pressure, cardiac index, and left ventricular stroke work were decreased significantly only at the 0.5 mg/kg dose level, while systemic and pulmonary vascular resistance and stroke index were unchanged. Heart rate ($p <0.01$) and the arterial systolic pressure-rate product ($p <0.05$), an indirect index of myocardial oxygen consumption, were decreased throughout the study period. Thus, the hemodynamic response resembles that seen in normal humans (Figs. 4–4 and 4–5).

Hypotension may be caused either by a direct dilator effect on the systemic vascular bed (Katz and Bigger, 1970), central suppression of sympathetic tone, or histamine release. Any of these, if excessive, may necessitate the use of a vasopressor. The incidence of severe hypotension appears to be related to the rate of morphine infusion; it is uncommon if morphine is injected at a rate not exceeding 5 mg/min.

Despite these disadvantages, the use of intravenous narcotics has added an important element of safety for induction of anesthesia in patients with chronic heart failure, probably because the blood volume increase associated with congestive failure counteracts some of the central and peripheral effects of narcotics. Loss of consciousness generally requires doses of intravenous morphine in excess of 2 mg/kg or fentanyl in excess of 50 mμg/kg. It would appear reasonable to use lower doses of narcotics and ensure loss of consciousness using ventilation with oxygen and an inhalational anesthetic (N_2O or halothane).

It is important to note that addition of nitrous oxide (60 percent inspired) to morphine analgesia (1 mg/kg) in two groups of patients, one with valvular heart disease, and the other with coronary artery disease, result-

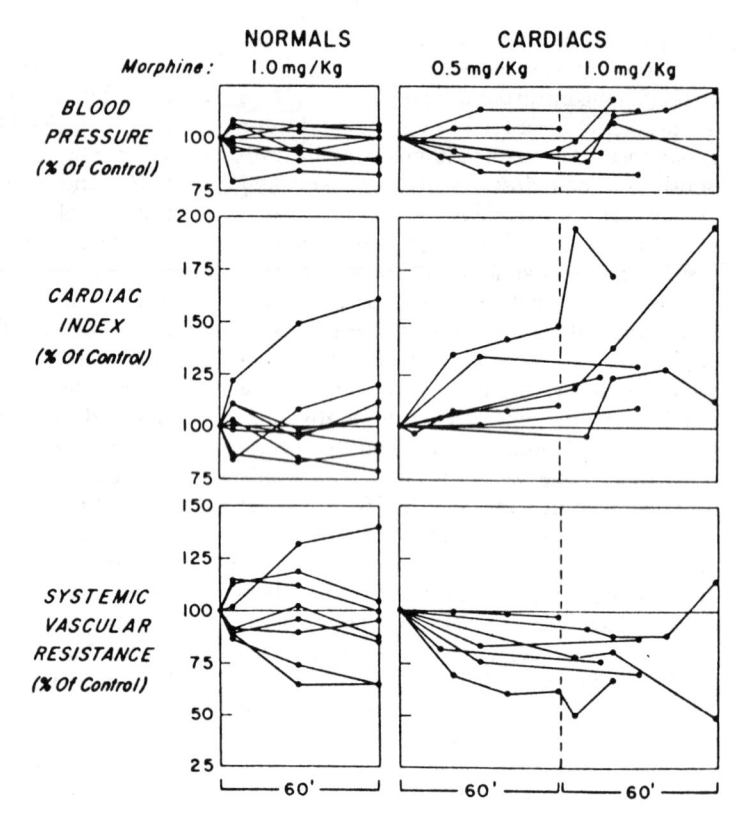

Figure 4–3. Hemodynamic effects of large doses of intravenous morphine. There was no statistically significant change in blood pressure, cardiac index, or systemic vascular resistance in patients without heart or lung disease. However, cardiac index increased and systemic vascular resistance decreased in each of a group of patients with aortic valve disease who required surgical correction. *(Reproduced with permission from Lowenstein E, Hallowell P, Levine F H, Daggett W M, Austen W G, and Laver M B. Cardiovascular response to large doses of intravenous morphine in man. N Engl J Med 281:1389–1393, 1969.)*

ed in cardiovascular depression in both groups (Stoelting and Gibbs, 1973; Wong et al., 1973; Lappas et al., 1975a). Mean arterial pressure and stroke volume index decreased, but less dramatically than the cardiac index. Although control values for some of these measurements were different in the two groups, the percentage of depression was comparable. A decrease in heart rate was seen in each group but was significant only in patients with coronary artery disease (Fig. 4–6). We also have found that nitrous oxide lowers LV contractility (Δ_P/Δ_T max), reduces arterial blood pressure, and constricts the pulmonary vasculature in the presence of pulmonary hypertension (Lappas et al., 1975a). The latter results in an increased right ventricular (RV) afterload and may influence profoundly the hemodynamic performance if abnormal RV function is present. Patients with pulmonary hypertension, regardless of etiology or RV dysfunction, secondary valvular disease, or coronary artery disease, are best not anesthetized with this drug. Because of its low solubility and demonstrated ability to cause enlargement of trapped gas bubbles, we prefer not to use it after discontinuation of extracorporeal circulation.

Halothane, a volatile anesthetic, found early acceptance in anesthesia for cardiac surgery at a time when most operations were intended to correct congenital heart defects. The choice was predicated by the fact that halothane is potent, nonexplosive, and can be administered with oxygen alone. These reasons explain why it remains the most common anesthetic used in congenital heart surgery. Its properties include myocardial depression, slight reduction in heart rate, and little effect on the systemic vascular resistance in normal

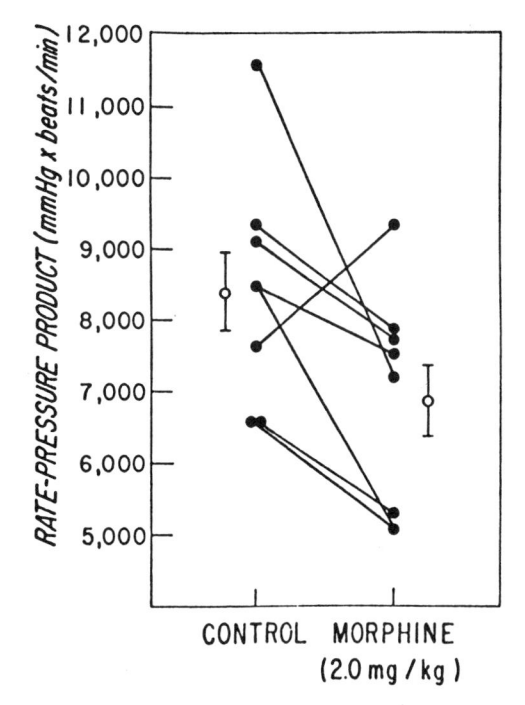

Figure 4–4. The heart rate-arterial systolic pressure product, which reflects myocardial oxygen consumption, decreased significantly following the intravenous administration of morphine at a rate of 5 mg/min (total dose: 2 mg/kg) in eight patients with coronary artery disease and normal ventricular contractility. *(Reproduced with permission from Lappas D G, Geha D, Fischer J E, Laver M B, and Lowenstein E. Filling pressures of the heart and pulmonary circulation of the patient with coronary artery disease after large intravenous doses of morphine. Anesthesiology, 42:153–159, 1975.)*

subjects (Eger et al., 1970). Recent prospective studies have substantiated the long-held fear that second exposures (within short periods) to the anesthetic may lead, on occasion, to hepatocellular necrosis, substantiated by liver biopsy in certain patients (Trowell et al., 1975; Wright et al., 1975). In patients with valvular heart disease, halothane (end tidal concentration: 0.55 percent) caused no significant change in mean arterial pressure, mean pulmonary artery pressure, heart rate, cardiac index, or systemic vascular resistance; mean left and right atrial pressures decreased slightly, as did the calculated pulmonary vascular resistance when compared with values obtained at cardiac catheterization (Stoelting et al., 1972) (Fig. 4–7). Addition of 60 percent nitrous oxide to the inspired mixture produced no significant change in the hemodynamic values measured (Fig. 4–8). This is at variance with Smith et al. (1970), who found peripheral vasoconstriction when 70 percent nitrous oxide was added to halothane in volunteers not having surgery. Stoelting et al. (1972) postulated that this difference in findings may have resulted from (1) differences in the halothane-nitrous-oxide concentrations used, (2) a small decrease in body temperature secondary to general anesthesia, (3) surgical stimulation, (4) altered peripheral vascular reactivity in patients with heart failure (Zelis et al., 1968), or (5) an increased arterial halothane concentration following addition of nitrous oxide (second gas effect) and (6) the use of d-tubocurarine.

These discrepancies emphasize again the need to recognize that the action of drugs in the critically ill may differ substantially from the effects noted in fit volunteers (Dowdy and Kaya, 1968).

Muscle Relaxants

The choice of muscle relaxants for cardiac surgery is determined more by their cardiovascular effects than by their neuromuscular blocking properties. Reversal of a nondepolarizing muscle blockade at the end of the operation is rarely necessary, as most patients are ventilated electively postoperatively. Usually, the effect of the relaxant has worn off by the time extubation is contemplated.

Succinylcholine, a rapidly acting, depolarizing muscle relaxant, may be administered in a single dose for intubation or by continuous infusion for sustained paralysis. Bradyarrhythmias may follow its administration, which may be prevented by the prior injection of atropine. The arterial blood pressure may rise following succinylcholine infusion, the result of release of endogenous catecholamines. Succinylcholine also causes a release of

Figure 4–5. Left ventricular stroke work index (LVSWI) plotted against balloon-occluded pulmonary arterial pressure ($\overline{PA}_O$) before and after administration of morphine 0.5, 1.0, 1.5, and 2.0 mg/kg BW to eight patients with coronary artery disease and normal ventricular contractility. Data from this study are superimposed on the normal left ventricular function curve. *(Reproduced with permission from Lappas D G, Geha D, Fischer J E, Laver M B, and Lowenstein E: Filling pressures of the heart and pulmonary circulation of the patient with coronary artery disease after large intravenous doses of morphine. Anesthesiology 42:153–159, 1975.)*

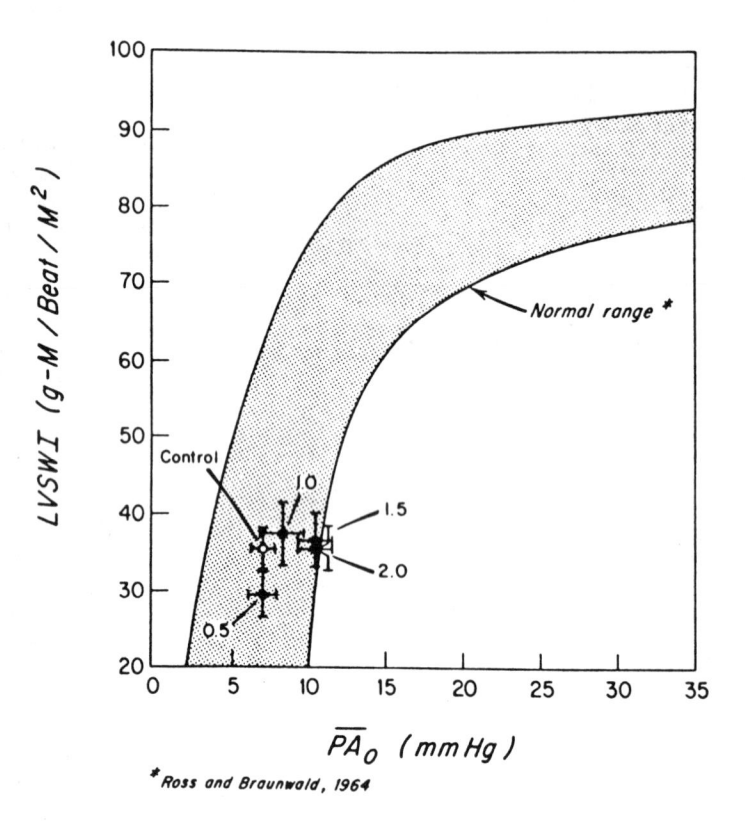

* Ross and Braunwald, 1964

Figure 4–6. Effect of nitrous oxide (60 percent N₂O with oxygen) on hemodynamic function during open heart surgery (mean ± S.E.M.). Sequential measurements were made during and after N₂O administration. The point of the skin incision is shown, and measurements were repeated two minutes later. Control values (zero min) were obtained 30 minutes after the start of the morphine infusion.

MAP = mean arterial pressure; HR = heart rate; CI = cardiac index; SVI = stroke volume index; SVR = systemic vascular resistance; and CVP = central venous pressure.

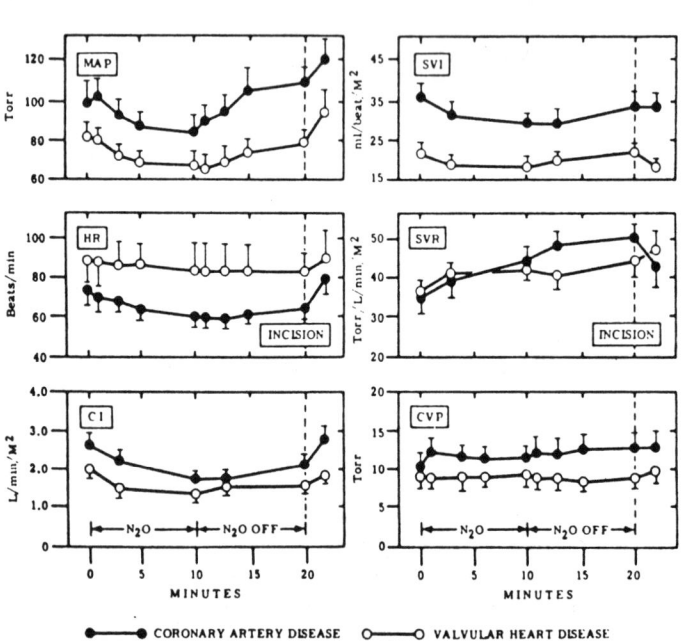

● CORONARY ARTERY DISEASE   ○ VALVULAR HEART DISEASE

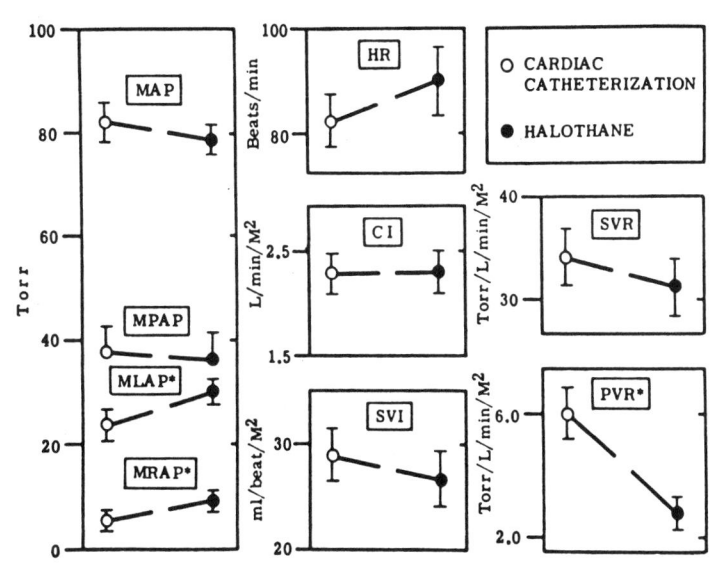

Figure 4–7. Data obtained during cardiac catheterization (patients breathing ambient air spontaneously) were compared with those obtained during administration of halothane (0.55 percent end-tidal) in 40 percent oxygen with controlled ventilation and the thorax open. MLAP at time of cardiac catheterization was estimated from pulmonary capillary wedge pressure. MLAP and MRAP increased, while PVR decreased significantly after halothane administration.

Asterisk indicates a p value <0.01; MAP, mean arterial pressure; MPAP, mean pulmonary arterial pressure; MLAP, mean left atrial pressure; MRAP, mean right atrial pressure; HR, heart rate: CI, cardiac index; SVI, stroke volume index; SVR, systemic vascular resistance; PVR, pulmonary vascular resistance; CVP, central venous pressure. *(Reproduced with permission from Stoelting R K, Reis R R, and Longnecker D E. Hemodynamic response to nitrous oxide-halothane in patients with valvular heart disease. Anesthesiology 37:430–435, 1972.)*

potassium from muscle. If the serum potassium is already raised, as in the presence of chronic renal failure or with muscle wasting secondary to neurologic disease, it is wise to avoid the drug.

D-tubocurarine, a commonly used nondepolarizing muscle relaxant, may cause hypotension by ganglionic blockade by increasing vascular capacitance or by the release of histamine. Hypotension, the result of a reduction in both systemic vascular resistance and cardiac output, usually can be avoided by incremental administration (Fig. 4–9). D-tubocurare has little effect on heart rate; allegedly, it also has an antiarrhythmic effect.

Gallamine, a relaxant with a slightly shorter duration of action than d-tubocurarine, may produce tachycardia, an increase in cardiac output, and a decrease in systemic vascular resistance, with a rise in mean arterial pressure and fall in central venous pressure following a bolus of 1 to 2 mg/kg injected intravenously. The tachycardia, which follows the injection of gallamine, can be minimized by slow incremental administration.

Pancuronium, a nondepolarizing muscle relaxant, was thought initially to have little or no effect on cardiovascular performance, but more recent experience has shown that it does increase heart rate without a change in stroke volume, thereby increasing cardiac output and mean arterial blood pressure (Fig. 4–10). Premature ventricular contractions have been reported to follow its administration. The latter has not been a problem in our experience. However, nodal rhythm has been nota-

Figure 4–8. Effect of nitrous oxide on intraoperative hemodynamic function obtained in eight patients during open heart surgery (aortic and/or mitral valve replacement). Control values were obtained during administration of halothane (0.55 percent end-tidal) in 40 percent oxygen (mean ± S.E.M.). Nitrous oxide (60 percent) was substituted for nitrogen at zero time and administered for 15 minutes and then discontinued; all measurements were repeated 10 minutes later during administration of halothane in 40 percent oxygen. No significant change was caused by the addition of nitrous oxide. (Reproduced with permission from Stoelting R K, Reis R R, and Longnecker D E. Hemodynamic responses to nitrous oxide-halothane in patients with valvular heart disease. Anesthesiology 37:430–435, 1972.)

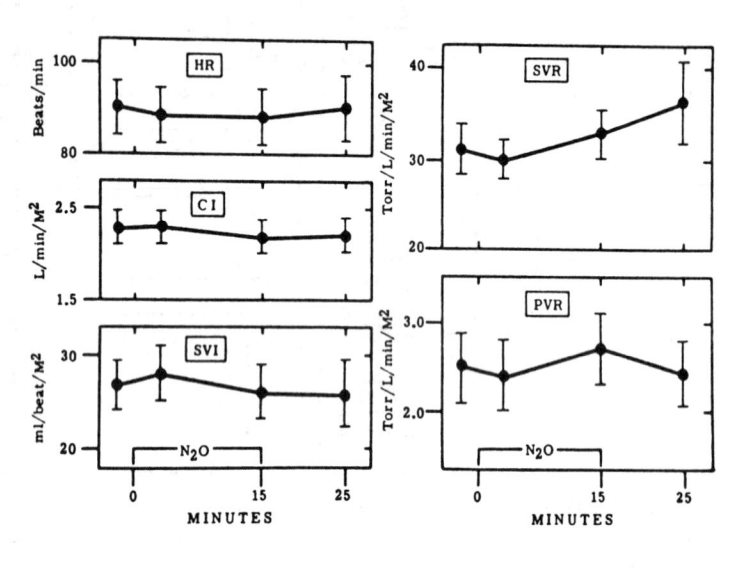

bly frequent and occasionally troublesome.

Figures 4–9 and 4–10 summarize the cardiovascular effects of pancuronium, d-tubocurarine, and gallamine following bolus injections of moderate to large doses. If one of these drugs is chosen, its potentially harmful, cardiovascular side effects can be minimized by slow administration.

Maintenance of Anesthesia

In cardiac surgical patients, modified autonomic nervous system activity, including basal tone of both capacitance and resistance vessels, may result from abnormal heart function (Chidsey et al., 1965) or may be drug-induced (e.g., digitalis therapy or chronic beta blockade). This alteration in autonomic activity may culminate in an exaggerated response, leading to hypotension or hypertension (Bland et al., 1973; Cohn, 1973). For this reason, intraoperative control of hemodynamic function requires careful, direct monitoring of systemic and pulmonary vascular pressures.

In the early days of anesthesia for cardiac surgery, emphasis was placed on the avoidance of an overdose with depressant anesthetics. Practice required that patients with myocardial failure be maintained at a level of anesthesia light enough to allow for an appropriate sympathetic stimulus elicited by surgical stimulation to maintain arterial blood pressure (Chidsey et al., 1965). Although light levels of general anesthesia are deemed desirable for preventing the myocardial depressant effects of anesthetics, the resulting intact sympathetic responses magnify the discrepancy between myocardial oxygen supply and demand when coronary vasculature is compromised by disease. In patients with coronary artery disease, coronary blood flow to the myocardium supplied by a narrow vessel may be affected sufficiently to initiate de novo ischemia, and, if sustained, myocardial infarction.

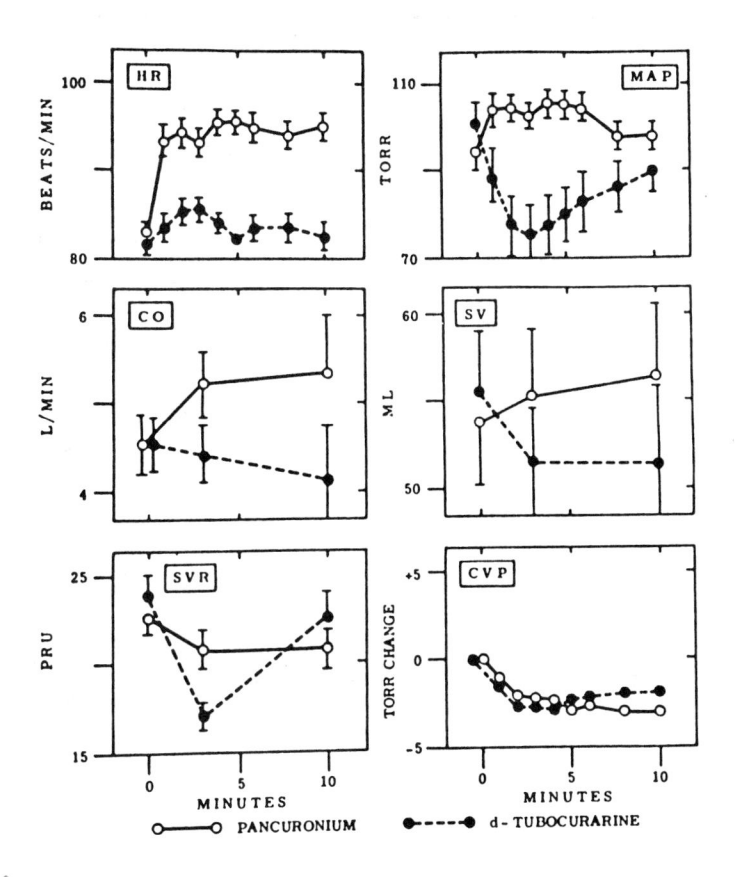

Figure 4–9. Effect of two nondepolarizing muscle relaxants, d-tubocurare (dTc) and pancuronium, on hemodynamic performance during open heart surgery (mean ± S.E.M.). Pancuronium 0.08 mg/kg and dTc 0.4 mg/kg ($n = 10$) were administered at zero time. Pancuronium increased significantly heart rate, mean arterial pressure, and cardiac output ($p <0.01$). Administration of dTc to these patients resulted in a small increase in heart rate ($p <0.05$), a decrease in mean arterial blood pressure ($p <0.01$), cardiac output at 10 minutes ($p <0.01$), and systemic vascular resistance at 3 minutes ($p <0.01$). The decrease in central venous pressure caused by both drugs was insignificant.

HR indicates heart rate; MAP, mean arterial pressure; CO, cardiac output; SV, stroke volume; SVR, systemic vascular resistance; and CVP, central venous pressure. *(Reproduced with permission from Stoelting R K. The hemodynamic effects of pancuronium and d-tubocurarine in anesthetized patients. Anesthesiology 36:612–615, 1972.)*

The massive sympathetic discharge elicited upon stimulation by endotracheal intubation or surgical stimulation causes an increase in resistance vessel tone, an increase in heart rate and myocardial contractility, and a decrease in peripheral venous compliance. Venoconstriction results in a central redistribution of blood volume, while arterial vasoconstriction may cause arterial hypertension. A marked rise in left ventricular end-diastolic pressure (LVEDP) secondary to an increase in afterload and heart rate may accompany intraoperative stimulation (Fig. 4–11). The problem is readily recognized and treated when arterial blood pressure rise is brisk. In fact, when LV failure is prominent, systemic arterial pressure may change little or not at all, while LVEDP (indirectly measured as the pulmonary capillary wedge pressure) may increase enormously due to the elevated afterload (Fig. 4–12).

Optimal therapy during induction of anesthesia and the operation includes control of those factors that promote myocardial oxygen consumption, including heart rate, systemic and pulmonary vascular resistance (right and left ventricular afterload), and pulmonary capillary wedge pressure. In this regard, it is mandatory to continuously monitor arterial pressure and heart rate. When available, certain measurements (such as ventricular filling pressures and cardiac output), which allow

Figure 4–10. Hemodynamic effects (mean ± S.E.M.) following 1 mg/kg (open circles) or 2 mg/kg (solid circles) gallamine. Three minutes after gallamine (1 mg/kg), heart rate and cardiac index had increased significantly ($p < 0.05$). After 10 and 20 minutes, cardiac index was no longer significantly different from control, but the sustained increase in heart rate resulted in a decreased stroke volume index ($p < 0.05$). Three minutes after gallamine (2 mg/kg), there was a significant decrease in systemic vascular resistance in addition to the increase in heart rate and cardiac index. Cardiac index decreased after three minutes but remained significantly above control after 10 and 20 minutes.

HR indicates heart rate; MAP, mean arterial pressure; CI, cardiac index; SVI, stroke volume index; SVR, systemic vascular resistance; CVP, central venous pressure. *(Reproduced with permission from Stoelting R K. Hemodynamic effects of gallamine during halothane-nitrous oxide anesthesia. Anesthiology 39:645–647, 1973.)*

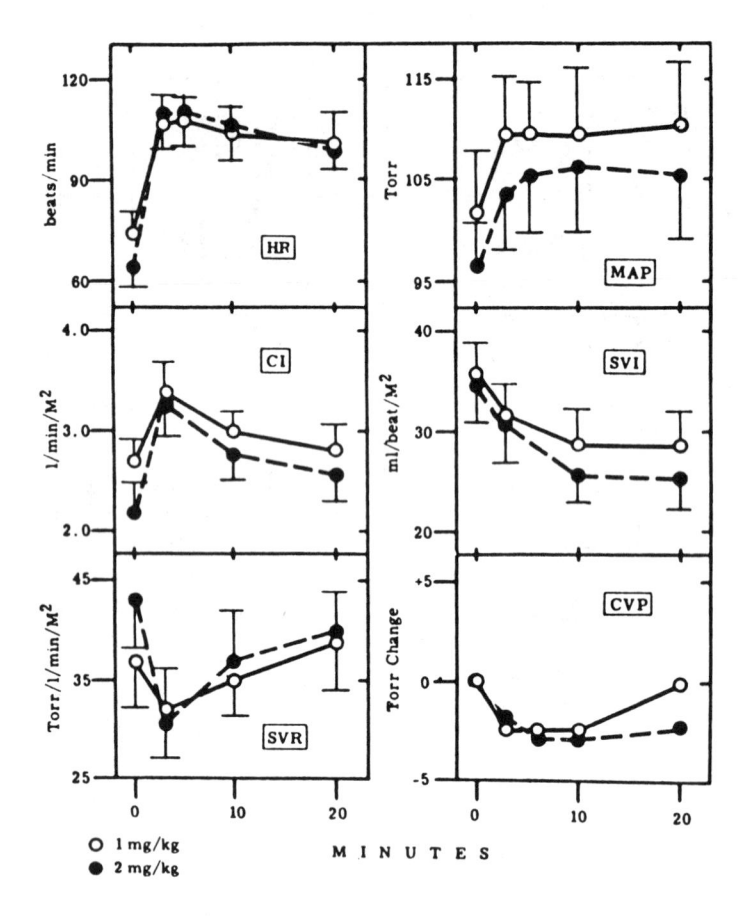

deductions regarding ventricular performance to be made, are also enormously helpful. In addition, a controlled level of myocardial depression is desirable in the patient with coronary artery disease to counteract the influence of sympathetic stimuli that augment myocardial oxygen consumption (Bland and Lowenstein, 1976).

In the patient with normal left ventricular function, halothane may be used to prevent this response by deepening the level of anesthesia. However, an attempt to do so in patients with left ventricular failure or dyskinetic left ventricular wall motion usually results in intolerable myocardial depression. As an alternative, drugs with vasodilating properties but little or no direct effect on the myocardium have been used successfully. (Kotter et al., 1977; Zelis et al., 1968). These drugs include: droperidol (Inapsine), trimetaphan (Arfonad), nitroglycerin, phentolamine (Regitine), and sodium nitroprusside (Nipride) (McDowall et al., 1974; Vesey et al., 1974; Lappas et al., 1976; Lappas et al., 1977). Nitroprusside has proved to be most satisfactory, since its effects are short-lived and moment-to-moment control is possible.

The availability of short-acting vasodilators for intravenous infusion has added an important dimension to the control of intraoperative hypertension (Fig. 4–13). The response to vasodilator therapy with sodium

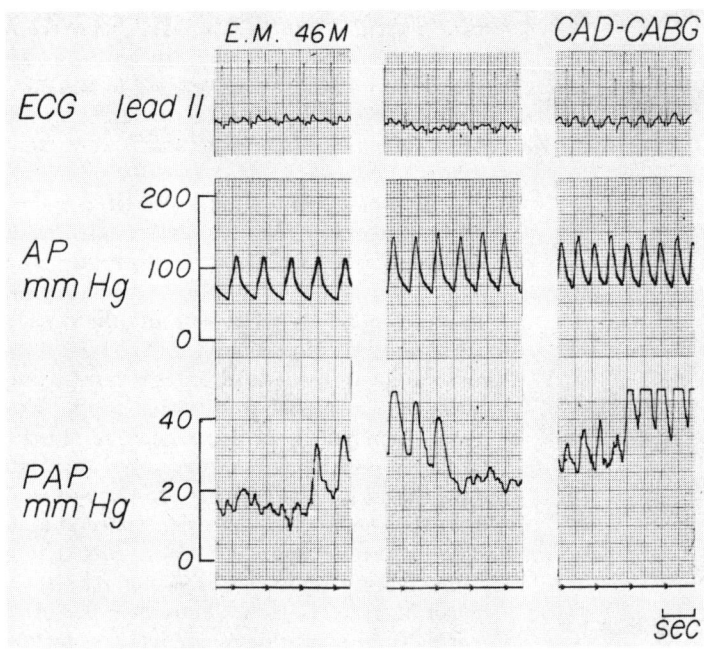

Figure 4-11. Hemodynamic response to surgical stimulation of a 46-year-old male with coronary artery disease (CAD) during coronary artery bypass grafting (CABG). The first section is a recording taken after anesthesia but before surgical stimulation. The second and third sections illustrate hemodynamic changes, 1 minute and 3 minutes, following sternotomy. Systemic arterial pressure (AP), pulmonary artery pressure (PAP), and heart rate increased. Pulmonary capillary wedge pressure, which is recorded in the PAP tracing, increased progressively from 15 mm Hg to 30 mm Hg approximately. The increase in wedge pressure and the appearance of pulsus altermans in the AP tracing suggest transient left ventricular dysfunction. These changes were subsequently reversed by an infusion of sodium nitroprusside (not shown).

nitroprusside differs between patients who have elevated LVEDP and those who have normal LVEDP (Lappas et al., 1976). In the former, vasodilation increases stroke volume and cardiac output, and decreases systemic vascular resistance. In patients with normal LVEDP, decreased peripheral vascular resistance produces a marked reduction in venous return, thereby causing systemic hypotension and tachycardia. Nitroprusside, because of its direct effect on the smooth muscle of the vascular bed, causes arterial and venous dilation. Nitroglycerin is also a direct vasodilator that primarily affects venous capacitance vessels (Ogilvie, 1978).

The combination of nitroglycerin to decrease systemic venomotor tone (Kotter et al., 1977) or diminish return to the right heart by redistribution between a slow and fast compartment (Ogilvie, 1978) with an alpha-agonist such as phenylephrine or methoxamine has proven effective. In our experience, the intraoperative use of a nitroglycerin-phenylephrine combination has proven extremely effective as long as each drug is infused at a rate intended to achieve a specific end point, i.e., low filling pressure with nitroglycerin and an appropriate aortic diastolic pressure with the alpha-agonist (Fig. 4-14).

An increase in heart rate heightens the oxygen demand-supply imbalance in the presence of coronary artery disease. The critical heart rate resulting in intraoperative ischemia varies substantially from patient to patient. Ischemia occurring after an increase in heart rate must be treated either with small quantities of intravenous propranolol or with a deeper level of general anesthesia. We recommend the administration of repeated intravenous doses of propranolol 0.25 mg (not to exceed a total of 0.05 mg/kg).

A decrease in systemic arterial pressure during anesthesia is common. Depending on the nature of underlying heart disease, cor-

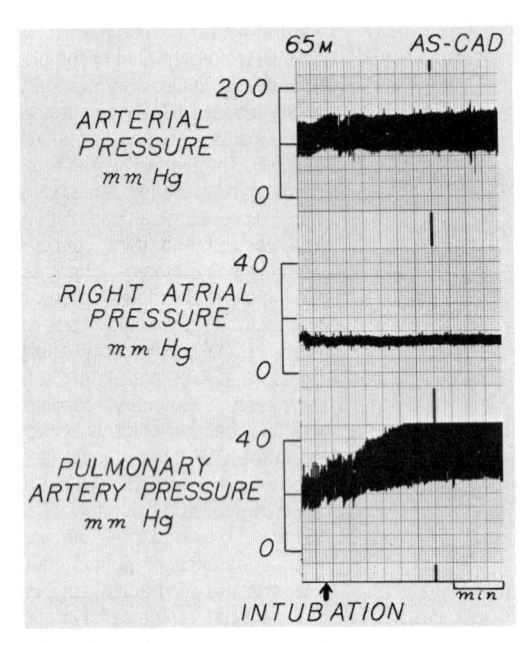

Figure 4–12. Effect of intubation, on arterial, right atrial and pulmonary artery pressures in a 65-year-old male undergoing open heart surgery for aortic stenosis (AS) and coronary artery disease (CAD). Note the significant change in pulmonary artery pressure while arterial pressure shows minimal change. These changes were reversed by an infusion of nitroglycerin (30 mμg/min).

rective measures include the infusion of alpha-agonist drugs to counteract the vasodilation induced by the anesthetics or drugs with both alpha- and beta-agonist properties to support ventricular function.

When left ventricular filling and left ventricular afterload have been adjusted to optimal levels, yet cardiac output and arterial pressure remain inadequate, augmentation of contractility with inotropic drugs is recommended (Lappas et al., 1977). The drug or combination of drugs chosen depends on the hemodynamic effects desired. Norepinephrine, epinephrine, isoproterenol, dopamine, and dobutamine, a new synthetic catecholamine, are widely used cardiac-stimulating drugs. They act on the cardiovascular system by activating the adrenergic receptors. Two major receptors have been identified in the cardiovascular system, alpha and beta receptors. Stimulation of alpha receptors causes an increase in vascular tone leading to vasoconstriction. Stimulation of beta receptors leads to an increase in heart rate and in contractility.

Norepinephrine stimulates both α- and β-adrenergic receptors, causes vasoconstriction, and increases myocardial contractility. The actual effects, however, vary with the condition of the individual patient and the dosage administered. Norepinephrine is known to possess a powerful α-adrenergic stimulating action that constricts vessels that supply kidneys, splanchnic viscera, and skeletal muscle, reducing regional flow to these areas although cardiac output is augmented. In patients who have pulmonary hypertension, norepinephrine may worsen the hemodynamic situation by increasing pulmonary vascular resistance, which aggravates right ventricular performance. Norepinephrine is used to restore arterial blood pressure mainly by increasing peripheral vascular resistance. It is less arrhythmogenic than other catecholamines.

Epinephrine is an endogenous catecholamine possessing α- and β-adrenergic receptor action, also. In small doses, a biphasic effect is observed with initial arterial vasodilation and subsequent vasoconstriction. Epinephrine has a direct effect on the cardiac β-adrenergic receptors, causing an increase in heart rate and in myocardiac contractility. Isoproterenol is a selective β-adrenergic receptor agonist with potent inotropic and chronotropic effects on the heart. Isoproterenol causes systemic and pulmonary arterial vasodilation. Dopamine is an endogenous catecholamine that possesses β-adrenergic action, causing increase in heart rate and myocardial contractility. Small doses stimulate dopaminergic receptors in the kidney, leading to an increase in kidney blood flow and an increase in urine output. In larger doses, dopamine causes vasoconstriction. (See Chapter 22.)

Finally, dobutamine, a new synthetic catecholamine with marked adrenergic stimulating action on the heart, has a strong β-adre-

ANESTHESIA FOR CARDIAC SURGERY 59

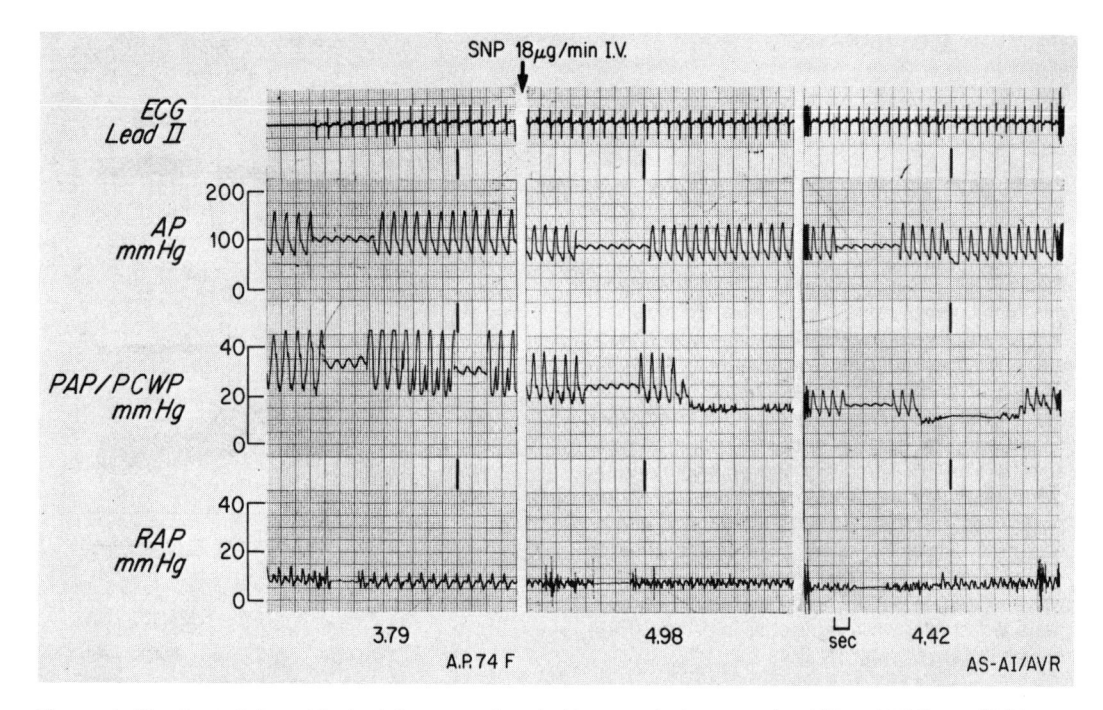

Figure 4–13. Acute left ventricular failure associated with systemic hypertension (AP = 165/70 mm Hg) in a 74-year-old female undergoing aortic valve replacement (AVR) for severe aortic insufficiency (AI) and stenosis (AS). Note the pronounced "v" waves on the first section of the pulmonary artery (PAP) pulmonary capillary wedge pressure (PCWP) tracing. Baseline cardiac output is 3.79 liters/min. With the infusion of sodium nitroprusside (SNP), the hypertension was controlled by reduction in peripheral vascular resistance. This was associated with a decrease in PCWP, disappearance of the "v" waves (middle and third sections) on the PCWP tracing, and an increase in cardiac output to 4.98 liters/min. With time PCWP and right atrial pressure (RAP), decreased further, resulting in a fall in cardiac output to 4.42 liters/min. Since heart rate did not change, the decline in cardiac output, can be attributed to diminished stroke volume. The importance of maintaining an optimal level of ventricular filling pressure (PCWP, RAP) to maintain good ventricular function is obvious.

nergic effect and no effect on alpha receptors, causes vasodilation, and increases myocardial contractility. The combined use of inotropic and vasodilator drugs is preferred for therapy of low-output syndrome to offset a peripheral and perhaps pulmonary vasoconstriction associated with the drugs intended to improve myocardial contractility.

The treatment of right ventricular failure by afterload reduction should be considered when pulmonary hypertension is present, particularly in the reactive form, usually secondary to mitral valve disease. We have preferred a constant infusion of phentolamine (starting dose 1.5 µg/kg/min) to sodium nitroprusside for the treatment of this condition, as it appears to provide a more stable situation when its use is required for a period of days into the postoperative period. The dramatic effect of phentolamine on pulmonary hypertension is shown in Figure 4–15. Long-term infusion of high doses of sodium nitroprusside are to be avoided because of their potential toxicity.

Judicious use of intraoperative electrical pacing has contributed greatly to the support of hemodynamic function. Nodal rhythm, a common result of anesthesia, may cause a fall in arterial blood pressure (Fig. 4–16). Restoration of appropriate atrial function can be

Figure 4–14. Hemodynamic effects of phenylephrine and nitroglycerin (TNG) in a patient with coronary artery disease (CAD) anesthetized in preparation for myocardial revascularization (CABG). An infusion of phenylephrine was started to treat the hypotension of 80/50 mm Hg. Note that phenylephrine caused an increase in systemic arterial pressure (AP) to 105/70 mm Hg and pulmonary artery pressure (PAP) from 30/12 to 40/17 mm Hg. At this point nitroglycerin infusion was started and continued until pulmonary artery pressure returned to normal levels. Arterial pressure continued to rise and was restored to 120/75 mm Hg. Heart rate (HR) remained stable, while right atrial pressure (RAP) decreased slightly with TNG.

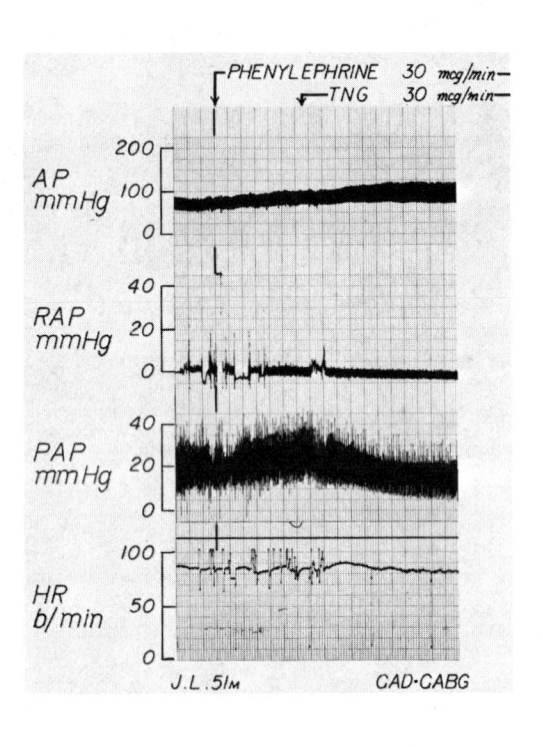

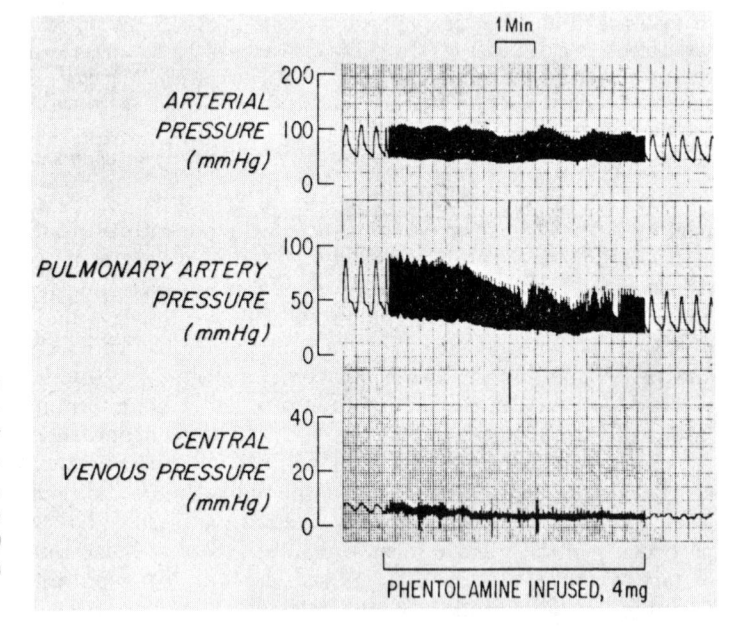

Figure 4–15. The hemodynamic effects of phentolamine in a 69-year-old female shortly after cessation of cardiopulmonary bypass for mitral valve replacement. The pulmonary artery pressure decreased from 90/40 to 55/20 mm Hg, with a minimal reduction in systemic arterial pressure.

ANESTHESIA FOR CARDIAC SURGERY

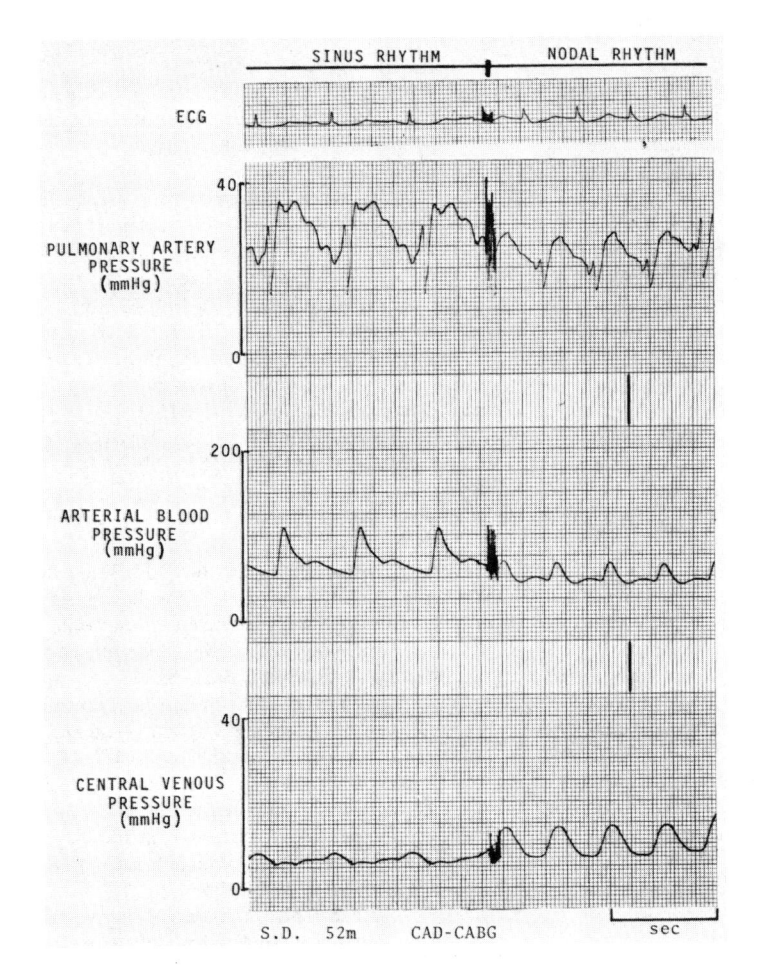

Figure 4-16. Hemodynamic changes associated with supraventricular arrhythmia in a 52-year-old male with coronary artery disease (CAD) during operation for coronary artery bypass grafting (CABG). Note the precipitous drop in arterial blood pressure as the patient's heart rhythm changed from sinus to nodal. Prominent "v" waves also appeared in the central venous pressure tracing.

achieved by pacing the atrium at a faster rate. Although atropine may serve the same purpose, it provides little controlability. Atrial pacing may be used to obtain optimal heart rates and suppress ventricular premature beats when they occur in conjunction with a slow heart rate. Ventricular pacing is obviously necessary in addition whenever atrioventricular dissociation or block is present. We do not employ isolated ventricular pacing except in patients with atrial fibrillation and high degree of AV block, as seen with digitalis toxicity. The hemodynamic benefits of sequential atroventricular pacing are so overwhelming (except in the presence of aberrant AV conduction with occasional diminution of the P-R interval) that ventricular pacing alone has no place in our therapeutic armamentarium. Occasionally, atrial flutter may be treated by rapid atrial pacing (up to 500 stimuli/min) to delay AV conduction and reduce the ventricular response. However, in this condition an electrical shock (35 to 45 joules) applied directly to the atria is preferred if the chest and pericardium are open.

REFERENCES

Bland J H L, Laver M B, Lowenstein E: Vasodilator effect of commercial 5% plasma protein fraction solutions. JAMA 224:1721-1724, 1973.

―――, Lowenstein, E.: Effect of halothane on myo-

cardial ischemia. Anesthesiology 45:287–293, 1976.
Boudoulas H, Lewis R P, Kates R E, Dalmangas G: Hypersensitivity to adrenergic stimulation after propranolol withdrawal in normal subjects. Ann Intern Med 87:433, 1977.
Chidsey C A, Braunwald E, Morrow A G: Catecholamine excretion and cardiac stores of norepinephrine in congestive heart failure. Am J Med 39:442–451, 1965.
Cohn J M: Blood pressure and cardiac performance. Am J Med 55:351–361, 1973.
Dalton B: Anesthesia for cardiac surgery. Anesthesiology 36:521–522, 1972.
Deutsch S, Dalen S E: Indications for prophylactic digitalization. Anesthesiology 30:648–652, 1969.
Dowdy E G, Kaya K L: Studies of the mechanism of cardiovascular responses to ketamine. Anesthesiology 29:931–943, 1968.
Egbert L D, Battit G E, Welch C E: Reduction of postoperative pain by encouragement and instruction of patients. N Eng J Med 270:825–827, 1964.
Eger E I II, Smith N T, Stoelting R K, Cullen D J, Kadis L B, Whitcher C E: Cardiovascular effects of halothane in man. Anesthesiology 32:396–409, 1970.
Faulkner S L, Hopkins J Y, Boerth R C, Young J L, Jr, Jellet L B, Nies A S, Bender H W, Sland D G: Time required for complete recovery from chronic propranolol therapy. N Eng J Med 289:607–609, 1973.
Ghia J, Andersen N B: Pulmonary function and cardiopulmonary bypass. JAMA 212:593, 1970.
Johnson L W, Dickstein R A, Freuhan C T, Kane P, Potts J L, Smuylan H, Webb W R, Eich R H: Prophylactic digitalization for coronary artery bypass surgery. Circulation 53:819, 1976.
Katz A M, Lappas D G, Lowenstein E: Cardiorespiratory effects of morphine scopalomine premedication in adult cardiac surgical patients. Abstracts of A.S.A. Scientific Meeting, 1974, p 225.
Katz R L, Bigger J T: Cardiac arrhythmias during anesthesia and operation. Anesthesiology 33:193–201, 1970.
Kotter V, von Leitner E R, Wunderlich J, Schroder R: Comparison of hemodynamic effects of phentolamine sodium nitroprusside and glyceryl trinitrate in acute myocardial infarction. Br Heart J 39:1196–1204, 1977.
Lappas D G, Buckley M J, Laver M B, Daggett W M, Lowenstein E: Left ventricular performance and pulmonary circulation following addition of nitrous oxide to morphine during coronary artery surgery. Anesthesiology 43:61–69, 1975a.
_____, Gayes J M: Intraoperative monitoring in anesthetic management of the patient with cardiovascular disease. Int Anesthesiol Clin 17:157–173, 1979.
_____, Geha D, Fischer J E, Laver M B, Lowenstein E: Effect of large doses of intravenous morphine upon filling pressures of the heart and pulmonary circulation of patients with coronary artery disease. Anesthesiology 42:153–159, 1975b.
_____, Lowenstein E, Waller J, Fahmy N R, Daggett W M: Hemodynamic effects of nitroprusside infusion during coronary artery operation in man. Circulation 54 (Suppl III):III-4, 1976.
_____, Powell J W, Daggett W M: Cardiac dysfunction. Anesthesiology 47:117–135, 1977.
Lockey E, Ross D N, Longmore D B, Sturridge M F: Potassium and open-heart surgery. Lancet 1:671–675, 1966.
Lowenstein E, Hallowell P, Levine F H, Daggett W M, Austen W G, Laver M B: Cardiovascular response to large doses of intravenous morphine in man. N Eng J Med 281:1389–1393, 1969.
_____, Whiting R B, Bittar B A, Sanders C A, Powell W J Jr: Local neurally mediated effects of morphine on skeletal muscle vascular resistance. J Pharmacol Exp Ther 180:359–367, 1972.
McFadden E R Jr, Ingram R H Jr: Relationship between diseases of the heart and lungs. In Braunwald E (ed): Heart Disease, A Textbook of Cardiovascular Medicine. Philadelphia, W B Saunders, 1980, pp 1894–1896.
McDowall D G, Keaney M P, Turner S M, Lane J R, Okuda Y: The toxicity of sodium nitroprusside. Br J Anaesth 46:327–332, 1974.
Myers M G, Wisenberg G: Sudden withdrawal of propranolol in patients with angina pectoris. Chest 71:24–28, 1977.
Nies A S, Shand D G: Clinical pharmacology of propranolol. Circulation 52:6–12, 1975.
Ogilvie R I: Effect of nitroglycerin on peripheral blood flow distribution and venous return. J Pharmacol Exp Ther 207:372–380, 1978.
Robinson B F: Relation of heart rate and systolic blood pressure to the onset of angina pectoris. Circulation 35:1073–1083, 1967.
Smith N T, Eger E I, Stoelting R K, Whayne T F, Cullen D, Kadis L B: The cardiovascular and sympathomimetic responses to the addition of nitrous oxide to halothane in man. Anesthesiology 32:410–421, 1970.
Stanley T H, Gray N H, Stanford W, Armstrong R: The effects of high dose morphine on fluid and blood requirements in open-heart operations.

Anesthesiology 38:536–541, 1973.

―――, Stanford W, Armstrong R, Cline R: The effect of morphine anesthesia on blood requirements during and after valve replacement and coronary artery bypass grafting. Ann Thorac Surg 17:368–376, 1974.

Stoelting R K: Hemodynamic effect of gallamine during halothane-nitrous oxide anesthesia. Anesthesiology 39:645–647, 1973.

―――: The hemodynamic effects of pancuronium and d-tubocurarine in anesthetized patients. Anesthesiology 36:612–615, 1972.

―――, Gibbs P S: Hemodynamic effects of morphine and morphine nitrous oxide in valvular heart disease and coronary artery disease. Anesthesiology 38:45–52, 1973.

―――, Reiss R R, Longnecker D E: Hemodynamic response to nitrous oxide-halothane and halothane in patients with valvular heart disease. Anesthesiology 37:430–435, 1972.

Trowell J, Peto R, Smith A C: Controlled trial of repeated halothane anesthetics in patients with carcinoma of the uterine cervix treated with radium. Lancet 1:821–827, 1975.

Vesey C J, Cole P V, Linnell J C, Wilson J: Some metabolic effects of sodium nitroprusside in man. Br J Med 2:140–142, 1974.

Wong K C, Martin W E, Hornbein T F, Freund F G, Everett J: The cardiovascular effects of morphine sulfate with oxygen and nitrous oxide in man. Anesthesiology 38:542–549, 1973.

Wright R, Eade O E, Chisholm M, Hawksley M, Lloyd B, Moles T M, Edwards J C, Gardner M J: Controlled prospective study of the effect on liver function of multiple exposures to halothane. Lancet 1:817–820, 1975.

Zelis R, Mason D T, Braunwald E: A comparison of the effects of vasodilator stimuli on peripheral resistance in normal subjects and in patients with congestive heart. J Clin Invest 47:960, 1968.

5. Open Intracardiac Operation Employing Extracorporeal Circulation

ROBERT S. LITWAK   STANLEY GIANNELLI

Unquestionably, the single most important advance in the surgical management of heart disease has been the development of predictable methods of performing open intracardiac operations employing cardiopulmonary bypass. Comroe and Dripps (1974) have clearly described the bases for this accomplishment, which lay in more than 150 years of diverse investigations. Nevertheless, the extraordinary contributions of the late John H. Gibbon, Jr. and his co-workers (among them his wife, Mary) over a period of 16 years are preeminent in having brought clinical cardiopulmonary bypass to successful fruition in 1953. It is beyond the scope of this chapter to review the fascinating and important history of temporary cardiopulmonary substitution, but the reader is referred to reviews by Meade (1961), Galletti and Brecher (1962), Eloesser (1970), and Johnson (1970) for such background.

With proper use of existing equipment, a well-executed operation, and thoughtful postoperative care, an imposing list of cardiac abnormalities now can be corrected unhurriedly with considerable certainty that the patient will recover and be improved.

EQUIPMENT

The basic components required for extracorporeal circulation (ECC) include an oxygenator (more properly termed a gas exchange device or artificial lung, since carbon dioxide is eliminated from the blood as oxygen is introduced), a reservoir (frequently an integral part of the oxygenator) into which venous blood flows, a pump to return oxygenated blood to the patient, two aspirating systems (one of which clears the operative field of blood while the other decompresses the left heart), a filter for removal of potential embolic material, a temperature controlling device (heat exchanger), and interconnecting tubing.

Since the surfaces of these components all have direct contact with blood, they have varying capacities to activate processes of thrombosis (Salzman, 1971). Although considerable progress has been made in improving blood-compatible surfaces, no completely reliable nonthrombogenic material has yet been described. Accordingly, all current methods of extracorporeal circulation require hemostatic inhibition with heparin. However, heparin does not prevent adhesion or deposition of platelets on pump-oxygenator surfaces, events that invariably lead to platelet microemboli.

The following is a necessarily brief discussion of apparatus currently in wide clinical use. For more comprehensive reviews, the reader is referred to Clowes (1960), Galletti and Brecher (1962), Nose (1973), and Ionescu (1981).

Tubing

Either medical grade polyvinylchloride (PVC) or silicone elastomer tubing is used in the extracorporeal circuit. Both have been demonstrated to be reasonably biocompatible with blood. The mechanical surface forces are somewhat less at the blood-silicone elastomer interface than are present when PVC is employed; consequently, the alterations in the formed and nonformed blood elements may be somewhat fewer. Silicone elastomer tubing should be used in that segment of the circuit that is in contact with the pump heads.

Pumps

Nonpulsatile Pumps. Although a variety of pumps have been devised for cardiopulmonary bypass (CPBP), the most commonly employed type in use is the roller pump, because of its simplicity, reliability, and ease of operation (Fig. 5–1). The pump tubing is positioned within a horseshoe-shaped housing, and rollers compress the tubing so that blood is continuously propelled forward. The flow pattern produced is essentially nonpulsatile. Blood trauma is reduced when the rollers are adjusted to be minimally nonocclusive and the rotational speed is relatively slow. Therefore, it is desirable to use tubing of relatively large internal diameter (ID) to avoid excessive roller speeds. Since clinical perfusions require flow rates per minute varying from 0.5 liter (infants) to almost 6 liters (adults), it is convenient to use one-quarter-inch (6.4 mm) ID tubing for infants and three-eighths- (9.5 mm) to one-half-inch (12.7 mm) ID tubing for larger children and adults. Commonly, the virtually occlusive roller pump is used as a flowmeter, since calibration is accomplished

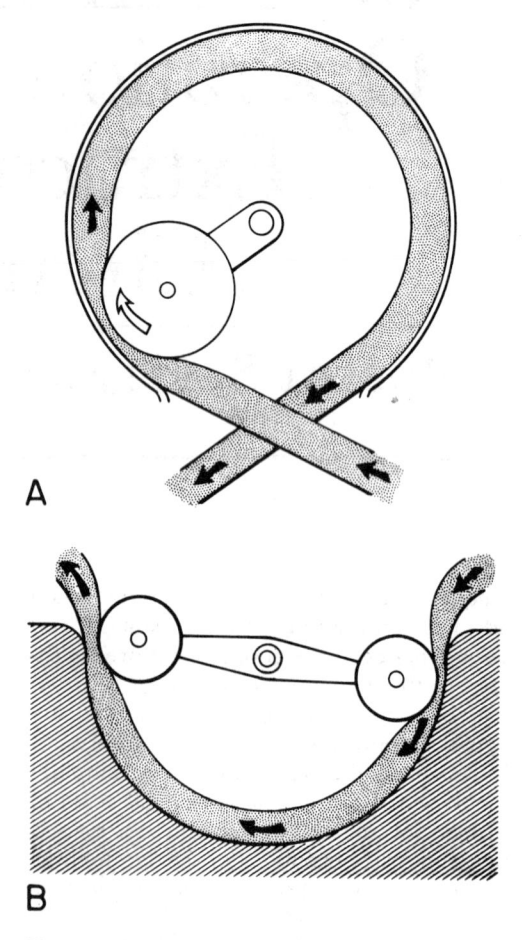

Figure 5–1. Roller pump design with one (**A**) and two (**B**) rollers.

by simply multiplying the known constant pump tubing displacement volume by the roller revolutions per minute. The relationship is essentially linear within the levels of outflow resistance encountered in clinical perfusions.

Pulsatile Pumps. Early experimental studies of ECC included extensive efforts to reproduce the normal pulse contour. Pulsatile pumps are more complex and can be more traumatic to blood. A later section of this chapter discusses both the theoretical and established advantages of pulsatile perfusion. Currently, however, roller pumps are used in essentially all open heart operations.

Coronary Perfusion Pumps. When the aortic valve is exposed and normal coronary blood flow interrupted for a considerable time, the method most commonly employed to protect the myocardium prior to widespread use of hypothermic cardioplegia involved cannulation of each coronary ostium and perfusion of each artery with separate roller pumps that were set to deliver up to 200 ml/min at line pressures below 120 mm Hg. Each pump system was designed so that sudden marked elevations in line pressure (possibly caused by cannula kinking or impingement on the coronary arterial wall) would automatically stop the driving motor (McGoon et al., 1965).

One of the authors (Gianelli et al., 1976) has employed a gravity-regulated system of constant pressure coronary perfusion. This more closely resembles the normal pattern of coronary perfusion, in which flow occurs primarily during diastole when myocardial wall tension is reduced. Under these conditions, total coronary flow (at the same mean perfusion pressure) is two to three times greater when gravity flow is employed compared to continuous pumping throughout the cardiac cycle. In the latter system, perfusion of the constricted coronary vascular bed of the hypertrophied left ventricle during systole elevates mean coronary perfusion pressure at relatively low flow rates. There is clinical evidence that the increased coronary flow with gravity perfusion is accompanied by better preservation of myocardial function.

Gas Exchange Devices ("Oxygenators")

Concepts. "Gas exchange device" defines the sharp performance limitations of existing artificial lungs. The natural lung is a complex organ. While gas exchange is unquestionably its single most important life-support function, several important nonrespiratory metabolic functions have recently been described. Inability of current mechanical "lungs" to perform these latter functions may have important and adverse consequences during ECC. For example, bradykinin is almost entirely inactivated during a single passage through the intact lung. The recent demonstration that active bradykinin is present during ECC probably reflects the inability of the patient's bypassed lungs to perform the inactivation function at this time.

All gas exchange devices employ the same basic principle for gas exchange as that in natural lungs: blood is brought into proximity with the oxygenating gas and is distributed in a thin layer to facilitate gaseous diffusion. The simplest approach is to create a thin blood layer that is in direct contact with the gas, either by creating the layer around a bubble of gas or thinly filming the blood on a surface over which the gas passes. A more complex and physiologically superior method is to interpose a permeable membrane between the gas and the blood layer, thereby simulating normal in vivo conditions of gas exchange.

The diffusion of a given quantity of oxygen across biologic liquid and tissue interface is 15 to 20 times slower than that for carbon dioxide. Therefore, it is apparent that the overriding physical problem for natural and artificial lungs is the delivery of enough oxygen to the blood. Galletti (1962, 1972) has compared the design and performance characteristics of the natural and artificial lung. The differences are striking. The natural lung has an enormous alveolar-capillary surface area (50 to 100 m^2), which allows a 5-micron monocorpuscular film of blood to be exposed to a partial pressure of oxygen approximating 100 mm Hg for only 0.1 to 0.3 second. Despite the fact that diffusion of oxygen through the plasma to the red cells is rapid, it is not instantaneous, and, in the natural lung, accounts for at least 20 percent of the time required for oxygen uptake. In contrast to the normal lung, where the thinness of the blood film spread over a huge area accounts for the efficient gas exchange, mechanical gas exchange devices have a relatively diminutive gas exchange surface area; layers of blood 20 to 60 times as thick (100 to 300 microns in sheet and disc oxygenators) are exposed to a partial pressure of oxygen seven times higher (700 mm Hg) over a time period 30 to 100 times longer (3 to 30 seconds) than conditions prevailing in the natural lung.

The thickness of the blood layer and the small exchange surface area make it impossible for current gas exchange devices to effect adequate oxygen uptake by the blood through the physical process of diffusion alone. How then does a mechanical device increase its efficiency so that blood oxygenation is improved? The answer is turbulence. This increased "stirring" enhances mixing between the varying layers of a thick column or film of blood so that the oxygen-blood interface is increased. In addition, some of the widely used artificial lungs have a priming volume larger than that of the natural lung, allowing a longer period of exposure to oxygen within the mechanical device for each volume of blood delivered to the patient per unit of time.

Elimination of the more diffusible carbon dioxide is no problem for the normal lung. However, circumstances prevail in gas exchange devices that tend to limit carbon dioxide exchange, although it is generally true that elimination of the gas will be adequate as long as oxygen uptake is satisfactory. However, this may not always be the case. When 100 percent oxygen is delivered to an artificial lung, the pressure gradient of oxygen from the liquid to the gas phase will be 12 to 14 times as large as the carbon dioxide pressure gradient. Because of its far greater solubility, carbon dioxide will still diffuse faster than oxygen but by no means as rapidly as in the natural lung. Indeed, the time required for carbon dioxide to diffuse across the plasma and red cell membrane in a gas exchange device will be at least 50 percent of the time required for the diffusion of oxygen (Galletti and Brecher, 1962).

It is also important to appreciate that high inflow volumes of pure oxygen may create conditions analogous to hyperventilation. In such cases hypocapnea can be avoided by use of a 2 percent carbon dioxide and 98 percent oxygen mixture.

Three types of gas exchange devices (hereafter termed oxygenators for brevity and because the term is commonly used) are currently in clinical use and are discussed below.

Gas Dispersion (Bubble) Oxygenators (Fig. 5–2).

Arterialization of venous blood is accomplished by passage of oxygen bubbles through the blood, a technique first employed by experimental physiologists almost a century ago. The gas (generally 98 percent oxygen and 2 percent carbon dioxide) is introduced through a manifold at the base of a vertical oxygenating column through which passes venous blood. The manifold discharges 3- to 7-mm bubbles into the blood, thereby creating foam and, in the process, permitting oxygen uptake and carbon dioxide elimination by the blood. The continuous inflow of both venous blood and gas into the oxygenating column creates forward and upward movement of the blood foam, which then surges into a coalescence and settling chamber. Here the foam is broken up by bringing the minute bubbles into contact with a polymethylsiloxane compound (Antifoam A, Dow Corning Corp.) lightly applied to special sponges, which thereby provide an enormous blood contact surface. This method of defoaming was first described by Clark et al. (1950) and solved a major problem, contributing to the first successful clinical use of a simple helical coil bubble oxygenator by DeWall et al. (1956).

It is important to limit the gas-blood flow ratio if excessive hemolysis is to be avoided and protein denaturation kept at a minimum. As discussed elsewhere, the latter alteration is largely the consequence of the direct exposure of blood to gas (Lee et al., 1961). Although earlier bubble oxygenators required gas-blood flow ratios as high as 4:1 to achieve adequate oxygen uptake, several current models allow effective gas exchange with ratios as low as 0.75:1.

Currently, efficient and disposable bubble oxygenators (Fig. 5–2, right) are the most widely employed of all gas exchange devices and provide satisfactory gas exchange for more than five hours.

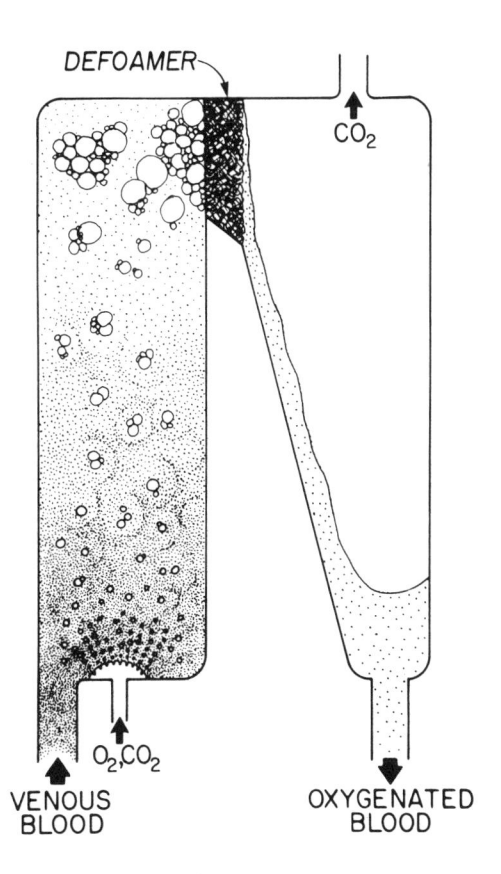

Blood Film Oxygenators (Fig. 5-3). These devices accomplish gas exchange by the layering of blood on planar surfaces. Two configurations were widely employed in the past. Gibbon et al. (1953) developed a device in which venous blood was filmed by gravity in an oxygen-rich atmosphere on a series of stationary vertical screens or sheets, each of which allowed satisfactory gas exchange of 230 to 250 ml of blood per minute. The number of screens or sheets required was proportional to the calculated perfusion rate.

A second type of filming device used in earlier years was the rotating disc oxygenator (Fig. 5-4), composed of a series of round planar or slightly convoluted plates mounted on a central shaft. The discs rotated within an enclosed, horizontally disposed, cylindrical housing in which a blood level was maintained. Venous blood entering at the bottom

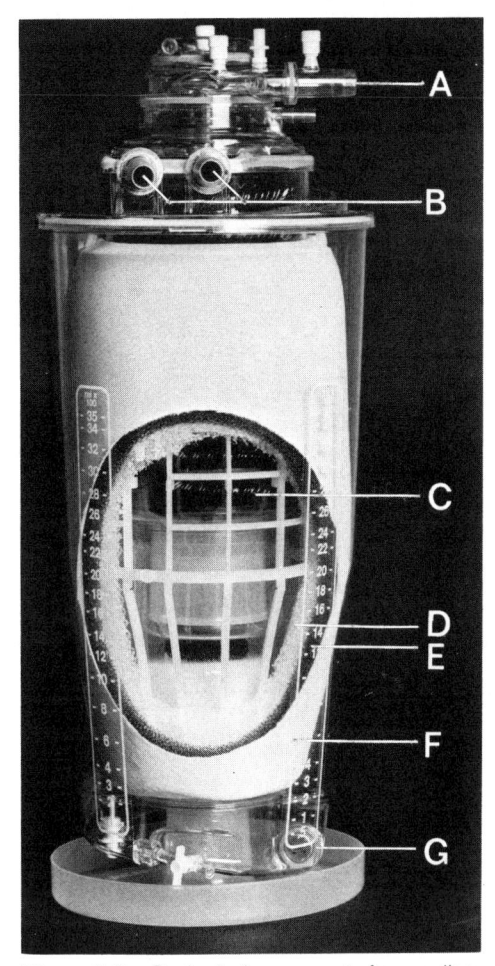

Figure 5–2. Basic design concept of a gas dispersion ("bubble") oxygenator (left). A modern gas dispersion oxygenator (Bentley BOS-10S) at right. For demonstration purposes a portion of the defoaming system (D, E, F) has been removed to reveal the self-contained helical exchanger (C). The inflow and outflow water ports are at B. Both venous blood (A) and cardiotomy return enter and are "oxygenated" at the top. This feature eliminates the need for a long bubble mixing column (common to earlier gas dispersion systems) and permits lower gas to blood flow ratios since high gas flow is not needed to propel venous blood up a bubble column. The oxygenated blood flows downward over the heat exchanger and initiates contact with the defoamer layers at the base, thereby minimizing blood contact with the defoamer. The arterial reservoir outlet is at G (right).

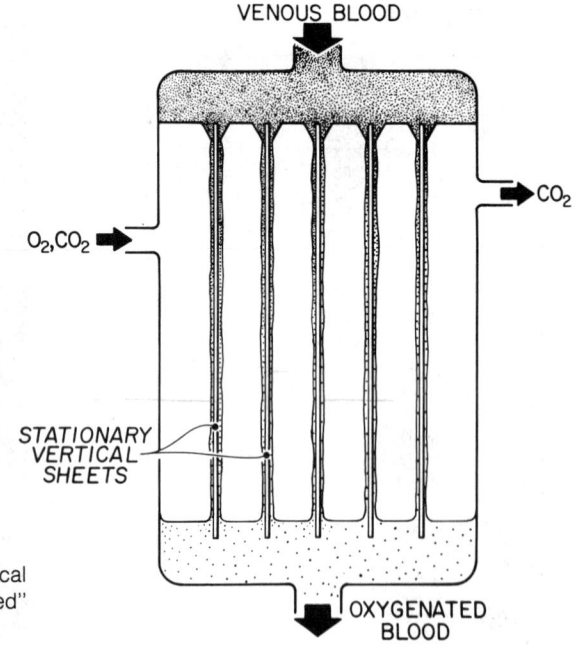

Figure 5–3. Design concept of a stationary vertical sheet oxygenator. The venous blood is "arterialized" as it flows down the sheets in thin films.

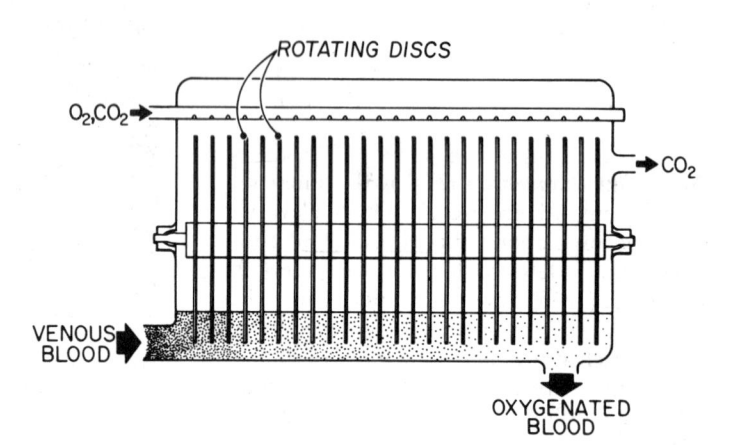

Figure 5–4. Design concept of a rotating disc oxygenator. The venous blood is filmed on the rotating discs, thereby effecting gas exchange.

of one end of the oxygen-enriched cylinder was filmed on the rotating discs, thereby permitting gas exchange. Arterialized blood exited from the other end. As in the previous type of filming device, the number of discs employed was proportional to the anticipated perfusion rate.

Membrane Oxygenators. This design (Fig. 5–5) most closely simulates the human lung because there is separation of blood from the ambient gas. Thus, protein denaturation and other adverse alterations associated with direct blood-gas interfaces are minimized. Venous blood is directed between two extremely thin semipermeable membranes across which gas exchange occurs. Currently, the membranes are fabricated largely from silicone elastomers, and the speed of oxygen and carbon dioxide transfer is theoretically effi-

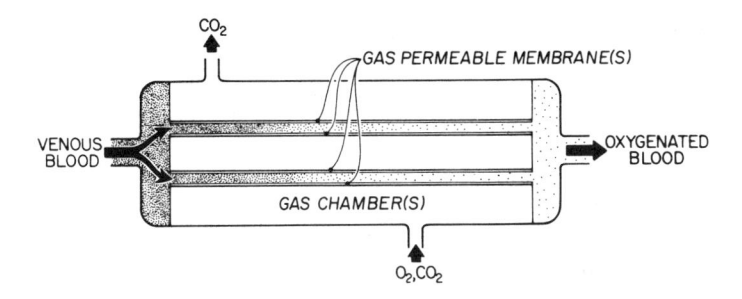

Figure 5-5. Design concept of a membrane oxygenator. Simulating the human lung, there is no direct gas-blood interface.

cient. However, in actual use the transfer rate is much slower, primarily because of the thickness of the blood film, which may vary from 150 to 300 microns. Although membrane oxygenators have been used successfully since 1958 (Clowes and Neville), they have not yet been demonstrably superior in reducing morbidity and mortality of patients undergoing intracardiac operations. Undoubtedly, this is primarily a tribute to man's capacity to withstand the traumata of conventional direct blood-gas interfacial oxygenators over a relatively short time course of several hours.

Currently, several excellent membrane oxygenators are commercially available that give promise of being widely accepted for routine open heart operations during the next few years. They are compact, require no more priming volume than bubble units, allow convenient perfusion of patients of all sizes, and are remarkably trouble-free.

Heat Exchangers

The deliberate induction of hypothermia during perfusion and the necessity to reverse this state in a controlled fashion prior to discontinuance of bypass has led to the development of efficient heat exchangers that operate on the physical principle of conduction. Although numerous designs are now in use, the method of Brown et al. (1958) is basic to almost all of them (Fig. 5-6). Blood (either in tubes or a thin annular chamber) is surrounded by a jacket through which circulates rapidly flowing heat-transferring water at temperatures carefully regulated with an automatic mixing valve.

At high perfusion rates, body temperature can be lowered rapidly, since the thermal

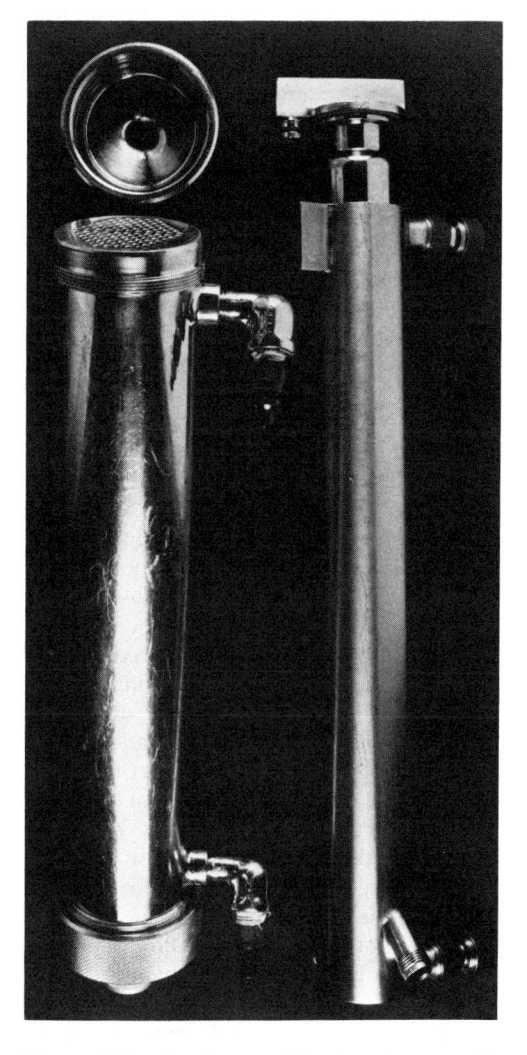

Figure 5-6. Two types of heat exchangers. By passing through either separate tubes (left) or a common annular chamber (right), the perfusate is warmed or cooled by a contiguous water jacket.

gradient between the blood and chilled water is relatively large. However, rewarming the patient during perfusion must proceed more slowly, since the temperature in the heat exchanger must not exceed 42C (preferably 40C) because of possible thermal blood trauma. Further, heated oxygenated blood delivered to a still cool patient has the capacity to release bubbles, since the solubility of oxygen in plasma falls as the blood temperature rises. Studies by Donald and Fellows (1960) indicate that limiting the temperature differential of blood above body temperature to 10C avoids bubble production. In practice, a 15-degree difference has not been accompanied by discernible clinical problems. Usually, patients can be rewarmed at rates between 0.5 and 1.5C per minute.

Cardiotomy Suction and Left Heart Vents

During total cardiopulmonary bypass (CPBP) a significant amount of blood continues to enter the heart and must be recovered and returned to the heart-lung machine to minimize blood usage. During operations within the right heart with intact septa, the primary source of blood in the operative field is the coronary venous return, which approximates 5 to 10 percent of total systemic blood flow. In the presence of cyanotic heart disease with right to left shunting and sharply diminished pulmonary blood flow (such as tetralogy of Fallot), an extensive aortopulmonary collateral system delivers large volumes of blood to the precapillary pulmonary circulation so that the blood either refluxes through the pulmonary artery trunk into the right heart or proceeds through the pulmonary venous circulation to the left heart, where it crosses a septal defect and appears in the right heart operative field. In severe cases, 30 to 40 percent of total systemic blood flow can return to the heart by these various channels.

During operations within the left heart, blood in the operative field derives primarily from the bronchial arterial circulation. Additionally, when the ascending aorta is intact, slight distortion of the aortic annulus by retractors can result in reflux of blood into the left ventricle through an otherwise competent aortic valve.

Removal of blood from within the heart is accomplished with a cardiotomy sucker system. An intracardiac suction tip is connected to a length of tubing and a roller pump. The speed of the pump is governed by the volume of blood returning to the heart. The cardiotomy aspirate is gently pumped into a settling chamber, thence through a filter, eliminating bubbles and particulate debris before the blood is returned to the inflow side of the oxygenator. Cardiotomy suction systems are a major source of blood trauma, and it is important that injudicious aspiration, which produces surging and frothing of blood, be avoided.

When the cardiac septa are intact, elective cardiac asystole or poor cardiac contractility would quickly be followed by disastrous left ventricular distension caused by blood entering the left heart from any of the sources described above. To avoid this, a venting system is employed that involves the same equipment components as the cardiotomy suction system. Although venting is feasible from a catheter located in the left atrium, optimal left heart decompression is accomplished with a multiperforated catheter positioned in the left ventricle. The left heart vent system also provides a means of evacuating air from the left heart before discontinuing perfusion.

Filters

Current methods of CPBP with ECC result in the production and release of varying numbers of particulate, lipid, and gaseous emboli which, when excessive, can adversely affect postperfusion subsystem performance and clinical outcome (discussion of these problems will be found later in this chapter).

A major advance in the reduction of quantity and size of emboli delivered to the patient has been the development of effective blood filters employed during the perfusion. Two basic configurations of filters (Figs. 7A,B) are currently in wide clinical use: a screen type filter (Pall Corp.) (Fig. 7A), in which the grid sizes are uniform (40 microns), and the

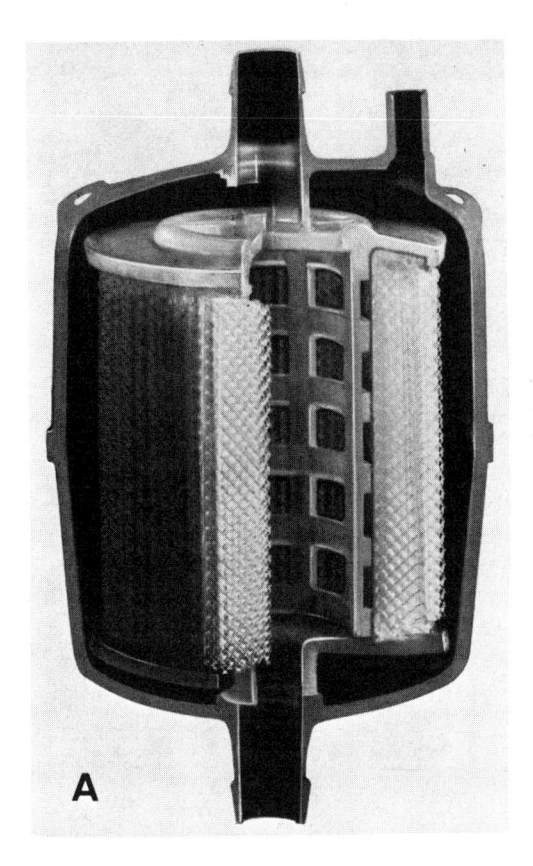

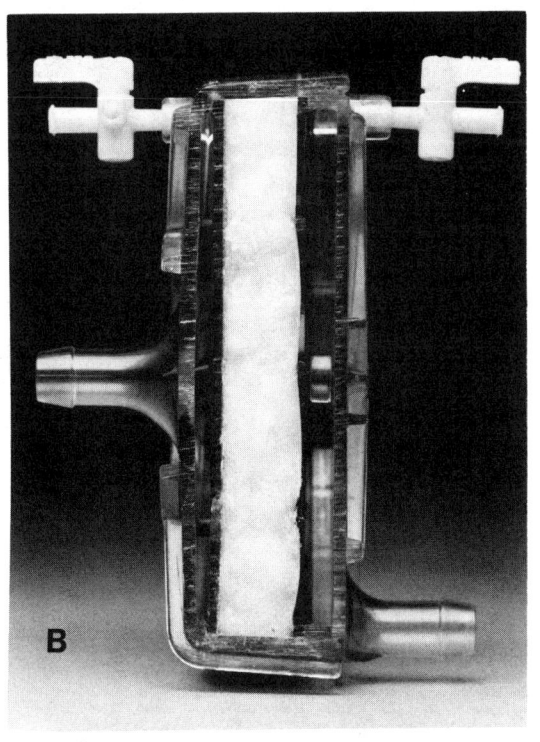

CARDIAC OPERATION WITH EXTRACORPOREAL CIRCULATION

Figure 5–7. **A.** Cutaway view of a polyester screen (Pall) filter. **B.** Cutaway view of a polyester wool (Pioneer Viggo) filter.

Swank (Fig. 7B) polyester (Dacron) wool filter (Pioneer Viggo, Inc.), which functions by adsorption of microparticles to a large surface area of packed polyester wool (Figs. 8A,B). Solis et al. (1974) documented that both filter types effectively reduce the volume of microemboli derived from cardiotomy suction blood (the major source of particulate and lipid debris), the polyester wool filter proving to be somewhat more efficient. Use of ultrapore filters has virtually eliminated the hazard of cerebral nonfat particulate emboli and reduced but not eliminated introduction of lipid emboli (Hill et al., 1970; Clark et al., 1975).

Although there is unequivocal evidence that filtration of cardiotomy return blood is essential, the advantages and possible disadvantages of arterial blood filtration throughout perfusion require further clarification. There is evidence that use of an arterial filter is accompanied by lower platelet and white blood cell counts, although these rise to satisfactory levels after bypass is terminated. Since there is the possibility that an arterial filter might become occluded with enough debris to produce proximal line pressures high enough to cause line disruption, it is advisable to insert two filters in parallel with pressure gauges appropriately positioned to detect unacceptable pressure gradients across the filter (above 250 mm Hg). Selective use of either filter is permitted by clamping the inlet line of one of them.

SAFETY DEVICES

It has been estimated that accidents associated with pump-oxygenator use (malfunction or human error) occur approximately once in

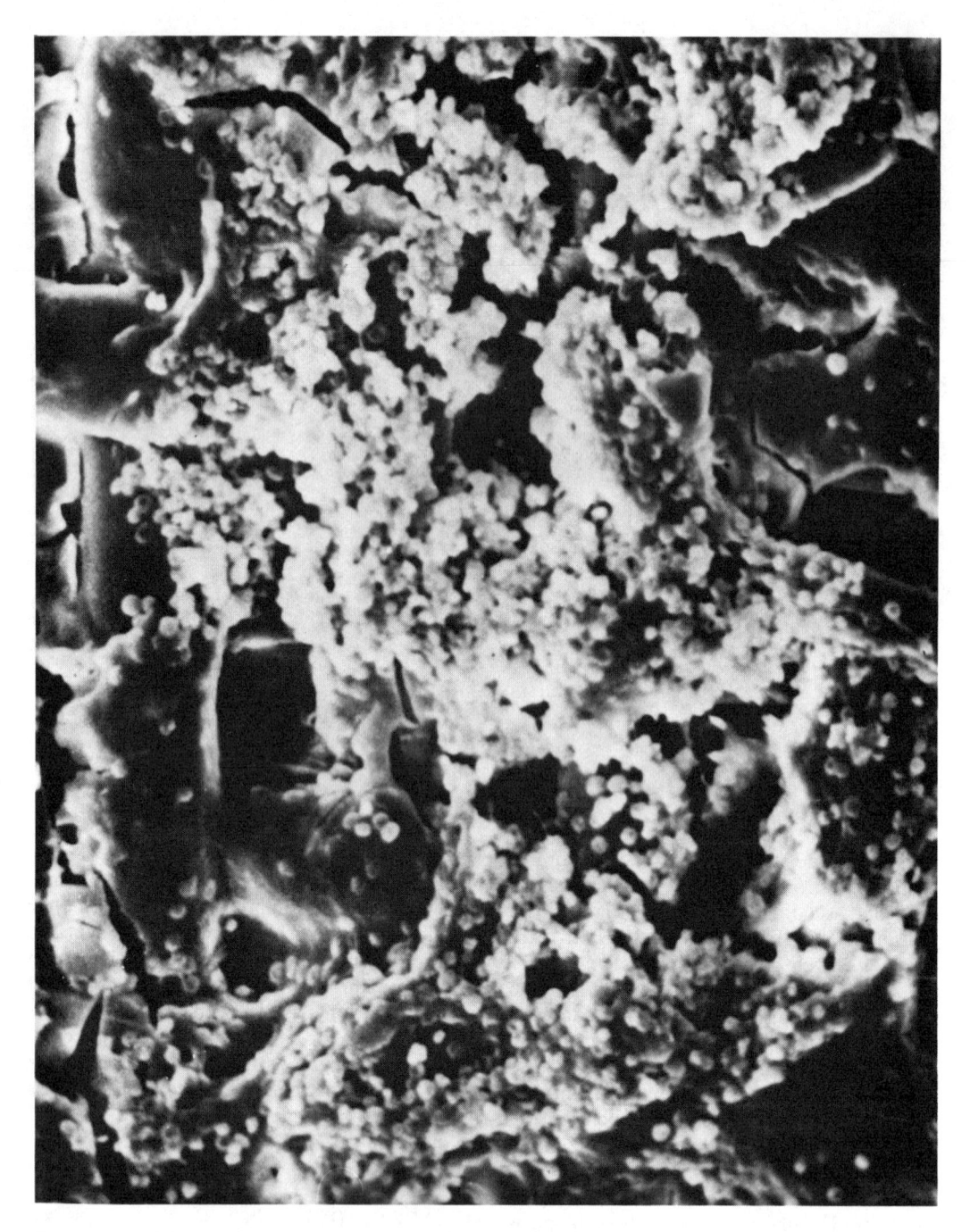

Figure 5–8. A. Scanning electron micrograph of microaggregated debris trapped by the 40-micron Pall screen filter.

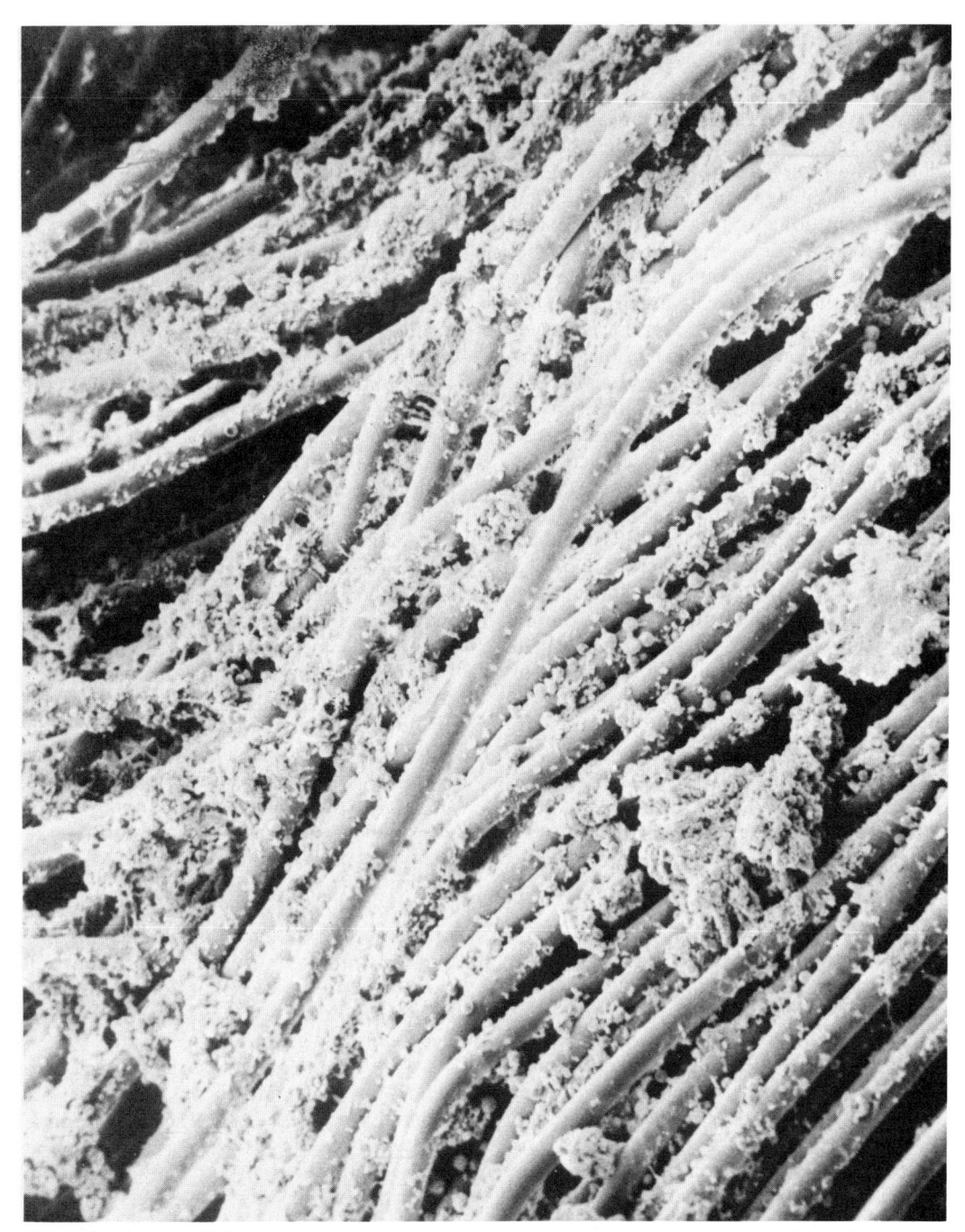

Figure 5–8 (cont.). **B.** Scanning electron micrograph of micraggregated debris adherent to the polyester wool fibers of a Swank (Pioneer Viggo) filter.

every 300 cases, with one patient per thousand suffering permanent injury or death (Stoney et al., 1980). High on the list of disastrous occurrences is massive air embolism, most frequently caused by either inattention to the reservoir level or reversal of the pump head tubing connected to the left ventricular vent (Mills and Ochsner, 1980). The first of these accidents should be preventable by use of a photosensor on the oxygenator reservoir, which both alarms and shuts off the arterial pump if a low blood level is detected. Several major manufacturers of heart-lung machines now include a low-level alarm and shutoff device as mandatory equipment. In addition to a low-level sensing device, it also seems prudent to routinely place a mechanical shutoff valved device* at the outlet of the oxygenator. The valve remains open as long as it is filled with perfusate, but will close if air enters the valve chamber, thereby blocking the ingress of air into the arterial line.

In their survey of 71 miscellaneous pump-oxygenator accidents, Stoney et al. (1980) found that a frequent cause of air embolism (25 percent) was the accidental reversal of the pump head tubing connected to the left ventricular vent. They wisely recommend that large and distinctive arrows be added to each pump head to clearly designate proper flow direction.

THE PERFUSATE

There are two interrelated considerations for constitution of the priming fluid: its volume and composition. Once ECC is instituted, the patient's blood and the priming solution mix to form the perfusate. Therefore, constitution of the prime must be undertaken with an appreciation of what the resultant perfusate will be. Moreover, since the perfusate remains in the patient's circulating blood mass after ECC, its composition must also take into consideration requirements of the postperfusion period as well.

---

*Delta Medical Industries, Costa Mesa, CA.

Volume of the Priming Solution

The first requirement of the prime must be to insure that the volume is adequate. There are two reasons for maintaining adequate volume in the ECC. First, enough perfusate should be available to ensure that the oxygenator is not drained to a dangerously low level, allowing air to be sucked into the arterial line should there be a sudden decrease in venous return. With a flow rate of 5 liters per minute, almost 100 ml of perfusate per second will be drained from the oxygenator if the venous return is suddenly totally occluded. Second, the number of gaseous microemboli in the perfusate leaving the oxygenator increases markedly as the volume is reduced, since there is a proportional diminution of residence time of the perfusate within the oxygenator (which acts as a settling chamber for the elimination of gas emboli). Thus, with higher systemic flow rates greater perfusate volume should be maintained in the oxygenator to reduce gaseous microemboli.

Pump-Oxygenator Prime

An ideal priming solution would perform all of the functions of autologous blood without imposing any of the disadvantages inherent in using such a perfusate with existing perfusion systems. It must be appreciated that regardless of the "ideal" nature of any prime, the circulating perfusate is exposed to the traumata of relatively noninert materials and direct and often turbulent blood-gas interfacial phenomena. Even when membrane oxygenators are employed, the former problem will exist in all cases where cardiotomy blood is recovered, defoamed, filtered, and reintroduced into the patient.

For the present, it is perhaps sufficient to define perfusate criteria on which there is general agreement. An acceptable priming solution is one that provides for oxygen and carbon dioxide transport and unloading, buffering, normal electrolyte levels, osmotic pressure to retain adequate fluid volume relationships within and between intravascular and extravascular compartments, and, finally, restoration of normal coagulation following perfusion.

Total Autologous Blood Prime

Although autogenous blood drawn over a period of several days to several weeks preoperatively has been used for the entire prime in open heart operations, this has been almost always in unusual investigational circumstances—usually to compare an autogenous prime with another method. For obvious logistical reasons, a fully autogenous blood prime is impractical. Moreover, hemodilution techniques make this no longer necessary.

Total Homologous Blood Prime

The early open heart operations generally employed primes consisting of homologous blood that usually had been drawn within 48 hours of surgery. Both heparin and citrate (most commonly ACD: acid-citrate-dextrose solution) stored blood have been widely used in the past as the sole priming solution. Although the logistical problems were somewhat eased with the development of a method of using buffered ACD blood for perfusion (Foote et al., 1961), difficulties remain in providing sufficient bank blood for a busy open heart program.

Decisions about the use of homologous blood in the prime require consideration of three questions. First, what are the adverse affects of homologous blood when administered in conventional blood transfusion? Second, are there harmful immunologic effects from mechanisms other than red cell incompatibility? Third, is deliberate reduction of the perfusate hematocrit desirable; if it is, how much (if any) of the priming volume should consist of homologous blood?

The Effects of Homologous Blood Transfusion.

Use of a stored whole blood prime has been aptly characterized by Zwart and Kolff (1974) as a massive blood transfusion delivered when bypass is started and possessing all of the intrinsic risks of such an infusion. Problems potentially associated with use of multiple units of homologous blood include reactions that may contribute to the still poorly understood homologous blood syndrome in humans, serum hepatitis, cytomegalovirus infections, and a host of difficulties related to various methods of blood storage—increased organic acid load, decreased performance and augmented breakdown of formed elements which result in particulate debris, cellular aggregates, and deviations of nonfilterable chemical species in the plasma component of the stored blood (increased potassium and adenosine diphosphate, decreased ionized calcium and magnesium in ACD preserved blood). Some, but by no means all, of these distortions can be favorably modified at the time the blood is used. Additionally, there is evidence that the adverse effects of the pump-oxygenator are greater when a whole blood perfusate is employed than with other priming methods. Formed element destruction is greater (Schrek and Neville, 1964), and it has been suggested that increased interfacial protein denaturation also occurs.

Immunologic Effects of Homologous Blood Administration.

Although data are sparse and space considerations do not permit an extensive review of the theoretical immunologic implications of homologous blood administration, there is evidence that massive homologous blood exchange during ECC can be accompanied by significant hemodynamic and pathophysiologic derangements (Gadboys et al., 1962). Simple admixture of two freshly drawn samples of human plasma of the same ABO-Rh groupings initiated activation of the fibrinolytic system in over 50 percent of the cases (Gianelli et al., 1965). This study was prompted by the observation that the fibrinolytic system was already activated in the homologous blood prime prior to initiation of ECC. In a similar in vitro mixing study, Schrek and Neville (1964) showed that upon admixture of two freshly drawn samples there was reduced survival time of neutrophiles and some lymphocytes underwent transformation into lymphoblastic cells.

Rabelo et al. (1973) studied the effects of different perfusion primes on the lung in three groups of patients undergoing open heart surgery. A total nonblood prime was employed in one group, autogenous blood in the second group, and homologous blood in the third (the perfusate hematocrits in the latter two groups were similar). Light and electron microscopy study revealed that only those patients perfused with homologous blood demonstrated significant postperfusion alterations in lung morphology, consisting of leukocyte migration to the capillaries, alveolar septa and spaces, vacuolization of type II (granular) pneumocytes, desquamation of alveolar epithelial cells, numerous free lamellar bodies within the alveoli, and interstitial edema. Additional ultrastructure studies by Ratliff et al. (1973) of lung biopsies of patients perfused with a large prime disc oxygenator (presumably primed totally or in part with homologous blood) demonstrated that sequestration of polymorphonuclear leukocytes within the alveolar vasculature was associated with injury to the pulmonary parenchyma. Severe damage to endothelial and membranous pneumocytes was observed only in the presence of large numbers of polys or fragments of them in the alveolar vessels.

These observations strongly support the concept that the presence of homologous blood in the perfusate is deleterious. Further, they suggest that many of the benefits attributed to hemodilution per se may in fact be related to the absence or reduction of homologous blood.

Hemodilute and Bloodless Prime

At present, virtually all groups performing open heart surgery have abandoned total homologous blood prime for various methods of hemodilution. Two reasons prompted this decision, the first being the obvious logistical advantages, since much less blood was required. A second reason, the possible physiologic benefit, is still unproven and largely based on favorable clinical experience.

When the priming volume of the extracorporeal perfusion system is small relative to the patient's blood volume (as generally pertains with most of the currently available disposable oxygenators when used in adults), it is generally permissible to completely fill the unit and tubing connections with a nonblood priming solution. Clinical use of a completely nonblood prime was first reported by Panico and Neptune (1960). Since then the contributions of Zuhdi et al (1961), Cooley et al. (1962), DeWall et al. (1962), and others have demonstrated the clinical efficacy of this method.

Perfusate Hematocrit. As early as 1954, Gollan et al. demonstrated that at markedly reduced temperatures it was possible to sustain life in the experimental animal with a perfusate virtually devoid of hemoglobin. Oxygen transfer was achieved solely through the physically dissolved gas. This extraordinary experiment indicated what might have been inferred by reflecting on the response of patients recovering uneventfully after experiencing blood loss. Moore's remarks (1974) are pertinent:

> For many generations of surgeons between Lester and Landsteiner, over a period of about 60 years, every postoperative patient had a stabilized posthemorrhagic hemodilutional anemia. Sometimes it was normovolemic, but it must have been hypovolemic on a great many occasions. Not so surprisingly, many of those patients got along well.

When the relative volumes of the pump-oxygenator and patient are such that hemodilution results in a severe reduction of the mixed perfusate hematocrit (below 20) at normothermia, metabolic acidosis is the inevitable result because of diminished oxygen-carrying capacity and reduced buffering capability of the diluted red cell mass. The acidosis occurs despite maintenance of high perfusion rates (Cruz and Callaghan, 1966). Use of buffering agents and hypothermic reduction of body metabolism are helpful in somewhat ameliorating the problem during perfusion. However, use of any method that *severely* reduces the perfusion hematocrit cannot be a physiologic asset and is inadvisable.

When the perfusate hematocrit approximates 25 (after complete mixing of prime and patient), the oxygen transport capacity of the diluted perfusate remains at acceptable levels, presumably through the mechanism of reduced perfusate viscosity and vascular resistance, so that blood flow is proportionately augmented (Replogle and Merrill, 1970). When both flow rate and intravascular volume of hemodilute perfusate are adequate, evidence suggestive of increased tissue extraction of oxygen (widening of the arteriovenous oxygen difference) is not consistently observed unless the hematocrit drops below 20. For a comprehensive discussion of this and other aspects of hemodilution physiology, the reader is referred to Messmer et al. (1972) and Messmer and Schmid–Schönbein (1972).

Hemodilution and Intravascular Volume. A basic principle of hemodilution is that, while the patient's blood is maximally diluted at the onset of ECC, the diluent tends to be lost from the perfusate, both into the interstitial space and the urine, as ECC continues. At the conclusion of ECC, some or all of the perfusate left in the extracorporeal circuit usually is slowly infused into the patient in anticipation of continued urinary losses. Regardless of the presence of higher molecular weight colloids, intravascular volume can be sharply reduced during hemodilution perfusion if the concentrations of electrolyte or crystalloid (particularly glucose) are high enough to make the priming solution hyperosmolar.* Under these conditions, increased water and solute excretion ensues (osmotic diuresis), with a proportionate loss of volume from the intravascular compartment.

It is essential that potassium supplementation be sufficient to sustain normal perfusate levels of this cation during and after perfusion in anticipation of the marked kaliuresis that commonly occurs (Paton et al., 1964; Obel et al., 1967). Magnesium loss is also increased (Scheinman et al., 1971) and, with coexisting hypokalemia, may seriously affect myocardial and perhaps (in the instance of hypomagnesemia) cerebral function.

---

*The colligative (osmotically active) character of a solution depends on the number of solute particles in a given fluid volume and not on the size or molecular weight of those particles.

Composition of the Hemodiluting Prime. Both noncolloid- and colloid-containing solutions have been employed as total or partial primes to achieve hemodilution. Basic to most blood dilution techniques has been the use of various combinations of crystalloids (generally glucose) and/or one or more electrolytes. These noncolloidal solutions are satisfactory provided that the perfusion times are predictably short. When more lengthy periods of bypass are anticipated (beyond 90 minutes), it is useful to include colloid in the perfusate (either donor blood or albumin) because of the limited intravascular residence times of the noncolloidal solutions. Addition of relatively nondiffusible colloid inhibits the permeation of water, ions, and small molecular species into the interstitial tissues.

The combination of ECC equipment with low priming volumes and hemodilution has made it possible to frequently eliminate use of donor blood both during perfusion and the subsequent hospital course (Cooley et al., 1966). Operative and postoperative use of homologous donor blood can be significantly reduced by a combination of hemodilution perfusion and subsequent administration of autologous whole blood that had been drawn before or during the early operative phase (Cuello et al., 1967).

Overview. The widespread use of hemodilution has significantly reduced demands on blood banks and permitted open intracardiac operations to be performed with little or no homologous blood. Despite the absence of quantitative data from randomized prospective studies, there can be no doubt that hemodilution perfusion improves the physiologic state during CPBP over that achieved with whole blood. The relative viscosity of the dilute perfusate is reduced, an important factor particularly when the hypothermic perfusion is employed. Other advantages ascribed to hemodilution perfusion include reduced postperfusion renal and pulmonary dysfunction. Finally, the incidence of postoperative bleeding has been shown to be lower when hemodilution has been used.

PHYSIOLOGIC REQUIREMENTS AND CHARACTERISTICS OF SATISFACTORY WHOLE BODY PERFUSION

Ideally, one seeks to reproduce with mechanical CPBP conditions existing in healthy, intact people, a concept in accord with the philosophy of Sir Francis Bacon: "We cannot command nature except by obeying her" (Gollan, 1966). To date, perfusion developments have roughly approximated, but not duplicated, the normal physiologic state; for this reason there are time limitations for the safe conduct of open heart surgery (four to six hours). Fortunately, the vast majority of intracardiac procedures are completed in one third of that time. Nevertheless, because existing perfusion techniques do have time limits they impose on the body's subsystems a series of distortions that are physiologically acceptable as long as bypass time is not excessive. Beyond that time, the derangements progressively resemble the characteristics of shock (Clowes, 1960).

The essential requirement of temporary ECC is that it satisfactorily replace the heart and lungs for a limited time. The need of the tissues for oxygen and the necessity for removal of carbon dioxide and other metabolic end products require that blood flow, gas exchange, and perfusion pressure be sufficient for such purposes.

Oxygen Consumption and Perfusion Rate

Oxygen Requirements. Since oxygen is the most flow limited of all molecular species necessary to sustain tissue viability, ECC flow rates must be based on calculations of total body oxygen consumption requirments. Because of size and mass differences among individuals, measurements of oxygen consumption and blood flow are generally normalized by the use of such values as calculated surface area or body weight. Thus, at basal conditions in adults, cardiac output approximates 3 liters/min/m² with an oxygen uptake of 125 ml/min/m². In this state, the mixed venous blood contains 14.8 ml O₂/100 ml blood, is 73 percent saturated, and the arteriovenous difference is 4.1 ml O₂/100 ml blood.

Although both surface area and weight have been widely used in physiologic studies and clinical practice, it is essential to appreciate that neither one possesses the high degree of predictive accuracy often reverently ascribed to them, particularly surface area (Taylor and Tiede, 1952; Krovetz, 1965). Nevertheless, there is an obvious practical necessity for a convenient means of calculating blood flow requirements, and the evidence is incontrovertible that physiologically stable perfusions in people of all ages can be accomplished based on either surface area or weight. However, in determining perfusion rates, it is important to note that the per kilogram relationship between oxygen consumption and increasing body mass is not linear.

As can be seen from Figure 5–9, basal oxygen requirements per kilogram are substantially higher in infants and children than adults. Between one and three weeks of age the minimal oxygen consumption of babies in

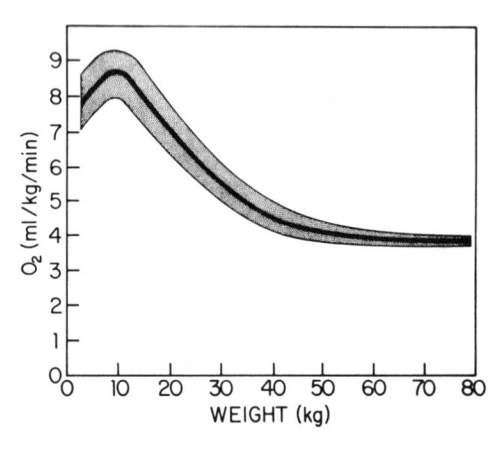

Figure 5–9. Relationship of basal oxygen consumption to body weight. The stippled area on either side of the solid line represents the confidence interval for 80 percent of the normal population. The decrease in oxygen consumption per kilogram that occurs with growth is apparent. (Modified from Clark, 1958, and Galletti and Brecher, 1962.)

a thermoneutral environment (36C) approximates 7.6 ml/kg/min; this figure rises to 9 ml/kg/min at two months. It has been suggested that the relatively high rate of oxygen consumption per unit body weight in babies may be due to the metabolic requirement of a brain that is disproportionately large in relation to body weight. Whatever the reason, it is apparent that oxygen use during the period of rapid growth and development is twice the approximate 4 ml/kg/min basal requirement of adults.

Perfusion Rate. Theoretically, to satisfy the levels of oxygen use cited previously, perfusion rates equivalent to normal basal cardiac index (3 liters/min/m^2) would be required. Expressed in terms of flow rate per kilogram of body weight at normothermic conditions, this would approximate 200 ml/kg/min in infants averaging 5 kg. Larger patients would require somewhat lower per kilogram flow rates: 170 ml/kg/min in small children averaging 10 kg, 135 ml/kg/min in larger children averaging 20 kg, and 85 ml/kg/min in a 60-kg adult (Peirce, 1969).

However, it is somewhat difficult to maintain these normal basal rates of blood flow through the full range of patients undergoing CPBP because of a combination of factors (cannula size limitations, subtle distortions of intravascular volume, and altered venous return mechanisms). Moreover, the requisite high flows would impose a considerable increase in blood trauma, since the number of passes of blood through the pump-oxygenator per unit time would be increased. Except in specific clinical situations, such as normothermic infant perfusions (rarely performed today), experience has shown that somewhat lower flow rates are satisfactory: 2.4 liters/min/m^2 in children and 2.2 liters/min/m^2 in adults (McGoon et al., 1960).

When the oxygen-carrying capacity of the blood is reduced, as is the case with diluted perfusate (hemodilution), one of two procedural modifications must be employed if metabolic demands are to be met: either the perfusion rate must be increased, or, more conveniently, total body oxygen consumption must be lowered by perfusion hypothermia (Gollan et al., 1954; Brown et al., 1958).

Oxygen Uptake. Despite several decades of experience with CPBP in humans, information remains incomplete concerning the precise relationships between oxygen availability, oxygen consumption, and perfusion flow rate. This is largely because of methodological problems inherent in obtaining direct measurements of oxygen consumption under anesthesia and of perfusion conditions where it is not yet possible to discern whether a steady state exists. A number of studies indicate that current anesthetic methods employed in patients induced without excitement tend to slightly reduce whole body oxygen consumption, particularly when muscle relaxants are used.

Information concerning whole body oxygen consumption in patients undergoing intracardiac operations has been almost entirely based on indirect calculations using the product of the perfusion flow rate and arteriovenous oxygen difference. Although this method lacks the accuracy of direct measurement of whole body oxygen consumption using analysis of expired air, the data have proven to be clinically useful. As indicated earlier, perfusion rates of 2.2 to 2.4 liters/min/m^2 permit oxygen uptake levels of the order of 130 ml/min/m^2 (McGoon et al., 1960; Levin et al., 1960), which begin to approach requirements in resting and intact anesthetized people (Gump et al., 1970). At these levels of flow, when the oxygen-carrying capacity of the blood is normal (undiluted perfusate) and oxygenator gas exchange is adequate, acid-base stability is reasonably well-maintained, and systemic mixed venous oxygen content and saturation are normal.

When normothermic perfusions are conducted at flow rates below 1.5 liters/min/m^2 for more than a brief period, progressive metabolic deterioration becomes apparent. Despite fully saturated arterial blood, the oxygen tension of venous blood falls, reflecting increased oxygen extraction by inadequately perfused tissues. This is accompanied by a rise in hydrogen ion and organic acids, evidence of hypoxic acidosis.

As will be discussed, the use of hypothermia in combination with moderate hemodilution allows lowering of perfusion flow rates without the patient incurring significant tissue hypoxia and metabolic acidosis.

Perfusion Temperature: Induced Hypothermia

There is no advantage in maintaining normal body temperature when the patient is initially placed on CPBP and during most of the intracardiac portion of the procedure. As will be discussed in a later section, some degree of perfusion hypothermia is routinely employed. Indeed, in the past several years there has been a trend to sharply reduce perfusion temperature, both as a means of keeping the myocardium cold and also allowing the surgeon to reduce the flow rate for a varying period of time.

The demonstration by Bigelow, Lindsay, and Greenwood (1950) that the oxygen consumption of a homoiotherm could be lowered by hypothermia and then reversed without incurring an oxygen debt formed the basis for the use of body temperature reduction in cardiac surgery. The reader is referred to excellent historical and physiologic surveys by Gollan (1959, 1965), Galletti and Brecher (1962), Zuhdi (1972), Swan (1973), and Rittenhouse et al. (1974) for comprehensive discussions of this important adjunct to cardiac surgery.

The decrease in oxygen consumption as the temperature is lowered conforms to van't Hoff's law, which states that the reaction rate is reduced two- to threefold for each 10C fall. With regard to mammalian tissues, this translates into a reduction in metabolic rate of approximately 7 percent per degree lowering of temperature. Experimentally, it has been shown that oxygen consumption is reduced by approximately 50 percent at 28 to 30C, 80 percent at 20C, and 90 percent at 10 to 15C. The practical implications are considerable, since perfusion flow rates may be significantly reduced at lower temperatures, and it is possible to totally discontinue perfusion for periods of up to 45 to 60 minutes when patients (primarily infants) are cooled between 15 and 18C, thereby permitting a precise repair in a bloodless field. In former years, preliminary surface cooling was employed to minimize the requisite period of supplemental perfusion hypothermia to attain the low body temperature levels to allow circulatory arrest for a significant time period. More recently, the simplicity, efficacy, and safety of profound hypothermic perfusion methods have led to abandonment of the time-consuming and cumbersome preperfusion surface cooling.

Several physiologic considerations are important in safely conducting perfusion cooling, particularly when profound hypothermic levels are desired. First, the delivery of adequate volumes of blood to the tissues is a problem, since the viscosity of whole blood goes up about 5 percent per degree centigrade of lowered temperature, primarily because of the inertial influence of the formed elements (Gollan, 1965). For example, because lowering the perfusion temperature from 37C to 12C more than doubles the viscosity of undiluted blood, microcirculatory flow may be inadequate. By reducing the hematocrit with hemodilution, this problem is considerably ameliorated.

Second, once the hypothermic blood is in the capillaries, the mechanism of oxygen transfer from the red cells to the tissues is compromised by a shift to the left of the oxygen dissociation curve. What does this shift to the left mean? In the colorfully descriptive words of Gollan (1965), "the bright red arterial blood of the hypothermic [subject] evokes a false sense of security because the oxygen is glued to hemoglobin and cannot come off." This condition is further enhanced by respiratory alkalosis. What can be done about this? Again, Gollan's commentary is without parallel in its lucidity: "We would like to shift [the oxygen dissociation curve] to the right to induce the greedy hemoglobin to release more oxygen to the needy tissues. A famous trio of physiologists, Bohr, Hasselbach, and Krogh, have shown that this can be done by increasing the carbon dioxide tension, and by honoring only the first violinist we speak of the 'Bohr effect.' . . ." In practical terms, oxygen unloading to the cells is improved by adding 3 to 7 percent carbon dioxide to the gas mixture entering the oxygenator during perfusion cooling.

Third, perfusion cooling and rewarming must be precise. It is important to appreciate that perfusion cooling does not reduce the tissue temperature of all components of the body at a uniform rate. Organs such as the brain, kidney, and heart which receive relatively high blood flow per unit mass, will have a more prompt temperature reduction while areas receiving less blood flow (muscle, skin) will lag behind considerably in the temperature fall. It is apparent that shivering must be avoided, since cooling will be even slower and the metabolic expenditure considerable. Perfusion rewarming can be accomplished without the development of metabolic acidosis, provided that the flow rate is maintained high enough and rewarming continued for an adequate period, since the high blood-flow organs will rewarm considerably faster than the muscle mass or skin.

Perfusion Pressure

The analogy of Ohm's law provides a convenient basis for an appreciation of the relationships between blood flow, perfusion pressure, and vascular resistance.

$$I = E/R \text{ (Ohm)}$$

where blood flow (I) is equal to the quotient between the pressure
head necessary for flow (E) and the resistance (R) of the vasculature.

Simple algebraic rearrangement makes it apparent that perfusion pressure (the arteriovenous pressure difference) is directly related to the product of vascular resistance (R) and blood flow (I).

The organizational arrangements of the vascular supply to the organs of the body are such that, with a single exception (the liver), they are parallel with one another. The combination of functionally parallel vascular arrangements and local resistance autoregulation of vascular beds, the latter influenced by a host of unknown and some known local factors, including oxygen tension, products of metabolism (hydrogen ion, organic acids, and carbon dioxide), and other moieties (such as norepinephrine and epinephrine), accounts for the remarkable "set point" stability of the systemic arterial pressure in humans despite transient changes in regional vascular resistances or cardiac function.

During open intracardiac surgery, the systemic arterial pressure is influenced by factors relating to alterations in vascular response accompanying anesthetic and operative trauma and, above all, by the controllable characteristics of the whole body perfusion: the flow rate, the partition of perfusate volume between the heart-lung machine and the patient, perfusate viscosity, and perfusion temperature. On occasion, an anatomic factor that adversely affects maintenance of satisfactory levels of systemic arterial pressure during perfusion is the presence of one or more large arterial communications, which permit excessive runoff (such as an improperly managed patent ductus arteriosus or the large bronchial arterial collateral circulation in patients with tetralogy of Fallot).

In the usual clinical situation, the systemic arterial pressure is an approximate linear function of perfusion flow rate. At the onset of perfusion, despite maintenance of the flow at or even above the calculated level, there is often a moderate fall in the mean arterial pressure. Factors etiologic to this transient hypotensive event are still incompletely understood, although the nature of the priming perfusate appears to play a dominant role: (1) dilution of blood with crystalloidal solutions and consequent reduction of perfusate viscosity; (2) adverse biochemical constituency of stored blood used for priming in which levels of hydrogen ion, organic acids, and potassium are inordinately high; (3) possible subtle anaphylactoid reactions, particularly when whole blood primes are employed (Gadboys et al.,

1962); and (4) introduction of room temperature perfusate that suddenly cools the vascular tree with possible temporary interference of sympathetic vasomotor activity.

During total bypass at an unchanging flow rate under normothermic or moderate hypothermic conditions, the arterial pressure gradually rises, indicative of increasing peripheral vascular resistance. In the era when normothermic whole blood perfusions were employed at unchanging flow rates of 2.2 to 2.4 liters/min/m^2, the mean arterial pressure early in the procedure averaged between 50 and 60 mm Hg and steadily rose to 75 to 80 mm Hg within the next 60 to 90 minutes, a reflection of the increasing systemic vascular resistance. Reduction of perfusate viscosity with hemodilution tends to lower the perfusion pressure despite concomitant use of moderate perfusion hypothermia (28 to 32C), which has the opposing effect of slightly increasing the perfusate viscosity. Perfusions conducted under these conditions employing the flow rates cited above generally are accompanied by arterial pressures that may be as low as 35 mm Hg in the early moments but gradually stabilize with pressures of 55 to 60 mm Hg as the procedure continues. Accumulating experience indicates that these reductions in mean arterial pressure are usually well-tolerated provided that adequate levels of systemic blood flow are maintained. However, it is apparent that sustained decrements in perfusion pressure below 55 mm Hg are dangerous. Even relatively brief reduction of perfusion pressure below this level can result in sharp diminution of blood flow to loci distal to fixed high-resistance atherosclerotic obstructions, circumstances likely to occur in older patients.

Distribution of Systemic Blood Flow

In intact man the magnitude of blood flow to organs varies widely, since two conditions must be satisfied, the first being the obvious necessity to support metabolic needs, and, second, the unique functional role of each organ. Hence, there is no direct relationship of blood flow to the weight or intrinsic metabolic state of a particular organ. For example, the kidneys normally receive approximately one quarter of the cardiac output although they are less than one percent of body weight. In this instance, less than 5 percent of blood flow is used for metabolic requirements and more than 95 percent used to subserve renal secretory and excretory functions. Oxygen extraction is, therefore, small and is reflected in a narrow arteriovenous oxygen difference. On the other hand, the heart, which weighs about the same as the kidneys, has a myocardial blood flow of only one twentieth of its total output at basal conditions, but because oxygen extraction is high, coronary venous blood is markedly desaturated and the arteriovenous oxygen difference is the widest of any organ of the body.

People could not long survive if it were not for a tightly integrated system that both controls and regulates regional blood flow, efficiently altering the volume of blood distributed to the organs in proportion to changing metabolic and functional requirements. Factors controlling these partitions may be local, systemic, or both, depending on the particular organ. Local controls generally involve metabolic factors such as temperature, Po_2, and Pco_2, whereas systemic controls are exerted by the nervous and endocrine subsystems. The efficiency of the integrative system becomes readily apparent when consideration is given to what would happen if, for example, all vascular beds were to simultaneously dilate to the same degree they do when the areas they supply are active. In this situation, Peterson (1965) has estimated that the required total flow would approach 40 liters per minute, a level far above the maximal attainable cardiac output (25 liters per minute).

There has been no systematic study in man of the distribution of systemic blood flow under conditions imposed by whole body perfusion, since existing methods of study of organ and regional flow are not readily applicable to patients. Information obtained from animals subjected to CPBP has shed some light on this question, but caution must be exercised in directly extrapolating to man conclusions drawn from these studies, since the importance of species difference cannot be overstated.

Much of the available data have been developed in canine studies, and, when compared to humans, dogs are known to differ significantly in the vascular configuration and supply of certain organs, particularly the brain and liver, and in the response to homologous blood perfusion. For example, homologous blood exchange in dogs usually causes hepatic vein constriction with resultant splanchnic visceral engorgement. However, when six to eight units of homologous blood were employed in humans to prime a disc oxygenator extracorporeal circuit, one of the authors (S.G.) demonstrated that the hepatic wedge pressure did not rise and systemic blood volume was found to be similar at the beginning of and prior to the conclusion of ECC. There is some evidence, however, that homologous blood administration during open heart surgery can be associated with isotopically measured hypovolemia, the cause of which may be anaphylactoid (Gadboys et al., 1962).

Studies of blood flow distribution during whole body perfusion of primates (Rhesus monkeys) using the radionuclide microsphere method would appear to more closely reflect blood flow partition as it probably occurs in man (Lees et al., 1971; Rudy et al., 1973). Using a whole blood perfusate at normothermic high flow conditions, blood flow has been shown to increase to many of the abdominal viscera (stomach, intestines, spleen, pancreas, and adrenals), limb bones, and skin. Significant decreases in total flow to the kidneys and brain have been observed. It is noteworthy that, unlike results with whole blood perfusion, when hemodilution is employed (hematocrit 25) with other perfusion conditions unchanged, blood flow to the brain apparently does not decrease during perfusion.

In summary, available experimental data suggest that conventional methods of high flow whole body perfusion are accompanied by substantial deviations in the distribution of blood flow to various organs and tissues. These alternations become further exaggerated when lower perfusion rates are employed and argue persuasively for use of high rates of blood flow in patients undergoing open intracardiac operations. Despite the realtive safety of existing perfusion methods in humans over a limited time (four to six hours), it is apparent that until acceptable investigative techniques can be developed that will allow precise simultaneous measurement of blood flow distribution and subsystem performance during clinical CPBP conditions, understanding of man's responses to perfusion will remain incomplete and decisions about optimal methods of support open to question.

Pulse Contour. Current methods of CPBP generally involve use of roller pumps that generate virtually a flat (nonpulsatile) arterial wave form, a major deviation from normal physiologic conditons. For many years, it has been suggested that use of pumps that would develop a pulsatile arterial pressure contour would improve the distribution of blood flow to vital organs and tissues, thereby mitigating some of the adverse effects of conventional bypass techniques that become manifest when perfusion times are excessive. This concept is based on experimental observations of the isolated kidney made over half a century ago, when it was shown that renal function was better when pulsatile perfusion was employed.

Studies in various animal species in which the effects of CPBP with a pulsatile pumping mode have been compared with nonpulsatile perfusion have produced conflicting results (Boucher et al., 1974; Mavroudis, 1978). Critical analysis of the value of pulsatile flow in CPBP has been complicated by the difficulties inherent in isolating pulsatile flow as the single variable to be perturbed and the still relatively inexact methods of measuring organ flow and subsystem performance. The preponderant weight of evidence suggests that pulsatile flow does appear to increase overall tissue perfusion as reflected by: (1) relatively lower peripheral vascular resistance;

(2) increased oxygen uptake; and (3) reduced lactate buildup. In addition, possible indication of more normal organ function may be inferred from observations of lessened deterioration of renal performance (increased urinary output, higher endogenous creatinine clearance, lower tissue and renal venous renin levels) when pulsatile flow is employed (Many et al., 1969; Jacobs et al., 1969). Recent studies in man, in which pulsatile and nonpulsatile modes were compared during CPBP, demonstrated lower vasopressin levels and systemic vascular resistance, higher flow rates, and increased urinary output when pulsatile flow was employed (Levine et al., 1978).

Despite the unquestioned physiologic advantage of pulsatile flow, it does not appear to be essential for the usual case of open heart surgery in which the perfusion period is limited to a few hours. Moreover, certain potential problems are associated with the method. When blood is pulsed through an arterial cannula that has a cross-sectional area eight to ten times smaller than the aorta, both the pressure gradient across and the velocity of flow through the cannula rise sharply during the systolic phase, thereby increasing the probability of hemolytic jet effects, shearing of adjacent atherosclerotic plaques, as well as possible cannula leaks and dislocation. In summary, since nonpulsatile flow is not associated with intolerable subsystem distortions and the renal alterations are largely transient, a strongly persuasive argument cannot yet be made to routinely employ the pulsatile mode, particularly since the potential problems accompanying its use cannot be ignored.

Oxygen and Carbon Dioxide Tensions

Comroe (1974) observed that "the 'wisdom of the body' has decided that [at sea level] an alveolar P_{O_2} of about 100 torr* and a P_{CO_2} of about 40 torr best meet the needs of the body for O_2 supply, CO_2 removal, and regulation of blood acidity . . . and [there are] remarkable mechanisms [that] regulate ventilation to keep alveolar P_{O_2} and P_{CO_2} at or near these levels. . . ." Considerable evidence is available indicating that substantial deviations above or below these alveolar gas tension norms (which closely approximate systemic arterial values) are accompanied by measurable distortions of metabolic performance and regional blood flow of many organs and tissues. Since certain types of oxygenators, particularly the commonly used gas dispersion ("bubble") type, have the capacity to sharply increase arterial blood P_{O_2} to levels that may reach 600 mm Hg and markedly drop P_{CO_2} far below the desired 40 mm Hg, it is pertinent to briefly discuss these matters.

Oxygen. In humans, the biochemical hallmark of low blood and tissue P_{O_2} persisting for more than a brief time is the appearance of life-threatening metabolic (hypoxic) acidosis. Presumably because of autoregulatory mechanisms, the oxygen tension of the brain is the last to fall during experimental low flow perfusions (Schwartz et al., 1958). It is also pertinent that inordinately high alveolar and arterial P_{O_2} have adverse effects, particularly on the brain. The classic studies of Kety and Schmidt (1948) documented the fall in cerebral blood flow that follows breathing 100 percent oxygen. It must be acknowledged that, as yet, no experimental or clinical evidence clearly incriminates persistently high arterial P_{O_2} levels as a cause of cerebral dysfunction following conventional CPBP. Indeed, Clark et al. (1958) did not observe any untoward responses in animals or patients undergoing perfusion with arterial P_{O_2} levels approaching 600 mm Hg. Nevertheless, there is no discernible advantage of maintaining this level of gas tension, and, until evidence is presented to the contrary, the data cited previously suggest the advisability of avoiding excessively high perfusion tensions of oxygen.

Carbon Dioxide. The critical importance of carbon dioxide to the body economy was first documented by Haldane and his colleagues

---

*In recent years respiratory physiologists have elected to use the term "torr" (after Torricelli) instead of "millimeters of mercury." For all practical purposes the terms are synonymous.

before the turn of the last century, when they observed that the ventilatory volume in humans was exquisitely sensitive to changes in carbon dioxide tension and relatively insensitive to alterations in oxygen tensions. Gollan (1965), in his discussion of the role of carbon dioxide during perfusion, provides us with August Krogh's characterization (1910) of the physiologic role played by this moiety:

> Even a relatively small decrease in the carbon dioxide content of the blood and tissues may produce the most strange and deleterious effects on the entire organism. It has been the important result of recent investigations that carbon dioxide can no longer be regarded as a mere waste product for the organism to get rid of; rather it must be accepted as one of the essential factors governing the processes of life.

The reciprocal actions of arterial oxygen and carbon dioxide tensions on regional blood flow are well-known and are particularly important in relation to cerebral blood flow during whole body perfusion. An increase in arterial Po_2 and a concomitant decrease in Pco_2 reduce cerebral blood flow, while, conversely, a decrease in arterial Po_2 and increase in Pco_2 tend to increase flow. Obviously, local autoregulation plays a key role in this control mechanism.

The implications for management of gas exchange during perfusion are clear. If the artificial lung is "hyperventilated" with oxygen in a fashion that maintains arterial Po_2 at the expense of a sharp decrease in Pco_2 (as can readily happen with gas dispersion oxygenators), cerebral blood flow would be expected to fall. Suggestive evidence supporting this concept was developed by Wollman et al. (1966) in patients undergoing intracardiac surgery. Cerebral blood flow was estimated from arterial-jugular vein oxygen difference. There was a general tendency for patients with lower arterial Pco_2 levels to have lower estimated cerebral flows, and there was a direct and consistent relationship in each patient between rising arterial Pco_2 levels and increasing estimated cerebral blood flow. In these studies, no reliable relationships could be demonstrated between the perfusion pressures employed and estimated cerebral flow. Summarizing, in the usual clinical perfusion conditions, cerebral vascular reactivity and flow are importantly influenced by arterial Pco_2 levels.

Apart from causing substantial reductions of cerebral blood flow, severe hypocarbia during perfusion may result in alkalosis, which, in turn, causes a shift of the oxygen dissociation curve to the left (the Bohr effect), thereby impeding oxygen delivery to the tissues by making more difficult the unloading of oxygen from the red cells. The message is clear: severe hypocarbia during perfusion must be avoided at all costs.

Acid-Base Balance

Physiologic conduct of whole body perfusion is reflected by maintenance of satisfactory acid-base conditions. Two decades ago investigative and clinical studies demonstrated the frequent tendency toward development of metabolic acidosis during cardiopulmonary bypass. The cause was shown to be of hypoxic origin due to either insufficient oxygenation of the blood in the heart-lung apparatus or inadequate oxygen delivery to the tissues. With adequate blood oxygenation, metabolic acidosis was still commonly observed at low flow rates but was significantly less when higher flow rates were employed (Kirklin et al., 1956; Clowes et al., 1958). For this reason, Moore (1958) proposed the term "hypoxic acidosis" to define conditions created by low perfusion rates, i.e., reduced tissue levels of oxygen with accumulation of acid metabolites.

As presently conducted, CPBP is still generally accompanied by a slight but tolerable tendency toward metabolic acidosis, provided that bypass time is not excessive. Perfusions carried out at flow rates of 2.0 to 2.4 liters/min/m^2 under conditions of moderate hemodilution and hypothermia (30C) are accompanied by a modest rise in arterial blood concentrations of lactate and pyruvate and a slight fall in pH (Moffitt et al., 1969). Apart from the metabolic alterations imposed by essentially nonpulsatile perfusions at the above flow rates, other factors contribute to the acidemic tendency. These include the acid metabolites in any priming blood, use of large amounts of crystalloidal diluent and glucose, as well as ventilator- or oxygenator-induced deviations from normal blood CO_2 tensions.

When perfusion times are inordinately lengthy (more than six hours), as occasionally occurs when a patient coming to the operation with severe cardiac decompensation requires extended postrepair support, the imperfect character of current methods of mechanical cardiopulmonary bypass becomes apparent. Despite maintenance of seemingly "physiologic" perfusion conditions, acidosis becomes increasingly prominent, and, as discussed earlier, the metabolic picture begins to manifest a striking resemblance to that observed in shock.

In most clinical circumstances, the mild metabolic acidosis accompanying anesthesia, surgery, and perfusion disappears within the first few postoperative hours when performance of the cardiovascular and pulmonary subsystems is satisfactory. Inadequate performance of these two subsystems following perfusion results in progressive life-threatening acid-base derangement.

SUBSYSTEM FUNCTIONAL ALTERATIONS ASSOCIATED WITH EXTRACORPOREAL CIRCULATION

Although most patients do not appear to suffer any clinically apparent early or late ill effects as a consequence of CPBP per se when it is properly conducted, this is primarily because of the capacity of the body's subsystems to continue to perform adequately despite the usual perfusion traumata. The resulting alterations are generally transient and physiologically tolerable. Nevertheless, it is important to appreciate that these circumstances are, within broad limits, time-related, despite the major improvements in perfusion equipment and techniques over the past decade. A tolerable functional derangement can become a clinically apparent *complication* if CPBP (particularly with a direct gas-blood interface) is continued for an exceedingly long period.

Underlying Factors

Methods and Biocompatibility. There are a number of reasons why ECC would be expected to impose pathophysiologic distortions of organ function that are both greater and frequently different from those accompanying major operations performed without CPBP. Clearly, perfusate distortions and the abnormal hemodynamics accompanying ECC impose potentially adverse conditions. The "physiologic" flow rates usually employed are, in reality, marginal in relation to normal levels of blood flow. Additionally, the usual nonpulsatile pumping mode and the frequently present subnormal perfusion pressures almost certainly create deranged partition of blood flow to various areas of the body. It must also be remembered that employment of the ECC circuitry per se eliminates the lungs as effective "in line" organs, so that their important but still incompletely understood non-gas exchange functions (endocrine, for example) are sharply modified. Finally, the precision of application of perfusion methods, the length of bypass, and volumetric management at the end of perfusion all varyingly influence subsystem alterations associated with CPBP.

A major factor in perfusion pathophysiology is the combined effects of imperfect biocompatibility of materials employed in ECC fabrication and areas of stagnation, high flow velocity, and angulation in various components of the devices. The result is a complex of adverse changes involving the perfusate that contribute to morbidity and, rarely, mortality. The causes of these alterations are multiple and still incompletely identified. It has long been known that direct exposure of blood to both the surfaces and unfavorable geometry of the ECC device as well as a gaseous interface result in plasma protein denaturation and damage (lethal and sublethal) of the blood formed elements. These derangements are enhanced when bubble or film oxygenators are employed and by the severe trauma imposed by excessive and unskilled use of strong cardiotomy suction with resultant severe foaming. The cardiotomy blood aspirate may also include pericardial fat, fragments of muscle, calcium, bone wax, and thromboplastin from incised tissues.

These and other factors combine to produce a host of alterations after CPBP in the delicate balance that normally exists between the coagulation and fibrinolytic systems. Reductions and fibrinogen (Factor I), prothrombin (Factor II), platelets, proaccelerin (Factor V), and antihemophilic globulin (Factor VIII) are commonly observed. Some degree of firbrinolytic activity may be measurable after perfusion, the extent of the abnormal state of the plasminogen-plasmin system being central to the production of fibrin degradation products. When severe, the clinical expression of all these changes is inappropriate bleeding after bypass.

Microemboli

Varying amounts of fibrinogen are adsorbed on to the blood contacting surfaces of all available ECC devices. As a result, platelets tend to adhere to some of these areas and ultimately form platelet-fibrin aggregates in which white and red cells can become enmeshed, conglomerate, and then embolize. The presence of these particulate microemboli has been documented by measurement of the screen filtration pressure (SFP), the driving pressure required to force a blood sample through a micropore filter with known pore size (Swank and Porter, 1963). Swank's initial studies of human CPBP demonstrated that the microaggregates in the donor bank blood used to prime the ECC were trapped in the systemic capillary beds.

Subsequently, Ashmore et al. (1968) described the formation of platelet-fibrin aggregates in a disc oxygenator when blood was exposed to oxygen. Under these conditions, the SFP of the oxygenated blood prior to bypass was high. That direct blood-gas interfacial phenomena play a role in this result is strongly suggested by Ashmore's observations that when oxygen was not directly passed through the oxygenator (when compressed air was used in a bubble oxygenator instead of oxygen or when a membrane oxygenator was employed), the SFP did not rise significantly. Further, it was noted that the SFP would rise promptly as soon as the patient's blood and the ECC priming perfusate were mixed, suggesting the presence of some moiety in the homologous priming blood that caused microaggregates to form.

Ashmore's study did not allow conclusions to be drawn about the possible relationship between increased SFP-defined microaggregation and clinical outcome. In this regard, it is important to appreciate that even when membrane oxygenators are used some platelet microaggregates are generated, but there is evidence suggesting that these may somehow disaggregate, return to the circulation, and presumably do not produce microembolic tissue damage (see Bartlett and Gazzaniga, 1978, for a thorough review of these important matters). Unlike such separable platelet masses, it is the fibrin-reinforced consolidated platelet plugs with enmeshed white and red cells that lodge in the microvasculature and cause damage.

Two other forms of microemboli associated with ECC are (1) fat that largely derives from lipid-laden pericardial blood aspirated by the cardiotomy suckers (Hill et al., 1969) and (2) microbubbles. Gaseous microemboli have been shown to be formed in the cardiotomy suction, by bubble oxygenators, and at sites of turbulence at the gas-blood interface in the reservoirs of extracorporeal circuits employing all types of oxygenators. Most of these gaseous microemboli data have been derived from ultrasonic probes placed into various tubing sites in the extracorporeal circuit (Kessler and Patterson, 1970). Two factors have been shown to cause marked increases in gaseous emboli production by bubble oxygenators: (1) allowing the blood level to fall to a low level in the oxygenator reservoir; and (2) increasing the gas to blood flow ratio through the oxygenator.

The lethal potential of gaseous and particulate microemboli has long been recognized, since neurologic damage presumed to be of such etiology was a disturbingly common feature of early experimental and clinical perfusions. The important studies of Hill et al. (1969) and Aguilar et al. (1971) subsequently confirmed the high incidence (85 percent) of significant neuropathologic lesions in patients dying after open heart surgery. Apart from hemorrhage and evidence of ischemic neuronal damage, the frequent presence of emboli was particularly disturbing. Fat emboli were present in almost 80 percent of the brains. Particulate emboli of both the fibrin-platelet or polarizable crystalline (presumably silicone) varieties were observed in 20 and 12 percent, respectively. Nine percent of the brains contained other types of particulate emboli, such as calcium.

It is apparent that these observations were carried out on a biased sample of the total operative experience of the investigators, i.e., those patients who died. During the period that these studies encompassed (the early to late 1960s), low cardiac output was a dominant cause of death in patients undergoing open heart surgery. Therefore, it is highly probable that, in addition to the specific trauma of ECC, the brains were subjected to varying periods of reduced flow, hypoxia, and acidosis. Despite these limitations, the autopsy findings confirmed that emboli of significant size and volume were being delivered to the patient by the ECC device and represented a major hazard of the method.

These observations, and previous studies by Swank and Hain (1952), suggested the need for some type of microfiltration with a small pore diameter (approximately 20 μ) rather than the relatively large-mesh wire filters (orifices of 100 to 150 μ) that previously had been in common use (and were employed in perfusing the patients whose brains had been shown to contain large numbers of emboli at necropsy). As discussed in an earlier section, after the introduction of microfilters in 1968, the incidence of cerebral nonfat microemboli in the brains of those dying after open intracardiac operation fell precipitously. The elimination of lipid emboli remains a problem. Although there is evidence that microfilters do remove some fat emboli, considerable amounts still can pass through.

Volumetric and Body Compositional Changes

Multiple factors associated with use of ECC result in a series of volumetric and compartmental changes that can contribute to both morbidity and mortality.

Acute Postperfusion Changes in Blood Volume.
In the earlier developmental years of open heart surgery, isotopic measurements of plasma volume (PV) and red cell volume (RCV) incidated consistent and statistically significant reductions of both from preperfusion values up to 48 hours after the operation. These measurements were made at a time when blood infusion at the termination of CPBP and thereafter was governed by (1) volume-for-volume replacement of all measured blood losses in an attempt to maintain the preoperative "normovolemic" state (Litwak et al., 1961) or (2) infusion of blood in amounts necessary to maintain *right* atrial pressure at approximately 12 mm Hg (Cleland et al., 1966). Subsequent studies by Pacifico et al. (1970), in which postperfusion blood administration was guided by *left* atrial and systemic arterial pressures, revealed only modest reductions in PV and RCV that did not differ significantly from preoperative measurements.

Acute Changes in Compartmental Water.
Detailed studies by Cleland et al. (1966) and Pacifico et al. (1970) indicate a predictable pattern of acute changes of body water after CPBP. The studies document a significant increase in the volume of both extracellular water (ECW) and interstitial fluid (ECW-PV). On the other hand, measurements of total body water (TBW) and calculations of intracellular water (TBW-ECW) do not reveal any sharp deviations from preoperative data. However, it is important to appreciate that the

method of determining intracellular water volume is crude, and important studies by Flear et al. (1969) and others indicate that cells do swell after major surgical trauma.

ACUTE CATION CHANGES. Total exchangeable sodium is significantly increased after ECC, presumably because of the patient's uptake of sodium (along with water) during perfusion. Despite the virtual absence of sodium administration, the increase in exchangeable sodium persists until at least the third postoperative day and implies minimal excretion of the cation during this period.

Total exchangeable potassium and both the amount and concentration of calculated intracellular potassium are all significantly decreased. It is probable that the multiple traumata of surgery and ECC create conditions in which sodium moves into and potassium out of the cell (Flear et al., 1969; Pacifico et al., 1970). The secondary renal excretion of potassium in the first 48 hours after perfusion is considerable (50 to 100 mEq/24 hours). The therapeutic implications of these data are apparent and are discussed in Chapters 6 and 14.

Despite addition of moderate amounts of calcium or magnesium to the priming perfusate, plasma levels of both cations tend to decrease with the onset of ECC, primarily but not solely as the result of perfusate dilution, and tend to remain slightly low throughout the perfusion (Turnier et al., 1972; Moffitt et al., 1973). As yet, there is no convincing evidence that in the usual circumstances these moderate ionic alterations are causally related to cardiac contractile or arrhythmic problems during or after the operation.

LEUKOCYTE AND PLATELET ALTERATIONS. The concentration of all types of white blood cells falls (particularly the granulocytes) with the start of ECC, initially because of dilutional factors. During the usual relatively short clinical perfusion, the leukocyte count remains low because of the multiple factors associated with perfusion traumata. However, as early as the fourth postperfusion hour the concentration of white cells has begun to increase significantly, the rise predominantly caused by immature granulocytes. Ryhänen et al. (1979) found that the total number of polymorphonuclear neutrophils and stab cells had significantly increased (relative to preoperative measurements) in early postperfusion measurements (second postoperative day) and remained high for 14 days when the study was terminated. In contrast, the patients manifested a significant lymphopenia in the early studies, which approximated preoperative levels by the seventh postoperative day. There was a significant increase in atypical lymphocytes in the early studies, which remained high through the two-week study period. The alterations were not significantly influenced by the two types of oxygenators (bubble or membrane) employed.

The phagocytic activity of circulating leukocytes is decreased during clinical ECC (Silva et al., 1974). However, the relationship between this observation and the occurrence of subsequent infection has not been established.

Paralleling the leukocyte changes is a sharp decrease in circulating platelets with the start of ECC. The platelet count remains low as long as perfusion is continued, the sharpest reductions not surprisingly being seen in long perfusions in which bubble oxygenators are used and prolonged (or excessive) cardiotomy suction is employed. In humans, the platelet count generally remains low for several days postoperatively, generally returning to normal by the third to fifth day.

Interesting information has been developed by deLeval et al. (1972) in their perfusion studies of platelet kinetics in dogs. They demonstrated that a substantial percentage of the thrombocytopenia was due to sequestration of the platelets within the liver during the course of perfusion, with subsequent reentry of the same platelets following discontinuance of cardiopulmonary bypass. Whether similar events occur in humans is not yet known.

Subsystem Distortions

Cerebral Function. At present, it is rare for patients undergoing uncomplicated open intracardiac operations employing CPBP to manifest gross evidence of cerebral dysfunction after surgery. Nevertheless, a host of clinical studies makes it clear that the still imperfect character of current perfusion methods does inflict some trauma on the brain. Despite this, it seems that the neuronal and glial cells can tolerate the usual magnitude of these insults so well that overt cerebral functional performance appears normal. Geha et al. (1969) documented that brain metabolism is normal during ECC and remains so even during induced severe hypocapnea and alkalosis.

When neurologic deficits are clinically apparent, the cause is commonly embolic (particulate, lipid, or air). Other factors associated with heightened probability of postoperative cerebral dysfunction include (1) inordinately lengthy periods of CPBP (beyond six hours), particularly if bubble oxygenators are employed, and (2) prolonged periods of hypotension during perfusion (perfusion pressure less than 50 mm Hg), particularly in older patients in whom the presence of cerebrovascular disease is more likely. A strong correlation has been observed between use of gas exchange devices with a direct blood-gas interface and transiently abnormal brain function. Using an ultrasonic method for detection of microemboli, Carlson et al. (1973) found much higher counts (shown by other studies to be predominantly microbubbles) and an increased incidence of minor cerebral dysfunction when bubble oxygenators were employed. Use of an ultrapore filter as a bubble trap in the arterial line of bubble oxygenators reduced both the number of microbubble counts and the incidence of neurologic dysfunction. The lowest counts and fewest clinically detectable neurologic and psychologic abnormalities have been observed when patients are perfused with membrane lungs.

The incidence of transient postoperative behavioral changes (confusion, disorientation, delirium, and depression), which used to occur not infrequently (Lee et al., 1970; Frank et al., 1972), has been sharply reduced as a result of a number of perfusion-related improvements: ultrapore filtration, improved gas exchange devices (effective bubble oxygenators permitting lower gas-blood flow ratios, and simple to use membrane oxygenators), as well as hemodilution. Additional discussion of neurologic and behavioral problems associated with open heart surgery will be found in Chapters 16 and 17.

Pulmonary Subsystem. Serious postoperative pulmonary dysfunction was common in the early years of open heart surgery performed with ECC and was referred to as "pump lung." Typically, the lesion was characterized by a large alveolar-arterial oxygen gradient and diffuse bilateral patchy "atelectatic" areas on the thoracic radiogram. The patients exhibited profuse, often blood-tinged tracheobronchial secretions, and the work of breathing was sharply increased (Dammann et al., 1963). Early investigations incriminated inadequate left heart decompression as a major factor in promoting the "pump lung" syndrome. This mechanistic etiology was lent further support by the observations that patients with advanced cardiac disease and those with low cardiac output (hence, those with inordinately elevated pulmonary venous pressures) frequently showed evidence of "pump lung." However, as valid as these mechanical and cardiac dysfunctional etiologies were (and are), other major perfusion-related causes slowly became apparent.

At the time that serious postperfusion pulmonary dysfunction was first being recognized (Muller et al., 1958), all of the patients were being perfused with equipment that incorporated crude bubble oxygenators requiring high gas-blood flow ratios or large nondisposable rotating disc or vertical screen gas exchange devices that required careful cleaning before the unit could be used again. The priming perfusates almost invariably consisted solely of large amounts of homologous blood, the volumes generally equalling the blood volume of an adult and exceeding the volumes of children by two- to four-fold ratios. Moreover ultrapore filtration of the priming blood either before it entered the heart-lung machine or during conduct of the perfusion was not employed. Persuasive evidence is now at hand indicating that all of these factors were instrumental in promoting the frequency and lethal potential of "pump lung."

Perhaps more than any other organ, the lung reacts adversely to a large number of perfusion-related distortions that are believed to be collectively etiologic to "pump lung." The reader is referred to the excellent surveys of Kouchoukos and Karp (1976) and Pennock et al. (1977) for a comprehensive discussion of these matters. In part, these provocative factors include protein denaturation, uncharacterized "toxic" substances associated with formed element destruction, anaphylaxis, and particulate microembolism. Thus, it is not surprising that "pump lung" would have become manifest as frequently as it did in earlier years with bypass techniques described above, which, in retrospect, must be considered to have been rather primitive.

First, the still poorly understood effects of protein denaturation (Lee et al., 1961; Dobell et al., 1965) must have been considerable because of the extensive direct gas-blood interfacial traumata inherent with use of the available ECC equipment. This problem must have been further aggravated if cleaning methods failed to remove all foreign substances from components of the circuit that were to be reused, thereby exposing the patient to release of toxic factors that had vasoactive and other adverse effects (Hollenberg et al., 1963).

Second, as emphasized earlier (see Perfusate section), the human lung is a target organ in the anaphylactoid response to exchange of large volumes of homologous blood (Gadboys et al., 1962; Schrek and Neville, 1964; Nahas et al., 1965). The study of Rabelo et al. (1973), previously cited, documented by light and electron microscopy significantly abnormal histologic findings in the lungs of a majority (but not all) of the patients perfused with a homologous blood prime, whereas no structural alterations were observed in those perfused with either autologous or asanguineous prime. This important study separates the rheologic from the immunologic aspects of hemodilution on lung morphology. It also demonstrates that the adverse alterations accompanying homologous blood exchange are not always discernible every time homologous blood is administered. Indeed, a wealth of clinical evidence indicates that significant pulmonary functional distortions generally occur only when large volumes of homologous blood are administered. Thus, it may be concluded that homologous blood exchange is but one of a number of factors, albeit an important one, that can damage the lung during ECC.

Third, in the early years of clinical ECC, it is a certainty that lack of effective ultrapore filtration of the blood contributed substantially to the development of postperfusion pulmonary dysfunction. In a critical study, Connell et al. (1973) evaluated the pulmonary ultrastructure of patients having CPBP both with and without Dacron wool filtration. Lung biopsies of those patients not having ultrapore filtration exhibited extensive occlusion of the pulmonary microcirculation by aggregates of disintegrating leukocytes and widespread degenerative changes in the cellular and noncellular components of the interalveolar septa. In severely damaged areas, the capillary endothelium was focally swollen and frequently ruptured, thereby exposing the underlying interstitium to cytoplasmic fragments, including lysosomal granules. Similarly, type I alveolar epithelial cells generally were swollen and occasionally ruptured. In those areas where cellular discontinuity of the alveolar epithelium was present, protein exudates were observed in the interstitial and alveolar air spaces. On the other hand, lung biopsies of patients having Dacron wool filtration of the priming perfusate, cardiotomy suction, and arterial line were essentially unchanged from the prebypass morphology.

Currently, the occurrence of florid, life-threatening "pump lung" is rare, undoubtedly because of the combined influences of (1) advances in perfusion technology and procedures (disposable low prime bubble oxygenators of improved design permitting low gas-blood flow ratios, disposable and efficient membrane lungs, effective ultrapore filters, hemodilution with consequent reduction or elimination of homologous blood prime) and (2) improved anesthesiologic and operative methods and postoperative care. Nevertheless, evidence of mild postperfusion pulmonary dysfunction is still commonly observed for the first 24 to 48 hours after the operation. During this period, patients will frequently exhibit widened alveolar-arterial oxygen gradients indicative of foci of nonventilated (atelectatic) but perfused (venous admixture) alveoli. In the usual postoperative situation, pulmonary compliance is essentially unchanged unless complicating circumstances exist, such as significant elevation of pulmonary vascular resistance, advanced left ventricular dysfunction, or the need for prolonged (four or more hours) of postrepair circulatory support.

Cardiovascular Subsystem. Properly conducted CPBP in man (with or without moderate hemodilution) does not per se significantly affect myocardial function over the period of time required for intracardiac corrective procedures. There is experimental evidence that severe hemodilution (hematocrit 18) results in myocardial edema, reduced compliance, and depressed left ventricular performance (Foglia et al., 1978). The clinical implications of these data are apparent. But, apart from these avoidable circumstances, cardiac performance alterations are largely related to the adequacy of myocardial protection during surgery and the nature and completeness of the repair.

Renal Subsystem. Renal performance is adversely affected by measures in the operating room beginning even before perfusion and further distorted during CPBP (Mielke et al., 1965, 1966). Both glomerular filtration rate (GFR) and renal blood flow (RBF) are reduced with the start of anesthesia and surgery, presumably related to decreased cardiac output and increased ADH secretion. Urinary output falls, and, with the start of CPBP, transient anuria is common. As bypass continues, urinary output slowly begins and can be brisk, particularly if the perfusate is hyperosmolar and the perfusion pressure is maintained at or above 60 mm Hg. The urine is dilute and the per minute excretion of sodium and potassium is increased.

GFR remains low during perfusion and, contrary to the suggestion of some investigators, is not solely consequent to the effects of anesthesia and sternotomy, since it rises in the postperfusion period while the patient is still anesthetized (Kahn et al., 1968). RBF is also reduced during CPBP, and, in experimental animals, there is a preferential shift of flow from the cortex to the medulla. It has been suggested that CPBP is accompanied by renal afferent arteriolar vasoconstrictive phenomena that are responsible for both the reduced partition of blood to the kidney and the relative cortical ischemia. The magnitude of these changes is significantly diminished if diuresis is promoted during CPBP (Engelman et al., 1974). In the usual circumstances, all of the renal functional alterations are transient and return to normal within several days after the operation.

It is gratifying that currently employed methods of hemodilution perfusion have made perfusion-related acute tubular necrosis and life-threatening renal failure rare events. Almost invariably, patients having serious renal dysfunction following open-heart surgery are those known to have had significant preoperative impairment of renal function in combination with advanced cardiac pathology. In these patients, any tendency toward postperfusion low cardiac output markedly increases the potential for the early onset of acute tubular necrosis. (An expanded discussion will be found in Chapter 14.)

Hepatic Subsystem. When current ECC methods are properly employed, clinically significant perfusion-related hepatic damage is rare, apart from an occasional case of serum hepatitis. Mechanical occlusion of hepatic veins by an improperly positioned inferior vena caval cannula can result in intrahepatic hemorrhage and major liver damage. In general, significant hepatocellular dysfunction in the postoperative period is restricted to those patients coming to the operation with abnormal hepatic function secondary to far-advanced cardiac disease.

OPERATIVE MANAGEMENT

General Considerations

Operative Protocols. Successful conduct of cardiac surgery is best accomplished by experienced personnel who follow a carefully laid out plan in which the activities of the anesthesiologist, surgeons, nurses, perfusionists, and technicians are programmed for maximum coordination. The plan should include anticipation of possible adverse events so that such contingencies can be managed calmly and thoughtfully.

The fundamental value to science of the written protocol has long been established. It follows that a serious attempt to optimize surgical care mandates the necessity for a written plan of management. A surgical group of outstanding competence and experience has turned to the use of a written set of rules for operative conduct to ensure proper sequencing of essential details (Kirklin et al., 1976). As the operative stages proceed, the anesthesiologist reads the plan aloud to ensure that each step is followed. While some experienced surgical groups might not be inclined to employ such an approach in commonly performed operations, the value of the method is clear when new or rare procedures are being carried out and certainly in the training of residents.

Anesthetic Conduct. The critical importance of proper preoperative analgesia and smooth anesthetic induction and management has become increasingly apparent, particularly in the era of myocardial revascularization. Apart from the long-established observation that cardiac output may fall significantly under anesthesia, it is now clear that even transient agitation or systemic pressure changes (hypotension or hypertension) during induction may be followed by serious ventricular arrhythmias and myocardial infarction. These and other matters are discussed elsewhere in this text.

Intraoperative Monitoring and Related Measures

BEFORE AND DURING BYPASS. Our surveillance procedures are patterned after those described by Kirklin et al. (1976). Lead II of the electrocardiogram is continuously monitored and recorded. Access for continuous monitoring of systemic arterial pressure and periodic checks of blood gas and electrolyte data is provided by insertion of a plastic needle into the radial artery (percutaneously when possible or by direct exposure of the vessel in infants and obese adults). Unless the patient is critically ill, the arterial line is inserted immediately after endotracheal intubation. The anesthesiologist then inserts a plastic needle into the external jugular vein, a procedure facilitated by temporarily lowering the head end of the operating table. Pressure measurements from this site approximate superior vena caval pressures and are particularly important during bypass in making certain that drainage into the superior vena caval cannula is unimpeded.

The increasing employment of profound levels of perfusion hypothermia demands continuous monitoring of body temperature with a thermistor. Because of the closer correlation of the nasopharyngeal or tympanic membrane measurement to brain temperature, we prefer following the body temperature from either of these areas rather than using the rectal measurement, which can be unreliable, particularly during cooling.

Although only a crude reflection of renal blood flow, urinary output is continuously measured with an indwelling bladder catheter.

Whenever possible, following exposure of the heart a small catheter should be inserted into the left atrium via the right superior pulmonary vein to allow continuous monitoring of left ventricular filling pressures throughout all phases of the operation. Although the importance of measuring left atrial pressures during separation from and following bypass is now widely appreciated, it is essential to recognize the great value of these measurements during the operative repair, since inadequate left heart decompression can be avoided and subsequent "inexplicable" pulmonary and cardiac complications related to this etiology avoided.

Ten minutes after the onset of bypass and every 30 minutes thereafter, it is our practice to obtain blood-gas, acid-base, and electrolyte measurements to be certain that all is proceeding properly. As suggested earlier in this chapter, if the perfusion has been conducted with precision the data will be predictably satisfactory, and, apart from the need to add modest increments of potassium during the run, no other intervention resulting from these measurements will be required.

MEASURES FOLLOWING BYPASS. When perfusion has been discontinued, a fine catheter is inserted into the right atrium for continuous pressure measurement. If desired, a second catheter is inserted to facilitate postoperative drug infusion and indicator injection to measure cardiac output. Whenever severe elevation of pulmonary artery pressure persists in the presence of satisfactorily low left atrial pressure after perfusion, it is essential that assessment of the elevated lesser circulation resistance be followed carefully in the postoperative period. Accordingly, in infants and children, a fine catheter is passed across the pulmonary valve into the pulmonary artery trunk by means of an oblique right ventricular mural puncture. A pledgeted mattress suture at the insertion site aids in establishing a nidus for clots to "discourage" bleeding when the catheter is subsequently removed. In adults, we elect to wait until the patient reaches the postoperative care unit, at which time a thermistor-bearing Swan-Ganz catheter is passed into the pulmonary artery so that thermodilution cardiac output measurements can be obtained in addition to the pulmonary artery and wedge pressures.

An obvious and serious deficiency of intraoperative monitoring technology has been the lack of a convenient and reliable means of obtaining frequent measurements of cardiac output in the operating room immediately after intracardiac repair. One approach has been the use of an electromagnetic flow meter, which can be positioned around the ascending aorta, passed through the chest wall, and used during the postoperative period as well. Closed chest removal of the device is apparently simple (Williams et al., 1971). Recently, we and several other groups have found it convenient to insert a fine (2F) thermistor into the pulmonary artery trunk for thermodilution output measurements. The method has provided reliable data and has been extremely useful in promptly indicating directional changes of cardiac output in relation to both time and therapeutic interventions in the early postperfusion period when the sternum is still open.

Establishment and Conduct of Cardiopulmonary Bypass
Preliminary Steps

THE HEART-LUNG MACHINE. It is advisable to have the pump-oxygenator in the operating room with all tubing components deployed between the operating table and the bypass unit and the entire system primed before the surgical incision is made. In the unusual circumstance in which sudden severe deterioration of cardiac performance occurs during the early phase of the surgical procedure, these anticipatory arrangements permit emergency cannulation to be performed and perfusion established without delay.

PRIMING PERFUSATE. As discussed previously (see earlier discussion dealing with pump-oxygenator primes), hemodilution perfusion is routinely employed. Usually a total asanguineous prime (predominantly or completely crystalloid) is permissible in adults since the mixed (patient and heart-lung machine) perfusion hematocrit will virtually always exceed 20. Obviously this does not consistently obtain in perfusion of infants and small children, and it is frequently necessary to add some blood to the diluent to achieve the desired mixed hematocrit (DMH). When a short normothermic perfusion is anticipated, a DMH of 30 is selected. When moderate hypothermic levels (28 to 32C) are to be employed, the DMH is calculated to be 25. If lower perfusion temperatures are to be used, a DMH of 20 is sought.

Estimation of the DMH is conveniently obtained by the use of the formula (slightly modified) of Kirklin et al. (1976). Required for the calculation is knowledge of the priming volume of the pump-oxygenator system (PVpo) to be used, the patient's estimated blood volume (BVp) and hematocrit (Hp). With this information it is possible to determine whether and what volume of bank blood (assumed hematocrit 0.38) is needed to be added to the diluent to achieve the DMH. Thus*:

Bank blood to be added =
$$\frac{(DMH \cdot [BV_p + PV_{po}]) - [BV_p \cdot H_p]}{0.38}$$

In addition to adults, some cyanotic children with hematocrits will also have a zero or even negative calculated volume of blood "to be added" because of a large red cell mass relative to the PVpo. In such cases, the entire prime will be acellular diluent.† When the calculated volume of bank blood (V_{bb}) to be added‡ is a positive number, the required diluent volume (DV) quite obviously will be:

$$DV = PVpo - V_{bb}$$

CARDIAC AND GREAT VESSEL EXPOSURE. Unless special circumstances prevail, the heart is approached through a median sternotomy. When the parietal pericardium is densely adherent to the epimyocardium (reoperation, pericarditis), mobilization of the heart and great vessels is limited to those areas that are required to establish partial bypass. Once perfusion has been established (32C), necessary additional mobilization can be carried out safely. On rare occasions, it is necessary to establish partial bypass before exposing the heart (see later cannulation discussion).

HEPARIN ADMINISTRATION. There is no more singularly critical consideration in the successful conduct of ECC than maintenance of proper levels of anticoagulation with heparin. Although it would be desirable to manage heparin administration with a uniform dosage program that would be suitable for all patients, the studies of Bull et al. (1975a) clearly indicate that this is not feasible because of wide variations in individual heparin dose responses. The amount of heparin required to produce an arbitrary prolongation in the clotting time may vary threefold from patient to patient. Moreover, the rate at which administered heparin disappears from the blood has a fourfold variability among patients. In part, this is related to the fact that heparin metabolism is temperature-dependent, slowing during hypothermic perfusion and becoming more rapid during rewarming (Wright et al., 1964). Finally, the addition of blood or other perfusate to the extracorporeal circuit will varyingly affect the heparin level.

---

*All volumetric data should be expressed in ml. Estimation of a patient's blood volume is calculated as 8 percent of body weight (kg). All hematocrit data (the DMH and the equation denominator, i.e., the assumed bank blood hematocrit) are expressed as percentages.

†Each liter of acellular prime is anticoagulated with 5,000 units of sodium heparin.

‡Each 500-ml bag of ACD or CPD blood must be converted for use in the heart-lung machine by addition of the following constituents in the following order:

ACD or CPD blood	500 ml
Sodium herparin (3,000 units)	3 ml
Sodium bicarbonate (20mEq)	20 ml
Calcium chloride (10%)	5 ml
	528 ml

The calculated volume of bank blood to be added is "rounded off" to the nearest 100 ml.

For all these reasons, it is essential to control heparin levels throughout the perfusion. A simple means of doing this is the sequential measurement of the activated coagulation time (ACT), employing the automated Hemochron method.* A Hemochron ACT of 90 to 100 seconds corresponds to a normal Lee-White clotting time. Guided by the data of Bull et al. (1975a), we attempt to maintain a Hemochron ACT of 450 to 500 seconds during normothermic perfusion.

Our protocol for heparin management is as follows. A baseline ACT is obtained as the thoracic incision is made. After establishing cardiac exposure, heparin (200 units/kg) is administered to the patient as the *initial heparinizing dose*. After allowing two minutes for mixing, we determine a second ACT. Without waiting for the results of the second ACT, one can safely proceed with aortic and vena caval cannulations, since, despite the patient-dosage variability, it has been our experience that the *initial heparinizing dose* consistently provides safe anticoagulation levels for this purpose (generally an ACT approximating 300 seconds). Not only is the patient heparinized, but also the priming perfusate (regardless of whether dilute blood or a completely asanguineous prime is employed) with 3,000 units/liter. By the time all cannulations and connections to the heart-lung machine have been made, the second ACT is available. If the ACT were to be less than 200 seconds (a situation we have rarely experienced), an additional heparin increment of 100 units/kg is administered before commencing bypass.

With the start of ECC, it is essential that a higher ACT be immediately attained, and the additional heparin load of the perfusate will indeed be shown to have lengthened the ACT substantially when a blood sample is drawn five minutes after the start of bypass. Additional ACT data are obtained every 20 minutes thereafter until completion of perfusion. Should blood be added during the run, 3,000 units of heparin are added for each 500 ml of blood. If moderate to profound levels of hypothermia are employed, it is wise to maintain an ACT of at least 600 seconds, since the subsequent rewarming phase (with its more rapid neutralization of heparin) can be accompanied by an alarmingly rapid fall in the ACT to potentially dangerous levels (less than 300 seconds). Guided by the ACT data and the anticipated time until perfusion is expected to be terminated, heparin in increments of 25 to 50 units/kg is administered to maintain a safe ACT level during rewarming (between 450 to 500 seconds).

Cannulation

ARTERIAL CANNULATION. This is always performed first, and, with rare exceptions (see peripheral cannulation discussion), the ascending aorta is used since it is more convenient and permits insertion of larger cannula sizes. Two purse-string sutures are placed in the aortic wall, allowing sufficient area (1.5 to 2 cm) to avoid occlusion of the innominate artery when the cannula is inserted. The sutures are fed through lengths of narrow tubing to facilitate controlled tightening of the purse-strings (this snaring method is used in venous cannulation as well). The purse-stringed area of the aortic wall is excluded with a side-biting clamp, the wall incised, and the cannula inserted. Occasionally, when the aortic wall is diffusely calcified, it is safer to avoid use of a side-biting clamp and insert the cannula through a direct aortic stab incision.

An appropriately sized cannula is selected (Table 5-1) that will have a pressure gradient of less than 100 mm Hg at the anticipated flow rate. This will minimize turbulence and associated blood trauma. The cannula itself is fitted with a snug plastic collar (Fig. 5-10) so that only a short length of cannula will lie within the aortic lumen. Since major cerebral damage can occur if the cannula is inadvertently inserted into the innominate artery, it is essential that the cannula be carefully positioned and fixed so that the tip is clearly away from the orifice of this vessel.

Hemochron Model 400, International Technidyne Corp., Edison, N.J.

CARDIAC OPERATION WITH EXTRACORPOREAL CIRCULATION

TABLE 5-1 PRESSURE GRADIENT ACROSS ARTERIAL CANNULA (mmHg)*

Cannula Size (French)	Flow (Liters per Minute)										
	0.5	1.0	1.5	2.0	2.5	3.0	3.5	4.0	4.5	5.0	5.5
10	55	115	185								
12	40	75	135	185							
14	30	55	100	135	190						
16		30	50	65	90	120	145				
18			35	45	50	70	90	100	120	140	
20				35	45	60	70	80	95	110	125
22					40	45	60	65	75	85	95
24					35	40	50	55	65	75	85

*Data obtained at 30C and hematocrit of 20. The numbers have been rounded off to the nearest 5 mm Hg.

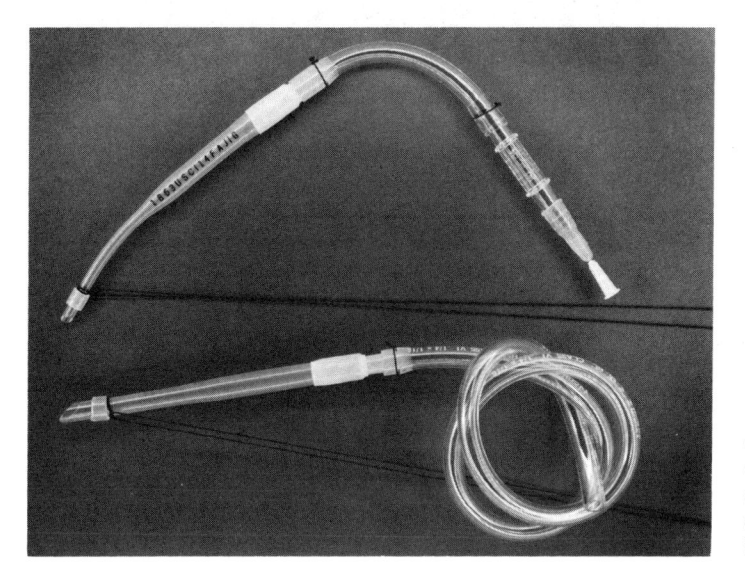

Figure 5-10. Arterial cannulae. Both have a snug but adjustable plastic collar. The upper cannula (used for infants and small children) requires little volume to fill it and is vented with a No. 25 hypodermic needle. The lower cannula is employed in adults.

SYSTEMIC VENOUS CANNULATION. Unless special circumstances exist, this is accomplished through the right atrium. A wide variety of cannula types are available (Fig. 5-11), the only critical factor being the necessity for the cannula selected to have sufficient internal diameter to allow unimpeded venous return of the predicted maximal perfusion rate. When single venous cannulation is to be employed, tubing with internal diameters of three-sixteenths to one-quarter inch (infants and small children) and three-eights to one-half inch (adults) will be satisfactory. When each vena cava is to be cannulated separately, the cannula sizes will be dictated by caval diameters. In practical terms, the largest cannula that can be *readily* inserted (external diameter slightly less than each caval diameter) is selected.

Figure 5-12 diagrams the major factors governing the rate of venous return from the patient to the extracorporeal circuit. As in all fluid systems, the venous return (Q) is directly related to the pressure head, or the driving

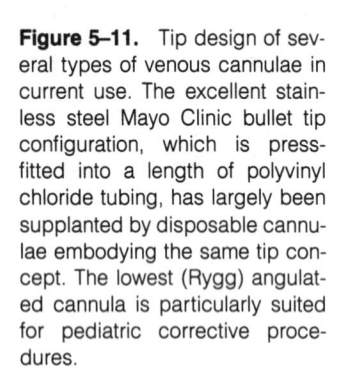

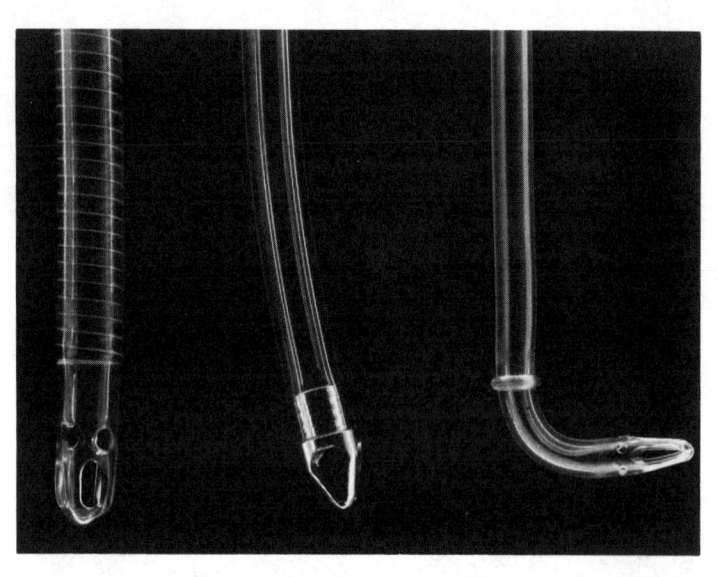

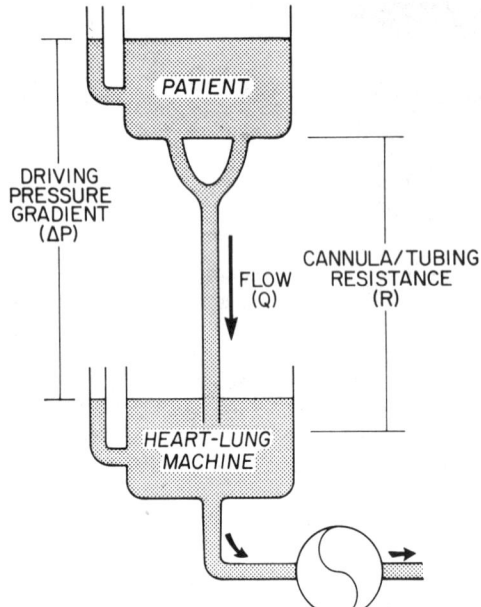

Figure 5-11. Tip design of several types of venous cannulae in current use. The excellent stainless steel Mayo Clinic bullet tip configuration, which is press-fitted into a length of polyvinyl chloride tubing, has largely been supplanted by disposable cannulae embodying the same tip concept. The lowest (Rygg) angulated cannula is particularly suited for pediatric corrective procedures.

Figure 5-12. Major factors influencing venous flow into the heart-lung machine. The flow rate (Q) from the patient is a direct function of the driving pressure gradient (ΔP) and an inverse function of the resistance (R) imposed primarily by the venous cannulae and tubing. Factors affecting ΔP and R are detailed in the text. (Drawing modified from Kirklin, JW, and Theye, RA. Whole body perfusion from a pump oxygenator for open intracardiac surgery. In *Surgery of the Chest*. Philadelphia: Saunders, 1962, p 696.)

pressure gradient (ΔP), and inversely related to the outflow resistance imposed primarily by the cannula and tubing components leading from the patient (R). Thus:

$$Q \propto \frac{\Delta P}{R}$$

It follows that the venous return can be increased by either raising the driving pressure gradient or reducing the outflow resistance, or both. Measures that increase the pressure gradient include (1) raising the systemic venous pressure slightly by addition of perfusate (thereby increasing venous volume) or (2) increasing the negative pressure (siphon) effect. The latter is determined by the vertical distance between the orifices of the venous drainage cannulae to the blood level in the oxygenator (assuming that gravity flow is being used to effect venous return).

In practice, the measures just described are the ones that are taken to increase venous return during open heart surgery, since those circuit arrangements tending to minimize outflow resistance (large diameter and appropriately short venous drainage cannulae and tubing connections leading to the venous reservoir of the oxygenator) will have been established before the start of perfusion.

In an intact subject, approximately 60 percent of the blood volume will be in the systemic veins while only 15 percent will reside in the arterial system, the remaining 25 percent being distributed between the capillaries (5 percent) and the heart and pulmonary vessels (combined volumes 20 percent). The venous system, being both more capacious and distensible than the arteries, plays a primary reservoir role in systemic blood volume changes during ECC. Deliberately increasing the inflow of perfusate into the patient will result in an increase in systemic venous volume followed by a rise in the venous return to the extracorporeal circuit (provided that there is no obstruction to outflow of blood from the patient). At the higher flow rate a new equilibrium will soon be established between venous return to the ECC and arterial inflow. There will, however, be a varyingly increased systemic venous blood volume at the higher flow rate, which is reflected by a proportional volume loss from the extracorporeal circuit. Thus, as flow rate is increased, additional priming fluid must be added to the ECC to maintain a satisfactory level in the oxygenator.

In practical terms, as long as the negative (siphon) gradient is large enough and outflow resistance of the venous drainage tubing system minimal, increasing the systemic arterial inflow will be accompanied by a relatively small increase in venous volume and little or no rise in venous pressure. However, if the arterial inflow rate continues to be increased, a point is reached where the resulting heightened systemic venous return volume cannot be delivered to the oxygenator because of the fixed diameters of the caval cannulae and venous drainage tubing. Under these conditions, systemic vascular volume will rise appreciably with a consequent elevation of systemic venous pressure.

The inferior vena cava (IVC) is cannulated through a purse-stringed site on the lateral right atrial wall close to the atrial-caval junction. The tip of the cannula is advanced into the IVC for only one to two centimeters to avoid inadvertent entrance into a hepatic vein. The superior vena cava (SVC) is usually cannulated through the right atrial appendage, care being taken to avoid traumatizing the sinoatrial node with the purse-string suture. Again, the cannula is introduced only a short distance into the SVC, since it is possible to partially or totally occlude the left innominate vein if too long a length is inserted.

Special circumstances necessitate modification of the usual systemic venous cannulation procedures. When venous switching operations are performed for transposition of the great arteries (Mustard or Senning), it is important to keep the right atrium free of cannulation sites. In these circumstances it is necessary to cannulate the IVC at the atrial-caval junction and the SVC directly. In neonates or those with multiple systemic venous anomalies, it is helpful to maintain an uncluttered operative field by means of perfusion-induced profound hypothermia and circulatory arrest. For such procedures, a single large venous cannula is inserted into the right atrium through the appendage. During the period of circulatory arrest the cannula is removed and is reinserted before reestablishing perfusion.

PERIPHERAL CANNULATION OF THE CRITICALLY ILL PATIENT. Rarely, the patient's preoperative hemodynamic state is so precarious that it is inadvisable to open the sternum in the absence of circulatory support. This is accomplished by establishing partial CPBP by means of femoral vein and arterial cannulations. If necessary, the procedure can be carried out prior to anesthetic induction in an adequately sedated patient. Using local infiltration anesthesia, the vessels are exposed, heparin is administered, the artery and vein cannulated, and partial CPBP commenced at 37C. Anesthesia is induced and, concomitantly, the perfusion temperature is reduced to 32C. The sternotomy is now carried out and cardiac exposure achieved. The SVC is cannulated in the usual manner and total bypass readily achieved by tightening a pericannular SVC snare and completely occluding the IVC at the atrial-caval junction with a snare.

In the fortunately rare situation in which an attempt to open the sternum has been accompanied by brisk bleeding because of subjacent, densely adherent structures, peripheral bypass as described above is promptly instituted. Profound perfusion cooling (12C) is begun and maintained until elective circulatory arrest is permissible. The sternotomy is then completed and the bleeding site identified and repaired. With the bleeding controlled and, if deemed permissible, perfusion at a low flow rate is reinstituted and maintained as additional cardiac exposure is obtained. The SVC is then cannulated and total bypass established (described above), and the flow rate and temperature conditions appropriate for correction of the cardiac lesion are instituted.

RECOVERY OF INTRACARDIAC BLOOD. During open operations, adequate visualization requires that intracardiac blood be gently removed from the operative field and returned to the pump-oxygenator. Additionally, left heart decompression must be carefully carried out in the vast majority of intracardiac operations. This is essential in all procedures involving the left heart and whenever the ascending aorta must be cross-clamped. In the first instance, specially designed cardiotomy suckers are employed that have shields that minimize the tendency for delicate structures to occlude the suckers. Left heart venting is frequently accomplished with an angulated multiple-holed catheter, which is usually inserted into the left atrium in the region of the right superior pulmonary vein. Whenever the operation does not involve the mitral valve, the catheter is advanced directly from the left atrium into the left ventricle. Whenever the left ventricle is to be incised, as in aneurysmectomy, the decompression catheter can be inserted directly into that chamber.

It has long been established that the intracardiac suction system can be highly traumatic to the recovered blood. There are two primary causes. First, the blood almost certainly will contain considerable lipid and other debris, particularly if the pericardial sac has been used as a blood collection and aspiration site, as it commonly is. For this reason it is important to interpose an ultrapore filter between the intracardiac blood recovery collecting chamber and the oxygenator. Second, if inappropriately high suction is employed, air as well as blood may be introduced into the system, and foaming will result. Therefore, it is important that frequent verbal exchange take place between the surgeon and perfusionist so that the aspirating pumps are adjusted to minimize such foaming.

Perfusion Techniques

TEMPERATURE. As described earlier, control of perfusion temperature is efficiently maintained by a heat exchanger that is located either on the venous or, more commonly, on the arterial inflow side of the heart-lung machine. Mild hypothermia (30 to 32C) usually is employed as CPBP is initiated to allow for a brief period of perfusion discontinuance should mechanical failure occur in the early minutes of bypass. This temperature level is maintained during short intracardiac procedures (repair of atrial septal defect, etc.). More substantial temperature reductions are usually employed for lengthier repairs.

The exact level of perfusion hypothermia employed varies with the specific requirements of the operative repair. Use of hypothermic cardioplegia is facilitated by concomitant perfusion cooling (12 to 20C) to optimize cardiac cooling and, in particular, to make certain that the endocardium is not selectively rewarmed by bronchial circulation blood returning to the left heart. Hypothermic perfusion (25C) allows reduction of the flow rate, if necessary, in cyanotic patients in whom a profuse bronchial arterial return has obscured the operative field; diminution of the bronchial return pari passu with the lowered flow rate permits better visualization and facilitates the repair. Additionally, when aortopulmonary shunts (such as a Potts or Waterston anastomosis) cannot be safely mobilized and closed before commencing the definitive repair, profound perfusion hypothermia allows a brief period of low flow (0.5 liters/min/m^2) or total circulatory arrest, enabling the pulmonary artery to be entered and the connections closed.

Finally, the use of circulatory arrest in neonates and infants undergoing intracardiac repair of complex anomalies requires profound temperature reduction to safely permit a lengthy period of arrest. The heat exchanger temperature is lowered to 12C and perfusion cooling is continued until the nasopharyngeal temperature has been lowered to 18C. Available data indicate that these conditions permit circulatory arrest for 45 minutes. However, detailed information about late intellectual function in the children who underwent 45 to 60 minutes of total circulatory arrest is not yet available. Hence, caution would dictate that the method be used highly selectively when no known alternative is deemed to be advisable.

As discussed previously (see heat exchanger discussion), rewarming must be performed with precision, care being taken to limit the blood-body temperature gradient to a maximum of 15 degrees to avoid microbubble production. During rewarming the highest permissible heat exchanger temperature is 42C.

PERFUSION RATE. Flow rates of 2.2 to 2.4 liters/min/m^2 at mild to moderate hypothermic conditions have been demonstrated to satisfactorily perfuse the microcirculation and maintain physiologic stability of all subsystems for four to six hours. If venous return is insufficient to maintain such a flow rate and there is no apparent mechanical impediment to blood flow, perfusate is added to improve the situation. If venous return exceeds 2.4 liters/min/m^2, the blood is sequestered in the oxygenator and subsequently slowly returned to the patient after bypass discontinuance.

The use of moderate hypothermia (28 to 30C) allows deliberate moderate reduction of flow rate (1.6 to 1.2 liters/min/m^2) for brief periods (10 to 15 minutes) to facilitate intracardiac exposure. The advantages of reduced or no flow in improving operative conditions in infants and children have been discussed previously. During profound perfusion hypothermia (≤20C), flow rates of 1.2 liters/min/m^2 are permissible for 90 minutes. As previously suggested, occasional operative circumstances require even greater flow reduction. Kirklin et al. (1976) have pointed out the advisability of attempting to maintain a low perfusion rate of 0.5 liters/min/m^2 rather than proceeding to total circulatory arrest, whenever possible. This approach appears to be intrinsically safer in that it provides some blood flow to the brain and other vital organs. Moreover, during total circulatory arrest air may enter and be entrapped in the aorta and subsequently embolize to the brain when the perfusion is restarted.

High flow rates (2.2 to 2.4 liters/min/m^2) are maintained during both the cooling and rewarming phases of the perfusion.

SYSTEMIC ARTERIAL PRESSURE. With the start of CPBP, despite high flow rates, the perfusion pressure tends to fall sharply for a brief period but thereafter begins to rise. During perfusion at normothermia (and even with moderate hypothermia), it is advisable to maintain the systemic arterial mean pressure no lower than 55 mm Hg so as to be reasonably certain that all vital organs (particularly the brain and kidneys) are being adequately perfused. This is especially important in older patients, since focal atherosclerotic stenoses otherwise may sharply limit both flow and perfusion pressure distal to the stenotic vasculature. When the flow rate is satisfactory but the mean perfusion pressure remains inordinately low, it is helpful to cautiously begin a low-dose infusion of a predominantly alpha agonist such as levarterenol, methoxamine, or phenylephrine.

Since the peripheral vascular resistance tends to rise progressively during nonpulsatile CPBP (McGoon et al., 1960), it is not surprising that, not infrequently, the systemic mean arterial pressure may rise to an inappropriately high level (over 100 mm Hg), particularly during the rewarming period of the perfusion. It is important to promptly reduce the pressure to acceptable levels (60 to 80 mm Hg) with a vasodilating drug, since there is heightened probability of intracerebral bleeding in a heparinized hypertensive patient. Although halothane and chlorpromazine were formerly used for this purpose, we now use a sodium nitroprusside infusion as the agent of choice to lower the pressure, since the drug's action is both immediate and readily controllable.

In several centers, *pulsatile flow* has been used recently as a preferential mode of pumping because of its physiologic advantages. Despite this, the potential problems associated with its use, discussed earlier (see *Pulse Contour*), and the fact that the vast majority of patients undergoing open intracardiac operation do beautifully with the nonpulsatile flow pattern unquestionably are the two reasons why the routine use of pulsatile flow has not been widely employed.

Bregman et al. (1977) and Kaplitt and Tamari (1977) have described simple methods of achieving pulsatile flow during CPBP with a device in series with the arterial roller pump. However, the major advantage of the method would seem to be its capacity to provide pulsatile diastolic augmentation and systolic afterload reduction in the period *immediately after* discontinuing CPBP and until aortic decannulation has been carried out.

Myocardial Preservation. At present there is no known method that predictably provides absolute protection of the diseased or congenitally malformed heart during open intracardiac operations. The following is a necessarily brief discussion of methods employed to limit the extent of damage during surgery.

CORONARY PERFUSION. Technical considerations aside, the ideal method of maintaining myocardial integrity during cardiac repair in man, employing CPBP, would be provision of *physiologic* perfusion of both coronary arteries through an intact aortic root with the heart beating slowly. A large number of experimental and clinical reports have documented that myocardial damage is generally minimal when these conditions prevail. This is not the case when the perfused heart is allowed to remain in ventricular fibrillation for prolonged periods, particularly if left ventricular hypertrophy or coronary artery occlusive disease is present. The classic report of Najafi et al. (1969) and numerous clinical and investigative reports since then have described the lethal potential of the severe subendocardial hemorrhagic necrosis that frequently is encountered with protracted ventricular fibrillation (Hottenrott et al., 1973, 1974).

Even in those operations in which it is possible to keep the heart beating while perfusing it through the intact aortic root (for example, isolated mitral valve replacement), technical considerations relating to maintenance of adequate intracardiac exposure commonly require pulling on retractors, which unquestionably imposes trauma on the myofibrils, adjacent vasculature, and conduction system. For these reasons, clinical experience in former years demonstrated the utility of combining moderate hypothermia (28 to 32C) and brief periods (10 to 15 minutes) of myocardial ischemia (aorta crossclamped). Each ischemic period was preceded by at least three minutes of coronary perfusion. While hardly optimal (and presently superceded by hypothermic cardioplegic methods to be described later), results with the technique were generally acceptable. Currently, use of the method largely is confined to repair of complex congenital anomalies that require either intraoperative determination of the location of the cardiac conduction system or confirmation of the persistence of sinus rhythm in the beating heart after suturing near the atrioventricular node or bundle.

In operations such as aortic valve replacement, where the aortic root must be open, continuous perfusion of the coronary arteries with individual catheters or hand-held cannulae cannot be viewed as achieving truly physiologic conditions, although, when properly performed, the clinical results have been impressive (McGoon et al., 1965). Nevertheless, data developed by Sapsford et al. (1974) indicate that although hospital mortality is low, measurable (and occasionally severe) myocardial damage can be encountered with the method, particularly in those hearts with severe left ventricular hypertrophy.

The differences between the physiologically normal relationships of coronary blood flow and perfusion pressure in the beating heart have been contrasted with those obtained with continuous, steady flow coronary perfusion by a roller pump during aortic valve replacement (Gianelli et al., 1976). The data indicate that with the usual type of continuous pump perfusion of the coronary arteries in a beating heart, the perfusion pressure within the coronary arteries can be excessively high during ventricular systole and significantly lower than the mean perfusion pressure during diastole.

The consequence of these clearly unphysiologic relationships would be a relatively low level of coronary blood flow which might prove to be significantly inadequate, particularly in patients with severe left ventricular hypertrophy. Moreover, the pistonlike effect of the roller pump forcing blood into a reduced coronary vascular bed during systole (which, at that moment, represents a high resistance locus) can produce severe myocardial hemorrhagic infarction. Indeed, these changes accompanied by deteriorating functional performance have been experimentally produced by Brown et al. (1969) in isolated canine hearts perfused at excessively high (160 mm Hg) pressures.

Using an alternative method of gravity flow coronary artery perfusion (in effect, establishing an open, distensible, and self-regulating system during both ventricular systole and diastole), Gianelli et al. (1976) documented an almost twofold increase in mean left coronary artery blood flow at comparable mean perfusion pressures during aortic valve replacement, with peak diastolic flow rates of 600 ml/min having been achieved in several patients. Although enzymatic and other precise indices of myocardial damage were not uniformly available, there were no hospital deaths and no clinical infarctions, nor were positive inotropic drugs employed in the series.

Even if one accepts the probability that the latter method of coronary perfusion closely approximates physiologic conditions, the occasional reports of coronary ostial damage, the cumbersome presence of cannulae in the aortic root during aortic valve replacement, prolongation of aortic crossclamp time, and the overall suboptimal visibility and operating conditions within or on a beating heart—all of these factors detract from continued widespread use of the technique, now that alternative acceptable and simpler methods of myocardial protection are available.

HYPOTHERMIA AND GLOBAL ISCHEMIC ARREST. The fall in tissue oxygen consumption pari passu with temperature reduction has been discussed earlier (see Perfusion Temperature: Induced Hypothermia). Greenberg and Edmunds (1961) documented the concept that myocardial hypothermia would extend the permissible period of ischemia during CPBP when they showed experimentally that the same percentage return of left ventricular function obtained with 10 minutes of global ischemia at 37C could be realized with ischemic times three and six times longer at temperatures of 18C and 10C, respectively. These and other experimental data (Fuhrman et al., 1950; Gott et al., 1962) provided the basis for clinical use of cold ischemic arrest, which, in turn, offered the advantage of improved operating conditions in a motionless and virtually bloodless heart.

Myocardial cooling has been accomplished in three basic ways. First, local cooling of the heart, as originally described by Shumway and colleagues in 1959 (see Griepp et al., 1973), has been employed clinically for two decades. The method consists of initially flooding the pericardial sac with two liters of 4C saline after the aorta has been cross-clamped, followed by a continuous drip of the cold solution on the heart at a rate of 100 to 150 ml/min. The heart remains immersed in a cold pool, the desired fluid level being maintained by gentle suction. Topical cooling is combined with low-flow CPBP (40 to 50 ml/kg/min) and moderate systemic hypothermia (31 to 33C), measures intended to minimize rewarming of the heart by blood returning to the left heart. Although reports indicate that the method has been satisfactory in the hands of a number of groups, this has not been the consistent case for other surgeons, almost certainly because the reduction in myocardial temperature can be relatively small and unpredictable (Stiles et al., 1977), allowing large transmural thermal gradients to exist with consequent significant myocardial damage.

A second method of local cardiac cooling has been the continuous or intermittent selective cannula introduction into the coronary arteries of cold perfusate (4 to 12C) delivered from a separate cooling circuit off the arterial limb of the heart-lung machine, while the rest of the body is perfused at 30C. Although this method is not used widely, clinical results (i.e., survival) have been satisfactory. However, it is apparent that all of the previously described technical problems associated with coronary perfusion are operative.

Finally, profound levels of perfusion hypothermia (core cooling) may be used to cool the entire body, including the heart. In a randomized study of two methods of myocardial preservation in patients undergoing aortic valve replacement, Sapsford et al. (1974) documented that when the myocardial temperature had been lowered to approximately 22C, a 45-minute period of cardiac ischemia was permissible. Isoenzyme and electrocardiographic evidence of myocardial necrosis was no greater than that observed in a cohort having coronary perfusion.

Since myocardial metabolism, albeit low, is not nil even at sharply reduced temperatures, it follows that inappropriately prolonged global cardiac ischemia will be accompanied by myocardial damage whenever the cellular requirements for oxygen and substrates exceed their availability. The nature and extent of the damage correlates directly with ischemic time (Jennings et al., 1960). When myocardial perfusion is reestablished, restoration of structural integrity and cardiac function is inversely related to the ischemic time. For reasons discussed earlier, myocardial hypothermia prolongs the period of permissible ischemia, but there are strict time limitations that, when exceeded, will result in severe, irreparable damage. Under these circumstances, reestablishment of blood flow to the myocardium is accompanied by sudden and massive extension of cardiac injury, the so-called *reperfusion injury* (Shen and Jennings, 1972; Whalen et al., 1974).

It is probable that severe reperfusion injury is merely a reflection of a crime that already has been committed (i.e., irreversible damage) during the ischemic period (see Hearse, 1977, for a detailed review). In such a state, the myocardial cell membrane has lost the ability to exclude calcium, which now rushes into the interior of the cell along a 10,000-fold concentration gradient (Maloney and Nelson, 1975). There is explosive cell swelling, mitochondrial rupture, the permanent deposition of intramitochondrial calcium phosphate particles, and the development of severe, irreversible myocardial contracture (Jennings and Ganote, 1976), the latter condition aptly characterized by Cooley et al. (1972) as "stone heart." Diastolic filling is impossible, and death of the patient is the inevitable result.

In its milder, generally tolerable form, reperfusion injury is characterized by cellular and mitochondrial edema. Functionally, there is a reduction in ventricular compliance. These morphologic and performance alterations are largely reversible, but do require continued cardiopulmonary bypass support during the reparative period.

HYPOTHERMIC CARDIOPLEGIA. More than a quarter of a century ago, Melrose et al. (1955) first reported their experimental investigations dealing with the feasibility of electively arresting the heart with potassium citrate. Their brief communication began:

> The goal of cardiac surgeons must be the unhurried correction of cardiac abnormalities under direct vision.... A most valuable contribution ... to the whole problem of intracardiac surgery would be made if the heart could be arrested and re-started at will, suffering no damage during periods of arrest and cessation of coronary blood-flow.

The goal envisioned by Melrose and his co-workers, though not yet completely attained, has been brought much closer to a clinical reality by recent developments in and application of hypothermic cardioplegic techniques.

Applied clinically, the Melrose method was soon abandoned because of severe early and late myocardial injury (Waldhausen et al., 1960), now believed to have been primarily the result of the hyperosmotic character (Gay and Ebert, 1973) and extremely high potassium concentration (greater than 200 mEq/liter) of the solution (Tyers et al., 1975). These initial results understandably dampened further investigative enthusiasm for elective cardiac arrest for almost a decade. Indeed, it was not until Bretschneider (1964), Kirsch et al. (1972), and other European surgeons had demonstrated the clinical efficacy and safety of cardioplegic arrest that worldwide interest in the method was rekindled.

In the past several years, there has been a veritable explosion of investigative and clinical studies that have sought to characterize the essential requirements of elective cardioplegic techniques. These reports notwithstanding, questions remain about the importance of including specific ions and their amounts, optimal temperature, pH, and osmolality, the need for colloid to maintain onconicity and for buffering, and the utility of substrates such as glucose (with or without insulin) or the desirability of an oxygenated (blood) infusate. For an overview of these areas of concern, the reader is referred to the reports of Hearse et al. (1974, 1975, 1976, 1978, 1981), Follette et al. (1977, 1978), Clark et al. (1977), Buckberg (1979), Bretschneider (1980), and Preusse et al. (1981).

Although gaps in our knowledge currently exist, two important components of cardioplegic protection of the myocardium now appear to be beyond dispute. *First*, pharmacologic induction of immediate electromechanical asystole as the ascending aorta is cross-clamped establishes conditions in which the large energy-consuming reactions associated with ventricular contraction essentially are eliminated. This allows the available energy produced by the anaerobic metabolic pathway to be used to maintain integrity of the myocardial cell membrane during the ischemic interval so that appropriate transmembrane ionic gradients can be sustained. Although the composition of cardioplegic solutions has varied widely, almost all contain potassium in concentrations of 10 to 30 mM/liter to achieve prompt electromechanical asystole. These concentrations appear to be both safe and effective.

It is probably important to include two other cations in the cardioplegic formulation. Hearse et al. (1978b) suggest that, apart from its capacity to induce diastolic arrest of the heart, the presence of magnesium (optimal dosage was found to be 16 mM/liter) exerts a significant protective effect on the ischemic myocardium by incompletely understood mechanisms that presumably involve the ion's critical role in the energy-transferring reactions of the cell as well as reactions involved in oxidation, synthesis, and transport. Experimental studies indicate that a small amount of calcium also is essential (Jynge et al., 1977) to maintain structural integrity of the cell membrane. It has long been known that perfusion of isolated hearts with calcium-free solutions is immediately followed by severe myocardial damage when a perfusate containing the ion is then introduced into the experimental preparation (see Hearse et al., 1978a, for a comprehensive discussion). Although conclusive data from human studies are lacking, it would seem advisable to include approximately 2 mM/liter of the cation in the cardioplegic formulation, an amount that is known to prevent cell damage in experimental preparations.

Since the speed of metabolic processes is a direct function of temperature, a *second* uncontroversial aspect of the cardioplegic method is that the cardiac infusate must be cold. Indeed, it has been established that combining hypothermia with pharmacologic cardioplegia is additive in protecting the myocardium (Hearse et al., 1975). Although some experimental information concludes that hearts perfused below 10C recover less well after the ischemic interval (Tyers et al., 1977), other studies (Shragge at al., 1978) and an expanding clinical experience suggest that a cardioplegic infusate temperature of 4C is well-tolerated. Indeed, it is becoming increasingly clear that the safety of the method lies more in maintaining the heart uniformly cold and less in the exact constituency of the cardioplegic solution.

Our clinical experience has been with the St. Thomas' Hospital cardioplegic solution (Hearse et al., 1976; Braimbridge et al., 1977; Jynge et al., 1977). A thermistor is inserted in a ventricular area believed to be at risk of inadequate protection (such as myocardium subserved by a severely obstructed coronary artery). Left heart venting is established and systemic cooling (12C) is begun. When the myocardial temperature has fallen to 22C (or earlier if ventricular fibrillation occurs), the ascending aorta is crossclamped and the cold (4C) cardioplegic solution is infused with a delivery pressure at the coronary ostia controlled between 40 to 50 mm Hg (no higher).

The infusion is carried out either through a large-diameter (13 gauge) needle or, with the aortic root open, with coronary perfusion cannulae if any aortic regurgitation is present. The infusion volume varies from 1000 to 1500 ml in adults (the larger volume being used in the presence of marked cardiomegaly, severe ventricular hypertrophy or when the fall in myocardial temperature has been insufficient); a proportionately lower volume is utilized in infants and children. If regional myocardial temperature reduction remains suboptimal in the presence of severe obstructive coronary artery pathology in patients undergoing bypass grafting, the artery is entered at the projected anastomotic site and an additional 100 to 150 ml of solution is infused distally at low pressure through a short plastic intravenous cannula (Mindich et al., 1981). A right atrial purse-string is loosened so that the cold coronary effluent will cool the epicardial surface of the heart. In adults with adequate renal function, this fluid can be returned to the heart-lung machine, but this should not be done in pediatric cases because of the potential danger of high serum potassium levels. Myocardial temperatures of 5 to 9C can be anticipated with this method. Supplemental topical cardiac cooling (described earlier) is now instituted and maintained with 4C Ringer's solution, with a multiple-hole catheter placed over the exposed areas of the right atrium and right ventricle. The perfusion temperature may now be raised to between 20 and 28C, depending on the anticipated length of the ischemic period.

Reinfusion of cold cardioplegic solution (in a volume identical to the original infusion) is carried out every 30 minutes during the crossclamp interval. Additional reinfusion criteria include: (1) the earlier reappearance of electromechanical activity; or (2) elevation of myocardial temperature over 14C.

Release of the aortic crossclamp must be precisely coordinated with properly timed prior perfusion rewarming such that the myocardium-perfusate gradient does not exceed 15 degrees while, on the other hand, avoiding premature rewarming, which would inappropriately heat the still ischemic heart via both the bronchial and noncoronary collateral circulations. Just before removing the crossclamp, the flow rate is transiently reduced to lower the systemic arterial pressure to approximately 50 mm Hg. This condition is maintained for two minutes, a maneuver that is believed to minimize myocardial edema, which is more prone to occur (in experimental animals) at postischemic perfusion pressures of 100 mm Hg (Engelman et al., 1975). Generous aortic root venting to avoid air embolism and proper cardiac chamber decompression with maintenance of low left ventricular filling pressures (4 mm Hg or less) to avoid myofibril overstretching are both essential.

There can be no doubt that hypothermic cardioplegic arrest represents a major advance in myocardial protection. However, even when it is properly conducted (in accordance with currently available information), reestablishment of blood flow to the myocardium following the ischemic interval is still commonly accompanied by discernible derangement in cardiac function.* This typically includes evidence of reduced ventricular compliance (presumably due to myocardial edema) and some impairment of contractility. Fortunately, these alterations are usually transient, but may take 20 to 30 minutes to become maximally manifest after discontinuance of bypass.

On the assumption that some degree of transient myocardial reperfusion injury will have occurred, a substantial period of essentially total bypass is continued after the cardiac repair (even in the presence of apparently satisfactory ventricular contractility) to allow myocardial cellular and subcellular organelles an adequate period of time for reparative processes to be completed. At present, no conclusive information allows logical decisions to be made about necessary supplemental support periods. Empirically, we provide a *minimum* total support time of 15 to 20 minutes for each hour of aortic occlusion. Obviously, those patients coming to the operation with advanced left ventricular dysfunction generally will require longer periods of postarrest support. Profitable use can be made of the supplemental support period by insertion of atrial and ventricular pacing wires, pericardial drainage catheters, etc.

Available information suggests that aortic crossclamp periods up to 120 minutes are permissible. Provided that the technique has been meticulously employed, the magnitude of measurable myocardial structural damage is small (Conti et al., 1978), and early and late cardiac functional performance is generally not adversely affected (Ellis et al., 1978a, 1978b).

Avoidance of Air Embolism. A bitter lesson every cardiac surgeon learns sooner or later is the propensity for air to remain stubbornly locked within the recesses of the heart and pulmonary veins and ultimately embolize to the brain or coronary arteries. This may happen even after considerable efforts have been made to rid the chambers of air (Fishman et al., 1969; Taber et al., 1970; Padula et al., 1971). Therefore, whenever the heart has been opened, systematic and vigorous steps must be taken to eliminate air. As a prelude to the process, it is absolutely essential that a capacious aortic root vent be established.

As cardiac chamber or aortic root closure is being completed, suction on the left heart venting catheter is temporarily slowed or discontinued so that blood fills the left heart and begins to spill out of the aortic vent site. (If the right heart has been opened, one or both caval tapes are momentarily loosened to fill these chambers during the latter moments of closure.) The pulmonary veins, left atrium, and left ventricle are manually compressed to dislodge any air. Only now is the ascending aortic crossclamp gradually released. Simultaneously, left heart vent decompression is resumed at a rate sufficient to maintain low (2 to 4 mm Hg) left atrial pressures.

As the heart begins to contract, the aortic crossclamp is temporarily closed to achieve obligatory egress of any trapped air through the aortic root vent. Immediately, the pulmonary veins and cardiac chambers are once again alternately compressed and released by the surgeon's hand, while the anesthesiologist fully inflates the lungs. Only after these measures are completed is the crossclamp again released. As a precaution, the open clamp is not removed from the aorta because of the possible need to suddenly occlude the vessel at the slightest sign (or sound) of air. With the

---

The derangements associated with myocardial reperfusion involve complex metabolic and structural alterations that adversely affect cardiac performance. Depending on the extent of the ischemic damage, the changes vary from transient reversible distortions (manifested principally by myocardial edema with reduced compliance) to irreversible damage with cellular death. Alterations indicative of severe reperfusion damage include loss of membrane integrity with calcium phosphate bodies within the mitochondria as well as disruption of these organelles, vascular endothelial damage, and both fragmentation and hypercontraction of myofibrils. Comprehensive discussions of factors etiologic to and characteristic of reperfusion damage in the cardiac surgical postischemic period will be found in the papers of Engelman et al. (1976), Hearse (1977), and Lucas et al. (1980).

heart now beating vigorously, copious venting is continued through the aortic root for at least three minutes. During this period the pulmonary veins and cardiac structures are manipulated for a third time, as described above. Following this the aortic root vent is closed with a previously placed purse-string suture and perfusion discontinuance measures are begun.

Discontinuance Measures. With the repair completed, all suture lines checked for bleeding, and the heart beating satisfactorily, a systematic protocol is followed that seeks to assess and optimize performance of all subsystems before perfusion discontinuance. As described previously, temporary atrial and ventricular pacing wires (two each) will have been routinely inserted earlier during perfusion rewarming. If, for whatever reason, a left atrial catheter was not positioned prior to the repair, it is now introduced through the left heart vent insertion (left atrial) site as the vent is being withdrawn. In this regard, it is important to momentarily release the caval tapes before withdrawing the vent to make certain that the left atrial pressure will be high enough to avoid the inadvertent trapping of air as the vent mattress suture is being tied.

Ventilation is now reinstituted and heart rate optimized by pacing, if necessary. Partial bypass is established by releasing the caval tapes. With stable and satisfactory cardiovascular, serum electrolyte, blood-gas, and acid-base variables, the perfusion flow rate is gradually reduced to 50 percent of the predicted flow rate by partially occluding the venous line. If all remains well, one caval cannula is now removed and the other withdrawn into the right atrium. With maintenance of satisfactory conditions, the perfusion flow rate is further reduced, appropriate adjustments of ventricular filling pressures are carried out, and bypass discontinued. Because of the possible delay in the maximal manifestation of reperfusion dysfunction, it is prudent to maintain atrial pressures as low as possible (consistent with acceptable hemodynamic conditions) soon after perfusion discontinuance in anticipation of reduced ventricular compliance and inappropriate elevation of filling pressures.

With continued hemodynamic stability, decannulation is carried out and protamine sulfate administered to neutralize the circulating heparin, ideally with the use of the dose-response curve of Bull et al. (1975b) as the means of determining the protamine dose. An alternative method that has proven effective in practice is determining the *total* amount of heparin administered (both priming perfusate and patient) and administering 1 mg of protamine for every 100 units of heparin given throughout the perfusion. Since approximately 1.3 mg of protamine are required to neutralize each 100 units of heparin, this admittedly empirical prescription is not likely to cause bleeding related to protamine excess. Regardless of the method employed, periodic determination of the ACT is used to determine what is interpreted to be residual heparin effect.

In those unusual circumstances where cardiac performance is clearly suboptimal, a supplemental period of perfusion support is maintained (ideally by reestablishing total bypass). During this period, preparations are made to measure cardiac output.

After a varying period of supplemental support, another attempt is made to discontinue perfusion without the need for ventricular filling pressures to be raised to excessively high levels. If discontinuance now proves to be possible, prompt and sequential measurements of cardiac output, together with knowledge and appropriate control of preload, afterload, and heart rate, will make it possible for logical decisions to be made about the continued adequacy of cardiovascular subsystem performance. In the rare event that perfusion support still cannot be terminated, one is forced to resort to positive inotropic agents and, if necessary, mechanical supportive measures, such as intraaortic balloon counterpulsation. These matters are discussed in Chapter 9.

REFERENCES

Aguilar MJ, Gerbode F, Hill JD: Neuropathologic complications of cardiac surgery. J Thorac Cardiovasc Surg 61:676, 1971.

Allardyce DB, Yoshida SH, Ashmore PG: The importance of microembolism in the pathogenesis of organ dysfunction caused by prolonged use of the pump oxygenator. J Thorac Cardiovasc Surg 52:706, 1966.

Andersen MN, Mendelow M, William OG: Relationship of respiratory alkalosis to metabolic acidosis during extracorporeal circulation. Surgery 53:730, 1963.

Ashmore PG, Svitek V, Ambrose P: The incidence and effect of particulate aggregation and microembolism in pump oxygenator systems. J Thorac Cardiovasc Surg 55:691, 1968.

Bartlett RH, Gazzaniga AB: Extracorporeal circulation for cardiopulmonary failure. Curr Probl Surg 15:1-96, 1978.

Bigelow WG, Lindsay WK, Greenwood WF: Hypothermia: its possible role in cardiac surgery: an investigation of factors governing survival in dogs at low body temperature. Ann Surg 132:849, 1950.

Boucher JK, Rudy LW Jr, Edmunds LH Jr: Organ blood flow during pulsatile cardiopulmonary bypass. J Appl Physiol 36:86, 1974.

Braimbridge MV, Chaven J, Bitensky L, Hearse DJ, Jynge P, Cankovic-Darracott S: Cold cardioplegia or continuous coronary perfusion? Report on preliminary clinical experience as assessed cytochemically. J Thorac Cardiovasc Surg 74:900, 1977.

Bregman D, Bowman FO, Parodi EN, Haubert SM, Edie RN, Spotnitz HM, Reemtsma K, Malm, JR: An improved method of myocardial protection with pulsation during cardiopulmonary bypass. Circulation 56 (Suppl II) :II–157, 1977.

Bretschneider HJ: Myocardial protection. Thorac Cardiovasc Surg 28:295, 1980.

———: Veberlebungszeit und wiederbelebungszeit des herzens bei normo- und hypothermie. Verh Dtsch Ges Kreislaufforsch 30:11, 1964.

Brown AH, Braimbridge MV, Niles NR, Gerbode F, Aguilar MJ: The effect of excessively high perfusion pressures on the histology, histochemistry, birefringence, and function of the myocardium. J Thorac Cardiovasc Surg 58:655, 1969.

Brown IW Jr, Smith WW, Emmons WO: An efficient blood heat exchanger for use with extracorporeal circulation. Surgery 44:372, 1958.

Buckberg GD: A proposed "solution" to the cardioplegic controversy. J Thorac Cardiovasc Surg 77:803, 1979.

Bull BS, Kropman RA, Huse WM, Briggs BD: Heparin therapy during extracorporeal circulation. I. Problems inherent in existing heparin protocols. J Thorac Cardiovasc Surg 69:674, 1975a.

———, Huse WM, Brauer FS, Korpman RA: Heparin therapy during extracorporeal circulation. II. The use of a dose-response curve to individualize heparin and protamine. J Thorac Cardiovasc Surg 69:685, 1975b.

Carlson RG, Lande AJ, Landis B, Rogoz B, Baxter J, Patterson RH Jr, Stenzel K, Lillehei, CW: The Lande-Edwards membrane oxygenator during heart surgery. J Thorac Cardiovasc Surg 66:894, 1973.

Clark, LC Jr: Optimal flow rate in perfusion. In Allen JG (ed): Extracorporeal Circulation. Springfield, Ill, Thomas, 1958, pp 150–163.

———, Gollan F, Gupta VB: The oxygenation of blood by gas dispersion. Science lll:85, 1950.

Clark RE, Margraf, HW, Beauchamp RA: Fat and solid filtration in clinical perfusions. Surgery 77: 216, 1975.

———, Ferguson TB, West PN, Schuchleib RC, Henry PD: Pharmacologic preservation of the ischemic heart. Ann Thoracic Surg 24:307, 1977.

Cleland J, Pluth JR, Tauxe WN, Kirklin JW: Blood volume and body fluid changes soon after closed and open intracardiac surgery. J Thorac Cardiovasc Surg 52:698, 1966.

Clowes GHA Jr, Neville WE: The membrane oxygenator. In Allen JG (ed): Extracorporeal Circulation. Springfield, Ill, Thomas, 1958, pp 81–100.

———, ———, Sabga G, Shibota Y: The relationship of oxygen consumption, perfusion rate and temperature to the acidosis associated with cardiopulmonary circulatory bypass. Surgery 44:220, 1958.

Comroe JH: Physiology of Respiration, 2nd ed. Chicago, Ill, Year Book, 1974, p 20.

Connell RJ, Page US, Bartley TD, Bigelow JC, Webb MC: The effect on pulmonary ultrastructure of Dacron-wool filtration during cardiopulmonary bypass. Ann Thorac Surg 15:217, 1973.

Conti VR, Bertranou EG, Blackstone EH, Kirklin, JW, Digerness SB: Cold cardioplegia versus hypothermia for myocardial protection: random-

ized clinical study. J Thorac Cardiovasc Surg 76:577, 1978.
Cooley DA, Beall AC Jr, Grondin P: Open heart operations with disposable oxygenators, five percent dextrose prime and normothermia. Surgery 52:713, 1962.
———, Bloodwell RD, Beall AC Jr, Hallman GL: Cardiac valve replacement without blood transfusion. Am J Surg 112:743, 1966.
———, Reul GJ, Wukasch DC: Ischemic contracture of the heart: "stone heart." Am J Cardiol 29:575, 1972.
Cruz AB Jr, Callaghan JC: Hemodilution in extracorporeal circulation: large or small non-blood prime? J Thorac Cardiovasc Surg 52:690, 1966.
Cuello L, Vasquez E, Rios R, Raffucci FL: Autologous blood transfusion in thoracic and cardiovascular surgery. Surgery 62:814, 1967.
Dammann JF Jr, Thung N, Christlieb II, Littlefield JB, Muller WH Jr: The management of the severely ill patient after open-heart surgery. J Thorac Cardiovasc Surg 45:80, 1963.
de Leval M, Hill JD, Mielke CH, Bramson M, Smith C, Gerbode F: Platelet kinetics during extracorporeal circulation. Trans Am Soc Artif Intern Organs 18:355, 1972.
DeWall RA, Lillehei CW: Simplified total body perfusion: reduced flows, moderate hypothermia and hemodilution. JAMA 179:430, 1962.
———, Warden HE, Gott VL, Read RC, Varco RL, Lillehei CW: Total body perfusion for open cardiotomy utilizing the bubble oxygenator. J Thorac Surg 32:591, 1956.
Dobell ARC, Mitri M, Galva R, Sarkozy E, Murphy D: Biologic evaluation of blood after prolonged recirculation through film and membrane oxygenator. Ann Surg 161:617, 1965.
Donald DE, Fellows JL: Relation of temperature, gas tension and hydrostatic pressure to the formation of gas bubbles in extracorporeally oxygenated blood. Surg Forum 10:589, 1960.
Egeblad K, Osborn JJ, Burns W, Hill JD, Gerbode F: Blood filtration during cardiopulmonary bypass. J Thorac Cardiovasc Surg 63:384, 1972.
Ellis RJ, Born M, Feit T, Ebert PA: Potassium cardioplegia: early assessment by radionuclide ventriculography. Circulation 58(Suppl I) :I-57, 1978a.
———, Sullivan R, Gertz E, Van Dyke E, Ebert PA: Mild ventricular dysfunction following cold K(+) cardioplegia (abstr). Circulation 58(Suppl II) :II-98, 1978b.
Engelman RM, Adler S, Gouge TH, Chandra R, Boyd AD, Baumann FG: The effect of normothermic anoxic arrest and ventricular fibrillation on the coronary blood flow distribution of the pig. J Thorac Cardiovasc Surg 69:858, 1975.
———, Chandra R, Baumann FG, Goldman RA: Myocardial reperfusion, a cause of ischemic injury during cardiopulmonary bypass. Surgery 80:266, 1976.
———, Gouge TH, Smith SJ, Stahl WM, Gombos EA, Boyd AD: The effect of diuretics on renal hemodynamics during cardiopulmonary bypass. J Surg Res 16:268, 1974.
Fishman NH, Carlsson E, Roe BB: The importance of the pulmonary veins in systemic air embolism following open-heart surgery. Surgery 66:655, 1969.
Flear CTG, Pickering J, McNeill JF: Observations on water and electrolyte changes in skeletal muscle during major surgery. J Surg Res 9:369, 1969.
Foglia RP, Lazar HL, Steed DL, Follete DM, Manganaro AJ, Deland E, Buckberg GD: Iatrogenic myocardial edema with crystalloidal primes: effects on left ventricular compliance, performance and perfusion. Surg Forum 29:312, 1978.
Follette DM, Fey K, Mulder DM, Maloney JV Jr, Buckberg GD: Prolonged safe aortic cross-clamping by combining membrane stabilization, multidose cardioplegia, and physiological reperfusion. J Thorac Cardiovasc Surg 74:682, 1977.
———, Mulder DG, Maloney JV Jr, Buckberg GD: Advantages of blood cardioplegia over continuous coronary perfusion or intermittent ischemia: experimental and clinical study. J Thorac Cardiovasc Surg 76:604, 1978.
Foote AV, Trede M, Maloney JV Jr: An experimental and clinical study of the use of acid-citrate-dextrose (ACD) blood for extracorporeal circulation. J Thorac Cardiovasc Surg 42:93, 1961.
Frank KA, Heller SS, Kornfeld DS, Malm JR: Long-term effects of open-heart surgery on intellectual functioning. J Thorac Cardiovasc Surg 64:811, 1972.
Fuhrman GJ, Fuhrman FA, Field J: Metabolism of rat heart slices, with special reference to effects of temperature and anoxia. Am J Physiol 163:642, 1950.
Gadboys HL, Slonim R, Litwak RS: Homologous blood syndrome. I. Preliminary observations on its relationship to clinical cardiopulmonary bypass. Ann Surg 156:793, 1962.
Galletti PM: The mechanics of cardiopulmonary bypass. In Cardiac Surgery, 2nd ed. New York, Appleton-Century-Crofts, 1972, pp 103–121.
Gay WA Jr, Ebert PA: Functional, metabolic and

morphologic effects of potassium-induced cardioplegia. Surgery 74:284, 1973.

Geha AS, Malt SH, Nara Y, Bave A: Effect of cardiopulmonary bypass on cerebral metabolism. J Thorac Cardiovasc Surg 61:200, 1969.

Gervin AS, McNeer JF, Wolfe WG, Puckett CL, Silver D: Ultrapore hemofiltration during extracorporeal circulation. J Thorac Cardiovasc Surg 67:243, 1974.

Gianelli S Jr, Conklin EF, Potter RT, Bonfils-Roberts EA, Mazzara JT, Moreno AH: Constant-pressure coronary artery perfusion during aortic valve operations. Ann Thorac Surg 22:347, 1976.

——, Grossi CE, Rousselot LM, Vastola JW, Ayers SM: Spontaneous fibrinolysis induced by *in vitro* admixture of human plasma. Ann Surg 161:89, 1965.

——, Mahajan DR, Navarre JR, Pratt GH: Anaphylactic-like reactions: a complicating factor in experimental extracorporeal circulation. Arch Surg 82:713, 1961.

Gibbon JH Jr, Miller BJ, Fineberg C: An improved mechanical heart-lung apparatus. Med Clin North Am 37:1603, 1953.

Gollan F: Criteria and requirements of adequate body perfusion. In Brest AN (ed): Heart Substitutes: Mechanical and Transplant. Springfield, Ill, Thomas, 1966, pp 105–115.

——: Carbon dioxide, waste product or elixir? J Mount Sinai Hosp 32:132, 1965.

——, Hoffman JE, Jones RM: Maintenance of life of dogs below 10C without hemoglobin. Am J Physiol 179:640, 1954.

Gott VL, Bartlett M, Long DM, Lillehei CW, Johnson JA: Myocardial energy substances in the dog heart during potassium and hypothermic arrest. J Appl Physiol 17:815, 1962.

Greenberg JJ, Edmunds LH Jr: Effect of myocardial ischemia at varying temperatures on left ventricular function and tissue oxygen tension. J Thorac Cardiovasc Surg 42:84, 1961.

Griepp RB, Stinson EG, Shumway NE: Profound local hypothermia for myocardial protection during open-heart surgery. J Thorac Cardiovasc Surg 66:731, 1973.

Gump FE, Kinney JM, Price JB Jr: Energy metabolism in surgical patients: oxygen consumption and blood flow. J Surg Res 10:613, 1970.

Hearse DJ: Reperfusion of the ischemic myocardium. (Editorial). J Mol Cell Cardiol 9:605, 1977.

Hearse DJ, Braimbridge MV, Jynge P: Protection of the ischemic myocardium. New York, Raven, 1981.

——, Humphrey SM, Bullock GR: The oxygen paradox and the calcium paradox: two facets of the same problem. J Mol Cell Cardiol 10:641, 1978a.

——, Stewart DA, Braimbridge MV: Myocardial protection during ischemic cardiac arrest: the importance of magnesium in cardioplegic infusates. J Thorac Cardiovasc Surg 75:877, 1978b.

——, ——, ——: Myocardial protection during ischemic arrest: possible deleterious effects of glucose and mannitol in coronary infusates. J Thorac Cardiovasc Surg 76:16, 1978C.

——, ——, ——: Cellular protection during myocardial ischemia: the development and characterization of a procedure for the induction of reversible ischemic arrest. Circulation 54:193, 1976.

——, ——, ——: Hypothermic and potassium arrest: metabolic and myocardial protection during elective cardiac arrest. Circ Res 36:481, 1975.

——, ——, Chain EB: Recovery from cardiac bypass and elective cardiac arrest: the metabolic consequences of various cardioplegic procedures in the isolated rat heart. Circ Res 35:448, 1974.

Hill DG, Sönksen PH, Braimbridge MV: Levels of plasma insulin and glucose after open heart surgery. J Thorac Cardiovasc Surg 67:712, 1974.

Hill JD, Aguilar MJ, Baranco A, de Lanerolle P, Gerbode F: Neuropathological manifestations of cardiac surgery. Ann Thorac Surg 7:409, 1969.

——, Osborn JJ, Swank RL, Aguilar MJ, de Lanerolle P, Gerbode F: Experience using a new Dacron wool filter during extracorporeal circulation. Arch Surg 101:649, 1970.

Hollenberg M, Pruett R, Thal A: Vasoactive substances liberated by prolonged bubble oxygenation. J Thorac Cardiovasc Surg 45:402, 1963.

Hottenrott CE, Maloney JV Jr, Buckberg G: Studies of the effects of ventricular fibrillation on the adequacy of regional myocardial flow. III. Mechanisms of ischemia. J Thorac Cardiovasc Surg 68:634, 1974.

——, Towers B, Kurkji HJ, Maloney JV, Buckberg G: The hazard of ventricular fibrillation in hypertrophied ventricles during cardiopulmonary bypass. J Thorac Cardiovasc Surg 66:742, 1973.

Jacobs LE, Klopp EH, Seamone W, Topaz SR, Gott VL: Improved organ function during cardiac bypass with a roller pump modified to deliver pulsatile flow. J Thorac Cardiovasc Surg 58:703, 1969.

Jennings RB, Ganote CE: Mitochondrial structure and function in acute myocardial ischemic injury. Circ Res 38(Suppl I):80, 1976.

———, Sommers HM, Smyth GA, Flack HA, Linn H: Myocardial necrosis induced by temporary occlusion of a coronary artery in the dog. Arch Path 70:68, 1960.

Jynge P, Hearse DJ, Braimbridge MV: Myocardial protection during ischemic cardiac arrest: a possible hazard with calcium-free cardioplegic infusates. J Thorac Cardiovasc Surg 73:848, 1977.

Kahn M, Goodman B, Litwak RJ, Gadboys HL: High flow whole body hemodilution perfusion: acid-base, renal, electrolyte and body fluid alterations. J Mount Sinai Hosp 35:111, 1968.

Kaplitt MJ, Tamari Y: Clinical experience with the Tamari-Kaplitt pulsator: a new device to create pulsatile flow or counterpulsation during open heart surgery (abstr). Am J Cardiol 39:260, 1977.

Kessler J, Patterson RH: The production of microemboli by various blood oxygenators. Ann Thorac Surg 9:221, 1970.

Kety SS, Schmidt CE: The effects of altered arterial tensions of carbon dioxide and oxygen on cerebral blood flow and cerebral oxygen consumption of normal young men. J Clin Invest 27:484, 1948.

Kirklin JW, Donald DD, Harshbarger HB, Hetzel, PS, Patrick RT, Swan HJC, Wood EH: Studies in extracorporeal circulation. I. Applicability of Gibbon-type pump-oxygenator to human intracardiac surgery; 40 cases. Ann Surg 144:2, 1956.

———, Lell WA, Baxley JG, Appelbaum A: Cardiopulmonary bypass for cardiac surgery. In Gibbon's Surgery of the Chest, 3rd ed. Philadelphia, Saunders, 1976, pp 846–866.

Kirsch U, Rodenwald G, Kalmar P: Induced ischemic arrest: clinical experience with cardioplegia in open-heart surgery. J Thorac Cardiovasc Surg 63:121, 1972.

Kouchoukos NT, Karp RB: Functional disturbances following extracorporeal circulatory support in cardiac surgery. In Ionescu MI, Wooler GH (eds): Current Techniques in Extracorporeal Circulation. London, Butterworths, 1976, pp 245–296.

Krovetz LJ: The physiological significance of body surface area. J Pediatr 67:841, 1965.

Lee WH Jr, Brady MP, Rowe JM, Miller WC Jr: Effects of extracorporeal circulation upon behavior, personality, and brain function: Part II; Hemodynamic, metabolic and psychometric correlation. Ann Surg 173:1013, 1970.

———, Krumhaar D, Fonkalsrud EW, Schjeide OA, Maloney JV Jr: Denaturation of plasma proteins as a cause of morbidity and death after intracardiac operations. Surgery 50:29, 1961.

Lees MH, Herr RH, Hill JD, Morgan CL, Ochsner AJ III, Thomas C, Van Fleet DL: Distribution of systemic blood flow of the rhesus monkey during cardiopulmonary bypass. J Thorac Cardiovasc Surg 61:570, 1971.

Levin MB, Theye RA, Fowler WS, Kirklin JW: Performance of the stationary vertical-screen oxygenator (Mayo-Gibbon). J Thorac Surg 39:417, 1960.

Levine FH, Philbin DM, Coggins CH, Emerson CW, Austen WG, Buckley MJ: Plasma vasopressin levels and urinary sodium excretion during cardiopulmonary bypass: a comparison of pulsatile and nonpulsatile flow. Surg Forum 29:320, 1978.

Litwak RS, Gadboys HL, Kahn M, Wisoff BG: High flow total body perfusion utilizing diluted perfusate in a large prime system. J Thorac Cardiovasc Surg 49:74, 1965.

———, Gilson AJ, Slonim RJ, McCune CC, Kiem I, Gadboys HL: Alterations in blood volume following "normovolemic" total body perfusion. J Thorac Cardiovasc Surg 42:477, 1961.

Lucas SK, Kanter KR, Schaff HV, Elmer EB, Glower DD Jr, Gardner TJ: Reduced oxygen extraction during reperfusion: a consequence of global ischemic arrest. J Surg Res 28:434, 1980.

Maloney JV Jr, Nelson RL: Myocardial preservation during cardiopulmonary bypass: an overview. J Thorac Cardiovasc Surg 70:1040, 1975.

Many M, Giron F, Birtwell WC, Deterling RA Jr, Soroff HS: Effects of depulsation of renal blood flow upon renal function and renin secretion. Surgery 66:242, 1969.

Mavroudis C: To pulse or not to pulse. Ann Thorac Surg 25:259, 1978.

McGoon DC, Moffitt EA, Theye RA, Kirklin JW: Physiologic studies during high flow, normothermic, whole body perfusion. J Thorac Surg 39:275, 1960.

———, Pestana C, Moffitt EA: Decreased risk of aortic valve surgery. Arch Surg 91:779, 1965.

Melrose DG, Dreyer B, Bentall HH, Baker JBE: Preliminary communication: elective cardiac arrest. Lancet 2:21, 1955.

Messmer K, Sunder-Plassmann L, Klövekorn WP, Holper K: Circulatory significance of hemodilution: rheological changes and limitations. Adv

Microcirc 4:1, 1972.

Mielke, JE, Hunt JC, Maher FT, Kirklin JW: Renal performance during clinical cardiopulmonary bypass with and without hemodilution. J Thorac Cardiovasc Surg 51:229, 1966.

———, Maher FT, Hunt JC, Kirklin JW: Renal performance of patients undergoing replacement of the aortic valve. Circulation 32:394, 1965.

Mills NL, Ochsner JL: Massive air emoblism during cardiopulmonary bypass: causes, prevention and management. J Thorac Cardiovasc Surg 80:708, 1980.

Mindich BP, Jurado RA, Estioko MR, Litwak RS: Administering cold cardioplegia in patients undergoing coronary artery bypass grafting. Ann Thorac Surg 31:188, 1981.

Moffitt EA, Rosevear JW, Townsend CH, McGoon DC: Myocardial metabolism in patients having aortic valve replacement. Anesthesiology 31:310, 1969.

———, Tarhan S, Goldsmith RS, Pluth JR, McGoon DC: Patterns of total and ionized calcium and other electrolytes in plasma during and after cardiac surgery. J Thorac Cardiovasc Surg 65:751, 1973.

Moore FD: Discussion. In Allen JG (ed): Extracorporeal Circulation. Springfield, Ill, Thomas, 1958, p 498.

Muller WH Jr, Littlefield JB, Dammann JF Jr: Pulmonary parenchymal changes associated with cardiopulmonary bypass. In Allen JG (ed): Extracorporeal Circulation. Springfield, Ill, Thomas, 1958, pp 336–341.

Nahas RA, Melrose DG, Sykes MK, Robinson B: Postperfusion lung syndrome: effect of homologous blood. Lancet 2:254, 1965.

Najafi H, Henson D, Dye WS, Javid H, Hunter J, Callaghan R, Eisenstein R, Julian OC: Left ventricular hemorrhagic necrosis. Ann Thorac Surg 7:550, 1969.

Neville WE, Colby C, Peacock H, Kronkowski TC: Superiority of buffered Ringer's lactate over heparinized blood as total prime of the large volume disc oxygenator. Ann Surg 165:206, 1967.

———, Kontaxis A, Gavan T, Clowes GHA: Postperfusion pulmonary vasculitis and its relationship to blood trauma. AMA Arch Surg 86:176, 1963.

Obel IWP, Marchand P, Du Plessis L: Biochemical changes associated with the use of haemodilution with 5% dextrose in water and mannitol for open-heart surgery. Thorax 22:180, 1967.

Osborn JJ, Swank RL, Hill JD, Aguilar MJ, Gerbode F: Clinical use of a Dacron wool filter during perfusion for open heart surgery. J Thorac Cardiovasc Surg 60:575, 1970.

Pacifico AD, Digerness S, Kirklin JW: Acute alterations of body composition after open intracardiac operations. Circulation 41:331, 1970.

Padula RT, Eisenstat TE, Bronstein M, Camishion RC: Intracardiac air following cardiotomy: location, causative factors and a method for removal. J Thorac Cardiovasc Surg 62:736, 1971.

Panico FG, Neptune WB: A mechanism to eliminate the donor blood prime from the pump-oxygenator. Surg Forum 10:605, 1960.

Paton BC, Rosenkrantz JG, Blount SG: Clinical and physiological results of perfusion with diluted blood. Circulation 29(Suppl I) :I–63, 1964.

Pennock JL, Pierce WS, Waldhausen JA: The management of the lungs during cardiopulmonary bypass. Surg Gynecol Obstet 145:917, 1977.

Peterson LH: Control and regulation of the cardiovascular system. In Physiologic Controls and Regulations. Philadelphia, Saunders, 1965, pp 308–333.

Preuss CJ, Gebhard MM, Bretschneider HJ: Myocardial "equilibration processes" and myocardial energy turnover during initiation of artificial cardiac arrest with cardioplegic solution—reasons for a sufficiently long cardioplegic perfusion. Thorac Cardiovasc Surg 29:71, 1981.

Prince AM, Szmuness W, Millian SJ, David DS: A serologic study of cytomegalovirus infections associated with blood transfusion. N Engl J Med 284:1125, 1971.

Rabelo RC, Oliveira SA, Tanaka H, Weigl DR, Verginelli, G, Zerbini EJ: The influence of the nature of the prime on postperfusion pulmonary changes. J Thorac Cardiovasc Surg 66:782, 1973.

Ratliff NB, Young WG Jr, Hackel DB, Mikat E, Wilson JW: Pulmonary injury secondary to extracorporeal circulation: an ultrastructural study. J Thorac Cardiovasc Surg 65:425, 1973.

Replogle RL, Merrill EW: Experimental polycythemia and hemodilution—physiologic and rheologic effects. J Thorac Cardiovasc Surg 60:582, 1970.

Rittenhouse EA, Mohri H, Dillard DH, Merendino, KA: Deep hypothermia in cardiovascular surgery. Ann Thorac Surg 17:63, 1974.

Rudy LW Jr, Heymann MA, Edmunds LH Jr: Distribution of systemic blood flow during cardiopulmonary bypass. J Appl Physiol 34:194, 1973.

Ryhänen P, Herva E, Hollmen A, Nuutinen L, Pihlajaniemi R, Saarela E: Changes in peripheral blood leukocyte counts, lymphocyte subpopulations, and in vitro transformation after heart valve replacement. J Thorac Cardiovasc Surg 77:259, 1979.

Salzman EW: Nonthrombogenic surfaces: critical review. Blood 38:509, 1971.

Sapsford RN, Blackstone EH, Kirklin JW, Karp RB, Kouchoukos NT, Pacifico AD, Roe CR, Bradley EL: Coronary perfusion versus cold ischemic arrest during aortic valve surgery: a randomized study. Circulation 49:1190, 1974.

Scheinman MM, Sullivan RW, Hutchinson JC, Hyatt KH: Clinical significance of changes in serum magnesium in patients undergoing cardiopulmonary bypass. J Thorac Cardiovasc Surg 61:135, 1971.

Schrek R, Neville WE: *In vitro* studies on the danger of use of mixed bloods for open heart surgery. Ann Surg 160:275, 1964.

Schwartz SI, De Weese JA, Niguadula FN, Gabel PV, Mahoney EB: Tissue oxygen "tension" at various flow rates of extracorporeal circulation. Surg Forum 9:151, 1958.

Shen AC, Jennings RB: Kinetics of calcium accumulation in acute myocardial ischemic injury. Am J Pathol 67:441, 1972.

Shragge BW, Digerness SB, Blackstone EH: Complete recovery of myocardial function following cold exposure. Circulation 58 (Suppl II):II-97, 1978.

Silva J Jr, Hoeksema H, Fekety FR: Transient defects in phagocytic functions during cardiopulmonary bypass. J Thorac Cardiovasc Surg 67:175, 1974.

Solis RT, Noon GT, Beall AC Jr, DeBakey ME: Particulate microembolization during cardiac operation. Ann Thorac Surg 17:332, 1974.

Stiles QR, Hughes RK, Lindesmith GG: The effectiveness of topical cardiac hypothermia. J Thorac Cardiovasc Surg 73:176, 1977.

Stoney WS, Alford WC Jr, Burrus GR, Glassford DM Jr, Thomas CS Jr: Air embolism and other accidents using pump oxygenators. Ann Thorac Surg 29:336, 1980.

Swan H: Clinical hypothermia: a lady with a past and some promise for the future. Surgery 73:736, 1973.

Swank RL, Hain R: The effect of different sized emboli on the vascular system and parenchyma of the brain. J Neuropathol Exp Neurol 11:280, 1952.

———, Porter G: Disappearance of the microemboli transfused into patients during cardiopulmonary bypass. Transfusion 3:192, 1963.

Taber RE, Maraan BM, Tomatis L: Prevention of air embolism during open-heart surgery: a study of the role of trapped air in the left ventricle. Surgery 68:685, 1970.

Tarhan S, Moffitt EA: Anesthesia and supportive care during and after cardiac surgery. Ann Thorac Surg 11:64, 1971.

Taylor HL, Tiede K: A comparison of the estimation of the basal cardiac output from a linear formula and the "cardiac index." J Clin Invest 31:208, 1952.

Turnier E, Osborn JJ, Gerbode F, Popper RW: Magnesium and open-heart surgery. J Thorac Cardiovasc Surg 64:694, 1972.

Tyers GFO, Todd GJ, Niebauer IM, Manley NJ, Waldhausen JA: The mechanism of myocardial damage following potassium citrate (Melrose) cardioplegia. Surgery 78:45, 1975.

———, Williams EH, Hughes HC, Todd GJ: Effect of perfusate temperature on myocardial protection from ischemia. J Thorac Cardiovasc Surg 73:766, 1977.

Waldhausen JA, Braunwald NS, Bloodwell RD, Cornell WP, Morrow AG: Left ventricular function following elective cardiac arrest. J Thorac Cardiovasc Surg 39:799, 1960.

Whalen DA, Hamilton DG, Ganote CE, Jennings RB: Effect of a transient period of ischemia on myocardial cells. I. Effects on cell volume regulation. Am J Pathol 74:381, 1974.

Williams BT, Sancho-Fornos S, Clarke DB, Abrams LD, Schenk WG Jr: Continuous long-term measurement of cardiac output after open-heart surgery. Ann Surg 174:357, 1971.

Wilson GM, Edelman IS, Brooks L, Myrdew JA, Harken DE, Moore FD: Metabolic changes associated with mitral valvuloplasty. Circulation 9:199, 1954.

Wollman H, Stephen GW, Clement AJ, Danielson, GK: Cerebral blood flow in man during extracorporeal circulation. J Thorac Cardiovasc Surg 52:558, 1966.

Wright JS, Osborn JJ, Perkins HA: Heparin level during and after hypothermic perfusion. J Cardiovasc Surg 5:244, 1964.

Zuhdi N: Hypothermic and hemodilution techniques. In Cardiac Surgery, 2nd ed. New York, Appleton-Century-Crofts, 1972, pp 159–181.

———, McCollough B, Carey J, Greer AE: Double helical reservoir heart-lung machine designed for hypothermic perfusion. AMA Arch Surg 82:320, 1961.

RECOMMENDED READING

Clowes GHA Jr: Extracorporeal maintenance of circulation and respiration. Physiol Rev 40:826, 1960.

Comroe JH Jr, Dripps RD: Ben Franklin and open heart surgery. Circ Res 35:661, 1974.

Eloesser L: Milestones in chest surgery. J Thorac Cardiovasc Surg 60:157, 1970.

Galletti PM, Brecher GA: Heart-Lung Bypass: Principles and Techniques of Extracorporeal Circulation. New York, Grune and Stratton, 1962.

Gollan F: Physiology of Cardiac Surgery: Hypothermia, Extracorporeal Circulation and Extracorporeal Cooling. Springfield, Ill, Thomas, 1959.

Ionescu MI: Techniques in Extracorporeal Circulation, 2nd ed. London, Butterworths, 1981.

Johnson SL: The History of Cardiac Surgery 1896–1955. Baltimore, The Johns Hopkins Press, 1970.

Meade RH: A History of Thoracic Surgery. Springfield, Ill, Thomas, 1961.

Messmer K, Schmid-Schoenbein H (eds): Hemodilution: Theoretical Basis and Clinical Application. Basel, Karger, 1972.

Nose Y: Manual on Artificial Organs. Vol. II. The Oxygenator. St. Louis, Mosby, 1973.

Peirce EC II: Extracorporeal Circulation for Open-Heart Surgery. Springfield, Ill, Thomas, 1969.

Zwart HHJ, Kolff WJ: Extracorporeal circulation for open heart surgery. In Blades B (ed): Surgical Diseases of the Chest, 3rd ed. St. Louis, Mosby, 1974, pp 664–701.

6. Patient Surveillance And General Care

Roy A. Jurado John J. Osborn

The clinical response to cardiac surgery is largely determined by the degree to which cardiovascular hemodynamics are improved by the operation. The magnitude of this improvement must be sufficient to favorably balance against the operative trauma and preexisting cardiac and related pathology. These factors are particularly apparent in open intracardiac operations employing extracorporeal circulation. At best, whole body perfusion currently is associated with a series of varyingly significant deleterious changes of organ system morphology and function. The postperfusion state generally is accompanied by some measurable reduction in cardiac performance (Boyd et al., 1959; Kirklin and Theye, 1963), relative instability of the intravascular and extravascular compartments (Carr et al., 1960; Kaplan et al., 1960; Litwak et al., 1961; Gadboys et al., 1962; Cleland et al., 1966), and a ventilation-perfusion defect (Osborn et al., 1962; Dammann et al., 1963; Hedley-Whyte et al., 1965). The nature and magnitude of these alterations are discussed in Chapter 5. Precise application of perfusion techniques and a maximally corrective cardiac procedure with minimal myocardial and pulmonary trauma are two of the basic elements of survival. The third element, postoperative care, primarily is designed to sustain and improve cardiac and respiratory function to avoid the disastrous effects of hypoxic acidosis (Moore, 1958), the most common cause of death following intracardiac operations. Additionally, the prevention and proper management of complications in the postoperative state are equally important objectives of care.

The fundamental intent of patient monitoring after cardiac surgery is the rapid and accurate acquisition of information about the performance of vital organ systems to ascertain whether convalescence is proceeding smoothly. Although the ultimate desideratum is a continuous comprehension of intracellular metabolic function, at present this cannot be accomplished. Therefore, other determinants must be employed by which it is possible to make certain deductions about such cellular function and to measure factors known to directly influence the stable state. Thus, the electrocardiogram permits discernment of heart rate, rhythm, and conduction characteristics. Adequacy of systemic blood flow and oxygen supply relative to tissue oxygen demand is inferred by sequential measurements of systemic arterial and atrial pressures, cardiac output, plasma oxygen and carbon dioxide gas tensions, hydrogen ion concentration, and body temperature. These and other measurements will be discussed in detail later.

The extent of monitoring is governed by the nature and severity of the cardiac lesion, coexisting pulmonary, renal, or hepatic pathology, and the technique and adequacy of the operative repair. One must also consider the influence of the trauma of extracorporeal circulation in further modifying the factors enumerated above. Certain closed intracardiac operations, such as mitral commissurotomy or juxtacardiac procedures such as division of an uncomplicated patent ductus arteriosus, generally do not require extensive postoperative monitoring, since the magnitude of the surgical and anesthesia trauma generally is insufficient to produce marked deterioration of cardiac or other organ function. As the pathologic and surgical complexity increases there is proportionately greater potential for significant cardiac and pulmonary dysfunction to occur, particularly after open intracardiac operations employing extracorporeal circulation. Logically, more extensive monitoring is employed in the postoperative management of these patients. It is imperative that monitoring be adjunctive in nature and must never substitute for careful bedside observation and analysis by the physician and nursing staff. Proper use of such techniques permits frequent quantitation of vital signs without unduly disturbing the patient. One should remember that an important part of convalescence is rest. One must skillfully balance periods when the patient is necessarily turned and examined with periods of quiet inactivity. This precept is particularly important in the postoperative care of infants and children.

THE CARDIAC SURGICAL INTENSIVE CARE AREA

A well-organized and well-equipped area is essential for the proper care of postoperative cardiac surgical patients. The intensive care unit concept satisfies this requirement by ensuring the concentration of well-trained staff and specialized equipment in one hospital area, thereby facilitating the care of critically ill patients. Details of intensive care unit design have been reviewed by Farrier et al. (1964) and Kinney (1966). More recently, the Committee on Guidelines of the Society of Critical Care Medicine outlined the general concepts of critical care unit design (Downes et al., 1972).

The specific requirements and available resources vary from one institution to another and the ideal setup is not always achievable. However, certain concepts are universally applicable. Design must provide for maximum surveillance and easy access to the patient, and the open, multiple-bed layout best answers this need. Although it is important to provide privacy to the patients, this is not an overriding consideration. Ample bedside space should be available (minimum floor space of 200 net square feet per bed in open, multiple-bed areas) to accommodate the necessary bulky equipment and personnel frequently required when an emergency arises. Individual isolation rooms must be provided for patients with communicable disease as well as for patients requiring reverse isolation. It has been suggested that isolation beds should be provided with a minimum floor space of 250 square feet per bed (Downes et al., 1972). Geographically, the unit should be in close proximity to the operating theater; this allows for rapid and expeditious bidirectional transport of patients, while permitting prompt treatment of those complications that might require operative intervention.

The unit should possess simple but precise monitoring equipment, ventilators, equipment for delivery of humidified oxygen, nebulizers, direct current defibrillators, pacemakers, hypothermia equipment, calibrated infusor pumps, blood-warming equipment, proper transfusion and infusion equipment, chest drainage and resuscitation equipment, calibrated urine collection receptacles, tracheostomy and emergency thoracotomy instruments, portable operating room lights, and a bedscale. Ideally, facilities for prolonged circulatory assistance and respiratory support should be available as well. Each bed should be provided with separate and multiple electrical, oxygen, and vacuum outlets.

A round-the-clock laboratory service must be provided for performance of rapid measurements of blood gas, pH, levels of glucose and electrolytes, and plasma and urine osmolality, as well as for carrying out routine hematologic, urine, and microbiologic studies. The ideal situation would be to have this laboratory situated adjacent to the intensive care unit, so as not to waste time and staff in transporting samples to and from the central hospital laboratories, which may be at some distance from the intensive care unit. Facilities for cardiac output measurement and routine pulmonary function tests as well as pulmonary artery catheterization should be available. Unit-based x-ray facilities must be provided and be comprehensive enough to cover most of the x-ray requirements in that area; this is necessary because critically ill patients usually do not tolerate even temporary disconnection from their life-support systems and monitoring devices, much less transportation to a remote area.

Ample ancillary space must be available next to the unit for storage of equipment, sterilization, utility rooms, kitchen, waiting rooms for relatives, office space, conference room, nurses' lounge, and sleeping rooms for physicians on call.

Maintenance of the highest possible degree of operational precision requires, above all, a stable, meticulous, well-trained, competent, and well-motivated medical, nursing, and paramedical staff working under the guidance of a medical director. It is advisable for the nursing table of organization to include a head nurse, an assistant head nurse per shift, and a staff complement permitting an overall nurse-to-patient ratio per eight-hour shift of 1:2, while maintaining a 1:1 ratio for the sickest patients. One auxiliary aide should be available for every four patients. Inhalation therapists, chest physiotherapists, biomedical electronic technicians, biomedical engineers, equipment technicians, and electrical safety officers should be made part of the critical-care team to free the bedside nurse to perform his or her specific functions. The quality of care can be further improved if the unit avails itself of the services of consultants from other disciplines, including medical cardiology, neurology, renal and metabolic diseases, infectious diseases, psychiatry, bronchoesophagology, physical medicine, radiology, and peripheral vascular surgery. A unit secretary is invaluable to carry out the numerous, time-consuming clerical duties associated with such an area. Finally, a unit manager is essential to relieve the nurses of some of the administrative load.

TRANSFER OF THE PATIENT FROM THE OPERATING ROOM

One of the most dangerous postoperative periods is the interval between the operation's termination and arrival of the patient in the intensive care area. During this time, hemodynamic and respiratory functional adequacy cannot be carefully measured and optimally controlled. Thus, any tendency of the staff to "let down" at this time can be lethal. The situation requires rapid but gentle transfer of the patient from the operating room with constant observation for signs of deterioration. At all times, careful attention is paid to ensuring airway patency and a satisfactory ventilatory pattern. The confusion of moving can be minimized by bringing the intensive care bed into the operating room and shifting the patient at that point. All monitoring and infusion catheters and electrocardiogram leads are checked after the patient has been transferred to his or her bed. If indwelling arterial and venous pressure lines have been used during surgery and are to be used in the postoperative period, they are filled with a dilute saline-herapin solution and occluded with a sterile end plug so that a direct connection to the transducer can be made immediately when the patient reaches the intensive care area.

The bed is adjusted so that the patient is in moderate semi-Fowler's position. Oxygen is routinely administered to all patients during transfer and is facilitated by a portable tank attached to the bed. The patient's electrocardiogram and pulse are monitored continuously. The ECG waveform is displayed on a portable battery-operated oscilloscope. Some portable monitors that incorporate a DC defibrillator as an integral part of the unit are now commercially available and are extremely useful. Pleural and mediastinal catheters are allowed to drain freely by gravity. An obvious but often overlooked detail is the need for the intensive care nursing staff to have sufficient prior knowledge of the approximate time of the patient's arrival so that everything will be in readiness. Patient transfer should be effected by the same team of physicians and nurses directly involved in the conduct of the operation.

ADMISSION TO THE CARDIAC SURGICAL INTENSIVE CARE AREA

Admission of the patient to the intensive care area requires the coordinated activity of a reception team of nurses and physician staff. A well-organized and disciplined effort by such a group may be life-saving for a critically ill patient. Immediately upon the patient's arrival, first considerations are directed toward prompt evaluation and support of the cardiorespiratory state. The quality and rate of the arterial pulse and airway patency are checked and appropriate connections made to visualize the electrocardiogram and arterial and atrial pressures. Pleural or mediastinal suction drainage is reestablished and ventilatory assistance initiated, if required. When respiratory assistance is not employed, well-humidified oxygen is administered either by face mask, tent, or nasal cannula, depending on the practice of the unit. If the patient is placed in an oxygen tent, the tent temperature is adjusted to maintain normothermic body conditions. Urinary catheter drainage is reestablished, a rectal thermistor inserted, and the patency of pleural or mediastinal drainage catheters ensured by frequent milking.

The patient's position in bed is adjusted according to his or her general condition. Unstable patients are allowed to remain flat in bed. When the patient's condition permits, he or she should be placed in a semi-Fowler's position with the head gatched up to 30 to 45°; this particular position promotes better pleural and pericardial drainage and improves ventilatory function by allowing the abdominal contents to fall away from the diaphragm. As in all postoperative situations, a common source of respiratory embarrassment is gastrointestinal distention. If this condition is clinically evident, nasogastric intubation and decompression are carried out. The tube is connected to an open plastic collection bag positioned at a level above the stomach, thereby minimizing loss of gastrointestinal contents while acting as an effective gas vent.

A quick but systematic "head-to-toe" evaluation is carried out, and a clinical baseline relative to the patient's overall condition is established.

EARLY GENERAL CARE

Patient Examination

A member of the physician staff must be in constant attendance in the immediate postsurgical hours and thereafter should be immediately available. A conscious attempt should be made to coordinate the required frequent periods of examination with nursing tasks (such as turning the patient and intramuscular injection of medications) so that adequate periods of rest are ensured. As previously mentioned, it should never be forgotten that rest is one of the indispensable components of convalescence and is of vital importance in the recovery of critically ill patients, particularly infants and children. After the hectic activity associated with reception has subsided, clinical assessment of the patient's general state can proceed in a more leisurely fashion.

Cardiovascular Subsystem. The pulse rate is recorded, which ordinarily would suffice for patients in regular sinus rhythm. The character of the pulse is also noted. For patients in atrial fibrillation, both apical (heart) and peripheral rates should be recorded and the corresponding pulse deficit noted. All peripheral arterial pulses are palpated. Asymmetry of pulses may indicate significant arterial obstruction (e.g., thromboembolism), while symmetrical diminution in pulse volume may indicate low cardiac output or peripheral vasoconstriction.

The fullness of the peripheral veins is noted; collapse of these veins may indicate hypovolemia. The temperature and color of the skin, especially of the face and the upper and lower extremities, as well as the capillary refill time are noted. A warm, pink skin generally indicates adequate blood flow. A prolonged capillary refill time, local cyanosis, and cold skin are indicative of diminished perfusion.

Auscultation of the heart is an essential ingredient in patient evaluation. The examiner should note the character of the heart sounds, the presence or absence of murmurs, the presence of a diastolic gallop, and the presence or absence of other adventitious sounds. Muffled heart tones may suggest a significant pericardial collection, while a diastolic gallop may indicate ventricular failure. On the other hand, one should remember that pericardial friction rubs are quite common after cardiac surgery.

Respiratory Subsystem. The position of the trachea relative to the midline is checked, which yields an important piece of information in determining presence or absence of mediastinal shift. Proper endotracheal tube position is established by noting the symmetry of the chest excursions and the character of breath sounds on both sides. Because of the anatomic orientation of the right main stem bronchus, not infrequently an endotracheal tube of improper length slips down to preferentially ventilate the right lung at the expense of the left. This could give rise to serious respiratory embarrassment, making early recognition and correction mandatory. The diagnosis of an improperly positioned endotracheal tube can usually be confirmed by chest roentgenography (Fig. 6–1).

A careful note is made of the nature and equality of the chest expansion, for this gives valuable information about the adequacy of ventilation. The presence of atelectasis, pneumothorax, significant pleural fluid collection, and left heart failure with pulmonary congestion or edema may also be suggested by careful examination.

In patients who are breathing spontaneously, the character and rate of the respirations may yield a valuable diagnostic clue and should therefore be carefully recorded. Rapid, shallow breathing with dilatation of the alae nasi suggests either atelectasis, inadequate analgesia with incisional splinting, or poorly compliant lungs, as seen in pulmonary hypertension and left heart failure with left atrial hypertension.

Central Nervous Subsystem. A cursory neurologic check can usually be performed reliably and with relative ease in the immediate postanesthetic state. The level of consciousness, pupillary reactions, and gross motor and sensory functions are noted. Unconsciousness or stupor, particularly when associated with discrete lateralizing signs of motor deficit, suggest cerebral damage from particulate embolism during surgery. Restlessness and anxiety in an otherwise conscious patient without lateralizing signs may be manifestations of a low cardiac output state. On the other hand, restlessness and delirium when associated with inappropriate jerky motor activity, with or without frank seizures, are usually indicative of the presence of a more diffuse type of central nervous system dysfunction, as seen following intraoperative air embolism. When cerebral dysfunction is suspected, a full neurologic evaluation is conducted (Chapter 16).

Renal Subsystem. Hourly measurement of the urinary output yields a fairly reliable index of kidney function and, indirectly, of cardiac performance as well. Indwelling urinary catheters are routinely inserted after anesthetic induction in all patients undergoing intracardiac operations employing extracorporeal circulation. This is especially important if dilute hyperosmolar priming solutions are used, since they are often associat-

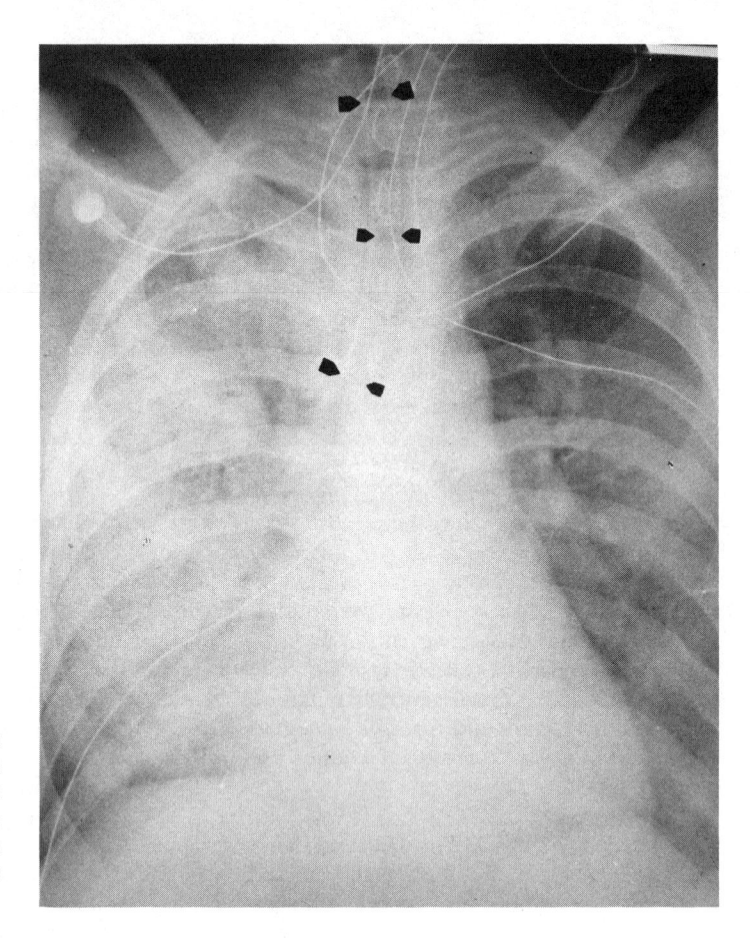

Figure 6–1. Postoperative chest roentgenogram showing slippage of an endotracheal tube into the right main stem bronchus in a patient who underwent repair of a posttraumatic ascending aortic aneurysm.

ed with large urine volumes during and after perfusion. Catheter drainage is continued postoperatively until cardiovascular and renal functional stability is ensured. The color, volume, and specific gravity of the urine are recorded hourly, while routine daily checks of the urine osmolality relative to that of plasma are made. In general, the passage of adequate volumes (minimum of 15 ml/hr/m^2) of clear, amber, hyperosmolar urine is indicative of adequate cardiorenal function.

Hemoglobinuria, when it occurs after extracorporeal circulation, indicates that significant formed element destruction has occurred. If only modest hemolysis has taken place the urine will remain clear, since plasma haptoglobin, an alpha 2 glycoprotein, stoichiometrically binds hemoglobin. This molecular complex is too large to be filtered by the kidney and is taken up by the reticuloendothelial system. Andersen et al. (1966) studied a series of patients after open heart surgery and found that hemoglobin appeared in the urine only when plasma hemoglobin levels significantly exceeded the binding capacity of haptoglobin.

Other Subsystems. Gaseous distension of the gastrointestinal tract, specifically of the stomach, is a common postoperative occurrence, especially in patients who require continuous assisted ventilation. The condition can be recognized readily, and treatment consists of prompt nasogastric intubation and aspiration.

The presence or absence of peristaltic sounds, hepatic enlargement, and ascites is also noted to serve as a basis for subsequent comparison.

Radiologic and Laboratory Examination

A portable thoracic roentgenogram should be obtained shortly after the patient's arrival in the postoperative care unit. Additional examinations should be made for the next two to three days and more frequently if clinically indicated.

A number of laboratory determinations should be obtained routinely after cardiac surgical procedures. After open operations these should include a complete blood count (including a platelet count), urinalysis, and measurements of hemoglobin, hematocrit, blood urea nitrogen, and serum electrolytes. If renal dysfunction is suspected the serum creatinine level should be determined in addition to measurements of plasma and urine osmolality. Microchemical methods should be used whenever possible in following infants and children. These examinations are performed for the first two postoperative days and on the fifth and seventh days. Patients undergoing closed cardiac operations generally do not require more than the usual postoperative laboratory profile that would be used in a routine thoracic surgical case, unless a complication occurs.

Temperature

Body temperature is measured continuously with a rectal thermistor. Frequently, the patient may have a subnormal temperature for the first hour or two. Covering the patient with a light blanket will minimize additional heat loss. Above all, shivering must be avoided, since the oxidative metabolic consequence of such muscular activity is enormous (Horvath et al., 1956). In addition to reducing cutaneous heat loss, small increments of opiate and chlorpromazine are helpful in management of this problem.

Additional information about the patient's hemodynamic status may be obtained if, in addition to core temperature, precise measurements of peripheral skin temperature are made. Earlier studies made by Joly and Weil (1969) suggest that continuous monitoring of the great toe temperature may yield valuable objective and prognostic information on the severity of shock, provided proper instrumentation is employed and appropriate corrections for changes in ambient temperature are applied. This technique is a refinement of the widespread clinical practice of "feeling the patient's skin"; it appears so appealingly simple and deserves further investigation.

Blood and Fluid Recording; Postoperative Bleeding

A careful record is kept of blood and fluid intake and output. Plasma, if administered, is considered to be blood in the calculations. One should remember that the arithmetic relationship between blood loss and administration cannot be used as the primary means of achieving and maintaining optimal intravascular volume. However, such a record is of assistance in following the pattern of blood loss, particularly in the occasional patient where significant volumes of blood are being put out through the drainage catheters. Excessive blood loss beyond four to six hours generally indicates the need for reoperation to search for a site of bleeding and removal of clots. It is therefore essential that a continuing effort be made to keep the catheters open lest a sudden reduction in measured blood loss be misconstrued.

The rate, amount, and pattern of blood loss and the patient's hemodynamic status are closely monitored. Chest x-rays are taken frequently. The possibility of "hidden" blood collections in the mediastinum or open pleural spaces and the ever-present danger of cardiac tamponade should always be borne in mind. The possibility of a coexisting coagulation defect should also be investigated.

Bleeding after *closed* cardiac operations is generally the result of insecure surgical hemostasis. Continued blood loss after whole body perfusion may also have the same cause; not infrequently, however, it can be associated with disturbances in the coagulation mechanism. When extracorporeal circulation has been employed and bleeding continues, the existence of a coagulation defect must be considered, although this possibility should *not* delay surgical reexploration in the presence of clear-cut indications. If hemodynamic stability can be maintained while a coagulation investigation is carried out, reoperation may be deferred when a hematologic defect has been recognized and treated or alternatively eliminated as a cause of the bleeding. If, on the other hand, the clinical situation is deteriorating, immediate reoperation is undertaken.

The following conditions are considered indications for immediate reoperation: (1) when signs of cardiac tamponade are present; (2) when blood loss is excessive or the bleeding pattern suggests insecure surgical hemostasis; and (3) when significant collection of blood occurs in open pleural spaces or mediastinum. Cardiac tamponade is an acute life-threatening situation that demands emergency action; it is considered an absolute and overriding indication for prompt surgical exploration. Blood loss is considered excessive if one or more of the following criteria are met: (1) the hourly estimated blood loss (HEBL) for a single hour exceeds 12 percent of the calculated blood volume (CBV); (2) the HEBL exceeds 10 percent of the CBV for two consecutive hours; (3) the HEBL exceeds 7.5 percent of CBV for three consecutive hours; (4) the cumulative blood loss at the end of the fifth hour $\geq$ 30 percent of the CBV; or (5) the cumulative blood loss at the end of the sixth hour $\geq$ 35 percent of the CBV. The pattern of bleeding is also an important consideration. For example, a sudden increase in blood drainage ($\geq$ 300 ml/hr), occurring in a patient who had no more than modest amounts of bloody drainage previously, may be ominous, especially if the blood is bright red and warm (suggesting active arterial bleeding). The above guidelines have been helpful in adult patients (body weight $\geq$ 50 kg), but should be modified for use in infants and small children.

Significant collections of extravasated blood in the mediastinum are likely to be accompanied by early or late tamponade. In addition, there is a potential danger of bypass graft compression in patients undergoing direct myocardial revascularization procedures. Bloody collections in open pleural spaces, although not posing an immediate threat to life, are generally associated with brisk hemorrhage. Significant hemothoraces interfere with early attainment of cardiorespiratory stability and are associated with late morbidity if not evacuated properly.

As mentioned previously, the presence of a coagulation defect should be ruled out; this will be discussed later in this chapter. In addition, a more detailed discussion of coagulation problems associated with whole body perfusion will be found in Chapter 15.

Fluid and Electrolyte Management

Administration of water and electrolytes after cardiac surgery is influenced by the general effects of anesthetic and surgical events on the kidney and further modified by preexisting cardiorenal dysfunction, which often requires that the patient enter the operating room in varying degrees of sodium, water, and nitrogen retention with or without potassium depletion. Water and electrolyte requirements may be additionally modified if whole body perfusion is employed because of the attendant volumetric, fluid compartment, and electrolyte changes (Chapter 5).

Sturtz et al. (1957) have recommended a basic fluid regimen that may be used with safety in virtually all postoperative cardiac surgical patients. These investigators have shown that a reasonable estimate can be made of daily obligatory water loss (the amount of water that would be lost on a postoperative day if a patient received no water) plus insensible and abnormal losses (nasogastric suction, diarrhea, visible perspiration) minus the metabolic water (the water of oxidation and the preformed water of catabolized tissue). This study, performed on children after whole body perfusion, led to a recommendation that the daily water need could be satisfied by the administration of 500 ml of fluid per m² on the first postoperative day and 750 ml per m² on each of the next two days. Experience has shown that somewhat more liberal fluid volumes may be administered to these patients with safety (Strauss et al., 1961; Mielke and Kirklin, 1966).

Electrolyte administration in the postoperative period should reflect anticipated sodium conservation and potassium loss by the renal tubules. Although sodium loss via all routes is relatively small for at least several days after surgery, it is not entirely negligible, especially if nasogastric decompression and drainage are used. Urinary loss of potassium after cardiac surgery generally is sufficient to require appropriate substitution therapy, especially if extracorporeal circulation has been employed in which the priming perfusate did not contain potassium. Under such circumstances, significant hypokalemia may be observed, which can provoke ventricular arrhythmias (Ebert et al., 1965; Obel et al., 1965, 1967). The potential for such events is further increased in patients who have either had intensive preoperative diuretic and digitalis therapy or who develop respiratory alkalosis during the course of postoperative assisted or controlled ventilation. A daily electrolyte regimen, applicable to pediatric and adult patients who have undergone either closed or open cardiac operations, consists of 5 percent dextrose in water solution administered in the volume described above and containing 40 mEq of sodium per liter, 20 mEq of potassium per liter, and 40 mEq of chloride per liter. A similar solution has been used by Humphreys et al. (1964).

Our own experience has shown that a more stringent postoperative maintenance fluid prescription schedule is not only safe but may actually reduce the incidence of significant pulmonary dysfunction in critically ill patients with severely impaired cardiac performance. The preferred intravenous solution is 5 percent dextrose in water. For adults, we have followed the program in Table 6–1. We have not found it necessary to use a sodium-containing solution since significant amounts of this essential electrolyte are almost invariably administered through other routes (heparinized intravenous "flush" fluids, drugs such as sodium penicillin, etc.). It must be remembered that the calculated total 24-hour fluid requirement is exclusive of blood and colloids required for optimal control of ventricular preload and maintenance of hemodynamic stability. The fluid prescription schedule used for children and infants is described in Chapter 19. A more comprehensive discussion of renal function and water and electrolyte management is given in Chapter 14.

Respiratory Management

Some degree of respiratory functional impairment is almost uniformly observed after all types of thoracic (Maier and Cournand, 1943) and cardiac surgery. Impaired respiratory gas exchange is almost invariably present in patients who have undergone corrective surgery with cardiopulmonary bypass; this is usually mild, and is most often characterized by arterial oxygen unsaturation caused by increased venous admixture (Fordham, 1965; McClenahan et al., 1965). Measurements of alveolar-systemic arterial oxygen gradients after open heart surgery reveal progressive widening, with a peak about 48 hours after the operation (Geha et al., 1966). A variety of factors contribute to such pulmonary dysfunc-

TABLE 6–1 SUGGESTED DAILY FLUID MAINTENANCE SCHEDULE FOR ADULT PATIENTS UNDERGOING OPEN INTRACARDIAC OPERATIONS*

Day of Operation	500 ml/m²/24 hours†
Postoperative Day 1	500 ml/m²/24 hours
Postoperative Day 2	750 ml/m²/24 hours
Postoperative Day 3	1000 ml/m²/24 hours

*Calculations based on body surface area in square meters (m²).
†Preferred intravenous fluid preparation is 5 percent dextrose in water; supplemental potassium added as necessary.

tion. In the first place, pulmonary function is frequently impaired in patients requiring cardiac surgery (Weintraub et al., 1965). Second, incisional pain and central depression (from the combined effects of anesthetic agents and postoperative sedation) both help to promote hypoventilation, retention of tracheobronchial secretions, and obstructive atelectasis (Dammann et al., 1963). Third, there is the varying but significant influence of extracorporeal circulation (Schramel et al., 1959; Tomin et al., 1961; Osborn et al., 1962; Neville et al., 1963).

The most commonly observed morphologic change in the postperfusion lung is the presence of numerous scattered regions of atelectasis (Tomin et al., 1961; Osborn et al., 1962; Hedley-Whyte et al., 1965a) with nonventilated but perfused alveoli. However, the anatomic basis for this physiologic phenomenon (i.e., arterial hypoxemia) may be considerably more complex than this, as suggested by others (Neville et al., 1963; Nahas et al., 1965; Williams et al., 1965; Awad et al., 1966; Veith et al., 1968; Panossian et al., 1969; Wilson et al., 1971). Loss of pulmonary surfactant has been described (Gardner et al., 1962; Mandelbaum and Giammona, 1964) and a moderate reduction in diffusing capacity has also been demonstrated (Howatt et al., 1962; Ellison et al., 1963). In addition, the data reported by Osborn et al., (1962) indicate that there is ventilation of some nonperfused alveoli. Other adverse factors include pleural effusion, pneumothorax, pulmonary emboli, pulmonary infection, and increased pulmonary capillary permeability (Kirklin, 1964).

The interaction of all these factors ultimately leads to an impairment of respiratory gas exchange and to an increase in the energy cost of breathing in the postoperative period (Christlieb et al., 1963; Thung et al., 1963). Moreover, since the postoperative metabolic demands are increased (Carlston et al., 1954), alveolar ventilation must be augmented in proportion to the increased oxygen demand. Although such functional alterations are frequently present in the total absence of clinical and radiologic signs, the net result is a situation where ventilatory reserve is reduced while metabolic demands are increased.

Preventive Measures. A more comprehensive discussion of measures routinely employed to prevent the development of postoperative respiratory failure is given in Chapters 12 and 13. However, some of these principles need reemphasis.

Certain operative measures will reduce the incidence and magnitude of postoperative respiratory problems. Transpleural procedures should be avoided whenever possible by approaching the heart through a midline sternal incision with careful preservation of the intact pleural spaces (Sullivan et al., 1966; Ghia and Andersen, 1970). During the course of open heart surgery, proper conduct of perfusion is mandatory, and adequate left heart decompression and intermittent pulmonary insufflation should be employed (Edmunds and Austen, 1966).

Patients deemed to be in satisfactory cardiorespiratory stability and who do not require mechanical ventilation are placed on a program of frequent deep breathing, coughing, chest physiotherapy, and turning from side to side. Well-humidified oxygen is administered for 24 to 48 hours by tent or plastic facehood. Failure to maintain adequate humidification during oxygen therapy contributes significantly to impairment of bronchial ciliary activity, with resultant thickening and drying of secretions. Normally, inspired air is warmed and fully saturated with water by the time it reaches the bronchi, and one must attempt to reproduce these conditions in the postoperative patients. Since the absolute amount of water held by any gas is determined by its temperature, it is essential that humidification devices be heated to approximately 55C (Wells et al., 1963). Maximal delivery of well-humidified gas to the alveoli is further ensured by reducing the water particle size to one micron or less by ultrasonic nebulization (Herzog et al., 1964). Indeed, such nebulization is so efficient that one must be aware of the possibility of overloading the patient with water (Bendixen et al., 1965;

Sladen et al., 1968). Proper humidification of inspired gases reduces the viscosity of secretions, prevents encrustation, and helps minimize postoperative atelectasis. Intermittent positive pressure breathing of humidified oxygen mixtures, when it is properly conducted in a well-trained and cooperative patient, also assists in raising secretions and reducing atelectasis.

Careful attention must be given to maintenance of adequate pleural drainage, if it has been employed. Portable thoracic roentgenograms are obtained immediately after the operation, the following morning, and thereafter as dictated by clinical events. In all patients who have had open heart surgery or who may have respiratory problems, systemic arterial blood gas measurements should be made shortly after their arrival into the intensive care area, two to four hours later, and on the following morning. If assisted ventilatory techniques are employed, additional studies may be required to ensure maintenance of proper gas tensions, particularly the carbon dioxide tension, which may be inordinately lowered by such methods.

Spontaneous vs. Mechanical Ventilation. With the complexity of cardiac operations and the acceptance of patients for surgery with highly limited cardiopulmonary reserve, frequent use of mechanical ventilatory methods to reduce or eliminate the postoperative work of breathing has gained wide acceptance (Bjork and Engstrom, 1957; Dammann et al., 1963; Clowes et al., 1964; Hill et al., 1965; Lefemine and Harkens, 1966; Provan and Austen, 1966; Pontoppidan et al., 1970). Indeed, Lowenstein and Bland (1972) advise a period of mechanical ventilation prior to extubation in virtually all adult patients undergoing open heart surgery. Since the postoperative state is attended by a reduction in ventilatory reserve, an increase in metabolic rate with a rise in the energy cost of breathing, and almost invariably by a reduction—albeit transient—in cardiac output, such a program would seem rational. This allows for a period of adequate ventilation and oxygenation while permitting a leisurely and unhurried assessment of the patient's cardiorespiratory status under optimal conditions.

In practice, patients are mechanically ventilated for 12 to 18 hours (generally overnight) and their ability to maintain satisfactory spontaneous respiration is evaluated the following morning. Immediate extubation and spontaneous ventilation are allowed only if at the end of the operative procedure: (1) the patient is awake, alert, and the anesthetic state fully reversed; (2) hemodynamic stability is maintained in the absence of supportive measures; (3) the prospects for early reoperation (i.e., for postoperative bleeding) are nil; and (4) the criteria for weaning from and termination of mechanical ventilation and for extubation are satisfied otherwise (Chapter 12).

In specific circumstances where cardiac or pulmonary function is considered borderline, it has been our practice to insert a nasotracheal tube prior to discontinuance of anesthesia. If the tube cannot be passed with ease, the patient is reintubated with a fresh orotracheal tube. Ventilatory assistance is carried out until the patient is alert and unassisted breathing can be maintained for a prolonged period with hemodynamic stability and satisfactory arterial gas tensions. If necessary, the endotracheal tube may be kept in place for as long as seven days. Laryngeal and tracheal damage is minimized by using a loose-fitting endotracheal tube (Lindholm, 1969) with a large-volume, low-pressure inflatable cuff (Cooper and Grillo, 1969). Beyond that period, the likelihood of permanent vocal cord injury increases, secretion removal becomes quite difficult, and the danger of tube obstruction by crusts increases. Tracheostomy is performed in such a situation; a plastic cannula with a large-volume, low-pressure inflatable cuff is inserted and mechanical ventilation continued.

For patients on mechanical ventilation, use of large tidal volumes with careful expansion of all pulmonary parenchyma has been shown to be effective in avoiding or minimizing postoperative atelectasis (Bendixen et al.,

1963). Tidal volumes of 10 to 15 ml/kg and respiratory rates of 10 to 15 breaths per minute are normally employed. Tidal volumes less than 7 ml/kg lead to progressive atelectasis (Hedley-Whyte et al., 1965b) and often to a distressing feeling of suffocation. If, on the above regimen, the arterial carbon dioxide tension ($Paco_2$) is below 35 mm Hg, an appropriate length of tubing is added between the ventilator and the endotracheal tube to serve as additional mechanical dead space. In the rare instance when a very high physiologic dead space causes carbon dioxide retention and hypercarbia, the respiratory rate is increased, maintaining a constant tidal volume, to lower $Paco_2$ to the desired level.

Synchronization and proper phasing with the ventilator may be difficult at the outset because of attendant hypoxemia and hypercarbia or patient apprehension. Sedation and temporary manual hyperventilation with 100 percent oxygen are helpful in establishing ventilatory control. Rarely, it may be necessary to resort to use of small increments of muscle relaxants (i.e., curariform and related agents). The inspired oxygen concentration (F_{IO_2}) is then adjusted to maintain a satisfactory arterial oxygen tension (Pa_{O_2}) of approximately 100 to 120 mm Hg.

Volume-limited vs. Pressure-limited Ventilators. Both volume- and pressure-limited ventilators are satisfactory in most circumstances if properly used. Although much has been written about the unique superiority of one type of ventilator over another, it is apparent that successful use of ventilatory equipment is largely a function of the patience and skill of the attendant staff and their knowledge of the mechanical properties and limitations of the equipment, as they apply to the ventilatory requirements of a particular patient.

Pressure-limited ventilators are driven by an air or oxygen source, and a peak pressure is set by a valving mechanism. The inspired gas mixture is delivered into the patient's lungs until this peak pressure is reached, when the inspiratory valve closes and the expiratory valve opens. The volume of inspired gas delivered into the patient is a function of the forces opposing the applied pressure (i.e., elasticity of the lungs, chest, and abdominal walls, the tone of the smooth muscles of the bronchi, the striated muscles of the diaphragm and abdominal wall, and the resistance to air flow in the respiratory tract).

In volume-limited ventilators, the inspired gas mixture is delivered by means of a piston pump. The volume of gas delivered is determined by setting the stroke volume of the piston, and the resultant peak pressure is dependent on the mechanical properties of the lungs and chest wall. The term *compliance* expresses the relationship between volume and pressure ($\Delta V/\Delta P$) and defines the change in lung volume per unit change in airway pressure.

Volume-limited ventilators are particularly useful when there are severe derangements in lung mechanics and compliance is poor or constantly fluctuating. Pressure-limited ventilators have the serious limitations of uncertain gas volume delivery (specifically when compliance is changing) and inadequate maximum inspiratory pressure in patients with markedly abnormal lung mechanics. In addition, when these ventilators are driven by oxygen, excessive concentrations of oxygen (greater than 90 percent) frequently occur even with the air mix (Venturi) valve turned on (Pontoppidan and Berry, 1967). The inspired oxygen concentrations may be lowered by using compressed air to drive the ventilator; even so, inspired oxygen concentrations are frequently unpredictable and close monitoring of F_{IO_2} and Pa_{O_2} is required. A more precise mixing valve may provide the most predictable way of regulating the F_{IO_2} in pressure-limited ventilators. In comparison, volume-limited ventilators provide a more reliable regulation of inspired oxygen concentrations.

Another important desideratum in a ventilator is a simple means of setting the rate and the ratio of inspiratory to expiratory time. (I:E). In pressure-limited ventilators, the pressure-volume relationship in the system (i.e., tracheobronchial tree, lungs, chest, and abdominal walls) largely determine the rate and the I:E ratio. For this reason, the settings will vary with changes in lung and chest wall mechanics and may, therefore, be difficult to control. To optimize venous return and cardiac filling, an I:E ratio of 1:2 to 1:3 is normally required. Some of the currently available volume-limited ventilators have this desirable feature.

Care of the Patient on Mechanical Ventilators. Careful observation of chest wall excursions, periodic auscultation of the lungs, monitoring of the arterial and atrial pressure fluctuations associated with respiratory cycling, and frequent checks of acid-base and blood-gas tension changes are the fundamental essentials for proper use of all ventilators. Management of a patient having mechanical ventilation through an endotracheal tube or cuffed tracheostomy cannula demands constant staff attendance and care. The cardiac and pulmonary dysfunction in these critically ill patients leaves but a slim margin of safety. The principles of respiratory care discussed previously are studiously employed: proper humidification, periodic position change and chest physiotherapy, and proper tracheobronchial toilette. Provisions should also be made for periodic manual and automatic hyperinflation (sighing) to minimize or prevent atelectasis. Despite the apparent adequacy of fixed ventilation volumes and pressures provided by respirators, there is a definite tendency for patients to develop foci of atelectasis and increased air flow resistance unless frequent hyperinflation is used.

Multiple checks of acid-base balance, gas tensions, and daily portable thoracic roentgenograms and electrolyte measurements are obtained. Tracheal aspirate cultures are obtained every other day. The emotional trauma associated with use of ventilators is considerable. The patient cannot speak and often is acutely aware of the precarious situation that might arise from a mechanical ventilator failure if the attending staff should momentarily absent themselves from the bedside. If possible, one arm should be left free so that messages may be written. A small bell left at the patient's hand is also comforting. Above all, gentle and calm reassurance is most important. In general, the more the patients know about their therapy the more comfortable and cooperative they will be. Occasionally it may be necessary to administer small increments of sedatives or tranquilizing agents to patients who cannot be reassured.

Weaning the patient from the respirator should be initiated as soon as possible consistent with cardiopulmonary stability, since prolonged therapy coupled with high inspiratory oxygen concentrations can produce life-threatening pulmonary lesions, characterized by congestion, edema, intraalveolar hemorrhage, and a fibrinous "hyaline membrane" exudate. Later parenchymal alterations include interlobular septal edema and fibrosis and hyperplasia of the alveolar lining cells (Nash et al., 1967). The principles and techniques of patient weaning will be discussed in Chapter 12.

Reduction of Factors Conducive to Hypermetabolism and Increased Oxygen Consumption

Oxygen consumption has been shown to increase after all major operations (Carlston et al., 1954), and this may be further augmented by hyperpyrexia, shivering, and apprehension. Elimination or reduction of those factors that contribute to increased energy expenditure will proportionally relieve the heart of the need to perform unnecessary work. Almost invariably, the trauma of surgery is associated with a moderate febrile response in the postoperative period. Roe (1966a) noted an association between intraoperative hypothermia and postoperative fever and suggested that a central thermoregulatory disturbance was responsible. Other more obvious factors are pre- and postoperative dehydration, wound trauma, blood infusion, and atelectasis. Mild hyperpyrexia immediately after surgery generally requires no therapy and will subside in two to four days. Severe temperature elevations following cardiac surgery require prompt management because of their attendant energy cost on the body in general and the heart in particular. DuBois (1936) showed that there is an approximately 13 percent rise in metabolic rate per one degree centigrade rise in body temperature. Pulmonary ventilation must increase in proportion to the increased oxygen demand. Cardiac output changes are variable but may increase up to 183 percent of afebrile measurements, and alternate early vasoconstrictive and late vasodilative responses are observed (Altschule et al., 1945; Bradley et al., 1945; Cranston, 1959).

Therapy of severe hyperthermic states is directed toward immediate fever reduction and elimination of the cause, if possible. Surface cooling by fluid evaporation of an alcohol-ice mixture is reasonably effective although somewhat disadvantageous, since the dressings and catheter sites must be protected from the cooling liquid and effective therapy requires continuous fluid application and therefore constant attention by at least one nurse or aide. A much more convenient method is the use of a hypothermia mattress. Coolant fluid is circulated through coils in the mattress, which is kept at 5 to 10C, thereby providing a substantial thermal gradient between the skin and mattress. Small intravenous increments of chlorpromazine (25 to 50 mg) aid in reducing or preventing shivering and cutaneous vasoconstriction. Temperature reduction should be controlled so that hypothermic levels are avoided, thereby minimizing the dangers of increased ventricular irritability that accompany such conditions. Salicylates have long been used for their antipyretic effect. They reduce temperature principally by inducing sweating, although they also appear to have a direct effect on the hypothalamus (Guerra and Brobeck, 1944). Although salicylates can themselves increase metabolic rate and oxygen consumption, the thermal reduction accompanying such therapy usually overrides their metabolic effects (Roe, 1966b). Nevertheless, circulatory alterations consequent to the fever may not be favorably affected despite the temperature fall (Roe, 1966a).

Mechanically assisted or controlled ventilation can significantly reduce the metabolic cost of breathing, as emphasized by Dammann et al., (1963). Normal humans expend 1 to 2 percent of their total oxygen consumption in performing the work of breathing (Bartlett et al., 1958), whereas postoperative cardiac surgical patients may have a twentyfold increase (Thung et al., 1963). Thus, in such patients with limited cardiac reserve, ventilatory assistance or control will reduce the energy expenditure of breathing and proportionally relieve the heart of the need to perform unnecessary work. Application of such techniques is discussed in the previous section and in Chapters 12 and 13.

Analgesia

It is essential that postoperative incisional pain be reduced to a tolerable level. Failure to do so will frequently result in the patient adopting a shallow and rapid respiratory pattern, which minimizes thoracic excursions and promotes retention of secretions. Proper analgesia must be individualized to blunt the pain while the patient remains alert. Morphine sulfate has proven to be satisfactory for patients of all ages and appears to offer a maximal sedative effect with minimal evidence of central depression. It is preferable that small increments of narcotic be administered relatively frequently. Morphine sulfate does not depress the myocardium and can be used safely in patients with marginal cardiac function. (Lowenstein et al., 1969); in fact, it may actually increase cardiac output, presumably by decreasing the afterload (Jurado et al., 1973). However, extreme caution must be exercised in its use in hypovolemic patients, since profound hypotension can ensue secondary to intravascular volumetric shifts due to alterations in vascular capacitance induced by the drug.

Infants often require no analgesia but

may be given 0.5 mg of morphine if restlessness persists. Doses of 1 to 2 mg in children and 3 to 5 mg in adults have proven satisfactory. It may be necessary to repeat these increments every one or two hours, as individually prescribed by the physician staff.

Postoperative Antibiotic Therapy
The rationale for preventive antibiotic management is discussed in Chapters 3 and 18. The antibiotic program instituted preoperatively is maintained in the postoperative period until the fifth postoperative day. The first postoperative dose of antibiotic is administered soon after the patient's arrival in the intensive care unit. It has been our practice to give cefazolin 1 gm IV or IM every six hours for adults. Infants and children are given a combination of penicillin (10,000 units/kg/day) and gentamicin (5 to 7.5 mg/kg/day in three divided doses). Adult patients with known allergy to cephalosporin are skin-tested to penicillin. If penicillin cross-sensitivity is ruled out, a combination of penicillin (600,000 units daily) and gentamicin (3 mg/kg/day) is used. The adult patient who is allergic to both penicillin and cephalosporin is given a combination of vancomycin (2 gm/day) and gentamicin (3 mg/kg/day), provided renal function is normal. Children who are allergic to penicillin are skin-tested to cephalosporins. If cephalosporin cross-sensitivity is ruled out, cefazolin (80 to 160 mg/kg/day) is given as the sole coverage. A combination of vancomycin and gentamicin may also be used in children with normal renal function at dosages adjusted to weight and age.

ASSESSMENT OF CARDIOVASCULAR SUBSYSTEM PERFORMANCE

Survival after cardiac surgery is, above all, dependent on the ability of the myocardium to alter its response to demands made on it. While a detailed discussion of the factors affecting cardiac output is beyond the scope of this chapter, it is apparent that the output of the heart is regulated by an interplay of rate and stroke volume. The latter is largely governed by myocardial distensibility, contractility, and outflow resistance. Both rate and stroke output are subject to a variety of neural, humoral, hormonal, and metabolic influences that serve to further modify the cardiac response at any given time. Analysis of cardiac performance, therefore, must involve observations and deductions that take these multiple factors into consideration. It is not possible to dissociate a discussion of postoperative cardiovascular function from such relevant factors as respiratory and renal function, fluid and electrolyte alterations, and acid-base balance, since they obviously are equally pertinent and interrelated.

Assessment of cardiovascular subsystem performance after intracardiac operations often can be satisfactorily accomplished by thoughtful appraisal of the patient's clinical appearance, electrocardiograms, urinary output, and blood pressure. Indeed, these observations alone generally suffice after closed cardiac surgery and differ little from the postoperative routine followed in general surgical patients. In open intracardiac surgery, these procedures often are supplemented by more extensive hemodynamic, blood-gas, and acid-base measurements. Table 6–2 summarizes the physiologic values routinely monitored after open intracardiac surgery.

Clinical Observations
Complicated equipment or measurements are not required to deduce that cardiac performance is satisfactory in a patient returning from the operating room who is alert, calm, breathing easily, and has a readily palpable and full pulse at an acceptably normal rate. Observations of the pulse rate, skin and mucus membrane color, nail-bed color, and capillary refill time, the level of consciousness, onset of restlessness, and alterations in ventilatory rate, rhythm, and volume are all important and simple means of assessing both cardiac and pulmonary function. Careful analysis of these

TABLE 6-2 OUTLINE OF CARDIOVASCULAR VALUES CONVENTIONALLY MONITORED AFTER OPEN INTRACARDIAC SURGERY

Measurements and Observations	Information derived
ELECTROCARDIOGRAM	Myocardial electrical phenomena: rate, rhythm, conduction, disturbances, ischemia
HEMODYNAMIC MEASUREMENTS	
Arterial Pressure	
Systolic	Upstroke of waveform: contractility Afterload
Diastolic	Pulse pressure (difference between systolic and diastolic pressure)
Mean	Effective perfusion pressure
Atrial Pressures	
Mean Left Atrial Pressure (LAP)*	Left ventricular filling pressure† Left ventricular end-diastolic pressure (LVEDP)† Left ventricular preload
Mean Right Atrial Pressure (RAP)	Right ventricular filling pressure† Right ventricular end-diastolic pressure (RVEDP)† Right ventricular preload
Cardiac Output	Actual measure of effective systemic blood flow
Other Measurements and Observations	

Clinical Appearance
  Sensorium, capillary refill time
  venous filling, skin temperature
Urinary Output
Acid-Base Measurements
	Indirect measures of the adequacy of systemic blood flow

*Pulmonary capillary wedge (PCW) pressure may be substituted for LAP.
†Assumes normal atrioventricular valve function.

signs may permit earlier recognition of clinical deterioration than some of the more quantitative measurements of a changing state. This will be discussed in more detail in a later section of this chapter.

Electrocardiographic Observations

A variety of operative circumstances influence cardiac rate and conduction in the postoperative period, and it therefore is important to continuously observe myocardial electrical phenomena. Moreover, proper control of both cardiac rate and rhythm is one of the important keystones in the maintenance of a satisfactory level of cardiac performance.

Hemodynamic Measurements

Measurement of Arterial and Atrial Pressures. Thoughtful use of arterial and atrial pressure measurements provides vital information about the postoperative cardiovascular state. These measurements are a function of three factors: cardiac output, blood volume, and vascular resistance. The integrative capacity of the cardiovascular system is such that changes in one, two, or even all three variables may occur without any significant systemic arterial pressure alteration until a relatively late stage of deterioration is reached. Atrial pressure measurements, on the other hand, are more sensitive aids in judging the effec-

PATIENT SURVEILLANCE AND GENERAL CARE

tiveness of cardiac output and whether optimal intravascular volume is present (Rehder et al., 1962; Kirklin and Theye, 1963; Fishman et al., 1966).

The rationale for use of such measurements is largely based on the experimental work of Berglund (1954), who showed that cardiac output could be maintained only if an adequate ventricular filling pressure existed. In turn, the filling pressure of the right and left ventricles at equal outputs depended on (1) the pressure-volume characteristics at end diastole (distensibility), (2) the work response to diastolic volume (contractility), and (3) the work required to overcome arterial resistance. Ventricular output equality therefore is regulated by volumetric shifts between the systemic and pulmonary vascular beds, thereby altering the filling pressure and adjusting the stroke work of both ventricles. Since the distensibility, contractility, and outflow resistance of the right and left ventricles differ in both normal and diseased states, it is clear that the functional dynamics of each ventricle can be inferred only by pressure measurements made in the ipsilateral atrium. Thus, right atrial pressures do not reliably reflect left ventricular function.

It has been our practice to directly measure arterial, right atrial (central venous), and left atrial pressures in all patients after open intracardiac surgery. For the reasons outlined above, left atrial pressure measurements in the absence of mitral valve disease provide invaluable insight into left ventricular function and should be used routinely in those patients for whom low cardiac output problems are anticipated (Fishman et al., 1966). Moreover, central venous (right atrial) pressure monitoring has been shown to be of limited value and, at worst, could be misleading as an indicator of left ventricular function in disease states affecting primarily the left ventricle (Forrester et al., 1971).

Figure 6–2 graphically illustrates the ventricular function curves under normal conditions and that of the left ventricle following acute infarction. Normally, the left ventricular end-diastolic pressure (equivalent to mean

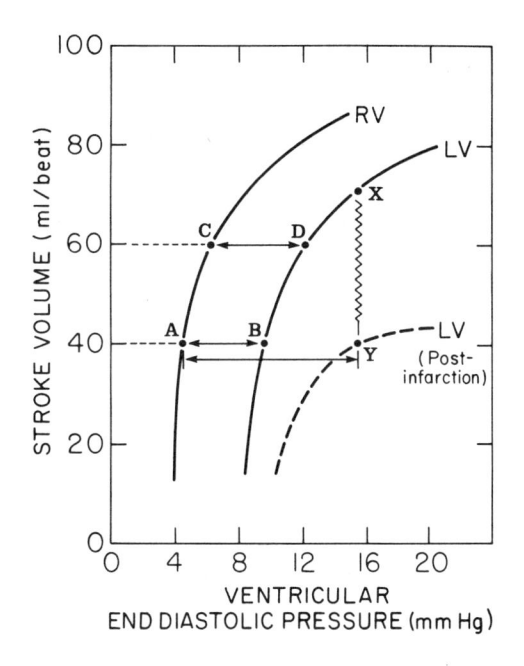

Figure 6–2. Simultaneously recorded Frank-Starling curves of the right ventricule (RV) and left ventricle (LV) in a patient who subsequently sustained an anterior wall myocardial infarction. Idealized LV function curve from the same patient after infarction is also shown for comparison.

left atrial pressure—LAP) is higher than the right ventricular end-diastolic pressure (equivalent to mean right atrial pressure—RAP) at a given level of forward flow, resistance, and work response to diastolic volume. This is primarily because of the inherent differences in compliance characteristics between the left and right ventricles, with the latter being more compliant than the former. The disparity widens up to the point (line AB vs. line CD in Fig. 6–2) where the horizontal limbs of both function curves begin to plateau. In the presence of left ventricular dysfunction, as occurs in myocardial infarction, the disparity is even greater (line AY vs. line AB in Fig. 6–2), and the left ventricular function curve is shifted to the right (line AY) and downward (wavy line XY). In the latter situation, the same level of stroke volume is, up to a point, attained at a higher left ventricular end-diastolic pressure with no appreciable change in right ventricular end-diastolic pressure.

Clearly, the implication is that the patient may already have substantially elevated left heart pressures, and, therefore, be at risk for developing pulmonary edema, while right heart pressures remain within the limits of normal. This has been the observation of several workers among critically ill patients (Forrester et al., 1970 and 1971) and in experimental animals as well (Hood et al., 1970; Kumar et al., 1970). This is in accord with our experience in patients recovering from open repair of acquired heart conditions.

Figure 6–3 shows the sequential changes in hemodynamic measurements during the early postoperative hours in a patient who recovered uneventfully after aortic valve replacement. There was a distinct disparity between LAP and RAP measurements immediately after repair, with the difference narrowing down with time. In contrast, the changes depicted in Figure 6–4 are those from a patient who succumbed following aortic valve replacement. The atrial pressure measurements remained widely disparate until death supervened on the sixtieth postoperative hour from a markedly reduced cardiac output.

In certain instances, however, RAP may be a more useful measurement to follow. This is particularly so in patients expected to have significant right ventricular dysfunction postoperatively—as happens following total correction of tetralogy of Fallot wherein extensive resection and reconstruction of the right ventricular outflow tract are required. Figure 6–5 shows the sequential changes in hemodynamic measurements in an 8-year-old boy who had ligation of a left Blalock-Taussig shunt and total repair of tetralogy of Fallot requiring extensive resection of hypertrophied septal and parietal muscular bands and

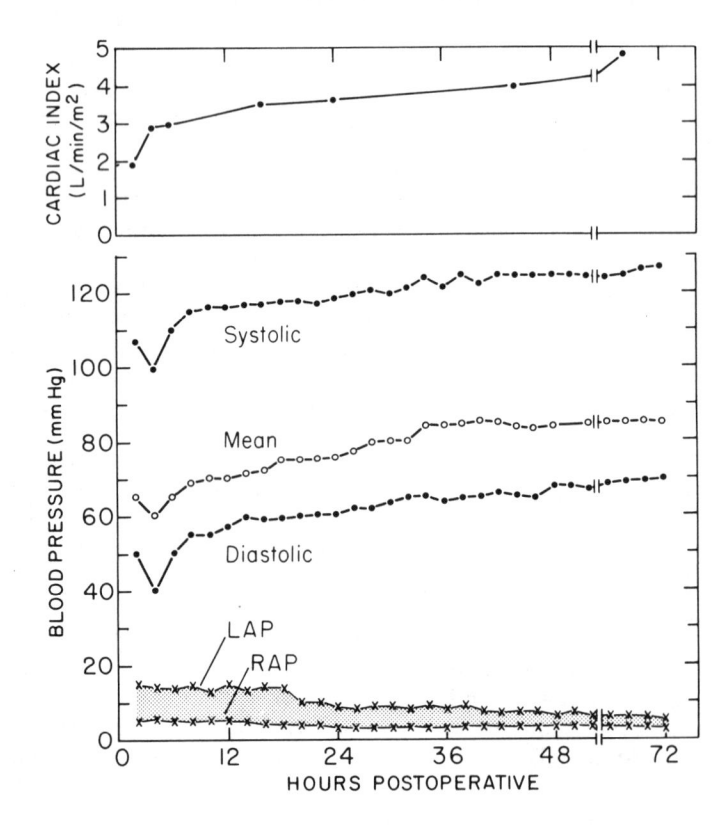

Figure 6–3. Hemodynamic changes in a patient recovering from aortic valve replacement illustrating "typical" disparity between left and right ventricular filling pressures. See text. (LAP = left atrial pressure; RAP = right atrial pressure.)

PATIENT SURVEILLANCE AND GENERAL CARE 137

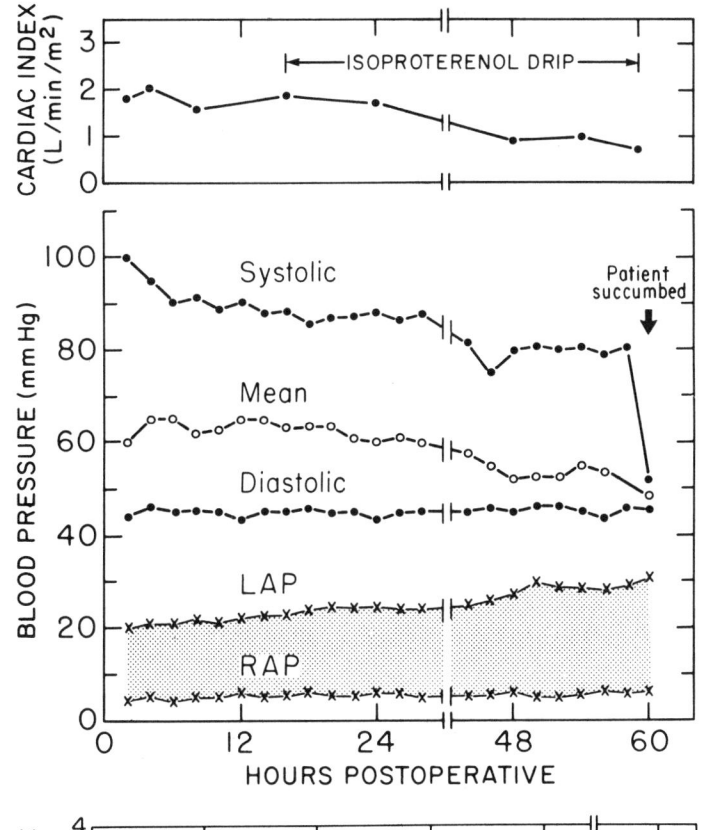

Figure 6–4. Hemodynamic changes in a patient who succumbed from severe left ventricular dysfunction following aortic valve replacement. Note markedly elevated filling pressures in the left compared to the right heart throughout the postoperative interval. (LAP = left atrial pressure; RAP = right atrial pressure.)

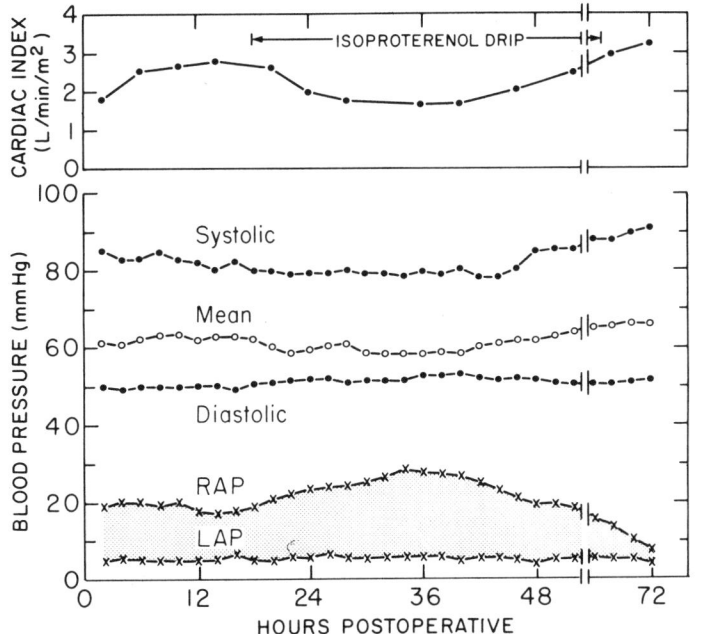

Figure 6–5. Hemodynamic changes after total correction of tetralogy of Fallot entailing extensive resection of right ventricular myocardium and outflow tract reconstruction with a pericardial gusset. Note that, in contrast to the normal pattern, filling pressures in the right heart are consistently higher than those in the left. (RAP = right atrial pressure; LAP = left atrial pressure.)

reconstruction of the outflow tract area using a pericardial gusset. The patient required inotropic and ventilatory support for 48 hours, during which time an enlarged, tender liver became palpable. The RAP remained higher (or had to be maintained at these levels to maximize systemic output) than LAP during the first two postoperative days.

The above examples point clearly to the importance of simultaneous right and left atrial pressure measurements in critically ill patients. In the absence of a direct left atrial line, a balloon-tipped, flow-directed catheter can be positioned easily in the pulmonary capillary wedge (PCW) position to monitor PCW pressure (Swan et al., 1970). Measurements of PCW pressure correlate closely enough with measurements of left ventricular end-diastolic pressure to be of value (Forrester et al., 1970).

Estimation of Cardiac Output. The performance of the cardiovascular system is assessed primarily in terms of *cardiac output* (systemic blood flow in liters per minute) *in relation to the function of the other organs and subsystems and to the metabolic requirements of a particular patient.* The cardiac output in normal people at rest averages 3.5 liters per minute per square meter of body surface area (range 2.5 to 4.4 liters/min/m² BSA). In the postoperative state (taking normal people convalescing normally from major surgery or major trauma), the cardiac output is elevated appropriate to the elevated oxygen consumption. Under the latter conditions, a cardiac index of 3.0 liters/min/m² or greater can be considered normal or adequate, provided the patient is not septic (Kirklin, 1971).

Present methods of assessing cardiovascular subsystem performance routinely include: (1) direct mensuration of arterial blood pressure and atrial pressures; (2) analysis of the character of the arterial pressure waveform; (3) observation of the cardiac rate and rhythm; (4) observations of the patient's clinical appearance, i.e., cerebration, skin color, and temperature, venous filling, and capillary refill time; (5) observations of urine flow and chemistry; and (6) obtaining of acid-base measurements. The information derived from these observations allows fairly reliable, albeit *indirect*, estimations of cardiac output to be made by deductive processes. In this regard these techniques represent a distinct advance over more traditional methods (e.g., feeling the pulse and repeated measurements of blood pressure by cuff manometry).

Thus, in the absence of a direct measurement, cardiac output may be assumed to be adequate in patients who are awake with full peripheral pulses, warm skin, pink finger- and toenail-beds, and who are able to maintain normal systemic arterial pressures at low atrial pressures (and therefore low ventricular filling pressures), continue to steadily produce an adequate volume of urine that is hyperosmolar relative to plasma, and have no major blood-gas or acid-gas deviations. In general, such patients have a cardiac index of 3.0 liters/min/m² or greater (Table 6–3). On the other extreme is the patient who appears anxious and perhaps disoriented, whose peripheral pulses are weak or absent, finger- and toenail-beds blue with delayed capillary refill time, skin of the feet cool, arterial blood pressure that may be *low, normal,* or *elevated,*

TABLE 6–3 CLINICAL SIGNS OF ADEQUATE CARDIOVASCULAR SUBSYSTEM PERFORMANCE*

Awake, reacted patient

Full peripheral pulses; good venous filling; rapid capillary refill time

Warm skin; pink fingernail and toenail beds

Ability to maintain *normal* systemic arterial pressure at *low* atrial and, therefore, *low* ventricular filling pressure

Production of an adequate volume of urine (15 ml/hour/m²) that is *hyperosmolar* relative to plasma

Absence of acid-base deviation

*Cardiac index generally > 3.0 liter/min/m².

and who may be oliguric (urine output less than 15 ml/hr/m^2). This patient generally has the classic signs of low cardiac output and will generally have a cardiac index less than 2.2 liters/min/m^2 (Table 6–4). Other patients distribute themselves normally between the two extremes.

The limitations of *indirect* methodology are apparent and underscore the importance of *direct* mensuration of cardiac output in certain clinical situations. Since the introduction of indicator-dilution techniques (Dow, 1956; Fox et al., 1957), other methods have been employed clinically (Berger et al., 1976). Unfortunately, such measurements are not performed when they should be or not systematically when they are. Discussions of the methodology, advantages, and disadvantages of currently employed methods of cardiac output measurement are given in Chapter 21. Irrespective of the particular method employed, one should remember that: (1) there is *not a necessary relation between the adequacy of cardiac performance and the level of cardiac output; neither is there a necessary relation between the arterial blood pressure and the level of cardiac output;* (2) cardiac output data should always be interpreted in the light of the patient's general metabolic activity as reflected in acid-base determinations and in measurements of mixed venous oxygen levels and total oxygen consumption, if the latter were available; and (3) the trend of the values obtained over a period of time correlated with the patient's clinical condition may be much more informative than any one isolated measurement.

Blood-Gas and Acid-Base Measurements

Properly conducted cardiac operations, including those in which extracorporeal circulation has been employed, should not be associated with more than minimal and transient deviations in acid-base balance. Development of postoperative metabolic acidosis is generally the *result* of reduced cardiac output rather than the primary etiologic agent, and, therefore, first considerations should be focused on prevention of acidosis by appropriate methods of support and augmentation of cardiac performance. Nevertheless, once present, metabolic (nonrespiratory) acidosis can itself further compromise cardiovascular function (Clowes et al., 1960; Darby et al., 1960; Campbell et al., 1958; Gerst et al., 1966). The deleterious effects of severe hypoxia and nonrespiratory acidosis on cardiac performance are well-known (Clowes et al., 1960, 1961). Respiratory acidosis may further complicate the picture and additionally reduce cardiac output and tissue perfusion. Clowes et al. (1961) have shown that at equivalent hydrogen ion concentration a greater depression of cardiac performance is observed with metabolic (nonrespiratory) than respiratory acidosis.

TABLE 6–4 CLINICAL SIGNS OF INADEQUATE CARDIOVASCULAR SUBSYSTEM PERFORMANCE*

Anxious, disoriented, perhaps semicomatous patient

Peripheral pulses weak or absent; poor venous filling; slow capillary refill time

Cool skin; blue fingernail and toenail beds

Systemic arterial pressure may be *low, normal,* or *elevated*

Oliguria (< 15 ml/hour/m^2)

Significant base deficit

*Cardiac index generally < 2.2 liters/min/m^2.

Properly conducted whole body perfusion should not be associated with significant alterations in buffer base and hydrogen ion concentration (McGoon et al., 1960; Litwak et al., 1965; Moffitt et al., 1967). Measurable but generally mild respiratory dysfunction is observed after closed and open intracardiac surgery. This latter problem will be discussed in Chapter 13. It is apparent, therefore, that postoperative acid-base relationships should be stable and relatively normal, provided that cardiac output is satisfactorily maintained.

Postoperative blood-gas and acid-base measurements are performed at frequent intervals after open intracardiac surgery. It has been our practice to routinely obtain such data at two-hour intervals for the first six hours postperfusion and on the following morning. More frequent observations may be necessary in critically ill patients, especially those requiring prolonged artificial ventilation or those with significant associated pulmonary dysfunction. For years, we have employed the method of Astrup (1960) to determine arterial carbon dioxide tension, pH, buffer base, standard bicarbonate, and base excess, using the normogram of Siggaard-Andersen and Engel (1960). Arterial oxygen tension is determined with a Clark electrode adapted to the Astrup apparatus.

More recently, we have adopted the "double pH method" described by Peirce (1962, 1967) to define acid-base relationships. A discussion of blood-gas and acid-base relationships is given in Chapter 7.

The oxygen saturation of mixed venous blood as a reflection of tissue oxygen levels has been used as an index of adequacy of cardiac output (Boyd et al., 1959; McArthur et al., 1962). However, it is apparent that postoperative alterations in metabolic rate (Sturridge et al., 1964), hemoglobin, and arterial oxygen content can all profoundly affect this measurement. It is therefore not surprising that Kirklin and Theye (1963) observed significant variability in the relationship between mixed venous oxygen saturation and cardiac output.

Recognition of Impaired Cardiac Performance

As suggested in the preceding section, it is extremely desirable to have quantitative estimates of cardiac output, especially in seriously ill patients. For the moment, it will be helpful to recall certain established concepts. Thus, cardiac output can be defined by the following relationships:

CO (ml/min) = SV (ml/beat) × HR (beats/min)

where CO is cardiac output; SV, stroke volume; and HR, heart rate.

Stroke volume or stroke output (ventricular output per heartbeat in ml), on the other hand, is determined by the interplay of three factors: (1) *preload,* which in turn is a function primarily of venous return (ventricular filling) and myocardial distensibility and compliance; (2) *contractility;* and (3) *afterload* (outflow resistance). Stroke volume is, generally, *directly* related to the stretch of the ventricular fibers at the end of diastole (preload) and to myocardial contractility, and *inversely* to the load-resisting shortening of ventricular fibers (afterload).

Applying Ohm's law to the dynamics of blood flow, the following relationship can be expressed:

Flow (CO) = $\dfrac{\text{Pressure}}{\text{Resistance}}$

or more precisely,

Flow (CO) = $\dfrac{\text{"Inlet" pressure minus "outlet" pressure}}{\text{Resistance}}$

A working knowledge of the aforementioned concepts is essential to the understanding and recognition of the various pathophysiologic alterations encountered in clinical practice. Table 6–5 outlines the different conditions that may bring about a reduction in stroke output and summarizes the distinguishing characteristics of each. Perhaps one of the most commonly used therapeutic maneuvers is to attempt to increase stroke volume and cardiac output by increasing intravascular volume and, therefore, ventricular end-diastolic pressure and volume, taking advantage of the Frank-Starling phenomenon (see Fig. 6–2). This usually is effective unless the ventricular end-diastolic pressure (similar to mean atrial pressure measured on the ipsilateral side) is already elevated (that is, over 15 to 18 mm Hg) and unless ventricular compliance is markedly decreased or intrapericardial pressure severely increased.

When cardiac output is low, atrial pressures high, systemic arterial pressure low or normal, the problem can be said to be one of

TABLE 6–5 A GUIDE TO THE DIAGNOSIS OF A REDUCED STROKE VOLUME

Primary Problem	Mean Atrial Pressures (Ventricular End-Diastolic Pressures)	Systemic Arterial Pressure	Systemic Arterial Pressure Waveform	Remarks
Contractility (Diminished)	High*	Low	Slow upstroke. Wide-based curve.	Rule out tamponade (myocardial restriction).
Preload (Reduced intravascular volume)	Low	Low	Sharp, rapid upstroke, rapid decay.	Pronounced "respiratory swing" may be present.†
Preload (Diminished myocardial distensibility; reduced compliance)	High*	Low	Narrow pulse pressure. Paradoxical pulse may be present. Upstroke may be rapid and sharp.	Must be differentiated from diminished contractility.
Afterload (Increased)	Normal or High	High	Normal upstroke; narrow-based curve. Pulse pressure may be reduced if diastolic pressure significantly elevated	If true cardiac output known, calculated arterial resistance is high. Arterial pressure may be normal.

*Mean atrial or ventricular end-diastolic pressure greater than 15 to 18 mm Hg.
†Variation in arterial pressure observed during respiration; peak systolic arterial pressure decreases whenever intrathoracic pressure becomes more positive; may sometimes be difficult to differentiate from pulsus paradoxus.

diminished myocardial contractility if pericardial tamponade is absent. The presence of reduced myocardial contractility calls for the use of an inotropic agent, while tamponade calls for prompt release of high intrapericardial pressure. When cardiac output is low, systemic arterial pressure high, atrial pressure normal or slightly elevated, and systemic arteriolar resistance high, the problem is most likely one of increased left ventricular afterload, and the therapeutic implications are apparent. It must be remembered, however, that two or more conditions may coexist. Moreover, compensatory mechanisms may become operative and unused reserves harnessed, rendering interpretation of physiologic data and selection of appropriate therapy complex. A more comprehensive treatment of this subject is given in Chapter 9.

Summarizing, attainment of satisfactory circulatory stability after cardiac surgery demands: (1) maintenance of optimal pressure-volume relationships within the heart; (2) support of myocardial contractility; (3) reduction of outflow resistance; and (4) optimal control of cardiac rate and rhythm. These factors are influenced by the nature and extent of preoperative myocardial dysfunction and intraoperative events, particularly after open heart surgery. Proper attention to details of perfusion, myocardial support, and a precise, minimally traumatic anatomic repair are the essential elements of cardiac function basic to survival.

ASSESSMENT OF VENTILATORY AND RESPIRATORY FUNCTION

Close postoperative monitoring of respiratory function is one of the essential elements in the care of the cardiac surgical patient. In general, the level of surveillance required is governed by the nature and severity of the cardiac lesion, the technique and adequacy of the operative repair, the duration of cardiopulmonary bypass, if it was employed, the quality of cardiac performance postrepair, and the presence of preexisting or coexisting pulmonary, renal, hepatic, or central nervous system pathology. Obviously, patients who have greater potential for or already are known to have significant cardiac or pulmonary dysfunction require more intensive surveillance. The sophistication of monitoring techniques and equipment used or of the measurement methods employed is largely determined by the resources available in a particular hospital. However, certain minimum requirements must be met to maintain acceptable standards of care. A comprehensive discussion of respiratory monitoring techniques and measurement methods is beyond the scope of this chapter and can be found in the publications of Pontoppidan et al. (1970), Osborn et al. (1968), Dammann et al. (1969), Peters and Hilberman (1971), and Turney et al. (1972).

The terms *ventilation* and *respiration* frequently are used interchangeably, for they generally are synonymous, but to many there is a subtle difference between them. Ventilation may be considered the mechanical movement of air into and out of the lung in a cyclic fashion, whereas respiration often refers to the exchange of oxygen and carbon dioxide in the lung and at the cellular level. The primary function of the lung is respiration, to supply the body with oxygen and to remove the waste product of metabolism, carbon dioxide. To fulfill this function, the lung must have adequate ventilation and perfusion, with the latter function controlled largely by a different subsystem.

The basic elements of respiratory monitoring include careful assessment of: (1) ventilation, lung mechanics, and ventilatory reserve; (2) blood-gas exchange; (3) cardiovascular subsystem function as it relates to pulmonary perfusion and gas transport; and (4) identification of other physiologic disturbances that are potentially deleterious to pulmonary function. Table 6–6 outlines the respiratory function measurements routinely monitored after open intracardiac surgery: this is the suggested basic minimum and includes tests that are readily available and easily performed. Cardiovascular function is monitored in the manner described in the previous section. In certain specific circumstances where respiratory insufficiency is suspected or has supervened, additional measurements may be required to gain a better insight into the nature and magnitude of the pulmonary dysfunction (Table 6–7). Such tests generally require special equipment and expertise, and, therefore, may not be readily available.

Central to all of the above is a carefully taken history and frequent examination of the patient, with particular attention to the cardiorespiratory system. In addition, chest roentgenograms and bacteriologic cultures of the tracheobronchial secretions are taken periodically. Careful accounts of daily fluctuations in body weight and changes in fluid and electrolyte balance are useful. Spot checks on the plasma protein concentration also are performed.

Measurements of respiratory rate, tidal volume, minute volume, peak airway pressure, inspiratory force, inspired oxygen concentration, arterial oxygen and carbon dioxide tensions, alveolar-arterial oxygen tension difference (when $F_{IO_2} = 1$), hemoglobin, and hematocrit can be performed with relative

TABLE 6–6 SUGGESTED OUTLINE OF RESPIRATORY FUNCTION VALUES TO BE MONITORED AFTER OPEN INTRACARDIAC SURGERY

Ventilation, Ventilatory Reserve, and Lung Mechanics
   Respiratory rate (f)
   Tidal volume (V_T)
   Minute volume
   Vital capacity (VC)
   Inspiratory force
   Peak airway pressure (P)
   Effective compliance (V_T/P)
   Mechanical dead space

Blood-Gas Exchange
   Inspired oxygen concentration F_{IO_2}
   Arterial oxygen tension (Pa_{O_2}) on mechanical ventilation
   Pa_{O_2} on spontaneous ventilation
   Arterial carbon dioxide tension (Pa_{CO_2}) on mechanical ventilation
   Pa_{CO_2} on spontaneous ventilation
   Alveolar-arterial oxygen tension difference (A-aD_{O_2}) when $F_{IO_2}=1$ and on ambient inspired oxygen concentration
   Hemoglobin and hematocrit

Perfusion
   See Table 6–7.

ease. Effective compliance is easily calculated by dividing the expired tidal volume by the peak airway pressure and provides a rough index of lung "stretchability." In the presence of airway disease, dynamic compliance measurements may be more meaningful, but are more difficult to obtain. As lung compliance decreases, respiratory rate rises while the tidal volume goes down; patients on volume-limited ventilators will show a rising peak inspiratory pressure.

Measurements of vital capacity, inspiratory force, and functional residual capacity (FRC) provide insight into the adequacy of ventilatory reserve, while timed vital capacity (FEV_1) measurements yield useful information in the presence of airway obstruction. Vital capacity and timed vital capacity measurements and estimations of inspiratory force require special equipment that is readily available. The determination of FRC, on the other hand, entails a more complicated setup. Similarly, special instrumentation is required for measurements of P_{ACO_2}, V_D/V_T, $\dot{V}_{O_2}$, and $\dot{V}_{CO_2}$. Right heart and pulmonary arterial

TABLE 6–7 SUGGESTED OUTLINE OF SPECIAL RESPIRATORY FUNCTION MEASUREMENTS TO BE PERFORMED ON SPECIFIC INDICATIONS AFTER OPEN INTRACARDIAC SURGERY

Ventilation, Ventilatory Reserve, and Lung Mechanics
   Dynamic compliance
   Functional residual capacity (FRC)
   Timed vital capacity (FEV_1)

Blood-Gas Exchange
   Arterial oxygen content (Ca_{O_2})
   Mixed venous oxygen content ($C\bar{v}_{O_2}$)
   Arteriovenous oxygen content difference
   Pulmonary end-capillary oxygen content (Cc'_{O_2})
   Right-to-left shunt ($\dot{Q}_S/\dot{Q}_T$)
   Alveolar (end-tidal) carbon dioxide tension (P_{ACO_2})
   Arterial to end-tidal P_{CO_2} difference
   Physiologic dead space-to-tidal volume ration (V_D/V_T)
   Oxygen consumption ($\dot{V}_{O_2}$)
   Carbon dioxide production ($\dot{V}_{CO_2}$)

Perfusion
   Pulmonary artery pressure
   Pulmonary capillary wedge pressure
   Cardiac output
   Pulmonary vascular resistance
   Plasma proteins; plasma oncotic pressure

catheterization to measure chamber pressures and to obtain mixed venous blood can now be readily accomplished using specially designed balloon-tipped, flow-directed catheters. Mean pulmonary capillary oxygen content may be calculated using alveolar P_{O_2} (either calculated or measured) with the assumption that hemoglobin is fully saturated, a condition that is reasonably satisfied if $P_{AO_2}, > 350$ mm Hg.

The ability to measure the oxygen and carbon dioxide tensions on both sides of the "alveolo-capillary membrane" is of considerable importance, for it provides valuable information about the adequacy and efficacy of blood-gas exchange. In the final analysis, respiratory function is measured in terms of the effectiveness of oxygenation and carbon dioxide removal. The efficacy of oxygenation is generally expressed by the alveolar-arterial oxygen tension difference (A-aD_{O_2}) and the degree of venous admixture (amount of right-to-left shunt) relative to cardiac output ($\dot{Q}_S/\dot{Q}_T$). The effectiveness of CO_2 removal, on the other hand, is expressed in terms of the arterial-to-end tidal carbon dioxide tension difference and the physiologic dead space to tidal volume ratio (V_D/V_T).

The interested reader is referred to standard texbooks of applied respiratory physiology and to the excellent monograph of Pontoppidan et al. (1970) for further elucidation. A detailed discussion of postoperative respiratory management can also be found in Chapter 12.

ASSESSMENT OF RENAL FUNCTION

Renal Response to Operative Trauma and Cardiopulmonary Bypass

The kidneys play a dominant role in the body's response to all forms of trauma, including surgery. An understanding of renal functional mechanisms and the derangements associated with major surgery is essential to proper postoperative water and elecrolyte administration. A detailed discussion of renal homeostasis following trauma is beyond the scope of this chapter and will be found in the publications of Moore et al., (1952, 1956), Elkinton and Danowski (1955), Hayes et al., (1957), Moore (1958a, 1959), Wilkinson (1960), deWardener (1961), Bland (1963), Kinney and Moore (1963), and Bartter (1964).

A measurable alteration of renal regulation accompanies all major surgery and is attributable in part to the combined effects of anesthesia and operative trauma (Coller et al., 1943; Habif et al., 1951; Hayes et al., 1957, 1959). Induction of anesthesia is associated with a marked reduction of renal blood flow and glomerular filtration, which is sustained throughout surgery (DeWardener, 1955). These alterations appear to be related to reduced cardiac output and neurogenically induced intrarenal vasoconstriction. Renal blood flow and glomerular filtration are further depressed in the presence of hypovolemia and may additionally be impaired by severe acid-base imbalance. Preoperative apprehension, fluid restriction, anesthesia, trauma, and hypovolemia all promote an excessive secretion of antidiuretic hormone (ADH). These pre- and intraoperative factors create a situation in which there is consistent reduction in the functional capacity of the kidneys to effectively clear nitrogen, hydrogen ion, and fixed acid radicals, three of the catabolic consequences of surgery. There is generally a prompt increase in both renal blood flow and glomerular filtration immediately after the operation. In the presence of adequate cardiac output and blood volume, these measurements will have returned to preoperative levels within 24 hours.

The adverse influence of anesthesia and surgery may also introduce a defect in maximum renal concentrating ability. Gullick and Raisz (1960) have observed a consistent intraoperative fall in urinary osmolality in spite of the ADH stimulating factors outlined above. Postoperatively, there is generally a distinct rise in urine osmolality, although several days may elapse before a normal concentrating capacity is apparent. In the presence of hemodynamic stability, the continued excretion of small volumes of a dilute urine beyond 48 hours may be the first signal of serious tubular dysfunction.

The volume of urine excreted in the postoperative antidiuretic phase is largely a function of the solute in the glomerular filtrate and is therefore primarily a measure of renal blood flow rather than tubular function (Kinney and Moore, 1963). Since glomerular filtration is, within limits, dependent on renal blood flow, the observation of satisfactory hourly urinary flow suggests that an adequate level of cardiac output is present. *The most common cause of a diminishing urinary volume after cardiac surgery is reduced cardiac output, which is frequently observed before there is a noticeable change in systemic arterial pressure or pulse rate.* Such a situation demands a thorough search for and elimination of the cause(s) of low output as the first consideration.

Renal excretion of sodium and water is sharply reduced after major surgical trauma. Depressed glomerular filtration with or without hypovolemia tends to provoke enhanced proximal tubular reabsorption of sodium, water, and urea, a "slow flow syndrome." Increased mineralocorticoid secretion further enhances the sodium retention, which may be observed for periods of up to six days after surgery. The sodium excretion then rises, and a negative sodium balance may be apparent during the second week. In addition to the enhanced proximal tubular reabsorption, elevated levels of circulating ADH promote a further increase in distal tubular reabsorption. Both factors, i.e., proximal and distal, cause a sharp curtailment of the kidney's ability to excrete a water load. The duration of this defect has been shown to directly correlate with the magnitude of the operative trauma (Hayes et al., 1957, 1959). Significant intolerance of a water load after surgery may be observed for two to three days in patients who presumably had normal cardiovascular and renal function preoperatively and even longer in patients with known cardiorenal disease, especially if congestive heart failure has been present.

It should be borne in mind that survival after trauma is largely dependent on the ability of the kidneys to conserve sodium and water, for this is one of the basic mechanisms by which the extracellular volume is maintained, which, in turn, sustains cellular metabolic exchange. If postoperative replacement consists of nonelectrolyte-containing fluids, an excess of water tends to be retained in relation to sodium, creating hypotonicity, which is reflected by hyponatremia. Oxidative metabolism provides an additional endogenous source of sodium free water, which further contributes to the hypotonicity.

In contrast to the renal retention of sodium and water, a marked elevation of potassium excretion is observed postoperatively for a period of one to two days and occasionally longer. Although the mechanisms governing potassium excretion are multiple, tissue damage, release of intracellular potassium, mineralocorticoid secretion, and "slow flow" are some of the factors that facilitate tubular secretion of the cation. Operative and postoperative hyperventilation sufficient to produce alkalosis potentiates this tubular loss, as does administration of steroid hormones and diuretics.

The preceding discussion has briefly reviewed what might be termed the normal renal response to operative trauma. It is apparent that the ability of the kidneys to effect the necessary postoperative homeostatic adjustments may be significantly compromised by factors commonly present in patients undergoing cardiac surgery: associated hepatic and renal disease, cardiac failure, drug-induced electrolyte derangements, and low cardiac output. Ordinarily operations performed with *properly conducted* whole body perfusion do not impose a uniquely deleterious influence on postoperative renal function unless excessively prolonged circulatory support, measured in hours, is required after completion of the intracardiac repair. This is not to say that use of extracorporeal circulation does not per se produce a measurable defect of kidney performance during the perfusion, for such is the case. There is usually a depression of glomerular filtration beyond that seen in the preperfusion period and a fall in the rate of solute-free water absorption (T^{c}H$_2$O). The rate of urine flow may be large, since it varies directly with the solute load (Goodman et al., 1965; Porter et al., 1966; Kahn et al., 1968) and perfusion pressure (Mielke et al., 1965, 1966), but the osmolality is depressed below normal at all rates of urine flow. Thus, use of hemodilution techniques employing hyperosmolar solutions tends to promote an osmotic diuresis despite the reduced glomerular filtration rate. Generally there is a prompt improvement in renal function in the postperfusion and immediate postoperative periods, although untoward consequences of perfusion such as excessive hemolysis, low cardiac output, and acidemia may alter the recovery pattern. To summarize, in the usual postperfusion circumstance, despite the possible preoperative existence of moderate renal disease or congestive heart failure with associated nitrogen retention, morbidity and mortality rarely result from primary renal failure. As previously discussed, renal alterations are functional rather than organic, and azotemia is more commonly prerenal and related to reduced cardiac output.

Evaluation of Renal Function

The adequacy of renal performance traditionally has been monitored by serial determinations of urine output and specific gravity, as well as blood urea nitrogen (BUN), serum potassium, and serum creatinine. All of these indices, however, have distinct limitations.

A *urine volume* that is inappropriately low ($<$ 15 ml/hr/m^2) or high ($>$ 40 ml/hr/m^2) deserves further investigation, but urinary volume, taken by itself, is an unreliable guide in assessing renal function. An abnormally low urine volume may occur if there is significant reduction in cardiac output from whatever cause, normal kidneys notwithstanding. Moreover, abnormally high urine volumes have been seen in patients with established acute renal failure (Baxter et al., 1964; Vertel and Knochel, 1967). While changes in *BUN and creatinine levels* are reliable indices of established renal function impairment, they are inadequate for early detection of acute renal failure. BUN and creatinine values are not significantly altered until approximately two thirds of renal function has been lost; moreover, these measurements are affected by a number of extrarenal disturbances. *Serum potassium* measurements are simple and universally available, but may likewise not be a sensitive enough indicator of incipient or mild renal failure.

The *quality of the urine* provides more insight into the status of renal function. Table 6–8 outlines certain indices of renal performance that are considered practical and useful in clinical practice. Tubular concentrating ability is most frequently assessed by measurements of urine specific gravity. Determinations of *specific gravity,* however, represent a poor substitute for *urine osmolality (tonicity).* Whereas urine osmolality (U$_{osm}$) indicates total solute concentration, specific gravity is only roughly related to osmolality in most clinical settings (Schoen et al., 1959). Moreover, specific gravity measurements are affected by the presence of albumin, dextran, and other high molecular weight substances that may be excreted in the urine (Baxter et al., 1964; Vertel and Knochel, 1967; Kassirer, 1971). Measurements of the *ratio of urinary to plasma osmolality* provide a better index of renal tubular concentrative capacity. In general, U$_{osm}$/P$_{osm}$ ratios of 1.7 or greater indicate good concentrating ability, while U$_{osm}$/P$_{osm}$ ratio of 1.2 is considered diagnostic of significant renal damage (Porter and Starr, 1969). One must, however, be aware of certain pitfalls in the interpretation of renal concentrative function studies, which have been reviewed by Kassirer (1971).

Baek et al. (1973) showed that measurements that indicate rate of removal of solutes from plasma may be more sensitive as indices of renal concentrative power, especially in the presence of oliguria. Specifically, they proposed that free water clearance measure-

TABLE 6–8 SUGGESTED OUTLINE OF RENAL FUNCTION TESTS TO BE MONITORED AFTER OPEN INTRACARDIAC SURGERY

Routine Tests

A. *Blood*
   1. Urea nitrogen (BUN)
   2. Na^+, K^+, Cl^-
   3. Creatinine
   4. Plasma osmolality (P_{osm})

B. *Urine*
   1. Volume* (UV)
   2. Specific gravity*
   3. Urine osmolality (U_{osm})

C. *Derived Measurements*
   1. U_{osm}/P_{osm} ratio
   2. Osmolar clearance $C_{osm} = \dfrac{(U_{osm} \times UV)}{P_{osm}}$
   3. Free water clearance $C_{H_2O} = UV - C_{osm}$)

D. *Special Tests†*
   Urinary Na^+, K^+
   Urinary creatinine
   Urinary urea nitrogen (UUN)
   Creatinine clearance
   UUN/BUN ratio

*Tests performed hourly until cardiorenal functional stability attained.
†Performed only when renal failure anticipated or suspected; all other tests done daily unless otherwise clinically indicated.

---

ments may be valuable in the early detection of acute renal failure. *Free water clearance* (C_{H_2O}) is derived from standard osmolar clearance (C_{osm}) measurements and is calculated as the difference between urine volume (UV) and osmolar clearance (see Table 6–8). C_{H_2O} values between -25 and -100 ml/hr are considered normal, whereas values closer to zero are said to be indicative of renal damage.

Measurements of *urinary sodium concentration* have been employed clinically to assess renal tubular reabsorptive capacity. A urinary sodium level of 40 mEq/liter or greater usually indicates significant organic tubular damage (Franklin and Merrill, 1960; Porter and Starr, 1969). The simplicity of the test accounts for its widespread use, but problems related to correct interpretation may limit its usefulness. Urinary sodium excretion is affected by a wide variety of factors, including the normal "metabolic" response to the stress of major surgery, sodium loading, sodium depletion, and changes in cardiac output and renal blood flow.

Estimation of *glomerular filtration rate (GFR)* may provide additional useful information, although its value is limited in the presence of severe oliguria. Calculations of GFR require measurements of serum and urinary creatinine and 24-hour urinary volume. Other tests employed clinically to assess renal function include serial measurements of urinary urea nitrogen (UUN) concentration (Selmonosky, 1969) and calculations of UUN/BUN ratios (Perlmutter et al., 1959; Porter and Starr, 1969). Urinary urea nitrogen values range between 1500 and 2500 mg %. A rapid and sustained fall in urinary urea concentration (Selmonosky, 1969) and a UUN/BUN ratio of 14 or less (Perlmutter et al., 1959; Porter and Starr, 1969) are considered to be indicative of renal failure.

The pathophysiology and diagnosis of acute renal failure are discussed in Chapter 14.

ASSESSMENT OF OTHER SUBSYSTEMS

Evaluation of Hepatic Function

Transient hepatic dysfunction occurring soon after cardiac surgery is not uncommon. The incidence of bilirubinemia (serum bilirubin greater than 1.5 mg %) has been reported to be as high as 76 percent in patients undergoing open intracardiac surgery (Robinson et al., 1967), but the incidence of clinical jaundice (generally associated with a serum bilirubin level of 3 mg % or greater) is estimated to be between 8.6 and 13 percent (Lockey et al., 1967; Sanderson et al., 1967).

A number of factors are important in the genesis of postoperative hepatic dysfunction. Severe preoperative congestive heart failure is an important predisposing factor, especially if accompanied by significantly deranged liver function (Kinglsey, 1966; Lockey et al., 1967; Robinson et al., 1967). Similarly, the type of cardiac lesion requiring correction appears to be an important determinant (Lockey et al., 1967; Robinson et al., 1967; Sanderson et al., 1967). For instance, the incidence of postoperative jaundice is higher in patients with acquired mitral valve disease (both as an isolated lesion or in association with aortic or tricuspid disease) than in those undergoing an operation for congenital heart or isolated acquired aortic lesions. This is not surprising, since mitral valve disease is frequently accompanied by right atrial hypertension, which in turn could cause hepatic congestion. The trauma of surgery, anesthesia, and extracorporeal circulation may further aggravate preexisting liver damage. Moreover, the increased pigment load from increased destruction of traumatized red blood cells, which occurs almost invariably during perfusion and early after surgery, may be detrimental. Following the operation, the occurrence of prolonged periods of low cardiac output may lead to progressive hepatic and renal failure (Mundth et al., 1967).

Fortunately, in most instances, postoperative hepatic dysfunction is transient and self-limited. In most cases, a benign, transitory rise in serum bilirubin, alkaline phosphatase, and the serum glutamic and pyruvic oxalecetic transaminases occurs during the first three postoperative days, with return to normal within a week. The occurrence of jaundice around the fifth to the seventh day or shortly thereafter usually is ominous. The latter pattern generally is seen in patients who have had severe congestive failure preoperatively and low cardiac output postoperatively; often there is associated renal dysfunction with a rising BUN level, and the prognosis generally is poor.

Hepatic function is monitored by serial determinations of serum bilirubin, prothrombin time, and alkaline phosphatase levels. Alterations in serum glutamic pyruvic and oxalacetic transaminase (SGPT, SGOT) levels may be misleading, as both measurements are affected by damage to other tissues, notably to the heart muscle from surgical resection and other causes. In certain instances, determinations of liver specific enzymes like isocitric dehydrogenase and lactic dehydrogenase isoenzyme 1 may be more informative (Kingsley, 1966). Determinations of serum albumin levels may be helpful in cases of prolonged illness. In most clinical settings, the above-mentioned tests are usually adequate for assessing hepatic function.

Evaluation of Central Nervous Subsystem Function

Disturbances of cerebral function after cardiac surgery, especially if extracorporeal circulation was employed, are usually secondary to organic brain damage. The clinical manifestations may take the form of psychiatric or neurologic disturbances of varying degrees of severity. The syndrome may become apparent shortly after discontinuance of general anesthesia or its appearance and recognition may be delayed for hours or even days.

A baseline neurologic check is routinely made by the attendant staff shortly after the patient's return to the intensive care unit. The level of consciousness, pupillary reactions, and the status of gross motor and sensory functions are recorded. A careful note of any involuntary or seizure activity is made. A check on the patient's neurologic state should be made part of the daily assessment of the patient's status. If neurologic dysfunction is suspected, a full and complete investigation is indicated. A more detailed discussion of neuropsychiatric problems following cardiac surgery can be found in Chapters 16 and 17.

Evaluation of Hematologic Function

A well-taken clinical history will help identify those patients who are likely to develop postoperative bleeding. In addition, patients undergoing cardiopulmonary by-pass will have had a preoperative coagulation screening performed (see Chapter 3).

Significant bleeding is perhaps the single most important hematologic disorder encountered in the early postoperative period. A full coagulation screen is performed if an abnormality in the hemostatic mechanism is suspected. Determinations of bleeding time, clotting time, thrombin time, prothrombin time, partial thromboplastin time, platelet count, and fibrinogen and Factor VIII (antihemophilic globulin) levels are helpful. Tests for fibrinolytic activity and fibrin split products are also important.

Exclusive of inadequate hemostasis, the most frequent cause of postperfusion bleeding is unneutralized heparin, which can be assessed by repetitive determinations of the activated coagulation time. If significant residual heparin activity is documented, supplemental protamine in an amount equivalent to the original heparin dose should be slowly administered in three divided increments over a 30-minute period (see Chapter 5). Although excess protamine can produce an anticoagulant effect, this dosage is generally substantially below that required for such a response.

Reduced levels of fibrinogen and platelets are rare causes of bleeding after perfusion, but fibrinolytic activity commonly is present (von Kaulla and Swan, 1958) and is a definite cause of postoperative hemorrhage (Kevy et al., 1966). Indeed, Kevy et al. have shown that plasminogen activator liberation is recognized after sternal division and before perfusion has commenced. They have therefore advised for open heart cases the prophylactic use of an inhibitor of plasminogen activation, epsilon aminocaproic acid (150 mg per kg), beginning immediately after sternotomy with continued infusion of the drug over a subsequent four-hour period. Fibrinolysis is effectively controlled by this regimen. Hypofibrinogenemia and thrombocytopenia are treated effectively by fresh whole blood. Alternatively, concentrated fibrinogen and platelet concentrates can be administered, although the former may lead to a thrombotic calamity and its use should be restricted to severe fibrinogen depletion (Salzman and Britten, 1965). Other disorders of the coagulation mechanism encountered postoperatively will be discussed in Chapter 15.

LATER CARE

Feeding

Until the return of peristalsis, no fluids are permitted to be taken by mouth except small increments of water given occasionally to partially assuage thirst. With return of bowel sounds a gradually increased feeding program is instituted, consisting of clear liquids followed by gelatins, custards, and soups. If well-tolerated, the diet is expanded to a semi-soft and finally a full diet. A one-gram sodium diet is prescribed for all patients who had a history of congestive heart failure before surgery.

Ambulation

A graduated program of arm and leg motion in bed, leg dangling, followed by short out-of-bed periods in a chair is begun once the thoracic drainage catheters and arterial and central venous pressure lines have been removed. The exact timing is individually dictated by the patient's capabilities and desires; the ambulatory program should not be rushed. Generally, patients who have had closed cardiovascular procedures are permitted out of bed on the first or second postoperative days and those who have had open cardiac operations are allowed out of bed between the second and fourth days. With gentleness and skill, one can often encourage a patient having prolonged assisted ventilation through a cuffed tracheostomy tube to leave his or her bed initially for a short time and later for progressively longer intervals.

Anticoagulation Therapy

Patients who have undergone prosthetic valve replacement are generally maintained on a strict anticoagulant regimen unless an overriding contraindication exists. Oral warfarin sodium is prescribed on the day the thoracic drainage catheters are removed (generally the second or third postoperative day); a one-stage Quick prothrombin time is drawn before administration of the drug. The initial dose is usually 20 mg, but a smaller amount is prescribed if hepatic dysfunction is present or suspected, which may be either primary or secondary to chronic heart failure. Therapy initially is controlled by daily prothrombin time determinations, with frequency reduced as stabilization occurs. Satisfactory anticoagulation range is deemed to be approximately twice the control level. Stabilization periods vary; considerable fluctuation can be seen for months after hospital dismissal and probably accounts for many of the thromboembolic complications of prosthetic valve replacement. Thus, prothrombin determinations ideally should be performed at two-week intervals, even in well-controlled patients. Imprecise anticoagulant therapy has been shown to provide virtually no protection against thromboembolic complications if maintained at less than optimal levels, and is also associated with a significant incidence of hemorrhagic complications if the therapeutic range is exceeded (Gadboys et al., 1967).

FUTURE PERSPECTIVES IN PATIENT MONITORING: THE ROLE OF DIGITAL COMPUTERS

Philosophy and Objectives

The primary objective of monitoring is the rapid and accurate acquisition of physiologic information by which it is possible to make certain deductions about the performance of the major subsystems. Such vital information is of inestimable value in following a patient's response to illness and evaluating the effect of therapy. After the operation, the information obtained allows accurate assessment of the patient's response to operative trauma and helps ascertain whether recovery is proceeding smoothly. Moreover, it provides valuable insight into changes in the patient's physiologic state and helps identify actual or potential crises.

Regardless of the techniques employed, monitoring in the critically ill must combine effective use of frequent direct observations by the attendant staff and precise quantitative measurements of vital physiologic functions made with the aid of reliable sensors and other electromechanical devices. The person-machine concept, as it relates to patient monitoring and as originally advanced by Maloney (1968), is now widely accepted.

Accurate bedside assessment of the function of almost every vital organ system in the critically ill has been made possible by the advent of modern instrumentation and the development of sophisticated measurement methods. The digital computer has played no small role in this area of endeavor. Measurement methods have been developed based on the use of unobtrusive physiologic sensors, with processing by digital computer and bedside display of numerical and graphic data. In designing such systems, the object has always been—and will always be—to yield the most information from the smallest number of physiologic sensors with the least possible disturbance of the patient.

The Role of Digital Computers

A comprehensive discussion of existing computer-based physiologic monitoring systems and their relative merits is beyond the scope of this chapter. The interested reader is referred to the original reports of Miller et al. (1966), Shubin and Weil (1966), Lewis et al. (1966), Siegel and del Guercio (1967), Mortensen and Anderson (1968), Sheppard et al. (1968), Warner et al. (1968), Osborn et al. (1968), Dammann et al. (1969) and the review made by Siegel (1977).

Currently operational computer-assisted monitoring systems differ in their approaches, in the algorithms and measurement methods employed, and even in their stated goals. However, a common initial objective appears to be the rapid acquisition of more physiologic information than is currently obtainable by conventional measurement methods. In the critical-care setting, the digital computer acquires and stores physiologic information. It then organizes and analyzes the information acquired and presents it in formats that are easily understood by the attendant staff. It can be programmed to identify abnormal patterns, recognize unfavorable physiologic trends, suggest diagnoses, warn the physician of potential crises, and, perhaps, enable the physician to better handle crises when they actually arise. The virtually continuous surveillance provided by the computer also has helped the clinician better understand heretofore inexplicable, sudden, untoward occurrences (Osborn et al., 1971). Moreover, by using simple rules of logic, the computer may also be relied on to initiate certain therapeutic interventions and terminate them when no longer indicated (Sheppard et al., 1968; Morgan et al., 1973).

There is now persuasive evidence that computer-based online physiologic monitoring is an extremely useful adjunct in the care of critically ill patients (Mortensen and Anderson, 1968; Sheppard et al., 1973; Osborn et al., 1968; Morgan et al., 1973; Jurado et al., 1977). Indeed, the digital computer has become a powerful clinical tool.

Description of a Computer-Based Monitoring System

In this section, we will briefly describe a measurement and monitoring system that has been in use at the Presbyterian Hospital of Pacific Medical Center (San Francisco) and at the Mount Sinai Medical Center (New York). The deployment of such a system in a clinical setting was first reported by Osborn et al. (1968).

The heart of the system consists of a central processing unit with a 48 K-word, 2-μ sec cycle time memory (IBM 1800 digital computer) supported by three 500,000 word-disk memories, a card read-punch unit, a line printer, a console keyboard printer, and a plotter. A typical bedside terminal inputs eight high-level analog signals, which are typically EKG, any three blood pressures (arterial, right and left atrial, or pulmonary artery or pulmonary capillary wedge), respiratory flow, respiratory pressure, partial pressures of oxygen, and carbon dioxide in both inspired and expired air. One or more low-level signals are monitored, typically body temperature, a 16-key keyboard, and a TV monitor. All communications with the system are performed via a 16-digit keyboard, and measurements are automatically made every 10 minutes and additionally on request. The analysis is done on 30 seconds of respiratory data and 10 seconds of cardiovascular data.

Body temperature signals are collected from a thermistor probe attached to the patient. The EKG signal is detected through standard paste-on electrodes. Respiratory flow and pressures are measured through a modified Fleisch pneumotachograph interposed in the respiratory line that feeds samples to a pressure gauge, a differential pressure transducer, and oxygen and carbon dioxide analyzers. Blood pressures are measured through catheters positioned in appropriate vascular chambers. Blood chemistry and cardiac output variables are read from semiautomatic test equipment operating on-line to the computer.

Using the above readings, the computer derives more than 20 additional values. The EKG gives heart rate and ectopic beat rate. The blood pressure signals provide systolic and diastolic pressures, pulse rate, rate of rise of arterial pressure per unit time, dp/dt (which is a rough index of ventricular contractility), and mean arterial, venous, and left atrial pressures. The respiratory flow and pressure are used to obtain respiratory mechanics data, such as respiratory rate, tidal and minute volume, lung compliance, nonelastic resistance, and work of inspiration. The flow and gas values supply oxygen uptake, carbon dioxide production, respiratory quotient, end-expiratory carbon dioxide tension (P_{ACO_2}) inspired, and alveolar oxygen concentrations. Combinations of data are used to obtain such measures as Fick cardiac output, alveolar-arterial oxygen gradient (A-aD_{O_2}), the physiologic dead space to tidal volume ratio (V_D/V_T), and shunt fraction ($\dot{Q}_S/\dot{Q}_T$). The stress laid on measurements of ventilatory and respiratory variables derives from the fact that pulmonary dysfunction is the second most common cause of death in patients undergoing intracardiac surgery (second only to low cardiac output). Several types of instrumentation may be interfaced with the system and used intermittently; the principal devices employed are a densitometer, an oximeter, and an indwelling intravascular thermistor. Blood-gas and chemistry data can be manually entered.

Figure 6-6 outlines the physiologic variables measured online. In addition to alphanumeric TV display (Fig. 6-7), graphic trend plots (Fig. 6-8) are readily available at the bedside terminals. Pressure-volume plots of inspiratory half-loops (Fig. 6-9) are also automatically generated. These have been extremely useful in following changes in lung mechanics and in the early recognition of airway obstruction. Messages and alarms are also displayed, generally triggering interventions and becoming exceedingly important when some trend toward instability is noted (Benis et al., 1980).

Hard-copy printouts of alphanumeric and graphic data are automatically generated once every 24 hours. They are available for staff review and become part of the patient's permanent hospital record. By taking over this clerical function, the computer frees the nurse of the burden and enables him or her to devote more time to direct patient care. Moreover, the system insures continuous acquisition of physiologic data during moments of crisis (as in cardiac arrest situations) when everyone else is busy "trying to do something" for the patient.

The Future

An area of great concern to us is the precision and reliability of computer-generated measurements made under varying physiologic conditions. A significant portion of our investigational efforts will be expended on improving measurement accuracy as newer techniques are developed. While the system just described can be considered advanced by most standards, additional programs are contemplated.

Although cardiac output currently can be measured with relative ease, this provides only a rough index of ventricular performance and pump efficiency. Beat-to-beat measurements of stroke volume and ventricular pressure combined with real-time analysis of myocardial contractility (Brody et al., 1973) and estimation of ventricular volumes employing ultrasonographic techniques may provide more meaningful information. Unfortunately, currently available methods of estimating stroke volume from the pressure pulse are not accurate enough (Jurado et al., 1973). Other methods (e.g., Doppler echocardiography), such as those described by Steingart et al. (1980) need to be looked into. Moreover, the methods employed for estimating myocardial contractility and ventricular volumes need further refinement and validation.

One of our short-term goals would be to improve our early warning system for prompt recognition of unfavorable physiologic trends.

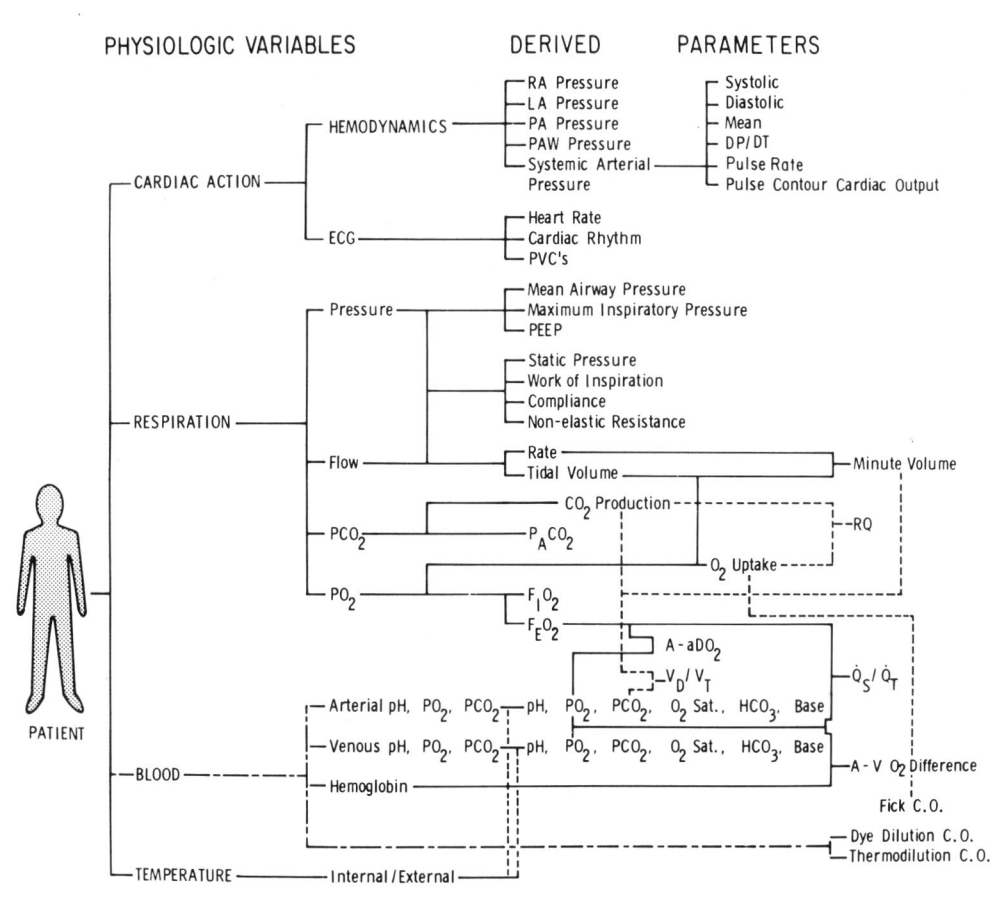

Figure 6–6. Schematic diagram of physiologic variables and derived parameters acquired, stored, and displayed by the computer. The solid lines indicate those variables and parameters automatically measured. The broken lines indicate those that are either measured intermittently or are manually entered. The dashed lines indicate computer-generated derived calculations. Additional details in text.

This will require complex program changes and new algorithms using multivariate and cross-correlation analyses and, perhaps, physiologic modeling techniques as well.

Currently employed techniques of automated care (Sheppard et al., 1968; Morgan et al., 1973) will amost undoubtedly be refined. We anticipate that algorithms similar to those used in automated care systems will be developed for the purpose of controlling ventilators and the operation of circulatory assist devices, in patients in whom these modalities are employed.

The human mind is still superior to the machine. Pattern recognition, interpretation of multiple variables, and differential diagnosis are exceedingly complex thought processes only one "computer" (the human brain) can perform well. This, however, presupposes prior training, experience, and usually a high order of intellect. Some evidence suggests that when there is a dearth of trained and experienced personnel, the computer might fill that void admirably (Sheppard et al., 1968). Moreover, even when experienced personnel are available, the problem of fatigue and the

```
SYS   103 1601    MV    10.9
DIA    72         I/E    1.7
MAP    83         MXIP  35
PAP    35         CMP   30
DPDT   1.1        RES    5
PR    121         PEEP
TMP   37.0 1549   FIO2  42
RR    12.8 1601
TVI   827         ECO2  34
TVO   854
```

Figure 6–7. Alphanumeric display of commonly used cardiorespiratory parameters. Since data are acquired at least once every ten minutes, information is no more than ten minutes old at any one time. (SYS = systolic pressure; DIA = diastolic pressure; MAP = mean arterial pressure; PAP = mean pulmonary artery pressure; DPDT = first derivative of the upstroke of arterial waveform; HR = heart rate; TMP = temperature; RR = respiratory rate; TVI = tidal volume in; TVO = tidal volume out; MV = minute volume; I/E = inspiratory-to-expiratory time ratio expression; MXIP = maximum inspiratory pressure; CMP = static compliance (lung and thorax); RES = nonelastic resistance; PEEP = positive end-expiratory pressure; F_{IO_2} = fraction of oxygen in the inspired breath; E_{CO_2} = end-tidal carbon dioxide tension. In this patient, left heart filling pressures were measured via balloon-tipped pulmonary artery catheter.)

difficulty of an individual in sustaining close attention for prolonged periods are real and have to be reckoned with. It would seem that the ideal critical care team would combine the strong attributes of people and digital computers. It is safe to predict that computational techniques will gain more widespread application in the care of the critically ill in the years to come.

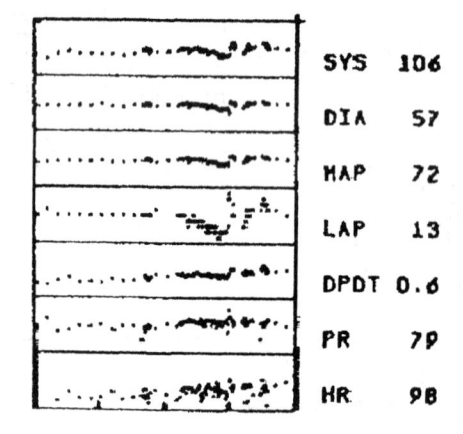

```
SYS   106
DIA    57
MAP    72
LAP    13
DPDT  0.6
PR     79
HR     98
```

Figure 6–8. Four-hour trend plot of cardiovascular paremeters are helpful in following directional changes. For legend to computer symbols, see Figure 6–6. (LAP = left atrial pressure; PR = pulse rate.)

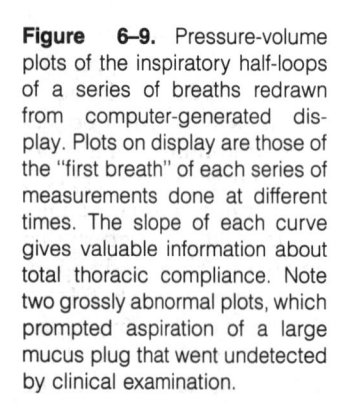

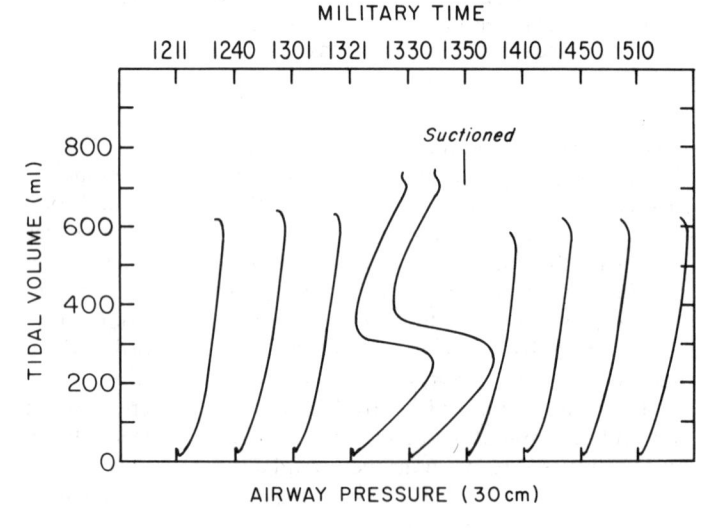

Figure 6–9. Pressure-volume plots of the inspiratory half-loops of a series of breaths redrawn from computer-generated display. Plots on display are those of the "first breath" of each series of measurements done at different times. The slope of each curve gives valuable information about total thoracic compliance. Note two grossly abnormal plots, which prompted aspiration of a large mucus plug that went undetected by clinical examination.

REFERENCES

Altschule MD, Freedburg AS, McManus MJ: Circulation and respiration during an episode of chill and fever in man. J Clin Invest 24: 878, 1945.

Andersen MN, Mouritzen CV, Gabrieli E: Mechanisms of plasma hemoglobin clearance after acute hemolysis: studies in open-heart surgical patients. Ann Surg 163: 529, 1966.

Astrup P, Siggaard-Andersen, OS, Jorgensen K, Engel K: The acid-base metabolism. A new approach. Lancet 1: 1035, 1960.

Awad JA, Lemieux JM, Lou W: Pulmonary complications following perfusion of the lungs. J Thorac Cardiovasc Surg 51: 767, 1966.

Bartlett RG Jr, Brubach HF, Specht H: Oxygen cost of breathing. J Appl Physiol 12: 413, 1958.

Bartter FC: Cardiac failure and hormonal control of fluid and electrolyte balance. Surg Gynecol Obstet 118: 767, 1964.

Baxter CR, Sedlitz WH, Shires GT: High output acute renal failure complicating traumatic injury. J Trauma 4: 567, 1964.

Bendixen HH, Egbert LD, Hedley-Whyte J, Laver MB, Pontoppidan H: Respiratory Care. St. Louis, Mosby, 1965, p 107.

———, Hedley-Whyte JJ, Laver MB: Impaired oxygenation in surgical patients during general anesthesia with controlled ventilation. A concept of atelectasis. N Eng J Med 269: 991, 1963.

Benis AM, Fitzkee HL, Jurado RA, Litwak RS: Improved defection of adverse cardiovascular trends with the use of a two-variable computer alarm. Crit Care Med 8: 341, 1980.

Berger RL, Weisel RD, Vito L, Dennis RC, Hechtman HB: Cardiac output measurement by thermodilution during cardiac operations. Ann Thorac Surg 21: 43, 1976.

Bjork VO, Engstrom CG: The treatment of ventilatory insufficiency by tracheostomy and artificial ventilation. J Thorac Cardiovasc Surg 34: 228, 1957.

Bland JH: Clinical Metabolism of Body Water and Electrolytes. Philadelphia, Saunders, 1963.

Boyd AA, Tremblay RE, Spencer FC, Bahnson HT: Estimation of cardiac output soon after intracardiac surgery with cardiopulmonary bypass. Ann Surg 150: 613, 1959.

Bradley SE, Chasis H, Goldring W, Smith HW: Hemodynamic alterations in normotensive and hypertensive subjects during the pyrogenic reaction. J Clin Invest 24: 749, 1945.

Brody WR, Arvin DE, Angell WW: Real-time analysis of myocardial contractility. Surgery 74:291, 1973.

Campbell GS, Houle GB, Crisps NW Jr, Weil MH, Brown EB Jr: Depressed response to intravenous sympathicomimetic agents in humans during acidosis. Dis Chest 33: 18, 1958.

Carlston A, Norlander O, Widman B: Observations on the postoperative circulation. Surg Gynecol Obstet 99: 227, 1954.

Carr EA, Sloan HE Jr, Tovar E: The clinical importance of erythrocyte and plasma volume determinations before and after open-heart surgery. J Nucl Med 1: 165, 1960.

Christlieb II, Dammann JF Jr, Thung NS, Muller WH Jr: Postoperative care in cardiac surgery: frequent determination of success or failure. Dis Chest 44: 47, 1963.

Cleland J, Pluth JR, Tauxe WN, Kirklin JW: Blood volume and body fluid compartment changes soon after closed and open intracardiac surgery. J Thorac Cardiovasc Surg 52: 698, 1966.

Clowes GHA Jr, Alichniewicz A, del Guercio LRM, Gillespie D: The relationship of postoperative acidosis to pulmonary and vascular function. J Thorac Cardiovasc Surg 39: 1, 1960.

———, Cook WA, Kurd Vujovic V: Patterns of circulatory response to the use of respirators. Circulation 30 (Suppl III): 62, 1964.

———, Sabga G, Kontaxis A, Tomin R, Hughes M, Simeone FA: Effects of acidosis on cardiovascular function in surgical patients. Ann Surg 154: 524, 1961.

Coller FA, Rees VL, Campbell KN, Iob LV, Moyer CA: The effects of ether and cyclopropane anesthesia upon renal function in man. Ann Surg 118: 717, 1943.

Cooper JD, Grillo HC: The evolution of tracheal injury due to ventilatory assistance through cuffed tubes: a pathological study. Ann Surg 169: 334, 1969.

Cranston WI: Fever: pathogenesis and circulatory changes. Circulation 20: 1133, 1959.

Dammann JF Jr, Thung N, Christlieb II, Littlefield JB, Muller WH Jr: The management of the severely ill patient after open-heart surgery. J Thorac Cardiovasc Surg 45: 80, 1963.

———, Wright DJ, Updike OL, Bowers DL: Assessment of continuous monitoring in the critically ill patient. Dis Chest 55:240, 1969.

Darby TI, Aldinger EE, Gadsden RH, Thrower WR: Effects of metabolic acidosis on ventricular isometric systolic tension and the response to epinephrine and levarterenol. Circ Res 8: 1242, 1960.

de Wardener HE: The Kidney: An Outline of Normal and Abnormal Structure and Function. Boston, Little, Brown, 1961, pp 205–211.

———, : Renal circulation during anesthesia and surgery. Anaesthesia 10: 18, 1955.

Dow P: Estimations of cardiac output and central blood volume by dye dilution. Physiol Rev 36: 77, 1956.

Downes J, del Guercio L, Grace WJ, Pontoppidan H, Waisbren BA: Guidelines for organization of critical care units. JAMA 222: 1532, 1972.

DuBois EF: Basal Metabolism in Health and Disease, 3rd ed. Philadelphia, Lea & Febeger, 1936.

Ebert PA, Jude JR, Gaertner RA: Persistent hypokalemia following open heart surgery. Circulation 31 (Suppl) 137, 1965.

Edmunds LH Jr, Austen WG: Effect of cardiopulmonary bypass on pulmonary volume-pressure relationships and vascular resistance. J Appl Physiol 21: 209, 1966.

Elkinton JR, Danowski TS: The Body Fluids—Basic Physiology and Practical Therapeutics. Baltimore, Williams & Wilkins, 1955.

Ellison LT, Yeh TS, Moretz WH, Ellison RG: Pulmonary diffusion studies in patients undergoing non-thoracic, thoracic and cardiopulmonary bypass procedures. Ann Surg 157: 327, 1963.

Farrier RM, Fink BR, Harmel MH, Steen S, Welkowitz W: Patient monitoring in the hospital. Ann NY Acad Sci 118 (Art 7): 387, 1964.

Fishman NH, Hutchinson JC, Roe BB: Controlled atrial hypertension: a method for supporting cardiac output following open-heart surgery. J Thorac Cardiovasc Surg 52: 777, 1966.

Fordham RMM: Hypoxaemia after aortic valve surgery under cardiopulmonary bypass. Thorax 20: 505, 1965.

Forrester J, Diamond G, Ganz V, Danzig R, Swan HJC: Right and left heart pressures in the actuely ill patient. Clin Res 18: 306, 1970.

———, ———, McHugh TJ, Swan HJC: Filling pressures in the right and left sides of the heart in acute myocardial infarction. A reappraisal of central venous pressure monitoring. N Engl J Med 285: 190, 1971.

Fox IJ, Brooker LGS, Heseltine DW, Esser HE, Wood EH: A tricarbocyanine dye for continuous recording of dilution curves in whole blood independent of variations in blood oxygen saturation. Proc Staff Meet, Mayo Clin 32: 478, 1957.

Franklin SS, Merrill JP: Medical progress: Acute renal failure. N Engl J Med 262:711, 1960.

Gadboys HL, Litwak RS, Niemetz J, Wisch N: The value of anticoagulants in preventing systemic embolization from prosthetic heart valves. JAMA 202: 282, 1967.

———, Slonim R, Litwak RS: The homologous blood syndrome: preliminary observations of its relationship to clinical cardiopulmonary bypass. Ann Surg 156: 793, 1962.

Gardner RE, Finely TN, Tooley WH: Effect of cardiopulmonary bypass on surface activity of lung extracts. Bull Soc Int Chir 21: 542, 1962.

Geha AS, Sessler AD, Kirklin JW: Alveolar-arterial oxygen gradients after open intracardiac surgery. J Thorac Cardiovasc Surg 51: 609, 1966.

Gerst PH, Fleming WH, Malm JR: Increased susceptibility of the heart to ventricular fibrillation during metabolic acidosis. Circ Res 19: 63, 1966.

Ghia J, Anderson NB: Pulmonary function and cardiopulmonary bypass. JAMA 212: 593, 1970.

Goodman B, Litwak RS, Gadboys HL, Brooks H, Kahn M: Renal function in highflow hemodilution perfusion. Circulation 32 (Suppl II): 100, 1965.

Guerra F, Brobeck JR: The hypothalamic control of aspirin antipyresis in the monkey. J Pharmacol Exp Ther 80: 209, 1944.

Gullick HD, Raisz LG: Changes in renal concentrating ability associated with major surgical procedures. N Engl J Med 262: 1309, 1960.

Habif DV, Papper EM, Fitzpatrick HF, Lowrance P, Smythe C Mc, Bradley SE: The renal and hepatic blood flow, glomerular filtration rate and urinary output of electrolytes during cyclopropane, ether and thiopental anesthesia, operation and the immediate postoperative period. Surgery 30: 241, 1951.

Hayes MA, Byrnes WP, Goldenberg IS, Greene NM, Tuthill E: Water and electrolyte changes during operation and convalescence. Surgery 46: 123, 1959.

———, Williamson RJ, Heidenreich WF: Endocrine mechanisms involved in water and sodium metabolism during operation and convalescence. Surgery 46: 353, 1957.

Hedley-Whyte J, Corning H, Laver MB, Austen WG, Bendixen HH: Pulmonary ventilation-perfusion relations after valve replacement or repair in man. J Clin Invest 44: 406, 1965a.

———, Pontoppidan H, Laver MB: Arterial oxygenation during hypothermia. Anesthesiology 26: 595, 1965b.

Herzog P, Norlander OP, Engstrom CG: Ultrasonic generation of aerosol for the humidification of inspired gas during volume-controlled ventilation. Acta Anaestheol Scand 8: 79, 1964.

Hill JD, Aguilar MJ, Baranco A, de Lanerolle P,

Gerbode F: Neuropathologic manifestations of cardiac surgery. Ann Thorac Surg 7: 409, 1969.

——, Main FB, Osborn JJ, Gerbode F: Correct use of respirator on cardiac patient after operation. Arch Surg 91: 775, 1965.

Hood WB Jr, Bianco JA, Kumar R, Whiting RB: Experimental myocardial infarction. IV. Reduction of left ventricular compliance in the healing phase. J Clin Invest 49: 1316, 1970.

Horvath SM, Spurr GB, Hutt BK, Hamilton LH: Metabolic cost of shivering. J Appl Physiol 8: 595, 1956.

Howatt WF, Talner NS, Sloan H, DeMuth GR: Pulmonary function changes following repair of heart lesions with the aid of extracorporeal circulation. J Thorac Cardiovasc Surg 43: 649, 1962.

Humphreys GH II, Blumenthal S, Bowman FO Jr, Malm JR, Singer DH, Sullivan SF: Immediate complications of thoracotomy for heart disease. Surg Clin North Am 44: 335, 1964.

Joly HR, Weil MH: Temperature of the great toe as an indication of the severity of shock. Circulation 35: 131, 1969.

Jurado RA, Fitzkee HL, de Asla RA, Lukban SB, Litwak RS, Osborn JJ: Reduction of unexpected life-threatening events in postoperative cardiac surgical patients: the role of computerized surveillance. Circulation 56 (Suppl): II–44, 1977.

——, Matucha D, Osborn JJ: Cardiac output estimation by pulse contour methods: validity of their use for monitoring critically ill patients. Surgery 74: 358, 1973.

Kahn M, Goodman B, Litwak RS, Gadboys HL: High flow whole body hemodilution perfusion: Acidbase, renal electrolyte and body fluid alterations J Mount Sinai Hosp 35:111, 1968.

Kaplan S, Edwards FK, Helmsworth JA, Clark LC: Blood volume during and after total extracorporeal circulation. Arch Surg 80: 31, 1960.

Kassirer JP: Clinical evaluation of kidney function —tubular function. N Engl J Med 285:499, 1971.

Kevy SV, Glickman RM, Bernhard WF, Diamond LK, Gross RE: The pathogenesis and control of the hemorrhagic defect in open heart surgery. Surg Gynecol Obstet 123: 313, 1966.

Kingsley DPE: Hepatic damage following profound hypothermia and extracorporeal circulation in man. Thorax 21: 91, 1966.

Kinney JM: The intensive care unit. Bull Am Coll Surg 51: 201, 1966.

——, Moore FD: Surgical metabolism in metabolism of body fluids. In Bland JH (ed): Clinical Metabolism of Body Water and Electrolytes. Philadelphia, WB Saunders, 1963, pp 337-359.

Kirklin JW: Circulation and cardiac failure. In Kinney JM, Egdahl RH, Zuidema GD (eds): Manual of Preoperative and Postoperative Care. Philadelphia, Saunders, 1971, pp 195–210.

——: Pulmonary dysfunction after open heart surgery. Med Clin North Am 48: 1063, 1964.

——, Theye RA:Cardiac performance after open intracardiac surgery. Circulation 28: 1061, 1963.

Kumar R, Hood WB Jr, Joison J, Norman JC, Abelmann WH: Experimental myocardial infarction. II. Acute depression and subsequent recovery of left ventricular function: serial measurements in intact conscious dogs. J Clin Invest 49: 55, 1970.

Lefemine AA, Harken DE: Postoperative care following open-heart operations: routine use of controlled ventilation. J Thorac Cardiovasc Surg 52: 207, 1966.

Lewis FJ, Shimizu T, Scofield AL, Rosi PS: Analysis of respiration by an on-line digital computer system: Clinical data following thoracoabdominal surgery. Ann Surg 164:547, 1966.

Lindholm CE: Prolonged endotracheal intubation. Acta Anaestheol Scand (Suppl XXXIII): 131, 1969.

Litwak RS, Gadboys HL, Kahn M, Wisoff BG: High flow total body perfusion utilizing diluted perfusate in a large prime system. J Thorac Cardiovasc Surg 49: 74, 1965.

——, Gilson AJ, Slonim R, McCune CC, Kiem I, Gadboys HL: Alterations in blood volume during "normovolemic" total body perfusion. J Thorac Cardiovasc Surg 42: 477, 1961.

Lockey E, McIntyre N, Ross DN, Brooks E, Sturridge MF: Early jaundice after open heart surgery. Thorax 22: 165, 1967.

Lowenstein E, Bland JHL: Anesthesia in cardiac surgery. In Norman JC (ed): Cardiac Surgery, 2nd ed. New York, Appleton-Century-Crofts, 1972, pp 75–102.

——, Hallowell P, Levine FH, Daggett WM, Austen WG, Laver MB: Cardiovascular response to large doses of intravenous morphine in man. N Engl J Med 281: 1389, 1969.

Maier HS, Cournand A: Studies of arterial oxygen saturation in the postoperative period after pulmonary resection. Surgery 13: 199, 1943.

Maloney JV Jr: The trouble with patient monitoring. Ann Surg 168:605, 1968.

Mandelbaum I, Giammona ST: Extracorporeal circulation, pulmonary compliance, and pulmonary surfactant. J Thorac Cardiovasc Surg 48: 881, 1964.

McArthur KT, Clark LC Jr, Lyons C, Edwards S: Continuous recording of blood oxygen saturation in open-heart operations. Surgery 51: 121, 1962.

McClenahan JB, Young WE, Sykes MK: Respiratory changes after open-heart surgery. Thorax 20: 545, 1965.

McGoon DC, Moffitt EA, Theye RA, Kirklin JW: Renal performance in patients undergoing replacement of the aortic valve. J Thorac Cardiovasc Surg 39: 275, 1960.

Mielke JE, Hunt JC, Maher FT, Kirklin JW: Renal performance during clinical cardiopulmonary bypass with and without hemodilution. J Thorac Cardiovasc Surg 51: 229, 1966.

———, Kirklin JW: Renal function during and after surgery. Med Clin North Am 50: 979, 1966.

———, Maher FT, Hunt JC, Kirklin JW: Renal performance in patients undergoing replacement of the aortic valve. Circulation 32:394, 1965.

Miller JM, Peters JJ, Devese IM: Experience with automated monitoring of physiologic functions. M Res Eng 5:6, 1966.

Moffitt EA, Sessler AD, Kirklin JW: Postoperative care in open-heart surgery. JAMA 199: 161, 1967.

Moore FD: Metabolic Care of the Surgical Patient. Philadelphia, Saunders, 1959.

———: Common patterns of water and electrolyte change in injury, surgery and disease. N Engl J Med 258: 277, 377, 427, 1958a.

———: Extracorporeal Circulation. Springfield, Ill, Thomas 1958b, p 498.

———, Ball MR: The Metabolic Response to Surgery. Springfield, Ill, Thomas, 1952.

———, McMurray JD, Parker HV, Magnus IC: Symposium: water and electrolytes. Body Composition. Total body water and electrolytes: intravascular and extravascular phase volumes. Metabolism 5: 447, 1956.

Morgan A, Anderson W, Bevilacqua R, Cohn L, Moore FD, Collins JJ Jr: Effects of computer-controlled transfusion on recovery from cardiac surgery. Ann Surg 178:391, 1973.

Mortensen JD, Anderson LH: Clinical experiences with computerized monitoring of cardiovascular variables in the postoperative thoracic patient. J Thor Cardiovasc Surg 56:510, 1968.

Mundth ED, Keller AR, Austen WG: Progressive hepatic and renal failure associated with low cardiac output following open heart surgery. J Thorac Cardiovasc Surg 53: 275, 1967.

Nash G, Blennerhassett JB, Pontoppiden H: Pulmonary lesions associated with oxygen therapy and artificial ventilation. N Engl J Med 276:368, 1967.

Nahas RA, Melrose DG, Sykes MK, Robinson B: Postperfusion lung syndrome: role of circulatory exclusion. Lancet 2: 251, 1965.

Neville WE, Kontaxis A, Gavin T, Clowes GHA Jr: Postperfusion pulmonary vasculitis: its relationship to blood trauma. Arch Surg 86: 126, 1963.

Obel IWP, Marchand P, DuPlessis LA: The biochemical effects of dextrose and water priming of the pump for open-heart surgery. S Afr Med J 39: 309, 1965.

———, ———, ———: Biochemical changes associated with the use of haemodilution with 5 percent dextrose in water and mannitol for open-heart surgery. Thorax 22: 180, 1967.

Osborn JJ, Beaumont JO, Raison JCA, Russell J, Gerbode F: Measurement and monitoring of acutely ill patients by digital computer. Surgery 64: 1057, 1968.

———, Popper RW, Kerth WJ, Gerbode F: Respiratory insufficiency following open heart surgery. Ann Surg 156: 638, 1962.

———, Raison JCA, Beaumont JO, Hill JD, Kerth WJ, Popper RW, Gerbode F: Respiratory causes of "sudden unexplained arrhythmia in postthoracotomy patients." Surgery 69: 24, 1971.

Panossian A, Hagstrom JWC, Nehlsen SL, Veith FJ: Secondary nature of surfactant changes in postperfusion pulmonary damage. J Thorac Cardiovasc Surg 57: 628, 1969.

Peirce EC II: A simplified approach to obtaining and recording acid-base information in surgical patients. Ann Surg 156:138, 1962.

———: Is acid-base balance important? Med Times 95:123, 1967.

Perlmutter M, Grossman SL, Rothenberg S, Dobkin G: Urine-serum urea nitrogen ratio: Simple test of renal function in acute azotemia and oliguria. JAMA 170:1528, 1959.

Peters RM, Hilberman M: Respiratory insufficiency: diagnosis and control of therapy. Surgery 70: 280, 1971.

Pontoppidan H, Berry PR: Regulation of inspired O_2 concentration during artificial ventilation. JAMA 201: 89, 1967.

_____, Laver MB, Geffin B: Acute respiratory failure in the surgical patient. Adv Surg 4: 163, 1970.

Porter GA, Kloster FE, Herr RJ, Starr A, Griswold H, Kimsey J, Lenertz H: Relationship between alterations in renal hemodynamics during cardiopulmonary bypass and postoperative renal function. Circulation 34: 1005, 1966.

_____, Starr A: Management of postoperative renal failure following cardiovascular surgery. Surgery 65:390, 1969.

Provan JL, Austen WG: The role of elective tracheostomy after open-heart surgery. Ann Thorac Surg 2: 358, 1966.

Rehder K, Kirklin JW, Theye RA: Physiologic studies following surgical correction of atrial septal defect and similar lesions. Circulation 26: 1302, 1962.

Robinson JS, Cole FR, Gibson P, Simpson JA: Jaundice following cardiopulmonary bypass. Thorax 22: 232, 1967.

Roe CF: Clinical significance of fever and hypothermia. Lecture outlines, postoperative course on pre- and postoperative care. Am Coll Surg Pub, p. 38, 1966a.

_____: Fever and energy metabolism in surgical disease. Monogr Surg Sci 3: 85, 1966b.

Salzman EW, Britten A: Hemorrhage and Thrombosis. A Practical Clinical Guide. Boston, Little, Brown, 1965, pp 144–147.

Sanderson RG, Ellison JH, Benson JA, Starr A: Jaundice following open heart surgery. Ann Surg 165: 217, 1967.

Schoen EJ, Young G, Weissman A: Urinary specific gravity versus total solute concentration: a critical comparison. I. Studies in normal adults. J Clin Lab Med 54: 277, 1959.

Schramel RJ, Cameron R, Ziskind MD, Adam M, Creech O Jr: Studies of pulmonary diffusion after open heart surgery. J Thor Cardiovasc Surg 38:281, 1959.

Selmonosky CA: Early detection of renal failure after cardiopulmonary bypass. Arch Surg 99:64, 1969.

Sheppard LC, Kouchoukos NT, Kirklin JW: The digital computer in surgical intensive care automation. Computer 6:29, 1973.

Shubin H, Weil MH: Efficient monitoring with a digital computer of cardiovascular function in seriously ill patients. Ann Intern Med 65:453, 1966.

Siegel JH: Computers and mathematical techniques in surgery. In Sabiston DC Jr (ed): Textbook of Surgery. Philadelphia, WB Saunders, 1977, pp 231-256.

_____, del Guercio L: The diagnosis and therapy of shock using physiologic correlates quantified with a bedside computer. Bull NY Acad Med 43:424, 1967.

Siggaard-Andersen OS, Engel K: A new acid-base nomogram. An improved method for the calculation of the relevant blood acid-base data. Scand J Clin Lab Invest 12: 177, 1960.

Sladen A, Laver MB, Pontoppidan H: Pulmonary complications associated with water retention during prolonged mechanical ventilation. N Engl J Med 279: 448, 1968.

Steingart RM, Meller J, Barovick J, Patterson R, Herman MV, Teichholz LE: Pulsed Doppler echocardiographic measurement of beat-to-beat changes in stroke volume in dogs. Circulation 62: 542, 1980.

Strauss J, Malm JR, Blumenthal S: Renal function after intracardiac operations involving total body perfusion. Bull NY Acad Med 37: 874, 1961.

Sturridge MF, Theye RA, Fowler WS, Kirklin JW: Basal metabolic rate after cardiovascular surgery. J Thorac Cardiovasc Surg 47: 298, 1964.

Sturtz GS, Kirklin JW, Burke EC, Power MH: Water metabolism after cardiac operations involving a Gibbon type pump-oxygenator. I. Daily water metabolism, obligatory water losses, and requirements. Circulation 16: 988, 1957.

Sullivan SF, Patterson RW, Malm JR, Bowman FO, Papper EM: Effect of heart-lung bypass on the mechanics of breathing in man. J Thorac Cardiovasc Surg 51: 205, 1966.

Swan HJC, Ganz W, Forrester J, Marcus H, Diamond G, Chonette D: Catheterization of the heart in man with the use of a balloon-tipped catheter. N Engl J Med 283: 447, 1970.

Thung N, Herzog P, Christlieb II, Thompson WM Jr, Dammann JF Jr: Cost of respiratory effort in postoperative cardiac patients. Circulation 28: 552, 1963.

Tomin R, Kontaxis A, Wittels B, Griggs R, Neville WE, Clowes GHA Jr: Pulmonary changes secondary to prolonged perfusion. Trans Am Soc Artif Intern Organs 7: 187, 1961.

Turney SZ, McCluggage C, Blumenfeld W, McAslan TC, Cowley RA: Automatic respiratory gas monitoring. Ann Thorac Surg 14: 159, 1972.

Veith FJ, Hagstrom JWC, Panossian A, Nehlsen SL, Wilson JW: Pulmonary microcirculatory response to shock, transfusion, and pump-oxygenator procedures. A unified mechanism underlying pulmonary damage. Surgery 64: 95, 1968.

Vertel RM, Knochel JP: Non-oliguric acute renal failure. JAMA 200: 598, 1967.

von Kaulla KN, Swan H: Clotting deviations during cardiac bypass: fibrinolysis and circulating anticoagulants. J Thorac Surg 36: 519, 1958.

Warner HR, Gardner, RM, Toronto AF: Computer-based monitoring of cardiovascular function in postoperative patients. Circulation (Suppl 2) 37:68, 1968.

Weintraub HD, Sullivan SF, Malm JR, Bowman FO Jr, Papper EM: Lung function and blood-gas exchange, before and after cardiac surgery. J Appl Physiol 20: 483, 1965.

Wells RE Jr, Perera RD, Kinney JM: Humidification of oxygen during inhalation therapy. N Engl J Med 268: 644, 1963.

Wilkinson AW: Body Fluids in Surgery, 2nd ed. Edinburgh, E. & S. Livingstone, 1960.

Williams WG, Manley RW, Drew C: Pulmonary circulatory arrest. Thorax 20: 523, 1965.

Wilson JW, Ratliff NB, Mikat E, Hackel DB, Young WG, Graham TC: Leukocyte changes in the pulmonary circulation. Chest 59 (Suppl 5): 36, 1971.

7. Concepts of Acid-Base Balance

E. Converse Peirce II

The key to a practical working knowledge of acid-base balance is an understanding of the hydrogen ion and its behavior in the body. Proper maintenance of the chemical reactions that are necessary at the cellular level entails careful regulation of the hydrogen ion activity. This is closely guarded by the body buffers which resist change in hydrogen ion activity and provide temporary storage or supply of hydrogen ions until compensatory mechanisms can act. The compensatory mechanisms comprise respiration, which controls the level of alveolar and arterial carbon dioxide tension, metabolism, which converts intermediary acids into carbon dioxide and water, and finally renal regulation of the excretion of hydrogen ions. Disease processes interfering with one or more of these compensatory mechanisms underlie most abnormal acid-base states. The addition of acid, as in blood transfusion, or the loss of acid or base from the intestinal tract may also produce primary abnormalities (Peirce, 1967).

THE SYSTEM OF NOTATION

There are three major facets to a workable system of acid-base balance:

1. Accurate measurement of two quantitative acid-base variables from which others may be derived mathematically, by use of a nomogram or by inspection.
2. A system of notation that makes possible the recording and communication of these measurements in such a way that the pattern of their change with time can be appreciated.
3. Sufficient clinical knowledge of the patient to permit a meaningful interpretation of the acid-base status over a useful period of time.

The multiplicity of current acid-base terms is in part a symptom of failure to develop a system that the majority of physicians can comfortably use. A principle problem is the method of notation. Most commonly, acid-base changes are measured in the arterial blood, and a system of two measured and one derived variable is used. Each variable is in a different unit of measurement and only one is a direct gauge of hydrogen ion activity (Table 7–1, Figs. 7–1 and 7–2). A system using noncommensurable variables that can be related to one another only mathematically and are commonly interpretable only by reference to a nomogram, is difficult to use. Each point in time must usually be considered separately, and the pattern of acid-base status as it changes with time is very difficult for many to follow. It is even more confusing if additional variables are gratuitously derived and given to the clinician (Gollan, 1966). Siggaard-Andersen (1960) has devised an ingenious way of plotting three noncommensurable variables against time, but in practice it is difficult to do.

The following pair of variables is commensurable, supplies the quantitative infor-

TABLE 7–1 A THREE-VARIABLE SYSTEM FOR ACID-BASE STUDIES WITH ARTERIAL BLOOD

Variable	Unit	Reason for Use
pH_A	$\dfrac{1}{\log aH^+}$	Overall acid-base status
Pa_{CO_2}	torr or mm Hg	Respiratory acid-base factor
Base excess	mEq/liter	Nonrespiratory acid-base factor

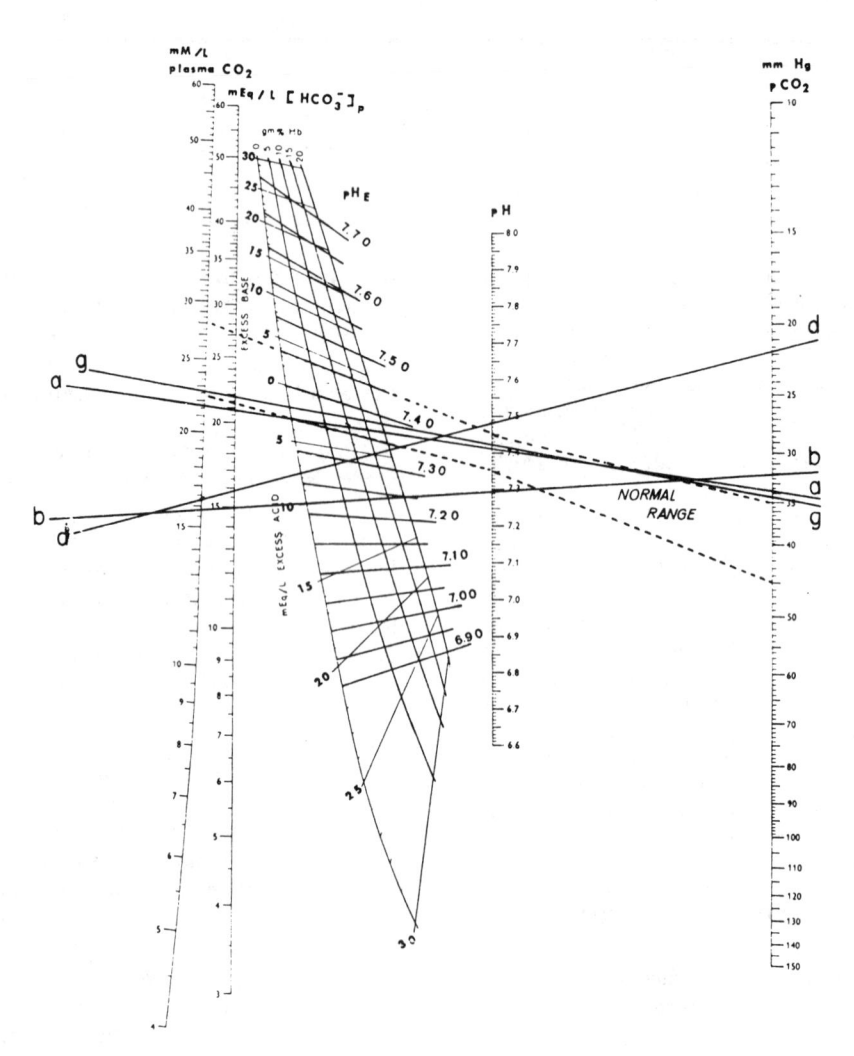

Figure 7–1. Although two noncommensurable acid-base variables can be used to derive other variables, if the hemoglobin and temperatures are known, they give an incomplete picture to most clinicians. It is necessary to derive additional values mathematically or with the aid of a nomogram, and this makes it difficult to follow a patient's acid-base status as it changes with time. This is illustrated by connecting values of the two measured variables on the Siggaard-Andersen nomogram. See Figure 7–4 for a clinical description. Note especially the difficulty of appreciating the effect of time.

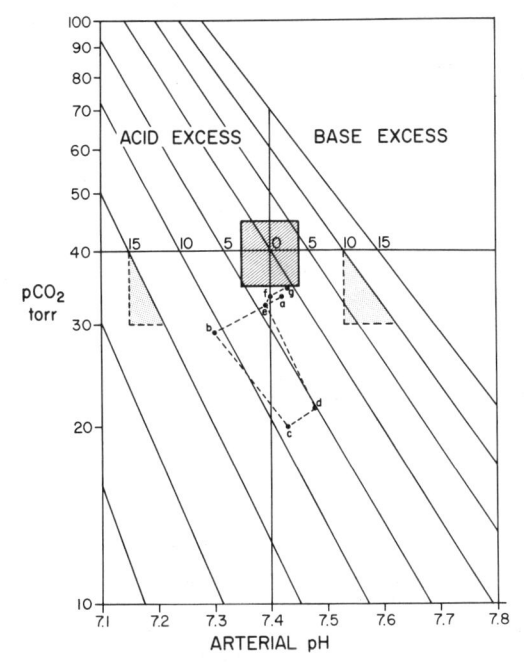

Figure 7-2. A display showing arterial pH$_A$, Paco$_2$, and base excess (on the isopleths). This provides a somewhat better idea of change than the use of the multivariable Siggaard-Andersen nomogram, but there is still no easy way of appreciating the effect of time. See Figure 7-4 for clinical explanation.

mation most needed by a clinician, and permits him or her to perceive at a glance a patient's acid-base status over an appropriate interval of time. Both variables are in units of hydrogen ion activity and no nomogram is needed for usual clinical work:

1. Hydrogen ion activity of the arterial blood in the form either of the arterial pH (pH$_A$) or in nanoequivalents per liter (Schwartz and Relman, 1963; Siggaard-Andersen et al., 1966; Davis, 1967). This represents the resultant of factors influencing hydrogen ion activity and is thus an overall measurement. It is the most important single acid-base variable. Tissue hydrogen ion activity is probably what is perceived by the carotid body and other chemoreceptors. Tissue measurements such as muscle pH may have special value but are more difficult to obtain (Smith et al., 1969). The Paco$_2$, plasma bicarbonate, etc. are also important in their own right, but the hydrogen ion activity probably takes precedence in regulation.

2. The hydrogen ion activity of the same arterial blood when the Paco$_2$ is returned to a normal mean arterial value of 40 torr (mm Hg). Deviations in this value from the normal range of the arterial pH or hydrogen ion activity represent the resultant of all nonrespiratory acid-base influences. This value is called the pH$_{40}$ to avoid any connotation of in vivo meaning. Names used earlier (see Table 7-2) have been discarded because they suggested how the value might be obtained or they had an in vivo connotation.

Since both the pH$_A$ and pH$_{40}$ are in units of hydrogen ion activity, each pair also delineates the Paco$_2$. If the values are the same, the Paco$_2$ is 40 torr. If the pH$_A$ represents a greater hydrogen ion activity than the pH$_{40}$ it must represent a greater Paco$_2$ and vice versa (Figs. 7-3 and 7-4). Any other usual quantitative measurement may be derived using the pH$_A$, pH$_{40}$, and the Hgb (Peirce, 1967).

THE NOMENCLATURE

Though a simple graphic display of the patient's acid-base course usually suffices, it is often desirable to express the condition in words. Here there are some important pitfalls (Table 7-2).

Measurement of the hydrogen ion activity in the blood may be expressed in pH units or in nanoequivalents per liter. It is frequently preferred, however, to use a directional term to express deviations from the normal range. For an increase in hydrogen ion activity, the term is acidemia, and for a decrease, alkalemia. Acidosis and alkalosis should not be used in reference to the hydrogen ion activity of blood, but only to indicate primary derangements of acid-base state (Siggaard-Andersen et al., 1966). An acidosis is a primary alteration that would result in an increase in hydrogen ion activity if there were no compensation. Thus an acidosis may be present without

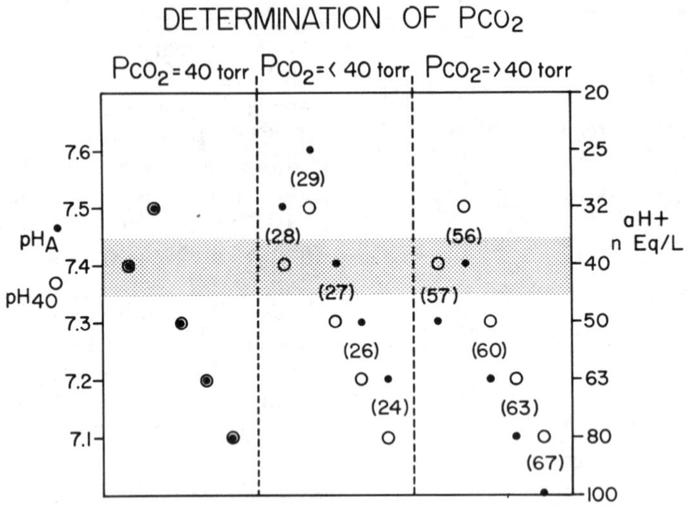

DETERMINATION OF PCO₂

Figure 7–3. Acid-base status determined by use of a two-variable system where the variables are commensurable. All data points are for a hemoglobin of 15 gm%. The arterial pH (pH$_A$) is corrected to the patient's temperature. Correction is not necessary for blood at a fixed Pco$_2$ as the pH$_{40}$. Where the pH$_A$ and the pH$_{40}$ are the same, the Paco$_2$ is 40 torr. This is true no matter how abnormal the pH$_A$ is. Where the pH$_A$ is higher than the pH$_{40}$ (representing a lower hydrogen ion activity for the pH$_A$), the Paco$_2$ is below 40 torr. Note that the lower the pH$_A$ the more the Paco$_2$, represented by a pH difference of 0.1 unit, is below 40 torr. Where the pH$_A$ is lower than the pH$_{40}$, the Paco$_2$ is greater than 40 torr. Again note that a pH difference of 0.1 unit represents a greater deviation from 40 torr when the pH$_A$ is low. Respiratory compensation for an acid base imbalance becomes progressively less effective as the hydrogen ion activity increases (pH$_A$ falls).

an acidemia. An alkalosis is a primary alteration that would result in a decrease in hydrogen ion activity if there were no compensation. Since more than one primary derangement can, and often does, exist at the same time, an alkalosis may be present when there is an acidemia or an acidosis when there is an alkalemia (Fig. 7–5). Primary derangements are respiratory or nonrespiratory. When possible, it is desirable to state what each nonrespiratory derangement is: metabolic (e.g., diabetic ketosis or lactic acidosis), renal, additive (ACD blood, antacid), or subtractive (upper or lower gastrointestinal loss).

A compensation is a return of hydrogen ion activity toward normal. This may be stated, for example, as respiratory compensation, metabolic compensation, or renal compensation. The rate of change is different from buffering and for the various compensations. This time-dependent quality is emphasized in Figure 7–6. One should remember that compensation by a diseased lung or kidney may not be possible, as they may literally be decompensated.

THE HYDROGEN ION AND HOMEOSTASIS

Significance

The level of hydrogen ion activity is one of the most carefully regulated variables of the internal environment. Major acid-base abnormalities, therefore, provide important clues to respiratory, circulatory, renal, and other derangements. Since the cause of the derangement may be more important than the hydrogen ion change, the deviation should usually not be corrected directly but, when possible, returned toward normal by treating the underlying cause. Some of the problems that

CONCEPTS OF ACID-BASE BALANCE

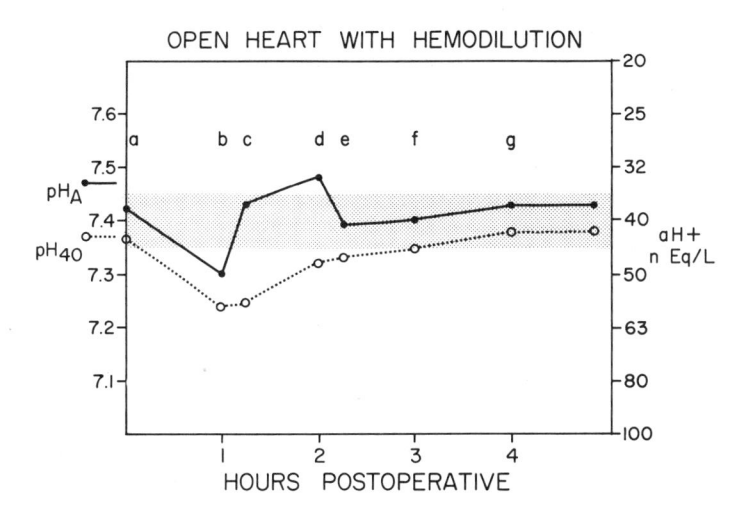

Figure 7-4. An early postoperative acid-base abnormality and its correction is illustrated. The pH_A is corrected to the temperature of the patient. During surgery (a) the pH values are within the normal range. One hour postoperatively (b) the central venous pressure, left atrial pressure, and hematocrit are all low. A falling pH_{40} suggests a low cardiac output. As nonrespiratory acidosis is at first uncompensated, the patient is placed on a respirator and blood is given concurrently to correct the low cardiac output. The $Paco_2$ is reduced from 32 to 22 torr and the pH_A is returned to the normal range (c). An hour later there is substantial reduction in the nonrespiratory acidosis, so that now there is a superimposed iatrogenic respiratory alkalosis (d). The respirator is adjusted (e) and the pH_A returned to the normal range (f) (g). The abnormalities of the pH pattern are easily appreciated and correction is shown much more clearly than in Figures 7-1 and 7-2, where the acid-base variables are noncommensurable and are not shown in relationship to time. The precise value of the $Paco_2$ is not clinically important in this instance, so the clinician need not be concerned with actual figures, only with the pattern.

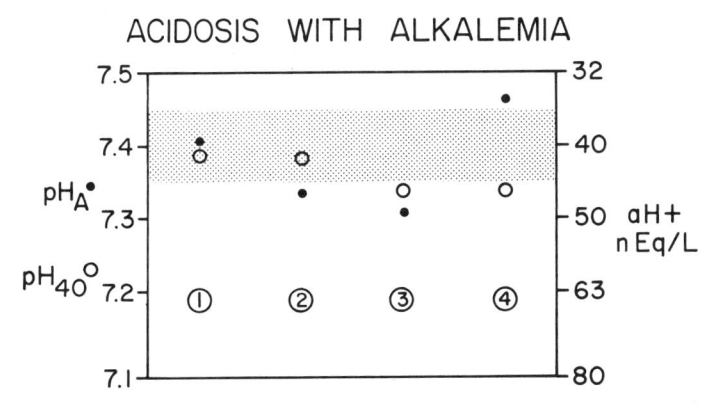

Figure 7-5. Mixed derangements: The reaction of the blood (acidemia or alkalemia) is determined by the net effect of the various primary abnormalities and compensations. It is thus possible to have an alkalemia in the presence of an acidosis, (1) pH values are within normal range. (2) Arterial pH is below the normal range, representing a respiratory acidosis with an acidemia. (3) Both the arterial and pH_{40} values are below the normal range. A renal failure has been added to the respiratory failure. There is now respiratory acidosis plus a renal acidosis with an acidemia. (4) The patient has been placed on a respirator and too vigorously ventilated. There is now a renal acidosis with an alkalemia.

TABLE 7–2 SOME DEFINITIONS FOR THIS PAPER

A. Description of the blood
  1. Overall acid-base factor
     a. Quantitative
        (1) pH_A, the arterial hydrogen ion activity (aH+) at the temperature of the patient. Normal range varies in different series but is approximately 7.35 to 7.45 (pH = 1/log aH+).
        (2) aH+ in nanoequivalents per liter (10^{-9} equivalents).
     b. Directional nonquantitative terms
        (1) Acidemia: pH_A below 7.35.
        (2) Alkalemia: pH_A above 7.45.
  2. Nonrespiratory (or noncarbonic) acid-base factor
     a. Quantitative
        (1) pH_{40}: The pH of arterial blood at a P_{CO_2} of 40 torr. Normal range assumed to be approximately the same as for the pH_A. May appropriately be outside the normal range because of compensation. Names used for the pH_{40} include: Reduced pH (Hasselbalch, 1916), metabolic pH factor (Peirce, 1959), nonrespiratory pH factor (Siggaard-Andersen, 1960), eucapnic pH (Peirce, 1962), eucarbic pH (Peirce, 1967).
        (2) Terms equivalent to the pH_{40} but in milliequivalents per liter rather than units of hydrogen ion activity include: Buffer base (Singer and Hastings, 1948), nonrespiratory acid (Peirce, 1959), base excess (Siggaard-Andersen, 1960), titratable acid (Siggaard-Andersen, 1966), fixed acid, noncarbonic acid, nonvolatile acid. Also used in much the same manner is the standard bicarbonate (Astrup et al., 1956, 1960). All of these values may be derived from the pH_{40} if the hemoglobin is known.
     b. Directional nonquantitative terms
        Hypobasemia and hyperbasemia are not generally used.
  3. Respiratory acid-base factor
     a. Quantitative
        Carbon dioxide tension of arterial blood at the temperature of the patient. This is frequently and appropriately outside the normal range because of compensation.
        (1) P_{CO_2} in mm Hg (or torr, in honor of Torricelli, a 17th century Italian physicist who described the mercury manometer). Arterial, Pa_{CO_2}; venous, $P\bar{v}_{CO_2}$.
        (2) The difference between the pH_A and the pH_{40}: (Semiquantitative by visual inspection and quantitative with a nomogram or mathematically).
            (a) pH_A and pH_{40} are equal: Pa_{CO_2} is 40 torr.
            (b) pH_A is greater than pH_{40}: Pa_{CO_2} is less than 40 torr.
            (c) pH_A is less than pH_{40}: Pa_{CO_2} is greater than 40 torr.
     b. Directional nonquantitative terms
        (1) Eucapnia: Pa_{CO_2} approximately 35 to 45 torr.
        (2) Hypocapnia: Pa_{CO_2} less than 35 torr.
        (3) Hypercapnia: Pa_{CO_2} greater than 45 torr.
B. Description of acid-base states in the patient
  1. Primary derangement: Initial acid-base alteration, usually qualified by mechanism as respiratory, renal, or metabolic.
     a. Acidosis: A primary derangement that would result in an increase in the hydrogen ion activity of the blood (pH_A) if there were no compensation.
     b. Alkalosis: A primary derangement that would result in a decrease in the hydrogen ion activity of the blood (pH_A) if there were no compensation.
  2. Mixed derangement: Two or more primary derangements.
  3. Compensation: A return of pH_A toward normal by a compensatory mechanism, eg., respiratory, metabolic, renal.

BUFFERING AND COMPENSATION

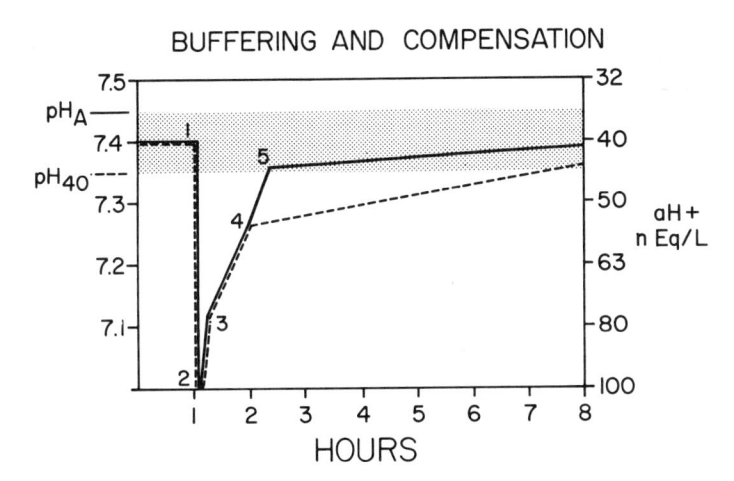

Figure 7-6. The dynamics of buffering and compensation for a nonrespiratory acidosis are illustrated for a hypothetical situation. The Paco$_2$ is held at 40 torr for the first two hours by hyperventilating a dog with 6 percent carbon dioxide in oxygen to keep the pH$_A$ and pH$_{40}$ values the same. At one hour, 25 mEq of HCl per liter of blood is added (1). Both pH values fall together to 7.0 (2). The change would be very much greater if it were not for the buffers of the blood, which act almost immediately. Extracellular buffering, other than blood, is a little less rapid but reduces the hydrogen ion activity fairly promptly and corrects the pH values to 7.1 (3). Intracellular buffering takes place more slowly and the pH values reach 7.27 (4). The dog is now allowed to ventilate on air without interference. The Paco$_2$ is promptly reduced and the pH$_A$ is brought within normal limits (5). Slow renal compensation gradually returns the pH$_{40}$ to the normal range. If an intermediary organic acid, such as lactic acid, rather than HCl, had been administered, metabolic compensation would have occurred also and the pH$_{40}$ would have been corrected more rapidly. Buffering and compensation are shown as though they have sequential effects. In reality, all buffering and compensatory effects would begin concurrently.

may occur with acidemia and alkalemia are of particular relevance to the thoracic surgeon and are shown in Table 7-3. Some, such as the effects of pH on oxygen-hemoglobin affinity, are well-known but still deserve careful study (Shappell and Lenfant, 1972).

It is generally taught that acidemia at first stimulates respiration but then produces respiratory failure when the acidemia is severe. If circulatory support is provided, as it is in total bypass, respiration is stimulated even with extreme acidemia (Peirce, 1961; see Fig. 7-11). Most deleterious effects of acidemia probably are caused by depression of cardiac function and are avoided during bypass. Acidemia need be of concern principally when bypass is being completed or in the post-bypass period. The possibility of reducing a high pulmonary vascular resistance (Enson et al., 1964; Barer et al., 1967), increasing renal blood flow (Kittle et al., 1965), or improving myocardial contractility are good reasons for trying to correct a serious acidemia.

As information accumulates, it appears likely, however, that alkalemia is a potentially more dangerous state than acidemia. Since alkalemia is not infrequently produced by the overzealous administration of alkali or by mechanical hyperventilation, its attendant risks deserve special emphasis. Good examples of the dangers are the leftward oxygen dissociation curve shift with potential "affinity hypoxia" (Fig. 7-7) and a reduction in serum potassium (Burnell et al., 1956) with potential muscle paralysis or cardiac problems.

TABLE 7-3 SOME PROBLEMS RELATED TO ABNORMALITIES OF HYDROGEN ION ACTIVITY

	Acidemia	Alkalemia
Heart	Reduced contractile force Slowing of rate Decreased catecholamine effects Harder to defibrillate	Increased rate May have reduced contractile force Arrhythmias
Arterioles	Decreased tone generally, but variable Increased pulmonary tone Less response to catecholamines	Variable and not well-studied
Respiration	Generally stimulates unless circulatory failure	May severely depress Apnea and hypoxia possible
Central Nervous System	Cortical depression Lethargy, coma Increased pain threshold Subcortical stimulation may cause convulsions	Cortical excitation Lethargy with seizures and coma possible but may be due to hypoxia
Sympathetic Nervous System	Activated with effects opposite to direct cardiac and arteriolar	Not well-studied System probably less active
Oxygen Dissociation Curve	Shifted to right O_2 uptake decreased O_2 release enhanced	Shifted to left O_2 more tightly bound May cause "affinity hypoxia"
Potassium	Plasma K^+ increase Intracellular K^+ reduced	Plasma K^+ decreased Intracellular K^+ increased

Hydrogen Ion Balance

Derangements resulting from excess acid are more frequently acute problems and generally easier to understand than are alkali or base deviations. Normal metabolism results in an excess acid production, which must be excreted by the lungs (carbon dioxide or carbonic acid) or kidneys (inorganic acids). Impairment of function of either of these organs may lead to acid retention. This may result also when intermediary metabolism is disturbed, as in diabetes, asphyxia, circulatory failure (Peirce, 1969b), or administration of large volumes of ACD blood. In such instances, substances that increase the hydrogen ion activity, such as keto acids, lactic acid, and citric acid, which are normally fully oxidized to carbon dioxide and water, accumulate (Huckabee, 1958; Peirce, 1962; Clowes, 1963; Peirce, 1967).

Alkaloses are, however, not infrequent during surgery and in the postoperative period (Table 7-4). Simple hyperventilation by mechanical means is probably an important cause of death due to "affinity hypoxia" and other serious side effects (Rotheram et al., 1964). A variety of conditions, such as septicemia, hepatorenal syndrome, and brain injury, may be accompanied by respiratory alkalosis, frequently with a concomitant nonrespiratory acidosis. Nonrespiratory alkaloses are more complex but of considerable importance. Addition alkalosis is frequent in alkali administration and occurs in a delayed form when large amounts of ACD blood are given (Lyons and Moore, 1966). There are 17 mEq of trisodium citrate in each unit of blood in addition to citric acid. As the citrate is metabolized, bicarbonate is generated to balance the sodium. This effect is accentuated by the

CONCEPTS OF ACID-BASE BALANCE

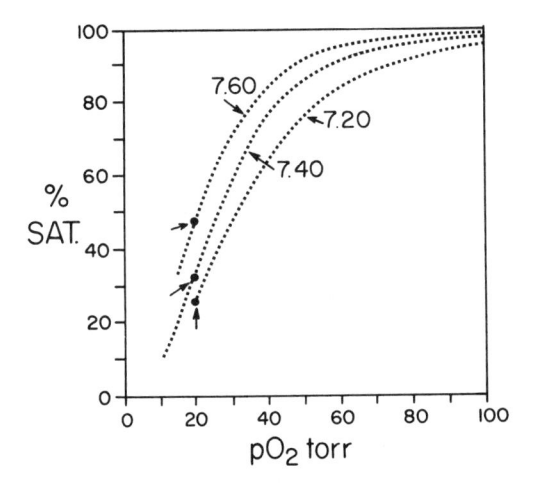

Figure 7-7. The effect of pH (Bohr) on the oxygen dissociation curve is illustrated. A rise in pH (decrease in hydrogen ion activity) increases the affinity of hemoglobin for oxygen. The principle effect is that less oxygen can be unloaded in the tissue at any given Po_2. An alkalemia can, therefore, significantly increase a preexisting hypoxia. This has been rather aptly called an "affinity hypoxia." A decrease in pH, such as occurs in conditions with decreased tissue perfusion, is somewhat compensated by the fact that more oxygen can be unloaded at any given Po_2. The decrease in oxygen-hemoglobin affinity also reduces the uptake of oxygen in the lungs at any given Po_2, but this change is relatively much less.

usual postoperative stress reaction, which results in maximum sodium and bicarbonate reabsorption from the renal tubule. The precise effect is not predictable from the number of transfusions (Miller et al., 1971). The administration of steroids, or the syndrome of hyperadrenalism, has the same effect.

Furosemide or ethacrynic acid may lead to an alkalosis by causing a loss of potassium, chloride, and hydrogen ions and reabsorption of bicarbonate. Nasogastric suction may cause severe losses of chloride and hydrogen with marked alkalosis. Chronic depletion of chloride and potassium may occur in long-standing respiratory insufficiency. Artificial ventilation for hypoxia may then unmask this depletion. Without chloride to reabsorb with sodium from the renal tubule or potassium to exchange for hydrogen ions, excess bicarbonate reabsorption and sometimes a "paradoxical aciduria" occurs (Refsum, 1961; Schwartz and Relman, 1967). Nonrespiratory alkalosis may occur in patients with liver failure. This is accentuated in the presence of bleeding varices (Sloop and Orloff, 1966).

A knowledge of the underlying mechanisms that may disturb hydrogen ion activity, coupled with its accurate measurement and

TABLE 7-4 SOME INTRAOPERATIVE AND POSTOPERATIVE CAUSES OF ALKALOSIS

Respiratory	Nonrespiratory
Intraoperative	**Intraoperative**
Mechanical hyperventilation	Administration of alkali
Hypothermia: Decreased CO_2 formed, solubility increased.	
	Postoperative
Postoperative	Administration of alkali
Mechanical hyperventilation	Blood transfusions in excess of 6 or 8 units
Brain injury or dysfunction	Diuretics as furosemide
Hepatorenal syndrome	Renal stress reaction
Septicemia	Steroid administration
	Nasogastric suction or vomiting
	Chronic respiratory insufficiency with low chloride or potassium
	Hepatic failure

intelligible recording, has the following advantages:

1. The cause of the disturbance may often be diagnosed.
2. The change in hydrogen ion activity with time will usually indicate whether the underlying problem is becoming more severe.
3. Methods of treatment may be determined rationally.
4. The results of treatment may be ascertained.

Body Buffers

Buffers are substances that resist change in hydrogen ion activity by taking up hydrogen ions when they are in excess and making them available when there is a deficit. Buffers, therefore, may be looked on as having a storage function for hydrogen ions. Buffers are both extracellular, principally in the blood, and intracellular. Blood buffers are predominantly bicarbonate (50 percent of total), the protein hemoglobin (30 percent), and the plasma protein (15 percent). Buffering by blood is rapid and achieved as soon as circulation of the blood has produced adequate mixing. The principle intracellular buffer is the protein myoglobin of muscle. It acts more slowly, but the exact rate of membrane equilibrium is not well-understood (see Fig. 7–6).

Hemodilution produces a relative deficiency of base by reducing the amount of buffer available per unit volume (Peirce, 1961). This dilutional acidosis need not be covered by the addition of alkali (Fig. 7–8).

Compensation

A useful clue to whether an acid-base deviation is a primary derangement or a compensation is the rule that a compensation tends to return the hydrogen ion activity toward normal but does not overshoot the mark. The position of the pH_A may, therefore, be of some assistance in formulating a diagnosis. As previously indicated, however, in mixed derangements the position of the pH_A may not be helpful. It follows, therefore, that a pH_A in the normal range may indicate one of three things:

1. A normal acid-base balance.
2. A compensated acid-base state.
3. The presence of two or more primary derangements that cancel each other out.

Respiratory Compensation

Respiratory adjustment of hydrogen ion activity takes place rapidly in patients with normally functioning lungs. This compensation is brought about by varying alveolar ventilation. Because of dead space effects, increasing or decreasing the depth of respiration is more effective than altering the rate. The precise numerical value of the $Paco_2$ is needed for the calculation of alveolar ventilation and other steady-state respiratory variables, such as the alveolar-arterial oxygen gradient (Altman and Dittmer, 1971), but is not otherwise of special clinical value. Respiratory compensation for an acidosis becomes less effective the more the

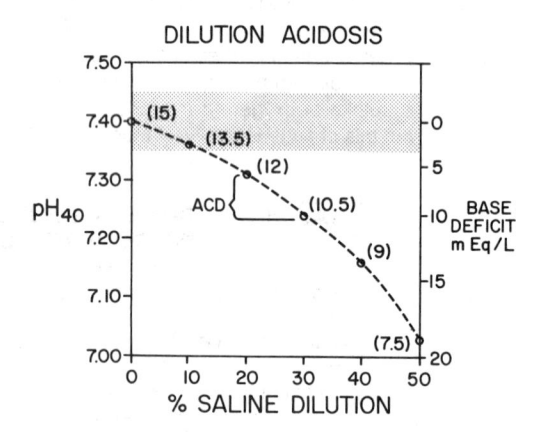

Figure 7–8. Dilution causes a reduction in buffer concentration and consequently produces an acidosis. When hemodilution is used for cardiac surgery, the pH_{40} will show a greater deviation from the normal range than is accounted for by any lactic acidosis or the acidosis caused by unbuffered banked blood. Alkali should not be given, however, for dilutional acidosis, as it is moderated by water redistribution and corrected by water elimination. Hemoglobin values (gm %) in parentheses. ACD shows range of dilution in ACD blood.

hydrogen ion activity is increased (see Figs. 7–2 and 7–3). Respiratory compensation for a decrease in hydrogen ion activity is of limited value, however, because arterial oxygen tension is diminished when alveolar ventilation is reduced, which may produce significant hypoxia in the patient. Respiratory compensation may be conspicuously limited in the postoperative cardiothoracic patient because of pain, sedation, pulmonary blood shunting, atelectasis, and retained secretions. In many instances, the patient will require mechanical ventilation, and the need for respiratory compensation must be considered in regulating the ventilator.

Metabolic Compensation
Lactic acidosis from decreased perfusion flow, dilutional acidosis, acidosis from the addition of ACD blood, and alkalosis from the addition of alkali are the principle early metabolic situations generally encountered in cardiothoracic surgery. Alkalosis should be especially avoided since it is dangerous. The problems of acidosis generally are corrected promptly if the cardiac output is adequate, so special postoperative attention should be given to maintaining adequate left heart filling pressures (Swan et al., 1970). The persistence of a nonrespiratory acidosis in the postoperative period generally suggests a low output syndrome, with the patient being unable to make a metabolic compensation (Ito et al., 1957). This effect may be obscured by development of a nonrespiratory alkalosis (see Table 7–4). In any event, metabolic compensation is limited to the metabolism of excess intermediary acids.

The lactic acidemia associated with low perfusion rates and the low cardiac output syndrome may roughly be correlated with oxygen debt. It is not ordinarily necessary to compute the "excess lactate" of Huckabee (1958), as the pyruvic acid usually is not much elevated (Knuttgen, 1962, Clowes, 1967, Peirce, 1967). Lactic acid is assumed to be distributed in the total body water (approximately seven times the blood volume). Oxgen debt amounts to 11.2 ml/mEq of lactic acid.

The total debt is, therefore, calculated as follows:

ml oxygen debt = mEq lactic acid × liters body water × 11.2.

It is apparent that a lactic acidosis of only 2.5 mEq per liter, which results in a pH_{40} of about 7.30, may represent as much as one liter of oxygen debt. Though a useful concept intellectually, the calculation of oxygen debt probably has little practical value at the present time. It should be emphasized also that correction of the acidosis with alkali does not abolish the oxygen debt but merely renders the repayment less urgent. Respiratory alkalosis may also be associated with an increase in lactate, probably indicating disruption of normal glucose metabolism (White et al., 1969).

Renal Compensation
The normal kidney not only excretes inorganic acids resulting from normal metabolism but may increase hydrogen ion excretion when carbon dioxide or other acids increase the hydrogen ion activity of the blood. The ability to excrete large amounts of hydrogen ion is accomplished by the following mechanisms:

1. Buffers, especially phosphate, are filtered and concentrated in the urine, permitting large amounts of hydrogen ion to be excreted with a relatively small change in the hydrogen ion activity of the urine.
2. Tubule cells produce ammonia, which diffuses into the tubules as the free base. Hydrogen ions are bound, forming ammonium ions, which diffuse poorly and are excreted.
3. The excretion of an acid urine increases the efficacy of the buffers and promotes back diffusion of carbon dioxide, thus enhancing the retention of base.

Renal compensation is slow, usually taking several days, and may be impaired postoperatively by stress and resultant high levels of aldosterone and antidiuretic hormone (ADH). Preoperative salt restriction, episodes of hypotension, and the presence of sepsis may decrease renal function and even precipitate acute renal failure. In alkalemia, hydrogen ions normally are retained, but a deficiency in chloride or potassium may prevent the retention of hydrogen ions and lead to a "paradoxical aciduria," which will aggravate the hydrogen ion deficit rather than correct it (Refsum, 1961; Schwartz and Relman, 1967).

Excretory problems resulting from a deficiency of free renal water or electrolyte, or excessive production of blood urea nitrogen, as in gastrointestinal bleeding, are thought of as prerenal. It frequently is difficult to distinguish prerenal and renal causes. The measurement of free water clearance may be helpful (Baek et al., 1972). Patients should have regular measurements of plasma and urine osmolality, and a urine approaching isosmolality should be a cause for careful evaluation. Cautious administration of pitressin will occasionally be helpful in demonstrating an inappropriate ADH level.

Temperature Correction

Temperature changes result in complex alterations in the solubility of carbon dioxide and oxygen, distribution of bicarbonate and other electrolytes across cell membranes, and shifts in the oxygen-hemoglobin dissociation curve. As the temperature is decreased in a blood sample, the Pco_2 and Po_2 fall, hydrogen ion activity decreases, and the pH rises. Since the cardiothoracic surgeon frequently uses hypothermia or must treat patients who have an elevation in temperature, understanding of the temperature correction is mandatory if the acid-base changes of the patient are to be followed intelligently. Fortunately, the pH at 40 torr (pH_{40}) changes very little with temperature and requires no correction in the clinical range (Brewin et al., 1955; Peirce, 1962). In addition, if the arterial pH is corrected, the relationship of the arterial and the pH_{40} values will be correct at the temperature of the patient, thus providing an automatic correction of $Paco_2$, which saves a good deal of trouble (Peirce, 1962, 1967). Since the hydrogen ion activity decreases as the temperature is lowered, the pH correction is added if the patient's temperature is below 37C, and is subtracted if the patient's temperature is above 37C. The temperature correction is shown in Figure 7–9; it amounts to approximately 0.015 pH units per degree centigrade (Rosenthal, 1948; Patterson and Sondheimer, 1966; Kent and Peirce, 1967). This correction should always be made for the arterial pH before it is charted.

The Effect of Hemoglobin Concentration

As seen in Figure 7–10, the conversion of pH_{40} to excess acid or base is affected by the hemoglobin value, since the hemoglobin constitutes approximately 30 percent of the blood buffer. For this reason, a given pH_{40} abnormality represents a greater change in acid or base when the hemoglobin value is high than when it is low. The hematocrit, or preferably the hemoglobin (approximately: hematocrit ÷ 3), should be measured each time acid-base values are determined. This will permit subsequent quantitative interconversions of various measurements without error.

Acute Steady-State Respiratory Changes

In the test tube, none of the values used to depict nonrespiratory changes in hydrogen ion activity are altered when the Pco_2 is varied. These values include the pH_{40}, the buffer base, the base excess, and the titratable acidity. For this reason they have been thought to be truly nonrespiratory. When the $Paco_2$ is varied in the patient, however, there is an alteration in the buffer content of the blood, and all of these "nonrespiratory" values do change. Increases in $Paco_2$ cause diffusion of sodium and bicarbonate from the vascular compartment, and decreases in $Paco_2$ have the opposite effect. These changes occur promptly and an acute steady state is reached in about 20 minutes (Goetter and Peirce, 1966; Arbus et al., 1969). When, subsequently, the blood sample is brought to a Pco_2 of 40 torr outside the body, it will have a different nonrespiratory value than would be the case if the Pco_2 was brought to 40 torr before the blood

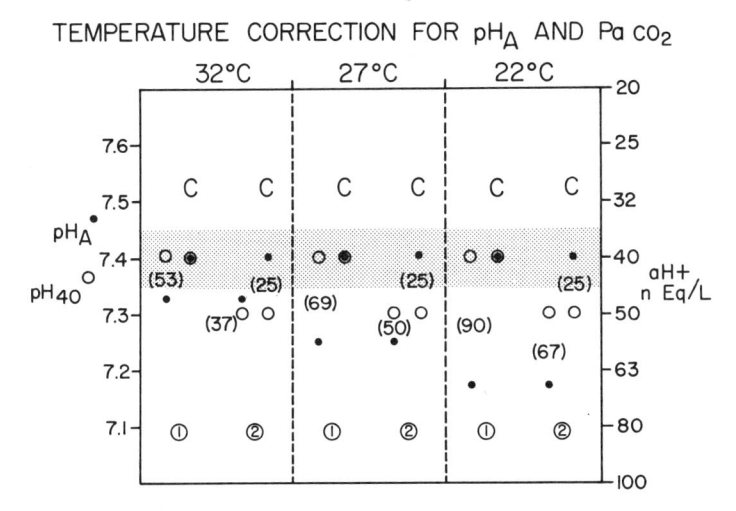

Figure 7-9. The pH_A and Pa_{CO_2} must be corrected to the patient's temperature to avoid serious error in acid-base evaluation. Data are shown for three different temperatures as read as 37C and as corrected to the patient's temperature (C). Hemoglobin for all examples is 15 gm%. The Pa_{CO_2} values are shown in parentheses. Example 1 at each temperature illustrates a normal acid-base status. Uncorrected, the pH_A appears abnormally low and the Pa_{CO_2} appears abnormally high. Example 2 at each temperature represents a compensated nonrespiratory acidosis. Uncorrected, the acidosis appears to be uncompensated at 32C. At lower temperatures, there appears to be a combined nonrespiratory and respiratory acidosis. If the pH_A is corrected to the patient's temperature, the Pa_{CO_2} can be read directly from the modified Siggaard-Andersen nomogram (Fig. 7-10) and need not be corrected separately. Note especially that the pH_{40} requires no temperature correction. Over an extremely wide range (shark to human) vertebrate blood has an almost constant pH at different temperatures, providing the Pa_{CO_2} remains constant (Kent and Peirce, 1967).

was removed. This correction for total body buffering of CO_2 is generally small enough so that it is not of much importance clinically. The fact that in vivo and in vitro values differ has been used, however, in attempts to discredit the Astrup method of acid-base measurement (Schwartz and Relman, 1963). This criticism is not warranted. The disagreement, if any, is with terminology and interpretation. The Astrup method of measurement is accurate and easy and produces data identical to those of any other good method of measurement.

Uncorrected, the pH_{40} tends to be deviated to the same side of the normal range as the arterial pH. For this reason, unless the pH_{40} is corrected for variations in total body buffering there will be an apparent nonrespiratory change with changes in P_{CO_2}. This effect is illustrated in Figure 7-11 and the correction is shown in Figure 7-12. The pH_{40} value can readily be corrected for the patient's P_{CO_2} before charting, but this is seldom desirable. It is better simply to accept the clinical fact that acute respiratory changes produce small nonrespiratory ones.

Chronic Respiratory Changes

Legitimate criticisms of nonrespiratory terms with an in vivo connotation are: (1) the possible incorrect identification of a compensation as a primary derangement; (2) failure to detect an acute derangement because of a preexisting chronic compensation; and (3) inevitable errors of interpretation in some instances when there are two or more opposing primary derangements. The second possibility is particularly likely to occur when chronic CO_2 retention has resulted in a substantial expansion of bicarbonate. Figure 7-13, for which

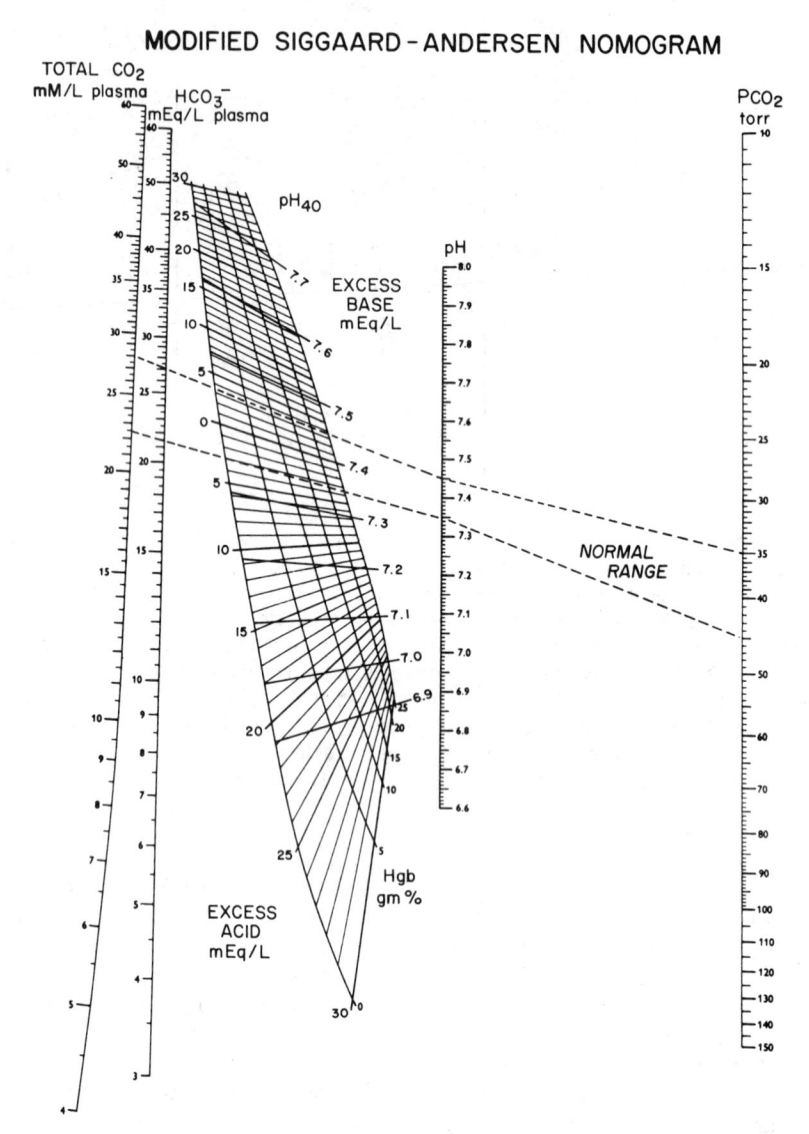

Figure 7-10. Siggaard-Andersen nomogram (1963) modified with permission. If any two acid-base values are measured, a straight edge placed through them will pass through other unmeasured values. The pH_{40} is shown to be a pivotal nonrespiratory value equivalent to the buffer base, the base excess, and the titratable acid. The behavior of blood in vitro can be demonstrated by rotating a straight edge about the intersection of the pH_{40} and the hemoglobin.

much data were drawn from Brackett et al. (1969), gives approximate 95 percent confidence limits for chronic $Paco_2$ values of 20 to 100 torr. Elimination of the compensation is slow when the $Paco_2$ is corrected, since bicarbonate must be excreted by the renal route.

Unless this relationship is well-understood, a low cardiac output state in a patient with chronic lung disease may go undetected, because the nonrespiratory acidosis is manifested not as a pH_{40} below the normal range but only as a deviation from the chronic pH_{40}

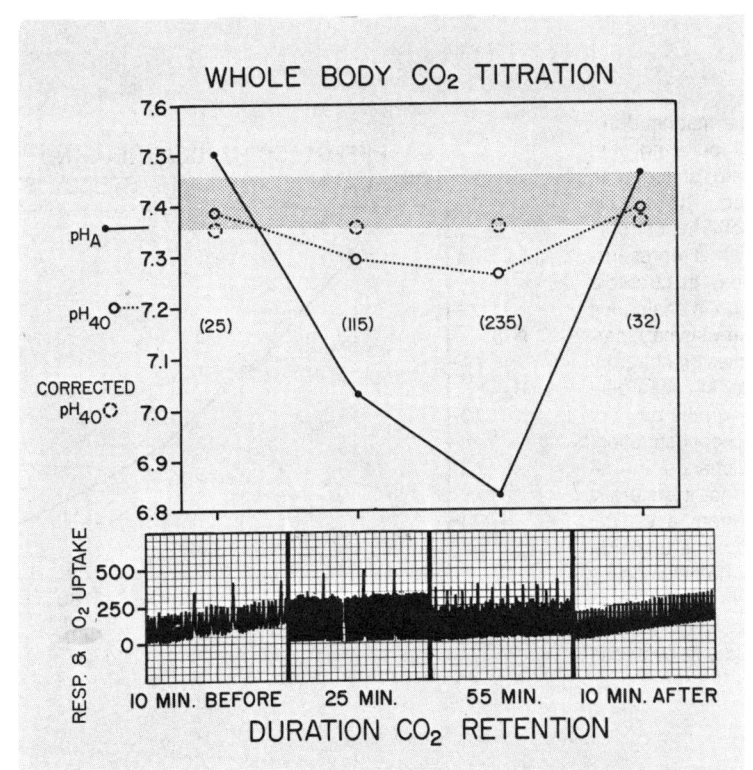

Figure 7-11. The effect of acute in vivo changes in Paco$_2$ are illustrated. Paco$_2$ values are shown in parentheses. Data are shown from a dog placed on total cardiopulmonary bypass and supported by an adequate extracorporeal flow but with the circuit lung ventilated by simple diffusion respiration so that Pco$_2$ rose in 55 minutes to 235 torr. The pH$_A$ fell to 6.84 and the pH$_{40}$ was reduced to 7.26 by actual loss of sodium bicarbonate from the blood to the extracellular space. Had the Paco$_2$ been brought back to 40 at any time, the pH$_{40}$ would have been at a constant value of 7.35. The change in pH$_{40}$ with Paco$_2$ demonstrates that respiratory changes do have effects usually considered nonrespiratory, which must be considered in evaluating the pH$_{40}$ measurement. The same is true for all other relatively nonrespiratory values such as buffer base, base excess, and titratable acidity. A corrected pH$_{40}$, not affected by changes in Paco$_2$ is shown (see Fig. 7–12).

$$pH_{40} \text{ (Corr)} = pH_{40} + k \log \frac{P_{CO_2}}{40}, \text{ where } k \cong 0.12.$$

confidence limit. Careful preoperative acid-base evaluation will largely prevent errors of this sort by detecting chronic elevations of the pH$_{40}$.

PHILOSOPHY OF TREATMENT

Use of Alkali

The simple correction of an acid-base imbalance is not a substitute for treating the underlying abnormality. In the case of the low cardiac output syndrome, treatment with alkali may be expected to improve myocardial function and enhance the effect of catecholamines, but the deviation of the pH$_{40}$ can then no longer be used easily as an index of circulatory integrity. The situation is somewhat analogous to attempting to assess the need for volume expansion in shock by the arterial pressure level after giving pressor drugs.

In general, if the arterial pH remains between 7.30 and 7.50, the hydrogen ion abnormality is insufficiently abnormal to require correction for the sake of correction alone. Attention should be directed to im-

Figure 7–12. The magnitude of change of blood buffering with acute steady state changes in Paco₂ is illustrated. The pH₄₀ is changed with both hypocapnia and hypercapnia. This represents a true gain or loss in titratable acidity. The change is analogous to that seen in the plasma bicarbonate that makes respiratory and nonrespiratory changes difficult to distinguish on the basis of the bicarbonate concentration. Fortunately, the change in the pH₄₀ is so small that it generally can be ignored from a clinical standpoint. A pH value unaffected by Paco₂ may be obtained by correcting the pH₄₀ according to the equation given in Figure 7–11. Corrected values are illustrated in Figure 7–11.

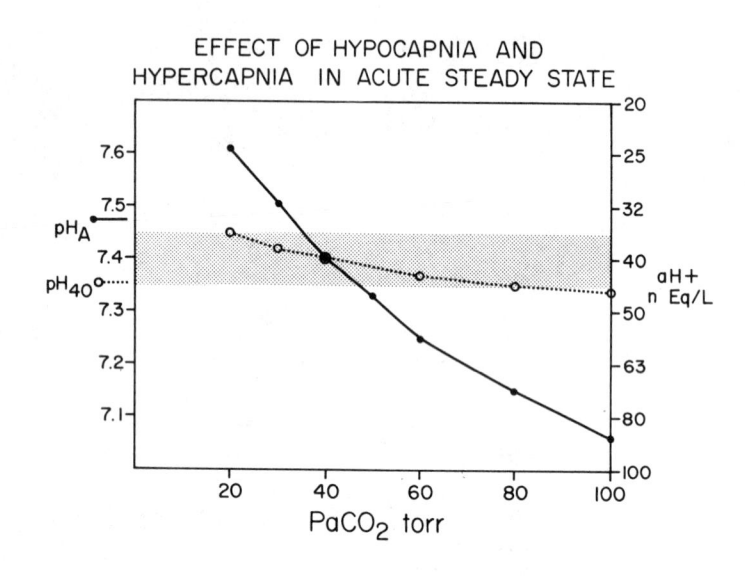

Figure 7–13. Confidence limits of approximately 95 percent are shown for chronic respiratory (Paco₂) effects. These values are largely taken from Brackett et al. (1969). Additional human values need to be obtained to clarify the confidence limits. Renal compensation produces an extension of base (NaHCO₃) at high chronic Paco₂ values. The opposite effect occurs with chronic reduction in Paco₂. It is important to recognize patients with renal compensation to avoid important errors of interpretation. A patient with an acute circulatory failure and a lactic acidemia might have a pH₄₀ within normal limits, though outside the chronic respiratory confidence span. It would be easy to misinterpret and fail to treat the circulatory failure.

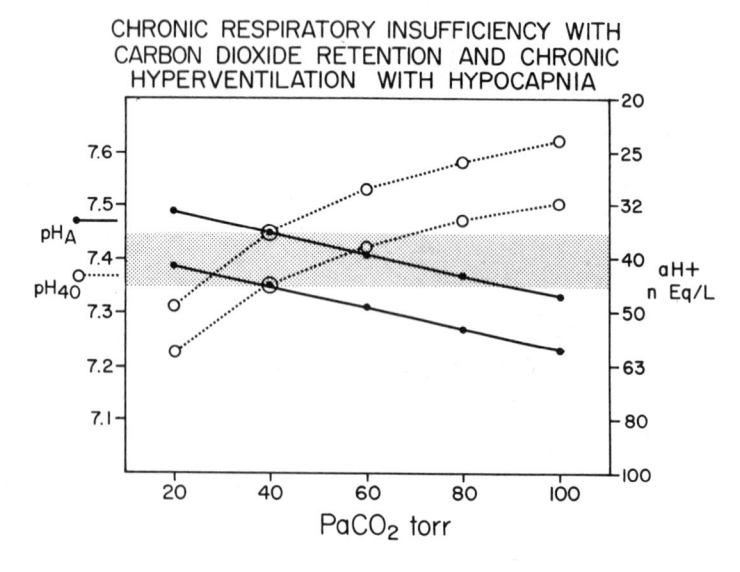

proving cardiac output, adjusting the ventilator, and giving appropriate fluids. When the abnormality is greater, or a trend toward progressive decompensation is apparent, correction will often be desirable. Attempts should always be made, however, to correct the underlying abnormal mechanisms at least concurrently.

The nonrespiratory abnormality denoted by the pH_{40} deviation is only what is seen in the blood and, therefore, represents the tip of the iceberg. The bulk of the imbalance, of indeterminate size, may lie in the extravascular extracellular space and the intracellular space. Any attempt to calculate the size of the entire acid-base imbalance on the basis of the blood value is an exercise in sophistry. If such a correction is attempted, the result may be disastrous to the patient. It is safer to make a correction of the blood abnormality alone. A pH_{40} of about 7.25 represents 10 mEq per liter of titratable acidity at a Pco_2 of 40 torr. An average adult would be expected to have a blood volume of about 5 liters, and an initial first correction would, therefore, require the administration of approximately 50 mEq of alkali or one 44.6 mEq ampoule of sodium bicarbonate IV. If a correction is elected, this amount of alkali should be given as rapidly as the situation warrants and another acid-base measurement made in 10 to 30 minutes, depending on the circumstances. An initial first correction for a pH_{40} of 7.10 would require approximately twice this dosage of alkali. Subsequent administration should be based on the results of the first injection and the condition of the patient. Unless circulatory failure persists, the total amount of alkali needed will usually be small, often only the initial dose (Peirce, 1961).

Two drugs are available for the treatment, by titration, of nonrespiratory acidosis. Sodium bicarbonate generally is effective in the therapy of acid-base disorders that accompany cardiac and great vessel surgery, but several possible advantages are offered by Tris buffer (THAM, Abbott) (Peirce, 1961, 1969a, 1969b). This material may be given without the addition of sodium. Its administration generally promotes diuresis, it crosses cell membranes readily, and it may be used in the presence of carbon dioxide retention, provided the patient is being carefully observed and a ventilator is available. Both drugs have the same potency, milliequivalent for milliequivalent. Tris buffer may be contraindicated in renal failure, subcutaneous infiltration may be very irritating, and, unfortunately, because it is supplied in single-dose containers of 150 mEq with 50 mEq of acetic acid (to reduce the alkalinity to pH 8.6), one container contains much more alkali than a standard ampoule of sodium bicarbonate.

In using alkali to reduce the acidosis of massive ACD blood administration one must remember that the final result may be an alkalosis. This can be moderated by undercorrecting the initial nonrespiratory acidosis (Miller et al., 1971).

Treatment with Acid

Although many factors may predispose to alkalosis in the postoperative period, the need to correct the hydrogen ion deficit by the administration of acid is unusual. Since an alkalemia is potentially dangerous, however, cautious use of ammonium chloride may occasionally be indicated in an attempt to relieve concomitant hiccoughs, tetany, arrhythmias, or central nervous system depression or hyperirritability.

A COMPOSITE EXAMPLE

Figure 7–14 illustrates a number of features of acid-base change in the perfused, postoperative cardiac patient. Data are a composite of several patients. For more dramatic examples see Peirce (1961, 1969a). The case is of a 50-year-old- man who had a triple vein graft for coronary insufficiency with moderate hemodilution (about 25 percent) and moderate hypothermia (to 31C). Data are limited to the time, pH_A, pH_{40}, temperature, and hematocrit. The pH_A values are corrected for temperature. The Pao_2 is omitted on purpose (though it is important), since it is not an

Figure 7–14. Acid-base changes during and following a triple coronary bypass using hemodilution and hypothermia are illustrated. A readily comprehensible pattern of change is shown by plotting pH_A and pH_{40} values. The pH_A is corrected to the patient's temperature. (1) Start of surgery. (2) Start of perfusion and cooling. (3) Begin warming. (4) Complete surgery, transport to intensive care unit, and place on a volume ventilator. (5) Add dead space. (6) Discontinue ventilator. See text for full explanation.

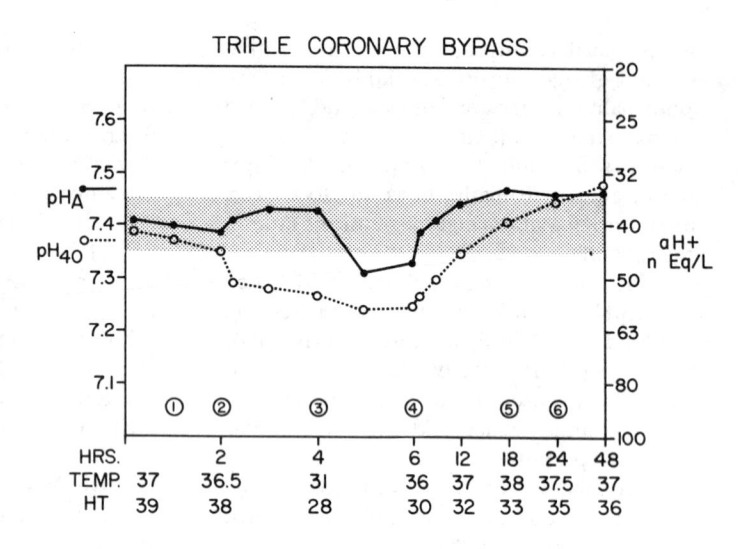

acid-base variable. It was at no time beyond reasonable limits. Only a few $Paco_2$ values are shown to avoid distracting attention from the pH pattern. The figure shows: (1) start of surgery; (2) start of perfusion and cooling; (3) begin warming; (4) complete surgery, transport to intensive care unit, and place on a volume respirator; (5) add dead space; (6) take off respirator. Patterns of significance include the following:

a. Initial situation: Acid-base status is within normal limits.
b. Perfusion acidosis: The low pH_{40} seen at start of perfusion (2) represents the effect of dilution, an incompletely buffered acid citrate load, and, since it persists for four hours, probably a moderately low flow state with some lactic acidosis. Alkali is not given to the patient on completion of surgery (4) and the progressive correction of the nonrespiratory acidosis indicates a satisfactory cardiac output.
c. Effect of hypothermia on $Paco_2$: Because of the increased solubility of CO_2 and its decreased metabolic production in hypothermia, the $Paco_2$ is low during cooling (2 to 3), which provides, in this instance, excellent respiratory compensation. With more rapid cooling, or hypothermia of greater depth, the addition of 3 to 5 percent CO_2 to the gas mixture is helpful in preventing serious alkalemia. An alkalemia would be a prominent feature in the present instance if there were no nonrespiratory acidosis.
d. Acidosis associated with warming: During the phase of warming (3 to 4), metabolic demands are increased and a low output cardiac state is usual. This is especially likely after valve replacement when there have been periods of myocardial hypoxia. As seen here, the pH_{40} is likely to fall further, indicating a progressive lactic acidosis. Respiratory compensation is less effective because now CO_2 is less soluble and more is being produced. For this reason the gas mixture should usually be switched to 100% oxygen.
e. Regulation of respirator: As the pH_{40} changes, the minute volume needs to be changed or the dead space adjusted to maintain a proper pH_A. At (5) it becomes clear that further reduction of the minute volume might result in atelectasis. As the pH_{40} has risen to a normal value, dead space is added and effectively increases the $Paco_2$.
f. Postoperative alkalosis: A tendency to nonrespiratory alkalosis with a rising pH_{40} is apparent at 24 hours. Possible causes of this are shown in Table 7–4. In this instance, the alkalosis most probably results from a combination of stress, the reconstituted ACD blood

used to prime, and some postperfusion ACD transfusion.

g. Respiratory compensation for a nonrespiratory alkalosis: At 48 hours a modest increase in $Paco_2$ is apparent, which tends to return the hydrogen ion activity toward normal. Since the patient is not obtunded, has a clear chest, and has good spontaneous respiration, this is assumed to represent a compensation. The surgeon must be alert to the possibility of fatigue or pulmonary complication in a patient so soon off a respirator, as one of these will frequently be the cause of an increased $Paco_2$. In this regard, the use of oxygen enrichment and/or sedation may significantly depress respiratory minute volume and favor CO_2 retention.

SUMMARY

Measurement and the convenient display of data relating to abnormalities of the hydrogen ion activity can provide important insights into many aspects of respiratory function, circulatory function, metabolism, renal function, and iatrogenic conditions of great importance to the cardiothoracic surgeon. The arterial pH indicates the net result of any acid-base imbalances, the pH of the same blood at a Pco_2 of 40 torr (mm Hg) provides a measure of nonrespiratory abnormalities and compensations, and the relation between these two pH values signals any deviation of the $Paco_2$ from 40 torr. To be most useful, the pH values are obtained at appropriate intervals and plotted against time, as the patient is a living organism, not a static chemical equation. Proper use of this notational system simplifies the clinician's job of interpreting the acid-base status of patients.

The physician must be alert to and correct for the prominent effects of temperature on arterial pH and $Paco_2$, and he or she must understand the potential confusion of chronic compensatory states. Generally, timely and properly interpreted acid-base information will permit steps to be taken to correct underlying respiratory and circulatory abnormalities. Should alkali or acid administration be necessary in uncompensated states to improve cardiac function and so forth, the correction should be done serially with only the abnormality of the blood being titrated at one time. Appropriately frequent acid-base measurements should be secured, as the amount of alkali or acid frequently will be much less than anticipated on a total body estimate. The special dangers of alkalemia are stressed. No cardiothoracic surgeon can be considered well-trained until he or she is able to use acid-base information comfortably and effectively.

REFERENCES

Altman P L, Dittmer D S: Respiration and Circulation, Biological Handbook. Bethesda, Md, Federation of American Societies for Experiment Biology, 1971, pp 127–128.

Arbus G E, Herbert L A, Levesque P R, Etsten B E, Schwartz W B: Characterization and clinical application of the "significance band" for acute respiratory alkalosis. N Engl J Med 280: 117–123, 1969.

Astrup P: A simple electrometric technique for the determination of carbon dioxide tension in blood and plasma, total content of carbon dioxide in plasma, and bicarbonate content in separated plasma at a fixed carbon dioxide tension (40 mm Hg). Scand J Clin Lab Invest 8: 33–43, 1956.

———, Jorgenson K, Siggaard-Andersen O, Engel K: The acid-base metabolism, a new approach. Lancet 1: 1035–1039, 1960.

Baek S, Brown R S, Shoemaker W C: Early prediction of acute renal failure with free water clearance. Surg Forum 23: 79–81, 1972.

Barer G R, Howard P, McCurrie J R: The effect of carbon dioxide and changes in blood pH on pulmonary vascular resistance in cats. Clin Sci 32: 361–376, 1967.

Brackett N C Jr, Wingo C F, Muren O, Solano J T: Acid-base response to chronic hypercapnia in man. N Engl J Med 280: 124–130, 1969.

Brewin E G, Gould R P, Nashat F S: An investigation of problems of acid-base equilibrium in hypothermia. Guy's Hosp Rep 104: 177–215, 1955.

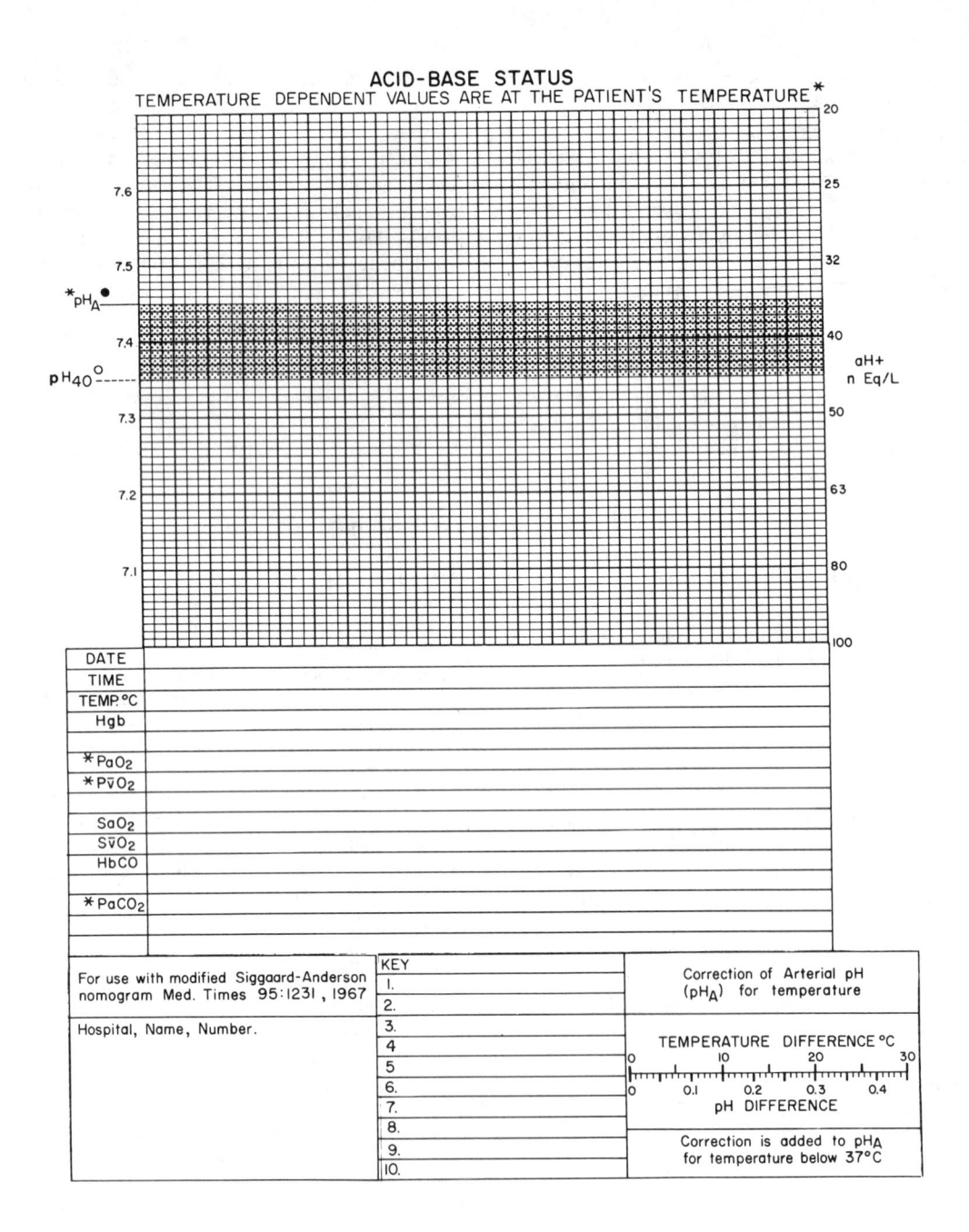

ACID-BASE STATUS
TEMPERATURE DEPENDENT VALUES ARE AT THE PATIENT'S TEMPERATURE*

pH values on vertical axis: 7.6, 7.5, 7.4, 7.3, 7.2, 7.1

*pH$_A$ •
pH$_{40}$ °

aH+ n Eq/L values: 20, 25, 32, 40, 50, 63, 80, 100

DATE										
TIME										
TEMP. °C										
Hgb										
*PaO$_2$										
*PvO$_2$										
SaO$_2$										
SvO$_2$										
HbCO										
*PaCO$_2$										

For use with modified Siggaard-Anderson nomogram Med. Times 95:1231, 1967

Hospital, Name, Number.

KEY
1.
2.
3.
4.
5.
6.
7.
8.
9.
10.

Correction of Arterial pH (pH$_A$) for temperature

TEMPERATURE DIFFERENCE °C
0   10   20   30
0   0.1   0.2   0.3   0.4
pH DIFFERENCE

Correction is added to pH$_A$ for temperature below 37°C

A simple format for recording acid-base and related variables which allows easy discernment of the patient's acid-base status as it changes with time. Acid-base status is determined by use of a two-variable system where the variables are commensurable.

Burnell J A, Villamil M F, Uyeno B T, Scribner B H: The effect in humans of extracellular pH change on the relationship between serum potassium concentration and intracellular potassium. J Clin Invest 35: 935–939, 1956.

Clowes G W A Jr: Metabolic responses to injury. Part II: acid-base balance. J Trauma 3:161–175, 1963.

Davis R P: Logland: A Gibbsian view of acid-base balance. (Editorial). Am J Med 42: 159–162, 1967.

Enson Y, Giuntini C, Lewis M L, Morris T Q, Ferrer M I, Harvey R M: The influence of hydrogen ion concentration and hypoxia on the pulmonary circulation. J Clin Invest 43: 1146–1162, 1964.

Goetter W E, Peirce E C II: Dependence of nonrespiratory parameters on Pco_2 (abstr). Fed Proc 25 (1): 264, 1966.

Gollan F: Criteria and requirements of adequate body perfusion. In Breast AN (ed): Heart Substitutes. Springfield, Ill, Thomas, 1966, pp 105–116.

Hasselbalch K A: Die "reduzierte" und die "regulierte" Wasserstoffzahl des Blutes. Biochem Z 74: 56–72, 1916.

Huckabee W E: Relationships of pyruvate and lactate during anaerobic metabolism. II. Exercise and formation of O_2 debt. J Clin Invest 37: 255–263, 1958.

Ito I, Faulkner W R, Kolff W J: Metabolic acidosis and its correction in patients undergoing open-heart operation. Cleve Clin Q 24: 193–204, 1957.

Kent K M, Peirce E C II: Acid-base characteristics of hibernating animals. J Appl Physiol 23: 336–340, 1967.

Kittle C F, Aoki H, Brown E B Jr: The role of pH and CO_2 in the distribution of blood flow. Surgery 57: 139–154, 1965.

Knuttgen H G: Oxygen debt, lactate, pyruvate, and excess lactate after muscular work. J Appl Physiol 17: 639–644, 1962.

Lyons J H Jr, Moore F D: Posttraumatic alkalosis: incidence and pathophysiology of alkalosis in surgery. Surgery 60: 93–106, 1966.

Miller R D, Tong M J, Robbins T O: Effects of massive transfusion of blood on acid-base balance. J A M A 216: 1762–1766, 1971.

Patterson R H Jr, Sondheimer H M: Assessing acid-base metabolism with samples of arterial blood obtained from hypothermic subjects. J Surg Res 6: 19–24, 1966.

Peirce E C II: Extracorporeal Circulation for Open Heart Surgery. Springfield, Ill, Thomas, 1969a, pp 53–58.

————: Pathophysiology of trauma. In Martin J D Jr (ed): Trauma to the Thorax and Abdomen. Springfield, Ill, Thomas, 1969b, pp 38–41.

————: Is acid-base balance important? Med Times 95: 1231–1256, 1967.

————: A simplified approach to obtaining and recording acid-base information in surgical patients. Ann Surg 156: 138–146, 1962.

————: Effects of 2-amino-1-hydroxymethyl-1, 3-propanediol (Tris) during cardiac bypass procedures. Ann N Y Acad Sci 92: 765–782, 1961.

————: A rapid quantitative method of determining metabolic and respiratory pH factors. Trans Am Soc Artif Organs 5: 265–272, 1959 and 6: 370–371, 1960.

Refsum H E: Hypokalemic alkalosis with paradoxical aciduria during artificial ventilation of patients with pulmonary insufficiency and high plasma bicarbonate concentration. Scand J Clin Lab Invest 13: 481–488, 1961.

Rosenthal T B: The effect of temperature on the pH of blood and plasma in vitro. J Biol Chem 173: 25–30, 1948.

Rotheram E B Jr, Sarar P, Robin E D: CNS disorder during mechanical ventilation in chronic pulmonary disease. J A M A 189: 993–996, 1964.

Schwartz W B, Relman A S: A critique of the parameters used in the evaluation of acid-base disorders. N Engl J Med 268: 1381–1388, 1963.

Schwartz W B, Relman A S: Effects of electrolyte disorders on renal structure and function. N Engl J Med 276: 383–458, 1967.

Shappell S D, Lenfant C J M: Adaptive, genetic, and iatrogenic alterations of the oxyhemoglobin-dissociation curve. Anesthesiology 37: 127–139, 1972.

Siggaard-Andersen O: Titratable acid or base of body fluids. Ann N Y Acad Sci 133: 41–58, 1966.

————: The Acid-Base Status of the Blood, 2nd ed. Baltimore, Williams & Wilkins, 1964, p 26.

————: Blood acid-base alignment nomogram. Scand J Clin Lab Invest 15: 211–217, 1963.

————: A graphic representation of changes of the acid-base status. Scand J Clin Lab Invest 12: 311–314, 1960.

————, et al.: Report of ad hoc committee on acid-base terminology. Ann N Y Acad Sci 133: 251–258, 1966.

Singer R B, Hastings A B: An improved clinical method for the estimation of disturbances of the acid-base balance of human blood. Medicine 27: 223–242, 1948.

Sloop R D, Orloff M J: An important syndrome of metabolic alkalosis in patients with cirrhosis, bleeding varices, and portacaval shunts. Surg Forum 17: 37–38, 1966.

Smith R N, Lemieux M D, Couch N P: Effects of acidosis and alkalosis on surface skeletal muscle hydrogen ion activity. Surgery 128: 533–538, 1969.

Swan H J C, Ganz W, Forrester J, Marcus H, Diamond G, Chonette D: Catheterization of the heart in man with use of a flow-directed balloon-tipped catheter. N Engl J Med 283: 447–451, 1970.

White J J, Mazur D, Kotas R V, Haller J A Jr: Excess lactate production due to hyperventilation and respiratory alkalosis. Surgery 66: 250–259, 1969.

8. Myocardial Energetics

Arnold M. Katz*

"The sum of all of the energies in an isolated system is constant."

The First Law of Thermodynamics

The First Law of Thermodynamics states that in a closed system energy is neither created nor destroyed, although changes in the nature of the energies in such a system are possible. It follows from this law that if energy is to appear in one portion of an isolated system, elsewhere in the system there must be a corresponding disappearance of energy. In the beating of the heart, where energy is caused to appear as blood is pumped under pressure into the aorta and pulmonary artery, the First Law of Thermodynamics requires that an appropriate amount of energy must disappear somewhere else. Thus, the generation of *mechanical work* by the myocardium represents the conversion into mechanical work of another form of energy, namely chemical energy available from the metabolism of foodstuffs. Like any other muscle, therefore, the heart is a *mechanochemical transducer* in that it converts chemical energy into mechanical energy. This fact must be constantly borne in mind by the physician who evaluates the cardiac patient preoperatively, by the surgeon who drastically alters myocardial function interoperatively, and by the team that works to restore and maintain circulatory function in the postoperative period.

The operation of the First Law of Thermodynamics requires that for any increase in the expenditure of mechanical energy by the heart, either more chemical energy must be made available to the myocardium or else a greater portion of the chemical energy released by the working myocardium must be converted into mechanical work and less be "wasted" as heat (i.e., an increase in mechanical efficiency). For this reason, the physician who is faced with a clinical situation where cardiac function is suboptimal must be aware of the possibility that the availability of chemical energy or the efficiency of its conversion into mechanical work may be impaired. In this chapter, several clinical problems will be examined from this standpoint. No attempt will be made to present a complete description of the mechanisms involved in these situations, this being a subject broad enough to warrant the writing of yet another textbook.[†] Instead, this discussion will focus on a limited number of general principles, the most important of which is that when faced with a patient with cardiac failure, the physician or surgeon must ensure that the supply of chemical energy to the myocardium is adequate to meet the re-

---

*Supported by Research Grants HL-22135 and HL-21812 from the United States Public Health Service, and a grant-in-aid from the American Heart Association.

†Katz, AM, Physiology of the Heart. New York: Raven Press, 1977.

quirements for the generation of mechanical energy. The cardiac surgical patient, like every known system in the universe, cannot evade the First Law of Thermodynamics!

THE HEART IS AN OBLIGATORY AEROBE

It is well-established that the heart derives energy for its mechanical performance primarily by the oxidation of a variety of carbohydrates, fats, and, to a much smaller extent, proteins. A much lesser ability to generate chemical energy by anaerobic metabolism has been known for half a century, but because this capacity for anaerobic energy production is not able to provide more than 5 percent of the energy needs of the mammalian heart, when deprived of oxygen the myocardium quickly ceases its contractile activity and the pumping of the heart becomes arrested.

The oxygen dependency of cardiac contraction is related to the high energy needs that are mandated by the sustained nature of the muscular action of the heart. Unlike most skeletal muscles, which contract intermittently and can rest between efforts, the heart muscle contracts without pause for a lifetime. Denied periods of recovery in which a depleted energy supply can be restored, the heart must, over any extended period of time, generate as much chemical energy from the metabolism of foodstuffs as it uses to maintain the circulation. It is thus a fundamental law of the heart that *the rate of expenditure of mechanical energy cannot exceed the rate of chemical energy production.* In the postoperative patient who is suffering from the inadequate mechanical output of a hypodynamic heart, for example, no inotropic agent can restore circulatory normality if the delivery of chemical substrates to the myocardium is lacking. Because a large variety of fats and carbohydrates, both endogenous and exogenous, can be oxidized by mitochondria, which fill about 40 percent of the myocardium (Figure 8–1), failure of the heart that is caused by inadequate energy production most commonly results from myocardial hypoxia. Myocardial hypoxia can, in turn, occur when oxygen delivery to the myocardium is reduced, or when energy demands become so great that they exceed the ability of the coronary circulation to deliver oxygen.

THE HYPOXIC HEART*

When the hypoxic myocardium fails, its contractile properties resemble closely those of the heart in a negative inotropic state. In the clinical approach to the patient with myocardial failure, therefore, the distinction between an unfavorable inotropic state induced by a deficiency in energy supply and that caused by hormonal abnormalities or the improper use of drugs cannot be made by any physiologic analysis of cardiac function, no matter how sophisticated. Instead, the correct clinical assessment can be made only by a judicious evaluation of the results of different modalities of therapy, both those intended to improve oxygen delivery to the myocardium and those designed to improve myocardial contractility.

The profound dependence of cardiac function on the continuing delivery of substrate, and especially of oxygen, is reflected in the rapid failure of the hypoxic myocardium. Soon after a coronary artery is occluded in the intact heart, systole is abbreviated, and less than a minute later the ischemic area of the myocardium bulges outward late in systole, being unable to overcome the pressure generated by the normally perfused regions of the ventricles. What mechanisms are responsible for this early "pump failure" remains uncertain. While the myocardium, like skeletal muscle, has the capacity to generate chemical energy in the absence of oxygen, anaerobic energy production in the mammalian heart is not adequate to provide sufficient ATP to sustain more than approximately 5 percent of normal contractile activity. This is because the pathways by which glucose and glycogen are

---

Katz, 1973a, 1978

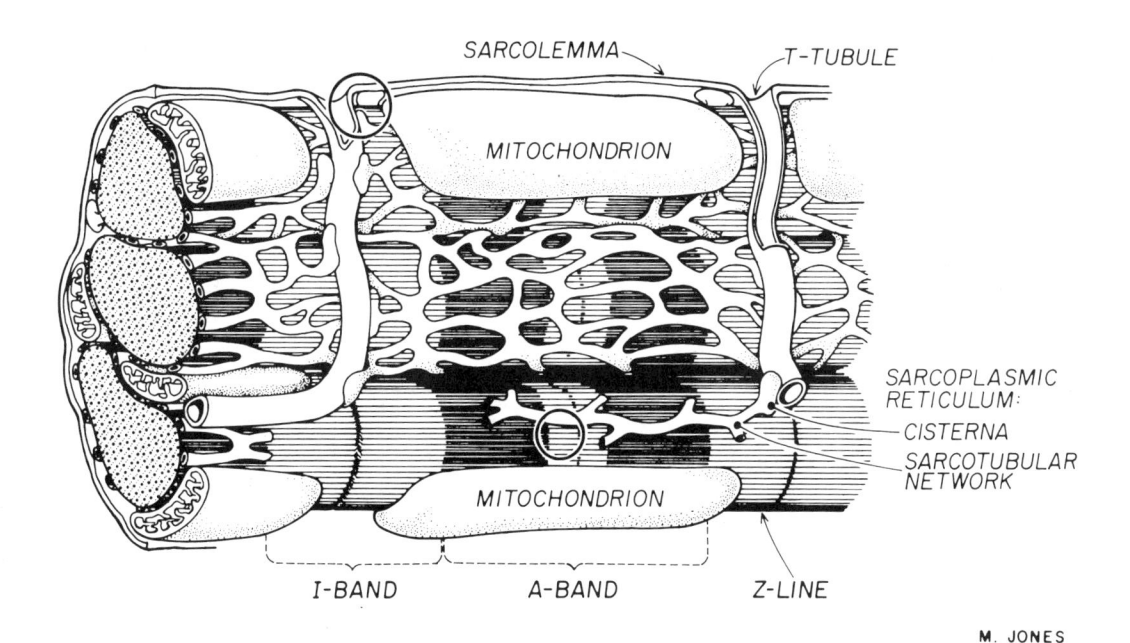

Figure 8–1. The myocardial cell. The *contractile proteins* are arranged in a regular array of thick and thin filaments (seen in cross-section at the left side of the figure). The *A-band* represents that region of the sarcomere occupied by the *thick filaments* into which thin filaments extend from either side. The *I-band* is the region of the sarcomere occupied only by *thin filaments,* which extend toward the center of the sarcomere from the *Z-lines,* which bisect each I-band. The *sarcomere,* the functional unit of the contractile apparatus, is the region between each pair of Z-lines and contains two half I-bands and one A-band. The *sarcoplasmic reticulum,* a membrane network that surrounds the contractile proteins, consists of the *sarcotubular network* at the center of the sarcomere and the *cisternae,* which abut the t-tubules and the sarcolemma. The *transverse tubular system* (t-tubule) represents an extension from the sarcolemma and carries the extracellular space into the myocardial cell. In contrast to the t-tubules of skeletal muscle, those of the myocardium can run in a longitudinal as well as in a transverse direction. *Mitochondria* are shown in the central sarcomere and, in cross-section, at the left side of the figure. Reprinted from Katz, 1975.

metabolized anaerobically to form lactic acid are inefficient, there being only two moles of ATP produced per mole of glucose consumed, instead of approximately 36 produced by oxidative metabolism.

Measurements of the contents of substrates and high energy phosphate compounds do not support the view that the contractile failure of the hypoxic myocardium is caused directly by a lack of ATP for conversion to mechanical energy. Instead, the curtailment of aerobic energy production appears to set into motion a series of events that impairs the processes by which the depolarization of the sarcolemma—the action potential—generates a signal that initiates the contractile process. The consequent reduction in myocardial contractility leads to an attenuation of the rate of liberation of mechanical energy. In this way, the heart curtails the most expensive of its energy-consuming reactions before the levels of high energy compounds are severely reduced. The functional significance of this response to myocardial ischemia is probably to delay the onset of irreversible consequences of severe depletion of these energy stores; namely, rigor and necrosis. To understand these mechanisms, it will be useful to review the complex role of adenosine triphosphate (ATP) in the chemistry of the contractile process (Katz, 1970; Katz and Tada, 1977).

Adenosine triphosphate has a dual role in muscle. On the one hand this high energy compound serves as the source of the chemical energy that is used in a number of energy-consuming reactions, notably those interactions between the contractile proteins that give rise to contraction. Yet higher concentrations of ATP also have the ability to dissociate the contractile proteins, an action that is the opposite of its primary role as a source of immediately available chemical energy for contraction. This second function of ATP, which reflects its "plasticizing effect," permits the muscle to be maintained in a state of relaxation in the absence of Ca^{2+}. High ATP concentrations also have an important regulatory role in a variety of biochemical reactions in the heart.

While ATP can induce either contraction or relaxation, the transitions from rest to contraction and from contraction to relaxation do not result from changes in the concentration of ATP within the heart. Instead, changes in intracellular calcium ion concentration represent the physiologic mechanism that permits the myocardial cell to use alternatively the "contraction-promoting" and "relaxing" actions of ATP in the cardiac cycle. These mechanisms will be examined in some detail later in this chapter; in the present context it is necessary only to indicate that a marked decline in ATP concentration could abolish its plasticizing effect, which requires higher ATP concentrations than the contraction-promoting action. Should such a drastic fall in ATP concentration occur in the hypoxic myocardium, the heart would go into a state of rigor (Katz and Tada, 1977) that could be reversed only if the metabolic processes responsible for ATP regeneration were to be restarted; for example, by the restoration of oxygen delivery to the hypoxic myocardium. Yet the ability to reestablish oxygen delivery to the heart that is in rigor is limited, if not altogether lost, because the forces compressing the coronary blood vessels (intramyocardial pressure) could exceed the ability of aortic pressure to reestablish flow to such region. For this reason, the failure of the hypoxic heart to contract while ATP levels are high enough to maintain plasticity (i.e., failure in diastole) has the advantage to the myocardium of allowing for restoration of function in the hypoxic heart should oxygen supply be reestablished.

THE ISCHEMIC HEART[*]

The effects of ischemia on the contractile performance of the heart are similar to those of hypoxia in that myocardial contractility rapidly declines and the heart is eventually arrested in a relaxed state. This rapid mechanical deterioration parallels the very rapid fall in the oxygen tension within the myocardium that follows coronary artery occlusion. Even though ischemia interrupts the delivery of carbohydrates and fats to the myocardium, mechanical failure occurs long before the intramyocardial stores of glycogen are exhausted; in fact, stores of fat actually increase in the severely ischemic myocardium. As is the case in hypoxic heart failure, the level of ATP is only slightly reduced when the ischemic heart fails.

Accumulation of extracellular K^+, which would diminish the normal transmyocardial potassium gradient, represents an alternative explanation for the failure of the ischemic heart. That loss of intracellular K^+ is probably not the primary mechanism responsible for the rapid decline in contractility is suggested by the finding that measurements of transcellular electrical potentials in the ischemic heart do not show a marked decrease in resting potential, such as would be expected to result from a loss of the normal potassium gradient across the cell membrane. Instead, the major effect of ischemia on the cardiac action potential is an abbreviation of the plateau phase. This finding is more likely to indicate a change in the calcium-dependent

---

[*]*Katz 1973b, 1978; Kübler and Katz, 1977.*

properties of the membrane than in those that reflect potassium gradients.

The ischemic heart, like the hypoxic heart, rapidly attenuates its contractile activity, so that both hypoxic and ischemic cardiac failure appear to result from negative inotropic mechanisms that are potentially reversible, at least in their early stages. The mechanism of these types of myocardial failure remains obscure, but the inescapable consequences of the First Law of Thermodynamics dictate that no inotropic agent, no matter how powerful, can have any lasting clinical value if cardiac failure is caused by a deficit in the delivery of oxygen to the myocardium. Thus, reversal of this type of myocardial failure can be achieved not by inotropic agents, but only by restoration of the normal balance between energy (oxygen) supply and demand.

CONTROL OF MYOCARDIAL CONTRACTILITY: "PHASIC" AND "TONIC" CONTROL MECHANISMS*

There is a growing body of evidence that changes in myocardial contractility can be brought about by two quite different biochemical mechanisms. The first, a "phasic mechanism," is capable of inducing rapid changes in contractility on a beat-to-beat basis, whereas the other, which can be considered a "tonic mechanism," requires hours or days to evolve. The tonic mechanism, which appears capable of influencing myocardial contractility as the result of changes in the chemical structure of certain of the heart's contractile proteins, is probably of less clinical significance in the cardiac surgical patient postoperatively than are the phasic mechanisms, which can effect rapid changes in myocardial contractility.

The tonic mechanisms appear to reflect the synthesis in the myocardium of contractile proteins that have an altered intrinsic rate of energy use. This rate, manifested in vitro as the intrinsic rate of ATP hydrolysis (ATPase activity) by *myosin*, one of the heart's contractile proteins, has been reported to increase in response to certain physiologic stresses, such as exercise. Conversely, myosin ATPase activity has been reported to be decreased in the chronically overloaded heart, especially after hypertrophy and the onset of heart failure. Although these observations are not yet universally accepted, their potential significance can be understood in terms of the First Law of Thermodynamics. In the case of the failure of the hypertrophied, overloaded heart, such as has been suggested to occur in response to abnormal pressure loads (e.g., aortic stenosis), volume loads (e.g., mitral insufficiency), and after the deletion of significant portions of working myocardium (e.g., ischemic heart disease), a reduction in the intrinsic rate of energy use might help satisfy the absolute requirement that in the heart the rate of energy production must be matched to the rate of energy expenditure. A slower rate of ATP use would help compensate for a deficit in the ability of the myocardium to generate ATP, when the deficit is caused by chronically increased demands for mechanical energy or when energy supply is chronically impaired. There is, in addition, some evidence that a reduction in myosin ATPase activity can improve mechanical efficiency in the tension-loaded myocardium, albeit at the expense of impairing the ability of the heart to achieve a high rate of energy expenditure when tension is low. Increasing the proportion of the energy available from ATP hydrolysis that can be used to develop tension could aid survival by the heart in the face of a sustained increase in the requirements for force generation.

The phasic mechanisms that permit myocardial contractility to be rapidly altered are probably of greatest importance in the responses of the myocardium to the negative inotropic actions of hypoxia and ischemia, and to the positive inotropic actions of drugs that enhance myocardial contractility. These phasic changes in myocardial contractility proba-

---

Katz, 1975.

bly reflect variations in the amount of calcium released to activate the contractile proteins in a complex series of events called *excitation-contraction coupling* (Katz, 1975). This process, in which the signal initiated by the action potential at the cell surface initiates the mechanical activity of the contractile proteins, leads to the mobilization and delivery of calcium ion (Ca^{2+}) to troponin, the Ca^{2+}-receptor located on the thin filament of the sarcomere. The potential sources, routes of delivery, and ultimate action of this Ca^{2+} will be considered at this point to provide some insight into the mechanisms of both the negative inotropic actions of hypoxia and ischemia and the positive inotropic actions of some of the drugs commonly used to strengthen the heartbeat.

EXCITATION-CONTRACTION COUPLING: THE DELIVERY OF Ca^{2+} TO THE CARDIAC CONTRACTILE PROTEINS*

While it is now well-established that Ca^{2+} is the chemical trigger that initiates the mechanical activity of the heart, the mechanisms by which Ca^{2+} is made available to the contractile proteins of the heart are complex and not yet fully understood. In the human heart, it is likely that two pathways participate in the delivery of Ca^{2+} to its receptor on the contractile proteins (Fig. 8–1). One of these is the movement of Ca^{2+} from the extracellular fluid into the interior of the cardiac muscle cell, and the other involves the movement of Ca^{2+} from an intracellular storage site in the sarcoplasmic reticulum to the cytosol immediately surrounding the contractile proteins, where it becomes available to bind to the troponin to initiate contraction.

The movement of Ca^{2+} from the extracellular space to the interior of the myocardial cell is probably effected by a large concentration gradient between the Ca^{2+} in the fluid bathing the cardiac muscle cell, which is the millimolar range, and the Ca^{2+} in the interior of the cell, where Ca^{2+} concentration is probably less than 0.1 µM in diastole and no more than 10 µM during systole. Thus, an inward movement of Ca^{2+} will readily occur when the cell membrane becomes permeable to Ca^{2+}. In diastole, the cell membrane is almost completely impermeable to Ca^{2+}, so that little or no Ca^{2+} is able to pass into the cell along this sizable concentration gradient. While the initial phase of the cardiac action potential, like that in nerve and skeletal muscle, involves the opening of "sodium channels," the characteristic plateau of the cardiac action potential is caused by an inward cationic current that is carried by Ca^{2+}. During the plateau of the cardiac action potential, specific calcium channels open briefly to allow a limited amount of Ca^{2+} to enter the cell. The Ca^{2+} entry during a single systole is much less than would be able to equalize the Ca^{2+} concentrations across the plasma membrane, but in the heart this influx of Ca^{2+} represents a significant contribution to the amount of Ca^{2+} available within the cell to activate the contractile proteins.

A great deal of evidence indicates that the Ca^{2+} derived from extracellular stores does not go directly to the contractile proteins; instead, the Ca^{2+} that enters during the plateau of the cardiac action potential is first retained in an intracellular storage site from which it becomes available for release during the following contractions. (Fig. 8–2) Thus, this Ca^{2+} entry increases the quantum of Ca^{2+} that is released to the contractile proteins in subsequent contractions, rather than going directly to the Ca^{2+} receptor of the contractile proteins. While the intracellular pool that receives the Ca^{2+} that enters the myocardium during systole has not yet been localized, it is reasonable to assume that this pool is within the heart's sarcoplasmic reticulum.

In most mammalian skeletal muscles, the sarcoplasmic reticulum (SR) is the source of virtually all of the Ca^{2+} that is delivered to the contractile proteins to initiate contraction, and reaccumulates this Ca^{2+} at the end of the contraction. While it has already been pointed out that Ca^{2+} entry from the extracellular

---

Fozzard and Gibbons, 1973; Katz, 1970, 1974, 1975; Katz and Repke, 1973; Weber and Murray, 1973; Reuter, 1974.

Figure 8–2. Calcium movements across the membranes of the sarcolemma and the sarcoplasmic reticulum. *Lower Diagram.* Release of calcium from the sarcoplasmic reticulum (SR) into the cytosol is probably largely responsible for the delivery of activator calcium to troponin, the calcium receptor of the contractile apparatus. This calcium appears to be derived primarily from stores in the subsarcolemmal cisternae (CISTERNA). Filling of these calcium stores from the extracellular space (EXTRACELLULAR) occurs across the sarcolemma and by way of the transverse tubular system (T-SYSTEM). A possible role of calcium stores in the mitochondria (MITOCH) is also illustrated, though this mechanism for delivery of calcium to the contractile proteins remains controversial. *Upper Diagram.* Schematic representation of enzyme and transport systems of the cardiac sarcolemma. Reading from left to right: *The calcium pump* (left) can transport calcium or sodium out of the cell, there being competition between these two cations for this efflux mechanism. *The sodium pump* (center) (Na + K ATPase) normally pumps sodium out of the cell in exchange for potassium. *Adenylate cyclase* (right) is responsible for the production of cyclic AMP. The binding of norepinephrine (NE) to the beta receptor (R) activates the catalytic component (C) of ADENYLATE CYCLASE to synthesize cyclic AMP (cAMP) from ATP.

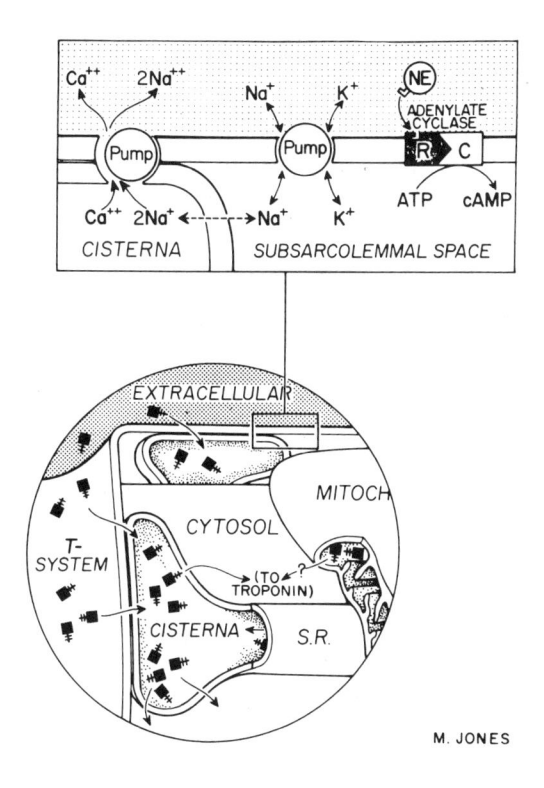

fluid contributes in an as yet incompletely understood manner to cardiac contraction, it is likely that in the heart the SR plays a similar role in both the initiation and termination of systole. Thus, the cardiac action potential probably triggers the release of Ca^{2+} from this intracellular store, and systole is terminated when Ca^{2+} is reaccumulated by the SR.

EXCITATION-CONTRACTION COUPLING: THE ACTION OF Ca^{2+} ON THE CARDIAC CONTRACTILE PROTEINS*

Although many details of the complex interaction between Ca^{2+} and the cardiac contractile proteins that initiates systole remain to be worked out, it is now clear that the contractile process itself results from the interactions between *myosin* and *actin;* two of the four named proteins of the contractile apparatus, and that Ca^{2+} control of the actin-myosin interactions requires the participation of two additional proteins: *troponin* and *tropomyosin.* The actomyosins made from actin and myosin alone have the ability both to liberate chemical energy and to undergo physiochemical changes that appear to represent an in vitro manifestation of the contractile process as it occurs in living muscle. *Myosin,* the major protein of the thick filament of the sarcomere (Fig. 8–3), catalyzes the hydrolysis of ATP, thereby serving as the "key" that unlocks the chemical energy of this nucleotide. Although the intrinsic ATPase activity of myosin is slow, it is accelerated by *actin,* which is the major protein of the thin filament.

Together, these two proteins can, under appropriate conditions, exhibit the properties

---

*Katz, 1970, 1974; Weber and Murray, 1973; Katz and Tada, 1977.

cally active "head" of the myosin molecule, which projects from the thick filament as the "cross-bridge," interacts with a site on the actin of the thin filament (Fig. 8–4). Thus, actomyosins made only of actin and myosin can, in vitro, exhibit the essential transducing function of muscle described at the beginning of this chapter. However, such two-protein actomyosins lack another salient feature of the contractile apparatus, namely, the ability to respond to the Ca^{2+} that normally effects excitation-contraction coupling.

The mechanism by which Ca^{2+} acts on the contractile proteins to initiate contraction involves a complex interaction with *tropomyosin* and *troponin*, two other proteins that are present, along with actin, in the thin filament of the sarcomere. The growing complexity of our knowledge of this control system is illustrated by the fact that troponin is now recognized to consist of three separate proteins, each of which serves a specific function in the control of the contractile process.

While it is clear that Ca^{2+} initiates contraction by an interaction with the regulatory proteins—tropomyosin and troponin—that involves the binding of Ca^{2+} to one of the components of troponin, this excitatory effect of Ca^{2+} does not represent a direct activating effect of the cation. Instead, Ca^{2+} acts to reverse an inhibitory effect of tropomyosin and the troponin complex on actomyosin that, in the absence of Ca^{2+}, "blocks" the actin-myosin interactions that give rise to tension and shortening. Stated simply, in the absence of Ca^{2+}, the tropomyosin-troponin complex inhibits contraction; Ca^{2+} initiates contraction by reversing this inhibition. Thus, if one adds the tropomyosin-troponin complex to an actomyosin composed only of highly purified actin and myosin under conditions where ATP would be rapidly hydrolyzed and the physicochemical changes that represent contraction would be seen, the regulatory proteins cause mechanochemical transduction to be inhibited and the actomyosin to remain in a state analogous to relaxation. This inhibitory effect can be reversed by the addition of small amounts of Ca^{2+}, an action that occurs when

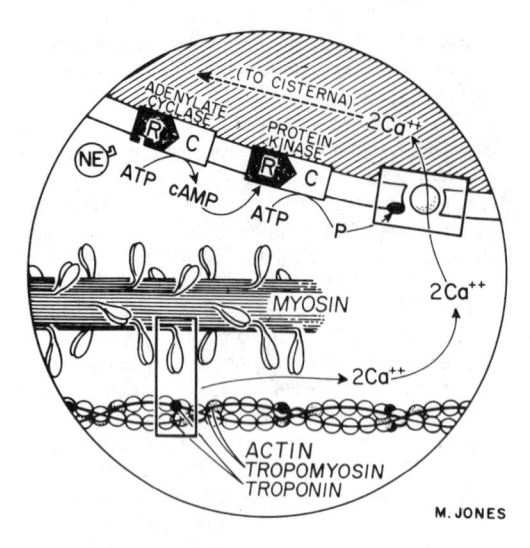

Figure 8–3. Diagrammatic representation of the contractile proteins and of enzymatic activities associated with the membranes of the sarcoplasmic reticulum. The *contractile proteins* (lower portion of diagram) are distributed between the thick filament (MYOSIN) and thin filament (ACTIN, TROPOMYOSIN, and the TROPONIN complex). Contraction takes place when the myosin cross-bridges of the thick filament interact with actin of the thin filament (see Fig. 8–4). The membrane of the *sarcoplasmic reticulum* (upper portion of diagram) has been found to contain key enzymes involved in the response of the cell to agents which, like norepinephrine (NE), cause cyclic AMP (cAMP) to be synthesized from ATP. These include ADENYLATE CYCLASE (left, see also Fig. 8–2) and PROTEIN KINASE (center), which catalyzes transfer of the terminal phosphate to ATP to various proteins, including those of the sarcoplasmic reticulum. Activation of the cyclic AMP-dependent protein kinase occurs when cyclic AMP binds to a receptor component (R), which, when not bound to cyclic AMP, prevents the actions of the catalytic component of protein kinase (C). Also shown is the calcium pump (right), which mediates the removal of calcium from troponin (see also Fig. 8–4) and its transport into the sarcoplasmic reticulum (see Fig. 8–6).

of tension generation and shortening that represent the conversion of the chemical energy derived from ATP into a form of mechanical work. These manifestations of the contractile process occur when the enzymati-

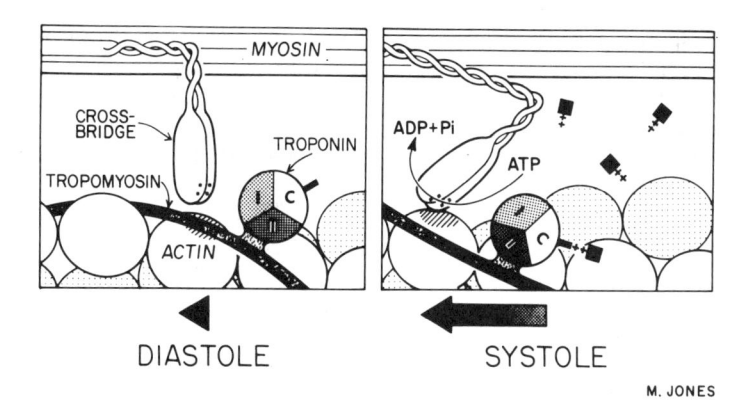

Figure 8–4. Schematic diagram illustrating current knowledge of the interactions of the heart's contractile proteins. **A.** Diastole. The potential interaction between the myosin cross-bridge and its light subunits (small rectangles) with the actin filament (represented as a polymer composed of two strands, each made up of a string of ovoid actin monomers) is inhibited by the regulatory proteins: tropomyosin and the troponin complex. The inhibitory effect of the regulatory proteins, which probably reflects a primary effect of tropomyosin to "block" active sites on actin, requires the three different components of the troponin complex: Troponin I, an interaction inhibitor; Troponin T, which binds the troponin complex to tropomyosin; and Troponin C, the Ca^{2+} receptor protein. **B.** Systole. Ca^{++} is delivered to the contractile proteins as a result of excitation-contraction coupling systems. This calcium binds to the Ca^{++}-binding component of troponin (Troponin C), thereby shifting the position of tropomyosin and abolishing the inhibitory effect of the regulatory proteins on the actin-myosin interaction.

Ca^{2+} binds to a high-affinity Ca^{2+}-binding site on one of the components of the troponin complex (see Fig. 8–4).

The phasic mechanism by which myocardial contractility is regulated, which appears to be the direct result of variations in the amount of Ca^{2+} released to the contractile proteins in systole, can be understood in terms of these complex interactions. Because the amount of Ca^{2+} delivered to the Ca^{2+}-binding site of troponin in the heart appears normally to be less than needed to activate all of these tension-generating interactions, any intervention that increases the amount of Ca^{2+} made available to the contractile proteins by the processes of excitation-contraction coupling will enhance contractility by increasing the number of active interactions between actin and myosin. Conversely, a reduction in the amount of Ca^{2+} that can be bound to troponin will have the opposite effect: to reduce myocardial contractility. To a large extent these variations in Ca-binding to troponin probably arise as the result of changes in the amount of Ca^{2+} delivered to the contractile proteins by the processes of excitation-contraction coupling. However, alterations in the Ca^{2+}-binding properties of troponin, which can arise either from changes in the molecular structure of troponin or in the ionic environment of this protein complex in the intact heart, may explain certain clinically observed abnormalities of myocardial function.

MECHANISM OF THE NEGATIVE INOTROPIC ACTION OF HYPOXIA OR ISCHEMIA

The preceding discussion of the basic mechanisms of cardiac contraction suggests a number of possible explanations for the prompt failure of the hypoxic and ischemic heart. These mechanisms will for convenience be considered either as a failure of the contractile proteins to respond to the Ca^{2+} made available during excitation-contraction coupling or as a defect in the process of excitation-contraction coupling that results in the delivery of a reduced amount of Ca^{2+} to the contractile proteins at the onset of systole.

Impaired Response of the Contractile Proteins to Ca^{2+}*

Myocardial contractility can be impaired by any mechanism that reduces the number of troponin molecules that are bound to Ca^{2+} during cardiac systole, even if Ca^{2+} delivery to the contractile proteins is normal. For example, failure of the troponin complex to undergo those changes that lead normally to the establishment of active actin-myosin interactions (see Fig. 8–4) could result from structural alterations of the troponin complex that cause a change in its Ca^{2+}-binding properties. Some evidence that myocardial ischemia alters the Ca^{2+} sensitivity of troponin is now available, although the reported changes appear to be in the direction of a loss of the ability of troponin to effect relaxation rather than an impairment of the contraction-promoting response to Ca^{2+}. These findings might be relevant to the contracture that occurs after prolonged hypoxia or ischemia. However, the role of such a loss in the Ca^{2+} sensitivity of troponin in explaining the rapid loss of contractility that occurs in the ischemic myocardium is not apparent.

Another mechanism that might explain the abrupt contractile failure that occurs duing hypoxia and ischemia is attributable to the state of acidosis that occurs when the myocardium turns from aerobic to anaerobic metabolism to meet energy needs (Poole-Wilson, 1978). As discussed earlier in this chapter, the initial response of the myocardium to oxygen deprivation includes a marked acceleration of anaerobic glycolysis. The resulting production of lactate is accompanied by the liberation of hydrogen ion, which is well-known to depress myocardial contractility. The mechanism of this negative inotropic effect may be triggered partly by the affinity of hydrogen ion for the Ca^{2+}-binding site on troponin. As a result, in the presence of increased levels of hydrogen ion, the response of troponin to Ca^{2+} will be reduced.

This action of hydrogen ion may result from a competition between H^+ and Ca^{2+} for the binding site on troponin that releases the inhibitory actin of the tropomysin-troponin complex on actin-myosin interaction. Thus, even when the delivery of Ca^{2+} by the processes of excitation-contraction coupling is normal, less Ca^{2+} would be bound to troponin in the acidotic heart and, therefore, fewer of the potential sites for actin-myosin interaction would be active. While evidence for this explanation remains incomplete, such a mechanism would provide the myocardium with a means by which the most expensive of its energy-consuming reactions would be attenuated in the face of a reduction in the delivery of oxygen, such as occurs when coronary artery perfusion is interrupted (Katz, 1973b, 1978).

Impaired Calcium Release by Sarcoplasmic Reticulum†

There is evidence that the calcium permeability of the sarcoplasmic reticulum decreases as pH is decreased, so that in the face of acidosis less Ca^{2+} would be delivered from the sarcoplasmic reticulum to the heart's contractile proteins. As has already been discussed, this negative inotropic effect could be initiated by the lactate produced when the hypoxic or ischemic heart uses its anaerobic pathways of energy production.

Imparied Calcium Entry into the Myocardial Cell‡

A major effect of both hypoxia and ischemia on the electrical response of the heart is abbreviation of the action potential, due primarily to a shortening of the plateau phase. In view of evidence that Ca^{2+} enters the myocar-

---

*Katz and Hecht, 1969; Schwartz et al., 1973; Fabiato and Fabiato, 1978.

†Fabiato and Fabiato, 1978; Dunnett and Nayler, 1979.
‡Katz, 1973b.

dium during this phase of the action potential (Reuter, 1974), it is possible that the negative inotropic effect of ischemia is caused in part by reduction of Ca^{2+} filling of intracellular stores.

Accumulation of Inorganic Phosphate*

The breakdown of phosphocreatine and ATP in the ischemic myocardium leads to the production of large amounts of inorganic phosphate, which could cause the precipitation of insoluble calcium phosphate salts. Such precipitates have been found in the mitochondria in the later stages of ischemic damage, but there is currently no direct evidence that this mechanism actually traps Ca^{2+} during the early pump failure of the ischemic heart.

Loss of a Regulatory Effect of ATP†

While a marked fall in ATP concentration appears unlikely to cause the early pump failure of the ischemic heart by depriving energy-utilizing systems of their substrate, a more moderate decrease in the myocardial concentration of this nucleotide could impair Ca^{2+} fluxes across the sarcolemma and sarcoplasmic reticulum by altering a regulatory effect of this nucleotide. Regulatory effects of ATP have been observed in passive as well as in active transport mechanisms, and in some cases do not require that chemical energy be liberated by ATP hydrolysis. Evidence that a minor fall could contribute to the negative inotropic state observed in ischemia is incomplete, but a growing number of biochemical studies suggest that a small decrease in cytosolic ATP concentration could slow the Ca^{2+} movements responsible for excitation-contraction coupling in the heart.

Accumulation of Lipids‡

A large literature indicates that a variety of fatty substances accumulate in and around the cells of the ischemic heart. These lipids are able to penetrate biological membranes, where they can exert a variety of effects. At low concentrations, a number of lipids have been shown to reduce membrane permeability and so could slow the Ca^{2+} movements responsible for excitation-contraction coupling. Higher concentrations of these lipids cause membrane disruption and thus might contribute to myocardial cell death after prolonged ischemia. Work in this important area is still in its early stages, however, so that the significance of lipid accumulation in the pathogenesis of ischemic cardiac damage cannot yet be adequately evaluated.

MECHANISM FOR THE POSITIVE INOTROPIC ACTIONS OF CARDIAC GLYCOSIDES§ AND β-ADRENERGIC AGONISTS∥

Although both cardiac glycosides and β-adrenergic agonists enhance myocardial contractility, there are a number of differences between the mechanical responses of the heart to these two classes of drugs. In the context of this discussion, the most significant of these differences is the marked decrease in contraction time caused by catecholamines, whereas the cardiac glycosides act to augment tension generation without attenuating the duration of systole. These findings suggest that the β-adrenergic agonists have an effect that speeds the relaxation process in cardiac muscle that is not shared by the cardiac glycosides.

Recent studies of the biochemical actions of agents like epinephrine indicate that they exert their action by initiating a cascade of enzymatic reactions (Fig. 8–5). The ability of these agents to bind to the *beta receptor,* and thereby activate the enzyme adenylate cyclase, is well-known (see Fig. 8–2). This enzyme, which catalyzes the formation of adenosine-3′,5′-phosphate *(cyclic AMP)* from ATP, is located on the plasma membrane of the cardiac muscle cell. A number of studies indicate

---

*Kübler and Katz, 1977; Katz, 1978.
†Kübler and Katz, 1977; Katz, 1978.
‡Katz and Messineo, 1981.

§Langer, 1972; Reuter, 1974.
∥Katz, 1975, 1979; Tsien, 1977.

```
β-adrenergic agonists           Other adenylate cyclase
         ↓                      activators (e.g., glucagon)
  β-receptor binding
              ↘               ↙
            Anenylate cyclase activation
                     ↓
              Increased cyclic AMP
                     ↓
            Activation of protein kinase
                     ↓
        Phosphorylation of sarcoplasmic reticulum
                     ↓
             Stimulation of calcium transport
                by sarcoplasmic reticulum
                     ↓
              Acceleration of relaxation
```

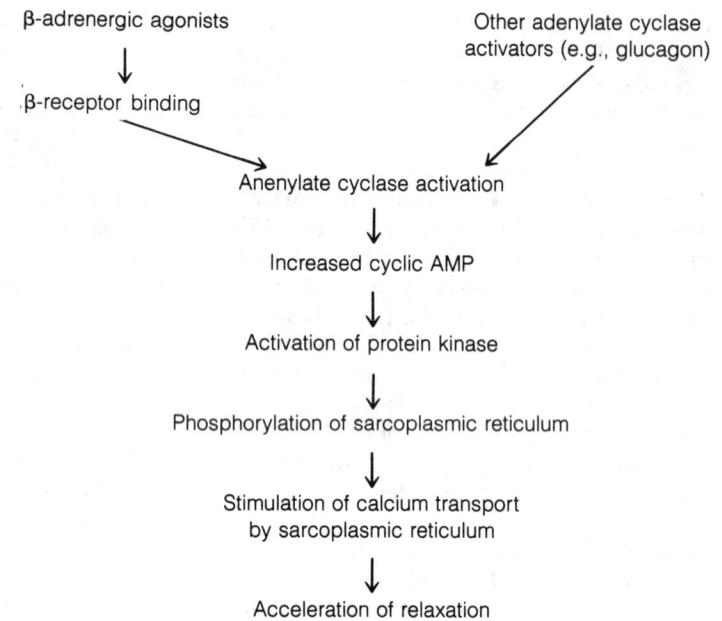

Figure 8–5. Schematic outline of positive inotropic actions of β-adrenergic agonists, cardiac glycosides, and glucagon.

that most actions of cyclic AMP in mammalian cells are mediated by yet another enzyme, *cyclic AMP-dependent protein kinase,* whose activity is increased by cyclic AMP. These protein kinases, which are found in a variety of cell types, are enzymes that catalyze the phosphorylation of proteins by transferring the terminal phosphate from ATP to the amino acid serine, thereby forming phosphoserine. Protein kinase-mediated phosphorylation has been described in a number of different proteins. One such protein, *phospholamban,* is found on the heart's sarcoplasmic reticulum (see Fig. 8–3). Concomitant with phosphorylation of phospholamban, the rate of calcium transport into the sarcoplasmic reticulum is increased, partly as the result of an increased Ca^{2+} affinity of the calcium pump (Fig. 8–6). The increased rate of relaxation that is seen in the intact heart under the influence of β-adrenergic agonists thus may be a manifestation of this increased rate of calcium transport into the sarcoplasmic reticulum.

A possible relationship between an increase in calcium transport rate into the sarcoplasmic reticulum and an augmentation of contractile force is less apparent. It appears to be more likely that the cascade of reactions that is initiated when β-adrenergic agonists bind to the beta receptor also leads to phosphorylation of the membranes that control calcium fluxes at the myocardial cell surface (see Fig. 8–2). Thus catecholamines have been shown to augment myocardial calcium stores by promoting an increased influx of Ca^{2+} during systole (Tsien, 1977). Glucagon, which activates adenylate cyclase by a mechanism different from that of the β-adrenergic drugs such as epinephrine, may set in motion the same sequence of events, leading ultimately to abbreviation of systole and enhanced contractility (Fig. 8–5).

The cardiac glycosides, unlike the agents just described that act to increase adenylate cyclase activity, exert their inotropic effect without shortening systole. This finding is in accord with a number of in vitro studies that have failed to identify an action of the cardiac glycosides on the membranes of the sarcoplasmic reticulum. Instead, the cardiac glycosides

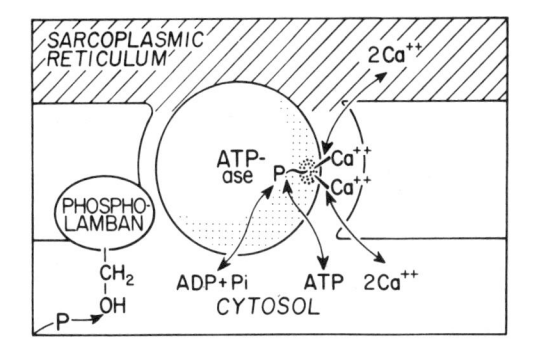

Figure 8-6. Calcium transport mechanism of the cardiac sarcoplasmic reticulum showing the ~100,000-dalton transport ATPase (large sphere) that transports two calcium ions from the cytosol to the interior of the sarcoplasmic reticulum for each molecule of ATP hydrolyzed. Also shown is phospholamban, a ~22,000-dalton protein that, when phosphorylated by the cyclic AMP-dependent protein kinase, increases the rate of calcium transport into the sarcoplasmic reticulum.

appear to enhance contractility by an action on the plasma membrane that increases intracellular calcium stores. A number of investigators have proposed a link between the inotropic effects of cardiac glycosides and their well-known action to inhibit the (Na$^+$ + K$^+$)-activated ATPase of the plasma membrane (see Fig. 8–2). This enzyme, which is believed to be a part of the sodium pump, participates in the active extrusion if the Na$^+$ that enters the myocardial cell during the action potential. Although there remains some question as to the existence of an invariable correlation between the positive inotropic actions of a number of different cardiac glycosides and their ability to inhibit (Na$^+$ + K$^+$)-activated ATPase, such a correlation generally is found.

Evidence from studies of the giant squid axon suggests one possible mechanism by which inhibition of the sodium pump could enhance myocardial contractility. In this nerve it was found that a cation exchange mechanism, which is distinct from the sodium pump that manifests the (Na$^+$ + K$^+$)-activated ATPase, can transport both Na$^+$ and Ca^{2+} out of the cell, and that these two cations compete for a single "carrier" site in the second cation pump (see Fig. 8–2). Thus, as both Ca^{2+} and Na$^+$ are available within the cell to be carried out of the cell, an increased amount of Na$^+$ available to the carrier within the cell would, by a simple chemical competition, cause a decrease in the efflux of Ca^{2+}. The action of cardiac glycosides to inhibit the sodium pump [i.e. the (Na$^+$ + K$^+$)-activated ATPase] could, by decreasing Na$^+$ efflux, increase the amount of Na$^+$ in a subsarcolemmal region of the myocardial cell and thereby reduce the amount of Ca^{2+} that is carried out of the cell by this second cation pump. The resulting retention of Ca^{2+} could enhance myocardial contractility by contributing to the filling of Ca^{2+} stores in the sarcoplasmic reticulum. This hypothesis, while attractive, is not yet fully documented, although attempts to define actions of cardiac glycosides directly on the heart's contractile proteins and the sarcoplasmic reticulum generally have yielded negative results.

HEART FAILURE*

The possible role that altered cellular function plays in the genesis of heart failure has been examined in a large number of studies carried out over the past two decades. It is common to define a continuum in the chronically stressed heart from "normal" through "hypertrophy" to "heart failure." Yet "hypertrophy" defines a complex process in the myocardium, rather than a single steplike change from normal. Furthermore, it has been clearly shown that a variety of subcellular systems behave differently during the early stages of hypertrophy than in the hypertrophied heart after prolonged overloading. The term "heart failure," in contrast, does not define the state of the myocardium, but instead refers to a pathophysiologic state of the circulation that can result from a readjustment of extracardiac homeostatic mecha-

---

Katz, 1973a, 1975.

nisms, such as salt and water retention by the kidney, as well as from impairment of cardiac function.

In an attempt to understand the abnormalities that are engendered by chronic overloading of the heart, it is useful to keep in mind three terms: circulatory failure, heart failure, and myocardial failure. *Circulatory failure* can be defined as an inability of the cardiovascular system to meet the needs of the body when the heart is normal. Thus, symptoms of congestive failure can be produced by overtransfusion, even when the heart is perfectly normal, and hypotension can be produced in normal people who hemorrhage. While not all cases of circulatory failure are the result of *heart failure*, it underlies most clinically encountered cases of circulatory failure. Yet the heart can fail when the myocardium is normal; for example, in cases with acute aortic insufficiency or left atrial myxoma. These conditions, in which heart failure is caused almost entirely by a mechanical abnormality, are different from those in which heart failure, and thus circulatory failure, results from disease of the heart muscle itself. The latter, which is true *myocardial failure*, is seen in conditions such as familial cardiomyopathy, toxic myocarditis, and myocardial ischemia.

Whereas the distinction between circulatory failure due to heart failure and that due to other, extracardiac, causes should pose no problem to the experienced—and alert—clinician, evaluation of the role of myocardial failure in patients with structural damage to the heart is much more difficult. In most cases in which a valvular abnormality causes chronic overloading of the heart, as in chronic aortic stenosis, it is likely that myocardial failure slowly evolves until a situation develops where repair of the underlying mechanical defect cannot restore the patient's health. Similarly, in the postoperative cardiac patient, great care must be exercised to distinguish between circulatory failure (e.g., inadequate or excessive replacement of blood), heart failure (e.g., inadequate repair of a defect), and myocardial failure (e.g., acidosis, hypoxia, persistence of chronic myocardial failure). At this time, quantification of the "myocardial factor" in such patients remains extremely difficult, and careful clinical judgments about the state of the myocardium may still be as valid as those based on complex and elaborate invasive techniques.

While the possibility remains that further efforts to quantify the mechanical characteristics of the human myocardium may provide more useful tools for the clinician than the variety of contractility "indices" that are currently available, adequate assessment of the intrinsic condition of the myocardium probably will require better definition in the hearts of these patients of the many specific biochemical and biophysical variables discussed in this chapter. At the present time, however, the means for such an evaluation seem remote. Yet it must be remembered that before 1940, the possibility that cardiologists could apply directly to their patients the hemodynamic concepts evolved in the laboratory by people such as Carl Wiggers seemed equally remote.

A number of biochemical abnormalities have been identified in the chronically overloaded, hypertrophied heart, but it is not now possible to distinguish between those abnormalities that are responsible for the deterioration in cardiac function and those that may represent a part of the compensatory response to the long-standing increase in loading. Although the late development of fibrosis is clearly detrimental to function, certain more subtle changes, such as the possible synthesis in the overloaded heart of a myosin with low ATPase activity, may be part of the compensatory mechanism. For these reasons, evaluation of patients with myocardial failure is complicated not only by problems in the quantification of myocardial function, but also by our lack of understanding of the significance of abnormalities in specific subcellular functions. Thus, we must look ahead not only for better means to evaluate myocardial function in the patient with cardiac disease, but also for the new knowledge that will permit the cardiologist and cardiac surgeon to understand the significance of the many abnormalities in these patients. As these goals are reached, one can, with confidence, predict that we will be in a position to define more accurately the balance between energy production and energy use in the diseased heart and the abnormalities responsible for these imbalances. With this knowledge, we can expect that new and more effective means will be developed for the prevention and treatment of myocardial failure.

REFERENCES

Dunnett J, Nayler WG: Effect of pH on calcium accumulation and release by isolated fragments of cardiac and skeletal muscle sarcoplasmic reticulum. Arch Biochem Biophys 198: 434, 1979.

Fabiato A, Fabiato F: Effects of pH on the myofilaments and the sarcoplasmic reticulum of skinned cells from cardiac and skeletal muscles. J Physiol (Lond) 276: 233, 1978.

Fozzard HA, Gibbons WR: Action potential and contraction of heart muscle. Am J Cardiol 31: 182, 1973.

Katz AM: Role of the contractile proteins and sarcoplasmic reticulum in the response of the heart to catecholamines: an historical review. Adv Cyclic Nucleotide Res 11: 303, 1979.

_____: The ischemic myocardium. Mechanism of early pump failure. Hosp Pract 13: 83, 1978.

_____: Physiology of the Heart, New York, Raven Press, 1977

_____: Congestive heart failure. Role of altered myocardial cellular control. N Engl J Med 293: 1184, 1975.

_____: Contractile proteins. In Langer GA, Brady A (eds): The Mammalian Myocardium. New York, Wiley, 1974, pp 51–80.

_____: The biochemical "defect" in the hypertrophied and failing heart: deleterious or compensatory? Circulation 47: 1076, 1973a.

_____: Effects of ischemia on the contractile processes of heart muscle. Am J Cardiol 32: 456, 1973b.

_____: The contractile proteins of the heart. Physiol Rev 50: 63, 1970.

_____, Hecht HH: The early pump failure of the ischemic heart. (Editorial). Am J Med 47: 497, 1969.

_____, Messineo FC: Lipid-membrane interactions and the pathogenesis of ischemic damage in the myocardium. Circ Res 48:1, 1981.

_____, Repke DI: Calcium-membrane interactions in the myocardium: effects of ouabain, epinephrine, and 3′,5′-cyclic AMP. Am J Cardiol 31: 193, 1973.

_____, Tada M: The "stone heart" and other challenges to the biochemist. Am J Cardiol 39: 1073, 1977.

_____, Tada M, Kirchberger MA: Control of calcium transport in the myocardium by the cyclic AMP-protein kinase system. Adv Cyclic Nucleotide Res 6: 453, 1975.

Kübler W, Katz AM: Mechanism of early "pump" failure of the ischemic heart: possible role of adenosine triphosphate depletion and inorganic phosphate accumulation. Am J Cardiol 40: 467, 1977.

Langer GA: Effects of digitalis on myocardial ionic exchange. Circulation 46: 180, 1972.

Poole-Wilson PA: Measurement of myocardial intracellular pH in pathological states. (Editorial). J Mol Cell Cardiol 10: 511, 1978.

Reuter H: Exchange of calcium ions in the mammalian myocardium: mechanisms and physiological significance. Circ Res 34: 599, 1974.

Schwartz A, Wood JM, Allen JC, Bornet ED, Entman ML, Goldstein MA, Sordahl LA, Suzuk M: Biochemical and morphological correlates of cardiac ischemia. I. Membrane systems. Am J Cardiol 32: 46, 1973.

Tsien R: Cyclic AMP and contractile activity in the heart. Adv Cyclic Nucleotide Res 8: 363, 1977.

Weber A, Murray JM: Molecular control mechanisms in muscular contraction. Physiol Rev 53: 612, 1973.

9. Analysis, Maintenance, and Support of Cardiac Function After Cardiac Surgery

Robert S. Litwak

Above all else, survival after cardiac surgery is dependent on the ability of the myocardium to constantly deliver enough unoxygenated blood to the lungs and oxygenated blood to the peripheral tissues to sustain functional and metabolic processes at satisfactory levels. Maintenance of optimal cardiovascular subsystem performance requires an exquisitely coordinated response of both the heart and blood vessels. Survey of the integrative mechanisms involved in cardiovascular control and regulation will be found in the reviews of Sarnoff and Mitchell (1962) and Folkow et al. (1965).

In healthy man the reserve capability of the cardiovascular subsystem to challenge is substantial. For example, cardiac output may approach five times basal levels in response to heavy exercise. However, in patients with heart disease, performance of the subsystem at rest may frequently be compromised to a point where all or most of the reserve capacity already may be in use. A metabolic challenge presented to such a patient over a sustained period results in death. Therefore, it is not surprising that patients coming to intracardiac operations with advanced myocardial dysfunction are at greater risk. Even in the best of circumstances (precise conduct of anesthesia and perfusion, physiologic repair, and excellent postoperative care), the higher total body oxygen consumption, which frequently exists in the early postoperative period, may exceed the oxygen transport capability of the cardiovascular subsystem.

As suggested by Kirklin (1970), analysis and proper management of any subsystem require knowledge of its *performance* at a given moment, as well as assessment of the *adequacy* of that performance. This, in turn, requires that the performance potential *(reserve capability)* of the subsystem be understood, with awareness of those reserves that are already in use. Use of this format provides a logical means of *analysis* of the cardiovascular subsystem, thereby establishing a basis for supportive management of patients who have undergone intracardiac operations.

CARDIAC PUMP PERFORMANCE

The output of the heart in an intact man is governed by an interplay of two functional components: *cardiac rate* and *stroke volume*. Both are subject to a variety of neural, humoral, and metabolic influences that modify the cardiac response at any given time. There is an exquisitely direct relationship between the metabolic state, as reflected by changes in the level of oxygen consumption and cardiac output. Figure 9–1 depicts the rise in cardiac output pari passu with the increase in oxygen consumption in response to exercise.

Above basal steady-state conditions, homeostatic adjustments of rate and stroke volume are accomplished through increased use of the reserve capacity of each. Even normal man's reserve capacity in response to severe stress has limitations of magnitude and time. Thus it follows that survival of a patient recovering from intracardiac surgery is threatened if maximal reserve use is required over a long period or if additional metabolic challenges suddenly occur that cannot be satisfied by further reserve recruitment. This concept is of obvious importance when reserve mechanisms are used either by the diseased cardiovascular subsystem to maintain satisfactory circulatory stability or are deliberately exploited as a therapeutic measure.

In accordance with the concept of systems analysis, this section will consider the performance of each of the two basic components of cardiac pump function as separate entities. This not only is a convenient framework for discussion, but also offers a systematic means of cardiovascular subsystem analysis and patient management. However, from a functional standpoint, it is important to recognize that the separation is an arbitrary one. The integrative negative feedback responses of the cardiovascular subsystem to changing conditions in intact people frequently involve concomitant or sequential adjustments of both rate and stroke volume.

Cardiac Rate

For years there has been controversy over the relative contributions of rate and stroke volume when cardiac output increases in response to the rising oxygen consumption accompanying exercise. Accumulating evidence from a number of studies in normal subjects indicates that both variables play a role, depending on the degree of exertion (Fig. 9-2). During mild exercise, the rise in cardiac output results almost totally from an increase in heart rate, with stroke volume remaining relatively unchanged. As exertion becomes increasingly severe, the reserve capacity of cardiac rate is ultimately reached (between 180 and 200 beats per minute in various studies). With maximal exertion and increasing oxygen consumption, the heart rate can rise no higher. An increase in stroke volume now is the means by which the necessary rise in cardiac output is achieved. The sequenced response of rate and stroke volume to varying stresses is a clear example of the integrative mechanism that affects cardiac output in normal man.

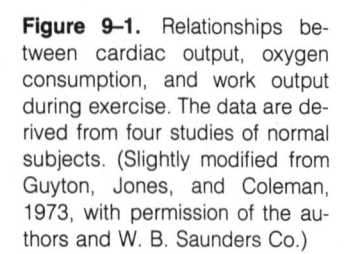

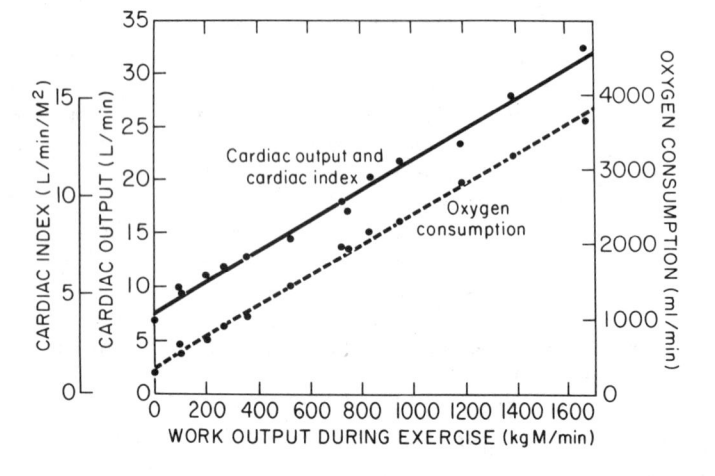

Figure 9–1. Relationships between cardiac output, oxygen consumption, and work output during exercise. The data are derived from four studies of normal subjects. (Slightly modified from Guyton, Jones, and Coleman, 1973, with permission of the authors and W. B. Saunders Co.)

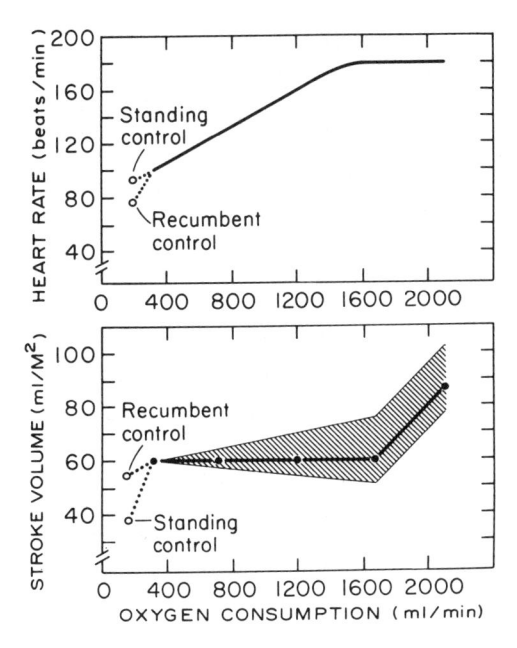

Figure 9-2. In normal, exercising man, the rise in cardiac output in response to an exercise-induced increase in oxygen consumption is met almost entirely by a proportional elevation of heart rate (above), stroke volume (below) remaining essentially unchanged. The shaded area indicates the slight exercise-related changes in stroke volume reported in some series as exercise proceeds. Only when exertion is severe and the reserve capacity of rate has been reached does stroke volume begin to rise sharply. (Adapted from Rushmer, 1976, with permission of the author and W. B. Saunders Co.)

The autonomic nervous system plays the primary role in the control and regulation of heart rate. Normally the parasympathetic nervous system exerts a dominant role. However, in the presence of congestive heart failure there is a significant defect in parasympathetic control. By maintaining or increasing the heart rate, the adrenergic component becomes the dominant factor in supporting the circulation. Eckberg et al. (1971) observed a significantly diminished response to atropine-induced elevations of cardiac rate in patients with heart disease compared with that seen in normal people.

These findings, coupled with the knowledge that myocardial catecholamine stores are depleted in heart failure, suggest a profound disturbance of control of the diseased heart's performance. The clinical implications are significant, since patients with heart disease frequently have only a limited capacity to increase cardiac output through the alternative mechanism of stroke volume. When this limitation is superimposed on abnormal rate control, the result may be a life-threatening inability to appropriately elevate cardiac output in response to a metabolic challenge.

The importance of heart rate in maintaining cardiac output is clearly apparent in patients whose rates are fixed and low, such as those in complete atrioventricular block. Although their cardiac output can be sustained by a rise in stroke volume, blood flow may be inadequate during periods of stress. Untreated, their prognosis is poor because of the early onset of severe heart failure imposed by the sharply increased energy requirements and inefficient energy use of the necessarily dilated heart. Moreover, these circumstances increase the potential for lethal ventricular arrhythmias.

Stroke Volume

The second variable controlling cardiac output is stroke volume. The heart is a volume displacement pump, and the amount of blood ejected per beat is a function of the extent of myocardial fiber shortening. Stroke volume is regulated by three determinants: (1) preload (ventricular end-diastolic volume); (2) afterload (the tension or load that the myocardium must develop during contraction); and (3) myocardial contractility.

Preload

THE FRANK-STARLING RELATIONSHIP. Within limits, the heart ejects a volume of blood per beat in direct proportion to its end-diastolic volume: an expression of the Frank-Starling relationship. With increasing diastolic volume there is myofibril lengthening and, during the succeeding systole, proportionately increased muscle shortening, so that a larger volume of blood is ejected. However (as will be discussed later), augmentation of ventricular volume beyond a critical point will no longer be accompanied by an increase in stroke output, since the peak of the Frank-Starling curve (the reserve capacity of the preload mechanism) will have been reached (Fig. 9–3).

An ultrastructural basis for the Frank-Starling relationship has been suggested (Sonnenblick et al., 1963, 1964; Braunwald et al., 1968; Sonnenblick, 1968, 1974). As ventricular filling pressure rises, there is an increase in sarcomere length, which, in turn, increases the number of sites for chemical interactions between adjacent myosin and actin filaments. The result is an augmentation of the force of contraction, an increase in muscle shortening, and a larger volume of blood ejected during that systole.

In animal experiments, sarcomere lengths have been correlated with diastolic filling pressure. At zero left ventricular filling pressure, diastolic sarcomere length is only 1.9μ; at filling pressures of 6 to 8 mm Hg the sarcomere is slightly longer (2.05μ to 2.15μ); and at still higher filling pressures (12 to 15 mm Hg), sarcomere length approximates 2.2μ. In this regard, it is pertinent that the force of myocardial contraction is greatest when sarcomere length averages 2.2μ. Thus, the rationale for preload augmentation in postoperative care (discussed later) is clear: ejection of ventricular volume is increased when the sarcomere is appropriately stretched. Consequently, a diastolic sarcomere length below 2.2μ reflects the morphologic basis for the physiologic reserve mechanism of the ascending limb of the Frank-Starling curve.

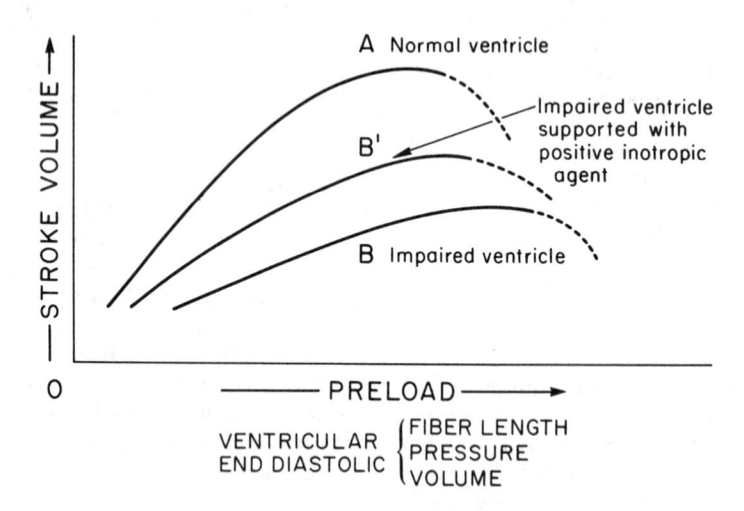

Figure 9–3. The Frank-Starling relationship and the influence of positive inotropic agents on the ventricular function curve. Within limits the stroke volume varies directly (but not necessarily linearly) with ventricular end-diastolic myofibril length, pressure, and volume. In a normal ventricle (**A**) preload augmentation will be accompanied by a larger increment in stroke volume than that observed with the same amount of volume augmentation of an impaired ventricle (**B**). Thus, the impaired ventricle can achieve an equivalent level of stroke volume only at the expense of higher filling pressures. Moreover, these ventricles tend to have limited capacity to increase stroke volume. Administration of a positive inotropic agent to the impaired ventricle allows a new ventricular function curve to be developed (**B**), in which an identical preload increment now results in a proportionately higher increase in stroke volume. The interrupted lines (descending limb) suggest the probable performance characteristics of the intact heart if volume loading were extreme.

With continued augmentation of preload, a point is reached where an additional modest increment will produce a disproportionately large elevation of resting wall tension, manifested by a sharp increase of ventricular end-diastolic pressure. The morphologic basis for this is the tendency of the cardiac muscle to resist stretch, i.e., low diastolic compliance. As a consequence, even when extreme elevations of ventricular diastolic pressure are suddenly imposed (in excess of 50 mm Hg) in the experimental animal, average sarcomere length is only slightly longer (Monroe et al., 1970). Despite this protective mechanism a point is reached where further stretching of the myofibril will not result in increased developed tension. This is also observed in animals with chronically dilated ventricles, and is attributed to slippage between myofibrils (Ross et al., 1971).

These findings indicate that sarcomeres are characteristically resistant to both acute and chronic overstretch and further imply that in clinical circumstances of marked left ventricular dilatation little or none of the Frank-Starling reserve mechanism is available for use. With continued deterioration of a heart—which was previously operating at the apex of its Frank-Starling curve—a pattern of performance suggestive of a descending limb (see Figure 9–3) could be anticipated. This condition is incompatible with prolonged survival. Although it has been argued that the descending limb is more theoretical than real in intact man, Ross and Braunwald (1964) have demonstrated its momentary existence in states of severe failure, employing interventions that transiently increase afterload.

For years investigators have debated the importance of the Frank-Starling law of the heart in the intact subject. The problem largely resides in the difficulty of distinguishing performance changes caused by altered preload (Frank-Starling) and those consequent to alterations in contractility. Specifically, the relationship between the initial length of the muscle and developed tension changes when myocardial contractility is modified by the autonomic nervous system. This can be clearly shown in a heart driven at a constant rate where sympathetic stimulation allows an increase in ventricular work at a lower filling pressure (Sarnoff et al., 1960a, 1960b). Thus, varying contractility conditions at any particular diastolic volume makes it possible for there to be a family of ventricular function curves (see Fig. 9–3), and, in Sarnoff's words (1955), "adds a third dimension to the Frank-Starling mechanism. This third dimensional adaptation is of importance not only in the responses of the normal organism but also in compensating for physiologic adversity."

Despite the inherent analytical difficulties, there is some evidence that the Frank-Starling relationship does play a role in the cardiac dynamics of intact man. When the performance of the autonomic nervous system is removed, it is possible to analyze more precisely changes in preload and pump function. In normal man with an intact autonomic nervous system, infusion of 1.5 liters of blood produces an increase in ventricular filling pressure but little or no change in stroke volume or cardiac output. Following autonomic blockade with trimethaphan (Arfonad), a similar blood infusion sharply increases left ventricular filling pressure, with an accompanying rise in both stroke volume and cardiac output (Frye and Braunwald, 1960; Braunwald et al., 1960, 1961). There is evidence that the atria as well as the ventricles perform in accordance with the Frank-Starling relationship, since the force of atrial contraction is a direct function of the pressure within that chamber at contractile onset (Braunwald and Frahm, 1961).

In summary, available evidence indicates that the Frank-Starling law does play a role in human cardiac regulation, the mechanism that permits independent regulation of the stroke volume of each ventricle so that, over the course of a few seconds, any small inequality in output between the ventricles is precisely adjusted.

In the failing heart, where contractility is diminished and end-diastolic volume increased (cardiac dilatation), the reserve capacity of the Frank-Starling mechanism is reduced. Compared to a normal curve, the function curve of the failing ventricle is characteristically flatter and lower in amplitude (see Fig. 9–3). Therefore, because of its reduced functional reserve, the failing ventricle can only increase its stroke output to a limited degree, and then only at abnormally high filling pressures. Administration of a positive inotropic agent to the failing ventricle creates a new set of conditions and a new function curve in which preload augmentation results in a proportionately higher increase in stroke volume when compared with the nontreated failing ventricle.

BLOOD VOLUME AND PRELOAD. At any level of its contractile state myocardial performance is influenced by factors affecting the magnitude and distribution of blood volume. For example, sarcomere length is reduced and stroke output adversely affected in hypovolemia (this and other functional and pathologic distortions affecting cardiac function will be discussed later).

At any level of intravascular volume, ventricular preload is influenced by the distribution of blood between the intrathoracic and extrathoracic compartments (Braunwald et al., 1968). Factors of clinical significance to patients undergoing or recovering from cardiac surgery include:

1. Body position. In the upright position gravitational forces result in blood pooling in the dependent portions of the body so that ventricular preload and stroke output are both reduced. In the supine position, ventricular end-diastolic volume is augmented and, in the absence of severe cardiac failure, stroke output is increased.
2. Intrathoracic pressure. Normally the mean intrathoracic pressure is negative and facilitates venous return to the heart. Circumstances that elevate intrathoracic pressure (positive pressure ventilation, pneumothorax) serve to impede venous return and can thereby reduce ventricular diastolic volume.
3. Systemic venous tone. Neurohumoral stimuli affect the tone of the systemic veins. Moderate elevation of systemic venous tone is usually observed for the first 48 hours after surgery (Reid et al., 1968), a negative feedback response (and a cardiovascular subsystem reserve mechanism) that reduces extrathoracic pooling so that intrathoracic blood volume is augmented and preload increased. Sympathomimetic drugs and digitalis exert similar effects on the systemic veins. Conversely, drugs such as nitroglycerine contribute to extrathoracic pooling and momentarily reduce preload.
4. Intrapericardial pressure. Normally the pericardium is relatively noncompliant and serves to inhibit ventricular overfilling. Elevation of intrapericardial pressure (effusion, postoperative tamponade) impedes ventricular filling, reducing stroke volume.

ATRIAL CONTRACTION AND PRELOAD. When normal atrial and ventricular electromechanical relationships exist, atrial contraction augments diastolic ventricular volume. Although by no means essential to ventricular filling, the atrial contribution to ventricular preload becomes significant during severe tachycardia if stenotic atrioventricular valve lesions exist or ventricular hypertrophy is present. In these two circumstances, loss of atrial systole (when atrial fibrillation occurs) reduces ventricular end-diastolic volume and cardiac output.

Afterload. The experiments of Otto Frank (1895) clearly demonstrated that stroke volume is significantly influenced by the resistance against which the ventricles must contract. Under normal conditions the dominant afterload factor affecting ventricular function is *arterial impedance* which, analogous to electrical impedance, has inertial, capacitive, and resistive components. Thus, the mass and viscosity of the blood, the physical characteristics of the arteries, and peripheral vascular resistance are major determinants of arterial impedance opposing ejection from either the left or right ventricle.

In isolated cardiac muscle experiments, where only afterload is changed (preload and the contractile state held constant), a reciprocal relationship between afterload and muscle shortening is demonstrable (Sonnenblick, 1966). These relationships are evidenced in the intact dog, where afterload elevation is accompanied by a fall in stroke volume; conversely, when afterload is reduced, stroke volume rises (Ross et al., 1966). Similar observations have been made in patients with cardiac disease (Ross and Braunwald, 1964).

The implications for postoperative management are apparent. For example, the augmented afterload accompanying a sustained rise in arterial impedance (frequently observed in the early hours after cardiac surgery) can adversely affect cardiac output by opposing and thereby diminishing myocardial fiber shortening and, therefore, stroke output. Viewed from the standpoint of an afterload reserve mechanism, autoregulatory mediated sudden elevation of systemic arteriolar resistance in response to brisk blood loss or other distortions offers a time-limited means of maintaining perfusion pressure. However, the physiologic "cost" exacted is high in terms of increased cardiac work requirements and the potential for decreased total systemic blood flow.

Geometric considerations also affect afterload. In accordance with Laplace's law, wall tension is related directly to the radius. Thus, in the dilated failing heart, myocardial wall tension, i.e., afterload, is increased. If, for example, the heart is considered simplistically to be a sphere and its diameter is doubled, the radii of curvature would be doubled and the total myocardial wall tension would be quadrupled to achieve the same intracavitary systolic pressure.

Myocardial Contractility. In intact man, if it were possible to keep preload and afterload constant, any change in stroke volume could be reliably attributed to a change in the contractile state of the myocardium. The problem, of course, is that man's cardiovascular subsystem changes from moment to moment, and the interacting variations in preload, afterload, and heart rate impose severe reliability problems for any derived index of contractility employed in analyzing this parameter in intact man. For example, simply increasing cardiac rate by atrial pacing provokes a positive inotropic response. Bowditch first observed expression of this phenomenon in the frog heart more than 100 years ago (1871). Moreover, the derived indexes of contractility are limited by nonuniformities of ventricular wall morphology and performance.

REGULATION OF MYOCARDIAL CONTRACTILITY. Braunwald et al. (1968) have enumerated the factors that modify myocardial force-velocity-length relations in intact man (Fig. 9–4). Inotropism is augmented by (1) increased cardiac sympathetic stimulation, which provokes a proportionate rise in the quantity of norepinephrine release and consequent myocardial beta receptor stimulation, (2) increased extracardiac catecholamine release by the adrenal medulla and other sympathetic ganglia, (3) a change in the force-frequency relationship in which, as described earlier, a rise in rate is accompanied by increased contractility, and (4) exogenous administration of drugs such as epinephrine, isoproterenol, cardiac glycosides, and calcium. Each of the first three mechanisms represents an intrinsic reserve function that serves to increase myocardial contractility, when necessary. Evidence for this can be found in congestive heart failure, where sympathetic activity is augmented and synthesis of norepinephrine increased in both the peripheral vasculature and the adrenal medulla (Braunwald et al., 1968; Kramer et al., 1968; Vogel and Chidsey, 1969).

Apart from the intrinsic contractility depression associated with ventricular failure, factors that tend to reduce contractility include (1) abnormalities of blood gases (hypoxia, marked hypercapnea), electrolytes (potassium), or the acid-base state (particularly metabolic acidosis), and (2) pharmacologic depressants such as halothane, quinidine, procaine amide, and propranolol.

MEASURING CONTRACTILITY. Since the most common cause of death after open intracardiac operations is low cardiac output

Figure 9-4. Major factors that modify the myocardial contractile state in man and how changes in the contractile state affect ventricular performance at any given level of ventricular end-diastolic volume. (Redrawn from Braunwald et al., 1968, with permission of the authors and Little, Brown and Co.)

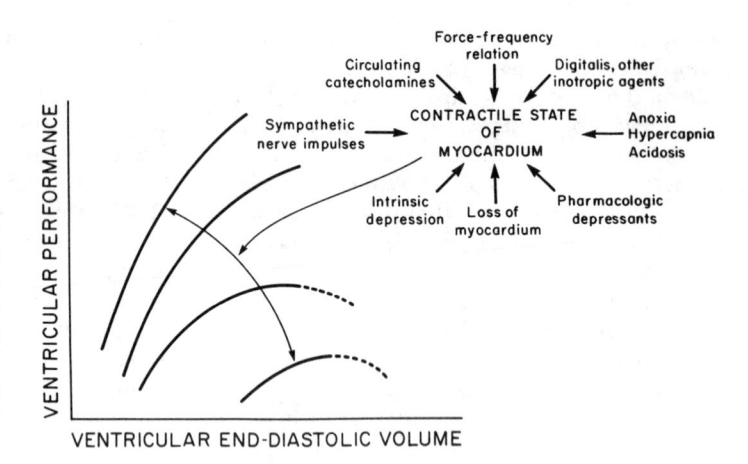

caused by sharply reduced myocardial contractility, the importance of frequent assessment of the contractile state is apparent. The problem is that determination of the level of contractility requires quantitation of the instantaneous relations between three variables: myocardial force, velocity, and fiber length. Study of these variables has been carried out in isolated cardiac muscle preparations (Sonnenblick, 1962) and carefully controlled animal experiments (Ross et al., 1966). Considerable effort has been made to apply these concepts to the study of intact man (Glick et al., 1965; Gault et al., 1968; Karliner et al., 1971; Peterson et al., 1973), but the methods are complex and their validity awaits verification. Moreover, the present time-consuming requirements of these studies exclude their use in areas where they are most critically needed—the cardiac operating room and intensive care unit.

FACTORS THAT ADVERSELY AFFECT MYOCARDIAL PERFORMANCE AFTER CARDIAC SURGERY

Four factors play dominant roles in adversely affecting the performance capability of the heart after intracardiac surgery: (1) the extent of preoperative cardiac dysfunction; (2) the combined traumata of operation—anesthesia, perfusion, and surgical manipulations; (3) uncorrected cardiovascular pathology; and (4) adverse postoperative events.

Preoperative Cardiac Dysfunction

Regardless of etiology, when cardiac pump function has been severely compromised for years, atrial and ventricular dysfunction frequently persists to varying degrees, despite satisfactory correction of all mechanical lesions. Therefore, a strong correlation prevails between the preoperative existence of advanced cardiac (specifically ventricular) dysfunction and heightened probability of death after intracardiac operation. Available methods of study do not allow precise differentiation of those derangements of cardiac pump function that may be immediately reversible by surgery from those that will persist despite satisfactory repair.

Preoperative determinants of abnormal pump function (Table 9-1) that predict heightened probability of mortality following cardiac surgery include: (1) marked cardiomegaly, particularly when accompanied by atrial or ventricular arrhythmias; (2) left ventricular end-diastolic volume greater than 150 ml/m^2; (3) systolic ejection fraction reduced below 0.3; (4) cardiac index less than 1.9 liters/min/m^2 in the presence of high ($\geq$ 18 mm Hg) left ventricular filling pressures; and

TABLE 9-1 PREOPERATIVE DETERMINANTS OF CARDIAC FUNCTION PREDICTIVE OF HEIGHTENED MORTALITY PROBABILITY AFTER CARDIAC SURGERY

Marked cardiomegaly

Cardiac index <1.9 liters/min/m^2

Left ventricular end-diastolic pressure ≥18 mm Hg

Left ventricular end-diastolic volume >150 ml/m^2

Left ventricular systolic ejection fraction <0.20

Severe elevation of pulmonary vascular resistance (>10 units)

---

(5) severely elevated pulmonary vascular resistance (> 10 units) (Kirklin and Rastelli, 1967; Litwak et al., 1969; Hammermeister and Kennedy, 1972; Appelbaum et al., 1976; Kirklin et al., 1976; Kouchoukos and Karp, 1976).

Pressure and Volume Overload. All hemodynamically significant obstructive, regurgitant, or septation abnormalities result in either ventricular pressure overloading, diastolic volume overloading, or a combination of both. The consequences of overloading are myocardial hypertrophy, dilatation, or both. These compensatory mechanisms have been shown to be frequently accompanied by a depressed contractile state that, if the pathophysiologic changes are severe, may not be improved by surgical elimination of the overload etiology. This is not surprising, since myofibril degeneration with fibrosis is the end result of hypertrophy. It is important to recall that, while hypertrophy classically is seen with pressure overload, it also is a component of the pathology of volume overload (Maron et al., 1975).

CONGENITAL HEART DISEASE. There is accumulating evidence that congenital cardiovascular lesions producing volume or pressure overloading on one or both ventricles can result in abnormal cardiac performance, which may persist to varying degrees after successful cardiac surgery. These data have been reviewed by Graham (1975).

In ventricular volume overload such as that produced by a ventricular septal defect, residual dilatation, hypertrophy, and depressed contractility have been observed in children with large left to right shunts who had proven surgical closure of their defects. It is of interest that the contractile state was normal postoperatively in those undergoing operative repair of a similar defect but who had substantially less pulmonary blood flow as a consequence of either previous pulmonary artery banding or the presence of pulmonary valve stenosis (Jarmakani et al., 1972).

Persistence of mild cardiac size and performance abnormalities may be detected in patients with right heart volume overload, e.g., secundum atrial septal defect. Following repair, increased right ventricular end-diastolic volume, occasionally depressed ejection fraction, and an abnormal cardiac output response to intense exercise may be observed in some of these patients (Epstein et al., 1973; Graham et al., 1973). Characteristically, infants with total anomalous pulmonary venous connection have small noncompliant left atria. Parr et al. (1975) have suggested that this abnormality and its subsequent inadequate reservoir function may be responsible in part for the small stroke volumes observed in these patients and thereby contribute to postoperative mortality.

Ventricular pressure overload such as that produced by hemodynamically significant aortic or pulmonary valve stenosis does not appear to be commonly accompanied by significant impairment of ventricular performance in the majority of children beyond infancy. However, when such overloading is severe enough to demand urgent surgical relief in neonates or infants, there is evidence that reduced diastolic compliance persists despite a successful operative result (Graham, 1975). Severe compliance reduction probably is a major factor in the outcome of those who succumb following repair of these lesions.

In tetralogy of Fallot, particularly the severe forms, impaired left ventricular function may be detected before and following the operation. In these patients, preoperative left ventricular end-diastolic volume tends to be diminished and in rare instances may be so small that systemic blood flow cannot be satisfactorily maintained after correction (Kirklin and Karp, 1970). Moreover, the preoperative left ventricular ejection fraction is often reduced and may persist postoperatively (Jarmakani et al., 1972). However, normal ejection fractions have been observed in postoperative studies of children who had been corrected before two years of age (Sunderland et al., 1973). The data suggest that the pattern of mild to moderate left ventricular dysfunction, so frequently persistent in older children after surgery, might be minimized or perhaps avoided by an earlier operation.

AORTIC VALVE DISEASE. Although cardiac index generally rises and left ventricular end diastolic pressure tends to fall after aortic valve replacement, evidence of persisting ventricular dysfunction has been documented with exercise studies (Ross et al., 1966). In one third of the patients, evidence of depressed left ventricular performance postoperatively was manifested by an abnormal response to exercise, in which left ventricular filling pressure rose while stroke volume either fell or remained constant.

Elegant studies (Figs. 9-5,6,7) by Gault et al. (1970) of patients who had undergone valve replacement for free aortic regurgitation clearly documented persistence of depressed ventricular function in all who had exhibited marked preoperative performance abnormalities, even though postoperative hemodynamic variables (cardiac index, left ventricular filling pressure) improved. In these patients evidence of reduced myocardial contractility persisted despite elimination of the regurgitant volume overload. Persistence of abnormal left ventricular diastolic pressure-radius (volume) characteristics was also observed. On the other hand, one patient, whose preoperative inotropic state had been normal, experienced not only the anticipated improvement in hemodynamic variables after surgery but also normal pressure-radius measurements, with persistence of the preoperative normal contractile state.

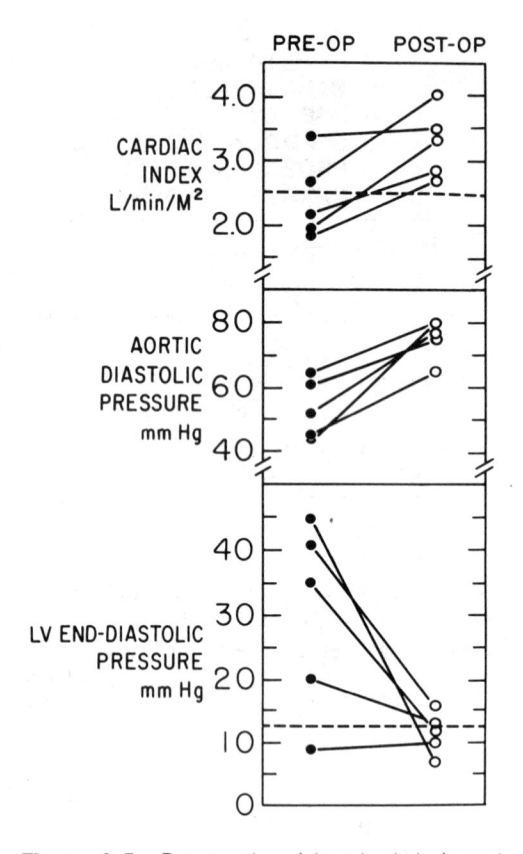

Figure 9-5. Preoperative (closed circles) and postoperative (open circles) hemodynamic data for five patients undergoing valve replacement for aortic regurgitation. Preoperatively, the left ventricular end-diastolic pressure (LVEDP) was elevated in each of four patients with depressed inotropic state. This variable fell to normal or near normal levels after surgery in each instance. A similar pattern of improvement is reflected in the postoperative rise in cardiac index (CI). In one patient with normal contractility LVEDP and CI were normal in both preoperative and postoperative studies. The dashed horizontal lines indicate the lower limit of normal for CI (2.5 liters/min/m²) and the upper limit of normal for LVEDP (12 mm Hg). (Redrawn from Gault et al., 1970, with permission of the authors and the American Heart Assn., Inc.)

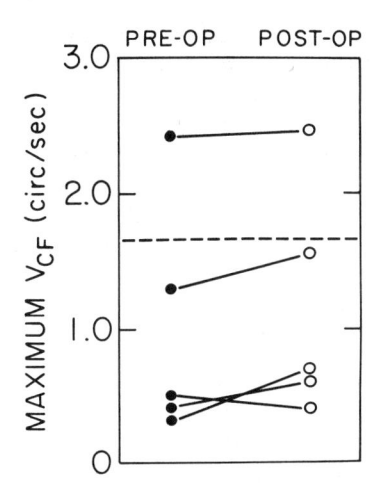

Figure 9-6. Maximum velocity of circumferential fiber shortening (maximum V_{CF}), circ/sec, is shown for each of the five patients preoperatively (closed circles) and postoperatively (open circles). The lower limit of normal for maximum V_{CF} (patients with normal ventricular function without valvular regurgitation) is shown by the horizontal dashed line. All four patients with preoperatively depressed inotropic state had postoperative maximum V_{CF} measurements that remained subnormal, whereas the measurement remained normal in the one patient coming to the operation with normal inotropic state. (Redrawn from Gault et al., 1970, with permission of the authors and the American Heart Assn., Inc.)

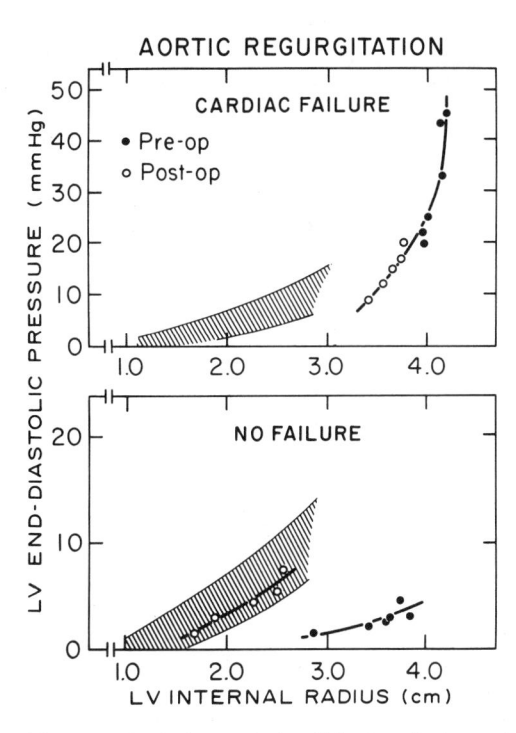

Figure 9-7. Left ventricular (LV) diastolic internal radius plotted against LV end-diastolic pressure (LVEDP) in two patients before (closed circles) and after (open circles) aortic valve replacement for aortic regurgitation. The shaded areas indicate the range of diastolic pressure-radius measurements in patients with normal LV function without valvular regurgitation. The upper plot depicts the data of a patient with preoperative depressed inotropic state. Postoperatively the LVEDP was reduced but the end-diastolic radius was only slightly smaller. The lower plot depicts the data of a patient with preoperative normal inotropic state. Postoperatively the diastolic pressure-radius curve moved sharply to the left into the normal range. LVEDP was unchanged despite the substantial reduction in radius. (Redrawn from Gault et al., 1970, with permission of the authors and the American Heart Assn., Inc.)

To summarize, available evidence indicates that patients with severe cardiac hypertrophy requiring aortic valve replacement may often have a depressed contractile state and restricted compliance. Diastolic reserve mechanisms are probably irreversibly lost, or at least reduced, in patients with severe aortic regurgitation and marked elevation of left ventricular filling pressure (Wisheart and Kirklin, 1973).

MITRAL VALVE DISEASE. Despite satisfactory hemodynamic correction, impairment of cardiac performance frequently is observed after mitral valve replacement. In the early postoperative period the decrement in cardiac output after mitral replacement with a ball valve tends to be significantly greater than that observed after aortic valve replacement with a similar prosthesis (Rastelli and Kirklin, 1966, 1967).

The extent of cardiac dysfunction persisting after mitral valve repair or replacement varies considerably and, in large measure, is related to the etiology of the valvular pathology. For example, as discussed later in the chapter, severe mitral regurgitation of chronic ischemic etiology generally is a component of extensive and largely irreversible left ventricular dysfunction, whereas the same degree of regurgitation of congenital or rheumatic origin may be accompanied by less severe cardiac performance abnormalities.

Myocardial and Coronary Artery Disease

MYOCARDIAL DISEASE. Persistent postoperative cardiac dysfunction after repair or replacement of rheumatic mitral valve pathology has been attributed in part to a "myocardial factor," which is believed to be a residual pathophysiologic derangement of the original rheumatic myocarditis. This is suggested by the observation that left ventricular performance is unimpaired in dogs after mitral valve replacement with a ball-valve prosthesis (Rastelli et al., 1967), while the same operation performed on humans occasionally is accompanied by lack of improvement in cardiac function despite correction of the valvular abnormality.

It is also pertinent that Hildner et al. (1972) detected preoperative left ventricular dysfunction in more than one third of patients with pure mitral stenosis, a lesion not accompanied by left ventricular systolic or diastolic overloading. These findings were believed indicative of intrinsic myocardial disease, possibly chronic rheumatic myocarditis. Further, this same study documented that there was lessened probability of postoperative improvement of contractility and that the frequency of unimprovement or worsening of the inotropic state was higher in patients having mitral than those having aortic valve replacement.

Hypertrophic obstructive cardiomyopathy, another type of myocardial disease occasionally requiring surgery, may present a low stroke volume and a preoperatively high left ventricular filling pressure. These abnormalities may persist postoperatively.

CORONARY ARTERY DISEASE. Significant occlusive coronary artery disease can exert an additive adverse effect on cardiac performance in patients with valvular heart disease (Befeler et al., 1970). When coronary artery disease was known to exist and revascularization procedures not yet widely performed, mortality in these patients was higher after isolated aortic or combined aortic and mitral valve replacement (Linhart and Wheat, 1967; Linhart et al., 1968; Coleman and Soloff, 1970). Moreover, in patients surviving replacements of the aortic valve, evidence of persistent myocardial dysfunction was commonly observed in those with concomitant coronary artery disease (Linhart and Wheat, 1967). A more recent analysis by Wisheart and Kirklin (1973) indicated that nearly one half of the late deaths after aortic valve replacement appeared to have been related to coronary artery disease. These data argue for concomitant coronary artery bypass when valve replacement is undertaken in patients who have significant coronary artery obstructions.

By far the most dominant factor contributing to hospital mortality of patients undergoing revascularization operations has been the preoperative existence of severe left ventricular dysfunction (Spencer et al., 1971; Loop et al., 1975), the consequence of either acute myocardial necrosis, chronic fibrosis, or both. Kouchoukos et al. (1974) noted a 15-fold increase in operative deaths (29 percent) when patients in congestive heart failure underwent coronary artery bypass procedures as opposed to the low risk of surgery for those not in failure.

Effects of Surgery

Anesthesia. Certain commonly used anesthetic agents, such as halothane and thiopental, tend to produce myocardial depression. In well-sedated patients these agents do not significantly increase catecholamine levels during anesthethic induction, so that contractility is depressed and cardiac output frequently reduced at this vulnerable period, particularly in patients with advanced cardiac dysfunction. Morphine anesthesia may be useful for these patients, since it does not seem to adversely effect myocardial contractility.

Cardiopulmonary Bypass. Although hard data derived from clinical experience are virtually nonexistent, evidence suggests that whole body perfusion, as presently practiced, can produce some degree of cardiac damage. Mechanical performance deteriorated in perfused canine isolated hearts maintained by disc oxygenators in contrast to hearts supported by cross-perfusion, in which no deterioration occurred (Brown et al., 1972). These studies were conducted without use of either microfilters in the circuit or membrane oxygenators. It is not known whether the adverse effects could have been ameliorated with these devices.

In humans, slight to moderate reduction of cardiac performance may become apparent soon after intracardiac surgery and may be maximal as late as 24 to 48 hours after surgery. An obvious and critical impediment to evaluating the adverse myocardial consequences of perfusion per se is the difficulty of separating its effects from the traumata associated with performance of the repair.

Interacting factors such as capillary damaging lysosomal enzymes, formed element, lipid and gaseous microemboli, hypoperfusion of the endocardial myocardium, and cellular and interstitial edema probably are all operative in transiently depressing both contractility and compliance.

Two additional perfusion-related factors can adversely affect cardiac performance. Relative instability of the intravascular and extravascular compartments is one of the characteristic aspects of cardiopulmonary bypass, as currently conducted. Even in the absence of overt bleeding postperfusion intravascular volume can be somewhat low. If repletion therapy is not appropriate, ventricular preload and stroke volume are reduced. Second, peripheral arteriolar resistance tends to rise slowly as perfusion continues. The increased afterload commonly persists for four to six hours postoperatively even when the general hemodynamic state is satisfactory.

Myocardial Injury during Surgery. Electrocardiographic studies, scintigraphic imaging, and detection of abnormal myocardial metabolic patterns and isoenzyme release all indicate that cardiac injury of varying severity frequently accompanies a variety of intracardiac operations performed with cardiopulmonary bypass, regardless of the method of myocardial preservation employed (Isom et al., 1973; Oldham et al., 1973; Sapsford et al., 1974; Klein et al., 1976; Kouchoukos and Karp, 1976). In a clinical setting it is difficult to systematically evaluate the factors etiologic to the injury, but they are probably multiple.

CARDIAC PATHOLOGY AND ISCHEMIA. Extensive hemorrhage and necrosis of presumed ischemic origin have been observed in patients presenting *severe left ventricular hypertrophy* who died in low cardiac output after open intracardiac surgery (Taber et al., 1967; Najafi et al., 1969; Buckberg et al., 1972). Clinical and experimental studies indicate that the inner myocardial zone is particularly vulnerable, even more so when there have been lengthy periods of ventricular fibrillation during bypass (Becker et al., 1973; Chiu, 1974). It is apparent that, when *occlusive coronary artery pathology* exists, there is heightened possibility of inadequate myocardial perfusion during the operation.

DAMAGE ASSOCIATED WITH CONDUCT OF REPAIR. Despite recent advances in myocardial protection, some degree of injury is necessarily inflicted on the myocardium as a consequence of the operative measures being employed on or within the heart. The insult of the surgical repair is superimposed on perfusion trauma and on a heart that is frequently at greater risk of compromise because of its intrinsic pathology (marked hypertrophy or coronary atherosclerosis or both).

Three factors varyingly contribute to the extent of surgically inflicted myocardial damage during the repair: (1) ischemia; (2) incisional and excisional trauma; and (3) technical complications. By far the most common and serious problem is the injury associated with *ischemia,* since, as indicated earlier, all current methods of myocardial protection are still not predictably optimal in all circumstances. For example, despite use of cold cardioplegia,

Conti et al. (1978) still found evidence indicating myocardial damage in approximately one fourth of the patients who had undergone coronary artery bypass grafting.

In previous years extensive damage of presumed ischemic origin was observed in both ventricles. Archie and Kirklin (1973) noted gross right ventricular subendocardial hemorrhage in patients dying after repair of tetralogy of Fallot and transposition of the great arteries. Perhaps the most extreme form of ischemia-induced myocardial injury has been the "stone heart" (Cooley et al., 1972), so described because the heart is "rock" hard and irreversibly frozen in tetanic contracture. It has been observed predominantly in patients with severe left ventricular hypertrophy having aortic valve replacement under conditions of normothermic cardiopulmonary bypass and anoxic cardiac arrest. Histologic examination of these hearts reveals widespread degeneration of myofibrils in hypercontracted muscle fibers (Baroldi et al., 1974). The "stone heart" has been characterized as myocardial rigor due to anoxic depletion of high energy phosphate stores in the hypertrophied myocardium (Katz and Tada, 1972).

As detailed in Chapter 5, reduction of cardiac energy requirements with hypothermia has been well-documented (Gott et al., 1962). Before the widespread acceptance of cold cardioplegia, hypothermia in combination with propranolol was shown to have reduced the clinical occurrence of the "stone heart" syndrome (Wukasch et al., 1973). Engelman et al. (1975) have shown that myocardial reperfusion itself can be accompanied by severe injury when multiple periods of anoxic arrest and reperfusion have preceded the final reestablishment of blood flow to the myocardium.

Cardiac incision or excision necessarily creates myocardial damage of different degrees. Even when properly executed, extensive incision or suturing of atrial or ventricular free walls or their septa may so compromise nodal tissue, internodal pathways, or bundle branches that cardiac performance may be damaged as a consequence of either arrhythmias or combined reduction of mechanical systolic efficiency and diastolic compliance. These findings are of particular importance when lengthy vertical ventriculotomy of either the right (Stirling et al., 1957; March et al., 1961) or left ventricle has been performed. It is apparent that extensive excision of either right or left ventricular myocardium, as typically required in repair of tetralogy of Fallot or hypertrophic obstructive cardiomyopathy, inflicts a traumatic insult of varying severity, with measurable reduction in cardiac performance almost always discernible immediately after the operation.

Although relatively unusual, *complications related to technical execution* can inflict extensive and life-threatening myocardial damage. Myocardial infarction caused by coronary artery injury can occur as a consequence of mural dissection (coronary cannulation for perfusion), division (anomalous coronary artery anatomy frequently seen in tetralogy of Fallot), or inadvertent suturing (particularly the left circumflex artery) during insertion of a mitral valve prosthesis. Particulate coronary artery embolization of fragments of calcium or thrombus is another cause of infarction. Inadvertent admission of as little as 0.1 ml of air into the coronary arteries (as can happen with incomplete venting of the left heart or aortic root) may depress ventricular function (Goldfarb and Bahnson, 1963). A variety of congenital cardiac lesions offer the potential for suture inclusion of or hemorrhage into the atrioventricular bundle, which can result in complete heart block. Fortunately, this complication has now become relatively rare because of increased knowledge of conduction pathway anatomy and intraoperative mapping techniques.

Suboptimal Conditions after Repair

Immediately after discontinuance of perfusion (and assuming that appropriate measures have been taken to optimize heart rate, rhythm, and stroke volume), three dominant factors affect the extent to which cardiac performance is impaired: (1) the magnitude of surgical trauma inflicted on the heart and the physiologic incompleteness of the repair; (2) residual cardiovascular pathology; and (3) the presence and nature of adverse postoperative events.

Factors Related to the Repair. As indicated previously, different degrees of cardiac dysfunction are intrinsic to the trauma of achieving a precise and complete repair. However, even a flawlessly executed repair may be physiologically imperfect. For example, in correction of severe forms of tetralogy of Fallot, extensive right ventricular outflow tract reconstruction may be required with a noncontractile patch of cloth or pericardium. This allows pulmonary regurgitation while also creating what, in effect, is a right ventricular "aneurysm," compromising right heart dynamics.

Valve replacement with many of the more widely used prostheses occasionally may not confer optimal physiologic conditions, an assertion supported by the following two examples. Ball valves possess considerable inertia, and tachyarrhythmias (above 150 beats per minute) can be accompanied by valve dysfunction. The sharply increased rate and the proportionately reduced diastolic period may, in the case of aortic prostheses, result in aortoventricular reflux because of failure of poppet seating. Similarly, after ball valve replacement of the mitral apparatus, left ventricular diastolic filling can be impeded at rapid rates, since poppet descent from its occluding position may be incomplete. Another type of valve, the ingeniously designed Bjork-Shiley prosthesis, permits a slight amount of reflux, which, while well-tolerated by a heart with some reserve, has at least the potential for adversely affecting performance in a patient with far-advanced left ventricular dysfunction.

It is apparent that cardiac performance can be severely compromised if an *inadequate repair* has been carried out (examples include incomplete relief of right or left ventricular outflow tract obstructions, incomplete closure of extracardiac or intracardiac shunts, and significant regurgitation after valve repair or replacement). When correctible residual lesions are present and cardiac performance is impaired, prompt reoperation should be considered.

Residual Cardiovascular Pathology. A second factor contributing to impaired cardiac function after surgical intervention is the presence of significant uncorrected cardiovascular pathology. Forward flow can be reduced as a consequence of increased afterload if vascular resistance remains distinctly elevated in either the pulmonary or systemic circulations. When these conditions prevail, forward flow is further impaired if there is associated residual regurgitation of the tricuspid or mitral valve. After mitral valve replacement with a ball valve, the presence of "mild to moderate" aortic regurgitation (which may have been judged insufficient to require concomitant valve replacement) can seriously impair cardiac performance, presumably as a result of the reflux volume impeding poppet descent during normal atrioventricular filling, while simultaneously inappropriately increasing the ventricular diastolic volume.

Comment has been made earlier about the adverse influence on cardiac performance of both nonbypassed coronary artery occlusive disease and advanced myocardial pathology (diffuse fibrosis, severe hypertrophy, and dilatation).

Adverse Postoperative Events. Even when preoperative cardiac performance has been satisfactory and the conduct of the open intracardiac procedure has been optimal, a number of usually tolerable and transient performance alterations of major subsystems may be detected. As discussed in Chapter 5, these are consequent to the multiple traumata of the operation (anesthesia, surgical exposure of the heart, perfusion, and the repair). It is pertinent to this and subsequent discussion to recall that the early postperfusion state of a "stable" patient frequently is accompanied by a rise in interstitial water, an unstable intravascular volume, mild derangement of the acid-base state and coagulation (Gralnick and

Fischer, 1971), as well as a tendency toward hypokalemia (Ebert et al., 1965). Therefore, this period is generally accompanied by some measurable reduction in cardiac performance (Kirklin and Rastelli, 1967) and a variable ventilation-perfusion defect (Osborne et al., 1962; Hedley-Whyte et al., 1965; Andersen and Ghia, 1970).

The usually mild and time-limited distortions just mentioned can be lethal in a postoperative patient with reduced or absent myocardial reserve. Regardless of cardiac pump function capability, the onset of significant adverse postoperative events in any patient after open intracardiac surgery can be life-threatening. Those conditions associated with the operation and etiologic to postoperative impairment of one or both of the two determinants of cardiac pumping capacity (i.e., rate or stroke volume) include: (1) development and persistence of abnormalities of heart rate or rhythm; (2) hypovolemia; (3) cardiac tamponade; (4) development and persistence of marked elevation of left ventricular afterload (increased impedance to ejection); and (5) factors contributing to significant reduction of myocardial contractility. These matters are discussed later in the chapter.

POSTOPERATIVE ANALYSIS OF CARDIOVASCULAR SUBSYSTEM PERFORMANCE

Concepts

As emphasized earlier, proper postoperative management of the cardiovascular subsystem always must be preceded by continual analysis. In practical terms, it is necessary to know whether (1) cardiac output and (2) both gas (particularly oxygen) transport and exchange mechanisms are adequate to sustain stable and satisfactory function of all organs and subsystems. Hence, analysis of (1) and (2) must always proceed together.

Adequacy of cardiac output does not necessarily have a direct relationship to the performance characteristics of the heart. It may be possible for the heart to maintain a satisfactory level of systemic blood flow at a given period but only through maximal use of energy-expending cardiac reserves, which, by their very nature, are time-limited (i.e., no reserve mechanism can be sustained at its highest physiologic limit of performance over a lengthy period of time).

Therefore, *analysis* of the cardiovascular subsystem requires assessment of both *performance* and *adequacy*, the latter relating to what might be termed the "clinical efficiency" of the subsystem's performance (i.e., the magnitude of *reserves* being used to achieve a particular level of systemic blood flow).

Subjective and Objective Information. There can be no disagreement that, to the extent possible, quantitative methods of assessing performance of all subsystems represent the sine qua non of optimal postoperative management. Kirklin (1973) has eloquently stated the case for this approach:

> Decisions are best made on [the basis of] numerical or objective data using well established rules of logic. We distrust subjective evaluations and intuitive judgments. . . . One of the most disillusioning things . . . has been the demonstration beyond doubt in our Intensive Care Unit that our ability to estimate the cardiac output from observation of the patient, palpation of his peripheral pulses, his blood pressure, his urine flow, and the like is extraordinarily poor.

This view is by no means intended to denigrate the value of careful observation of the patient, although the obvious limitation of this mode of evaluation lies in its dependence on the experience and accuracy of the observer. It is probable that convalescence is proceeding satisfactorily when a patient is alert and calm, breathing easily at an approximately normal rate and depth, has readily palpable and full peripheral arterial pulses in the absence of venous distension, pink nail-beds and mucous membranes, prompt "capillary" refill following release of momentary nail-bed compression, and warm skin. On the other hand, there is virtual certainty that systemic blood flow is inadequate when the patient is obtunded or restless, has weak peripheral pulses (often with systemic venous distension), blue nail-beds and mucous membranes, sluggish "capillary" refill, and cold skin.

When either of these two clinical extremes exists, one can be reasonably confident that quantitative assessment of the cardiovascular and pulmonary subsystems will document the clinical impressions. However, this is not the case when subsystem performance is changing and the general clinical state lies somewhere between the two extremes. Thus, routine quantitative evaluation of subsystem variables obviously is needed.

Measurements. The extent of quantitative monitoring obviously will vary with the magnitude of the cardiac procedure. After open intracardiac operation, analysis is facilitated by routinely measuring a number of pertinent variables. Adequate *hourly flow of urine* (15 ml/hr/m^2 or more) that is hyperosmolar relative to plasma suggests (but by no means proves) that systemic blood flow is satisfactory. Cardiac *rate* and *rhythm* are readily determined from the electrocardiogram. Systemic arterial pressure (a reflection of left ventricular *afterload*) and analyses of blood gases and the acid-base state are all accomplished with measurements and blood specimens obtained from an indwelling catheter in the radial (or occasionally brachial or femoral) artery.

Some groups have recommended insertion of a catheter into the pulmonary artery at the operation. Although there are specific circumstances in which it is desirable to have both knowledge of pulmonary artery systolic pressure (a reflection of right ventricular afterload) and availability of a means of drawing a mixed venous sample, routine pulmonary artery catheter insertion does not seem warranted. However, when the thermo-dilution method of cardiac output is to be employed, a 2.5 F thermistor is inserted through the right ventricular wall into the pulmonary trunk. Alternatively, in adults, a thermistor-tipped Swan-Ganz catheter is inserted via a peripheral vein. This permits the measurement to be made with convenience while additionally providing knowledge of pulmonary artery and pulmonary wedge pressures. Left and right atrial catheters positioned at the time of surgery permit measurement of transmural pressures in these chambers and provide a means of assessing the extent to which the Starling *preload* reserve mechanism is being used to maintain stroke volume. Currently there is no reliable means of clinically measuring *myocardial contractility*.

Postoperative *cardiac output measurements* are not performed routinely. However, these data are obtained sequentially in all patients who come to surgery with advanced cardiac dysfunction, those recovering from complex operative procedures of higher risk, and any patient whose cardiac performance, as judged by other criteria, is uncertain. Formulas have been developed for calculation of stroke volume and cardiac output from the contour of the systemic arterial pulse. However, in the early postoperative period the unpredictable arterial impedance changes, and their influence in altering the pulse contour makes the method unreliable (Kouchoukos et al., 1969) unless frequent recalibration with a standard cardiac output method is employed (Jurado et al., 1973). Fortunately, relatively simple, rapid, and reproducible indicator dilution methods for determining cardiac output at the bedside are available (thermodilution or indocyanine green techniques). These data, in combination with known preload and afterload measurements, allow useful deductions to be made about the myocardial contractile state.

Performance interdependency requires that the *pulmonary subsystem* (and particularly *oxygen transport*) be evaluated concurrently with the cardiovascular subsystem. These matters are discussed elsewhere (Chapters 3, 12, and 13) and are briefly mentioned here for completeness. Variables that are routinely measured include body temperature, blood hemoglobin concentration, hydrogen ion concentration, and gas tensions of systemic arterial blood. In the past, frequent use was made of mixed venous oxygen tension as an index of adequacy of cardiac output. However, the relationship is a crude one because the measurement is a reflection of not one but two interacting factors: oxygen transport mechanisms (including cardiac output) and oxygen consumption of perfused areas of the body. Since oxygen consumption of different organs varies considerably and the venous effluent volumes of underperfused areas of the body are low, it is not surprising that the mixed venous oxygen tension or saturation is not a sensitive index of adequacy of cardiac output.

However, for reasons that are at present unclear, it has been shown that after open intracardiac surgery there is significant correlation between mixed venous oxygen tension and cardiac index in infants and small children, while no clear relationship is demonstrable in adults undergoing mitral valve surgery (Parr et al., 1975; Appelbaum et al., 1976). Obviously, interpretation of mixed venous oxygen tension data would be much more useful if it were possible to conveniently measure total body oxygen consumption. However, *direct* measurement of oxygen consumption is difficult to obtain at the bedside. When an estimate of total oxygen consumption is desired, it is indirectly calculated by the Fick equation: arteriovenous oxygen difference multiplied by cardiac index.

POSTOPERATIVE MAINTENANCE AND SUPPORT OF CARDIAC FUNCTION

Continuing analysis of the cardiovascular subsystem and oxygen transport and utilization mechanisms makes it possible to conduct cardiac maintenance and supportive management systematically. Obviously the hemodynamic goal is maintenance of physiologically adequate levels of both systemic blood flow and perfusion pressure (cardiac index above 2.2 liters/min/m^2 and mean arterial pressure between 90 and 100 mm Hg in previously normotensive patients) at acceptably low levels of preload and arteriolar impedance.

Postoperative cardiac functional maintenance and support involves: (1) prompt detection and correction of dysfunction related to an inadequate repair (such as resuture of periprosthetic dehiscence after valve replacement) or other adverse events following the operation (excessive postoperative bleeding with or without cardiac tamponade, etc.); (2) "preventive" management of anticipated distortions that commonly accompany open intracardiac operations (such as the tendency toward hypovolemia, hypokalemia, mild pulmonary dysfunction, etc.); (3) optimizing cardiac rate, rhythm, and stroke volume and manipulating their reserves when necessary to attain satisfactory circulatory stability; and (4) aggressive use of pharmacologic and mechanical support methods when significant low cardiac output persists. The first two matters have been discussed elsewhere, and the following sections will deal primarily with the last two concerns.

Optimizing Rate and Rhythm: Dysrhythmia Problems*

Disturbances of cardiac rate and rhythm are commonly encountered after cardiac surgery and are prone to occur within the first 48 hours. Careful postoperative monitoring has documented that 75 percent of adult patients recovering from open cardiac procedures will experience at least one arrhythmic episode (Smith et al., 1972). In approximately 50 percent of patients the arrhythmia will not have been present preoperatively (Rose et al., 1975). Although the majority of arrhythmias tend to be transient and generally respond to therapy, their serious potential is apparent.

Factors commonly associated with or predisposing to arrhythmia development include advanced heart disease (particularly if marked cardiomegaly is present), renal dysfunction, cardiac incisional or ischemic trauma, perfusion or drug-induced hypokalemia, cardioactive drug toxicity (particularly digitalis preparations), acid-base imbalance, and hypoxemia.

As discussed in Chapter 10, fine epicardial electrodes implanted on the right atrium

---

*A comprehensive discussion of the diagnosis and management of these problems will be found in Chapter 10.

and either ventricle during the operation are effective means of both diagnosing complex postoperative arrhythmias and establishing cardiac pacing as a therapeutic measure.

Hemodynamic Consequences of Dysrhythmias

TACHYCARDIAS OR TACHYARRHYTHMIAS. When a regular or irregular cardiac rate exceeds 140 to 150 beats per minute in the adult recovering from cardiac surgery, stroke output may fall because of reduced diastolic filling time. As discussed earlier, hemodynamic deterioration is particularly likely to occur at these heart rates when valve prostheses with considerable inertia (such as ball valves) have been inserted, since poppet seating or opening may not be complete during the appropriate but abbreviated phase of the cardiac cycle. Additionally, tachyarrhythmias may impair myocardial perfusion because of the reduced length of diastolic coronary flow, circumstances particularly adverse in patients with coronary artery occlusive disease.

BRADYCARDIAS OR BRADYARRHYTHMIAS. Cardiac rates of 60 to 70 per minute in the adult may not be immediately accompanied by a fall in cardiac output if there is a compensatory rise in stroke volume. However, when diastolic volumes are sharply increased and cardiac rates remain low, the probability of the onset of serious reentrant arrhythmias is heightened. Moreover, in many circumstances after cardiac surgery, the rise in stroke volume that would normally occur as a compensatory (reserve) response to the low rate may be significantly limited if patients have marked ventricular hypertrophy (reduced diastolic compliance) or other coexisting abnormalities of preload, afterload, or contractility. For all these reasons, persistence of postoperative bradycardia, with or without accompanying arrhythmia, ultimately tends to be accompanied by significant cardiac output reduction and must be managed aggressively.

Postrepair Pacing and Cardiac Performance. As indicated earlier, the frequent occurrence of postoperative arrhythmias makes it advisable to routinely insert atrial and ventricular myocardial pacing wires during the operation. Apart from facilitating both diagnosis and pacing therapy, their presence permits more confident administration of cardiotonic or cardiac depressant drugs.

Postoperative cardiac rates of 65 to 70 (in the adult), which would not be considered particularly disadvantageous in other circumstances, frequently may be associated with reentrant arrhythmias and significant reduction in cardiac output. Rate augmentation with pacing to achieve ventricular rates of 90 to 100 beats per minute is helpful in suppressing these arrhythmias (Harris et al., 1968). When the ventricular rate is slow in the presence of atrial fibrillation, ventricular pacing is immediately effective in increasing and stabilizing the ventricular rate, significantly increasing cardiac output, and concomitantly reducing left ventricular filling pressurs (Litwak et al., 1968) (Figs. 9-8 and 9-9).

Atrial pacing is the procedure of choice in bradycardic patients in whom atrioventricular conduction is intact (Friesen et al., 1968). In such situations maintenance of normal electromechanical relationships between the atria and ventricles offers the advantage of the atrial contribution to ventricular filling, which generally results in a sharp rise in cardiac output in postoperative patients. If atrial pacing is not available in bradycardic patients with intact atrioventricular conduction, it is inadvisable to employ ventricular pacing, since cardiac output may be further depressed and ventricular filling pressures may rise (Wisheart et al., 1973), primarily because of loss of atrioventricular synchrony (Gilmore et al., 1963). Interestingly, the same hemodynamic derangements are demonstrable in subjects who have normal atrioventricular conduction during ventricular pacing (Samet et al., 1968).

The marked bradycardia generally accompanying *complete atrioventricular dissociation* obviously requires pacing to maintain an adequate ventricular rate. Fortunately, heart block related to surgical trauma is an unusual occurrence and may be transient. Although ventricular pacing itself can be effective, it establishes a rapid idioventricular rhythm. The hemodynamic consequence is distinctly

Figure 9-8. Effect of ventricular pacing on cardiac index in patients with bradycardia (slow atrial fibrillation) during the early post-operative period. Discontinuance of pacing (mean rate 97) and reappearance of slower rate (mean nonpaced rate 66) resulted in a 23.4 percent fall in the cardiac index. Resumption of pacing (rate deliberately set slightly higher: mean rate 109) promptly increased the cardiac index 28.3 percent above the nonpaced state. Addition of small increments of isoproterenol insufficient to significantly change the rate (mean 110) was associated with a further modest rise in cardiac index. (From Litwak et al., 1968, with permission of the C. V. Mosby Co.)

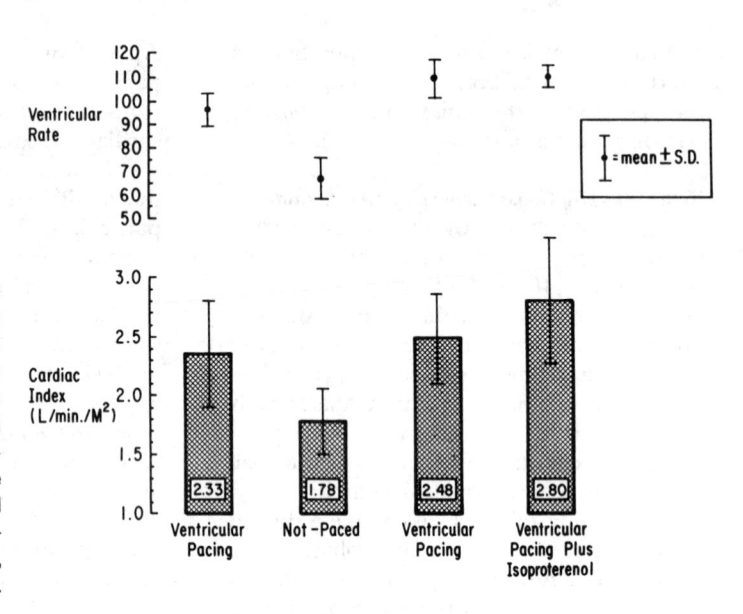

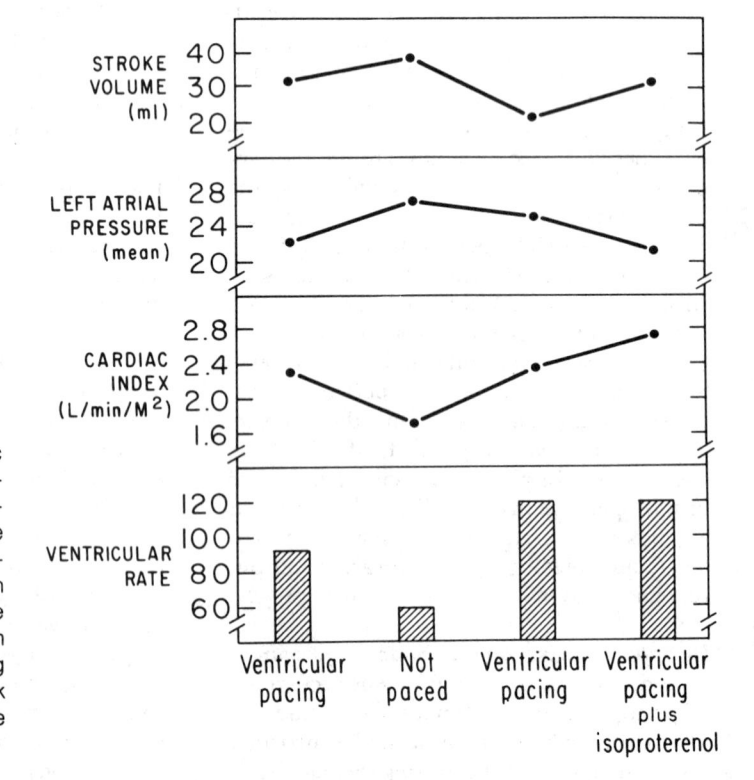

Figure 9-9. Hemodynamic changes associated with ventricular pacing in a 58-year-old patient with severe mitral valve disease, atrial fibrillation, and advanced myocardial dysfunction who underwent prosthetic valve replacement. The improvement in cardiac dynamics during pacing is evident. (Redrawn from Litwak et al., 1968, with permission of the C. V. Mosby Co.)

poorer than that achievable with sequential atrioventricular pacing, which allows retention of the atrial contribution to ventricular filling, increasing cardiac output significantly (Fields et al., 1973; Hartzler et al., 1977). The procedure merely requires intraoperative implantation of atrial as well as ventricular myocardial wires and their attachment to an appropriate pacing unit,* which first initiates atrial stimulation followed by sequenced ventricular stimulation with an appropriate delay period between the two.

Optimizing Ventricular Filling Pressures (Preload)

The two dominant factors affecting ventricular filling pressures (blood volume and adequacy of ventricular performance) have been discussed previously. Although neither of these two determinants is quantitatively defined by left and right atrial pressure data per se, these pressure measurements do allow useful deductions to be made about the adequacy of volume filling and cardiac performance. Since the performance characteristics of the left and right ventricle may be sharply different (particularly after cardiac surgery), it follows that the functional dynamics of each ventricle can be evaluated only by pressure measurements made in the ipsilateral atrium. Thus, left ventricular performance cannot be assessed reliably by right atrial pressures.

It is important to underscore the potential for development of hypovolemia after open intracardiac operations. Studies have shown that isotopically measured blood volume often is lower than would be anticipated from careful gravimetric determination of blood loss (despite volume-for-volume replacement of these losses). No predictable relationship can be demonstrated between the magnitude of the isotopic blood volume deficits, systemic arterial and central venous (or right atrial) pressure, or postperfusion hematocrit (Litwak et al., 1961; Gadboys and Litwak, 1963). Although understanding is still incomplete, factors contributing to the tendency toward hypovolemia include hemodilution perfusion with subsequent fluid loss from the intravascular compartment, arterial and venous capacitance vessel constriction, and inadequate blood replacement.

Preload Optimization of the Ventricular Performance-Volume Relationship. An adequate level of ventricular preload is best attained immediately after discontinuance of cardiopulmonary bypass by infusing perfusate from the pump-oxygenator into the patient until the mean left atrial pressure approximates 8 to 12 mm Hg. When preoperative left ventricular compliance has been sharply reduced because of either marked hypertrophy or extreme dilatation (or both) and poor performance conditions persist immediately after repair, slightly higher pressures (14 to 18 mm Hg) may be required in the operating room to maximize use of the Frank-Starling reserve mechanism. However, as discussed below, preload augmentation to these high levels must be done with caution, since cardiac performance may be adversely affected.

In the early postoperative period (with blood loss being replaced), left and right atrial pressures gradually fall, presumably because of the multiple factors of steadily improving myocardial function, water loss from the intravascular compartment, and beginning reduction of vasomotor tone (after some hours). Ordinarily the left atrial pressure exceeds the right atrial pressure except when right ventricular function has been impaired by ventriculotomy, excisional trauma (as in tetralogy of Fallot), elevated outflow resistance (after-load), or right coronary arterial air embolism.

When left atrial pressures are relatively low (less than 7 mm Hg) in the early hours after intracardiac repair, infusion of blood to increase atrial pressures moderately (3 to 5 mm Hg) will consistently increase stroke volume. However, there is relatively little response to blood administration when preinfusion ventricular filling pressures are in the

---

*Model 2020 bifocal pacemaker (American Pacemaker, Woburn, Mass.).

16 to 22 mm Hg range, undoubtedly because the sarcomere stretch (Frank-Starling reserve) mechanism is being used fully. Indeed, in an important study, Kouchoukos et al. (1971) found that in these conditions blood infusion was sometimes accompanied by a fall in stroke index, suggesting that the left ventricle was briefly performing on a descending limb of its function curve (Fig. 9–10).

Cardiac Tamponade. It is apparent that inappropriate bleeding with pericardiac accumulation of clotted and liquid blood can seriously impair cardiac performance postoperatively (see Chapter 15 for expanded discussion). Intrapericardial pressure rises, reducing both ventricular end-diastolic volume and stroke volume. The development of cardiac tamponade can be insidious, and its discovery can be disastrously late unless the possibility is constantly kept in mind.

Typically, early postoperative blood loss may be greater than usual, and component therapy with agents promoting clotting may be followed by sudden reduction or cessation of mediastinal tube drainage. This sequence may lead to the erroneous conclusion that vigorous bleeding has stopped. On the contrary, these events may signal the onset of tamponade, and, when accompanied by rising atrial pressures, disaster shortly may follow. Unequivocal evidence of low cardiac output, systemic arterial hypotension, and oliguria are not observed until relatively late. Successful

Figure 9–10. Comparison of the influence of blood infusion on cardiac index and stroke index soon after intracardiac surgery in adult patients with low and high mean left atrial pressures (LAP) prior to infusion. In those with preinfusion LAP less than 12 mm Hg, increasing preload resulted in a consistent and significant rise in both cardiac index (**A**) and the mean stroke index data of the entire group (**B**) However, when preinfusion LAP was 12 mm Hg or greater, blood infusion did not produce a significant augmentation of cardiac index (**C**), while mean stroke index declined significantly (**D**). Heart rate did not change significantly in either patient subgroup. As indicated above, Figures B and D reflect the mean trends in each patient subgroup and are derived from the data of Kouchoukos et al., 1971. (Figures A and C are redrawn, with modification, from Kouchoukos and Karp, 1976, with permission of the authors and Butterworth and Co.)

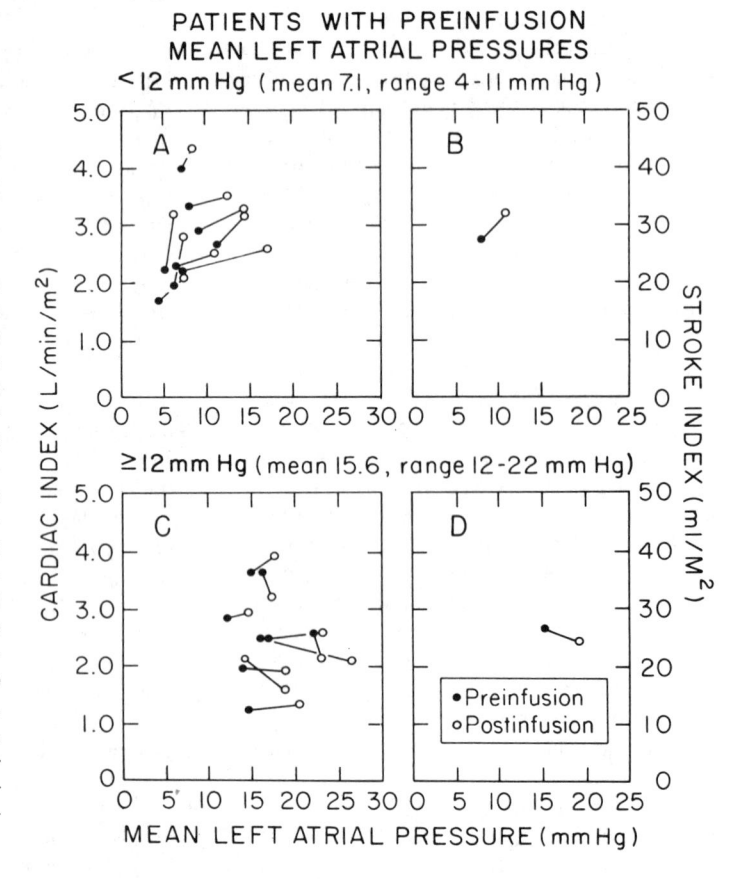

management is based on a high index of *suspicion*, early diagnosis, and prompt reoperation.

Optimizing Ventricular Afterload

When afterload is suddenly elevated in patients with left heart disease, stroke output falls (Ross and Braunwald, 1964). These observations have particular pertinence to patients recovering from open cardiac operations, since systemic arterial impedance is frequently elevated during the first six postoperative hours. It is apparent that left ventricular systolic wall tension must rise in these patients if stroke output is to be maintained. The hearts of patients with advanced dysfunction may not be able to attain the requisite wall tensions and assuredly cannot sustain these performance levels for long periods. When, in response to impedance elevation, the stroke output cannot be maintained, peripheral arteriolar resistance tends to rise even higher as a compensatory mechanism for reduced systemic blood flow. This establishes positive feedback conditions that, uncorrected, may be lethal. Severe postoperative elevations of systemic arterial pressure are particularly common in patients who have undergone either myocardial revascularization (Estafanous et al., 1973) or prosthetic replacement for stenotic lesions of the aortic valve (McQueen et al., 1972).

Management of Afterload Elevation. Optimizing cardiac performance in the postoperative period requires reducing severe systemic hypertension to acceptable levels. In patients with adequate cardiac output, lowering the inappropriately high pressure levels will reduce the potential for bleeding from suture lines and also provide for a more favorable myocardial oxygen supply-demand relationship (Buckberg et al., 1972). In postoperative infants and adults manifesting low cardiac output with elevated systemic arterial resistance and high ventricular filling pressures, afterload reduction will significantly increase cardiac index while atrial pressures are lowered (Fig. 9–11) (Kouchoukos et al., 1972; Benzing et al., 1976; Appelbaum et al., 1977).

Two methods of afterload reduction are available: pharmacologic means and intra-

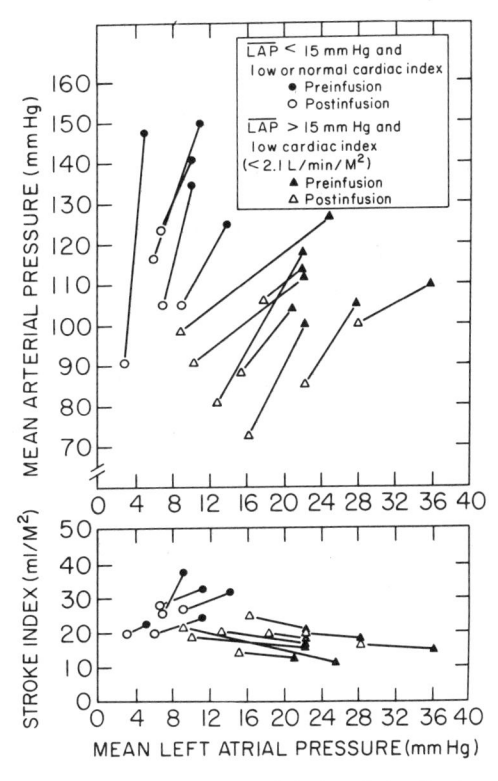

Figure 9–11. Response to infusion of trimethephan (Arfonad) into adult patients with elevated mean arterial pressures soon (within six hours) after intracardiac operations. Patients with low or normal cardiac index and mean left atrial pressure less than 15 mm Hg (circles) responded to the decrease in arterial pressure after infusion of Arfonad with a fall in stroke index and cardiac index (not illustrated), presumably due in part to a concomitant reduction in left ventricular filling pressure. Patients with low cardiac index and mean left atrial pressure greater than 15 mm Hg (triangles) responded to the Arfonad with significant reduction in mean arterial pressure and left atrial pressure with a significant increase of both stroke index and cardiac index (not illustrated). (Modified from Kouchoukos et al., 1972, with permission of the authors and the C. V. Mosby Co.)

aortic balloon counterpulsation. The latter procedure is discussed later in the chapter. Of the drugs currently available, sodium nitroprusside and Arfonad (trimethepan camsylate) appear to be the most convenient for clinical use. Both agents offer the advantages of rapid effect and brief duration of action. Simply varying the delivery speed of either agent using a mechanical infusing system can lower and control the arterial pressure.

Maintenance and Support of Myocardial Contractility

The Concept. There is a profound difference between the approach to postoperative management of myocardial contractility and the other determinants of cardiac performance. Rate, rhythm, and preload generally can be optimized without excessive physiologic cost to the heart, and afterload reduction significantly reduces myocardial energy expenditure. However, apart from the Bowditch effect (increasing rate to enhance contractility), the only direct and readily available means of augmenting the inotropic state is the use of pharmacologic agents. In effect, their use is analogous to whipping a tired horse. This is not to denigrate the importance of these drugs, for their proper use is invaluable for effective postoperative myocardial supportive care. What is proposed is that *maintenance* (optimizing) myocardial contractility is, by implication, *indirect,* involving proper perturbation of all other components so that the diseased and surgically traumatized heart functions at its maximal level of residual contractility. When contractility remains significantly impaired despite maintenance efforts, *supportive* measures must be invoked. This implies *direct* intervention with drugs that actuate the physiologically costly reserve mechanism of inotropic augmentation.

Maintenance (Optimization) of Residual Contractility. Earlier, factors adversely affecting postoperative cardiac performance (and particularly contractility) were reviewed. It will be recalled that, apart from intrinsically depressed inotropism associated with advanced myocardial disease, the other causes of postrepair reduction of contractility are primarily related to the effects of the operation (anesthesia, surgical and perfusion traumata, suboptimal repair) and postoperative events that either directly reduce contractility (myocardial infarction, hypoxia, severe acid-base or electrolyte imbalance, negative inotropic drugs) or circumstances that, by their prolonged presence, ultimately do so (protracted and marked afterload elevation or preload reduction, persisting hypermetabolic state). Therefore, it can be appreciated that optimizing myocardial contractility essentially begins in the operating room, and postoperative efforts are merely extensions of what has gone on before.

The major elements of optimization include: (1) a well-conducted operation with a precise, complete, and minimally traumatic repair; (2) prompt reoperation when significant residual correctible lesions are detected in the early postoperative period; (3) maintenance of satisfactory serum electrolyte balance and gas transport mechanisms (adequate oxygen uptake and carbon dioxide exchange, proper hemoglobin levels); (4) avoidance of procedural errors that commonly result in acid-base derangements (metabolic acidosis of perfusion origin, respiratory alkalosis from overly vigorous mechanical ventilation); (5) prompt detection and management of adverse postoperative events that impose severe distortions of rate, preload, or afterload (dysrhythmias, bleeding, tamponade, hypertension); and (6) reduction of factors conducive to hypermetabolism and increased oxygen consumption (therapy of severe hyperthermia and, when necessary, employment of mechanical ventilation to reduce the metabolic cost of breathing).

Pharmacologic Support (Augmentation) of Myocardial Contractility. Without exception, augmentation of myocardial contractility with pharmacologic agents is elected only after cardiac rate and preload reserve mechanisms have been appropriately exploited and any significant afterload elevation satisfactorily controlled. Therefore, the decision to enhance the inotropic state with drugs defines, per se, the existence of significantly impaired cardiac performance. This mandates that immediate preparations be made to carry out sequential measurements of cardiac output if this has not been done previously. Cardiac output data are one of three essential assessment criteria by which the response to and adequacy of therapy is judged, the other two variables being mean left atrial and systemic arterial pressures.

Three sympathomimetic amines have been widely used in patients who require augmentation of myocardial contractility after intracardiac surgery: isoproterenol, epinephrine, and dopamine (see Chapter 22 for pharmacologic details). *Isoproterenol* exerts moderate inotropic and powerful chronotropic effects and also tends to modestly reduce systemic arterial resistance. Although formerly used widely in the management of low cardiac output, it is no longer selected as the drug of choice since the other two agents have equally effective cardiotonic effects but far less tendency to provoke the tachycardias that frequently required that isoproterenol be discontinued. At present the drug is used in those unusual circumstances where the cardiac rate is low and pacing has not been effective, but only after dopamine and epinephrine have been employed unsuccessfully.

When the cardiac rate and mean systemic arterial pressure are both satisfactory, *dopamine* is selected; its positive inotropic effect is similar to epinephrine, while its pressor influence is somewhat less. On occasion, the substantial chronotropic effect of dopamine necessitates its discontinuance (Stephenson et al., 1976).

Epinephrine is employed when impaired myocardial contractility is accompanied by significant systemic arterial hypotension (mean pressure less than 90 mm Hg in previously normotensive adult patients), since, in addition to its positive inotropic effect, it activates peripheral arteriolar alpha receptors (with the usual adequate doses employed at these times), with a consequent rise in the systemic arterial pressure. Although epinephrine also has a distinct chronotopic effect, the frequency of its discontinuance because of marked tachycardia is somewhat less than that of dopamine.

Mechanical Support of Severely Impaired Left Ventricular Performance

When the previously described maintenance and supportive measures have failed to achieve satisfactory hemodynamic stability after cardiac repair, mechanical circulatory support is clearly indicated. Although a variety of ingenious methods of support have been described, discussion will be limited to consideration of currently available left ventricular support methods that currently appear to be clinically useful. For an overview of the history of, various approaches to, and problems accompanying cardiac and cardiopulmonary support, the reader is referred to the National Academy of Sciences—National Research Council publication (1966) and reviews by Sugg et al. (1967), Kolff and Lawson (1975), and Bregman (1976).

Goals. Postrepair mechanical support of the failing left ventricle has two major goals. The first of these is temporary maintenance of satisfactory levels of both systemic blood flow and pressure to sustain adequate performance of all body subsystems until cardiac recovery is sufficient to allow discontinuance of mechanical support. A second goal is reduction of the energy-consuming reactions of the heart to enhance myocardial recovery.

The energy-generating capacity of the myocardium is limited even in the normal heart (Katz, 1975). Therefore, conceptually, mechanical circulatory support must establish conditions where a greater amount of the available chemical energy reserves can be allocated to synthetic and reparative myocardial processes. Since a great deal of energy is used when intramyocardial tension is high, methods that reduce abnormally high outflow resistance (afterload) or inappropriately large left ventricular diastolic volume (preload) can play an effective role in facilitating recovery of the diseased, surgically traumatized, and failing left ventricle.

Intraaortic Balloon Counterpulsation. The concept of reducing afterload while simultaneously augmenting diastolic perfusion pressure with an appropriately timed "arterial counterpulsator" was first proposed by Clauss et al. (1961). The technique required bifemoral cannulation, and blood trauma was substantial. A practical approach to counterpulsation using an intraaortic balloon was introduced by Moulopoulos et al. (1962) and further developed by Kantrowitz et al. (1968), Buckley et al. (1973), and Bregman et al. (1974). Because of its relative simplicity of application, safety, and demonstrated effectiveness, intraaortic balloon counterpulsation (IABC) is the most widely used of all assist methods. Technical details concerning balloon deployment and management are discussed in Chapter 21.

In its proper position the intraaortic balloon lies immediately distal to the left subclavian artery. Balloon inflation and deflation (Fig. 9–12) are properly sequenced with the electrocardiogram so that at the onset of cardiac diastole the balloon suddenly inflates, causing both blood displacement in proportion to the balloon volume (volumes of adult-size balloons vary from approximately 20 to 40 ml) and elevation of the central aortic diastolic pressure. Because of the diastolic pressure augmentation proximal to the balloon, one of the few contraindications to IABC is the presence of aortic regurgitation. Balloon deflation is timed to occur immediately before the onset of ventricular systole, so that the end-diastolic and the succeeding systolic arterial pressures are both reduced. The primary physiologic effect of IABC in humans is reduction of afterload (Fig. 9–13), proportionately reducing external work-related energy-consuming reactions of the heart.

Changes in coronary blood flow in response to IABC have been variable. In patients suffering acute myocardial infarction and requiring IABC, Mueller et al. (1971) observed significant increases in coronary blood flow, while Leinbach et al. (1971) found either no significant change or a reduction in flow in the majority of patients. Myocardial lactate production tends to fall, and cardiac output rises modestly (500 to 900 ml/min) in these patients. Our experience and that of others (Berger et al., 1973; Buckley et al., 1973; Bregman et al., 1974; Parker et al., 1974) indicate that patients with impaired myocardial performance after open cardiac surgery exhibit a favorable hemodynamic re-

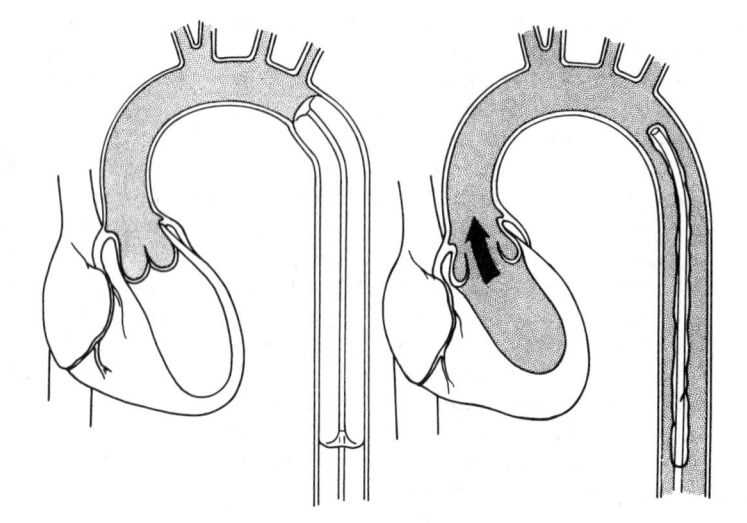

Figure 9–12. Intraaortic balloon performance is sequenced so that balloon suddenly deflates immediately before the onset of mechanical ventricular systole (right) and inflates at the onset of diastole (left).

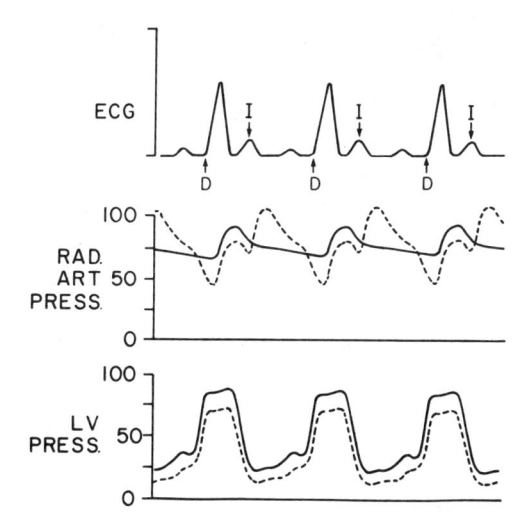

Figure 9-13. Comparison of radial artery and left ventricular dynamics before (solid line) and during (dashed line) intraaortic balloon counterpulsation. Balloon deflation is denoted by D and inflation by I. Systemic arterial and left ventricular systolic pressures are both reduced, while systemic arterial diastolic pressure is sharply augmented during counterpulsation. The favorable effect of the intervention on left ventricular filling pressure is also apparent.

sponse to intraaortic balloon counterpulsation, as reflected in a moderate increment in cardiac output (500 to 800 ml/min) and concomitant reduction of left ventricular filling pressure.

Reports from a number of centers clearly indicate that IABC is effective in permitting separation of approximately 75 percent of patients who are cardiopulmonary bypass-dependent. Analysis of several series indicates that between 40 and 70 percent of patients having IABC will be hospital survivors.

Left Heart Bypass

PHYSIOLOGIC CONSIDERATIONS. Despite the impressive salvage with IABC, a small number of patients cannot be weaned from cardiopulmonary bypass unless increments in systemic blood flow are provided that are substantially greater than that achieved with IABC. This can be accomplished with left heart bypass techniques.

In the past it was commonly believed that total left ventricular (LV) bypass was a virtual sine qua non for functional recovery of the ventricle to take place. The precept was based on experimental physiologic studies indicating that marked reduction in myocardial oxygen consumption ($M\dot{v}_{O_2}$) was achieved only when the LV was completely unloaded (Dennis et al., 1962b; Baird et al., 1963). In these studies, nonpulsatile total LV bypass was shown to reduce $M\dot{v}_{O_2}$ in the nontraumatized beating animal heart to about half the control level. At 50 percent partial LV bypass there was only an approximately 20 percent reduction in $M\dot{v}_{O_2}$.

Because of the response of $M\dot{v}_{O_2}$ to the mechanical support interventions in experimental animals, major efforts have been made to develop cardiac support devices that can totally bypass the LV. However, as Salisbury observed more than two decades ago (National Academy of Sciences—National Research Council publication, 1966), there is serious question about the extent to which experimental data derived from a normal animal heart can be extrapolated to a diseased human heart that has been traumatized by an operation. Moreover, no simple linear relationship exists between $M\dot{v}_{O_2}$ and cardiac work. The $M\dot{v}_{O_2}$ measurement reflects the summated requirements of nine oxygen-dependent factors (Braunwald, 1971). Depending on the state of the myocardium, a number of these factors can have varying oxygen requirements. For example, studies in patients with depressed hearts indicate that wall tension or fiber shortening work may be of less importance than the inotropic state in determining $M\dot{v}_{O_2}$ (Henry et al., 1973).

Therefore, this discussion is intended to question whether $M\dot{v}_{O_2}$ directional changes accompanying bypass of different percentages of left ventricular volumes *in the experimental animal* can be expected to provide insight per se into the subtle but significant changes in cardiac energetics that must exist during the mechanically supported recovery phase of the surgically traumatized human heart. It is entirely possible that a reduction in ventricular volume during partial left ventricular bypass, by lessening wall tension, could conceivably increase the amount of chemical energy made available for intracellular reparative processes. In these circumstances there might be no change or perhaps even an actual increase in measured $M\dot{v}_{O_2}$. Otherwise stated, it is reasonable to postulate that surgically depressed but still viable myocardial cells may use less oxygen than they normally would and that functional recovery of these cells would be reflected by increased oxygen uptake and consumption.

A parallel may be drawn between this situation and that observed in patients during septic shock, where the cellular defect is characterized by reduced oxygen use. It is of interest that Schenk et al. (1964) found that $M\dot{v}_{O_2}$ rose in some animals during partial left heart bypass. More recently, Wakabayashi et al. (1975) extended these observations and noted that $M\dot{v}_{O_2}$ fell sharply in ischemically induced cardiogenic shock but gradually increased under conditions of left heart bypass. As discussed later, left heart recovery has occurred in desperately ill patients undergoing varying degrees of partial left heart bypass, and it is apparent that total left heart bypass is not an absolute requirement. This assertion has practical importance, since the design requirements for total LV bypass systems are substantially more complex than those necessary for partial left heart bypass.

DIRECT LEFT VENTRICULAR DECOMPRESSION AND BYPASS. Appreciation that maximal reduction in $M\dot{v}_{O_2}$ could be accomplished in animals under conditions of total LV unloading has led to a number of approaches to attain this goal, several of which have been employed in preterminal cardiac patients. Bernhard et al. (1968, 1975), Norman et al. (1972, 1976), Peirce et al. (1977), and Berger et al. (1979) have used a pulsatile LV assist device in patients who could not be weaned from conventional bypass. The system (Fig. 9–14) consists of a bladder (ventricle) that is coupled to an inflow valved conduit

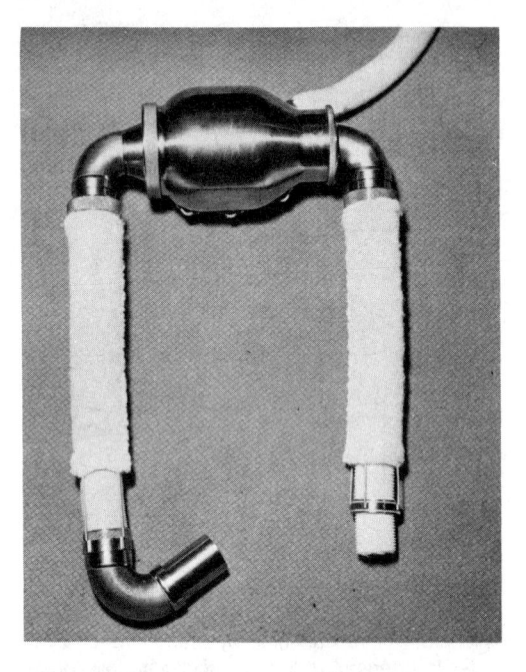

Figure 9–14. Temporary left ventricular assist device. The curved left ventricular nipple and valve-containing conduit (inflow) is attached to the pump housing, which delivers blood to the aorta via another valved outflow conduit. (From Bernhard et al., 1975, with permission of the authors and the C. V. Mosby Co.)

sutured to the apex of the LV and an outflow valved conduit sutured to the aorta. A pneumatic pump drive permits complete LV decompression with delivery of the blood into the aorta under conditions of sequenced counterpulsation.

Zwart et al. (1970) have used a transarterial LV bypass system that is simple and can be instituted and terminated without opening the chest. A thin-walled cannula is inserted into an axillary artery and passed retrograde through the aortic valve into the LV. Blood is sucked from the LV and returned via a femoral artery. This type of transarterial LV bypass system cannot be used when replacement of the aortic valve has been carried out with a prosthesis employing a central occluding poppet.

LEFT ATRIAL-SYSTEMIC ARTERY BYPASS. Clinical use of this means of left heart decompression and augmentation of systemic blood flow was first reported by Dennis et al. (1962a), who used an ingenious closed chest transatrial septal puncture method. Subsequently, Glassman et al. (1975) modified the procedure and used a large-sized flexible outflow catheter positioned in the left atrium with inflow achieved via a cannula positioned in a femoral artery. The system permits bypass flow rates up to 6 liters/min. Perhaps the earliest clinical reports of direct (open chest) left atrial cannulation with systemic arterial return were those of the 1963 experiences of DeBakey et al. (reported in 1966) and Spencer et al. (1965), which clearly showed the potential value of this mode of support.

The author and colleagues have developed a relatively simple *left heart assist device* (LHAD), which can be conveniently deployed in patients unable to be separated from conventional cardiopulmonary bypass (Litwak et al., 1973, 1976). An asset of the system (left atrial-ascending aorta partial bypass of the LV) is that it may be terminated without reentering the thorax to remove the cannulae, thereby eliminating the need for a second major procedure, an added risk to those critically ill patients who require circulatory support. Apart from special cannulae, the only other equipment necessary for the LHAD is a conventional calibrated roller pump.

The concept on which LHAD application is based derives from the common clinical experience that hemodynamic stability frequently can be achieved in "pump-dependent" patients when only a portion (25 to 50 percent) of total systemic blood flow (TSBF) is shunted around the LV. This clinical observation provoked the hypothesis that partial LV bypass, in reducing preload, could establish conditions favoring gradual cardiac recovery, while TSBF was concomitantly maintained at satisfactory levels. Therefore, our goal has not been to totally bypass the left ventricle but rather to regulate the flow rate of the LHAD, so that the combined output of the support system and the depressed LV approximates 2.5 liters/min/m^2 at acceptably low filling pressures ($\leq$20 mm Hg).

As suggested above, an impediment to clinical application of any assist system would be the need to carry out a second major operative procedure to separate the patient from the device. We reasoned that this could be obviated if cannulae could be developed that could be permitted to remain permanently in vivo when the support period had been concluded. Therefore, we elected to fabricate cannulae from two materials of established long-term biocompatibility in humans: silicone elastomeric tubing and polyester fabric (Fig. 9–15). The fabric skirts permit convenient suturing to the left atrium and ascending aorta. The distal ends of both cannulae are positioned subcutaneously in the right upper quadrant of the abdominal wall, where they connnect to an extracorporeal tubing loop and a calibrated roller pump (Fig. 9–16). Left ventricular bypass flow rates up to 5 liters/min are permitted by the system.

A key component that permits subsequent patient separation from the LHAD without thoracic reentrance has been the design of silicone elastomer obturators, each of which precisely fills a cannula lumen. When mated properly, axial and radial orientation of each obturator within its respective cannula allows the lumen to be filled and a smooth proximal surface presented to the blood flowing by. Thus, each obturator eliminates retention of a stagnant column of blood within the cannula and minimizes the danger of thromboembolism and infection. The occluded cannulae are allowed to remain permanently in situ.

The hypothesis that partial LV bypass is often sufficient to allow the diseased and surgically traumatized myocardium time to recover is supported by the observation that approximately two thirds of the patients have gradually recovered enough cardiac function to permit ultimate separation from the LHAD. Support times in these patients have varied from 1.75 to 21 days. Patients requiring three days or less of assistance had a more favorable prognosis than those needing more

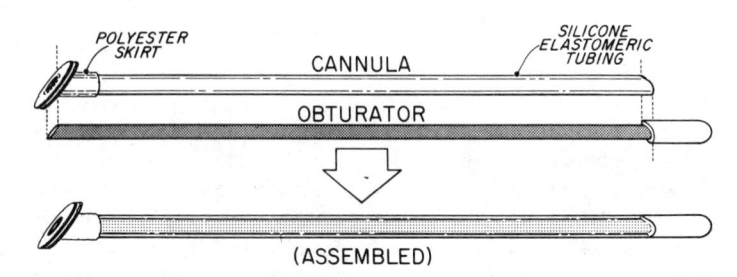

Figure 9–15. Design of left atrial and ascending aortic cannulae and obturators. The cannulae are sutured into place with double skirts, facilitating hemostasis. When circulatory assistance is discontinued, a precisely fitting obturator is slid into each cannula. Matching angularity of the obturator shoulder and distal cannula tip ensures proper mating of the two components, obliterating the entire cannula lumen. The occluded cannulae remain permanently implanted. (From Litwak et al., Postcardiotomy low cardiac output: Clinical experience with a left heart assist device. Circulation 1976, 54 [Suppl III], III–102, with permission of the American Heart Assn., Inc.)

Figure 9–16. The left atrial and aortic cannulae have been sutured into place and the distal tips positioned subcutaneously in the right subcostal area of the abdominal wall, where they connect to a tubing loop and roller pump (left). Separating the patient from the extracorporeal pump is accomplished by exposing the distal cannula tips in their subcutaneous location through a small skin incision (center). The pump connections are separated from the cannulae, the obturators are slid into place and secured, and the skin is closed (right). The insert depicts the concept of obliteration of each cannula lumen by an obturator. (From Litwak et al., Postcardiotomy low cardiac output: Clinical experience with a left heart assist device. Circulation, 54 (Suppl III):III–102, 1976, with permission of the American Heart Assn., Inc.)

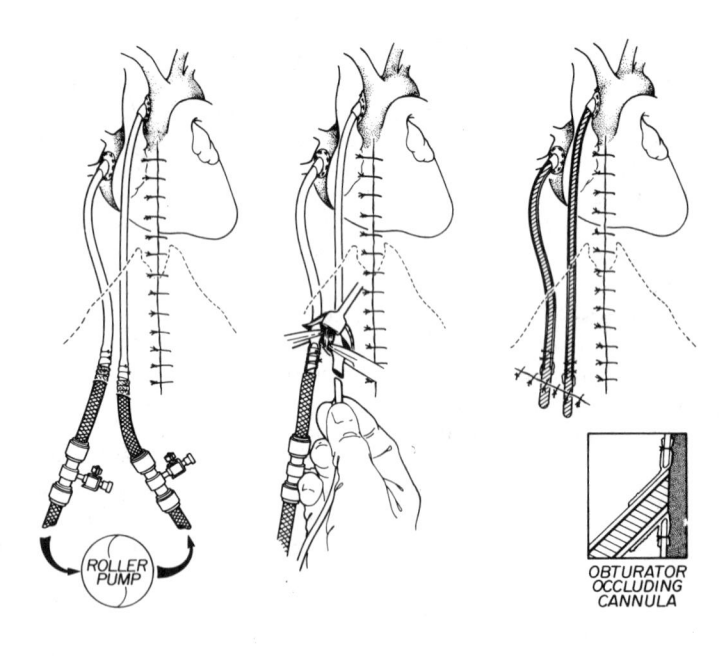

extended periods of support. Approximately one third of the patients have been dismissed from the hospital. Left ventricular support with the LHAD will rarely be required, but its capacity to reduce preload while substantially augmenting systemic blood flow may permit a critically ill patient to survive open intracardiac surgery when all other supportive measures have failed (Figs. 9–17 and 9–18).

A Systematic Plan for Postrepair Cardiac Management

The preceding discussions have emphasized the value of a systematic plan for cardiovascu-

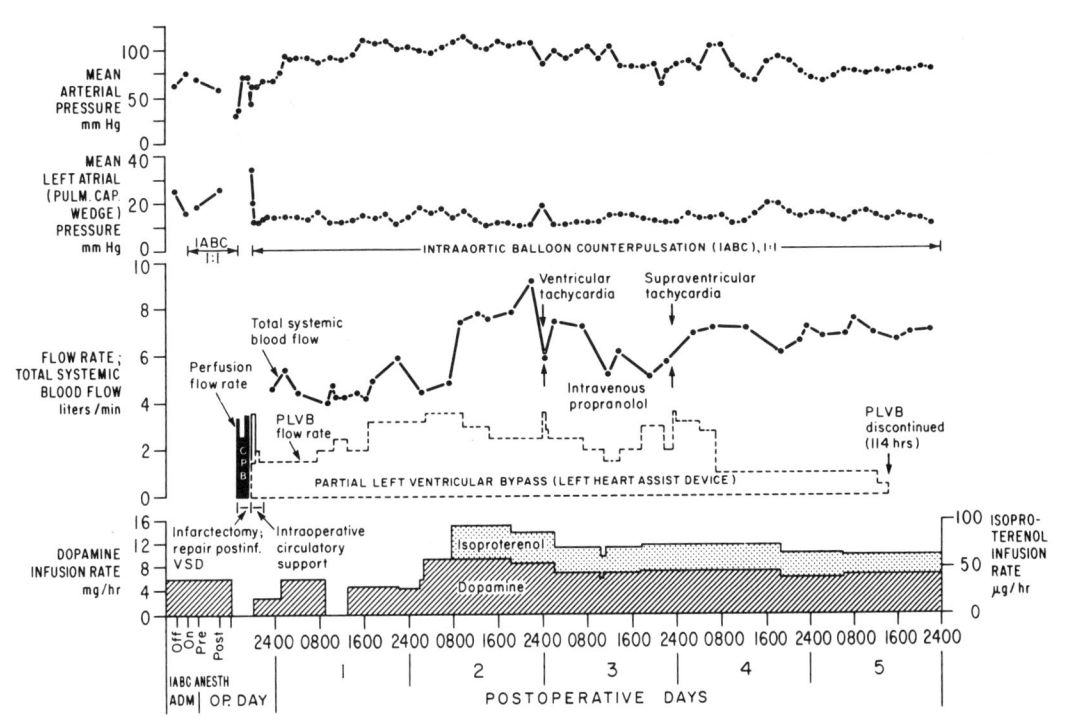

Figure 9–17. Perioperative course of a patient with postinfarction cardiogenic shock refractory to supportive therapy, including intraaortic balloon counterpulsation (IABC). After emergency infarctectomy and ventricular septal defect repair, the patient could not be weaned from cardiopulmonary bypass despite continued IABC, and support with LHAD was initiated. Hemodynamic stability was achieved promptly. Serial measurements showed increasing LV contribution to total systemic blood flow as the LHAD flow rate was slowly reduced. With improved cardiac performance LHAD support was terminated after 114 hours. (Adm=admission; Anesth=anesthesia; Op=operative; PLVB=partial left ventricular bypass; VSD=ventricular septal defect.) (From Litwak et al., 1976, with permission of Little, Brown.)

lar subsystem management during and after the operation (Table 9–2). This is particularly important for patients coming to the operation with advanced cardiac functional impairment, since postrepair persistence of dysfunction can be anticipated in these patients and requires substantial use of subsystem reserves. When serious postrepair depression of cardiac performance occurs in patients who came to surgery with adequate function, the cause must be ascribed to either technical operative problems or an adverse postoperative event (bleeding, cardiac tamponade, myocardial infarction, etc.). Whenever postoperative impaired cardiac performance is anticipated or suspected, proper management *demands* that sequential measurements of systemic blood flow be carried out in addition to the other more commonly used assessment procedures.

Operating Room Analysis and Management. During the weaning period from perfusion, the initial operative evaluation of cardiac performance involves one subjective component (visual judgment of contractility) and objective assessment of the adequacy of cardiac rate, rhythm, and the two readily measured variables affecting left ventricular stroke output: preload (mean left atrial pressure) and afterload (systemic arterial pressure).

A major advance in intraoperative and postoperative management has been the de-

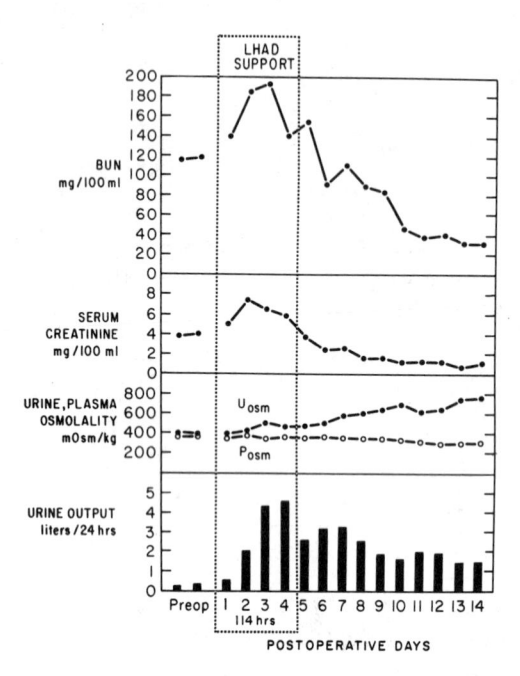

Figure 9–18. Perioperative pattern of renal performance in the same patient as in Fig. 9–17. Evidence of renal tubular dysfunction had been present preoperatively, a consequence of cardiogenic shock. After intracardiac repair with the patient supported by the LHAD, gradual improvement in renal function was observed. (Modified from Litwak et al., 1976, with permission of Little, Brown and Co.)

velopment of small (2.5F) thermodilution thermistor probes, which are passed through the right ventricular wall into the pulmonary artery trunk, allowing convenient measurement of cardiac output after bypass discontinuance. Theoretically, one would desire to use the system in all cases. However, we restrict use of the procedure to those patients in whom impaired cardiac performance is either present or anticipated.

When all variables affecting cardiac rate, rhythm, and stroke output have been optimized during partial bypass, and in the absence of quantitative measurements of blood flow, *significantly impaired cardiac performance* is considered to be present if the preload reserve mechanism has been used fully (mean left atrial pressure 20 mm Hg or higher) and the mean systemic arterial pressure is less than 80 mm Hg. When these adverse circumstances become manifest as perfusion flow rate is being reduced or shortly after discontinuance, partial or total bypass is reestablished and a systematic evaluation made of (1) the integrity and completeness of the operative repair, (2) adequacy of blood-gas tensions, electrolyte levels, and the acid-base state, and (3) the certainty that all cardiac reserve mechanisms have been appropriately exploited. If it has been possible to momentarily discontinue perfusion, baseline cardiac output measurements (see above) are performed.

With persistent evidence of significantly impaired cardiac performance during the supportive period of bypass, positive inotropic or afterload reducing agents are employed as indicated and their response assessed. If these drugs fail to allow discontinuance of perfusion after 30 minutes of support, *severe impairment of cardiac performance* is considered to be present, and an intraaortic balloon is inserted and perfusion slowly terminated, if possible. If IABC fails to achieve satisfactory hemodynamic stability, an additional 45-to 60-minute period of partial to total cardiopulmonary bypass support is employed, after which attempts are again made to wean the patient from perfusion. Failure of these efforts defines the presence of *critical (life-threatening) impairment of cardiac performance*, and a left heart bypass assist device is deployed. Fortunately, in the vast majority of cases postoperative management of impaired cardiac performance rarely demands mechanical support such as the LHAD.

Early Postoperative Analysis and Management. Patients coming to surgery with adequate cardiac function generally will not have routine postoperative measurement of cardiac output soon after the operation unless events in the operating room or shortly thereafter suggest the onset of significant myocardial dysfunction. In the usual favorable circumstances, postoperative adequacy of cardiac performance will be assessed primarily by evaluation of rate, rhythm, and measurement of both LV filling (mean left atrial) and systemic arterial pressures.

TABLE 9-2 A SYSTEMATIC APPROACH TO MAINTAIN AND SUPPORT THE CARDIOVASCULAR SUBSYSTEM IN THE EARLY POSTOPERATIVE PERIOD

Maintenance Measures

1. Institute "preventive" management of anticipated distortions commonly accompanying open intracardiac surgery:
   a. hypovolemia
   b. electrolyte imbalance
   c. mild deterioration of gas exchange.
2. Optimize (manipulation of reserves as necessary):
   a. cardiac rate and rhythm
   b. preload (Frank-Starling)
   c. afterload (pharmacologic reduction of inappropriately high impedance).
3. Eliminate factors conducive to hypermetabolism (shivering, etc.).

Supportive Therapy (Implies presence of significantly impaired cardiac performance. Therapy preceded by systematic review of adequacy of maintenance measures)

1. Early recognition and correction of:
   a. inadequate repair
   b. adverse postoperative event (bleeding, tamponade, etc.).
2. Pharmacologic augmentation of contractility.
3. Therapy for acid-base derangements.
4. Mechanical circulatory support.

While adequacy of cardiac performance cannot be determined with certainty in the absence of quantitative determination of systemic blood flow, the probability of adequacy is high when subjective assessment indicates that the patient is alert, breathing easily, and has warm, pink extremities, and objective data demonstrate a stable cardiac rhythm and physiologic rate in relation to age (obviously higher in infants and children), a mean systemic arterial pressure approximating 100 mm Hg (in previously normotensive patients), a mean left atrial pressure of 14 mm Hg or less, and urine that is hyperosmolar relative to plasma and secreted at a rate of 15 ml/hr/m^2 or more. It is again emphasized that if any evidence suggests the onset of impaired cardiac performance, it is imperative that these data be supplemented by measurements of cardiac output.

Impaired Cardiac Performance. When impaired cardiac performance is suspected or established, institution of appropriate therapy must be based on an analytical scheme that (1) attempts to quantitatively characterize the *extent* of performance impairment, (2) permits evaluation of *performance trends,* and (3) facilitates early detection of the dominant *cause* of the depressed performance.

As discussed previously, quantitative characterization of the magnitude of cardiac performance impairment requires measurement of cardiac output. Since heart rate and two of the three controlling variables of stroke volume are also known (i.e., preload and afterload), logical deductions can be made about the one remaining factor affecting stroke volume that currently cannot be satisfactorily quantitated: the contractile state.

When the presence of postoperative low

cardiac output (cardiac index < 2.2 liters/min/m^2) has been documented, systematic exploration of the following three questions offers a means of isolating the probable cause and allows prompt institution of appropriate management. Is the impaired cardiac performance caused by:

1. An adverse postoperative event (bleeding, tamponade, hypoxia, acid-base or electrolyte disturbance, myocardial infarction)?
2. An incomplete cardiac repair (residual and significant obstruction, regurgitation, shunt, etc.)?
3. Inadequate optimizing of cardiac rate, rhythm, preload, and afterload?

Questions 1 and 2 seek to identify factors associated with technical execution of the repair and sequelae that are potentially correctable. Therapeutic decisions about adverse postoperative events are generally more readily made than those involving question 2. When low cardiac output is believed to be primarily related to an incomplete cardiac repair, the extent of cardiac improvement and the performance trends determine the obviously critical decision for or against prompt reoperation.

If questions 1 and 2 can be eliminated as factors underlying the impaired cardiac performance, the dysfunction logically can be ascribed to suboptimal performance of one or more of the determinants of cardiac output. There must be certainty that proper measures (previously described) have been taken to optimize cardiac rate, rhythm, preload, and afterload. If objective data indicate that each of these factors have been optimized, it may be deduced that the underlying cause of the low cardiac output is impaired contractility, and appropriate supportive measures can be undertaken. Table 9–3, adapted (with slight modification) from Kouchoukos and Karp (1976), outlines a plan for early postoperative management of impaired cardiac performance in adults using only data derived from direct measurements.

MANAGEMENT WHEN CARDIAC INDEX IS UNDER 2.2 LITERS/MIN/M^2. Previous discussion has emphasized the high probability of mortality when the cardiac index is less than 2.2 liters/min/m^2. When rate and rhythm are satisfactory, but cardiac index is below the aforementioned level and the mean left atrial pressure is 14 mm Hg or less, the LV preload reserve mechanism can be exploited. Blood or albumin solution is administered (the latter is given if the hematocrit is 35 or above) regardless of the level of the mean systemic arterial pressure.

At higher LV filling pressures (mean left atrial pressure between 15 and 20 mm Hg), the preload reserve mechanism has already been fully used, and augmentation of contractility is indicated with a positive inotropic drug. If the mean systemic arterial pressure is low (under 90 mm Hg), epinephrine is used because of its dual salutary effect on both contractility and blood pressure. When the mean systemic arterial pressure is satisfactory (above 90 mm Hg), dopamine is administered instead.

When LV filling pressures are above 20 mm Hg and cardiac index is under 2.2 liters/min/m^2, either epinephrine or dopamine are employed, depending on the level of mean arterial pressure, as just discussed. If these agents fail to significantly increase the cardiac index and systemic hypotension persists, IABC should be instituted, although its effectiveness is considerably diminished if the systemic pressure is low. If the mean arterial pressure is above 90 mm Hg and both preload and cardiac index are at levels cited above, it is apparent that systemic arterial resistance will be elevated. Simultaneous use of two drugs is indicated: dopamine for its positive inotropic effect and either nitroprusside or trimethephan to reduce arterial impedance to LV ejection. If the hemodynamic response to these agents is unsatisfactory, IABC should be instituted promptly.

MANAGEMENT WHEN CARDIAC INDEX IS BETWEEN 2.2 AND 3.0 LITERS/MIN/M^2. Levels of systemic blood flow between 2.2 and 3.0 liters/min/m^2 are generally adequate for survival provided that oxygen transport and consumption remain at physiologic levels. However, it is obviously important that the

TABLE 9-3 SCHEMA FOR MAINTENANCE AND SUPPORT OF CARDIAC PERFORMANCE IN ADULTS DURING THE EARLY POSTOPERATIVE HOURS AFTER CARDIAC OPERATION

Cardiac Rate and Rhythm	Mean Left Atrial Pressure (mm Hg)	Mean Systemic Arterial Pressure (mm Hg)	Cardiac Index (liters/min/m^2) Under 2.2	2.2–3.0	3.0–3.5
Optimize with pacing and pharmacologic interventions as indicated (see text)	7 or less	Under 100	Blood or other colloid*	Blood or other colloid*	Blood or other colloid‡
		Over 100	Blood or other colloid* If response unsatisfactory add nitroprusside or trimethephan	Blood or other colloid*	Blood or other colloid‡
	8–14	Under 100	Blood or other colloid*	Blood or other colloid*	Blood or other colloid‡
		Over 100	Blood or other colloid* *plus* nitroprusside or trimethephan	Blood or other colloid* *plus* nitroprusside or trimethephan	—
	15–20	Under 80	Epinephrine	—	—
		Over 80	Dopamine†	—	—
		Under 80	Epinephrine If response unsatisfactory use intraaortic balloon counterpulsation	—	—
	Above 20	Over 80	Dopamine† *plus* nitroprusside or trimethephan If response unsatisfactory use intraaortic balloon counterpulsation	Nitroprusside or trimethephan	Furosemide

*Albumin solution given if hematrocrit is 35 or above.
†Isoproterenol may be used if dopamine has been ineffective and the cardiac rate remains low (i.e., pacing has been ineffective).
‡Blood volume augmented in anticipation of subsequent reduction of systemic arterial resistance and concomitant loss of intravascular volume through renal and other mechanisms.

cardiac index not fall, and for this reason either blood or albumin solution should be administered if the mean left atrial pressure is under 14 mm Hg. If LV preload is sharply elevated (above 20 mm Hg), cardiac index remains between 2.2 and 3.0 liters/min/m^2, and the mean systemic arterial pressure is above 90 mm Hg, arterial impedance reduction with either nitroprusside or trimethephan will generally reduce mean left atrial pressure and increase cardiac output.

MANAGEMENT WHEN CARDIAC INDEX IS OVER 3.0 LITERS/MIN/M^2. Despite these levels of cardiac output, suboptimal (impaired) cardiac performance is considered to exist if LV preload is high (above 20 mm Hg) or if distortions of oxygen transport mechanisms or general body metabolism require even higher levels of systemic blood flow that the heart is incapable of delivering. In the former situation the possibility of colloid or other fluid overload must be considered. Administration of a diuretic such as furosemide usually will reduce the mean left atrial pressure to more acceptable levels without significant reduction of the cardiac index. In the latter circumstances management obviously is directed at identifying and eliminating the factor (or factors) causing the need for the inordinately high levels of blood flow.

REFERENCES

Andersen N B, Ghia J: Pulmonary function, cardiac status and post-operative course in relation to cardiopulmonary bypass. J Thorac Cardiovasc Surg 59:474, 1970.

Appelbaum A, Blackstone E, Kouchoukos N T, Kirklin J W: Afterload reduction and cardiac output in infants early after intracardiac surgery. Am J Cardiol 39:445, 1977.

―――, Kouchoukos N T, Blackstone E, Kirklin J W: Early risks of open heart surgery for mitral valve disease. Am J Cardiol 37:201, 1976.

Archie J P Jr, Kirklin J W: Myocardial blood flow and cardiac surgery. In Kirklin J W (ed): Advances in Cardiovascular Surgery. New York, Grune and Stratton, 1973, p 189.

Åstrand P-O, Cuddy T E, Saltin B, Stenberg J: Cardiac output during submaximal and maximal work. J Appl Physiol 19:268, 1964.

Baird R J, La Brosse C J, Lajos T Z, Thomas G W: Effects of a selective bypass of the left ventricle. Circulation 27:835, 1963.

Baroldi G, Milam J D, Wukasch D C, Sandiford F M, Romagnoli A, Cooley D A: Myocardial cell damage in "stone hearts." J Mol Cell Cardiol 6:395, 1974.

Becker R M, Schizgal H M, Dobell A R C: Distribution of coronary blood flow during cardiopulmonary bypass in pigs: possible implications for left ventricular hemorrhagic necrosis. Ann Thorac Surg 16:228, 1973.

Befeler B, Kamen A R, Macleod C A: Coronary artery disease and left ventricular function in mitral stenosis. Chest 57:435, 1970.

Benzing G III, Helmsworth J A, Schrieber J T, Loggie J, Kaplan S: Nitroprusside after openheart surgery. Circulation 54:467, 1976.

Berger R L, Saini V K, Ryan T J, Sokol D M, Keefe J F: Intra-aortic balloon assist for postcardiotomy cardiogenic shock. J Thorac Cardiovasc Surg 66:906, 1973.

―――, Merin G, Carr J, Sussman H. A. Bernhard W F: Successful use of a left ventricular assist device in cardiogenic shock from massive postoperative myocardial infarction. J Thorac Cardiovasc Surg 78:626, 1979.

Bernhard W F, LaFarge C G, Robinson T, Yun I, Shirahige K: An improved blood-pump interface for left ventricular bypass. Ann Surg 168:750, 1968.

―――, Poirer V, LaFarge C G, Carr J G: A new method for temporary left ventricular bypass: preclinical appraisal. J Thorac Cardiovasc Surg 70:880, 1975.

Braunwald E: Regulation of the circulation. N Engl J Med 290:1124, 1420, 1974.

―――: Control of myocardial oxygen consumption: physiologic and clinical considerations. Am J Cardiol 27:416, 1971.

―――, Frahm C J: Studies on Starling's law of the heart. IV. Observations on the hemodynamic functions of the left atrium in man. Circulation 24:633, 1961.

―――, ―――, Ross J Jr: Studies on Starling's law of the heart. V. Left ventricular function in man. J Clin Invest 40:1882, 1961.

―――, Frye R L, Aygen M M, Gilbert J W Jr: Studies on Starling's law of the heart. III. Observations in patients with mitral stenosis and atrial fibrillation on the relationships between left ventricular end-diastolic segment length, filling, and the characteristics of ventricular contraction. J

Clin Invest 39:1874, 1960.
Bregman D: Mechanical support of the failing circulation. Curr Probl Surg 13(12):1, 1976.
———, Parodi E N, Malm J R: Left ventricular and unidirectional intra-aortic balloon pumping. J Thorac Cardiovasc Surg 68:677, 1974.
Brown A H, Niles N R, Braimbridge M V, Austen W G: Damage to isolated hearts by oxygenators. Ann Thorac Surg 13:575, 1972.
Buckberg G D, Towers B, Paglia D E, Mulder D G, Maloney J V: Subendocardial ischemia after cardiopulmonary bypass. J Thorac Cardiovasc Surg 64:669, 1972.
Buckley M J, Craver J M, Gold H K, Mundth E D, Daggett W M, Austen W G: Intra-aortic balloon pump assist for cardiogenic shock after cardiopulmonary bypass. Circulation 47, 48 (Suppl III):III-90, 1973.
Clauss R H, Birtwell W C, Albertal G, Lunzer S, Taylor W J, Fosberg A F, Harken D E: Assisted circulation. I. Arterial counterpulsator. J Thorac Cardiovasc Surg 41:447, 1961.
Chiu C J: The pathophysiology of intramyocardial pressure and blood flow distribution—a surgical perspective. J Surg Res 17:278, 1974.
Coleman E H, Soloff L A: Incidence of significant coronary artery disease in rheumatic valvular heart disease. Am J Cardiol 25:401, 1970.
Conti V R, Bertranou E G, Blackstone E H, Kirklin J W, Digerness S B: Cold cardioplegia versus hypothermia for myocardial protection: randomized clinical study. J Thorac Cardiovasc Surg 76:577, 1978.
Cooley D A, Reul G J, Wukasch D C: Ischemic contracture of the heart: "stone heart." Am J Cardiol 29:575, 1972.
DeBakey M E, Liotta D, Hall C W: Left heart bypass using an implantable blood pump. In National Academy of Sciences—National Research Council: Mechanical Devices to Assist the Failing Heart. Pub No 1283. Washington, D C, National Academy of Sciences Printing Office, 1966, p 223.
Dennis C, Carlens E, Senning Å, Hall D P, Moreno J R, Cappelletti R R, Wesolowski S A: Clinical use of a cannula for left heart bypass without thoracotomy: experimental protection against fibrillation by left heart bypass. Ann Surg 156:623, 1962a.
———, Hall D P, Moreno J R, and Senning Å: Reduction of the oxygen utilization of the heart by left heart bypass. Circ Res 10:298, 1962b.
Ebert P A, Jude J R, Gaertner R A: Persistent hypokalemia following open heart surgery. Circulation 31(Suppl):137, 1965.
Eckberg D L, Drabinsky M, Braunwald E: Defective cardiac parasympathetic control in patients with heart disease. N Engl J Med 285:877, 1971.
Engelman R M, Adler S, Gouge T H, Chandra R, Boyd A D, Baumann F G: The effect of normothermic arrest and ventricular fibrillation on the coronary blood flow distribution of the pig. J Thorac Cardiovasc Surg 69:858, 1975.
Epstein S E, Beiser G D, Goldstein R E, Rosing D R, Redwood D R, Morrow A G: Hemodynamic abnormalities in response to mild and intense upright exercise following operative correction of an atrial septal defect or tetralogy of fallot. Circulation 47:1065, 1973.
Estafanous F G, Tarazi R C, Viljoen J F, El Tawil M Y: Systemic hypertension following myocardial revascularization. Am Heart J 85:732, 1973.
Fields J, Berkovits B V, Matloff J M: Surgical experience with temporary and permanent A-V sequential demand pacing. J Thorac Cardiovasc Surg 66:865, 1973.
Folkow B, Heymans C, Neil E: Integrated aspects of cardiovascular regulation. In Hamilton W F, Dow P (eds): Handbook of Physiology, Section 2. Circulation, Vol III. Washington, DC, American Physiological Society, 1965, pp 1787—1823.
Frank O: Zur dynamik des herzmuskels. Z. Biol 32:370, 1895. Chapman C B, Wasserman E (trans). Am Heart J 58:282, 467, 1959.
Friesen W G, Woodson R D, Ames A W, Herr R H, Starr A, Kassebaum D G: A hemodynamic comparison of atrial and ventricular pacing in postoperative cardiac patients. J Thorac Cardiovasc Surg 55:271, 1968.
Frye R L, Braunwald E: Studies on Starling's law of the heart. I. The circulatory response to acute hypervolemia and its modification by ganglionic blockade. J Clin Invest 39:1043, 1960.
Gadboys H L, Litwak R S: The postperfusion hematocrit. J Thorac Cardiovasc Surg 46:772, 1963.
Gault J H, Covell J W, Braunwald E, Ross J Jr: Left ventricular performance following correction of free aortic regurgitation. Circulation 42:773, 1970.
———, Ross J Jr, Braunwald E: Contractile state of the left ventricle in man: instantaneous tension-velocity-length relations in patients with and without disease of the left ventricular myocardium. Circ Res 22:451, 1968.
Gilmore J P, Sarnoff S J, Mitchell J H, Linden R J: Synchronicity of ventricular contraction: observations comparing hemodynamic effects of atrial

and ventricular pacing. Br Heart J 25:299, 1963.

Glassman E, Engleman R M, Boyd A D, Lipson D, Ackerman B, Spencer F C: A method of closed chest cannulation of the left atrium for left atrial-femoral artery bypass. J Thorac Cardiovasc Surg 69:283, 1975.

Glick G, Sonnenblick E H, Braunwald E: Myocardial force-velocity relations studied in intact, unanesthetized man. J Clin Invest 44:978, 1965.

Goldfarb D, Bahnson H T: Early and late effects on the heart of small amounts of air in the coronary circulation. J Thorac Cardiovasc Surg 46:368, 1963.

Gott V L, Dutton R C, Young W P: Myocardial rigor mortis as an indication of cardiac metabolic function. Surg Forum 13:172, 1962.

Graham T P Jr: Myocardial performance after anatomic or physiologic corrective surgery. Prog Cardiovasc Dis 17:439, 1975.

——, Jarmakani J M, Atwood G F, Canent R V Jr: Right ventricular volume determinations in children: normal values and observations with volume or pressure overload. Circulation 47: 144, 1973.

Gralnick H, Fischer D: The hemostatic response to open-heart operation. J Thorac Cardiovasc Surg 61:909, 1971.

Hammermeister K E, Kennedy J W: Predictors of surgical mortality in patients undergoing myocardial revascularization. Circulation 49, 50 (Suppl): II–49, 1972.

Harris P D, Malm J R, Bowman F O Jr, Hoffman B F, Kaiser G A, Singer D H: Epicardial pacing to control arrhythmias following cardiac surgery. Circulation 37 (Suppl II):II-178, 1968.

Hartzler G O, Maloney J D, Curtis J J, Barnhorst D A: Hemodynamic benefits of atrioventricular sequential pacing after cardiac surgery. Am J Cardiol 40:232, 1977.

Hedley-Whyte J, Corning H, Laver M B, Austen W G, Bendixen H H: Pulmonary ventilation perfusion relations after valve replacement or repair in man. J Clin Invest 44:406, 1965.

Henry P D, Eckberg D, Gault J H, Ross J Jr: Depressed inotropic state and reduced myocardial oxygen consumption in the human heart. Am J Cardiol 31:300, 1973.

Hildner F J, Javier R P, Cohen L S, Samet P, Nathan M J, Yahr W Z, Greenberg J J: Myocardial dysfunction associated with valvular heart disease. Am J Cardiol 30:319, 1972.

Isom O W, Kutin N D, Falk E A, Spencer F C: Patterns of myocardial metabolism during cardiopulmonary bypass and coronary perfusion. J Thorac Cardiovasc Surg 66:705, 1973.

Jarmakani J M, Graham T P Jr, Canent R V Jr: Left ventricular contractile state in children with successfully corrected ventricular septal defect. Circulation 45, 46 (Suppl I):I–102, 1972a.

——, ——, ——, Jewett P H: Left heart function in children with Tetralogy of Fallot before and after palliative or corrective surgery. Circulation 46:478, 1972b.

Jurado R A, Matucha D, Osborn J J: Cardiac output estimation by pulse contour methods: validity of their use for monitoring the critically ill patient. Surgery 74:358, 1973.

Kantrowitz A, Tjønneland S, Krakauer J S, Phillips S J, Freed P J, Butner A N: Mechanical intraaortic cardiac assistance in cardiogenic shock. Arch Surg 97:1000, 1968.

Karliner J S, Gault J H, Eckberg D, Mullins C B, Ross J Jr: Mean velocity of fiber shortening: a simplified measure of left ventricular contractility. Circulation 44:323, 1971.

Katz A M: Congestive heart failure: role of altered myocardial cellular control. N Engl J Med 293:1184, 1975.

——, Tada M: The "stone heart": a challenge to the biochemist. Am J Cardiol 29:578, 1972.

Kirklin J W: Systems Analysis in Surgical Patients, with Particular Attention to the Cardiac and Pulmonary Subsystems (Macewen Memorial Lecture). Glasgow, University of Glasgow Press, 1970.

——: Postoperative intensive care after intracardiac operation with emphasis on respiratory care in infants. In Barret-Boyes B G, Neutze J M, Harris E A (eds): Heart Disease in Infancy: Diagnosis and Surgical Treatment. Edinburgh, Churchill-Livingston, 1973, p 307.

——, Karp R B: The Tetralogy of Fallot from a Surgical Viewpoint. Philadelphia, Saunders, 1970, p 119.

——, ——, Bargeron L M Jr: Surgical treatment of ventricular septal defect. In Sabiston D C Jr, Spencer F C (eds): Gibbon's Surgery of the Chest, 3rd ed. Philadelphia, Saunders, 1976, p 1032.

——, Rastelli G C: Low cardiac output after intracardiac operations. Prog Cardiovasc Dis 10:117, 1967.

Klein M S, Coleman R E, Weldon C S, Sobel B E, Roberts R: Concordance of electrocardiographic and scintigraphic criteria of myocardial injury after cardiac surgery. J Thorac Cardiovasc Surg 71:934, 1976.

Kolff W J, Lawson J: Status of the artificial heart and cardiac assist devices in the United States. Trans Am Soc Artif Intern Organs 21:620, 1975.

Kouchoukos N T, Karp R B: Functional disturbances following extracorporeal circulatory support in cardiac surgery. In Ionescu M I, Wooler G H (eds): Current Techniques in Extracorporeal Circulation. London, Butterworths, 1976, p 245.

———, Kirklin J W, Oberman A: An appraisal of coronary bypass grafting. Circulation 50:11, 1974.

———, ———, Sheppard L C, Roe P A: Effect of left atrial pressure by blood infusion on stroke volume early after cardiac operations. Surg. Forum 22:126, 1971.

———, Sheppard L C, Kirklin J W: Effect of alterations in arterial pressure on cardiac performance early after open intracardiac operations. J Thorac Cardiovasc Surg 64:563, 1972.

———, ———, McDonald D A, Kirklin J W: Estimation of stroke volume from central arterial pressure contour in postoperative patients. Surg Forum 20:180, 1969.

Kramer R S, Mason D T, Braunwald E: Augmented sympathetic neurotransmitter activity in the peripheral vascular bed of patients with congestive heart failure and cardiac norepinephrine depletion. Circulation 38:629, 1968.

Leinbach R C, Buckley M J, Austen W G, Petschek H E, Kantrowitz A R, Sanders C A: Effects of intra-aortic balloon pumping on coronary flow and metabolism in man. Circulation 43, 44 (Suppl I): I–77, 1971.

Linhart J W, de la Torre A, Ramsey H W, Wheat M W Jr: The significance of coronary artery disease in aortic valve replacement. J Thorac Cardiovasc Surg 55:811, 1968.

———, Wheat M W Jr: Myocardial dysfunction following aortic valve replacement: the significance of coronary artery disease. J Thorac Cardiovasc Surg 54:259, 1967.

Litwak R S, Gilson A J, Slonim R, McCune C C, Kiem I, Gadboys H L: Alterations in blood volume during "normovolemic" total body perfusion. J Thorac Cardiovasc Surg 42:477, 1961.

———, Koffsky R M, Jurado R A, Lukban S B, Ortiz A F Jr, Fischer A P, Sherman J J, Silvay G Lajam F: Use of a left heart assist device after intracardiac surgery. Ann Thorac Surg 21:191, 1976.

———, Kuhn L A, Gadboys H L, Lukban S B, Sakurai H: Support of myocardial performance after open cardiac operations by rate augmentation. J Thorac Cardiovasc Surg 56:484, 1968.

———, Lajam F, Koffsky R M, Silvay G, Shiang H, Geller S A, Pedersen F S: Obturated permanent left atrial and aortic cannulae for assisted circulation after cardiac surgery. Trans Am Soc Artif Intern Organs 19:243, 1973.

———, Silvay J, Gadboys H L, Lukban S B, Sakurai H, Castro-Blanco J: Factors associated with operative risk in mitral valve replacement. Am J Cardiol 23:335, 1969.

Loop F D, Berrettoni J N, Pichard A, Siegel W, Razavi M, Effler D B: Selection of the candidate for myocardial revascularization: a profile of high risk based on multivariate analysis. J Thorac Cardiovasc Surg 69:40 1975.

March H W, Ross J K, Weirich W L, Gerbode F: The influence of ventriculotomy site on the contraction and function of the right ventricle. Circulation 24:572, 1961.

Maron B J, Ferrans V J, Roberts W C: Myocardial ultrastructure in patients with chronic aortic valve disease. Am J Cardiol 35:725, 1975.

McQueen M J, Watson M E, Bain W H: Transient systolic hypertension after aortic valve replacement. Brit Heart J 34:227, 1972.

Monroe R G, Gamble W J, LaFarge C G, Kumar A E, Manasek F J: Left ventricular performance at high end-diastolic pressures in isolated, perfused dog hearts. Circ Res 26:85, 1970.

Moulopoulos S D, Topaz S, Kolff W J: Diastolic balloon pumping (with carbon dioxide) in the aorta: a mechanical assistance to the failing circulation. Am Heart J 63:669, 1962.

Mueller H, Ayres S M, Conklin E F, Gianelli S Jr, Mazzara J T, Grace W T, Nealon T F Jr: The effects of intra-aortic counterpulsation on cardiac performance and metabolism in shock associated with acute myocardial infarction. J Clin Invest 50:1885, 1971.

Najafi H, Henson D, Dye W S, Javid H, Hunter J A, Callaghan R, Eisenstein R, Julian O C: Left ventricular hemorrhagic necrosis. Ann Thorac Surg 7:550, 1969.

Norman J C: An intracorporeal (abdominal) left ventricular assist device (ALVAD): clinical readiness and initial trials in man. Bull Texas Heart Inst 3:249, 1976.

———, Whalen R L, Daly B D T, Migliore J, Huffman F N: An implantable abdominal left ventricular assist device (LVAD). Clin Res 20:

855, 1972.

Oldham H N, Roe C R, Young W G, Dixon S H: Intraoperative detection of myocardial damage during coronary artery surgery by plasma creatine phosphokinase isoenzyme analysis. Surgery 74:917, 1973.

Osborne J J, Popper R W, Kerth W J, Gerbode F: Respiratory insufficiency following open heart surgery. Ann Surg 156:638, 1962.

Parker F B Jr, Neville J F, Hanson E L, Webb W R: Intra-aortic balloon counterpulsation and cardiac surgery. Ann Thorac Surg 17:144, 1974.

Parr G V S, Blackstone E H, Kirklin J W: Cardiac performance and mortality early after intracardiac surgery in infants and young children. Circulation 51:867, 1975.

Peterson K L, Uther J B, Shabetai R, Braunwald E: Assessment of left ventricular performance in man: instantaneous tension-velocity-length relations obtained with the aid of an electromagnetic velocity catheter in the ascending aorta. Circulation 47:924, 1973.

Pierce W S, Donachy J H, Landis D L, Brighton J A, Rosenberg G, Migliore J J, Prophet G A, White W S, Waldhausen J A: Prolonged mechanical support of the left ventricle. Circulation 58 (Suppl I):I-133, 1977.

Rastelli G C, Kirklin J W: Hemodynamic state early after replacement of aortic valve with ball valve prosthesis. Surgery 61:873, 1967.

———, ———: Hemodynamic state early after prosthetic replacement of mitral valve. Circulation 34:448, 1966.

———, Tsakiris A G, Frye R L, Kirklin J W: Exercise tolerance and hemodynamic studies after replacement of canine mitral valve with and without preservation of chordae tendineae. Circulation 35 (Suppl):I-34, 1967.

Reid D J, Digerness S B, Kirklin J W: Changes in whole body venous tone and distribution of blood after open intracardiac surgery. Am J Cardiol 22:621, 1968.

Rose M R, Glassman E, Spencer F C: Arrhythmias following cardiac surgery: relation to serum digoxin levels. Am Heart J 89:288, 1975.

Ross J Jr, Braunwald E: The study of left ventricular function in man by increasing resistance to ventricular ejection with angiotensin. Circulation 29:739, 1964.

———, Covell J W, Sonnenblick E H, Braunwald E: Contractile state of the heart characterized by force-velocity relations in variably afterloaded and isovolumic beats. Circ Res 18:149, 1966.

———, Morrow A G, Mason D T, Braunwald E: Left ventricular function following replacement of the aortic valve: hemodynamic responses to muscular exercise. Circulation 33:507, 1966.

———, Sonnenblick E H, Taylor R R, Spotnitz H M, Covell J W: Diastolic geometry and sarcomere lengths in the chronically dilated canine left ventricle. Circ Res 28:49, 1971.

Samet P, Castillo C, Bernstein W H: Hemodynamic consequences of sequential atrioventricular pacing. Am J Cardiol 21:207, 1968.

Sapsford R N, Blackstone E H, Kirklin J W, Karp R B, Kouchoukos N T, Pacifico A D, Roe C R, Bradley E L: Coronary perfusion versus cold ischemic arrest during aortic valve surgery: a randomized study. Circulation 49:1190, 1974.

Sarnoff S J: Myocardial contractility as described by ventricular function curves: observations on Starling's law of the heart. Physiol Rev 35:107, 1955.

———, Brockman S K, Gilmore J P, Linden R J, Mitchell J H: Regulation of ventricular contraction: influence of cardiac sympathetic and vagal nerve stimulation on atrial and ventricular dynamics. Circ Res 8:1108, 1960a.

———, Gilmore P J, Brockman S K, Mitchell J H, Linden R J: Regulation of ventricular contraction by the carotid sinus: its effect on atrial and ventricular dynamics. Circ Res 8:1123, 1960b.

———, Mitchell J H: The control of the function of the heart. In Hamilton W F, Dow P (eds): Handbook of Physiology, Section 2. Circulation Vol I. Washington, DC, American Physiological Society, 1962, pp 489–532.

Schenk W G Jr, Delin N A, Camp F A, McDonald K E, Pollack L, Gage A, Chardack W M: Assisted circulation: an experimental evaluation of counterpulsation and left ventricular bypass. Arch Surg 88:327, 1964.

Smith R, Grossman W, Johnson L, Segal H, Collins J, Dalen J: Arrhythmias following cardiac valve replacement. Circulation 45:1018, 1972.

Sonnenblick E H: Myocardial ultrastructure in the normal and failing heart. In The Myocardium: Failure and Infarction. New York, H. P. Pub. Co., 1974, pp 3–13.

———: Correlation of myocardial ultrastructure and function. Circulation 38:29, 1968.

———: The mechanics of myocardial contraction. In Briller S A, Conn H L (eds): The Myocardial Cell: Structure, Function and Modification by Cardiac Drugs. Philadelphia, University of Pennsylvania Press, 1966, pp 173–250.

———: Force-velocity relations in mammalian heart muscle. Am J Physiol 202:931, 1962.

———, Spiro D, Cottrell T S: Fine structural changes in heart muscle in relation to length-tension curve. Proc Natl Acad Sci USA 49:193, 1963.

———, ———, Spotnitz H M: Ultrastructural basis of Starling's law of heart: role of sarcomere in determining ventricular size and stroke volume. Am Heart J 68:336, 1964.

Spencer F C, Eiseman B, Trinkle J K, Rossi N P: Assisted circulation for cardiac failure following intracardiac surgery with cardiopulmonary bypass. J Thorac Cardiovasc Surg 49:56, 1965.

———, Green G E, Tice D A, Wallsh E, Mills N L, Glassman E: Coronary artery bypass grafts for congestive heart failure. J Thorac Cardiovasc Surg 62:529, 1971.

Stephenson L W, Blackstone E H, Kouchoukos N T: Dopamine vs. epinephrine in patients following cardiac surgery: randomized study. Surg Forum 27:272, 1976.

Stirling G R, Stanley P H, Lillehei C W: The effect of cardiac bypass and ventriculotomy upon right ventricular function. Surg Forum 8:433, 1957.

Sugg W L, Webb W R, Cook W A: Collective review. Assisted circulation. Ann Thorac Surg 3:247, 1967.

Sunderland C O, Matarazzo R G, Lees M H, Menashe V D, Boncheck L I, Rosenberg J A, Starr A: Total correction of tetralogy of fallot in infancy: postoperative hemodynamic evaluation. Circulation 48:398, 1973.

Taber R E, Morales A R, Fine G: Myocardial necrosis and the postoperative low cardiac output syndrome. Ann Thorac Surg 4:12, 1967.

Vogel J H K, Chidsey C A: Cardiac adrenergic activity in experimental heart failure assessed with beta receptor blockade. Am J Cardiol 24:198, 1969.

Wakabayashi A, Kubo T, Gilman P, Zuber W F, Connolly J E: Oxygen consumption of the normal and failing heart during left heart bypass. J Thorac Cardiovasc Surg 70:9, 1975.

Wisheart J D, Kirklin J W: The long-term effects of aortic valve replacement on myocardial function. In Kirklin J W (ed): Advances in Cardiovascular Surgery. New York, Grune & Stratton, 1973, p 217.

———, Wright J E C, Rosenfeldt F L, Ross J K: Atrial and ventricular pacing after open heart surgery. Thorax 28:9, 1973.

Wukasch D C, Reul G J, Milam J D, Hallman G L, Cooley D A: The "stone heart" syndrome. Surgery 72:1071, 1973.

Zwart H H J, Kralios A, Kwan-Gett C S, Backman D K, Foote J L, Andrade J D, Calton F M, Schoonmaker F, Kolff W J: First clinical application of trans-arterial closed-chest left ventricular (TaCLV) bypass. Trans Am Soc Artif Intern Organs 16:386, 1970.

RECOMMENDED READING

Braunwald E, Ross J, Sonnenblick E H: Mechanisms of Contraction of the Normal and Failing Heart. Boston, Little, Brown, 1968.

Guyton A C, Jones C E, Coleman T C: Circulatory Physiology: Cardiac Output and Its Regulation. Philadelphia, Saunders, 1973.

National Academy of Sciences—National Research Council. Mechanical Devices to Assist the Failing Heart. Pub No 1283. Washington, D C, National Academy of Sciences Printing Office, 1966.

Rushmer R F: Cardiovascular Dynamics 4th ed. Philadelphia, Saunders, 1976.

Symposium on the regulation of the performance of the heart. Physiol Rev 35:91–168, 1955.

10. Electrophysiologic Considerations For the Cardiac Surgical Patient*

ALBERT L. WALDO   GERARD A. KAISER

Knowledge of the anatomy and electrophysiology of the specialized conduction system of the heart, and ability to diagnose, treat, and prevent cardiac arrhythmias is central to proper care of the cardiac surgical patient. This chapter will focus on these subjects from the point of view of the cardiac surgeon, and, in particular, will emphasize the use of electrophysiologic techniques that are largely unique to open heart surgical patients for the diagnosis, treatment, and prevention of arrhythmias.

THE ANATOMY OF SPECIALIZED CONDUCTION SYSTEM OF THE HEART

The Sinus Node
The sinus node (Hudson, 1960; James, 1961a; Merideth and Titus, 1968) is an ellipsoid-shaped structure and on the average is 1.5 cm long, 5 mm wide at its widest portion, 1.5 mm thick, and lies only 1 to 2 mm below the epicardium at the junction of the superior vena cava and right atrium (Fig. 10–1). The location of the sinus node is identified by two useful landmarks: (1) the lateral junction of the superior vena cava and atrium, for the node is situated just posterior to the crest formed by the edge of the atrial appendage at its junction with the superior vena cava; (2) the sinus node artery, which is a constant vessel supplying the sinus node and encircling the ostium of the superior vena cava.

The Internodal Pathways
Three specialized atrial internodal pathways (James, 1963; Merideth and Titus, 1968) leave the sinus node and course via different routes to the A-V node (see Fig. 10–1). The anterior internodal pathway leaves the sinus node at its anterior margin and courses leftward, anterior to the superior vena cava. At the anterior and superior margins of the atrial septum, the anterior internodal pathway turns inferiorly and posteriorly into the atrial septum, but also gives off a branch that continues in Bachmann's bundle. The anterior internodal pathway continues inferiorly through the atrial septum anterior to the fossa ovalis connecting with the superior and anterior aspects of the A-V node.

---

*Supported in part by USPHS NHLBI Program Project Grant HL11,310 and SCOR on Ischemic Heart Disease Grant 1P17HL17667 and by a grant-in-aid from the American Heart Association. Work performed during Dr. Waldo's tenure as the Otto G. Storm Established Investigator for the American Heart Association.

ostium (some fibers may also travel inferior to the coronary sinus ostium) and then anterior to the coronary sinus ostium to enter the posterior and inferior aspects of the A-V node.

Although there is still much to understand about these pathways, enough information is available to suggest some of their roles. First, although these pathways are not isolated along their course and do not consist entirely of Purkinje-like cells, they are pathways of rapid conduction. Second, the anterior internodal pathway seems to be the major pathway for conduction of the impulse from the sinus to the A-V node. Third, the branch of the anterior internodal pathway into Bachmann's bundle is the main pathway of conduction of the impulse from the sinus node to the left atrium. Fourth, these pathways may very likely be involved in the genesis of atrial arrhythmias, both automatic ectopic rhythms and reentrant rhythms. The consequences of traumatic interruption of these pathways during open heart surgery are discussed subsequently.

The A-V Node and His Bundle

Knowledge of the anatomy of the A-V node and His bundle (Kistin, 1949; James, 1961b; Truex and Smyth, 1965; Merideth and Titus, 1968; Massing et al., 1972; Massing and James, 1976) is essential for the cardiac surgeon, as so much cardiac surgery is concerned with pathology in and around the A-V junction. The atrioventricular (A-V) node is an oblong structure and averages about 6 mm in length, 3 mm in width, and 1 mm in thickness. It lies low in the interatrial septum just above the septal insertion of the tricuspid valve, just anterior to the ostium of the coronary sinus, just beneath the right atrial endocardium, and abutting the mitral annulus (see Fig. 10–1).

The anterior portion of the A-V node penetrates the central fibrous body and becomes the His bundle. The His bundle descends to the crest of the interventricular septum in the posterior margin of the membraneous septum (see Fig. 10–1). The length of the His bundle varies considerably but

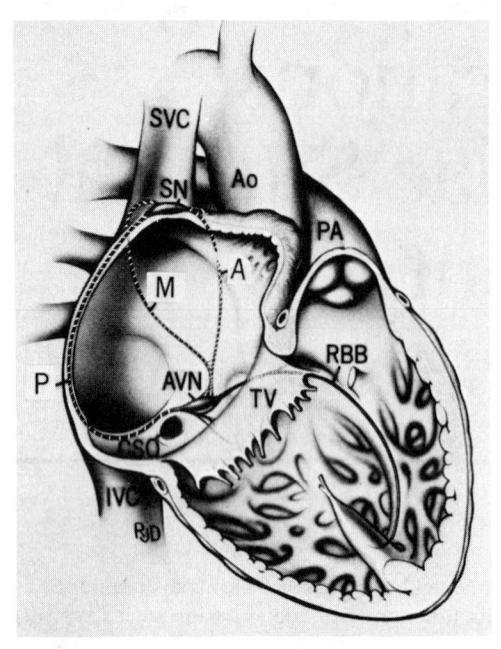

Figure 10–1. Drawing of the human heart illustrating the specialized conduction tissue. SN = sinus node; A = anterior internodal pathway; M = middle internodal pathway; P = posterior internodal pathway; AVN = atrioventriuclar node; HB = His bundle; RBB = right bundle branch; SVC = superior vena cava; IVC = inferior vena cava; AO = aorta; PA = pulmonary artery; CSO = coronary sinus oriface; TV = tricuspid valve. It should be emphasized that the pathways between the sinus and A-V nodes (the internodal pathways) are not discrete, isolated pathways, which is why they appear cross-hatched.

The middle internodal pathway leaves the superior and posterior margin of the sinus node and passes to the right of and posterior to the superior vena cava (see Fig. 10–1). It then enters the atrial septum initially superior and then anterior to the fossa ovalis, where it joins with the anterior internodal pathway to enter the A-V node together with it.

The posterior internodal pathway leaves the posterior and inferior margins of the sinus node and courses first via the crista terminalis and then through the eustachian ridge to the region of the coronary sinus ostium (see Fig. 10–1). There its fibers travel through the superior lip of the coronary sinus probably ranges from 7 to 15 mm, with an average of 11.3 mm. Its width also varies from 0.7 to 3.5 mm, with an average of 1.8 mm.

The Bundle Branches

The right and left bundle branches (Kistin, 1949; Hudson, 1965; Davies, 1971; Massing et al., 1972; Massing and James, 1976) are, of course, a continuation of the His bundle. The right bundle branch originates from the His bundle shortly after it reaches the muscular crest of the interventricular septum. It travels in a generally anterior and apical direction to the base of the papillary muscle. The proximal and distal portions of the right bundle branch usually lie just subendocardially. The midportion of the right bundle branch usually lies somewhat deeper in the interventricular septum. The length of the right bundle has been reported to range from 23 to 50 mm, with an average of 39 mm. Its width ranges from 0.3 to 2.7 mm, with an average of 1 mm.

The anatomy of the left bundle branch varies considerably from person to person. It leaves the left margin of the His bundle from much of the latter's course as a sheet of fibers and fans out over the endocardial surface of the left side of the interventricular septum. The left bundle also may originate as a very narrow stem (maximum 1.5 mm in cross-section) crossing from right to left through the inferior margin of the membranous septum (Massing and James, 1976). Although there are two relatively direct pathways to the anterior and posterior papillary muscle, the left bundle also spreads so diffusely to other portions of the left ventricle that it cannot be distinctly separated into an anterior and posterior fascicle.

Some Useful Reminders

Because so many of the techniques of various open heart surgical procedures involve potential damage to the specialized conduction system, several points bear emphasis:

1. Placing and securing the superior vena caval cannula involves potential damage to the sinus node.

2. The integrity of the posterior internodal pathway will be compromised by an atriotomy through the crista terminalis or the coronary sinus ostium.

3. The integrity of one or all of the internodal pathways may be compromised by an atrial septostomy or septectomy or by suture placement in the atrium (e.g., during the Mustard procedure).

4. The proximity of the A-V node to the coronary sinus ostium is an especially important consideration in surgery involving the coronary sinus (e.g., the Mustard procedure, repair of some types of anomalous pulmonary venous drainage).

5. The proximity of the left surface of the A-V node to the mitral annulus serves as a reminder of the hazard of trauma to the A-V node during mitral valve surgery.

6. The proximity of the noncoronary cusp of the aortic valve to the membranous interventricular septum serves as a reminder of the hazard of potential trauma to the His bundle and the left bundle branch during aortic valve surgery.

7. The relationship of the His bundle and proximal bundle branches to the membranous interventricular septum is especially important in surgery for repair of ventricular septal and endocardial cushion defects.

THE NATURE OF CARDIAC ARRHYTHMIAS

Cranefield et al., 1973, described arrhythmias as being "caused by an abnormality in the rate, regularity, or site of origin of the cardiac impulse or by certain disturbances in the conduction of the impulse such that the normal sequence of activation of the atria and ventricles is disturbed. Arrhythmias thus may be said to result from abnormalities of impulse initiation, impulse conduction or both." A detailed consideration of the genesis of cardiac arrhythmias will be found in the reviews of Hoffman and Cranefield (1964), Cranefield et al., (1973); Wit et al. (1974a;

1974b; 1974c); Hoffman et al. (1975), Cranefield (1977) and Hoffman and Rosen (1981).

Abnormalities of Automaticity

Cells that are capable of initiating impulses through the process of spontaneous self-excitation are said to be automatic, and this property of spontaneous self-excitation has been called automaticity. Automaticity is thought to be limited to the specialized conduction system of the heart. Therefore, while the sinus node is the normal pacemaker of the heart, potential pacemaker sites are located in the atrial internodal pathways, the distal A-V node (N-H region), and the His-Purkinje system. Anything that depresses the intrinsic rate of automaticity of the sinus node or enhances the intrinsic rate of automaticity of any of these sites can result in an arrhythmia. The most common ectopic automatic arrhythmia associated with open heart surgery is an A-V junctional rhythm, most often appearing transiently after repair of congenital heart defects.

Abnormalities of Impulse Conduction

Impulse conduction abnormalities are of two general types: (1) failure of propagation, and (2) slowed conduction with unidirectional block. Failure of propagation, usually readily appreciated in an ECG, results in arrhythmias associated with the various forms of block, complete heart block being one example. Slowed conduction with unidirectional block is the basis for reentrant rhythms, and its presence permits circus or reentrant excitation to occur and in many instances to become sustained. Therefore, the cardiac excitation that results during reentrant rhythms is not pacemaker-induced. Acknowledged or probable reentrant rhythms include coupled ventricular extrasystoles, paroxysmal atrial tachycardia, atrial flutter, and most forms of ventricular tachycardia.

Combined Abnormalities

Some arrhythmias are a combination of abnormalities of automaticity and conduction. An example of this combination is A-V dissociation, in which an enhanced A-V junctional automatic focus serves as the pacemaker of the ventricles in the presence of functional A-V block and usually (though not necessarily) somewhat depressed automaticity of the sinus node.

The importance of understanding the difference between automatic and reentrant rhythms becomes especially apparent in the treatment of tachycardias. As discussed subsequently in this chapter, reentrant tachyarrhythmias can be converted to normal sinus rhythm by interrupting the reentrant or circus movement with overdrive pacing or DC cardioversion. However, such treatment of automatic tachycardias is ineffective because after cessation of overdrive pacing or DC cardioversion the automatic focus will quickly reappear.

Triggered Activity

Recently, there has been an in vitro demonstration that abnormal rhythms may result from delayed after-potentials. These rhythms may be triggered by premature stimuli or rapid pacing, may be terminated by spontaneous or induced premature stimuli or rapid pacing, and may terminate spontaneously. While a clinical counterpart of these in vitro demonstrations has yet to be identified with certainty, it is likely that as more is learned about this arrhythmogenic mechanism, their clinical counterparts will indeed be found (Rosen and Reder, 1981).

PREOPERATIVE CONSIDERATIONS

A preoperative program designed to evaluate the prospective cardiac surgical patient comprehensively is discussed in Chapter 3. An essential part of this program is a complete medical history in which antecedent cardiac rhythms and drug therapy are carefully noted. Whenever possible, previous electrocardiograms should be obtained and reviewed. Preoperative baseline laboratory studies should include a standard 12-lead electrocardiogram containing a long rhythm strip from a lead demonstrating a good P wave (usually V1 or II) should any arrhythmia be present, and serum electrolytes (in particular Na^+, K^+, Ca^{++}) and blood chemistries (in particular, those reflecting renal and liver function), which, if abnormal, could influence the cardiac rhythm or cardiac drug therapy. Clearly, if any of these laboratory studies are abnormal and require further preoperative evaluation and correction, this should be accomplished. Whenever possible, digitalis preparations should be discontinued at least one day and preferably several days prior to surgery if the clinical condition permits it.

INTRAOPERATIVE CONSIDERATIONS

It is imperative that a logical plan of care be initiated in the operating room and continued postoperatively in which: (1) factors known to cause arrhythmias are eliminated or minimized; (2) means of making a precise arrhythmia diagnosis are provided; and (3) methods of appropriate management are understood and available.

Electrophysiologic Concepts and Techniques

Identification of the Specialized Cardiac Conduction System. It is essential that the cardiac surgeon know the anatomy and physiology of the specialized conduction system of the heart. This information is particularly vital in surgery for complex congenital lesions, and is of importance in some operations for acquired heart disease as well. Awareness of the anatomy of the specialized conduction system allows the surgeon to better plan incisions and suture lines and minimize traction trauma. Several studies (Reemtsma et al., 1960; Titus et al., 1963; Lev et al., 1964; Hudson, 1967; Tung et al., 1967; Kaiser et al., 1970a; El-Said et al., 1972; Isaacson et al., 1972) that have demonstrated surgical interruption of the sinus node, the atrial internodal pathways, the A-V node, the His bundle, and the bundle branches emphasize this point.

Perhaps this problem is best illustrated by the example of the surgical repair of endocardial cushion defects, where the integrity of the specialized A-V conduction system is particularly at risk, and where reported incidences of complete heart block range from 2 percent to 20 percent (Spencer, 1969). In a large series of patients undergoing total correction of this defect (81 cases), one group (Cooley and Hallman, 1966) reported 22 instances of early complete heart block, 17 of which were permanent. Furthermore, heart block was thought to be the direct cause of three of the six postoperative deaths. Another clinical series (Murphy et al., 1970) also emphasized that complete heart block was a contributing cause of death in 14 of 40 patients (35 percent) who developed it following repair of congenital lesions. In light of reports such as these, and particularly since surgical correction for less common but more complex congenital lesions is now performed with increasing frequency, it is apparent that techniques demonstrating the anatomic position of the cardiac conduction system during surgery would be helpful.

A reliable and easily used electrophysiologic technique is available to localize the A-V conduction system during open heart surgery (Kaiser et al., 1970a). The method uses atrial pacing to ensure a supraventricular rhythm and a hand-held probe electrode (Fig. 10-2) to localize the anatomic course of the His bundle and bundle branches. A stable sinus rhythm also will permit use of this technique. However, atrial pacing ensures unchanging antegrade conduction to the ventricles, thereby permitting beat-to-beat observation of changes in the P-R interval or QRS configuration that might result from surgical manipulation. The anatomical course of the His bundle and bundle branches is dilineated by the appearance of an electrogram recorded during the isoelectric portion of the P-R interval (Fig. 10-3). This technique has been used successfully to identify the specialized A-V conduction system and thereby avoid injury to it in corrective surgery for both congenital and acquired cardiac lesions (Kaiser et al., 1970a; Waldo et al., 1973, 1975a; Krongrad et al., 1974b, 1974c; Kupersmith et al., 1974; Kupersmith, 1976; Maloney et al., 1975; Dick et al., 1977). At present no reliable electrophysiologic technique is available to identify

Figure 10–2. Illustrated here are several electrodes that may be used during intraoperative electrophysiologic studies. On the right is the end of an exploring electrode probe containing three silver electrodes. The electrode probe is used to record electrograms from selected sites on the endocardium and epicardium during various intraoperative electrophysiologic studies. Also illustrated are three types of acrylic plaques, each containing five silver electrodes. The first and third plaques are designed to be placed in the region of the sinus node after securing them under the superior vena caval cannula tape. The middle plaque may be temporarily sutured to selected sites on the atrium or ventricle. The plaques may be used either to record electrograms or to pace the heart; to record atrial electrograms or to pace the atria to maintain a conducted atrial rhythm during His bundle studies; for recording or pacing during studies to identify A-V bypass (accessory) pathways; or to record during studies the sequence of ventricular activation during ventricular tachycardia.

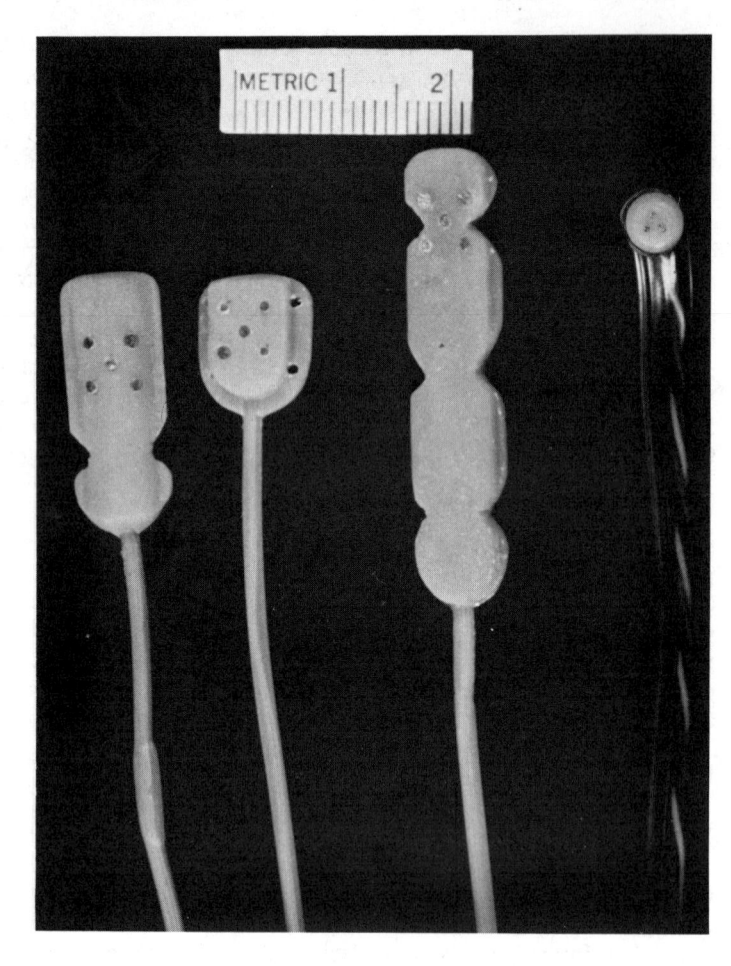

the sinus and A-V nodes directly. However, the A-V node may be assumed to be immediately posterior to the site of the most proximal His bundle. Recently, an electrophysiologic technique to identify the sinus node has been described (Hariman et al, 1980), and may prove useful to the surgeon in selected cases.

The mapping technique to identify the course of the specialized A-V conduction system must, of course, be performed in a beating heart during cardiopulmonary bypass. To map the His bundle in the A-V junction, the probe should be placed through a right atriotomy, initially just anterior to the coronary sinus ostium, and electrograms then should be recorded simultaneously with at least one electrocardiogram (see Fig. 10–3). An atrial electrogram or atrial pacing stimulus artifact also should be recorded through a bipolar electrode temporarily fixed to the right atrium. With an appropriate anatomic grid (Fig. 10–4) as a reference, the electrode probe then should be advanced anteromedially toward the membranous septum by increments of 5 mm, i.e., the probe diameter, to explore the region of the A-V junction. The proximal portion of the right bundle branch may be mapped by moving the electrode probe onto the right ventricular septum just distal to the membranous septum. For adequate delineation of the course of the right bundle branch,

ELECTROPHYSIOLOGIC CONSIDERATIONS 247

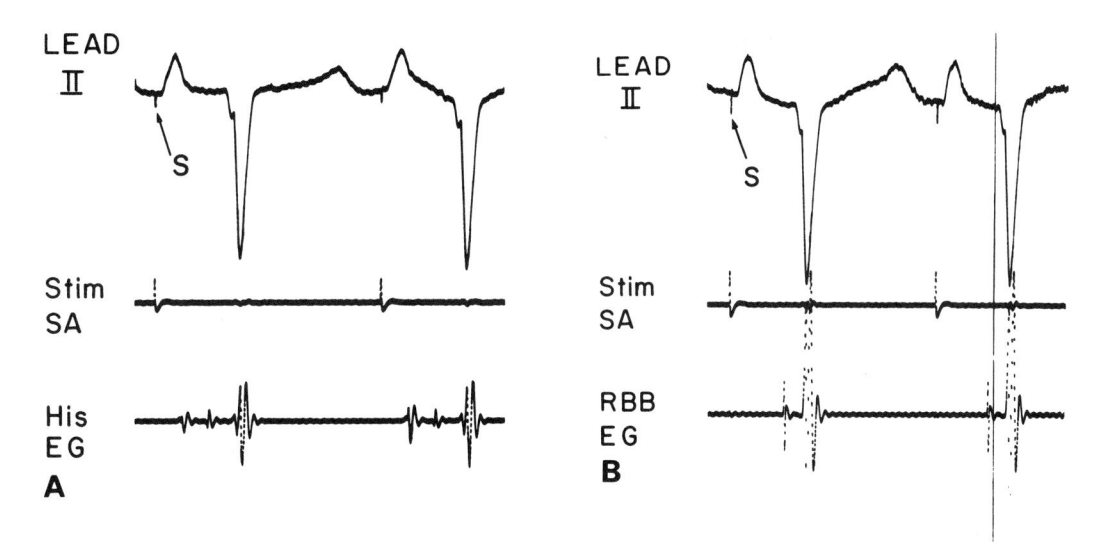

Figure 10-3. A. Lead II electrocardiogram (top trace) recorded simultaneously with the stimulus (Stim) artifact (middle trace) produced by pacing the atria from a plaque electrode in the region of the sinus node, and a bipolar electrogram (bottom trace) from an exploring probe electrode that has localized the bundle of His low in the right atrium (HB$_{EG}$) in a patient with an ostium primum defect. The first deflection in the His bundle electrogram represents atrial activation, the second deflection represents His bundle activation occurring during the isoelectric portion of the P-R interval, and the third deflection represents ventricular activation at that recording site. **B.** Records from same patient as in **A**. The bottom trace is a bipolar electrogram recorded from an electrode probe that has delineated the proximal right bundle branch (RBB$_{EG}$). The first deflection in the bottom trace is a right bundle branch electrogram, recorded during the isoelectric portion of the P-R interval, and the second deflection is the ventricular electrogram. Note the absence of a deflection representing atrial activation in this trace. S = stimulus artifact in the ECG. Paper recording speed is 100 mm/sec. *(Modified from Kaiser et al., 1970a).*

it often is necessary to place the electrode probe through a right ventriculotomy. Depending on the nature of the underlying heart defect, it may be possible to place the electrode probe distal to the His bundle to map the left bundle branch on the left ventricular septum. However, in unusual cases in which it is desirable to delineate the course of the A-V conduction system in the left ventricle, the mapping is best performed through an aortotomy or left ventriculotomy. Apart from the location of the electrode recording site distal to the membranous septum, no characteristic of the right or left bundle branch electrogram distinguishes it from a His bundle electrogram.

In the beating, blood-perfused heart, venous return of blood to the right atrium and right ventricle via the coronary sinus ostium and thebesian veins occasionally may obscure the recording field. In these cases, gentle suction in the region of the foramen ovale will permit adequate visualization of the field so that the electrode probe can be placed with precision. In other circumstances, either because the venous return of blood is so great that it obscures the field, or because there is an unacceptable danger of air entering the systemic circulation, it may be desirable to crossclamp the aorta before delineating the A-V conduction system (Waldo et al., 1975a). Delineation of the A-V conduction system during periods of aortic crossclamping is possible despite the cardiac ischemia produced, because A-V conduction usually is maintained for an acceptable period of time. When the

Figure 10-4. Four representative anatomical grids that may be used to aid in delineation of the specialized A-V conduction system. Circled numbers represent recording sites. Each site is the diameter of the recording electrode probe. The numbers used for each site are arbitrary and can be modified to meet individual requirements. In these grids, the free wall of the right atrium and the free wall of the right ventricle have been cut away to better visualize the right side of the atrial septum, the A-V junction, and the ventricular septum. Recording site 1 is at or minimally anterior to the coronary sinus ostium (CSO). **A.** Grid for mapping the A-V junction in the presence of an intact atrial septum. It also can be used with ostium secundum atrial septal defects or sinus venosus atrial septal defects. **B.** Grid for mapping the A-V junction in the presence of an ostium primum atrial septal defect. **C.** Grid for mapping the A-V conduction system in the right ventricle in the presence of a ventricular septal defect. In the presence of corrected transposition of the great vessels, it is critical to map anterior and superior to the ventricular septal defect. **D.** Grid for mapping the entire A-V conduction system in the presence of a complete endocardial cushion defect. SVC = superior vena cava; IVC = inferior vena cava; Ao = aorta; PA = pulmonary artery; PV = pulmonary vein; TV = tricuspid valve; RV = right ventricle; RA = right atrium. *(Modified from Krongrad et al., 1974b, 1974c.)*

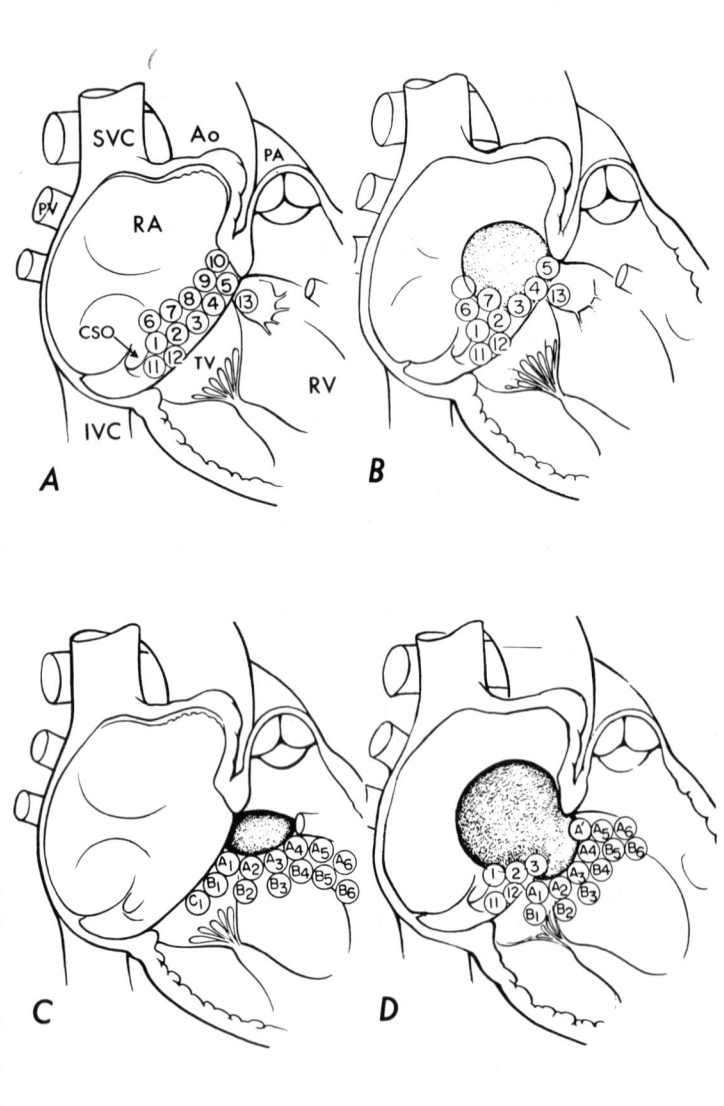

A-V block develops and makes further mapping meaningless, release of the aortic cross-clamp and reperfusion of the heart will allow recovery of A-V conduction. Then, an additional period of aortic crossclamping will permit further delineation of the A-V conduction system.

Recently, repair of congenital heart defects during hypothermic cardioplegic ischemic arrest has become widely used. Obviously, it is impossible to delineate the specialized A-V conduction system under these circumstances because the heart is not beating. If the surgeon wishes to perform the operative cardiac repair under these circumstances, yet wants to delineate the A-V conduction system electrophysiologically, it is appropriate first to map the A-V conduction system during a conducted rhythm under the conditions outlined above. After the surgeon has satisfactorily identified the course of the His bundle and bundle branches, hypothermic ischemic arrest then can be instituted.

It can never be overemphasized that care always must be taken not to apply undue pressure when placing the electrode probe on the cardiac tissue (Krongrad, et al., 1974c). It has been known for a long time that pressure applied to specialized conduction tissue will prolong conduction velocity and may produce heart block. Fortunately, should undue pressure inadvertently be applied during mapping, and prolonged A-V conduction or heart block appear, these changes almost always are transient. There is as yet no report of permanent abnormal A-V conduction secondary to the use of the mapping technique.

Special note should be made of the specialized A-V conduction system mapping studies in patients with corrected transposition of the great vessels with an associated ventricular septal defect (Kupersmith et al., 1974; Waldo et al., 1975a; Maloney, 1975; Dick et al, 1977). The A-V conduction system was not delineated in the right atrium and was found anterior and superior to the ventricular septal defect. This is in contradistinction to its usual location in the right atrium and posterior and inferior to most types of ventricular septal defects. However, when corrected transposition was present with dextrocardia (I,D,D), the A-V conduction system was located in the right atrium and coursed posterior and inferior to the ventricular septal defect. These observations highlight the value of His bundle mapping in complex congenital heart defects.

Other electrophysiologic studies have recently produced information that should provide a better understanding and interpretation of electrocardiographic patterns in several complex congenital lesions. For example, it has been established (Gelband et al., 1971) that the right bundle branch block pattern that occurs routinely in patients after open heart surgical correction of tetralogy of Fallot is caused by delayed right ventricular activation secondary to the vertical ventriculotomy and not by a lesion in the right bundle branch. The vertical ventriculotomy alone was always associated with significant prolongation of the time of right ventricular epicardial activation distal to the vertical incision, and the infundibular resection and repair of the ventricular septal defect were not associated with any additional changes in the electrophysiologic variables measured. Krongrad et al. (1974a) demonstrated that, in the presence of a right bundle branch block pattern produced by a vertical ventriculotomy, the main right bundle is intact. This was done by delineating the course of the right bundle branch all the way to the peripheral Purkinje fiber-ventricular muscle junction. More recently, Krongrad et al. (1974a) showed that the location and extent of the vertical ventriculotomy is critical for the development of the right bundle branch block ECG pattern. They postulated that the right bundle branch block pattern occurs when one of the major peripheral branches of the right bundle is interrupted.

A retrospective analysis of 251 patients undergoing correction of tetralogy of Fallot, ventricular septal defect, and pulmonic stenosis revealed a 100 percent incidence of a right bundle branch block pattern in the electrocardiograms of only those patients in whom a standard, long vertical ventriculotomy had been performed.

It is important to make the distinction between the pattern of right bundle branch block, which is relatively benign in terms of the long-term prognosis in patients undergoing surgical correction, and the pattern of right bundle branch block with left axis deviation immediately following surgical repair of tetralogy of Fallot. In this second group of patients, Wolff et al. (1972) have reported that complete heart block was 10 times more common, the incidence of serious arrhythmias 16 times more common, sudden death 6 times more common, and the late mortality 10 times more common than in those patients undergoing total repair of tetralogy of Fallot who did not develop this pattern.

These reports have been followed by a host of others (more than 15) dealing with the presence of a right bundle branch block pattern with or without associated abnormal left axis deviation in patients who have undergone surgical repair of ventricular septal defect of various types (Waldo, 1975). The reports and conclusions about the etiology and clinical significance of this postoperative ECG pattern are conflicting. What is clear, however, is that the distal His bundle and proximal right bundle branch are both at risk during these repairs. This again serves to underscore the importance of identifying the specialized A-V conduction system at surgery to prevent injury to it.

The importance of the specialized atrial internodal pathways in atrial conduction has been amply demonstrated (Eyster and Meek, 1913–1914; Bachmann, 1916; Eyster and Meek, 1916; Rothberger and Scherf, 1927; James, 1963; Vassalle and Hoffman, 1965; Wagner et al., 1966; Holsinger et al., 1968; Merideth and Titus, 1968; Waldo et al., 1968, 1970, 1971a, 1973, 1975a, 1977b; Narula et al., 1971). These studies strongly suggest that rapid conduction of the impulse from the sinus node to the A-V node occurs via these pathways, the preferential route being the anterior internodal pathway or both the anterior and middle internodal pathways (Eyster and Meek, 1916; Holsinger et al., 1968; Waldo et al., 1971a, 1973, 1975a, 1977b). It seems likely that lesions in these pathways may contribute to the genesis of arrhythmias. For instance, it has been demonstrated (Waldo et al., 1973) that all patients with endocardial cushion defects have prolonged time of conduction of the impulse from the sinus node to the A-V node. The location of the lesion in the atrial septum in these patients very likely disrupts or grossly distorts the anterior and middle internodal pathways. Since it has been demonstrated that these patients almost always have normal A-V nodal-His-Purkinje conduction, the increased P-R interval that they often manifest is due to the location of the atrial lesion.

One group (Bowman and Malm, 1965) has noted a very high incidence of postoperative arrhythmias following placement of a prosthetic mitral valve through an atrial septal incision that clearly had to interrupt the atrial internodal pathways. When the incision was restricted to the region of the foramen ovale, i.e., sparing the atrial internodal pathways, the incidence of postoperative arrhythmias decreased markedly. In total repair of transposition of the great vessels using the Mustard procedure, the atrial internodal pathways are especially at risk. In fact, recent electrophysiologic and pathologic studies (El-Said et al., 1972; Isaacson et al., 1972; Waldo et al., 1972a) have demonstrated that the sinus node and A-V node as well as the atrial internodal pathways may be damaged by this surgery. The high incidence of serious arrhythmias, which included tachycardias, bradycardias, and heart block, both in the immediate postoperative period and during the long-term follow-up period, seem clearly related to these lesions and again emphasize the importance of avoiding injury to the specialized conduction system during this repair. While it is not possible to avoid interrupting the middle and probably the posterior internodal pathways during this procedure, it has recently been shown (Waldo et al., 1972a) that the anterior internodal pathway can be preserved. Although there is some question as to whether interruption of the internodal pathways plays a role in the genesis of arrhythmias following the Mustard procedure, there is no question that during this procedure special care should be taken to avoid injury to the sinus and A-V node.

Identification of Areas of Myocardial Damage. The cardiac surgeon is more and more involved in the treatment of coronary artery disease and its complications. Surgical procedures such as placement of coronary artery bypass grafts, resection of left ventricular aneurysms, and infarctectomy for acute myocardial infarction associated with a ventricular septal defect have become a part of the cardiac surgery repertoire. In many instances, it would be helpful to the cardiac surgeon to be able to delineate discrete areas of damaged myocardium during these operations.

An electrophysiologic technique (Kaiser et al., 1969, 1970b) that permits identification of normal and abnormal myocardium can provide such help. The technique uses an electrode probe to record bipolar and unipolar electrograms from the myocardium during a conducted beat and its associated electrical complex. Figure 10–5 demonstrates typical electrograms recorded from normal and abnormal myocardium. Alterations from the normal ventricular electrogram are manifested by the appearance of Q wave in the unipolar electrogram and a decrease in amplitude and an increase in duration of the bipolar electrogram. The form of the abnormal electrograms is constant and reproducible. The technique requires only an electrode probe, which may be sterilized and connected to the standard cardiac operating room oscilloscope or graphic recorder.

Small discrete areas of damaged myocardium may be outlined accurately because the bipolar electrode records only from myocardium immediately beneath the probe contacts. This technique is most useful when employed during surgery for acute infarction with septal rupture and in cases of resection of akinetic areas of the left ventricle. In these instances, the limits of damaged myocardium may not be grossly apparent and the margins of the defect not distinct. In the case of a classical left ventricular aneurysm, the area to be resected usually is defined by fairly complete fibrous border, obviating the need for this technique, although the surgeon may want to know the status of the suture line. In left ventricular resection, electrograms provide information about the status of the myocardium at the line of resection, thus helping to minimize the occurrence of rupture of the myocardial repair.

Mapping of Arrhythmias

Wolff-Parkinson-White Syndrome (W-P-W). There is now a large experience (Sealy et al, 1976; Gallagher, 1978; Gallagher et al, 1981) with the surgical interruption of A-V bypass pathways to treat arrhythmias associated with this syndrome. There are at least two categories of W-P-W patients in whom this surgical procedure is indicated: (1) patients with clini-

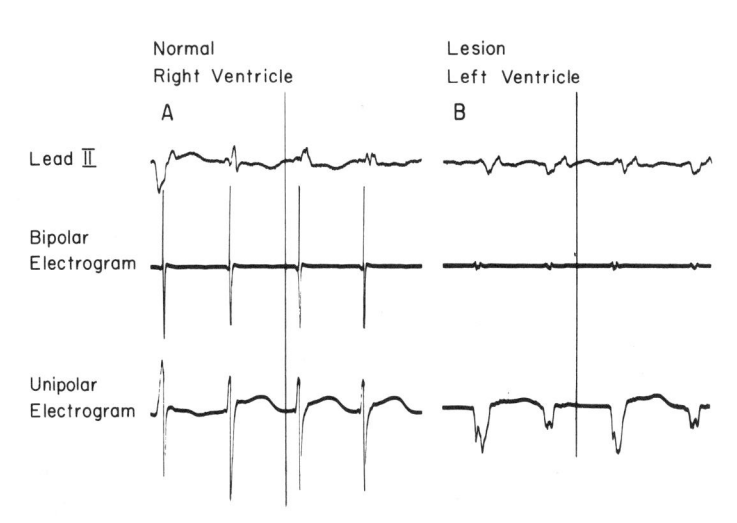

Figure 10–5. ECG lead recorded during open heart surgery simultaneously with a bipolar and unipolar electrogram from a patient with a history of myocardial infarction and mitral insufficiency. **A.** Control electrograms recorded from the right ventricle simultaneously with lead II. **B.** Electrograms recorded from the region of the anterior papillary muscle. Note the marked decrease in amplitude of the bipolar electrogram and the appearance of a Q wave in the unipolar electrogram in **B** when compared to the respective recordings in **A.** Paper recording speed 50 mm/sec. *(From Kaiser et al., 1969.)*

cally unacceptable and uncontrollable arrhythmias in which conduction over the A-V bypass pathway is central to the problem as in rapid ventricular response rates or frank ventricular fibrillation in response to atrial fibrillation, atrial flutter, or ectopic atrial tachycardia, or as in paroxysmal atrial tachycardia; and (2) patients coming to open heart surgery for other indications who also have the W-P-W syndrome.

The first category also includes patients with a so-called retrograde concealed A-V bypass pathway associated with intractable paroxysmal atrial tachycardia. In this forme fruste of the W-P-W syndrome, the A-V bypass pathway only conducts in a retrograde direction. Thus, these patients never exhibit a delta wave in the ECG, but because of the presence of retrograde conduction in the A-V bypass pathway, may manifest a narrow QRS complex paroxysmal atrial tachycardia, which is indistinguishable from that of patients with the W-P-W syndrome.

In the second category, it is important to demonstrate preoperatively, using standard cardiac electrophysiologic techniques during cardiac catheterization (Gallagher et al, 1978) where the A-V bypass is located, whether or not it is associated with provokable arrhythmias (e.g., paroxysmal atrial tachycardia) and whether or not it is capable of conducting impulses rapidly during atrial fibrillation or rapid atrial pacing. The latter is particularly important to assess because, should one of the common postoperative arrhythmias such as atrial fibrillation or atrial flutter occur, it may place the patient at risk for the development of ventricular fibrillation.

If the potential is demonstrated for involvement of the A-V bypass pathway in serious or life-threatening arrhythmias, it is strongly recommended that the bypass be identified at surgery and incised (Kluger et al., 1978). If the A-V bypass pathway is not involved in any clinically significant arrhythmia, it can probably be safely ignored at the time of surgery. If the bypass is involved only in arrhythmias considered relatively benign, such as paroxysmal atrial tachycardia, and if these arrhythmias can be pharmacologically controlled, the indication for interruption of the A-V bypass becomes elective. If, in the latter type of patient, the bypass appears to be easily accessible at surgery, an attempt to interrupt it probably should be made (Kluger et al., 1978).

The surgical interruption of the A-V bypass pathway requires careful application of intraoperative electrophysiologic techniques. Initial evaluation usually can be performed before initiation of cardiopulmonary bypass. An electrode should be sewn to a site on one of the atria and another to a selected site on one of the ventricles. These electrodes will be used both to introduce stimuli either to pace the heart or to initiate arrhythmias, and to record electrograms which will be used as reference recordings. The choice of sites for placement of the electrodes is determined largely by the type of thoracotomy and the location of the A-V bypass pathway, as determined from preoperative studies.

Prior to cardiopulmonary bypass and during a spontaneous or paced atrial rhythm in which a delta wave is present, an electrode probe is used to record electrograms from selected ventricular epicardial sites and the point of earliest ventricular epicardial activation is identified (the shortest atrial electrogram-to-ventricular electrogram interval). This point should be depolarized simultaneously with the onset of the delta wave in the ECG. The atria then are paced with threshold stimuli at selected sites along the A-V groove with an electrode probe, and the site that, when paced, results in the shortest stimulus artifact-to-onset of the delta wave interval is identified. Ventricular pacing then is initiated utilizing the previously placed ventricular electrode. If retrograde atrial activation is achieved, the electrode probe is used to record atrial electrograms from selected sites along the A-V groove and the earliest point of atrial activation is identified (shortest stimulus artifact-to-atrial electrogram interval). This study may not be possible because of depressed cardiac output associated with ventricular pacing or because a tachyarrhythmia is precipitated. However, for patients with a retrograde concealed A-V bypass pathway, this latter form of mapping is critical, and should be done even if it must be done during cardiopulmonary bypass.

Finally, if the patient has had a supraventricular tachycardia that reenters the atria by retrograde conduction over the accessory pathway (this information should be available from preoperative electrophysiologic studies), this arrhythmia may be precipitated again. During this latter tachyarrhythmia, using the electrogram recorded from the ventricular electrode as a time reference, one can identify the earliest point of atrial activation by recording atrial electrograms from selected sites adjacent to the A-V groove (shortest ventricular electrogram-to-atrial electrogram interval). Generally, the reentrant tachycardias are quite rapid and, shortly after their initiation, produce a degree of hypotension that is unacceptable. Therefore, this portion of the study usually must be performed during cardiopulmonary bypass. Again, this form of mapping is particularly important in patients with a retrograde concealed A-V bypass pathway.

At this point, if the patient is not already on cardiopulmonary bypass, the latter is initiated and the same mapping and pacing studies are performed endocardially following an appropriate atriotomy to permit visualization of the endocardial aspects of the A-V junction. The anatomic course of the A-V bypass pathway may be in close proximity to the normal A-V conduction system. This emphasizes the need to perform careful endocardial mapping and to identify the course of the His bundle. After the apparent location of the accessory pathway is identified, it can be cut. The incision should extend in the atrioventricular groove 2 to 3 cm to each side of the previously demonstrated site of earliest ventricular activation. After cardiopulmonary bypass is terminated but before removal of the bypass cannulae, attempts should be made to assess the efficacy of the procedure. Thus, the epicardial studies should be repeated to insure that there was successful interruption of the pathway. In addition, it is now known that more than one accessory A-V bypass pathway can be present in the Wolff-Parkinson-White syndrome, so that while the previously recognized AV bypass pathway may have been interrupted, another now may be evident. If during the repeat studies a delta wave is demonstrated, this suggests but does not prove the procedure was unsuccessful. In fact, the proof of success is failure to reprecipitate arrhythmias that use the A-V bypass pathway. It should be noted that cryosurgical ablation of the A-V bypass pathway recently has been utilized (Gallagher et al, 1979).

There also is an occasional role for surgical interruption of the His bundle for treatment of the reentrant tachycardia associated with the Wolff-Parkinson-White syndrome (Dreifus et al., 1968) or with a concealed retrograde A-V pathway. To perform this operation, the His bundle must be identified by the electrophysiologic techniques described earlier. If the His bundle is cut, the patient then maintains A-V conduction solely via an accessory A-V conduction pathway. The indications for cutting the His bundle are controversial. However, this technique is unacceptable if it has been demonstrated that the refractory period of the A-V bypass pathway is short, thereby permitting rapid conduction over it during atrial fibrillation, atrial flutter, or ectopic atrial tachycardia. Should surgical interruption of this bundle be performed, an appropriate permanent pacemaker system is virtually always required.

MAPPING OF VENTRICULAR TACHYCARDIA. As summarized recently (Waldo et al, 1981) intractable and life-threatening ventricular arrhythmias, i.e., ventricular tachycardia and ventricular fibrillation, may be amenable to surgical correction. Until very recently, ventricular arrhythmias associated with coronary artery disease with and without an associated left ventricular aneurysm, when approached surgically, were treated empirically with aortocoronary artery-saphenous vein bypass procedures or left ventricular aneurysmectomy or both. A review of reports of such surgical approaches confirms that this empirical approach was entirely hit-or-miss and without any clear reason for success or failure (Waldo et al, 1981). More recent studies (Wittig and Boineau, 1975; Fontaine et al., 1976, 1977; Moran et al., 1977; Gallagher, 1978; Guiradon et al, 1978; Harken et al, 1979; Josephson et al, 1979; Horowitz et al, 1980; O'Keefe et al, 1980; Arcineagas et al, 1980; Kehoe et al, 1981; Josephson et al, 1981) demonstrate that a more systematic approach to surgical treatment of these serious ventricular arrhythmias is possible and promising. While techniques, particularly intraoperative electrophysiologic and surgical ones, have already evolved considerably, they are still in their infancy. However, enough information is available to permit a systematic approach to be outlined for the surgical treatment of these arrhythmias.

Whenever possible, patients should undergo both a full standard cardiac catheterization with appropriate angiography (this may include coronary artery, left ventricular, and right ventricular angiograms) and a cardiac catheterization for cardiac electrophysiologic studies. The latter should identify the chamber of origin of the ventricular arrhythmia and the apparent mechanism of the arrhythmia. The catheterization also should carefully identify the characteristics of the ventricular tachycardia, particularly its initiation and termination, with cardiac pacing, as both may be critical during the surgery.

INTRAOPERATIVE SURGICAL TECHNIQUES

Ventricular Tachycardia Associated with Coronary Artery Disease

Guiraudon and colleagues (Guiraudon et al., 1978, 1978a; Fontaine et al., 1979; Guiraudon et al., 1981) initially tried epicardial mapping of the left ventricle in this group of patients but did not find the mapping sufficiently helpful. Therefore, Guiraudon designed an encircling endocardial ventriculotomy as an appropriate treatment in these patients (Fig. 10–6). This approach did not require mapping and was performed in the following manner: Either the ventricle is opened through a frank aneurysm or through the thin fibrous zone of the infarct scar, permitting examination of the entire endocardium. A transmural ventriculotomy is then performed from the endocardium perpendicular to the ventricular wall along the entire outer limit of the visible endocardial fibrosis. The perpendicular incision is made in the free wall to, but not through, the epicardium, thus sparing the epicardium and coronary vessels (Fig. 10–6). In the septum, the ventriculotomy is also made perpendicularly and made virtually through to the other cavity. The ventriculotomy is then repaired in a standard fashion using a running suture that is buttressed with strips of Teflon pledgets. The ventricle is then closed in the usual way.

Other techniques have been described which use endocardial as well as epicardial mapping to direct surgical treatment of ventricular tachyarrhythmias. Most prominent has been the technique advanced by the group at the University of Pennsylvania (Harken et al., 1979; Josephson et al., 1979; Horowitz et al., 1980) in which epicardial and endocardial mapping is performed using an anatomical grid during periods of ventricular tachycardia. The technique aims to identify the point of earliest activation relative to the onset of the QRS complex during the tachycardia (Fig. 10–7). Having identified the site of earliest ventricular activation during the ventricular tachycardia, the heart is then cooled using cardioplegic techniques, and direct resection of the tissue from the site of earliest activation ". . . to 2–4 cm beyond the edge of the aneurysmectomy border . . ." is performed, the resection being that of an endocardial layer 1 to 2 mm thick. When the site of earliest ventricular activation during the tachycardia is in the septum, ". . . 10–25 cm^2 of the septal endocardium is resected in the area of the earliest recorded electrogram."

Another technique (Arciniegas et al., 1981; Wiener et al., 1981; Klein et al., 1982) is to map the epicardium and the endocardium during a sinus or atrial paced rhythm and identify areas demonstrating delayed activation, fractionation, or double potentials (Fig.

ELECTROPHYSIOLOGIC CONSIDERATIONS

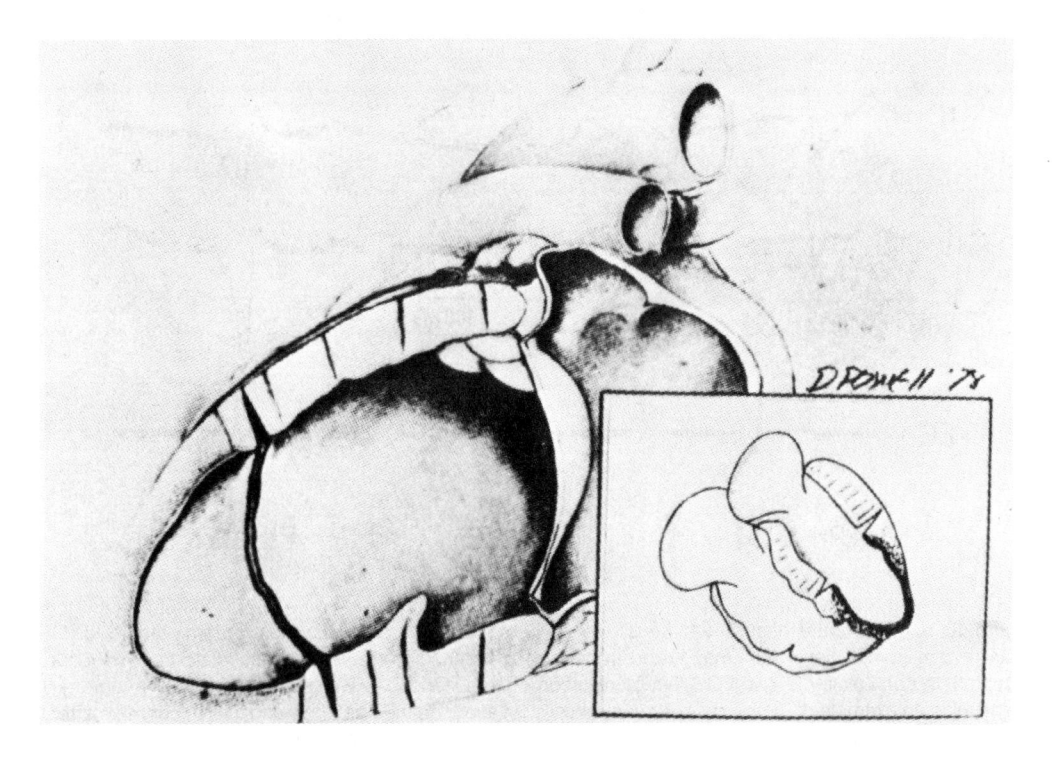

Figure 10–6. Diagrammatic illustration of the endocardial encircling ventriculotomy of Guiraudon. Note that a perpendicular incision is made in the endocardium to, but not through, the epicardium. This incision is then extended to encircle the edge of the endocardial fibrosis. *(From Guiraudon et al., 1978.)*

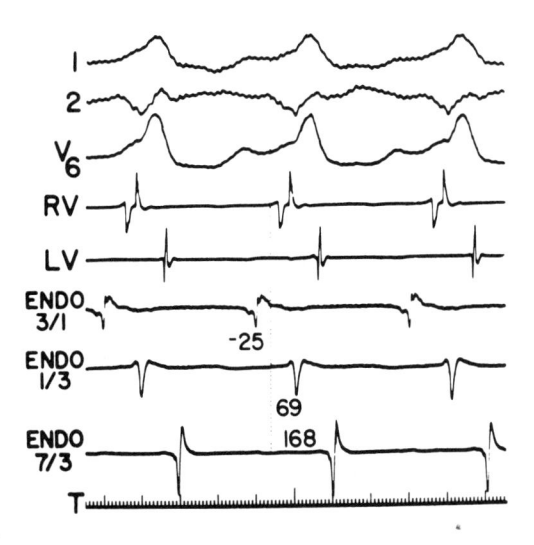

Figure 10–7. Recording during endocardial mapping from a patient during the period of ventricular tachycardia showing ECG leads I, II, and V_6 recorded simultaneously with the reference electrograms recorded from the right (RV) and left (LV) ventricles, and with electrograms recorded at three endocardial sites (ENDO 3/1, ENDO 1/3, ENDO 7/3). The bottom tracing (T) shows 10 ms and 100 ms time marks. The vertical dotted line indicates the onset of the QRS complex, and the activation times indicate the time from the onset of the QRS complex. Note the earliest endocardial activity occurred 25 ms before the onset of the QRS complex of the ECG leads. This site is identified as the earliest site of ventricular activation during ventricular tachycardia. *(From Josephson et al, 1979.)*

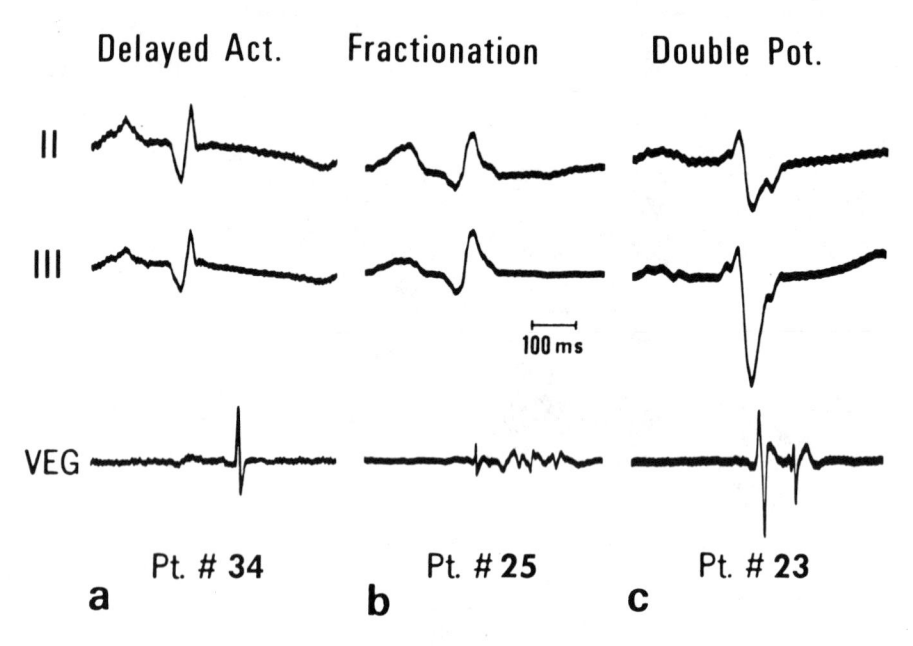

Figure 10–8. This figure illustrates three different types of bipolar ventricular electrograms recorded during sinus rhythm from patients who manifested spontaneous ventricular arrhythmias associated with myocardial infarction. In each example, two ECG leads are recorded simultaneously with the ventricular electrogram. The left panel is an example of locally delayed ventricular activation, defined as occurring 100 ms or more after the onset of the QRS complex in the ECG. In this example, the deflection in the ventricular electrogram occurs 150 ms after the beginning of the QRS complex. The middle panel is an example of fractionation of the ventricular electrogram. Note that the ventricular electrogram consists of small, multiphasic potentials distributed over a period of almost 200 ms, outlasting the duration of the QRS complex of the ECG. The right panel is an example of a double potential. Note that there are two clearly separated deflections for one ventricular beat, with the second deflection occurring beyond the duration of the QRS complex in the ECG. *(From Klein et al., in press.)*

10–8). Having identified these areas, they are then surgically excluded in some manner during a period of hypothermia. The exclusion consists of excision of all tissue when possible and/or resection of the endocardium as described above and/or performing a modified encircling endocardial ventriculotomy.

A third technique (O'Keeffe et al., 1980) utilizes ventricular pacing to identify the apparent site of origin of the tachycardia. Initially, spontaneous or induced ventricular tachycardia is recorded in as many ECG leads as possible at the time of open heart surgery. Then, utilizing standard electrophysiologic techniques, the ventricles are explored by pacing from selected epicardial and endocardial sites. When pacing from one site completely mimics the morphology of the ECG recorded during the spontaneous or induced tachycardia, this group considers that they have identified the site responsible for the tachycardia. Should the ventricular tachycardia not be precipitable during surgery, the QRS morphology of the ECG during pace mapping is compared to the QRS morphology obtained in the standard 12-lead ECG obtained prior to open heart surgery. When the responsible site is identified, the tissue surrounding that site is excised for a radius of 1–2 cm. Aneurysmectomy is also performed when appropriate.

More recently, Kehoe et al. (1981) have

suggested that endocardial resection may be performed quite satisfactorily without having to perform any sort of ventricular mapping. In a study in which they compared the results of two groups of patients, those who were mapped and those who were not, they demonstrated that the results with both groups were virtually identical.

In sum, there are several approaches to the surgical treatment of ventricular tachyarrhythmias, most of which require intraoperative mapping of some sort. However, it is uncertain whether intraoperative ventricular mapping will always be necessary to provide effective surgical treatment of ventricular tachyarrhythmias associated with coronary artery disease. It is suggested that while this approach to treatment remains largely investigational, one of the mapping techniques should be performed.

Ventricular Tachycardia Unassociated with Coronary Artery Disease

In this group of patients, in whom ventricular tachycardia can be precipitated by pacing techniques, intraoperative epicardial mapping has always shown the presence of delayed potentials (Fig. 10–9). This constant demonstration, regardless of the underlying cardiac abnormality, strongly suggests that it is in some important way associated with the generation of the tachycardia. It is a logical extension of this observation that these areas should either be excised or otherwise surgically excluded from the ventricles. Furthermore, if the tachycardia is precipitated, particularly in the patients with arrhythmogenic right ventricular dysplasia or Uhl's disease, mapping becomes critical in terms of denoting the point of epicardial breakthrough of right ventricular activation. This is because, as Fontaine and Guiraudon have shown in a series of papers and summarized recently (Waldo et al., 1981), a full thickness incision (ventriculotomy) at the point of earliest epicardial breakthrough during the ventricular tachycardia and/or at the site or sites where delayed potentials were recorded has provided successful treatment of the ventricular tachycardia. In addition, there have been several reports of

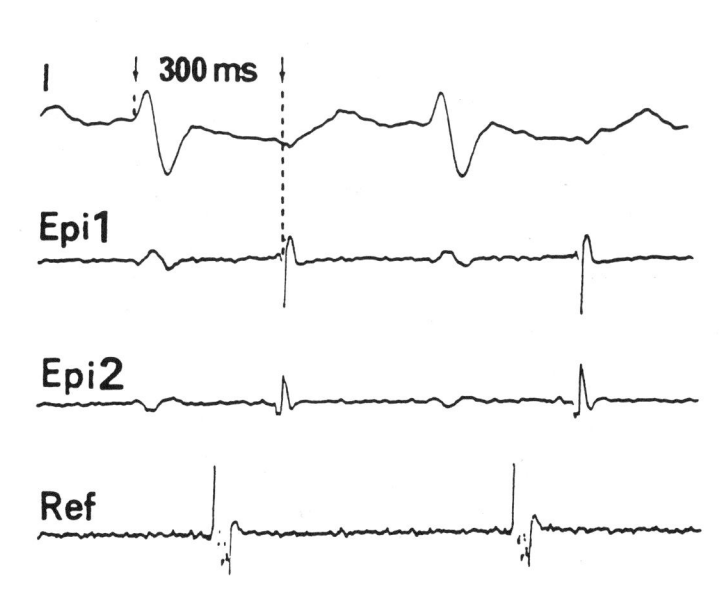

Figure 10–9. ECG lead I (top trace) recorded simultaneously with two epicardial ventricular electrograms recorded from an exploring electrode probe (traces EPI 1 and EPI 2) and a ventricular electrogram recorded from a reference electrode (Ref) sewn to the right ventricle (bottom trace) recorded during an epicardial mapping study in a patient with ventricular tachycardia. The electrograms recorded from both the probe electrode as well as the reference electrode occur considerably after the inscription of the QRS complex in the ECG. The electrogram highlighted by the dotted lines is recorded 300 msec after the beginning of ventricular depolarization and is clearly occurring during the T wave of the ECG. *(From Fontaine et al., 1976.)*

successful treatment using cryosurgical techniques (freezing) (Gallagher et al., 1978; Camm et al., 1979).

Intraoperative Arrhythmias

Etiologic Considerations. Arrhythmias that occur during (or after) cardiac surgical procedures almost invariably are the result of factors relating to the intraoperative methods and techniques employed and the degree of preexisting cardiac and pulmonary dysfunction. Anesthetic and surgical factors potentially etiologic to arrhythmias include alkalosis, acidosis, hypoxia, hypothermia, hypokalemia, perfusion-related particulate microemboli or air embolism, improper coronary perfusion, aortic crossclamping without coronary artery perfusion, and trauma accompanying placement of sutures, incisions, traction, or excision of tissue. If operative execution has been precise, most intraoperative arrhythmias are transient, generally of little or no consequence, and rarely require treatment.

Diagnosis and Treatment. The operative diagnosis and treatment of cardiac arrhythmias differ very little from that in the postoperative period, as discussed in the next section of this chapter (Postoperative Considerations). The reader is referred, therefore, to that section for a detailed discussion. The specific therapeutic problems with the operative and postoperative managment of long established atrial fibrillation (greater than one year) in patients undergoing surgery for mitral valve disease are discussed in Chapter 22. It is pertinent to reemphasize that consideration should always be given to defibrillating the atria in the operating room after the operative repair and then attempting to maintain an atrial rhythm with atrial pacing. Although the long-term prognosis for maintaining a spontaneous sinus rhythm in these patients is poor, the hemodynamic advantages in the early postoperative period are considerable (Woodson and Starr, 1968).

Implantation of Epicardial Electrodes. Prompt and accurate diagnosis and treatment of arrhythmias in the postoperative period are greatly facilitated by intraoperative implantation of temporary wire electrodes. Therefore, it is strongly recommended that temporary wire electrodes (Fig. 10–10) be placed routinely whenever possible on one of the atria (usually the right) and on one of the ventricles at the time of surgery, bringing the distal ends of each out through the anterior chest wall (Harris et al., 1967; Litwak et al., 1968; Waldo et al., 1971b, 1976a, 1976b, 1977a, 1978). Although there are a number of operative procedures in which one might anticipate little or no need for implantation of these electrodes, their potential use in the diagnosis and treatment of arrhythmias as well as the virtual absence of complications related to their presence justifies their routine use.

Ideally the wire electrodes should be placed as a pair, with the electrodes within each pair separated by a distance of 0.5 to 1.0 cm. A simple way to place the wires on the atria (Waldo et al., 1978) is to first make a loop in the atrial epicardium with a 5–0 silk suture. The Teflon-free end of the wire electrode is then bent to form a J hook, passed through the loop, and secured by tying the suture. This same technique may be used for the ventricular wire electrode placement. However, because of the thickness of the ventricular wall, the Teflon-free end may be implanted superficially in the ventricular myocardium. These electrodes will then serve to record electrograms or to pace the heart, should either be desirable. Bipolar electrodes are preferable to unipolar electrodes, particularly for the atria, for several reasons: (1) should one electrode come out, a unipolar electrode is still available for use; (2) bipolar electrodes, when properly placed, will record electrograms solely from the chamber in which they are implanted; (3) with unipolar pacing, pain usually is produced at the skin site of the indifferent electrode; and (4) with unipolar atrial pacing, the stimulus artifact so distorts the ECG that it may not be possible to be sure that atrial capture has been obtained, especially during rapid atrial pacing. Finally, it is important to appreciate that neither absence

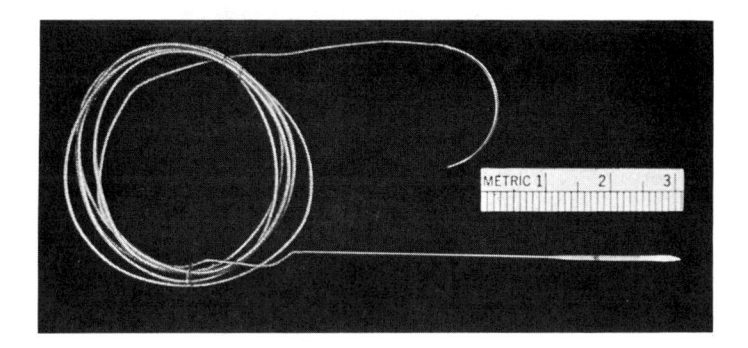

Figure 10–10. Stainless steel wire electrode (Davis and Geck No. 2597–63 0 Flexon) that can be used for the placement of temporary atrial and ventricular wire electrodes. The wire has a curved needle swedged onto one end and a straight needle swedged onto the other end. The wire is Teflon-coated except for about 2 cm immediately proximal to each of the needles. In preparation for placement of the wire electrodes on the right atrium, the curved needle along with the distal 1 cm of Teflon-free wire is cut off, leaving 1 cm of bared wire. After securing the wire electrode to the atrium, the straight needle is used to bring the wire electrode out through the anterior chest wall. The straight needle is then cut off along with the distal 1 cm of wire, leaving about a 1-cm portion of the wire bare of Teflon. When the ventricular wire electrode(s) is placed, the round, atraumatic needle may be used to implant the Teflon-free portion of the wire superficially in the myocardium, following which the needle is cut off. It should be noted that these wire electrodes also may be used for intraoperative studies in lieu of the plaque electrode demonstrated in Figure 10–2.

of preoperative arrhythmias nor presence of atrial fibrillation is a contraindication to placement of atrial epicardial electrodes (Waldo et al., 1976b, 1978).

POSTOPERATIVE CONSIDERATIONS

The previous discussion has attempted to make the point that arrhythmias appearing in the postoperative period may well have had the stage set earlier by a combination of factors existing preoperatively and those imposed during the operation. Proper preoperative preparation of the patient, physiologically sound operative conduct, and carefully executed postoperative care will minimize, but clearly will not eliminate, the problem of postoperative arrhythmias. For instance, patients with far-advanced myocardial dysfunction have a tendency to develop postoperative arrhythmias even under the best of management. Additionally, a number of factors commonly encountered after open heart surgery predispose to the development of arrhythmias. These include: (1) ventilatory problems, which produce hypoxia or respiratory alkalosis; (2) electrolyte imbalance; namely, hypokalemia during the early postperfusion period and, more rarely, hyperkalemia later postoperatively if severe renal dysfunction (either of a primary nature or secondary to low cardiac output) is present; (3) sterile pericarditis associated with pericardiotomy; and (4) drug toxicity.

Diagnosis and Management of Arrhythmias

Although some postoperative arrhythmias may prove to be transient and benign, the onset of any arrhythmia must be viewed as a potentially serious and even life-threatening event. Therefore, it is important to have established a plan that allows prompt diagnosis and institution of appropriate therapy. These measures are initiated in the operating room and are continued into the postoperative period. There are four elements of the program: (1) All factors previously discussed that are known to predispose to arrhythmias should be eliminated or reduced to an absolute minimum. Therefore, sequential measurements should be made of serum electrolytes, blood gases, and pH during the operation and particularly just before discontinuance of perfusion to be certain that all three values are in physiologically acceptable ranges. Correction of any abnormality should be accomplished before termination of bypass. Subsequent determinations should be made during the postoperative periods until they are normal and stable. These considerations are reviewed in detail in Chapters 3 and 9. (2) Temporary epicardial atrial and ventricular wire electrodes should be placed. (3) The patient's cardiac rhythm should be constantly monitored. (4) A condenser discharge (DC) cardioverter should be readily available and accessible.

Epicardial Electrodes in the Diagnosis of Cardiac Arrhythmias. It is universally recognized that the electrocardiogram is indispensable for the proper diagnosis of cardiac arrhythmias. However, it is also recognized that the ECG has its own limitations. Inability to demonstrate clear evidence of a P wave is probably the most often encountered limitation in the use of the ECG. Since the rate of atrial depolarization and its timing relative to ventricular depolarization is crucial to the correct diagnosis of cardiac arrhythmias, the importance of determining the presence of P waves and their relationship to QRS complexes is apparent. This ECG limitation is easily overcome by recording an atrial electrogram, preferably a bipolar atrial electrogram, simultaneously with an ECG (Fig. 10–11). In this manner, an accurate evaluation of most arrhythmias should be possible (Harris et al., 1967; Waldo et al., 1971b, 1972b, 1978; Wells et al., 1978; Waldo and MacLean, 1980).

For some arrhythmias, although the differential diagnosis of an arrhythmia may be narrowed by clearly identifying atrial activation and its relationship to ventricular activation, the diagnosis still may not be established. In such cases, the diagnosis can be established by pacing through the electrodes. A classical example would be a narrow QRS complex tachycardia with a ventricular rate of 150 beats/min. The differential diagnosis includes atrial flutter with 2:1 A-V block, sinus tachycardia, ectopic atrial tachycardia, sinus node reentrant tachycardia, A-V junctional tachycardia with retrograde conduction to the atria, and paroxysmal atrial tachycardia. Bipolar atrial electrograms recorded simultaneously or sequentially with an ECG will quickly

Figure 10–11. Monitored ECG (top trace) recorded simultaneously with a bipolar atrial electrogram (bottom trace) demonstrating atrial tachycardia with 2:1 A-V conduction. The routinely monitored electrocardiogram only suggested a sinus rhythm at 100 beats/min. However, when the bipolar atrial electogram was recorded simultaneously with the ECG, it was clear that an ectopic atrial tachycardia was present. Paper recording speed 25 mm/sec. *(From Waldo et al., 1978.)*

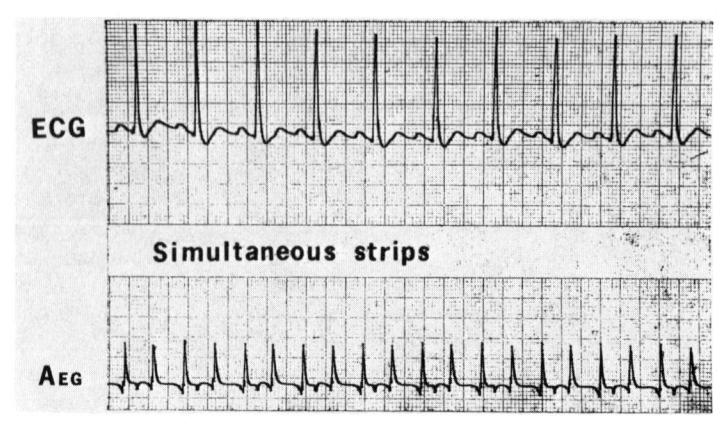

establish the presence or absence of atrial flutter.

However, if there is a 1:1 A-V relationship, there remain five possible diagnoses. Atrial pacing will permit a diagnosis: if it is an automatic rhythm (sinus tachycardia or A-V junctional tachycardia), after termination of pacing the rhythm will return promptly after a brief warm-up, and the relationship of the P wave to the QRS complex will determine if it is of sinus or A-V junctional origin; failure to interrupt it in the absence of overdrive suppression with warm-up will identify the rhythm as ectopic atrial tachycardia; interruption of the rhythm will identify it as either sinus node reentry or paroxysmal atrial tachycardia. To differentiate between the latter two then becomes somewhat academic, but if during the tachycardia the atrial electrogram occurred simultaneously with or just after the QRS complex, the diagnosis is most likely paroxysmal atrial tachycardia; if it occurred with a normal P-R interval, in the absence of W-P-W or a unidirectional retrograde A-V bypass pathway, it is most likely sinus node reentry. The latter, in fact, is probably an unusual postoperative rhythm.

Recording Atrial Electrograms. In most instances, it is preferable to record a bipolar atrial electrogram simultaneously with an electrocardiogram. However, should only a single-channel recording machine be available, it is possible to record an ECG and an atrial electrogram sequentially. The right arm, left arm, right leg, and left leg leads of the patient cable should first be applied to the appropriate limbs of the patient and an ECG recorded. Then, the right and left arm leads should be removed from the limb electrodes and each attached to one of the atrial wire electrodes. This may be done simply by using two alligator clips, one each to connect one of the limb leads with one of the atrial wire electrodes. Since lead I is a bipolar recording between the right arm and left arm leads, by moving the ECG lead selector on the recorder to the lead I position, a bipolar atrial electrogram will be recorded. By moving the ECG lead selector either to the lead II or lead III position, a unipolar atrial electrogram will be recorded because in each instance the recording will be made between an atrial wire electrode and the left leg; i.e., between the right arm lead attached to the wire electrode and the left leg (lead II) or between the left arm lead attached to a wire electrode and the left leg (lead III).

The bipolar atrial electrogram is usually the desirable electrogram to record because when the electrodes have been placed properly, it will demonstrate only atrial activity. The unipolar atrial electrogram will record both atrial and ventricular activity. On occasion, when only a single-channel recorder is available, the unipolar atrial electrogram may be useful in demonstrating the relationship of atrial to ventricular activation. However, a limitation of the unipolar atrial electrogram is that atrial events occurring simultaneously with ventricular events usually will be masked within the ventricular complex of the recording.

Epicardial Electrodes in the Treatment of Cardiac Arrhythmias—Cardiac Pacing. The treatment of many cardiac arrhythmias with cardiac pacing is now established as a rapid, reliable, and effective mode of therapy (Lister et al., 1960; Haft el al., 1967; Harris et al., 1967, 1968; Litwak et al., 1968; Hodam and Starr, 1969; Zeft et al., 1969; Gulotta and Aronson, 1970; DeSanctis, 1971; Vergara et al., 1972; Waldo et al., 1972b, 1977a, 1977b, 1978; Cooper et al., 1978; MacLean et al., 1978; Waldo and MacLean, 1980; Waldo et al., 1981). This is not to say that drugs have little or no place in the treatment of these arrhythmias. On the contrary, a combination of pacing and drug therapy may be required or drug therapy alone may prove most efficacious. The two major advantages of pacing over drug therapy are (1) the flexibility and convenience of immediacy of starting and stopping therapy and (2) avoidance of the side effects and toxic effects of drugs. It should be emphasized that initiation of pacing therapy requires the presence of a physician. This is particularly important when such therapy requires pacing the heart at rapid rates.

Diagnosis and Treatment of Postoperative Arrhythmias

Bradycardias. Bradycardia (rate less than 60 beats/min) and relative bradycardia (rates between 60 and 75 or 60 and 80 beats/min) are common postoperative rhythms. They are often associated with a low cardiac output and with rate-related supraventricular and ventricular arrhythmias. Ventricular extrasystoles that would not be present at a more rapid heart rate are the most obvious example of the latter. By the simple expedient of pacing the atria or ventricles at a more rapid rate than the spontaneous rate, it is possible to increase the cardiac output solely by this rate augmentation and at the same time to suppress the ventricular arrhythmia. If A-V conduction is intact, this is best accomplished by overriding the spontaneous heart rate by pacing the atria.

Supraventricular Tachycardias

PAROXYSMAL ATRIAL TACHYCARDIA (FIG. 10–12). Paroxysmal atrial tachycardia is a reentrant rhythm, the site of reentry most often being the A-V node. However, it recently has been recognized that in perhaps as many as 30 to 35 percent of cases of paroxysmal atrial tachycardia, the reentrant loop may include an A-V bypass pathway that will only conduct impulses in a retrograde direction, so-called unidirectional or retrograde W-P-W. And, of course, patients with classical W-P-W syndrome may manifest paroxysmal atrial tachycardia using the same mechanism. During these rhythms, the usual rate of both the atria and ventricles is between 180 and 200 beats/min, although the range is wider (about 130 to 220 beats/min). These rhythms are readily amenable to treatment with atrial pacing. Simply by capturing the atria at a rate faster than the spontaneous rate of the tachycardia, the tachycardia is interrupted. When pacing is then abruptly terminated, a spontaneous rhythm, usually a sinus rhythm, will ensue (see Fig. 10–12). Alternatively, once the atria have been captured by the pacemaker, the pacemaker rate may be quickly slowed from its "overdrive" rate (e.g., 200 beats/min) to a more normal rate (e.g., 100 beats/min). The rate required to interrupt this tachycardia is usually only a few beats faster than the spontaneous rate. However, particularly for cases of paroxysmal atrial tachycardia that involve reentry via a retrograde bypass pathway, the atrial pacing rate may have to exceed the spontaneous rate by 20 to 40 beats/min, in

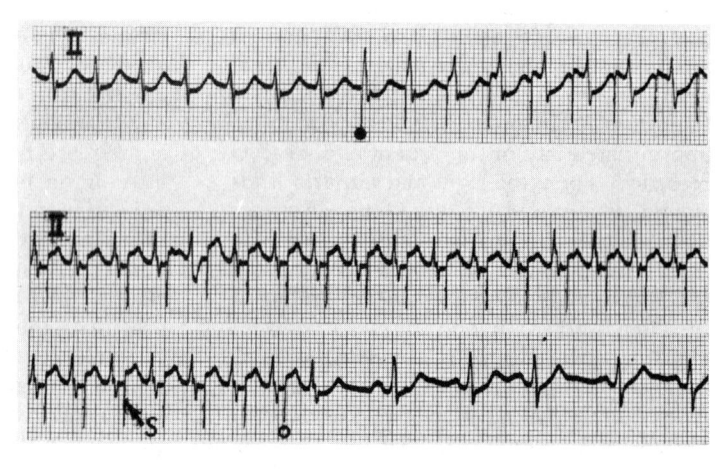

Figure 10–12. The top trace shows ECG lead II recorded during episodes of paroxysmal atrial tachycardia at a rate of 150 beats/min. Beginning with the eighth beat in this trace (black dot), rapid atrial pacing at a rate of 165 beats/min was initiated. In the middle trace, which begins 12 seconds after the last beat on the top trace, atrial capture is clearly demonstrated. In the bottom trace, which is continuous with the middle trace, when atrial pacing is abruptly terminated (open circle), sinus rhythm appears. S = stimulus artifact. Paper recording speed 25 mm/sec. *(From Cooper et al., 1978.)*

fact, usually to a rate that produces second-degree A-V block.

Since paroxysmal atrial tachycardia is most often precipitated by a premature atrial beat, it is usually worthwhile to attempt to suppress these beats. Pacing the atria at a rate the patient can tolerate that is significantly faster than the spontaneous sinus rate, usually up to 110 beats/min, may be effective. Another, more effective, technique is to pace the atria rapidly at rates between 180 and 230 beats/min to achieve 2:1 A-V conduction (Waldo et al., 1976b). This more rapid atrial pacing technique is more effective in suppressing the premature atrial beats, and allows a satisfactory ventricular rate. Of course, atrial pacing is only a temporizing measure and drug therapy must be added to the patient's regimen to suppress recurrent paroxysms of tachycardia. Quinidine or procainamide are the drugs of choice for long-term suppression of this arrhythmia. Digitalis, too, is often quite effective alone and occasionally is required in addition to either quinidine or procainamide.

ATRIAL FLUTTER. Recent studies of patients who have had open heart surgery have identified two types of atrial flutter, labeled Types I (classical) and II. Both types of atrial flutter resemble each other in that they are rapid, regular atrial rhythms (Fig. 10–13) (Wells et al., 1979). They differ from each other in that Type I atrial flutter can always be influenced by rapid atrial pacing from the high right atrium, i.e., from the usual atrial location of the temporary, epicardial atrial wire electrode, whereas Type II cannot be so influenced. The range of atrial rates of Type I atrial flutter is about 240 to 340 beats/min, and for Type II atrial flutter about 340 to 433 beats/min, the upper and lower limits for each probably being somewhat variable.

TREATMENT OF TYPE I ATRIAL FLUTTER. Type I atrial flutter may be treated with atrial pacing. The atria must be paced at a rate critically faster than the spontaneous atrial rate. Then, when the atrial pacing is abruptly stopped, a spontaneous sinus rhythm usually ensues. Alternatively, instead of abruptly stopping pacing, the pacing rate may be slowed to a clinically desirable rate, e.g., 110 beats/min, to maintain control of the heart rhythm. The critical pacing rate to interrupt Type I atrial flutter usually is between 115 and 125 percent of the spontaneous atrial flutter rate. When paced at rates short of the critical rate, the atrial flutter will be transiently entrained to the pacing rate, but will not be interrupted (Waldo et al., 1977a; Waldo et al, 1981). When pacing from the high right atrium, the hallmark of successful interruption of Type I atrial flutter is the appearance of positive, i.e., completely upright, atrial complexes in ECG leads II, III, and a VF (Fig. 10–14) (Waldo et al., 1977a, 1981).

Two additional factors are critical in

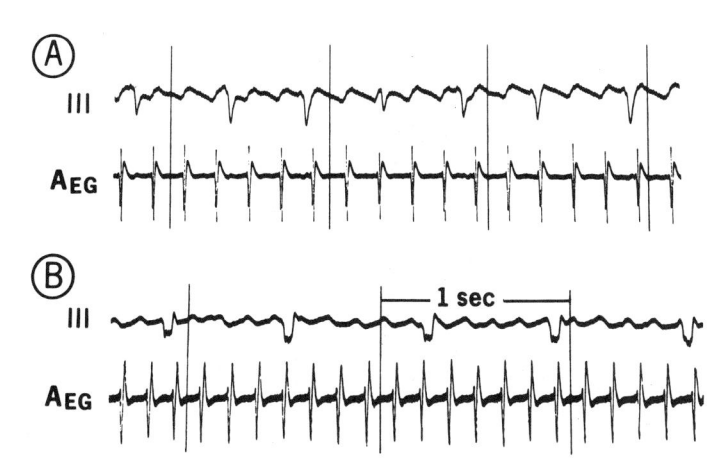

Figure 10–13. **A.** ECG lead III recorded simultaneously with a bipolar atrial electrogram, demonstrating Type I atrial flutter at a rate of 304 beats/min. **B.** ECG lead III recorded simultaneously with a bipolar atrial electrogram in another patient, demonstrating Type II atrial flutter with a regular atrial rate of 420 beats/min. Time lines are at one-second intervals. *(Modified from Wells et al., 1979.)*

Figure 10–14. A. ECG lead II (top trace) and a bipolar atrial electrogram (AEGbi); bottom trace recorded sequentially in a patient who had open heart surgery, demonstrating Type I atrial flutter at a rate of 260 beats/min with 2:1 A-V conduction (ventricular rate 130 beats/min). Paper recording speed 25 mm/sec. *(From Cooper et al., 1978.)*

B. ECG lead II recorded from the same patient as in **A**. Atrial pacing at a rate of 320 beats/min was initiated (top trace). With the onset of atrial pacing, the atrial complexes in the ECG that had been predominantly negative became predominantly positive and notched. The bottom trace is recorded several seconds after the top trace. Note that now, although the atrial pacing rate remains at 320 beats/min, the atrial complexes have become completely positive. Had the rapid atrial pacing been abruptly terminated at any time during the recording of the bottom trace, the spontaneous rhythm would have returned to sinus. However, in this patient, it was elected to slow the pacing rate (c.f.). Paper recording speed 25 mm/sec. S = stimulus artifact. *(From Cooper et al., 1978.)*

C. ECG lead II recorded from the same patient as in **A** and **B**. These three traces are continuous, and the top trace is continuous with the bottom trace of **B**. Having demonstrated that the atrial complexes were positive in lead II, the atrial pacing rate was slowed gradually to 120 beats/min. Note that atrial capture was maintained throughout the period of atrial pacing. Paper recording speed 25 mm/sec. S = stimulus artifact. *(From Cooper et al., 1978.)*

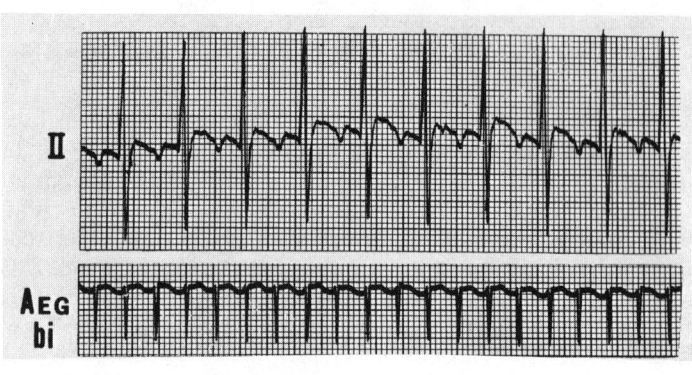

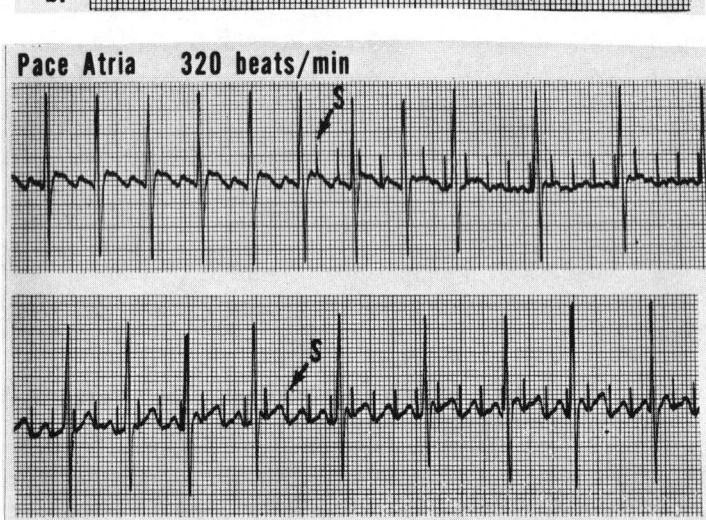

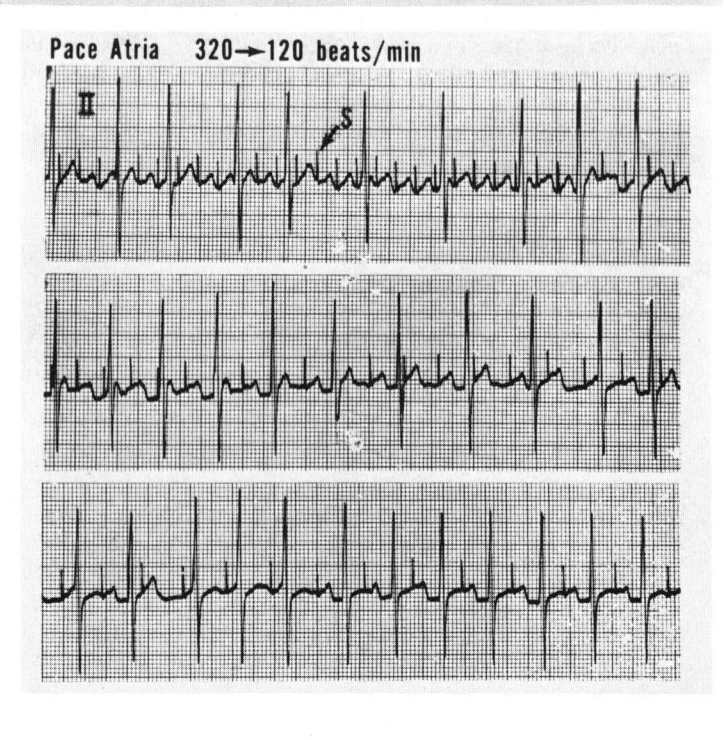

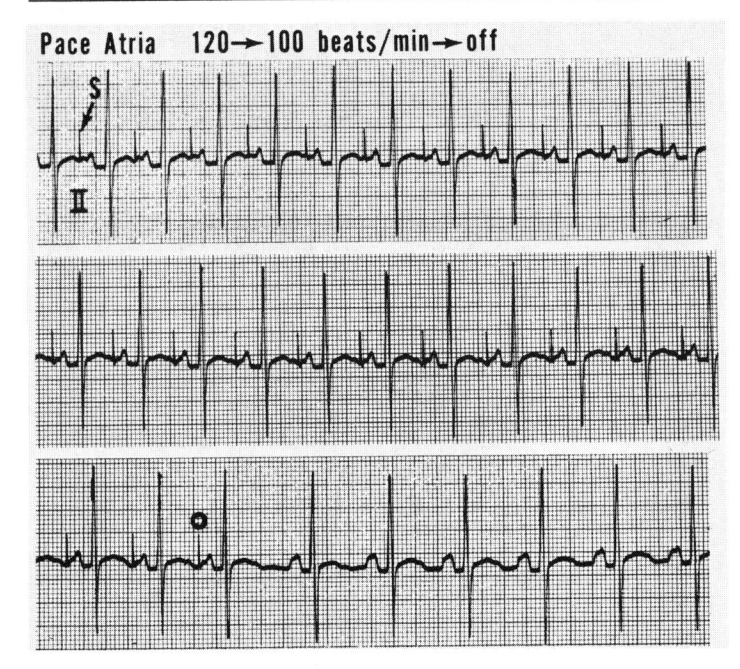

Figure 10–14 (Cont.)
D. ECG lead II recorded from the same patient as in **A, B,** and **C.** The three traces in this figure are continuous, and the top trace is continued from the bottom trace in **C.** The atrial pacing rate was slowed from 120 to 100 beats/min, and when the pacing was abruptly terminated (open circle), sinus rhythm was present.

properly using the technique of rapid atrial pacing to interrupt Type I atrial flutter. First, the required stimulus strength to obtain atrial capture is often surprisingly large, usually being 10 to 20 mA, and occasionally even higher (Plumb et al., 1981). Second, a critical duration of atrial pacing is required at the critical rate (Waldo et al., 1977a). The reported mean duration of pacing is 10 seconds, with a range of 2 to 22 seconds. However, the upper range of the critical duration of pacing probably extends to about 40 seconds.

Occasionally, rapid atrial pacing to treat Type I atrial flutter may precipitate atrial fibrillation. Atrial fibrillation in this circumstance is usually a more desirable rhythm than atrial flutter, as the ventricular response rate to atrial fibrillation is usually slower and is easier to control with digitalis (Waldo et al., 1976b). Furthermore, unless the preoperative rhythm was atrial fibrillation, the atrial fibrillation precipitated by rapid atrial pacing most often spontaneously reverts to sinus rhythm. In patients with recurrent Type I atrial flutter, it is desirable to precipitate and maintain atrial fibrillation deliberately by pacing the atria continuously at a rate greater than 450 beats/min. Precipitating atrial fibrillation permits easy control of the ventricular response with digitalis, while time and antiarrhythmic drug therapy permit suppression of the atrial flutter. This may require up to 72 hours of pacing, but it usually requires less than 35.

TYPE II ATRIAL FLUTTER. This rhythm cannot be treated with rapid atrial pacing from sites high in the right atrium (Wells et al., 1979). Therefore, it should be treated with a digitalis preparation just as one would treat atrial fibrillation.

ATRIAL FIBRILLATION. Atrial fibrillation is a rapid, irregular atrial rhythm. Atrial electrograms recorded from patients with atrial fibrillation are characterized by complexes having a myriad of sizes, shapes, polarities, and amplitudes, as well as a broad range of rates and beat-to-beat intervals (Wells et al., 1978). In fact, according to recorded bipolar atrial electrograms, the hallmark of atrial fibrillation is the characteristic beat-to-beat variability of these ranges.

Figure 10–15. ECG lead III recorded simultaneously with a bipolar atrial electrogram demonstrating three of the four types of atrial fibrillation. Type I atrial fibrillation (**A**) is characterized by discrete atrial electrograms having variable morphology, polarity, amplitude, and cycle lengths, but with an isoelectric interval between the recorded electrograms. Type II atrial fibrillation (**B**) differs from Type I atrial fibrillation only in that the interval between recorded electrograms is not isoelectric, but rather contains perturbations of the baseline. Type III atrial fibrillation (**C**) is characterized by absence of discrete atrial electrograms as well as absence of an isoelectric interval of any sort. Note that Type I atrial fibrillation and sometimes Type II atrial fibrillation can mimic atrial flutter. See text for discussion. Time lines at one-second intervals.

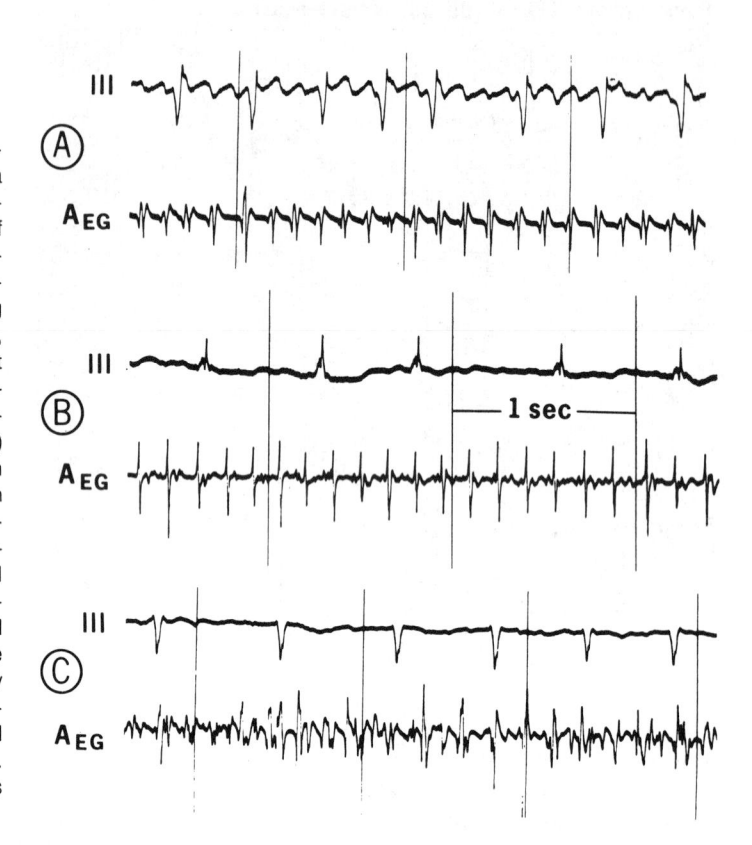

On the basis of the bipolar atrial electrogram morphology and the nature of the baseline between the atrial electrogram complexes, it is possible to separate four distinct types of atrial fibrillation. Type I atrial fibrillation is characterized by discrete atrial electrogram complexes of variable morphology separated by an isoelectric baseline free of perturbation (Fig. 10–15). Type II atrial fibrillation is characterized by discrete atrial electrogram complexes of variable morphology, but is different from Type I atrial fibrillation in that the baseline is not isoelectric, having perturbations of varying degrees (see Fig. 10–15). Type III atrial fibrillation is characterized by atrial electrograms that fail to demonstrate either discrete complexes or isoelectric intervals (see Fig. 10–15). Type IV atrial fibrillation is characterized by atrial electrograms consistent with Type III alternating with periods of atrial electrograms consistent with Type I and/or Type II (Fig. 10–16).

It is clear that not all atrial fibrillation is the chaotic type manifested by Type III. Some types of atrial fibrillation appear to be rather well-ordered. This fact is even reflected in the electrocardiogram in which coarse, rather discrete atrial complexes instead of an irregular baseline can be seen (see Fig. 10–13). The ability to distinguish atrial fibrillation from atrial flutter is particularly important because atrial flutter can be treated effectively with rapid atrial pacing whereas atrial fibrillation cannot.

The atrial rates as measured from atrial electrograms recorded during atrial fibrillation range widely (Wells et al., 1978). Surprisingly, rates as low as 263 beats/min have been documented. In fact, it is not unusual to find atrial rates of Type I or Type II atrial fibrillation within the range of rates associated with atrial flutter. Thus, should the rate of atrial fibrillation be rather slow, and the atrial electrogram relatively organized, it is important

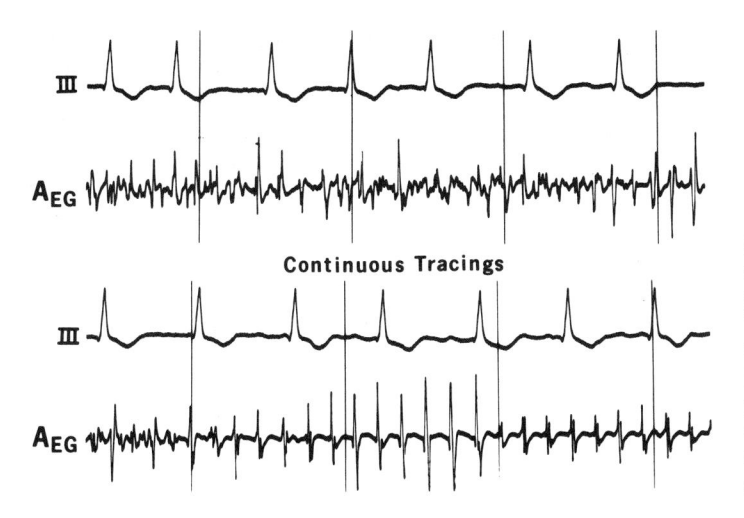

Figure 10–16. ECG lead III recorded simultaneously with a bipolar electrogram demonstrating Type IV atrial fibrillation, which is characterized by periods of Type III atrial fibrillation alternating with periods of either Type I or Type II atrial fibrillation. Time lines at one-second intervals. *(From Wells et al., 1978.)*

to distinguish this rhythm from atrial flutter.

ECTOPIC (NONPAROXYSMAL) ATRIAL TACHYCARDIA. Ectopic atrial tachycardia is a poorly understood rhythm that is generated in the atria and is characterized by an atrial rate ranging from about 130 to 240 beats/min, the more common rates being 180 to 220 beats/min. When the atrial rate is greater than 160 beats/min, it is usually characterized by second-degree A-V block. This is particularly helpful in the differentiation of this rhythm from paroxysmal atrial tachycardia. Another frequent, though not constant, characteristic of this rhythm that helps differentiate it from other supraventricular tachycardias with similar atrial rates is a remarkable beat-to-beat variability in atrial cycle length. This arrhythmia is not uncommon in adult patients immediately after open heart surgery, and in this situation is virtually never a consequence of digitalis toxicity. This point bears emphasis, because in other circumstances, this arrhythmia is a common manifestation of digitalis toxicity.

When present, this rhythm is commonly associated with 2:1 A-V conduction such that despite rapid atrial rates (e.g., 200 beats/min), the ventricular rate of 100 beats/min is clinically acceptable. Thus, therapy to interrupt the arrhythmia may not be required. In such circumstances, often over a period of several days, the rhythm will spontaneously revert to the preoperative rhythm (e.g., sinus rhythm or atrial fibrillation). However, the degree of A-V conduction may be variable or rapid atrial pacing may be employed to interrupt the rhythm. The pacing technique is similar to that described for Type I atrial flutter. Through use of the atrial wire electrodes, atrial pacing at a rate 10 beats/min faster than the intrinsic rate of the arrhythmia should be initiated. Pacing should be continued for at least 30 seconds and then should either be abruptly terminated or quickly slowed to a desirable atrial pacing rate (e.g., 110 beats/min). Should the rapid atrial pacing fail to interrupt the arrhythmia, rapid atrial pacing should be reinitiated, increasing the pacing rate in 5 to 10-beat increments until the arrhythmia has been interrupted. Such rapid atrial pacing may have one of three outcomes: (1) the arrhythmia may be interrupted with return to sinus rhythm; (2) the arrhythmia may be converted to atrial fibrillation; or (3) the arrhythmia may be converted to atrial flutter, usually Type I. Should the latter occur, this new rhythm should be treated in standard fashion for any Type I (classical) atrial flutter (see above).

During rapid atrial pacing to interrupt ectopic atrial tachycardia, the arrhythmia commonly is transiently entrained to the pacing rate until a sufficiently rapid pacing rate is achieved to which the arrhythmia cannot be entrained. Therefore, failure to interrupt the arrhythmia with rapid pacing at rates faster than the pacing rate should not be interrupted as indicating that this rhythm is pacing noninterruptable (Cooper et al., 1978). Finally, for some patients, particularly those with ectopic atrial tachycardia at rates resulting in 1:1 A-V conduction, simply pacing at rates producing 2:1 A-V conduction with acceptable clinical rates may prove the most desirable therapy (Fig. 10–17) (Waldo et al., 1976b).

Drug therapy of this arrhythmia usually is unsuccessful in the postoperative period. Rapid atrial pacing and "tincture of time" seem most effective. However, if the patient is receiving procainamide therapy, it should be discontinued, as it seems to potentiate rather than alleviate this arrhythmia. And, of course, should digitalis toxicity be suspected, the drug should be discontinued and the diagnosis confirmed by obtaining a serum digozin level.

SPONTANEOUS AUTOMATIC TACHYCARDIA (SINUS AND A-V JUNCTIONAL). Generally, sinus and automatic A-V junctional tachycardia in the postoperative period are transient and benign, and do not require special attention apart from seeking the cause of the tachycardia (e.g., fever, anemia, cardiac tamponade, hypovolemia as a cause of sinus tachycardia), and initiating appropriate therapy. Sinus and A-V junctional automatic tachycardias are not amenable to atrial pacing therapy. While they can be overdriven, as soon as the external pacemaker is stopped or slowed to a rate slower then the spontaneous rate, the spontaneous automatic pacemaker again becomes the rhythm of the heart.

On occasion, it may be desirable to overdrive an A-V junctional tachycardia to obtain the atrial contribution to cardiac output. This usually is possible simply by pacing the atria at a rate just faster than the A-V junctional rate. On occasion, the enhanced A-V junctional pacemaker responsible for the spontaneous tachycardia may be associated with significant antegrade A-V block such that atrial impulse produced by pacing the atria at a faster rate than that of the A-V junction will block proximal to the focus of the A-V junctional pacemaker and thus will not overdrive the A-V junctional rhythm. In such circumstances, it may be desirable to initiate A-V sequential pacing. This is performed by pacing the atria at a rate appropriately faster than the A-V junctional rate and then, using the ventricular

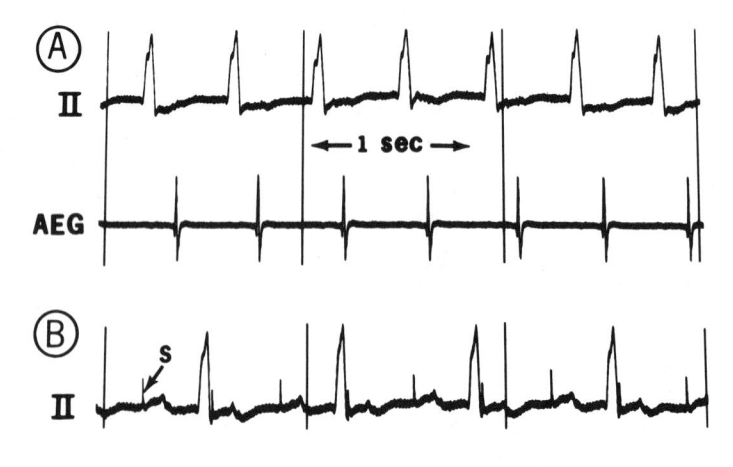

Figure 10–17. **A** shows ECG lead II recorded simultaneously with a bipolar atrial electrogram (A$_{EG}$), demonstrating an ectopic atrial tachycardia at a rate of 135 beats/min with 1:1 A-V conduction in a patient who had open heart surgery. Rapid atrial pacing could overdrive the arrhythmia but could not interrupt it. Drug therapy also failed to interrupt the arrhythmia. Therefore, as shown in **B**, continuous rapid atrial pacing at a rate of 180 beats/min was initiated. This produced 2:1 A-V conduction with a clinically satisfactory ventricular rate of 90 beats/min. Paper recording speed 50 mm/sec. S = stimulus artifact. Time lines are at one-second intervals. *(From Cooper et al., 1978.)*

wire electrode, pacing the ventricles after a short delay (i.e., creating a P-R interval). Usually the A-V junctional tachycardia is secondary to trauma to the A-V junction associated with the surgical procedure, and over a period of up to several days it will subside spontaneously. It is not really known whether drug therapy speeds this process or in fact is helpful in any way. However, a trial with virtually any of the standard antiarrhythmic drugs except propranolol may be helpful, as they all suppress ectopic automaticity (Waldo et al., 1976a). Digitalis is probably contraindicated because it enhances automaticity of the A-V junctional pacemaker.

Whenever an automatic A-V junctional tachycardia becomes life-threatening, generally because of marked hypotension and low cardiac output, ventricular paired pacing may be required (Cranefield, 1966; Cranefield and Hoffman, 1966; Resnikov, 1970; Waldo et al., 1976a; Waldo and MacLean, 1980, Waldo et al., 1981). In this mode of therapy, the ventricles are paced rapidly but every other beat is deliberately premature. In effect, ventricular pacing with ventricular bigeminy is produced. However, each premature beat is introduced early enough so that although ventricular activation occurs, there is no ejection of blood from the ventricles because ventricular contraction is ineffective. Thus, use of this mode of therapy, although the heart rate will still be rapid, will halve the effective heart rate because every other beat will be mechanically ineffective. For example, during ventricular paired pacing at a rate of 240 beats/min, while the electrical rate will be 240 beats/min, the mechanical rate will be 120 beats/min, a rate that should be hemodynamically satisfactory. It should be emphasized that this mode of therapy is potentially hazardous, for if inappropriately applied, it may not effectively halve the mechanical rate, resulting in an even faster ventricular rate than the spontaneous rate or in ventricular fibrillation. Also, primarily in adults, if applied for a prolonged period, it may be difficult to wean the patient from the ventricular paired pacing because cessation of the pacing may be associated with marked hypotension and impaired cardiac output.

Ventricular Tachycardia. Either intravenous lidocaine therapy or DC cardioversion is generally the treatment of choice for this arrhythmia. However, when not induced by a spontaneous automatic pacemaker, it may be effectively treated by rapid ventricular or even rapid atrial pacing (Fisher et al., 1978; MacLean et al., 1979). Atrial pacing will only be successful if 1:1 A-V conduction of each atrially paced beat occurs. The method of pacing is similar to that described for Type I atrial flutter. When the situation permits, ventricular pacing at a rate at least 10 beats faster than the spontaneous ventricular rate should be initiated, and after 5 to 15 capture beats, the ventricular pacing should be abruptly terminated. If the ventricular tachycardia has not been interrupted, the pacing should be repeated, increasing the pacing rate by increments of 5 to 10 beats/min. Generally, ventricular pacing at rates between 115 and 125 percent of the intrinsic rate is required to interrupt the tachycardia, although rates as high as 140 percent of the intrinsic rate have been reported (Fisher et al., 1978; MacLean et al., 1979). Rapid ventricular pacing at rates faster than the intrinsic rate of the tachycardia that fails to interrupt the tachycardia has merely transiently entrained the tachycardia (MacLean et al., 1981). As with rapid atrial pacing to interrupt Type I atrial flutter, ventricular pacing to interrupt ventricular tachycardia must achieve rates to which the ventricular tachycardia cannot be transiently entrained (MacLean et al., 1981; Waldo et al., 1981). It must be emphasized that whenever rapid ventricular pacing techniques are being used to treat ventricular tachycardia, one must be prepared to initiate prompt DC cardioversion should ventricular fibrillation be precipitated or in the event that rapid pacing may have provoked an even faster ventricular tachycardia than previously present.

Ventricular Fibrillation. This rhythm is incompatible with life and cannot be treated with ventricular pacing. Rapid treatment with DC cardioversion is mandatory and should be performed as quickly as possible.

Extrasystoles. As described above, ventricular extrasystoles are often easily suppressed simply by increasing the heart rate either with atrial or ventricular pacing. When rate augmentation alone is ineffective in suppressing the ventricular extrasystoles, the addition or substitution of either lidocaine, procainamide, quinidine, disopyramide, or phenytoin is necessary.

Atrial extrasystoles, too, often may be suppressed simply by increasing the atrial rate with atrial pacing. It is usually desirable to suppress atrial extrasystoles should they be frequent because they are the harbingers of atrial fibrillation, paroxysmal atrial tachycardia, ectopic atrial tachycardia, and atrial flutter. Often, the combination of atrial pacing plus either procainamide or quinidine administration is required for satisfactory suppression of the atrial extrasystoles. For some patients, to suppress the premature atrial beats it may be necessary to pace the atria at rapid rates, usually between 180 and 220 or 230 beats/min, which will effectively suppress the premature atrial beats and also produce 2:1 A-V conduction with a clinically acceptable ventricular rate (Waldo et al., 1976b).

Atrial Quiescence. Atrial quiescence (Fig. 10–18), a form of atrial standstill, is a rhythm in which there is no spontaneous atrial activity and in which the atria cannot be paced, i.e., the atria are inexcitable (Waldo et al., 1972b). During this rhythm, the ventricles are usually depolarized from an A-V junctional pacemaker. As the ensuing ventricular rate is usually less than 60 beats/min, ventricular pacing is required. The incidence of this arrhythmia after open heart surgery is not known, largely because it usually goes unrecognized and usually is transient, most often lasting not more than 24 hours. However, it is easily diagnosed

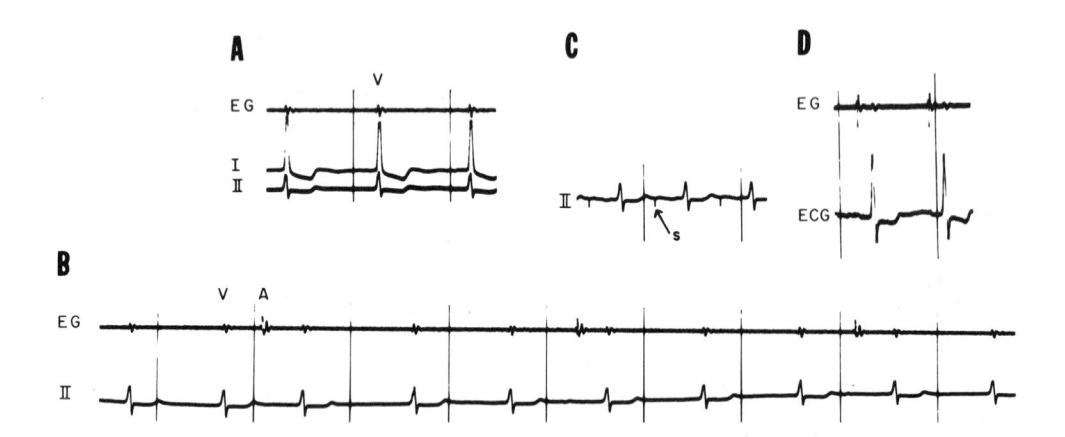

Figure 10–18. Rhythms recorded from a patient who had open heart surgery. In **A, B,** and **D,** a bipolar atrial electrogram (top trace) is recorded simultaneously with one or more ECG leads. In **A**, note the absence of a P wave in the ECG leads and the absence of any atrial activity in the atrial electrogram recording. Also, the atria could not be captured by pacing through the atrial epicardial wire electrodes. Thus, the diagnosis of atrial quiescence was established. An intravenous infusion of isoproterenol, 1 μg/min, was then initiated. About 15 minutes after the start of this infusion, slow, spontaneous atrial activity appeared along with evidence of antegrade conduction (**B**). The atria then could be captured by pacing through the atrial wire electrodes (**C**). Several hours later, when atrial pacing was no longer clinically necessary, the patient had a spontaneous atrial rhythm (**D**). EG = electrogram; A = atrial electrogram; V = ventricular electrogram (recorded through the atrial wire electrodes); S = stimulus artifact. Time lines are at one-second intervals. Paper recording speed 50 mm/sec. *(From Waldo et al., 1972b.)*

when there are no P waves in the ECG, an atrial electrogram cannot be recorded, and the atria cannot be paced. Administration of intravenous isoproterenol at a rate of 1 μg/min has been shown to restore atrial excitability with return of spontaneous atrial activity. The atria may then be paced to increase cardiac output, to treat bradyarrhythmias, and to suppress extrasystoles or tachyarrhythmias, thereby improving cardiac performance.

Condenser Discharge (DC) Cardioversion. This mode of therapy has an important place in the treatment of life-threatening reentrant tachyarrhythmias and in the treatment of reentrant tachyarrhythmias refractory to other modes of therapy. Its most urgent use is in the emergency management of ventricular tachycardia and ventricular fibrillation. It is also of great value in the treatment of paroxysmal atrial tachycardias and atrial flutter if atrial pacing is not possible and if drug therapy is either ineffective or would take too long to become effective. Atrial fibrillation usually is effectively treated with cardioversion, commonly in conjunction with quinidine or procainamide therapy. However, if atrial fibrillation has been of long standing prior to surgery (more than one year) or if the atria are very enlarged, the likelihood of converting atrial fibrillation to sinus rhythm and of maintaining the sinus rhythm for any substantial period of time is poor. Therefore, unless there are important reasons for attempting to convert atrial fibrillation to sinus rhythm, it is recommended that such patients not undergo elective cardioversion. For all instances of elective DC cardioversion, digitalis therapy should be stopped for as long as possible (in most instances, at least 36 to 48 hours) before the contemplated time of the procedure. Also, if the patient has been receiving digoxin therapy, a digoxin level should be obtained before the procedure to be certain that unacceptably high levels are not present, and serum potassium should be checked routinely.

Drug Therapy of Arrhythmias

A detailed review of the pharmacology and use of various antiarrhythmic agents is beyond the scope of this chapter. The reader is referred to several standard references (Hoffman and Bigger, 1971; Bigger and Hoffman, 1980) that deal with this subject adequately. However, it is pertinent to make some generalizations about drug use and some suggestions about administration. Additional comments appear in the previous sections.

The most commonly used anti-arrhythmic agents are quinidine, procainamide, disopyramide, lidocaine, phenytoin, and propranolol. The action on the heart of quinidine, procainamide, and disopyramide is essentially identical. Quinidine and disopyramide are excellent drugs, but are limited in that they should not be used parenterally. One advantage of procainamide over quinidine and disopyramide is that the latter two should not be used parenterally. Lidocaine is quite a useful drug, but one disadvantage is that it can only be used parenterally, and almost exclusively intravenously. Phenytoin is a drug whose usefulness is underappreciated, but when used with patience (it may require several days of oral medication to achieve the desirable therapeutic blood levels), it has an important place in the treatment of arrhythmias.

Propranolol rarely has a place in the acute treatment of postoperative arrhythmias, primarily because of its marked negative inotropic effects on the heart. Generally, propranolol's only use is to slow the ventricular response to rapid atrial arrhythmias in which there is a very rapid ventricular rate refractory to the usual forms of treatment, i.e., despite adequate digitalis therapy. In such instances, propranolol is administered to increase A-V block. However, verapamil, recently released in the United States, should supplant this role in most instances. Disopyramide and procainamide should be used with great caution, because renal excretion is their major route of elimination.

Phenytoin and lidocaine are converted to pharmacologically inactive metabolites primarily by the liver, with very little unaltered drug being renally excreted. Therefore, they may be preferable to disopyramide and procainamide in the treatment of arrhythmias in patients with significant renal impairment.

However, phenytoin and lidocaine should be used cautiously or not at all in patients with impaired hepatic function.

When drug treatment of a cardiac arrhythmia is required, an appropriate drug should be selected. It should be carefully administered, especially with regard to dosage, and its therapeutic efficacy should be evaluated only after it has received an appropriate clinical trial. In this regard, it is useful to obtain the blood concentration of the drug to determine whether it is in the desirable therapeutic range. Should the drug prove ineffective, its administration should be terminated and therapy with another drug initiated. If attempts at therapy with one drug at a time in appropriate doses at appropriate intervals has proven ineffective, combined drug therapy may then be tried.

While considerable progress has been made in understanding the cardiac actions of these antiarrhythmic agents, there is insufficient information about their effects when used in combination. As indicated above, the actions on cardiac tissue of procainamide, quinidine and disopyramide should be considered as essentially identical. The actions of phenytoin on cardiac tissues are considerably different and in some ways opposite to those of procainamide, quinidine and disopyramide. Until recently, lidocaine was thought to have effects on cardiac tissue largely similar to those of phenytoin, but it now appears that lidocaine has some actions similar to those of procainamide and quinidine as well. Propranonol has actions on cardiac tissue primarily like those of quinidine, but in some respects has actions similar to phenytoin and lidocaine. Because of these drugs' different actions on cardiac tissue, it should be anticipated that combination drug therapy in the treatment of arrhythmias may produce desirable (complementary or synergistic) effects, undesirable (antagonistic) effects, or indifferent effects. Unfortunately, at this time no reliable body of information exists to guide the physician in the use of drug combinations, and as should be apparent, treatment of cardiac arrhythmias with combinations of antiarrhythmic agents therefore is largely empirical.

When digitalis is being administered for the treatment of a supraventricular arrhythmia with an associated rapid ventricular rate (most commonly atrial fibrillation), it should be administered aggressively until the ventricular response to the atrial arrhythmia is slowed sufficiently or the rhythm reverts to sinus rhythm. This should be accomplished with intravenous administration of the appropriate dose every one to two hours. During this time, the ECG must be carefully monitored for ventricular rate as well as signs of digitalis toxicity. When a digitalis preparation is indicated in the treatment of an arrhythmia, digoxin, rather than other preparations, is recommended. It can be administered orally, intramuscularly, or intravenously (IV). When compared with other preparations, its time to the onset of action is rapid (20 to 30 minutes after IV administration; two hours after oral administration), time to onset of maximal action is relatively rapid (1.5 to 2 hours after IV administration; six hours after oral administration), and its duration of action is relatively short (44 hours half-life; two to seven days duration of action). The latter fact is particularly important should digitalis toxicity appear. Because digoxin is excreted by the kidneys, considerable care should be used when it is required in the presence of impaired renal function.

The following are some suggestions about administration of the drugs just described.

Lidocaine. After an initial intravenous injection of 1 mg/kg every three to five minutes if necessary to a total dose (in adults) of 200 to 300 mg, a constant intravenous infusion of 20 to 50 µg/kg/min should be administered. Doses lower than 20 µg/kg/min are usually ineffective and doses higher than 50 µg/kg/min lead to drowsiness, confusion, and seizures. Also, when a patient has been receiving a constant intravenous infusion of lidocaine for several hours, additional large injections of lidocaine are contraindicated because of the danger of elevating the blood lidocaine concentration to a level that, though transient, will produce seizures. Small injections, generally 10 to 25 mg in adults, may be given carefully if required. Also, since it takes about six hours to achieve a constant blood level after the initiation of a constant intravenous infusion, small additional injections may be required in the early period following initiation of this therapy.

It is a fortunate coincidence that a reasonably accurate estimate of the steady-state plasma concentration of lidocaine can be calculated by dividing the amount of drug infused each minute by a factor of 10. Thus, an infusion rate of 35 µg/kg/min would produce a steady state of 3.5 µg/ml of plasma. Since the usual therapeutic range of plasma concentrations of lidocaine is 2 to 5 µg/ml of plasma, one can then quite easily determine with acceptable accuracy the desired plasma concentration of lidocaine, the usual therapeutic infusion rate ranging from 20 to 50 µg/kg/min. Since lidocaine is primarily metabolized by the liver, it must be given carefully in the presence of any degree of hepatic failure. For instance, in the presence of severe right-sided congestive heart failure with congestion of the liver, usually appropriate doses of lidocaine may result in higher plasma levels than clinically desirable. Therefore, when the drug is administered to patients under these circumstances the appearance of drowsiness or confusion despite ostensibly appropriate dosage should be viewed as a manifestation of toxicity to lidocaine. Finally, lidocaine is generally ineffective in the treatment of supraventricular arrhythmias except when they are secondary to digitalis toxicity.

Procainamide. This drug is best given at least every four hours and more often every three hours to maintain therapeutic blood levels. For adults, the usual oral or intramuscular dose is 500 mg every three to four hours. For intravenous administration, 100 mg initially may be given *slowly* every five minutes up to a total of one gram. For maintenance of intravenous administration of procainamide, 20 to 80 µg/kg/min (1.5 to 5.0 mg/min) may be given. The effective plasma concentration of this drug is 5 to 10 mg/liter. Plasma levels about 10 mg/liter are associated with a significant incidence of toxicity, largely manifested as arrhythmia. Because procainamide's half-life is two to three hours, it should be anticipated that after its chronic oral administration, a steady-state plasma concentration will not be reached for 18 to 24 hours. Thus, adjustment of all doses should be made after at least an 18- to 24-hour trial on the initial dosage, unless there are clear and compelling reasons for doing otherwise. As 50 to 60 percent of procainamide is excreted in the kidneys in an unmetabolized form, it should be given with great care, if at all, in the presence of renal decompensation.

Quinidine. This drug should only be given orally. For adults, 300 to 400 mg every six hours usually is an adequate regimen to obtain therapeutically effective blood levels. The effective plasma concentration is 2.5 to 8.0 mg/liter, using the laboratory method that measures both quinidine and its metabolites. The drug may be therapeutically ineffective when the plasma concentration is at the lower end of the therapeutic range. Above the level of 8 mg/liter, there is a predictable incidence of quinidine toxicity, which manifests itself largely as cardiac arrhythmias. Since quinidine toxicity can produce many of the arrhythmias for which treatment with this drug has been initiated, it is recommended that arrhythmias that persist during quinidine administration or that appear later after quinidine administration be considered a potential manifestation of quinidine toxicity. In such circumstances, quinidine plasma levels should be obtained. Since the plasma half-life of quinidine is about six to seven hours, it will take about one and a half to two days to obtain a steady-state plasma concentration after chronic oral administration. This becomes especially important in manipulating the dosage to control arrhythmias.

It is recommended that the dosage not be adjusted until the drug has been given a trial at the originally selected dose for at least two days, unless there are clear and compelling reasons for doing otherwise. Similarly, it is recommended that the plasma concentration not be obtained for at least 36 to 48 hours after beginning chronic oral administration of the drug, unless one is considering the possibility of quinidine toxicity. Lastly, as 20 to 50 percent of quinidine is excreted in an unmetabolized form by the kidneys, care must be taken to adjust the dosage in the presence of renal disease.

Disopyramide. This anti-arrhythmic drug has become available only recently. It is quinidine-like in terms of its effects on the heart. However, at the time of this writing, in the United States it has only been approved for use in the treatment of ventricular arrhythmias. It holds promise of providing effective treatment for most supraventricular arrhythmias as well. One important effect of the drug, its anticholinergic action, has proved particularly troublesome for some patients, causing urinary retention, visual disturbances, and dry mouth. The usual dose of disopyramide is 100 to 200 mg administered orally every six hours. The drug can be given parenterally, but because of serious negative inotropic effects when administered in this fashion, especially when given intravenously, this should be avoided. Because the half-life of this drug is 6 to 7 hours (range 4 to 10 hours), it should be anticipated that, following the chronic oral administration of disopyramide, a steady-state serum concentration usually will not be reached for 36 to 48 hours. Thus, adjustment of oral dosage usually should be made only after a trial of therapy for at least 36 hours. As 50 percent of this drug is excreted in its unmetabolized form by the kidneys, it should be given only with great care, and then utilizing a reduced dosage schedule, in the presence of renal dysfunction. The effective serum concentration is 2 to 4 mg per liter.

Propranolol. As indicated above, propranolol is rarely a drug of first choice in the treatment of cardiac arrhythmias, especially during the postoperative period, when its marked negative inotropic effects on the heart are undesirable. Propranolol may be given orally or parenterally, usually every four to six hours. For the treatment of arrhythmias, the total oral daily dose varies between 10 and 100 mg. When administered intravenously, 1 mg/min to a total dose of 5 mg is an acceptable regimen. The effective therapeutic plasma concentration for treatment of arrhythmias with this drug is less than 100 ng/ml and usually between 40 and 60 ng/ml. Propranolol is primarily metabolized by the liver.

Digoxin. A reasonable and generaly safe digitalizing dose for patients is 0.9 mg/sq m of body surface area over a 24-hour-period for IV administration, and 1.6 mg/sq m of body surface area for oral administration (Kirklin, 1971). A reasonable method of administering digoxin intravenously to a patient not previously receiving the drug is to give one half to two thirds of the digitalizing dose initially, followed by one sixth of the digitalizing dose every two to four hours until five sixths of the total digitalizing dose has been administered or digitalis toxicity appears. Any sign of digitalis toxicity demands that additional doses be withheld. These doses only serve as a useful guide when digoxin is required in the treatment of supraventricular tachycardias, since control of ventricular rate is the end point for digitalization in this instance.

It is recommended that digoxin be administered intravenously when used to treat supraventricular tachycardias with a rapid ventricular response. Since the goal of digitalization in the treatment of atrial fibrillation is the ventricular rate, this rate and of course the patient's clinical circumstance should guide therapy. For instance, the initial digitalizing dose suggested above may be too large, especially if the ventricular rate is relatively slow (e.g., 100 to 120 beats/min) or if the patient has been receiving digoxin. For this rhythm, a suggested guide to the IV administration of digoxin after an initial dose is as follows: for ventricular rates greater than 160 beats/min give 0.375 to 0.50 mg; for ventricular rates between 140 and 160 beats/min give 0.25 to 0.375 mg; for rates between 110 and 120 beats/min give 0.125 to 0.25 mg. Occasionally, doses as small as 0.0625 mg may be indicated. Using this guide, one can give subsequent doses, if necessary, generally in a range of one to four hours.

It must be emphasized that the amount and frequency of administration of each dose must be somewhat flexible and should be largely determined by the clinical status of the patient as well as the ventricular rate. A satisfactory goal for the postoperative patient is 100 to 105 beats/min. Maintenance doses of digoxin may then be administered to maintain the rate at this level. These doses should be initiated about 6 to 12 hours after achieving the desired ventricular rate, although this time period may vary, depending on ventricular rate. Generally, maintenance digoxin ranges between 0.25 and 0.50 mg in adults, or one eighth of the estimated digitalizing dose. For children, 10 to 15 percent of the estimated digitalizing dose is usually required for a maintenance dose. The maintenance dose may be given in one single daily dose or in divided doses, e.g., twice daily.

ELECTRICAL SAFETY

It is appropriate to end this chapter with some words of caution. First, any electrodes sewn to the heart and brought out through the chest wall are a potential source for the induction of ventricular fibrillation should the electrode come into contact with a ground or stray current source. Therefore, when not in use, the electrode should be electrically isolated. This is perhaps most easily done by securing the electrodes beneath nonconductive tape. When the wire electrodes are being used to record electrical activity from the heart, an isolation device must be placed between the wire electrodes and the recorder, should the recorder itself not be isolated (Weinberg, 1967). Furthermore, when the heart is being paced through the wire electrodes, an isolation device must similarly be used, unless the pacing unit is battery-powered. If these simple procedures are followed at all times, the electrophysiologic techniques described in this chapter can be employed safely and should provide a useful and important clinical tool for improved patient care.

REFERENCES

Arciniegas JG, Klein H, Karp RB, Kouchoukos NT, James TN, Kirklin JW, Waldo AL: Surgical treatment of life-threatening ventricular tachyarrhythmias. Circulation 62:III-42, 1980 (abstr).

Bachmann C: Inter-auricular time interval. Am J Physiol 41:309–320, 1916.

Bigger JT Jr, Heissenbuttel RH: Clinical use of antiarrhythmic drugs. Postgrad Med 47:119–125, 1970.

―――, Hoffman BF: Antiarrhythmic drugs. In Gilman AG, Goodman LS, Gilman A (eds): The Pharmacological Basis of Therapeutics, 6th ed. New York, MacMillan, 1980, pp 761–792.

Bowman FO Jr, Malm JR: The transseptal approach to mitral valve repair. Arch Surg 90:329–331, 1965.

Camm J, Ward DE, Cory-Pearce R, Rees GM, Spurrell RAJ: The successful cryosurgical treatment of paroxysmal venticular tachycardia. Chest 75:621–624, 1979.

Cooley DA, Hallman GL: Atrial septal defect, ventricular septal defect. In Cooley DA, Hall GL (eds): Surgical Treatment of Congenital Heart Disease. Philadelphia, Lea & Febiger, 1966, pp 82–120.

Cooper TB, MacLean WAH, Waldo AL: Overdrive pacing for supraventricular tachycardia. A review of theoretical implications and therapeutic techniques. PACE 1:196–221, 1978.

Cranefield PF: Action potentials, after potentials and arrhythmia. Circ Res 41:415–423, 1977.

―――: Paired pulse stimulation and postextrasystolic potentiation of the heart: Prog Cardiovasc Dis 8:446–460, 1966.

―――, Hoffman BF: The physiologic basis and clinical implications of paired pulse stimulation of the heart. Dis Chest 49:561–567, 1966.

―――, Wit AL, Hoffman BF: The genesis of cardiac arrhythmias. Circulation 47:190–204, 1973.

Davies MI: Pathology of Conducting Tissue of the Heart. New York, Appleton-Century-Crofts, 1971, pp 40–47.

DeSanctis RW: Diagnostic and therapeutic uses of atrial pacing. Circulation 43:748–761, 1971.

Dick M III, van Praagh R, Rudd M, Fulkerth T, Castenada AR: Electrophysiological delineation of the specialized atrioventricular conduction system in two patients with corrected transposition of the great arteries in situs inversus [I,D,D]. Circulation 55:896–1900, 1977.

Dreifus LS, Nichols H, Morse D, Watanabe Y, Truex R: Control of recurrent tachycardia of

Wolff-Parkinson-White syndrome by surgical ligature of the A-V bundle. Circulation 38:1030–1036, 1968.
El-Said G, Rosenberg HS, Mullins CE, Hallman GL, Cooley DA, McNamara DE: Dysrhythmias after Mustard's operation for transposition of the great arteries. Am J Cardiol 30:526–532, 1972.
Eyster JAE, Meek WJ: Experiments on the origin and conduction of the cardiac impulse: VI. Conduction of the excitation from the SA node to the right auricle and A-V node. Arch Intern Med 18:775–799, 1916.
———, ———: Experiments on the origin and propagation of the impulse in the heart: the point of primary negativity in the mammalian heart and the spread of negativity to other regions. Heart 5:119–136, 1913–1914.
Fisher JD, Mehra R, Furman S: Termination of ventricular tachycardia with bursts of rapid ventricular pacing. Am J Cardiol 41:94–102, 1978.
Fontaine G, Guiraudon G, Frank R, Coutte R, Dragodanne C: Epicardial mapping and surgical treatment in six cases of resistant ventricular tachycardia not related to coronary artery disease. In Wellens HJJ, Lie KL, Janes MJ (eds): The Conduction System of the Heart. Philadelphia, Lea & Febiger, 1976, pp 545–563.
———, ———, ———, Vedel J, Grosgogeat Y, Cabrol C, Facquet J: Stimulation studies and epicardial mapping in ventricular tachycardia: study of mechanisms and selection for surgery. In Kulburtus HE (ed): Reentrant Arrhythmias. Mechanisms and Treatment. Baltimore, University Park Press, 1977, pp 333–350.
———, ———, ———: Mechanism of ventricular tachycardia with and without associated chronic myocardial ischemia: Surgical management based on epicardial mapping. In Narula OS (ed): Cardiac Arrhythmias. Electrophysiology, Diagnosis, and Management. Baltimore, Williams & Wilkins, 1979, pp 516–545.
Gallagher JJ: Surgical treatment of arrhythmias. Current status and future directions. Am J Cardiol 41:1035–1044, 1978.
———, Anderson RW, Kasell J, Rice JR, Pritchett ELC, Gault JH, Harrison L, Wallace AG: Cryoblation of drug-resistant ventricular tachycardia in a patient with a varient of scleroderma. Circulation 57:190–197, 1978a.
———, Oldham HN, Wallace AG, Peter RH, Kasell J: Ventricular aneurysm with ventricular tachycardia. Report of a case with epicardial mapping and successful resection. Am J Cardiol 35:696–700, 1975.
———, Pritchett ELC, Sealy WC, et al.: The preexcitation syndromes. Prog Cardiovasc Dis 10:285–327, 1978b.
———, Sealy WC, Cox JL, Kassell J: Results of surgery for preexcitation in 200 cases. Circulation 64:IV-146, 1981 (abstr).
———, ———, Anderson RW, Kasell J, Millar R, Campbell RWF, Harrison L, Pritchett ELC, Wallace AG: Cryosurgical ablation of accessory atrioventricular connections: A new technique for correction of the preexcitation syndrome. Circulation 55:471–479, 1977.
Gelband H, Waldo AL, Kaiser GA, Bowman FO Jr, Malm JR, Hoffman BF: Etiology of right bundle branch block in patients undergoing total correction of tetralogy of Fallot. Circulation 44:1022–1033, 1971.
Guiraudon G, Fontaine G, Frank R, Baehrel B, Bors V, Cabrol C: Encircling endocardial ventriculotomy. A new surgical treatment for life-threatening ventricular tachycardia resistant to medical treatment following myocardial infarction. Ann Thorac Surg 26:438–43, 1978.
———, ———, ———, Escande G, Etievent P, Cabrol C: Encircling endocardial ventriculotomy: A new Surgical treatment for life-threatening ventricular tachycardias resistant to medical treatment following myocardial infarction. Ann Thorac Surg 26:438–444, 1978.
———, ———, ———, Leandri R, Barra J, Cabrol C: Surgical treatment of ventricular tachycardia guided by ventricular mapping in 23 patients without coronary artery disease. Ann Thorac Surg 32:439–450, 1981.
Gulotta S, Aronson AL: Conversion of atrial tachycardia and flutter by atrial stimulation. Am J Cardiol 26:262–269, 1970.
Haft JI, Kosowsky BD, Lau SH, Stein E, Damato AN: Termination of atrial flutter by rapid electrical pacing of the atrium. Am J Cardiol 20:239–244, 1967.
Hariman J, Krongrad H, Boxer RA, Weiss MB, Steeg CN, Hoffman BF: Method for recording electrical activity of the sinoatrial node and automatic atrial foci during cardiac catheterization in human subjects. Am J Cardiol 45:775–781, 1980.
Harken AH, Josephson ME, Horowitz LN: Surgical endocardial resection for the treatment of malignant ventricular tachycardia. Ann Surg 190:456–460, 1979.
Harris PD, Malm JR, Bowman FO Jr, Hoffman BF, Kaiser GA, Singer DH: Epicardial pacing to control arrhythmias following cardiac surgery. Circulation 37 (Suppl II): 178–183, 1968.
———, Singer DH, Malm JR, Hoffman BF: Chroni-

cally implanted cardiac electrodes for diagnostic, therapeutic and investigational use in man. J Thorac Cardiovasc Surg 54:191–198, 1967.

Hodam RP, Starr A: Temporary postoperative epicardial pacing electrodes. Their value and management after open heart surgery. Ann Thorac Surg 8:506–510, 1969.

Hoffman BF, Bigger JT Jr: Antiarrhythmias drugs. In DiPalma JR (ed): Drill's Pharmacology in Medicine, 4th ed: New York, McGraw-Hill, 1971, pp. 824–852.

_____, Cranefield PF: The physiological basis of cardiac arrhythmias. Am J Med 37:670–684, 1964.

_____, Rosen MR, Wit AL: Electrophysiology and pharmacology of cardiac arrhythmias. III. The causes and treatment of cardiac arrhythmias. Part A. Am Heart J 89:115–122, 1975.

_____, _____: Cellular mechanisms for cardiac arrhythmias. Circ Res 49:1–15, 1981.

Holsinger JW Jr, Wallace AG, Sealy WC: Identification and surgical significance of the atrial internodal conduction tracts. Ann Surg 168:447–453, 1968.

Horowitz LN, Harken AH, Kastor JA, Josephson ME: Ventricular resection guided by epicardial and endocardial mapping for treatment of recurrent ventricular tachycardia. N Engl J Med 302:589–593, 1980.

Hudson REB: Surgical pathology of the conducting system of the heart. Br Heart J 29:646–670, 1967.

_____: Cardiovascular Pathology. Baltimore, Williams & Wilkins, 1965, pp 69–84.

_____: The human pacemaker and its pathology. Br Heart J 2:153–167, 1960:

Isaacon R, Titus JL, Merideth J, Feldt RH, McGoon DC: Apparent interruption of atrial conduction pathways after surgical repair of transposition of great arteries. Am J Cardiol 30:533–535, 1972.

James TN: The connecting pathways between the sinus node and A-V node and between the right and left atrium in the human heart. Am Heart J 66:498–508, 1963.

_____. Anatomy of the human sinus node. Anat Rec 141:109–139, 1961a.

_____. Morphology of the human atrioventricular node, with remarks pertinent to its electrophysiology. Am Heart J 62:756–771, 1961b.

Josephson ME, Harken AH, Horowitz LN: Endocardial excision: A new surgical technique for the treatment of recurrent ventricular tachycardia. Circulation 60:1430–1439, 1979.

_____, _____, _____: Long term results of endocardial resection for sustained ventricular tachycardia. Circulation 203:IV–768, 1981.

Kaiser GA, Waldo AL, Beach PM, Bowman FO Jr, Hoffman BF, Malm JR: Specialized cardiac conduction system; improved electrophysiologic identification techniques at surgery. Arch Surg 101:673–676, 1970a.

_____, _____, Bowman FO Jr, Hoffman BF, Malm Jr: The use of ventricular electrograms in operation for coronary artery disease and its complications. Ann Thorac Surg 10:153–162, 1970b.

_____, _____, Harris PD, Bowman FO Jr, Hoffman BF, Malm JR: New method to delineate myocardial damage at surgery. Circulation 39 (Suppl I): 83–89, 1969.

Kehoe R, Moran J, Loeb J, Sanders J, Lesch M, Michaelis L: Visually directed versus electrically directed endocardial resection in recurrent ventricular tachycardia. Circulation 64:321, 1981 (abstr).

Kirklin JW: Circulation and cardiac failure. In Kinney JM, Egdahl RH, Zuidema GD (eds): Manual of Preoperative and Postoperative Care. Philadelphia, Saunders, 1971, pp 195–210.

Kistin AD: Observations on the anatomy of the atrioventricular bundle (bundle of His) and the question of other vascular atrioventricular connections in normal human hearts. Am Heart J 37:849–867, 1949.

Klein HH, Karp, RB, Kouchoukos NT, Zorn GLJr, James TN, Waldo AL: Intraoperative electrophysiological mapping of the ventricles during sinus rhythm in patients with a previous myocardial infarction. Identification of the electrophysiological substrate for the generation of ventricular arrhythmias. Circulation, in press.

Kluger JD, Gillette PC, Duff DF, Cooley DA, McNamara DG: Elective mapping and surgical division of the bundle of Kent in a patient with Epstein's anomaly who required tricuspid valve replacement. Am J Cardiol 41:602–605, 1978.

Krongrad E, Hefler SE, Bowman FO Jr, Malm JR, Hoffman BF: Further observations on the etiology of the RBBB pattern following right ventriculotomy. Circulation 50:1105–1113, 1974a.

_____, Waldo AL, Bowman FO Jr, Hoffman BF, Malm JR: Electrophysiological delineation of the specialized A-V conduction system in patients with congenital heart disease. II. The distal His bundle and right bundle branch. Circulation 49:1232–1238, 1974b.

_____, _____, Kaiser GA, Bowman FO Jr, Hoffman BF, Malm Jr: Electrophysiological delineation of the specialized A-V conduction system in patients with congenital heart disease. I. The His Bundle. J Thorac Cardiovasc Surg 67:875–

882, 1974c.

Kupersmith J: Electrophysiological mapping during open heart surgery. Prog Cardiovasc Dis 19:167–202, 1976.

———, Krongrad E, Gersony WM, Bowman FO Jr: Electrophysiologic identification of the specialized conduction system in corrected transposition of the great arteries. Circulation 50:795–800, 1974.

Lev M, Fell EH, Arcilla R, Weinberg MH: Surgical injury to the conduction system in ventricular septal defect. Am J Cardiol 14:464–476, 1964.

Lister JW, Cohen LS, Bernstein WH, Samet P: Treatment of supraventricular tachycardia by rapid atrial stimulation. Circulation 38:1044–1059, 1968.

Litwak RS, Kuhn LA, Gadboys HL, Lukban SB, Sakurai H: Support of myocardial performance after open cardiac operations by rate augmentation. J Thorac Cardiovasc Surg 56:484–496, 1968.

MacLean WAH, Cooper TV, Waldo AL: Use of cardiac electrodes in the diagnosis and treatment of tachyarrhythmias. Cardiovasc Med 3:965–980, 1978.

———, Plumb VJ, Waldo AL: Transient entrainment and interruption of ventricular tachycardia. PACE 4:358–366, 1981.

Maloney JD, Ritter DG, McGoon DC, Danielson GK: Identification of the conduction system in corrected transposition and common ventricle at operation. Mayo Clin Proc 50:387–394, 1975.

Massing GK, James TN: Anatomical configuration of the His bundle and bundle branches in the human heart. Circulation 53:609–621, 1976.

———, Liebman J, James TN: Cardiac conduction pathways in the infant and child. Cardiovasc Clin 4:27–42, 1972.

Merideth J, Titus JL: The anatomic atrial connections between sinus and A-V node. Circulation 37:566–579, 1968.

Moran JM, Talano JF, Euler D, Moran JF, Montoya A, Pifarre R: Refractory ventricular arrhythmia: the role of intraoperative electrophysiological study. Surgery 82:809–815, 1977.

Murphy DA, Tynan M, Graham GR, Bonham-Carter RE: Prognosis of complete atrioventricular dissociation in children after open heart surgery. Lancet 1:750–752, 1970.

Narula OS, Scherlag BJ, Samet P, Javier RP. Atrioventricular block. Localization and classification by His bundle recordings. Am J Med 50:146–165, 1971.

O'Keeffe DB, Curry PVL, Prior AL, Yates AK, Deverall PB, Sowton E: Surgery for ventricular tachycardia using operative pace mapping. Br Heart J 43:116, 1980 (abstr).

Plumb VJ, Karp RB, James TN, Waldo AL: Atrial excitability and conduction during rapid atrial pacing. Circulation 63:1140–1149, 1981.

Reemtsma K, Delgardo JP, Creech O: Heart block following intracardiac surgery: localization of conduction tissue injury. J Thorac Cardiovasc Surg 39:688–693, 1960.

Resnikov L: Electrical slowing of the heart and post-extrasystolic potentiation. Med Clin North Am 54:247–259, 1970.

Rosen MR, Reder RF: Does triggered activity have a role in the genesis of cardiac arrhythmias? Ann Int Med 94:794–801, 1981.

Rothberger CJ, Scherf D: Zur Kenntnis der Erregungsausbreitung von Sinusknoten auf den Vorhf. Z Gesamte Exp Med 53:792–835, 1927.

Sealy WC, Gallagher JJ, Wallace AG: The surgical treatment of Wolff-Parkinson-White syndrome: evolution of improved methods for identification and interruption of the Kent bundle. Ann Thorac Surg 22:433–457, 1976.

Spencer FC: Atrial septal defect, anomalous pulmonary veins and atrioventricular canal. In Spencer FC (ed): Surgery of the Chest. Philadelphia, Saunders, 1969, pp 688–709.

Titus JL, Daugherty GW, Kirklin JW, Edwards JE: Lesions of the atrioventricular conduction system after the repair of ventricular septal defect. Circulation 28:82–88, 1963.

Truex RC, Smyth MQ: Recent observations on the human cardiac conduction system with special considerations of the atrioventricular node and bundle. In Taccardi B, Marchetti G (eds): Electrophysiology of the Heart. New York, Pergamon Press, 1965, pp 177–201.

Tung KSK, James TN, Effler DB, McCormack LJ: Injury of the sinus node in open heart operations. J Thorac Cardiovasc Surg 53:814–829, 1967.

Vassalle M, Hoffman BF: Spread of sinus activation during potassium administration. Circ Res 17:285–295, 1965.

Vergara GS, Hildner FJ, Schoenfeld CB, Javier RP, Cohen LS, Samet P: Conversion of supraventricular tachycardias with rapid atrial pacing. Circulation 46:788–793, 1972.

Wagner ML, Lazzara R, Weiss RM, Hoffman BF: Specialized conducting fibers in the interatrial band. Circ Res 18:502–518, 1966.

Waldo AL: Limitations of electrocardiograms. Chest 68:482, 1975.

———, Bush HL Jr, Gelband H, Zorn GL Jr, Vitikainen KJ, Hoffman BF: Effects of the canine P wave of the discrete lesions in the specialized atrial tracts. Circ Res 29:452–467, 1971a.

———, James TN: The cardiac conduction system. Electrophysiological mapping during cardiac surgery. Arch Intern Med 135:411–417, 1975.

———, Kaiser GA, Bowman FO Jr, Malm JR: The etiology of prolongation of the P-R interval in patients with an endocardial cushion defect: further observations on internodal conduction and the polarity of the retrograde P wave. Circulation 48:19–26, 1973.

———, Krongrad E, Bowman FO Jr, Kaiser GA, Husson GS, Malm JR: Electrophysiological considerations during total repair of transposition of the great vessels. Circulation 46 (Suppl II): 34, 1972a.

———, ———, Kupersmith J, Levine OR, Bowman FO Jr, Hoffman BF: Ventricular paired pacing to control rapid ventricular heart rate following open heart surgery: observations on ectopic automaticity. Report of a case in a four-month-old patient. Circulation 53:176–181, 1976a.

———, MacLean WAH, Cooper TB, Kouchoukos NT, Karp RB: The use of temporarily placed epicardial atrial wire electrodes for the diagnosis and treatment of cardiac arrhythmias following open heart surgery. J Thorac Cardiovasc Surg 76:500–505, 1978.

———, ———, Karp RB, Kouchoukos NT, James TN: Entrainment and interruption of atrial flutter with atrial pacing. Studies in man following open heart surgery. Circulation 56:737–745, 1977a.

———, ———, ———, ———, ———: Sequence of retrograde atrial activation of the human heart. Correlation with P wave polarity. Br Heart J 39:634–640, 1977b.

———, ———, ———, ———, ———: Continuous rapid atrial pacing to control recurrent or sustained supraventricular tachycardias following open heart surgery. Circulation 54:245–250, 1976b.

———, Pacifico AD, Bargeron LM Jr, James TN, Kirklin JW: Electrophysiological delineation of the specialized A-V conduction system in patients with corrected transposition of the great vessels and ventricular septal defect. Circulation 52:435–441, 1975a.

———, Ross SM, Kaiser GA: The epicardial electrogram in the diagnosis of cardiac arrhythmias following cardiac surgery. Geriatrics 26:108–112, 1971b.

———, Vitikainen KJ, Harris PD, Malm JR, Hoffman BF: Mechanism of synchronization in isorhythmic A-V dissociation: some observations on the morphology and polarity of the P wave during retrograde capture of the atria. Circulation 38:880–898, 1968.

———, ———, Hoffman BF: The sequence of retrograde atrial activation in the canine heart. Correlation with positive and negative retrograde P wave. Circ Res 37:156–163, 1975b.

———, ———, Kaiser GA, Bowman FO Jr, Malm JR: Atrial standstill secondary to atrial inexcitability (atrial quiescence); recognition and treatment following open-heart surgery. Circulation 46:690–697, 1972b.

———, ———, ———, Malm JR, Hoffman BF: The P wave and P-R interval: effects of the site of origin of atrial depolarization. Circulation 42:653–671, 1970.

Waldo Al, Wells JLJr, Cooper TB, MacLean WAH: Temporary cardiac pacing. Applications and techniques in the treatment of cardiac arrhythmias. Prog Cardiovasc Dis 23:451–473, 1981.

Waldo AL, Arciniegas JG, Klein H: Surgical treatment of life-threatening ventricular arrhythmias: The role of intraoperative mapping and consideration of the presently available surgical techniques. Prog Cardiovasc Dis 23:247–264, 1981.

Weinberg DI: Electrical safety in the operating room and at the bedside. In Segal BL, Kirkpatrick DG (eds): Engineering in the Practice of Medicine. Baltimore, Williams & Wilkins, 1967, pp 63–74.

Wells, JL Jr, Karp RB, Kouchoukos NT, MacLean WAH, James TN, Waldo AL: Characterization of atrial fibrillation in man. Studies following open heart surgery. PACE 1:426–438, 1978.

———, MacLean WAH, James TN, Waldo AL: Characterization of atrial flutter. Studies in man following open heart surgery using fixed atrial electrodes. Circulation 60:665–673, 1979.

Weiner I, Mindich B, Pitchon R: Determinants of ventricular tachycardia in patients with ventricular aneurysms: Results of intraoperative epicardial and endocardial mapping. Circulation 64:IV–88, 1981 (abstr).

Wit AL, Rosen MR, Hoffman BF: Electrophysiological pharmacology of cardiac arrhythmias. II. Relationship of normal and abnormal electrical activity of cardiac fibers to the genesis of arrhythmias. A. Automaticity. Am Heart J 88:515–524, 1974a.

———, ———, ———: Electrophysiology and pharmacology of cardiac arrhythmias. II. Relationship of normal and abnormal electrical activity of cardiac fibers to the gensis of arrhythmias.

B. Re-entry. Section I. Am Heart J 88:664–670, 1974b.

———, ———, ———: Electrophysiology and pharmacology of cardiac arrhythmias. II. Relationship of normal and abnormal electrical activity of cardiac fibers to the genesis of arrhythmias. B. Re-entry. Section II. Am Heart J 88:798–806, 1974c.

Wittig JH, Boineau JP: Surgical treatment of ventricular arrhythmias using epicardial, transmural, and endocardial mapping. Ann Thorac Surg 20:117–126, 1975.

Wolff GS, Rowland TW, Ellison RC: Surgically induced right bundle branch block with left anterior hemiblock; an ominous sign in postoperative tetralogy of Fallot. Circulation 46:587–594, 1972.

Woodson RD, Starr A: Atrial pacing after mitral valve surgery. Arch Surg 97:984, 1968.

Zeft HJ, Cobb FR, Waxman MB, Hunt NC, Morris JJ: Right atrial stimulation in the treatment of atrial flutter. Ann Intern Med 70:447–456, 1969.

RECOMMENDED READING

Bigger JT Jr, Hoffman BF: Antiarrythmic drugs. In Gilman AG, Goodman LS, Gilman A (eds): The Pharmacological Basis of Therapeutics. 6th Edition, MacMillan Publishing Company, New York, 1980, pp 761–792.

Hoffman BF, Bigger JT Jr: Antiarrhythmic drugs. In DiPalma JR (ed): Drill's Pharmacology in Medicine, 4th ed: New York, McGraw-Hill, 1971, pp 824–852.

Hudson REB: The conducting system. In Hudson REB (ed): Cardiovascular Pathology. Baltimore, Williams & Wilkins, 1970, Vol 3, pp S.57–S.142.

———: The conducting system. In Hudson REB (ed): Cardiovascular Pathology. Baltimore, Williams & Wilkins, 1965, pp 53–145.

James TN: Anatomy of the conduction system of the heart. In Hurst JW, Logue RB (eds): The Heart, 2nd ed. New York, McGraw-Hill, 1976, pp 47–58.

Marriott HJL: Practical Electrocardiography, 6th ed. Baltimore, Williams & Wilkins, 1976.

Waldo AL, MacLean WAH: Diagnosis and Treatment of Arrhythmias Following Open Heart Surgery—Emphasis on the Use of Epicardial Wire Electrodes. Mt. Kisco, NY, Futura, 1980.

Weinberg DI: Electrical safety in the operating room and at the bedside. In Segal BL, Kirkpatrick DG (eds): Engineering in the Practice of Medicine: Baltimore, Williams & Wilkins, 1967, pp 63–74.

11. Lung Function Following Open Heart Surgery

MYRON B. LAVER

The magnitude of impaired blood-gas exchange following open heart surgery is closely related to the adequacy of hemodynamic function. With few exceptions, limitation of pulmonary function results from acute or chronic congestive heart failure and its consequences. Occasionally, the chronic pulmonary venous hypertension of mitral valve disease may be associated with chronic bronchitis, particularly in the heavy smoker. In this setting, preoperative evaluation of lung function may not succeed in separating the respective contributions of heart or intrinsic lung disease, and a decision as to which component is most important postoperatively may not be possible.

Inappropriate hemodynamic function implies abnormal blood-gas exchange, and the years of experience with open heart surgery suggest that mechanical support immediately after the operation has supportive rather than therapeutic value.

Three factors determine the blood-gas exchange response to a change in airway pressure: lung geometry, cardiac output, and oxygen consumption. Manipulation of any or all of these variables will have a significant effect on the state of oxygenation. Each will be examined in detail in the sections to follow.

FACTORS THAT INFLUENCE OXYGENATION

Effectiveness of arterial oxygenation is determined by the relationship between ventilation and perfusion. Normally, alveolar ventilation at rest is 4 liters per minute and perfusion (or cardiac output), 5 liters per minute, with a resulting overall ratio of 0.8. This ratio must also equal CO_2 production ($\dot{V}co_2$) (ml/min) divided by O_2 consumption ($\dot{V}o_2$) (ml/min). If the amount of CO_2 produced per minute as determined by overall metabolic processes remains constant, an increase in ventilation will result in a transient excessive wash-out of CO_2, and $\dot{V}co_2$ will appear to rise as arterial Pco_2 declines. Once an equilibrium point is reached, $\dot{V}co_2$ will return to control values while arterial Pco_2 remains low. If minute ventilation increases but alveolar ventilation ($\dot{V}_A$) remains constant, the "efficiency" of ventilation will be reduced. The effect is tantamount to an addition of dead space.

Similarly, efficiency of oxygenation may be impaired by any process that influences lung geometry. Closure of a terminal air unit, or nonventilation, is associated with only slight diminution in perfusion, thereby adding a substantial quantity of mixed venous blood (right-to-left shunt, also known as venous admixture) to that portion of cardiac output that is being oxygenated. Expressed in simple terms, if one fourth of cardiac output or pulmonary blood flow remains unoxygenated, cardiac output must rise by 25 percent if oxygen uptake is to be maintained (Fig. 11-1).

Although the focus of therapy has been principally to sustain adequate arterial oxygenation with ventilator assistance, little will be gained unless the relationship between blood flow (cardiac output), oxygen uptake ($\dot{V}O_2$), and the arterial-mixed venous oxygen content difference (a=$\bar{v}O_2$) is clearly kept in mind. The major drawback of any measure intended to assess the appropriateness of oxygenation is our inability to define the limits of adequate oxygen demand as contrasted to O_2 uptake. This is a particularly difficult decision to make whenever changes in body temperature, sepsis, and autonomic activity are evident, as in the early postoperative period (Gump et al., 1971).

For example, a rise or fall in blood flow is commonly followed by a concomitant change in oxygen uptake in patients with acute respiratory insufficiency (Fig. 11-2). Most organs, such as the heart, kidney, brain, or liver, demonstrate a dependency of steady-state oxygen consumption on the Po_2 of its perfusate (Caldwell and Wittenberg, 1974). In fact, the myocardium may require greater quantities of O_2 per unit time in the face

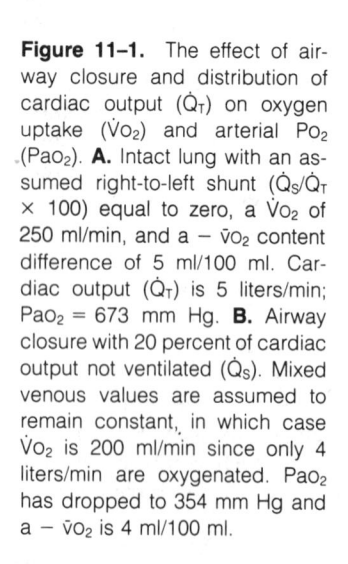

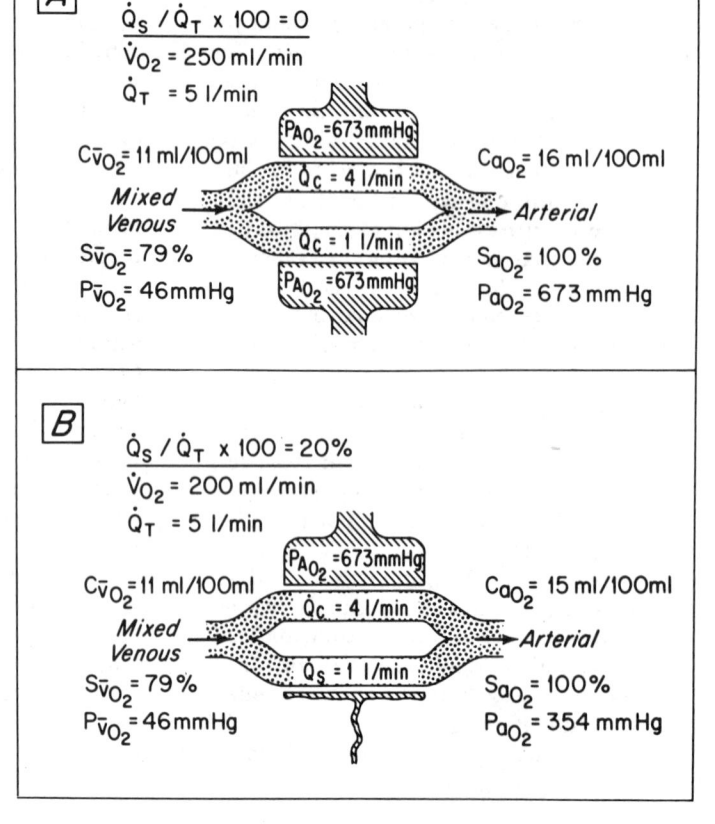

Figure 11-1. The effect of airway closure and distribution of cardiac output ($\dot{Q}_T$) on oxygen uptake ($\dot{V}O_2$) and arterial Po_2 (Pao_2). **A.** Intact lung with an assumed right-to-left shunt ($\dot{Q}_S/\dot{Q}_T \times 100$) equal to zero, a $\dot{V}O_2$ of 250 ml/min, and a $-\bar{v}O_2$ content difference of 5 ml/100 ml. Cardiac output ($\dot{Q}_T$) is 5 liters/min; Pao_2 = 673 mm Hg. **B.** Airway closure with 20 percent of cardiac output not ventilated ($\dot{Q}_S$). Mixed venous values are assumed to remain constant, in which case $\dot{V}O_2$ is 200 ml/min since only 4 liters/min are oxygenated. Pao_2 has dropped to 354 mm Hg and a $-\bar{v}O_2$ is 4 ml/100 ml.

C

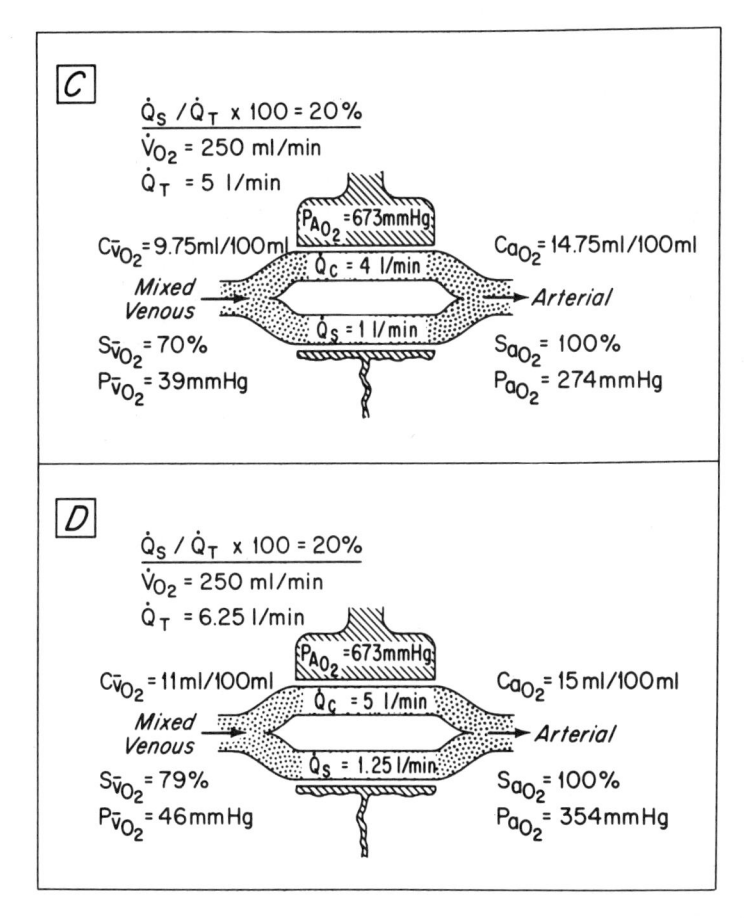

$\dot{Q}_S / \dot{Q}_T \times 100 = 20\%$
$\dot{V}_{O_2} = 250$ ml/min
$\dot{Q}_T = 5$ l/min
$P_{A_{O_2}} = 673$ mmHg
$C\bar{v}_{O_2} = 9.75$ ml/100 ml
$\dot{Q}_C = 4$ l/min
$Ca_{O_2} = 14.75$ ml/100 ml
Mixed Venous → Arterial
$\dot{Q}_S = 1$ l/min
$S\bar{v}_{O_2} = 70\%$
$Sa_{O_2} = 100\%$
$P\bar{v}_{O_2} = 39$ mmHg
$Pa_{O_2} = 274$ mmHg

D

$\dot{Q}_S / \dot{Q}_T \times 100 = 20\%$
$\dot{V}_{O_2} = 250$ ml/min
$\dot{Q}_T = 6.25$ l/min
$P_{A_{O_2}} = 673$ mmHg
$C\bar{v}_{O_2} = 11$ ml/100 ml
$\dot{Q}_C = 5$ l/min
$Ca_{O_2} = 15$ ml/100 ml
Mixed Venous → Arterial
$\dot{Q}_S = 1.25$ l/min
$S\bar{v}_{O_2} = 79\%$
$Sa_{O_2} = 100\%$
$P\bar{v}_{O_2} = 46$ mmHg
$Pa_{O_2} = 354$ mmHg

Figure 11-1 (Cont.) **C.** Airway closure as in **B**, but the mixed venous O_2 content ($C\bar{v}_{O_2}$) has dropped from 11 to 9.75 ml/100 ml and $\dot{V}_{O_2}$ is returned to 250 ml/min despite a constant $\dot{Q}_S/\dot{Q}_T \times 100$ and $\dot{Q}_T$. Pa_{O_2} has dropped further to 274 mm Hg because of the lower mixed venous O_2 content. **D.** Mixed venous O_2 content as in **A**, but $\dot{Q}_T$ has increased to 6.25 liters/min and distributed in a ratio of 4:1 between open and closed airway. $\dot{V}_{O_2}$ is 250 ml/min. Arterial Po_2 is 354 mm Hg, as in **B**.

The "adequacy" of oxygenation has generally been evaluated by calculation of the product between $\dot{Q}_T$ and arterial O_2 content ($C\bar{v}_{O_2}$). As the figures show, this product has little relevance, being reduced in **C** despite a normal $\dot{V}_{O_2}$ uptake and normal in **B** despite a reduction in $\dot{V}_{O_2}$. Oxygen uptake under these conditions is not equal to oxygen demand. The latter is extremely difficult to define.

of progressive arterial hypoxia (Powers and Powell, 1973).

Despite the complex morphologic basis of alveolar-capillary gas exchange (Weibel, 1973), practical criteria for evaluation of lung performance can be set whenever respiratory insufficiency is present or suspected (Pontoppidan et al., 1973; Wilson, 1974; Laver et al., 1975), but they must never be taken out of context of the patient's hemodynamic or metabolic status.

The relationship between cardiac output, $\dot{V}_{O_2}$, and arterial Po_2 (Pa_{O_2}) defined by the shunt equation* is shown in Figure 11-3. When the right-to-left shunt is of moderate

---

*The shunt equation quantifies the percentage of cardiac output ($\dot{Q}_T$) that perfuses the lung but is not oxygenated ($\dot{Q}_S$). It is expressed by the following formula, whose derivation is given elsewhere (Bendixen et al., 1965; Laver et al., 1975):

$$\frac{\dot{Q}_S}{\dot{Q}_T} = \frac{Cc_{O_2} - Ca_{O_2}}{Cc_{O_2} - C\bar{v}_{O_2}}$$

Cc_{O_2}, Ca_{O_2}, and $C\bar{v}_{O_2}$ are the pulmonary capillary, arterial, and mixed venous O_2 contents (ml/100 ml), respectively. This ratio is influenced by the inspired O_2 concentration, or $F_{I_{O_2}}$. Many authors refer to $\dot{Q}_S/\dot{Q}_T \times 100$ as the percent shunt when 100 percent O_2 is the inspired gas ($F_{I_{O_2}} = 1.0$) and prefer the designation $\dot{Q}_{VA}/\dot{Q}_T \times 100$ when $F_{I_{O_2}}$ is less than 1.0.

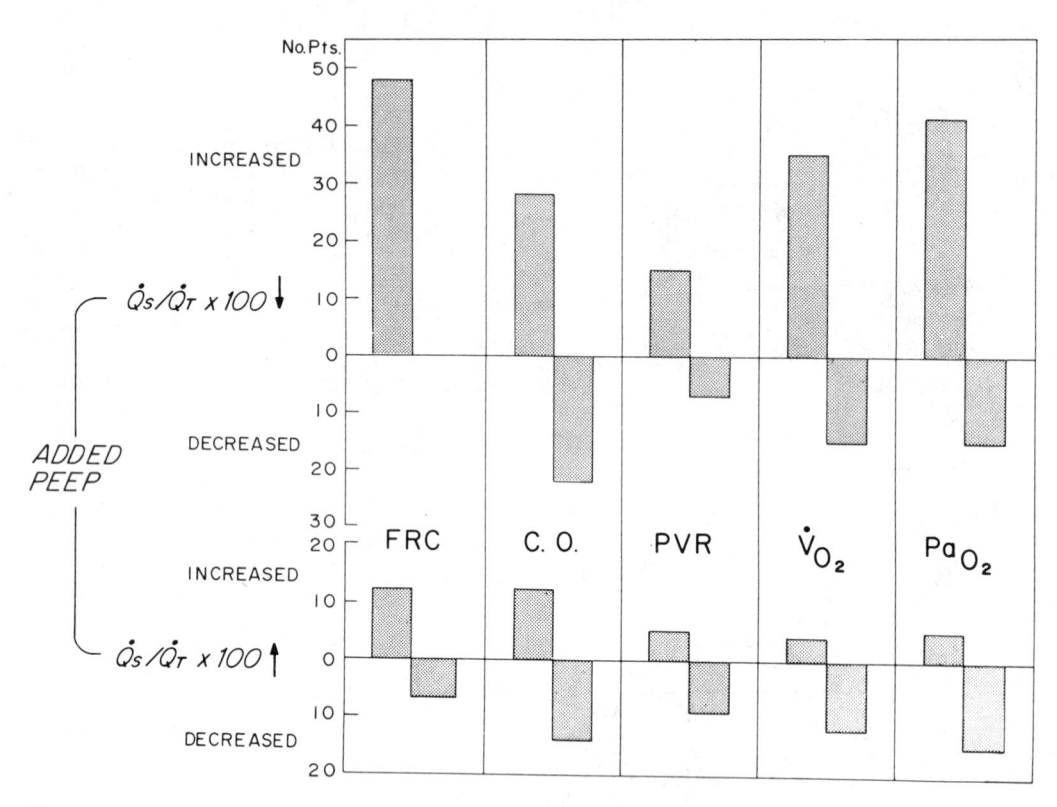

Figure 11–2. Effect of mechanical ventilation with PEEP on functional residual capacity (FRC), cardiac output (CO), pulmonary vascular resistance (PVR), O_2 uptake ($\dot{V}O_2$), and arterial P_{O_2} (PaO_2) in patients with acute respiratory insufficiency. The patients were divided into groups according to the response of $\dot{Q}_S/\dot{Q}_T \times 100$. When $\dot{Q}_S/\dot{Q}_T \times 100$ decreased (↓), FRC rose in all patients; the remaining measurements varied, increasing in some patients and decreasing in others. In a few patients, addition of PEEP caused $\dot{Q}_S/\dot{Q}_T$ to rise (↑). Variability in the response was maintained. Note that in well over half the patients, CO and $\dot{V}O_2$ rose upon an increase in airway pressure. *(Modified and reproduced with permission from Powers, S R, Jr, et al. Physiologic consequences of positive end-expiratory pressure (PEEP) ventilation. Ann Surg 178:265–272, 1973.)*

size (e.g., when 25 percent of cardiac output perfuses nonventilating alveoli), a rise in cardiac output from 2 to 4 or even 6 liters per minute will be accompanied by a striking rise in arterial P_{O_2} (determined during a period of breathing 100 percent oxygen). On the other hand, the effect of a rise in cardiac output on arterial P_{O_2} becomes increasingly limited as $\dot{Q}_S/\dot{Q}_T$ rises above 40 percent, a value not uncommon in acute respiratory insufficiency.

Close examination of Figure 11–1 presents certain intriguing relationships between the oxygenation function of the lung and the expected response by the cardiac output. We have indicated above that a loss of efficiency in oxygenation must be accompanied either by an increase in cardiac output or a *decrease* in the mixed venous oxygen content if the requirements of oxygen demand are to be met. A wealth of circumstantial evidence suggests that despite wide variability in individual organ venous O_2 contents, the mixed venous value can vary only within small limits. If this is indeed true, an increase in blood flow to nonventilated air units must be associated with a corresponding rise in cardiac output,

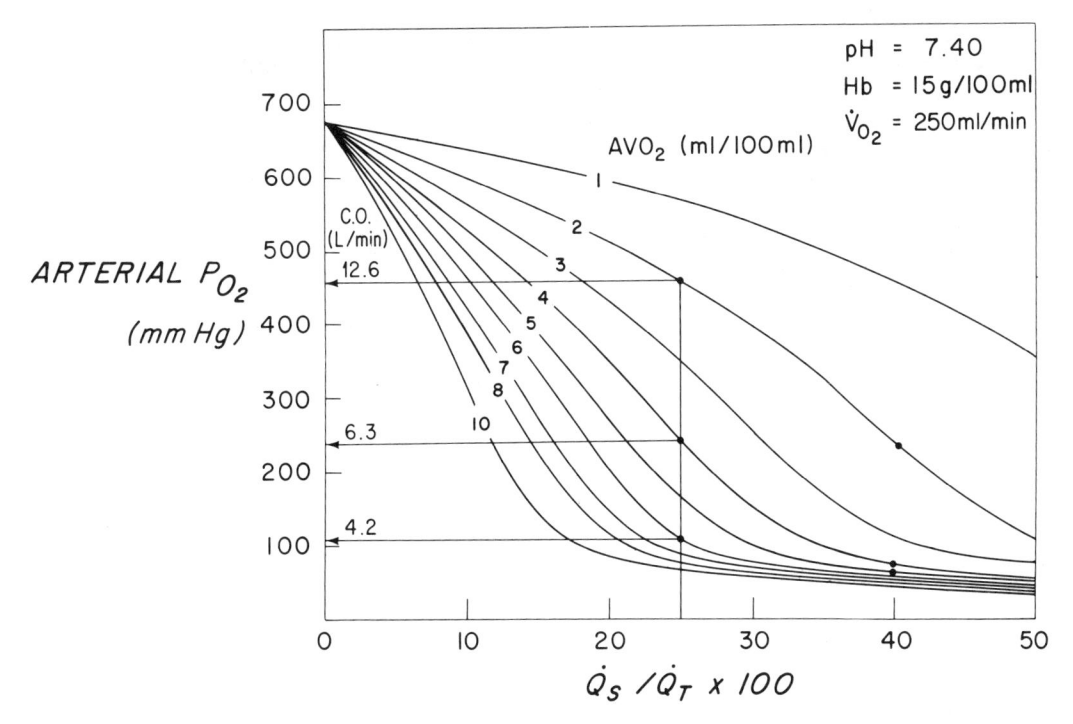

Figure 11-3. Effect of changes in cardiac output (reflected by a change in the $a - \bar{v}_{O_2}$ content difference with $\dot{V}_{O_2}$ remaining constant) on arterial P_{O_2} at a moderate and high $\dot{Q}_S/\dot{Q}_T \times 100$. When $Q_S/\dot{Q}_T \times 100$ is 25 percent, a rise in CO from 4.2 to 12.6 liters/min will increase Pa_{O_2} from 110 to 460 mm Hg. At $\dot{Q}_S/\dot{Q}_T \times 100$ of 40 percent, a rise in CO from 4.2 to 6.3 will have a minimal effect on Pa_{O_2}. If cardiac output rises to 12.6 liters/min, Pa_{O_2} will increase from approximately 70 to 230 mm Hg. *(Modified and reproduced with permission from Laver M B, & Austen W G: Lung function: Physiologic considerations applicable to surgery. In Sabiston, D C, Jr (ed), Davis-Christopher Textbook of Surgery. 10th ed. Philadelphia: Saunders, 1972.)*

the rise being regulated by the need to keep arterial blood fully oxygenated.

Such a relationship is easily recognized from the shunt equation, in which total blood flow ($\dot{Q}_T$) equals the sum of blood flow to ventilated ($\dot{Q}_C$) and nonventilated ($\dot{Q}_S$) portions of the lung. If all blood flow is oxygenated (i.e., when $\dot{Q}_T = \dot{Q}_C$), then

$$\dot{V}_{O_2} = \dot{Q}_C (Cc_{O_2} - C\bar{v}_{O_2})$$

where Cc_{O_2} is equal to O_2 content of pulmonary capillary blood, and $C\bar{v}_{O_2}$ is equal to O_2 content of mixed venous blood.

If oxygen uptake is to remain constant in the presence of respiratory failure in which blood flow is partitioned between ventilated and nonventilated lung, either total flow ($\dot{Q}_T$) must rise by the quantity not oxygenated ($\dot{Q}_S$) or the mixed O_2 content ($C\bar{v}_{O_2}$) must drop to account for the diminished $\dot{Q}_C$ (see Fig. 11-1). For example, assume that under normal circumstances $\dot{Q}_T = \dot{Q}_C = 5$ liters/min. If 20 percent of this flow is not oxygenated, flow to ventilated lung must rise by an equal amount, or from 4 to 5 liters/min to keep $\dot{V}_{O_2}$ constant. If distribution of blood flow remains constant, $\dot{Q}_S$ must also increase by an equivalent amount, or from 1 to 1.25 liters/min, and total flow ($\dot{Q}_S + \dot{Q}_C$) will be 6.25 liters/min. As a matter of fact, the change consists of a combination of a rise in blood flow with a decrease in the mixed venous O_2 content. The details of these arguments are shown in Figure 11–1.

Two important conclusions may be drawn from these considerations. First, that cardiac output must rise in the face of acute respiratory failure, and second, that this rise is possible only if conditions in the pulmonary vasculature continue to be such that a rise is possible, i.e., if pulmonary vascular resistance (PVR) remains low.* Preexisting high PVR, as in chronic mitral valve disease, precludes this response, and right, not left, ventricular function will determine appropriate adjustment to the hemodynamic consequences of postoperative respiratory failure.

As we have stated, the requirements of oxygen demand can be met by an appropriate increase in cardiac output combined with a decrease in the mixed venous O_2 content. When an increase in blood flow is impossible, the latter becomes an important adaptive mechanism, as in chronic congestive heart failure. Unfortunately, it does not appear as a potential source for compensation secondary to acute pulmonary dysfunction.

The causes of respiratory insufficiency soon after open heart surgery are listed in Table 11–1. Most frequently, these abnormalities are related to the presence of congestive heart failure or structural changes in the pulmonary vasculature secondary to congenital or acquired heart disease. A simplified diagram of vascular patterns that may ultimately affect blood flow is shown in Figure 11–4. Their presence may distort the $\dot{V}/\dot{Q}$ relationship to a point where the changes in oxygenation predicted by the acute appearance of left ventricular failure are no longer apparent. This is of particular importance in the patient with pulmonary hypertension and an elevated PVR secondary to chronic mitral valve disease (Harrison, 1958; Trichet et al., 1975).

An increase in right ventricular afterload (represented in part by pulmonary vascular resistance) precludes a spontaneous rise in RV stroke volume.

TABLE 11–1 CAUSES OF ACUTE RESPIRATORY INSUFFICIENCY AFTER OPEN HEART SURGERY

I. Hemodynamic
   A. Left ventricular dysfunction with left atrial hypertension
   B. Intrapulmonary bleeding
      1. After repair of tetralogy of Fallot
      2. Thoracic aortic aneurysm
   C. Sepsis:
      1. Extrapulmonary
      2. Intrapulmonary
   D. Severe vasoconstrictive pulmonary hypertension
   E. Massive blood transfusion
   F. Hypersensitivity response to infused white cells

II. Mechanical
   A. Inappropriate pattern of ventilation
   B. Limitation of diaphragmatic motion
      1. Phrenic nerve palsy
      2. Peritoneal dialysis

An acute rise in left atrial pressure will result in the accumulation of water, first in the extravascular compartment of the dependent lung, rising to the apex if pulmonary venous hypertension persists. When fluid passes into alveoli, their geometric stability is impaired, leading to a marked reduction in alveolar volume (Staub et al., 1967). A fluid-filled alveolus is perfused, not ventilated, and is a source of diminished arterial oxygenation (Burnham et al., 1972). Thus, acute left ventricular failure is characterized by arterial hypoxemia, treatable by improvement of left ventricular function and increased airway pressure to ensure patency of the jeopardized terminal air unit (Ayres, 1973; Trichet et al., 1975).

The patient with mitral valve disease and pulmonary hypertension may not exhibit this pattern. First, chronicity of pulmonary venous hypertension results in altered vascular histology, predominantly in the dependent lung (Harrison, 1958). Perfusion of the lung is reversed, with a major portion of blood flow to apex, not base. If high left atrial pressures

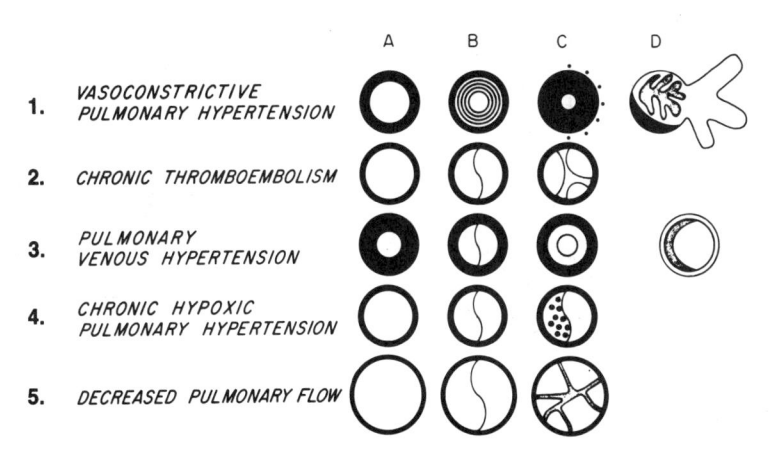

Figure 11–4. A simplified schematic representation of pulmonary vessels with characteristic lesions in several types of pulmonary vascular disease. Outer darkened circle is the medial layer of muscular pulmonary arteries; inner circles represent internal layer of these vessels. Vessel shown at right (**3D**) is representative of a pulmonary vein. **1** = vasoconstrictive pulmonary hypertension with medial hypertrophy (**A**), concentric laminar intimal fibrosis (**B**), necrosis with or without fibrinoid arteritis (**C**), and plexiform lesion (**D**). **2** = chronic thromboembolism with mild medial hypertrophy (**A**), eccentric intimal fibrosis (**B**), and intraluminal fibrous septa (**C**). **3** = pulmonary venous hypertension with severe medial hypertrophy (**A**), eccentric (**B**) or concentric (**C**) but nonlaminar intimal fibrosis with arterialization and intimal fibrosis of pulmonary veins (**D**). **4** = chronic hypoxic pulmonary hypertension with normal media (**A**), eccentric intimal fibrosis (**B**), and longitudinal muscle bundles in the intima (**C**). **5** = decreased pulmonary blood flow with wide arteries and medial atrophy (**A**), eccentric intimal fibrosis (**B**), and intraluminal fibrous septa (**C**). *(Reproduced with permission from Wagenvoort C A. Classifying pulmonary vascular disease. Chest 64:503–504, 1973).*

are maintained postoperatively, accumulation of additional water will probably appear in the dependent, lesser-perfused lung and the effect on arterial oxygenation will be modest at best. It is not uncommon to find an adult with chronic pulmonary hypertension who may be ventilator-dependent because of borderline hemodynamic function yet be capable of surprisingly good oxygenation with relatively low concentrations of inspired O_2. In these patients, measurement of the alveolar-arterial O_2 gradient does not provide a satisfactory criterion of adequate lung function.

In the normal adult, distribution of a normal spontaneous inspiration is controlled by the regional distribution of compliance (Lemelin et al., 1972) (Fig. 11–5). At end-expiration (upright lung), compliance of the dependent portion is higher than in the nondependent part because of the effects of gravity and the influence of abdominal contents on the diaphragm. An active inspiration (i.e., spontaneous) will be associated with preferential distribution of the inspirate to the dependent lung unless the gas flow rates are excesssively high (Bake et al., 1974). Since the dependent lung also receives a substantially greater blood flow, it is evident that although normal blood-gas exchange is characterized by inhomogeneity, it is maintained by close match of the $\dot{V}/\dot{Q}$ ratio.

Careful measurement of pleural pressures from the bottom to the apex of the lung has demonstrated the presence of a vertical gradient, which explains the regional distribution of a spontaneous tidal breath (Agostoni and Miserocchi, 1970) (Fig. 11–6). Muscle paralysis and mechanical ventilation cause this vertical gradient to disappear and are probably responsible for the altered distribution of

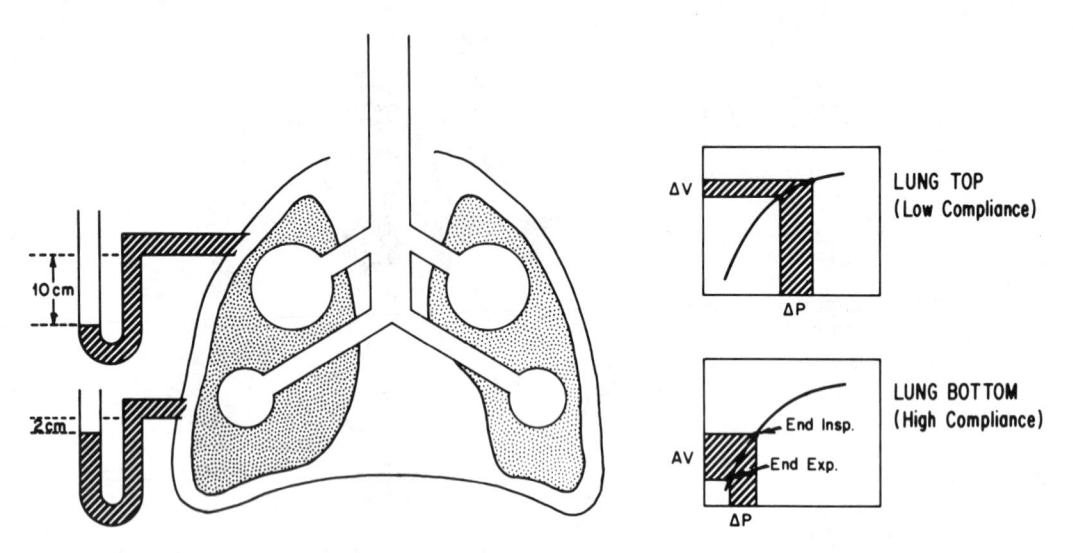

Figure 11–5. Distribution of transpulmonary pressures and compliance in an upright lung at end-expiration. At the base of the lung, pleural pressure is 2 cm H$_2$O below and at the apex, 10 cm H$_2$O below atmospheric pressure. Because of the higher transmural pressure, apical alveoli lie on the top portion of their volume/pressure curve (upper insert); their volume is large and compliance ($\Delta V/\Delta P$) is low. Basal alveoli, subject to a low transmural pressure, lie on the steep portion of their volume/pressure curve (lower insert); end-expiratory volume is low and compliance high. An inspiration generated from this point will be directed principally to the basal, high compliance airways. Basal airways are shown to be smaller than their apical counterpart at end-expiration.

ventilation demonstrated in this setting. For example, Rehder et al. (1971, 1972, 1973) found that the distribution of ventilation in anesthetized, paralyzed, and mechanically ventilated people without heart or lung disease was more even than in the awake person (Fig. 11–7). There appears to be no immediate explanation for this phenomenon, although, as shown by Bake et al, (1974), changes in inspiratory flow rate do alter the ventilation ratios between dependent and nondependent lobes of the lung. Changes in tone of chest wall muscles and diaphragm are probably important because of their effect on the distribution of pleural pressures (Agostoni and Miserocchi, 1970; Froese and Bryan, 1974).

Regardless of the operation, the most common cause of early inappropriate lung function after open heart surgery for acquired disease, be it valves or coronary arteries, is secondary to excessive intrapulmonary accumulation of liquid, be it water or blood. The most common cause of late disturbances is gram-negative infection.

Gross pulmonary edema is readily diagnosed by examination of the chest x-ray and arterial blood gases. It requires prompt intervention to prevent the catastrophic consequences of severe hypoxemia. Respiratory acidosis usually appears late and is a poor criterion for early detection of edema. Moderate levels of pulmonary venous hypertension may cause subtle regional changes in the distribution of ventilation and perfusion, not readily diagnosed by the chest x-ray or blood-gas analysis. Table 11–2 gives an example.

This patient had had multiple coronary artery bypass grafts for severe coronary artery disease and required extensive postoperative support, including diastolic augmentation with an intraaortic balloon. Although his left atrial (LA) pressure was in excess of 15 mm Hg, the chest film failed to document the

	Δ AP (cm H₂O)	Δ TPP (cm H₂O)
TOP	25	11.3
BOTTOM	25	15.6

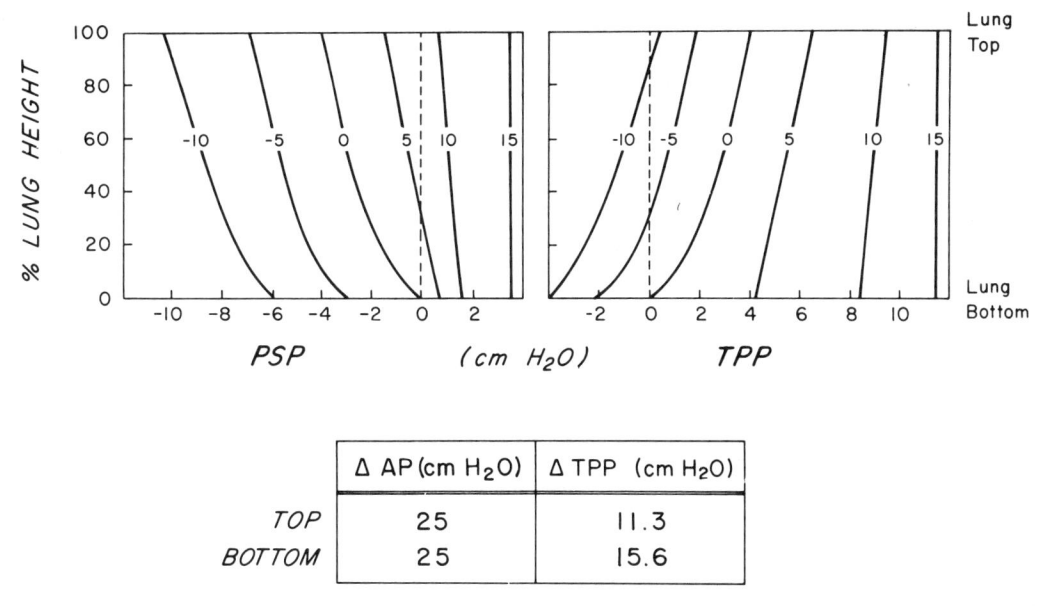

Figure 11-6. The relationship between changes in alveolar (AP) and transpulmonary pressures (TPP) during inflation are shown for the upright lung from top to bottom. Graph at left indicates the relationship between pleural surface pressure (PSP) and percent lung height. The isopressure lines (−10 to +15 cm H₂O) represent alveolar pressure. During mechanical inflation of the lung, AP rises from 0 to 15 cm H₂O. TPP for the lung top is obtained from the differences of values at points where isopressure lines for 0 and 15 cm H₂O cross the top of the right-hand box (i.e., 11.5 − 4 = 7.5 cm H₂O); similarly for the lung bottom (i.e., 11.5 − 0 = 11.5 cm H₂O). TPP changes during ventilation with extremes of negative and positive AP [i.e., 15 − (−10) = 25 cm H₂O] are shown below. *(Redrawn with permission from Agostoni, E, and Miserocchi, G. Vertical gradient of transpulmonary pressure with active and artificial lung expansion. J Appl Physiol 29:705-712, 1970.)*

presence of severe pulmonary edema. Arterial oxygenation was borderline, but a sample removed from the LA catheter indicated a Po₂ consistent with mixed venous blood. Injection of contrast medium into the catheter indicated that the sample was being withdrawn from the left lower pulmonary vein (LLPV), which was being ventilated very poorly. Although it was possible to improve matters considerably by appropriate mechanical ventilation with positive end-expiratory pressure (Falke et al., 1972), this case exemplifies the difficulties we face clinically when faced with the need to establish guidelines for appropriate therapy.

We have studied this problem of acute regional nonventilation after open heart surgery by inserting catheters into both the right upper and lower pulmonary veins shortly after completion of extracorporeal circulation. In most cases where nonventilation of the lower lobe was suggested by a low arterial Po₂, the chest x-ray failed to support the severity of regional nonventilation. In our experience, grossly inadequate ventilation of dependent lobes is frequent whenever left atrial pressure is maintained at a minimum of 15 mm Hg for 48 hours or longer and particularly in patients with a history of chronic congestive heart failure. Although the example chosen (see Table 11-2) was accompanied by a substantial decrease in arterial Po₂, this is not invariably the case, since intrinsic mechanisms within the lung do compensate for a chronic reduction in ventilation.

Nonventilation of terminal air units is associated with a marked reduction in blood

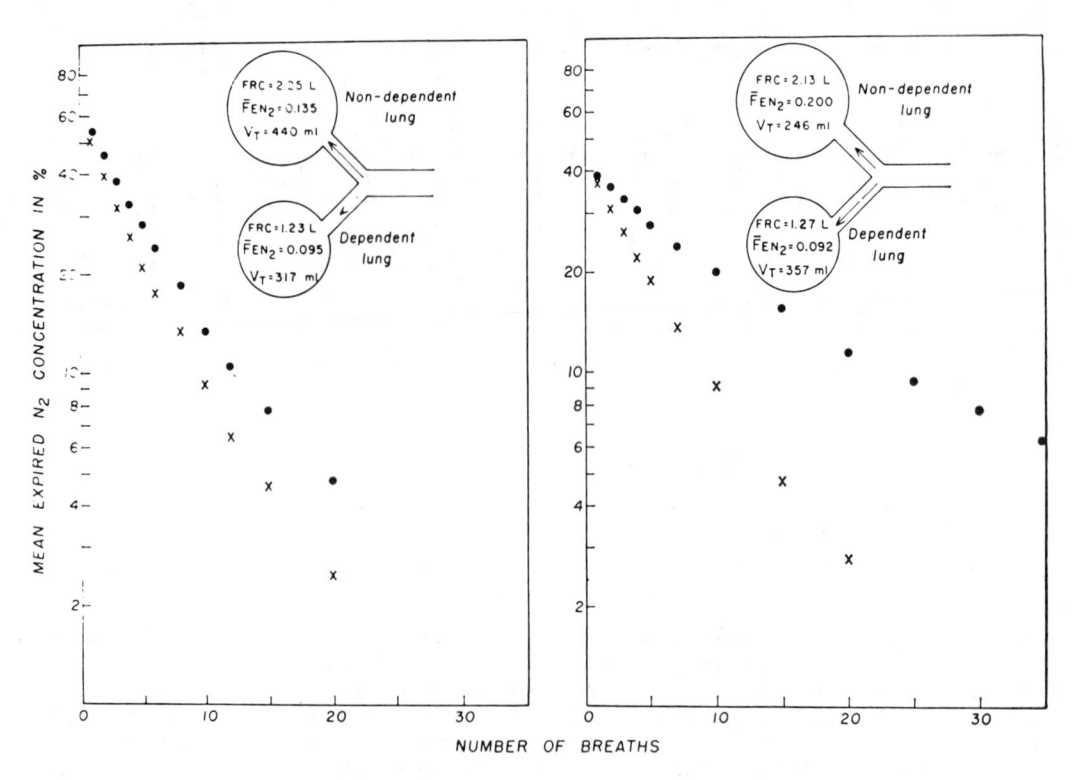

Figure 11–7. Nitrogen clearance curves determined at the mouth for dependent (×) and nondependent (·) lungs in normal adult volunteers awake and breathing spontaneously (right) and then paralyzed, anesthetized, and mechanically ventilated (left). Inserts indicate the respective values for functional residual capacity (FRC), mixed end-tidal N$_2$ concentration ($\bar{F}$EN$_2$) and tidal volume (V$_T$) of respective dependent and nondependent lungs. $\bar{F}$EN$_2$ values are for the tenth breath during the N$_2$ clearance measurements. Note that with muscle paralysis and mechanical ventilation, the dependent and nondependent lungs became similar (left) to those in the awake state. This was because of a significant increase in tidal ventilation (V$_T$) of the nondependent lung and documented by substantially lower $\bar{F}$EN$_2$ by the tenth breath. *(Reproduced with permission from Rehder, K, et al. The function of each lung of anesthetized and paralyzed man during mechanical ventilation. Anesthesiology 37:16–26, 1972.)*

flow (i.e., hypoxic pulmonary vasoconstriction or HPV). In most cases with little or no ventilation of the dependent lobes that we have studied, arterial Po$_2$ generally reflected more closely the blood draining nondependent lung, suggesting that blood flow to the nonventilated portion had been reduced (Table 11–3). Generally, an increase in airway pressure will improve gas exchange. However, on occasion the increase in airway pressure may increase blood flow rather than ventilation to a grossly collapsed lobe and decrease arterial Po$_2$ while increasing the calculated $\dot{Q}_S/\dot{Q}_T$ (Fig. 11–8).

A reduction in blood flow to a nonventilated lung may be regarded as a protective mechanism against excessive intrapulmonary right-to-left shunt and profound hypoxemia. Unfortunately, HPV can be blocked with drugs (Nomoto et al., 1974) and probably by high concentrations of oxygen. This explains why the measured $\dot{Q}_S/\dot{Q}_T \times 100$ has been found to increase upon ventilation with 100 percent O$_2$ in patients with acute respiratory

TABLE 11-2 DATA FROM A 65-YEAR-OLD MAN (WEIGHT 75 KG) WHO HAD RECEIVED TWO CORONARY ARTERY BYPASS GRAFTS

	F_{IO_2}	P_{O_2} (torr)	P_{CO_2} (torr)	pH	V_T(ml)	PEEP (cmH$_2$O)
8 minutes						
Radial artery	1.0	87	40	7.44	1,000	5
Left lower pulmonary vein		38	47	7.40		
15 minutes						
Radial artery	1.0	271	28	7.54	1,400	0
Left lower pulmonary vein		95	42	7.40		
45 minutes						
Radial artery	1.0	273	27	7.49	1,400	5
Left lower pulmonary vein		176	33	7.43		
24 hours						
Radial artery	1.0	248	30	7.58	1,400	5
Left lower pulmonary vein		182	34	7.53		

Reproduced with permission from Trichet B, Falke K, Togut A, and Laver M B. The effect of pre-existing pulmonary vascular disease on the response to mechanical ventilation with PEEP following open-heart surgery. Anesthesiology, 42:56-67, 1975.

TABLE 11-3 EFFECTS OF MECHANICAL VENTILATION WITH AND WITHOUT PEEP ON REGIONAL PULMONARY OXYGENATION FOLLOWING MITRAL VALVE REPLACEMENT IN A PATIENT* WITH SEVERE PULMONARY VASCULAR DISEASE†

	Supine						Right Lung Down		
	Without PEEP			8 CM H$_2$O PEEP			8 CM H$_2$O PEEP		
$F_{IO_2} = 1.0$; $V_T = 900$ ml	P_{O_2} (torr)	P_{CO_2} (torr)	pH	P_{O_2} (torr)	P_{O_2} (torr)	pH	P_{O_2} (torr)	P_{CO_2} (torr)	pH
Right upper pulmonary vein	309	25	7.63	427	30	7.57	‡	‡	‡
Right lower pulmonary vein	34	31	7.57	70	35	7.51	398	38	7.51
Radial artery	242	25	7.62	371	30	7.56	620	31	7.57

*59-year-old female; 61 kg.
†Preoperative Catheterization: PA 160/90 torr; PAP 105 torr; PVR 78 units; CI 0.7 l/min/m^2
‡Catheter inadvertently moved out of position; blood sample unavailable.
(Reproduced with permission from Trichet B, Falke K, Togut A, and Laver M B. The effect of pre-existing pulmonary vascular disease on the response to mechanical ventilation with PEEP following open-heart surgery. Anesthesiology, 42:52-67, 1975.

insufficiency (McAslan et al., 1973; Powers et al., 1973). In these cases, a decrease in calculated pulmonary vascular resistance also is apparent.

It is likely that both alveolar and mixed venous blood P_{O_2} and pH modulate HPV. For example, the peripheral vasoconstrictor response to lower body negative pressure disappears in the presence of arterial hypoxemia, only to reappear when P_{O_2} returns to normal levels (Heistad et al., 1972). Although hypoxemia is a potent vasoconstrictor of the pulmonary vasculature, we do not know whether selective reduction of blood flow to nonventi-

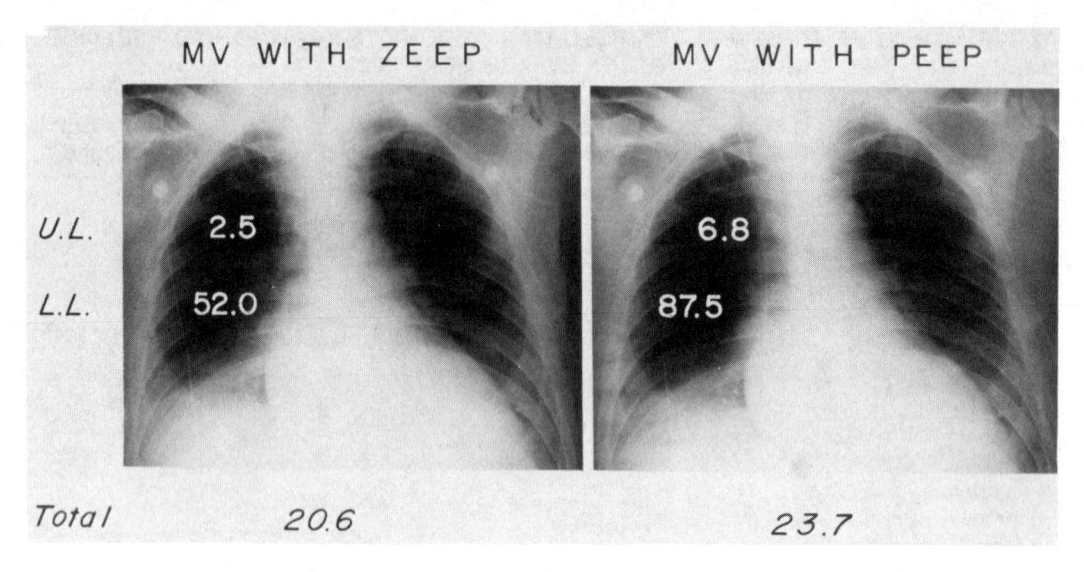

Figure 11–8. Regional distribution of oxygenation evaluated with pulmonary vein catheters inserted into upper and lower lobe veins at time of operation. After mitral valve replacement the patient was ventilated mechanically with zero end-expiratory pressure (MV with ZEEP). $\dot{Q}_S/\dot{Q}_T \times 100$ was calculated for the right upper (RUL) and right lower lobe (RLL) by measuring O_2 contents in pulmonary artery and respective pulmonary vein blood. A modification of the shunt equation was used:

$$\frac{\dot{Q}_S}{\dot{Q}_T} = \frac{Cc_{O_2} - Cpv_{O_2}}{Cc_{O_2} - C\bar{v}_{O_2}}$$

where $Cpv_{O_2} = O_2$ content of pulmonary vein blood. Data were obtained with the patient in a semirecumbent position. Chest x-ray demonstrated collapse of the RLL, substantiated by a $\dot{Q}_S/\dot{Q}_T \times 100$ of 52.0. Note (1) the low $\dot{Q}_S/\dot{Q}_T$ for the upper lobe and (2) the rise in $\dot{Q}_S/\dot{Q}_T \times 100$ for RLL when airway pressure was increased, suggesting a substantial rise in blood flow to this lobe.

lated parts of the lung is impaired or enhanced as Po_2 declines below a critical level. In any event, sampling of mixed venous blood must include the possible effect of hypoxemia and acidosis (i.e., mixed venous Po_2 less than 30 mm Hg and pH less than 7.25) as a potential source for pulmonary vasoconstriction and an attendant reduction in cardiac output. Whenever diminished blood flow results from increased right ventricular afterload, neither inotropic support of myocardial function nor an increase in intravascular volume is likely to augment stroke volume. In fact, the success of vasodilator therapy may be the result of pharmacologic influence on right rather than left ventricular afterload.

Diffuse nonventilation of one lung is a frequent consequence of left thoracotomy for resection of a dissecting thoracic aortic aneurysm. Retraction of the lung while the patient is heparinized and on left ventricular bypass may be followed by extensive bleeding into the lung parenchyma and marked opacification on the early postoperative chest roentgenogram. These changes are usually (but not always) preventable by the use of endobronchial tubes, which minimize the trauma by preventing expansion of the retracted lung during the operation.

Whenever extensive unilateral opacification is apparent in the postoperative chest x-ray, the choice of body position during mechanical ventilation may have a substantial effect on oxygenation. This complication can be derived from our earlier considerations on the distribution of $\dot{V}/\dot{Q}$ (Fig. 11–9). If the patient is ventilated with the opacified lung in a dependent position, oxygenation will be impaired maximally. Conversely, oxygenation will be optimal if the better lung is dependent, since both ventilation and perfusion will be matched to greatest advantage. A striking example of this disparity, though unrelated to open heart surgery, is shown in Figure 11-10. Extensive opacification of one lung occurred secondary to a prolonged period in the left lateral decubitus position. The patient required mechanical ventilation because of an obtunded sensorium secondary to an ingestion of barbiturates. As the numbers indicate, optimal oxygenation was achieved when the clear lung was dependent.

Although problems of oxygenation are common consequences of general anesthesia, thoracotomy, and extracorporeal perfusion, the immediate cause for their appearance is unclear (Andersen and Ghia, 1970; Ghia and Andersen, 1970; Froese and Bryan, 1974; Trichet et al., 1975). Changes in chest wall configuration, a rise in the position of the diaphragm, and altered abdominal muscle tone all play a role. Inadequate venting of the left ventricle and intermittent pulmonary venous hypertension during extracorporeal bypass are associated with perialveolar and ultimately intraalveolar accumulation of fluid (Staub et al., 1967).

After open heart surgery, most if not all patients demonstrate an elevation of their $\dot{Q}_S/\dot{Q}_T$ fraction (range: 8 to 15 percent of cardiac output). Neither the skill of the surgeon or the anesthetist, the duration of extracorporeal perfusion, nor the nature of the prime appears to prevent its occurrence. The consequences of extracorporeal perfusion, particularly its effects on the formed elements of the blood, have been held responsible for postoperative lung dysfunction, but the evidence to support this hypothesis is weak. Most studies suggest that the abnormalities recorded are little different from changes noted to follow thoracotomy or upper abdominal surgery.

Fortunately, enthusiasm for the term "pump lung" is waning, while arguments in favor of elective postoperative mechanical

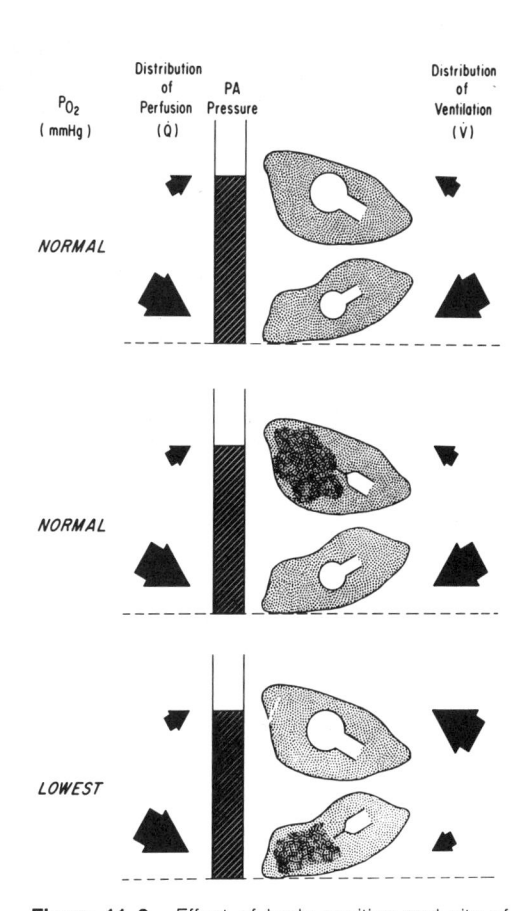

Figure 11-9. Effect of body position and site of airway collapse on arterial oxygenation. Distribution of perfusion undergoes only minor alteration secondary to an acute change of airway geometry. Normally, the dependent lung receives the major portion of blood flow and ventilation (top). If the nondependent lung contains areas of nonventilation, distribution of ventilation and perfusion remain unchanged but moderate hypoxemia will be present, the degree depending on the pulmonary artery pressure and the amount of blood flow to the nondependent lung (middle). If the lesser ventilated lung is dependent and if its compliance is also low, preferential ventilation of the upper lung will occur. Since distribution of perfusion remains unchanged, arterial hypoxemia will be severe (bottom). Arrow thickness reflects the relative magnitude of flow, be it blood or gas. (Reproduced with permission from Laver M B, and Austen, W G. Lung function: Physiologic considerations applicable to surgery. In Sabiston, D C, Jr, (ed), Davis-Christopher Textbook of Surgery. 10th ed. Philadelphia: Saunders, 1972.)

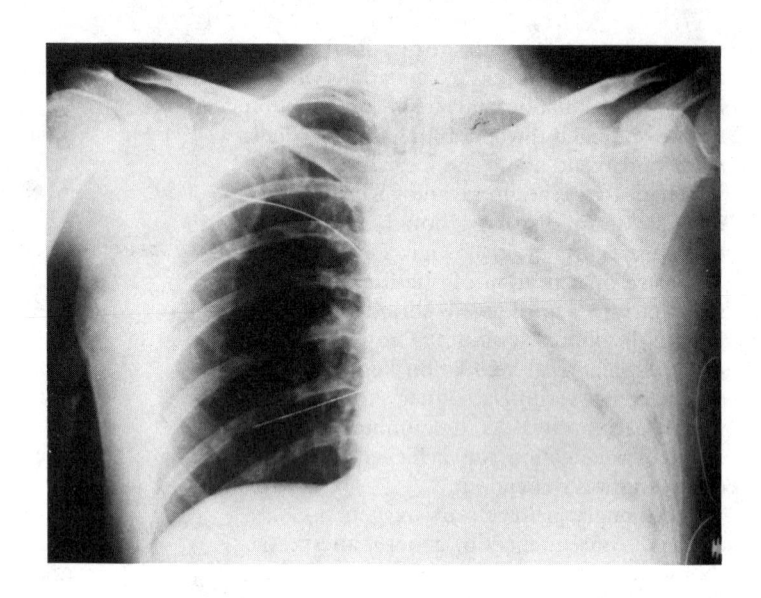

Figure 11-10. Effect of body position on arterial oxygenation during mechanical ventilation. Left lung was diffusely opacified, cause unknown. Arterial Po2 was lowest when the affected lung was dependent, i.e., with maximal blood flow but minimal ventilation. (Reproduced with permission from Laver, M B, Austen, W G, Wilson, R. Blood-gas exchange and hemodynamic performance. In Sabiston, D C, Jr, & Spencer, F C (eds), Surgery of the Chest. 3rd ed. Philadelphia: Saunders, 1975.)

26 y.o. ♀ STATUS p̄ BARBITURATE INTOXICATION ON VOLUME CONTROLLED VENTILATOR WITH 8cm H_2O PEEP

POSITION	$F_{I_{O_2}}$	Pa_{O_2} (mmHg)	Pa_{CO_2} (mmHg)	pH
Supine	0.43	82	26	7.56
R Side Down	0.43	141	28	7.52
L Side Down	0.43	70	31	7.51

ventilation are based entirely on the experience of the team charged with the patient's care. More specifically, a low morbidity with continuing support of lung function has shifted emphasis to the presence of an unstable hemodynamic situation (i.e., the need for high cardiac filling pressures or the presence of an elevated pulmonary vascular resistance) or excessive bleeding as prime indicators for ventilator assistance. In the presence of appropriate myocardial function and in the absence of pulmonary vascular disease, a strong argument can be made for early extubation and spontaneous ventilation. This is particularly true for patients with coronary artery disease and quasinormal left ventricular function.

Fortunately, the mechanism of impaired blood-gas exchange after open heart surgery, though poorly understood, is rapidly reversible and in most cases requires little therapy. Marshall and Wyche (1972) have recently reviewed this problem as it applies to the surgical patient without heart disease. Occasionally massive blood transfusion and embolization with particulate matter may play a role (Marshall et al., 1974; Soma et al., 1974). Use of proper filters has been recommended to prevent this syndrome (Cullen and Ferrara, 1974), but the evidence in favor is also inconclusive. Rarely, pulmonary edema may result from the presence of white blood cell antibodies in the recipient (Thompson et al., 1971). The characteristic response is an acute change in the radiologic appearance of the lungs, with an accompanying low arterial Po$_2$ and left atrial pressure.

Recent studies suggest that early postoperative lung dysfunction, unrelated to congestive heart failure, is caused by changes in the "closing volume." This is the volume (expressed in percentage of total lung capacity) at which airway closure becomes evident, and is measured by following the concentration at the mouth of a reference gas (such as radioactive xenon) during expiration after an inspiration to total lung capacity (TLC). An abrupt increase in concentration of the indicator gas as the end-expiration point is reached signals a change in the site from which the gas is expired because of sudden airway closure. For details, the reader is referred to other papers on the subject (Laver et al., 1975).

In the awake young adult, an abrupt increase in indicator gas concentration at the mouth (a point also designated as phase IV) is rarely apparent before end-expiration, and the "closing volume"* is said to be below functional residual capacity (FRC). In the older person, loss of elastic recoil is associated with a measurable CV before completion of a normal expiration, and CV is above FRC. Although most investigators have come to believe that the "phase IV concentration changes" are indicative of airway closure, opinion on the matter is not unanimous.

Hyatt and Rodarte (1975) have summarized recently the reasons for an alternative explanation. Theirs are cogent arguments that deserve serious consideration. It is beyond the purview of our analysis to present all the features of the controversy. Suffice it to say that in lieu of "closure," Hyatt and Rodarte consider the changes to be secondary to flow limitation when dynamic compression of the airways becomes apparent during expiration. In favor of this argument is the fact that an increased expiratory flow rate makes "closing volume" more difficult to detect. In fact, if expiratory flow is rapid enough, the signs associated with "closing volume" (i.e., phase IV) are no longer apparent.

From a practical point of view, it matters little which explanation is correct. The important points to realize are (1) that geometry of the airway and the pattern of emptying is altered by the aging process as well as by the severity of congestive heart failure, and (2) that early postoperative inappropriate oxygenation may be secondary to iatrogenic disturbances of a dynamic process whose existence we recognize but are unable to control and for whose appearance we do not have a very good explanation.

Slow postoperative recovery of hemodynamic function is likely to have the same effect on blood-gas exchange. If the situation is severe enough to require prolonged mechanical ventilation, the consequences of high airway pressure, sepsis, and poor "healing" (the result of a borderline cardiac output) may cause further deterioration of lung function. The ubiquity of respiratory failure in the critically ill patient has stimulated a plethora of terminology intended to characterize post mortem appearance. Blaisdell and Schlobohm (1973) have listed no less than 27 different names, none of which is helpful either with therapy or diagnosis. Common to all is progressive hypoxemia and the need for ventilator support occasionally with excessively high airway pressure, including positive end-expiratory pressure (PEEP) (Kirby et al., 1975) and an elevated inspired oxygen concentration.

Histologically, the changes in lung morphology are extensive, involving alveolar surface epithelium, interstitium, and the cap-

---

*"Closing volume" (CV) is defined as the volume of gas, above residual volume (RV), at which closure of terminal air units becomes apparent. "Closing capacity" (CC) is the sum of RV plus CV.

illaries. What is caused by disease rather than therapy is difficult to define. It hardly justifies the pathologic diagnosis of "respirator lung." Recovery, when it occurs, is slow. The chest x-ray may continue to appear abnormal and arterial Po_2 may be low long after the patient has been extubated.

We have indicated earlier that a measure of inefficient gas exchange is obtained by evaluation of the alveolar to arterial O_2 gradient (A-aDo_2) or, better still, calculation of $\dot{Q}_S/\dot{Q}_T \times 100$ during ventilation with 100 percent oxygen. Although this appears to have received universal acceptance, interpretation does require caution. First, if a substantial number of terminal air units have a very low ventilation-perfusion ratio ($\dot{V}/\dot{Q} = 0.01$), filling of these air units with pure oxygen may result in rapid absorption of gas, more rapidly than made available by ventilation, and closure may follow. As a result, measurements made during ventilation with 100 percent O_2 may indicate an excessively high $\dot{Q}_S/\dot{Q}_T$. On the other hand, the presence of small quantities of nitrogen (e.g., 20 percent) in the inspired gas may prevent full absorption of gas due to poor solubility of N_2 in whole blood (Markello et al., 1972; 1973) (for details see Fig. 11–11). Second, the previously elaborated dilator effect of O_2 (or the constrictor effect of

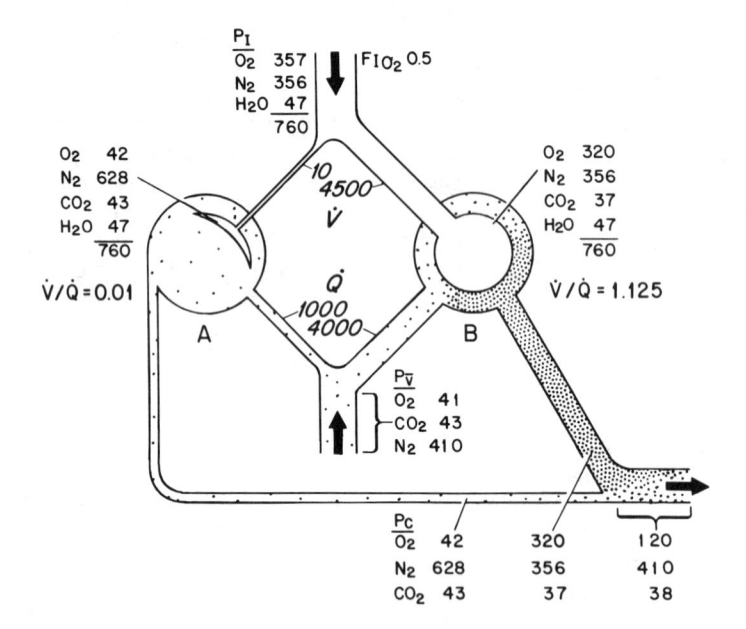

Figure 11–11. Effect of ventilation with high and low concentrations of oxygen on gas exchange in a two-alveoli lung with marked disparity of $\dot{V}/\dot{Q}$ ratios. Overall $\dot{V}/\dot{Q} = 4,500/5,000 = 0.9$; $\dot{V}/\dot{Q}$ to alveolus A = 10/1,000 = 0.01; $\dot{V}/\dot{Q}$ to alveolus B = 4,500/4,000 = 1.125. When ventilated with 50 percent O_2/50 percent N_2, alveolus A receives approximately 5 ml N_2 and 5 ml O_2/min. Because of the substantial blood flow to alveolus A, 5 ml O_2/min increases Po_2 of mixed venous blood from 41 to 42 mm Hg, not enough to fully saturate this blood. N_2 solubility in whole blood is low and N_2 content will rise by 1,000(628 − 410) (0.0015/100) = 3.3 ml N_2/min. Since this is only a fraction of the N_2 available, the additional nitrogen provided in the inspired gas will prevent closure of the alveolus. On the other hand, ventilation with 80 percent O_2 will provide only 2 ml N_2/min (0.2 × 10), less than the required amount, and closure is inevitable. *(Redrawn with permission from Pontoppidan H. The black box illuminated. Anesthesiology 37:1–3, 1972.)*

low mixed venous P_{O_2} combined with low pH) on the pulmonary vasculature and enhanced or diminished perfusion on nonventilated lung may confuse the issue in a similar manner.

Regardless of etiology, the increase in calculated pulmonary right-to-left shunt while oxygen is breathed is likely to be more prominent as respiratory failure becomes severe. Generally, measurement of the *change* in $\dot{Q}_S/\dot{Q}_T \times 100$ as $F_{I_{O_2}}$ is increased to 100 percent is a valuable, albeit limited, indicator of lung function. Since the use of pulmonary artery catheters is routine in patients with acute respiratory failure, samples should be obtained for measurement of P_{O_2}, pH, and hemoglobin, with calculation of O_2 content and $\dot{Q}_S/\dot{Q}_T \times 100$. Programmable pocket calculators are now available and can be used for this purpose.*

The subject of oxygen toxicity and the effect of ventilator therapy on lung morphology always invites discussion whenever the inspired O_2 concentration is elevated above ambient during ventilation for acute respiratory failure. We prefer not to enter into a lengthy controversy and refer the reader to recent reviews on the subject (Nash et al., 1971; Pontoppidan et al., 1973). Suffice it to say that awareness of its existence is important as well as the need for repeated monitoring of the inspired and arterial P_{O_2}. Generally, passion appears to have overcome reason when relevance is evaluated. There is no evidence that ventilation with 100 percent oxygen during the operation for periods up to 12 hours has a deleterious effect on lung function. Until such evidence is obtained and its physiologic importance demonstrated, discussion is a classic example of an exercise in futility. It is more likely that the occasional disasters reported are related to an inappropriate pattern of mechanical ventilation than a high concentration of O_2.

FACTORS THAT INFLUENCE CO_2 REMOVAL

Except for the patient with chronic obstructive lung disease (COLD), CO_2 removal is not a significant problem in acute respiratory failure until the advanced or terminal stages have been reached.

If tidal volume is not below the minimum required of 15 ml/kg, the most common cause for an increase in P_{CO_2} is an increased physiologic dead space produced by a marked diminution of the $\dot{V}/\dot{Q}$ ratio.† If $\dot{Q}_S/\dot{Q}_T \times 100$ is large, alveolar ventilation to ventilated terminal air units must be increased if arterial P_{CO_2} (Pa_{CO_2}) is to remain within normal limits.

The relationship between the whole blood venoarterial CO_2 content difference ($v-aC_{CO_2}$), $\dot{Q}_S/\dot{Q}_T$, and the arterial to alveolar P_{CO_2} gradient (a-$A_{P_{CO_2}}$) is shown in Figure 11-12. When cardiac output is low (i.e., $V_{A_{CO_2}}$ is large) and $\dot{Q}_S/\dot{Q}_T \times 100$ markedly increased (above 30 percent of cardiac output), a substantial increase in minute ventilation may be necessary to maintain Pa_{CO_2} at normal levels. Although P_{CO_2} is defined in the strict sense by alveolar ventilation, the *efficiency* of CO_2 removal must take into account CO_2 production ($\dot{V}_{CO_2}$) and the ratio of physiologic dead space to tidal volume (V_D/V_T). When $\dot{V}/\dot{Q}$ is outside the normal range of 0.8 to 1.0, the efficiency of ventilation is diminished. An increase in V_D/V_T above normal values of 0.35 to 0.40 requires a higher minute ventilation, as shown in Figure 11-13. During acute respiratory failure, the V_D/V_T ratio is frequently above 0.50. Common sources for this change are shown in Figure 11-14.

Problems with CO_2 homeostasis are rare after open heart surgery. If Pa_{CO_2} is abnormally high during mechanical ventilation,

---

Hewlett-Packard Model HP 67.

†*Impaired diffusivity or an "alveolar-capillary" block contributes little to the difficulties of gas exchange (Wagner and West, 1972).*

Figure 11-12. The effect of cardiac output (reflected by a change in the venoarterial CO_2 content difference (v − a Cco_2) and intrapulmonary shunt ($\dot{Q}_S/\dot{Q}_T$) on the arterial-alveolar CO_2 difference. As the shunt increases, greater ventilation will be required of blood exposed to ventilating surface in the lung to maintain arterial Pco_2 within normal limits. (Reproduced with permission from Bendixen H H, Egbert L D, Hedley-Whyte J, Laver M B, and Pontoppidan H. Respiratory Care. St. Louis: C.V. Mosby, 1965.)

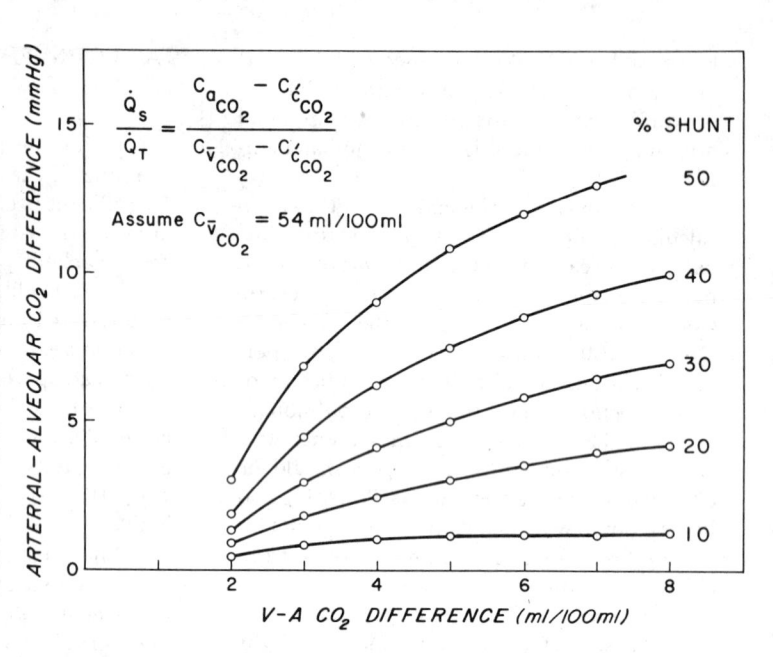

correction is achieved by an increase in respiratory frequency. If $Paco_2$ is excessively low (e.g., below 30 mm Hg), adjustment must be made either by decreasing the frequency of breathing or by the addition of mechanical dead space in the form of corrugated tubing inserted between the endotracheal tube and the Y-piece of the ventilator. A formula for calculation of the dead space required to achieve a desired rise in $Paco_2$ has been published (Suwa et al., 1968). It does not eliminate the need for repeated blood-gas analyses whenever a step change in ventilation is initiated.

Occasionally, the patient with protracted postoperative left ventricular failure may demonstrate a tendency to maintain a high arterial Pco_2 with a normal pH on spontaneous ventilation due to vigorous diuretic therapy with furosemide and extensive urinary loss of [H^+] (Goldring et al., 1968). This condition is best treated by the intravenous administration of hydrochloric acid (100 mEq of 1 N HCl diluted in 500 ml of 5 percent glucose in water) at a rate not to exceed 20 mEq per hour (Abouna et al., 1974).

EFFECT OF CHANGES IN AIRWAY PRESSURE ON HEMODYNAMIC PERFORMANCE

Although the effects of mechanical ventilation on hemodynamic performance have been well-studied in humans and experimental animals with normal lungs and in acute respiratory failure (Falke et al., 1972; Beach et al., 1973; Powers et al., 1973; Harken et al., 1974), information on the response elicited in the presence of heart failure is remarkably limited. After open heart surgery, changes in airway pressure may be associated with a hemodynamic response that, on first impression, appears paradoxical (Beach et al., 1973) but on close analysis can be recognized to form part of a predictable pattern whenever myocardial function is compromised. We have noted earlier that the need for prolonged postoperative ventilatory support is closely related to the magnitude of residual myocardial failure. Similarly, weaning from ventilator support will be found intimately related to (1) the state of right and left ventricular performance, (2) the patient's blood volume,

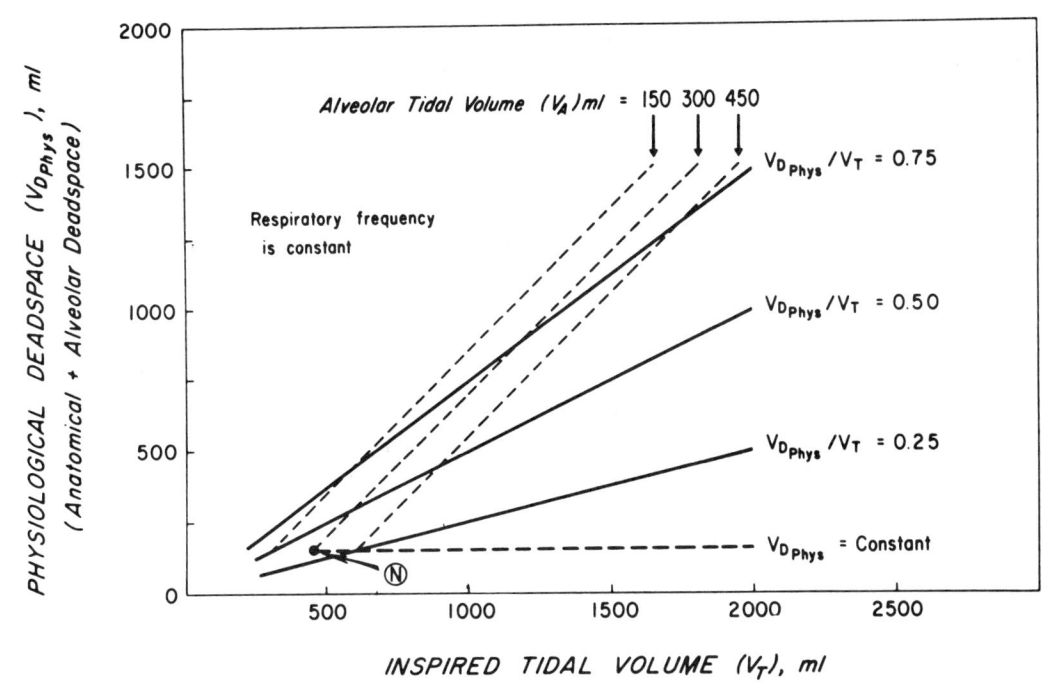

Figure 11-13. Effect of tidal volume on alveolar ventilation at constant $V_{D_{PHYS}}/V_T$ ratios. If $V_{D_{PHYS}}/V_T = 0.75$ and an increase in alveolar tidal volume from 150 to 300 ml is desired, the inspired tidal volume must also be doubled (from 400 to approximately 800 ml). Extensive experience with critically ill patients has shown that the average value for V_D/V_T during moderate respiratory failure is 0.6. Proper ventilation is achieved by increasing tidal volume (recommended value: 15 ml/kg BW) while keeping frequency in the normal range of 10 to 14 breaths per minute. (Reproduced with permission from Bendixen H H, Egbert L D, Hedley-Whyte J, Laver M B, and Pontoppidan H. Respiratory Care. St. Louis: C.V. Mosby, 1965.)

and (3) the state of the pulmonary vasculature.

The acute effects of initiating mechanical ventilation on thoracic venous inflow and right ventricular function are well-known, while the consequences of the reverse maneuver appear to have been generally ignored. It is fair to state that the problems of weaning from ventilator therapy are related to residual lung dysfunction, weak or discoordinate respiratory muscle function, and, finally, inability to cope with the "excessive work of breathing." Although these mechanisms are occasionally responsible, experience suggests they may be infrequent in the first few days after open heart surgery.

The interest of my colleagues and I in the problem coincided with the observation that patients with residual myocardial failure demonstrated a *decrease* in cardiac output and a *rise* in calculated pulmonary vascular resistance upon trial at spontaneous ventilation. Conversely, when airway pressure was increased, cardiac output remained unchanged or occasionally increased, a phenomenon already alluded to in Figure 11-2. An attempt to explain this paradoxical reaction has been made by several authors (Beach et al., 1973; Harken et al., 1974). We have sought to clarify this problem by performing (1) animal experiments in which mechanical ventilation was discontinued after induced hypervolemia

I. Permanent cessation of pulmonary capillary blood flow to ventilated unit

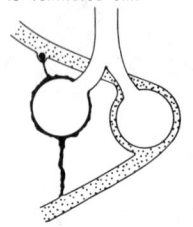

II. Marked regional variation between ventilation and perfusion of ventilated units

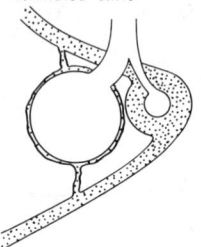

III. Perfusion of non-ventilated unit

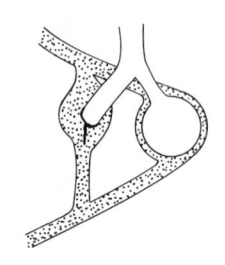

IV. Intermittent cessation of pulmonary capillary blood flow to ventilated units.

End Expiration   End Inspiration

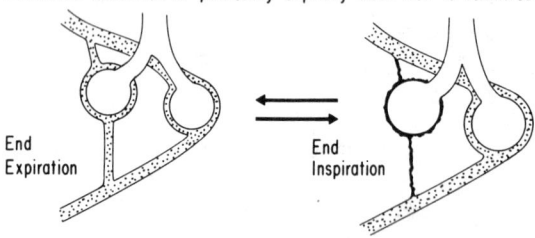

Figure 11-14. Potential sources of an increased physiologic dead space during and after surgery. The problem in every case is due to a marked deviation of $\dot{V}/\dot{Q}$ from normal. **I.** Permanent cessation of pulmonary capillary blood flow arises as a result of embolism or pulmonary artery hypotension. **II.** Marked regional variation between $\dot{V}/\dot{Q}$ is conspicuous in chronic obstructive lung disease and during thoracotomy. **III.** Perfusion of a nonventilated unit leads to an increase in arterial Pco_2 because mixed venous blood, with a high carbon dioxide content, raises the Pco_2 of the oxygenated and ventilated blood ("pseudo-dead space effect"). **IV.** Intermittent cessation of pulmonary capillary blood flow is common in acute respiratory failure when major portions of the lung have a low compliance, and ventilation with a high airway pressure distends excessively the high-compliance airspaces. *(Reproduced with permission from Laver, M B, and Austen, W G. Lung function: Physiologic considerations applicable to surgery. In Sabiston, D C, Jr, (ed), Davis-Christopher Textbook of Surgery. 10th ed. Philadelphia: Saunders, 1972.)*

(Qvist et al., 1975) and (2) studies of patients with or without elevated pulmonary vascular resistance and right ventricular failure on their response to changes in airway pressure (Trichet et al., 1975).

Qvist et al. subjected animals with normal lungs and normal ventricular function to mechanical ventilation with end-expiratory pressure (MV with PEEP). The initial decrease in cardiac output that occurred secondary to reduced right and left heart transmural pressures returned to control values when the animals were made hypervolemic by transfusion with whole blood (25 ml/kg body weight). Upon cessation of mechanical ventilation six hours later, transmural pressures and flow increased and remained well above control values (Fig. 11-15, top). If we examine this relationship on the Frank-Starling curve (Fig. 11-15, bottom), we note that on discontinuation of mechanical ventilation, the equilibrium point, which relates stroke work index to transmural pressure, was substantially higher than control and in fact nearly reached the point of ventricular failure, i.e., where further changes in transmural pressure no

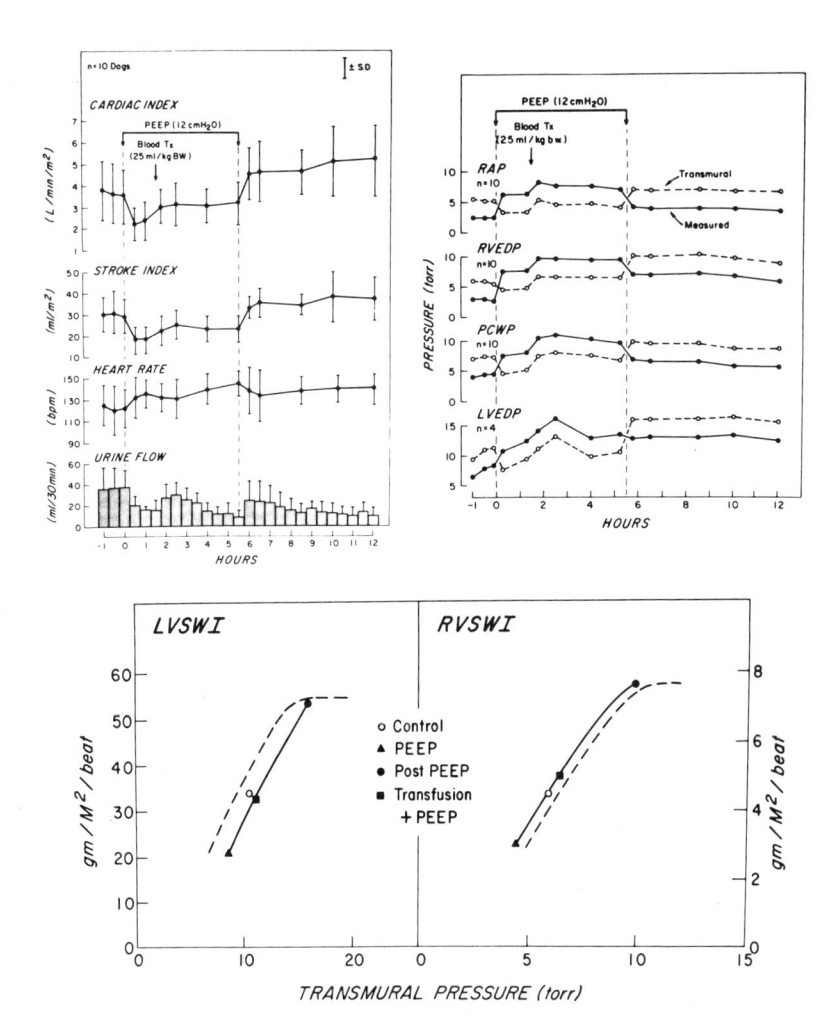

Figure 11-15. Effect of MV with PEEP and hypervolemia on hemodynamic function in anesthetized dogs. Transmural pressure was obtained as the difference between airway and pleural pressure. Addition of PEEP (12 cm H$_2$O) to MV resulted in a decrease of cardiac and stroke index, no significant change in heart rate, and a decrease in transmural pressures for all four heart chambers. Transfusion with 25 ml/kg BW of dog blood caused all variables to return to control values. After approximately six hours of MV with PEEP, the PEEP was removed and ventilation continued at zero end-expiratory pressure (MV with ZEEP). The reduction in airway pressure resulted in an RV and LVEDP that were significantly higher than before addition of PEEP (upper right panel) because of blood volume redistribution in the presence of hypervolemia. Using the Frank-Starling relationship (bottom panel) we note that addition of PEEP lowers stroke work indices as well as transmural pressures (▲). Transfusion during MV with PEEP caused this relationship to return to control values (■). Removal of PEEP caused both to rise significantly (●) to a point near the plateau or failure stage for both RV and LV. *(Reproduced with permission from Qvist J, Pontoppidan H, Wilson R S, Lowenstein E, and Laver M B. Hemodynamic responses to mechanical ventilation with PEEP. Anesthesiology 42:45–55, 1975.)*

longer cause an increase in stroke work index.

Turning to the postoperative period, Trichet et al. (1975) studied the response of patients with and without pulmonary hypertension to added PEEP during mechanical ventilation. Their data are summarized in Figure 11–16. None of these patients was in respiratory failure at the time of study, although some, particularly after mitral valve replacement (MVR), exhibited a markedly elevated left atrial pressure and calculated pulmonary vascular resistance (PVR). Patients with a normal PVR (i.e., after aortic valve replacement—AVR) demonstrated the predictable hemodynamic and blood-gas exchange response when PEEP was added to their ventilatory pattern: cardiac output fell and $\dot{Q}_S/\dot{Q}_T$ decreased. In patients with pulmonary hypertension and after MVR, added PEEP had relatively little effect on PVR, while cardiac output did not change despite a decrease in right and left atrial transmural pressures. How do we explain this phenomenon? Reference to Figure 11–17 will be helpful.

Let us assume that the patient being ventilated mechanically with PEEP has a right ventricle (RV) whose pump function is characterized by the flat portion of the Frank-Starling curve; let us also assume that this condition occurs in association with a state of hypervolemia and elevated ventricular filling pressures, a condition often induced to maintain an optimal arterial blood pressure. If PEEP is discontinued, the reduction in airway pressure results in increased venous inflow, an increase in transmural pressure (secondary to enhanced venous return), but no change in stroke volume. If pulmonary vascular disease is present with a decreased pulmonary vascular compliance, redistribution of blood into the lungs will cause a further decrease in vascular compliance, an increase in RV afterload, and the right ventricular function curve will shift to the right. As a consequence, stroke

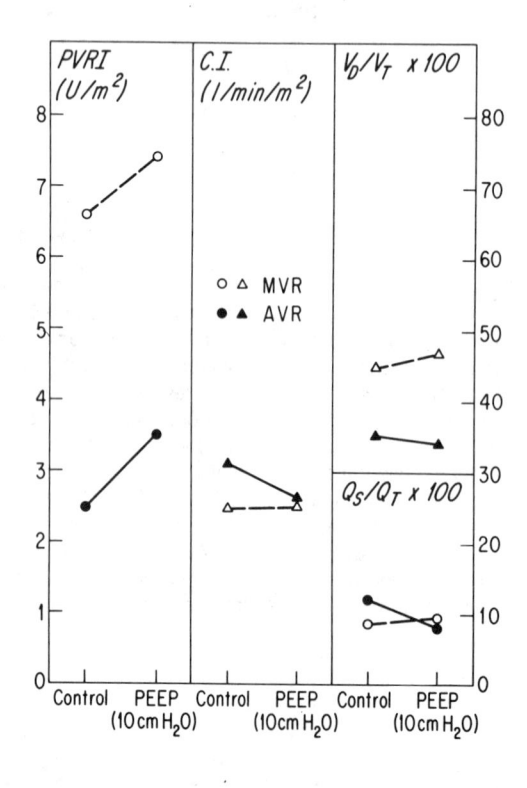

Figure 11–16. Effect of added PEEP (10 cm H$_2$O) during mechanical ventilation following mitral (MVR) and aortic valve replacement (AVR). Patients with MVR had a substantially higher PVRI (PA$_{mean}$ − LA$_{mean}$/C I) than patients with AVR. Upon addition of PEEP, cardiac index (C I) and $\dot{Q}_S/\dot{Q}_T$ × 100 decreased only in AVR patients. We attribute this to the abnormalities of the pulmonary vasculature present in patients with MVR in whom the distribution of pulmonary blood flow is reversed, the apices being preferentially perfused. The increase in airway pressure increased ventilation either to the poorly perfused dependent lung, or to the ventilated, well-perfused nondependent lobes where $\dot{Q}_S/\dot{Q}_T$ was low to begin with (see also Figure 11–8). The percentage of increase in PVRI was substantially less in MVR than AVR patients. None had a large $\dot{Q}_S/\dot{Q}_T$ × 100. It is likely that a high PVRI combined with marked hypervolemia may decrease markedly the compliance of the pulmonary vasculature when airway pressure is reduced and blood translocated to the lung. In this case, RV afterload would rise and cardiac output decrease despite a reduction in airway pressure. (Reproduced with permission from Trichet B, Falke K, Togut A, & Laver M B. The effect of pre-existing pulmonary vascular disease on the response to mechanical ventilation with PEEP following open-heart surgery. Anesthesiology 42:56–67, 1975.)

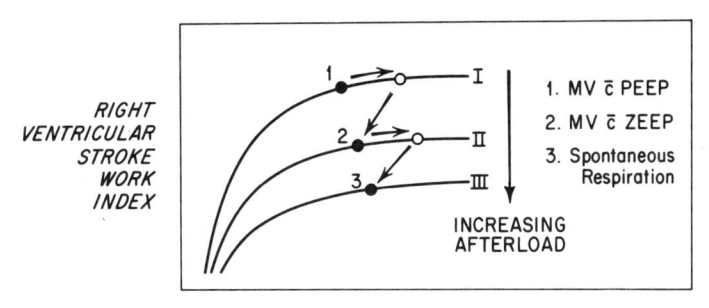

Figure 11-17. Plot of RVSWI [(RVP$_{systolic}$ − RVP$_{endiastolic}$) × stroke index] versus transmural pressure (TMP) at different levels of afterload produced by changes in airway pressure. We assume here that the right ventricle is in failure and on the flat portion of its Frank-Starling curve (point no. 1) during mechanical ventilation with PEEP. Upon removal of PEEP, additional blood returns to the right heart and TMP rises (see arrow). If pulmonary vascular compliance is low, further distention by an increased pulmonary blood volume will cause vascular compliance to fall (i.e., afterload rises). This shifts the RVSWI versus TMP relationship to the right (curve II) and RVSWI decreases (point no. 2). The decrease in TMP from curve I to II is due to the decrease in pleural pressure secondary to a reduction in airway pressure. The same mechanism comes into effect when the patient is allowed to breathe spontaneously (curve III). Thus, with each quantitative decrease in airway pressure, stroke index will decrease, not increase as expected with normal heart and lungs.

volume will decrease while measured transmural pressure will barely increase. Further reduction in airway pressure, as when an attempt at spontaneous respiration is made, can place an additional burden on the right ventricle.

None of the usually available measurements of blood flow or filling pressure is satisfactory for diagnosis of the complex mechanisms functioning in the patient with pulmonary hypertension. Clarification has been made possible by use of the gamma camera after intravenous administration of the isotope technetium-99m for visualization of both right and left ventricles during systole and diastole (Fig. 11-18). This technique, used with increasing frequency at the bedside, has provided greater appreciation of the degree of acute right ventricular dysfunction when pulmonary vascular resistance is abnormally high.

These considerations lead us to several important practical consequences. First, an ability to wean from ventilator therapy will be closely dependent on the adequacy of right ventricular function and the ability of the right ventricle to adjust to an increase in either pre- or afterload. The presence of right ventricular failure with an elevated PVR precludes discontinuation of mechanical ventilation, since a reduction in airway pressure will intensify the magnitude of RV dysfunction. Second, if weaning from the ventilator is unsuccessful, improvement of RV function by the administration of inotropic drugs is in order. If the problems of RV function are recognized early, weaning from mechanical ventilation must proceed prior to cessation of inotropic therapy. In addition, an attempt must be made to reduce PVR by drug therapy with vasodilators (e.g., nitroprusside).

As the data of Trichet et al. (1975) have demonstrated, oxygenation is not impaired in patients with a high PVR soon after surgery. In fact, these patients may be well-oxygenated at a relatively low inspired O$_2$ concentration (i.e., 40 percent) yet unable to tolerate periods of spontaneous ventilation. In other words, adequacy of arterial oxygenation fails to provide a proper criterion for the need of ventilator support. Since the lower or dependent lung portions are affected by chronic pulmonary venous hypertension, with the bulk of ventilation and perfusion diverted to the non-

Figure 11-18. Components necessary for obtaining a gated cardiac blood pool scan. Technetium-99m-tagged human serum albumin (^{99m}Tc-HSA) is given intravenously. The gamma camera collects counts that produce an image of the cardiac blood pool while the synchronizer allows collection of counts gated to the electrocardiogram, so that one image is collected during the QRS complex (end-diastole) and a second image during the later portion of the T wave (end-systole). The images displayed in this illustration were obtained in the 50-degree left anterior oblique projection. The left ventricle (right) and right ventricle and pulmonary outflow tract (left) are easily identified. The interventricular septum is also well defined. Comparison of diastole and systole reveals normal concentric contraction of both ventricles. *(Reproduced with permission from Wexler L F & Pohost G M. Hemodynamic monitoring: Noninvasive techniques. Anesthesiology 45:156–183, 1976.)*

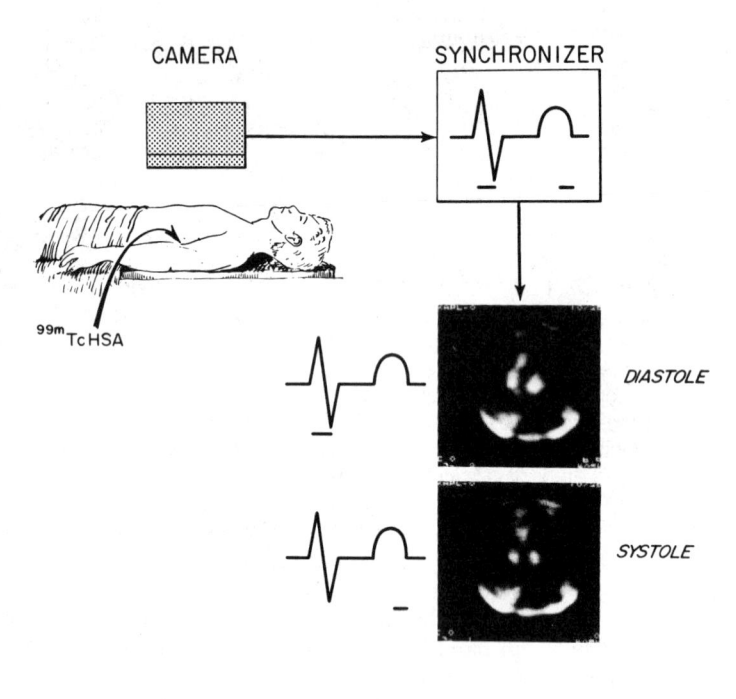

dependent lung, weaning may be extremely difficult, particularly when it is attempted in the presence of a low cardiac output.

It is likely that early use of vasodilator therapy to reduce right ventricular afterload and augment blood flow has more to offer when combined with conventional inotropy. Because of the low flow state, gram-negative sepsis is common and further deterioration of lung function is likely.

METHODOLOGY OF VENTILATOR SUPPORT

Details of methodology are beyond the scope of this chapter but are available elsewhere. Standards for optimal care have been published (Behnke et al., 1971; Pontoppidan et al., 1973).

Routine ventilator support during the first 24 hours after open heart surgery can be provided with either pressure- or volume-controlled ventilators. If "effective" compliance is high, i.e., ratio of tidal volume (ml) to peak inspiratory pressure (cm H_2O) is higher than 40, arterial Po_2 is in excess of 150 mm Hg when $FI_{O_2} = 0.5$, and the chest film is clear, use of a pressure-controlled ventilator will suffice. The volume-controlled ventilator is mandatory when compliance deteriorates and peak airway pressures in excess of 35 cm H_2O are required. We generally choose a tidal volume of 15 ml/kg BW and set the rate to maintain arterial Pco_2 within normal limits, adding mechanical dead space as required.

Early weaning is achieved by allowing the patients to breathe spontaneously through the endotracheal tube via a T-piece arrangement with added oxygen (Fig. 11–19). Stable arterial blood gases (Po_2 in excess of 150 mm Hg while the patient inspires 50 percent O_2), a forced expired vital capacity of 10 ml/kg BW, a cardiac index in excess of 2.5 liters/min/m^2, chest tube drainage less than 1 mg/kg/hr, lack of agitation, and a clear sensorium are signs that favor extubation. Occasionally, one may encounter a patient whose hemodynamic status, chest x-ray, arterial oxygenation, and sensorium are all within normal limits yet whose spontaneous ventilation through an endotracheal tube may be accompanied by a marked elevation in Pco_2 and corresponding decrease in arterial pH. For reasons that are not entirely clear, these patients may appear comfortable breathing through the endotracheal tube and, upon extubation, alveolar ventilation improves and arterial Pco_2 returns to normal.

If prolonged mechanical ventilation is required (i.e., over a period of days or weeks), every effort should be made to establish a pattern of intermittent spontaneous ventilation (also termed intermittent mandatory ventilation) except under the most precarious hemodynamic circumstances. When arterial Po_2 cannot be maintained above 100 mm Hg with less than 80 percent inspired O_2, ventilation (mechanical with continuous or intermittent positive end-expiratory pressure) is indicated. The amount of required positive pressure (i.e., MV with PEEP, CPAP) can only be determined by trial and error. We usually begin with 8 to 10 cm H_2O; less is rarely

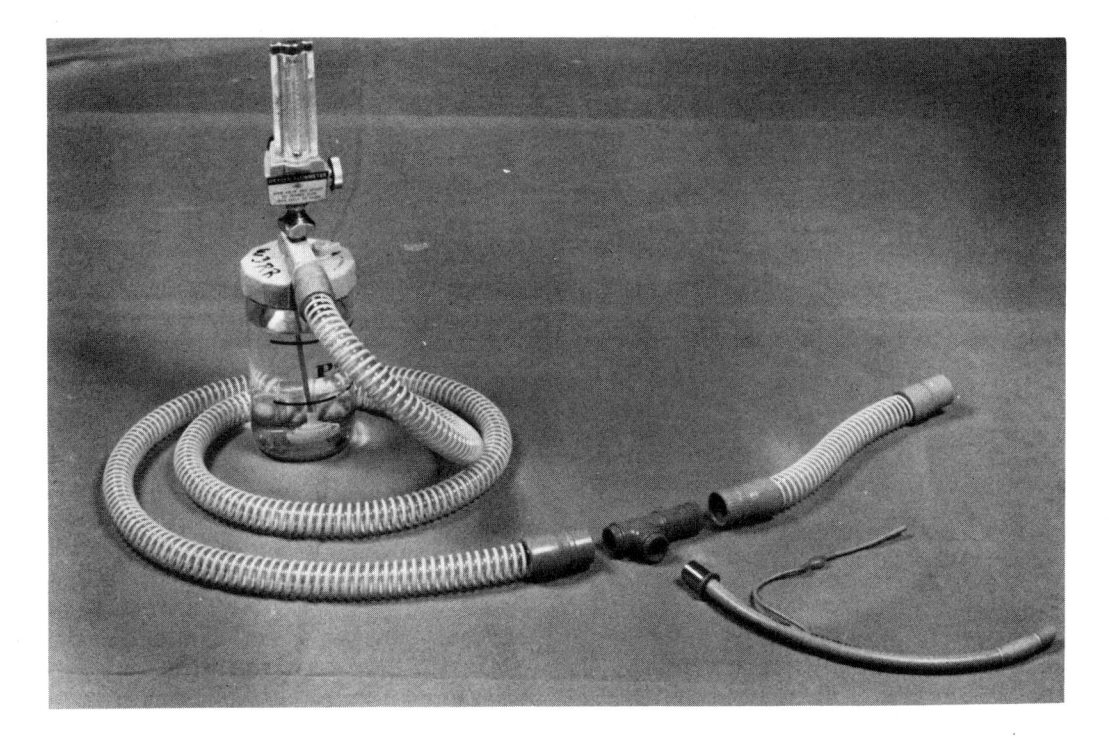

Figure 11–19. Arrangement for spontaneous respiration via an endotracheal tube with increased F_{IO_2}. The desired O_2 concentration is regulated at vaporizer. A small segment of corrugated tubing is added on the expiratory side of the T-piece to prevent excessive dilution of inspirate with ambient air. If the patient's tidal volume is large, gas flow must be increased and the corrugated tubing on the expiratory side lengthened. At gas flows in excess of twice minute ventilation, the tubing on the expired side will not act as a dead space. *(Reproduced with permission from Dalton B C, Hallowell P, Bland J H L, & Lowenstein E. A method for supplemental O_2 administration during weaning from mechanical ventilation. Anesthesiology 33:452–454, 1970.)*

effective. Considerably higher levels of PEEP (15 to 20 cm H₂O) may be required in the presence of profound pulmonary dysfunction. In our experience, there has been little or no need for PEEP in excess of 15 cm H₂O in patients whose respiratory failure followed open heart surgery.

Patients who have required prolonged ventilation with high airway pressures must be weaned by spontaneous respiration with decreasing amounts of PEEP (Civetta et al., 1972) (Fig. 11–20). Spontaneous ventilation without the benefit of PEEP accompanied by adequate gas exchange is an indication for extubation. In the patient with acute renal failure, mechanical ventilation should be considered and continued during peritoneal dialysis, irrespective of lung function. Infusion of the dialysate impairs diaphragmatic motion and limits gas exchange during attempts at spontaneous ventilation. Thorough chest physiotherapy must be included daily.

REFERENCES

Abouna G M, Veazey P R, Terry D B Jr: Intravenous infusion of hydrochloric acid for treatment of severe metabolic alkalosis. Surgery 75:194–202, 1974.

Agostoni E, Miserocchi G: Vertical gradient of trans-pulmonary pressure with active and artificial lung expansion. J Appl Physiol 29:705–712, 1970.

Andersen N, Ghia J: Pulmonary function, cardiac status, and postoperative course in relation to cardio-pulmonary bypass. J Thorac Cardiovasc Surg 59:474–483, 1970.

Ayres S M: Ventilatory management in pulmonary edema. Am J Med 54:558–562, 1973.

Bake B, Wood L, Murphy B, Macklem P T, Milic-Emili J: Effect of inspiratory flow rate on regional distribution of inspired gas. J Appl Physiol 37:8–17, 1974.

Beach T, Millen E, Grenvik A: Hemodynamic response to discontinuance of mechanical ventilation. Crit Care Med 1:85–90, 1973.

Behnke R H, Bristow J D, Carrieri V, Pierce J A,

Figure 11–20. Valveless system for spontaneous ventilation with positive end-expiratory pressure (PEEP) via an oro- or nasotracheal tube. Flowmeters deliver desired quantities of O₂ and compressed air to achieve an appropriate inspired concentration of oxygen. The 10-liter rubber bag, which acts as a reservoir, is compressed throughout the respiratory cycle to ensure maintenance of positive pressure. In practice, a second reservoir (not compressed) may be necessary to provide an adequate gas volume for a large inspirate, particularly if excessively high gas flow rates from the nebulizers are to be avoided. All tubing should be of as wide a bore as possible. *(Reproduced with permission from Wilson R, Pontoppidan H, in press.)*

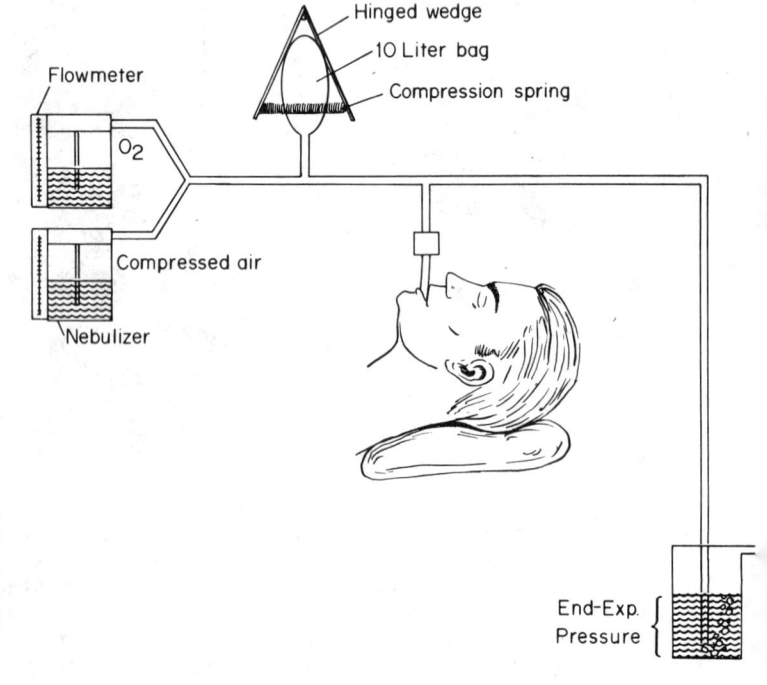

Sasahara A, Soffer A: Resources for the optimal care of acute respiratory failure. Study group on pulmonary heart disease. Circulation 43:A185–A195, 1971.

Bendixen H H, Egbert L D, Hedley-Whyte J, Laver M B, Pontoppidan H: Respiratory Care. St. Louis, C.V. Mosby, 1965.

Blaisdel F W, Schlobohm R M: The respiratory distress syndrome: a review. Surgery 74:251–262, 1973.

Burnham S C, Martin W E, Cheney F W Jr: The effects of various tidal volumes on gas exchange in pulmonary edema. Anesthesiology 37:27–31, 1972.

Caldwell P R B, Wittenberg B A: The oxygen dependency of mammalian tissues. Am J Med 57:447–452, 1974.

Civetta J M, Brons R, Gabel J C: A simple and effective method of employing spontaneous positive-pressure ventilation. J Thorac Cardiovasc Surg 63:312–317, 1972.

Cullen D J, Ferrara L: Comparative evaluation of blood filters. A study in vitro. Anesthesiology 41:568–575, 1974.

Dalton B C, Hallowell P, Bland J H L, Lowenstein E: A method for supplemental O_2 administration during weaning from mechanical ventilation. Anesthesiology 33:452–454, 1970.

Falke K, Pontoppidan H, Kumar A, Leith D E, Geffin B, Laver M B: Ventilation with end-expiratory pressure in acute lung disease. J Clin Invest 51:2315–2323, 1972.

Froese A B, Bryan A C: Effects of anesthesia and paralysis on diaphragmatic mechanics in man. Anesthesiology 41:242–255, 1974.

Ghia J, Andersen N B: Pulmonary function and cardio-pulmonary bypass. JAMA 212:593–597, 1970.

Goldring R M, Cannon P J, Heinemann H O, Fishman A P: Respiratory adjustment to chronic metabolic alkalosis in man. J Clin Invest 47:188–202, 1968.

Gump F E, Kinney J M, Price J B Jr: Energy metabolism in surgical patients: oxygen consumption and blood flow. J Surg Res 10:613–627, 1971.

Harken A H, Brennan M F, Smith B, Barsamian E M: The hemodynamic response to positive end-expiratory ventilation in hypovolemic patients. Surgery 76:786–793, 1974.

Harrison C V: The pathology of the pulmonary vessels in pulmonary hypertension. Br J Radiol 31:217–226, 1958.

Heistad D D, Abboud F M, Mark A L, Schmid P G: Impaired reflex vasoconstriction in chronically hypoxemic patients. J Clin Invest 51:331–337, 1972.

Hyatt R E, Rodarte J R: "Closing volume," one man's noise—other men's experiment. Mayo Clin Proc 50:17–27, 1975.

Kirby R R, Downs J B, Civetta J M, Modell J H, Dannemiller F J, Klein E F, Hodges M: High level positive end-expiratory pressure (PEEP) in acute respiratory insufficiency. Chest 67:156–163, 1975.

Laver M B, Austen W G: Lung Function: physiologic considerations applicable to surgery. In Sabiston D C Jr (ed.); Davis-Christopher Textbook of Surgery, 10th ed. Philadelphia, Saunders, 1972.

———, ———, Wilson R: Blood-gas exchange and hemodynamic performance. In Sabiston D C Jr, Spencer F C (eds): Surgery of the Chest, 3rd ed. Philadelphia, Saunders, 1975.

Lemelin J, Ross W R D, Martin R R, Anthonisen N R: Regional lung volumes with positive pressure inflation in erect humans. Resp Physiol 16:273–281, 1972.

Markello R, Olszowka A, Winter P, Farhi L: An up-dated method for determining $V_A/\dot{Q}$ inequalities and direct shunt using O_2, CO_2 and N_2. Resp Physiol 19:221–232, 1973.

———, Winter P, Olszowka A: Assessment of ventilation-perfusion inequalities by arterial-alveolar nitrogen differences in intensive care patients. Anesthesiology 37:4–15, 1972.

Marshall B E, Soma L R, Harp J R, Neufeld G R, Wurzel H A, Dodd O C: Pulmonary function after exchange transfusion of stored blood in dogs. Ann Surg 179:46–51, 1974.

———, Wyche M Q Jr: Hypoxemia during and after anesthesia. Anesthesiology 37:178–209, 1972.

McAslan T C, Matsjasko-Chiu J, Turney S Z, Cowley R A: Influence of inhalation of 100% oxygen on intrapulmonary shunt in severely traumatized patients. J Trauma 13:811–821, 1973.

Nash G, Bowen J A, Langlinais P C: Respirator lung: a misnomer. Arch Pathol Lab Med 91:234–240, 1971.

Nomoto S, Berk J L, Hagen J F, Koo R: Pulmonary anatomic arteriovenous shunting caused by epinephrine. Arch Surg 108:201–204, 1974.

Pontoppidan H: The black box illuminated. Anesthesiology 37:1–3, 1972.

———, Geffin B, Lowenstein E: Acute Respiratory Failure in the Adult. Boston, Little, Brown, 1973.

Powers E R, Powell W J Jr: Effect of arterial hypoxia

on myocardial oxygen consumption. Circ Res 33:749–756, 1973.

Powers S R Jr, Mannal R, Neclerio M, English M, Marr C, Leather R, Ueda H, Williams G, Custead W, Dutton R: Physiologic consequences of positive end-expiratory pressure (PEEP) ventilation. Ann Surg 178:265–272, 1973.

Qvist J, Pontoppidan H, Wilson R S, Lowenstein E, Laver M B: Hemodynamic responses to mechanical ventilation with PEEP. Anesthesiology 42:45–55, 1975.

Rehder K, Hatch D J, Sessler A D, Fowler W S: The function of each lung of anesthetized and paralyzed man during mechanical ventilation. Anesthesiology 37:16–26, 1972.

———, ———, ———, Marsh H M, Fowler W S: Effects of general anesthesia, muscle paralysis and mechanical ventilation on pulmonary nitrogen clearance. Anesthesiology 35:591–601, 1971.

———, Wenthe F M, Sessler A D: Function of each lung during mechanical ventilation with ZEEP and with PEEP in man anesthetized with thiopental-meperidine. Anesthesiology 39:597–606, 1973.

Soma L R, Neufeld G R, Dodd D C, Marshall B E: Pulmonary function in hemorrhagic shock. The effect of pancreatic ligation and blood filtration. Ann Surg 179:395–402, 1974.

Staub N C, Nagano H, Pearce M L: Acute pulmonary edema in dogs, especially the sequence of fluid accumulation in the lungs. J Appl Physiol 22:227–240, 1967.

Suwa K, Geffin B, Pontoppidan H, Bendixen H H: A nomogram for deadspace requirement during prolonged artificial ventilation. Anesthesiology 29:1206–1210, 1968.

Thompson J S, Severson C D, Parmely M J, Marmorstein B L, Simmons A: Pulmonary "hypersensitivity" reactions induced by transfusion on non-HL-A leukoagglutinins. N Engl J Med 284:1120–1125, 1971.

Trichet B, Falke K, Togut A, Laver M B: The effect of pre-existing pulmonary vascular disease on the response to mechanical ventilation with PEEP following open-heart surgery. Anesthesiology 42:56–67, 1975.

Wagenvoort C A: Classifying pulmonary vascular disease. Chest 64:503–504, 1973.

Wagner P D, West J B: Effects of diffusion impairment on O_2 and CO_2 time courses in pulmonary capillaries. J Appl Physiol 33:62–71, 1972.

Weibel E R: Morphological basis of alveolar-capillary gas exchange. Physiol Rev 53:419–495, 1973.

Wexler L F, Pohost G M: Hemodynamic monitoring: non-invasive therapeutic criteria. Anesthesiology 45:156–183, 1976.

Wilson R S: Acute respiratory failure: diagnostic and therapeutic criteria. Crit Care Med 2:293–304, 1974.

12. Concepts of Ventilatory and Respiratory Care

ROY A. JURADO   JOSEPH JAGUST
SIDNEY OWITZ

Some degree of pulmonary dysfunction is almost uniformly observed after all types of thoracic and cardiac surgery. Such functional alterations usually are transitory and frequently are present in the total absence of overt clinical and radiologic signs. A variety of factors are known to contribute to such dysfunction; these are briefly reviewed in Chapter 6 and discussed in greater detail in Chapter 13.

The nature of this functional impairment generally takes the form of *decreased oxygenation* and *ventilatory depression,* resulting in *arterial hypoxemia, alveolar hypoventilation,* and a *reduced ventilatory reserve.* Since postoperative metabolic demands invariably are increased (Carlston et al., 1954), the net result is an unfavorable alteration of supply (oxygen transport) and demand (oxygen consumption) relationships, setting the stage for impaired tissue exchange.

The main goal of therapy is to favorably alter and optimize ventilatory supply and demand relationships by: (1) preventing hypoventilation; (2) improving respiratory gas exchange; (3) optimizing the efficiency of the oxygen transport system; and (4) reducing metabolic needs and energy expenditure. The successful accomplishment of these objectives requires optimal support of ventilatory and circulatory functions and proper attention to the demands of tissue metabolism. This chapter is devoted to discussions of those concepts and management techniques considered important in the attainment of these objectives.

MANAGEMENT TECHNIQUES

At the end of the operation, a clinical decision is made whether to allow the patient to resume unassisted spontaneous ventilation or whether mechanical ventilatory assistance is required. This decision is arrived at after careful consideration of the following: (1) the severity of preexisting cardiorespiratory disease; (2) the patient's cardiorespiratory and neurologic status at operative termination; (3) the magnitude of the operative procedure; (4) the extent of anesthetic reversal; and (5) the probability of impaired performance of the cardiac or pulmonary subsystems in the early postoperative interval. Patients undergoing relatively minor, uncomplicated operative procedures and who have no significant preoperative cardiorespiratory impairment may be allowed to resume spontaneous ventilation soon after the end of the operation. On the other hand, the use of temporary mechanical ventilatory assistance is advisable for patients undergoing complicated operative repair requiring prolonged cardiopulmonary bypass and for those whose cardiac or pulmonary function is considered borderline or when the likelihood of impaired cardiopulmonary performance in the early postoperative hours is great.

If it appears likely that postoperative mechanical ventilatory assistance may not be necessary, the indwelling endotracheal tube (generally of the orotracheal type) is allowed to remain in place and the patient is transferred to the intensive care unit (ICU) with mechanical ventilation maintained manually. Complete anesthetic reversal and extubation ideally are deferred until after the patient is well-settled in the ICU and his or her vital functions carefully reassessed. This practice offers the advantage of complete control of respiratory function during the critical transfer period, when surveillance is perhaps at its lowest level. It also allows for a smoother transition from mechanical to spontaneous ventilation as soon as emergence from the anesthetic effect is completed.

However, if it appears likely that prolonged mechanical ventilatory assistance will be required postoperatively, the orotracheal tube is replaced with a nasotracheal tube prior to the patient's transfer to the ICU. A nasotracheal tube is preferred when ventilatory support will be required for more than 24 hours because it is much better tolerated by a conscious patient and it facilitates maintenance of oral hygiene. Additionally, the possibility of tube obstruction from biting is eliminated and the hazards of kinking are significantly reduced. Adequate ventilation can be delivered and proper pulmonary toilet maintained provided nasotracheal tubes of appropriate lumen size (≥ 7 mm internal diameter for adults) are used.

The patient is transported to the ICU accompanied by the anesthesiologist and surgeon. Manual ventilation is maintained with an Ambu bag using a well-humidified inspired gas mixture ($F_{IO_2} \cong 0.8$). A not uncommon occurrence at this point is vigorous and overenthusiastic hyperventilation. This should be avoided because of the increased likelihood of life-threatening arrhythmias associated with hypocarbia and hypokalemia—the latter a common occurrence following hemodilute perfusion. The risk of producing hypocarbia may be minimized by interposing a sufficient length of respiratory dead space tubing in the breathing circuit. Hypoventilation, on the other hand, is especially dangerous because of the possibility of hypoxia and hypercarbia.

Spontaneous Ventilation

Criteria for Early Extubation. In patients who have undergone simple operations and are doing very well after their return to the ICU, extubation may be carried out and spontaneous ventilation allowed if certain criteria are satisfied. These criteria (not arranged in the order of importance) are listed in Table 12-1. In brief, a neurologically intact patient with satisfactory and stable cardiopulmonary and other subsystems performance, without life-threatening complications (such as postoperative bleeding and arrhythmias), is a good candidate for early extubation.

Postextubation Management. After removal of the endotracheal tube, a well-humidified oxygen-rich mixture ($F_{IO_2} = 0.4$) is administered for 24 to 48 hours by facemask, nasal cannula, or tent. Adequate humidification of the inspired gas mixture is essential for the maintenance of normal bronchial ciliary activity and helps prevent thickening, drying, and crusting of secretions. Effective humidification is accomplished by passage of the inspired gas over a heated water bath to saturate it with water vapor. Alternatively, an ultrasonic nebulizer may be used, if it is available.

To prevent postoperative pulmonary complications, the patient is placed on a program of frequent deep breathing, coughing, chest physiotherapy, and turning from side to side. Frequent deep breathing and related maneuvers help break the pattern of shallow monotonous tidal ventilation without sighs so often seen in postoperative patients, which invariably leads to progressive alveolar collapse. Total lung capacity, functional residual capacity (FRC), residual volume, and lung compliance decrease while the work of

TABLE 12-1 CRITERIA FOR EXTUBATION AND ALLOWING SPONTANEOUS VENTILATION SOON AFTER CARDIAC SURGERY

1. Patient alert and completely responsive.
2. Cardiac pulmonary, and renal subsystems performance satisfactory.
3. Arterial blood-gas and acid-base values satisfactory. This usually means:
   a. Pao_2 of at least 100 mm Hg (Fio_2 of 0.4)
   b. $Paco_2$ between 35 and 45 mm Hg
   c. Absence of significant base deficit.
4. Absence of significant complications:
   a. postoperative mediastinal or chest drainage not excessive.
   b. life-threatening cardiac arrhythmias not present.
5. Criteria for weaning from and termination of mechanical ventilation satisfied otherwise.*

*See Weaning from Mechanical Ventilation and Table 12-2.

breathing is increased. Almost invariably, the result is arterial hypoxia caused by increased shunting and venous admixture (perfusion of nonventilated alveoli).

There is evidence that this train of events largely can be prevented and reversed if maximal inflations to total lung capacity are included in the respiratory maneuvers, either by positive pressure inflation or by voluntary maximal inspiration (Bartlett et al., 1973). Expiratory exercises, including coughing, blowing into a balloon or glove, and blowing out against resistance (blow bottles), may also be helpful if maximal lung inflations from deep inspiration are made part of the maneuvers. The use of commercially available equipment such as the incentive spirometer accomplishes the same objective. Chest physiotherapy and frequent position changes may facilitate clearing of tracheobronchial secretions and help prevent bronchiolar obstruction and atelectasis.

Criteria for Reinstitution of Mechanical Ventilation. After removal of the endotracheal tube, close surveillance is maintained and the patient is carefully observed for signs of deterioration of cardiorespiratory function. Early warning signs of difficulty frequently include tachypnea, flaring of the alae nasi, increased respiratory efforts with use of the accessory muscles of respiration, and diaphoresis. These circumstances, by themselves, may constitute indications for reintubation.

It must be remembered that measurements of arterial blood-gas tensions at this point may be misleading, since the delivery of an oxygen-rich inspiratory gas mixture and hyperventilation may help maintain relatively normal Pao_2 and $Paco_2$ values. In practice, the first arterial blood-gas analysis is performed one hour after extubation. If the $Paco_2$ is between 45 and 55 mm Hg or the Pao_2 is less than 80 mm Hg, the respiratory maneuvers described in the previous section are intensified and the blood-gas measurements are repeated in one hour. If the subsequent arterial blood-gas analysis set shows a persistent hypercarbia ($Paco_2 > 55$ mm Hg) or hypoxemia ($Pao_2 < 70$ mm Hg), reintubation with reestablishment of mechanical ventilation should be strongly considered.

At this point, clinical signs of advanced deterioration may become apparent. These generally include clouding of the sensorium, tachycardia, the development of arrhythmias, peripheral vasoconstriction, a decrease in the urine output, and, eventually, hypotension. On rare occasions, hypertension, tachycardia, and elevated intracardiac filling pressures associated with hypercarbia may predominate; this clinical picture generally is seen in patients who have been heavily sedated and in those who have significant, but largely unrecognized, pulmonary pathology. The appearance of signs of impaired cardiac performance is an overriding indication for reintubation and reinstitution of mechanical ventilatory assistance, regardless of the prevailing biochemical picture.

Elective Short-Term Mechanical Ventilation

Rationale. The use of temporary mechanical ventilation prior to extubation is deemed advisable in patients undergoing open intracardiac operations (Lowenstein & Bland, 1972). Such a practice would seem logical in the face of a number of unfavorable physiologic alterations that occur in the early postoperative period. First, there is a reduction in ventilatory reserve (see Chapter 6). Second, postoperative metabolic demands are increased (Carlsten et al., 1954). Third, the postperfusion state generally is accompanied by some measurable reduction in cardiac performance (Boyd et al., 1959; Kirklin and Theye, 1963).

Mechanical ventilation optimizes respiratory gas exchange and ensures proper ventilation and oxygenation during this period of relative cardiorespiratory instability. Moreover, it can significantly reduce the metabolic cost of breathing (Dammann et al., 1963), which may be increased as much as twenty times normal in postoperative cardiac surgical patients (Thung et al., 1963). Thus, by reducing the energy cost of breathing, mechanical ventilatory assistance proportionally relieves the heart of the unnecessary workload—a most important therapeutic adjunct in patients with reduced cardiac performance and limited reserve capacity.

If cardiopulmonary bypass has been employed, ventilatory assistance for a few hours after the operation is prudent. In practice, most patients are placed on mechanical ventilation for a period of 12 to 18 hours. While selection of this time period is purely arbitrary, there are pragmatic considerations. First, most operations are completed in the latter half of the day. Second, it may take as long as 4 to 12 hours before hemodynamic stability is attained. Third, when operations are prolonged (more than 4 to 6 hours), patients will have received significant amounts of respiratory depressant or muscle relaxant drugs and complete reversal of their effects may take several hours. Experience has shown that many patients will not be ready to resume spontaneous ventilation until the late evening of the operative day. Consequently, most of these patients are electively placed on mechanical ventilation overnight and extubated the following day. It is not considered good practice to extubate patients at night when the level of ICU surveillance may be less than optimal.

In patients requiring short-term (< 24 hours mechanical ventilation) an orotracheal tube is preferred.

Principles of Patient Management. Management of patients placed on elective overnight mechanical ventilation is similar to that of those who require more prolonged periods of ventilatory support. Thus, the established principles of respiratory care are meticulously followed: careful nursing, adequate sedation, proper humidification and tracheobronchial toilette, periodic position change, chest physiotherapy, and, above all, intelligent use of the ventilator. These principles will be discussed in greater detail under the sections that follow.

MANAGEMENT OF PATIENTS REQUIRING PROLONGED MECHANICAL VENTILATORY ASSISTANCE

Indications for Prolonged Mechanical Ventilatory Assistance

While most patients can safely resume spontaneous respiration within the first 24 hours after surgery, some will require mechanical support of ventilation for longer periods (i.e., from a few days to several weeks). This group includes those with (1) severe preexisting pulmonary pathology; (2) severe pulmonary resistive hypertension; (3) reduced postoperative cardiac performance with low cardiac output; (4) pulmonary edema; (5) acute respiratory insufficiency (see Chapter 13); and (6) acute cerebral dysfunction. The specific indications for mechanical ventilation can be broadly categorized as follows: (1) *hypoventilation;* (2) *increased work of breathing;* (3) *ventilation-perfusion ($\dot{V}/Q$) imbalance;* (4) *need for predictable delivery of high inspired oxygen concentrations* (F_{IO_2}); and (5) *need for special therapeutic modalities,* such as positive end-expiratory pressure (PEEP), continuous positive pressure ventilation (CPPV), and intermittent mandatory ventilation (IMV). Frequently, multiple specific indications coexist and therapy is designed accordingly.

In general, patients requiring prolonged mechanical ventilatory assistance have either marginal or reduced cardiopulmonary reserves. In such patients, it is essential to follow a carefully designed program of management. An example of such a program is outlined below.

Choice of Airway

For the reasons cited earlier, a nasotracheal tube is preferred in virtually all situations where it is anticipated that ventilatory support will be required for more than 24 hours. There are but a few exceptions to this rule. For example, if the patient's hemodynamic condition at operative termination is extremely unstable, it is wiser to allow the indwelling orotracheal tube to remain undisturbed and defer passage of a nasotracheal tube to a more propitious moment. In rare instances, unfavorable patient anatomy (e.g., narrow airways, septal abnormalities) may preclude atraumatic insertion of a nasotracheal tube of proper size and length. In most instances, however, a nasotracheal tube will have been passed and positioned before the patient's transfer to the ICU.

The nasotracheal tube can be safely left in place for as long as 7 to 10 days. Laryngeal and vocal cord injury can be minimized if a loose-fitting tube is used (Lindholm, 1969). Beyond this period, secretion removal becomes difficult, with increasing danger of tube obstruction by crusts. Moreover, the possibility of permanent vocal cord damage increases. Thus, when there is a great likelihood that mechanical ventilatory assistance may be required beyond this period, a tracheostomy is electively performed around the seventh day (see Special Problems).

Care of the Airway

Proper Positioning of the Airway. The proper size and length of the nasotracheal tube are determined prior to tube insertion. In making this decision, it is important to consider such factors as patient build and habitus, the probable size of the trachea and larynx, and the nasal anatomy. In general, small-diameter tubes (<7 mm, ID) are not satisfactory for use in most adults because of the greater possibility of obstruction from encrusted secretions. On the other hand, use of too large a tube increases the likelihood of local trauma (e.g., epistaxis, nasal necrosis, laryngeal and vocal cord injury). The nasotracheal tube should be of sufficient length so that final cuff position is situated just below the vocal cords, with the adapter-to-tube junction situated within 2 to 3 cm of the nostril. Use of too long a tube increases the likelihood of kinking and nasal necrosis from tube angulation and pressure; additionally, there is an enhanced possibility of accidental tube slippage and entry into one or the other main bronchus. With experience, selection of the appropriate tube can be made with dispatch.

The endotracheal tube is secured with strips of cotton tape tied around the tube at the level of the adapter-to-tube junction and then around the patient's neck below the ear. This may also be reinforced with narrow strips of adhesive tape applied in similar fashion. Once a secure tube position is obtained, it is good practice to place an indelible mark on

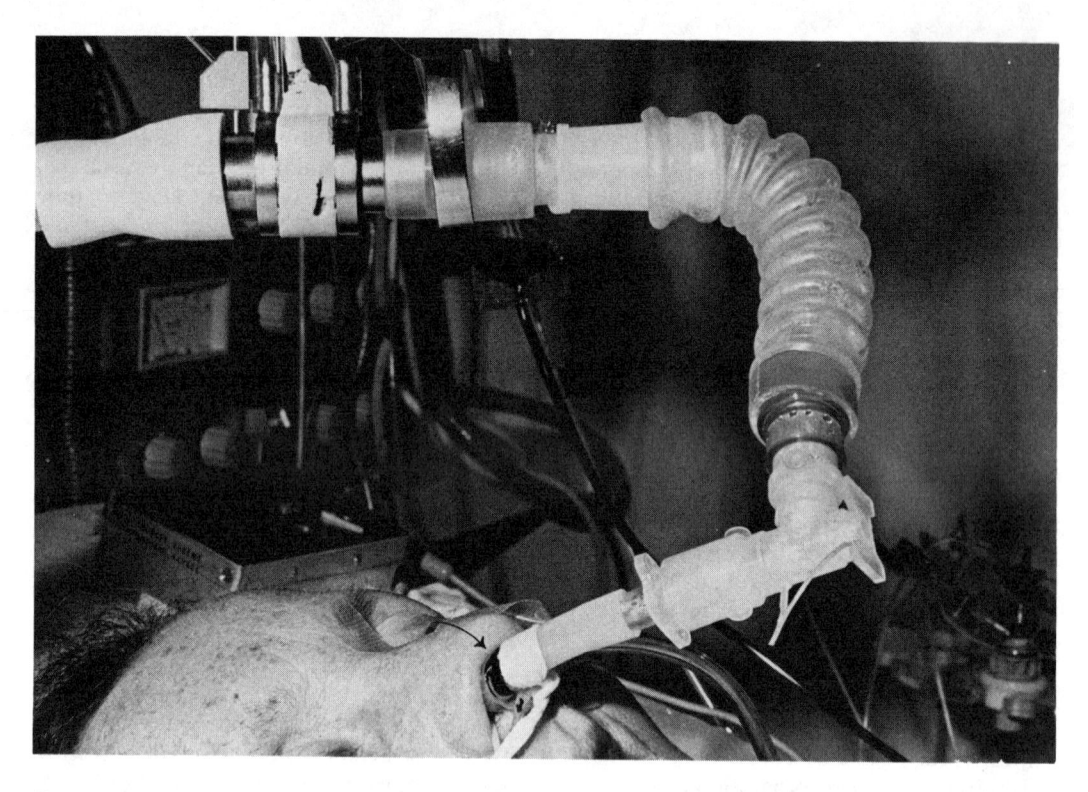

Figure 12-1. A method of securing an indwelling nasotracheal tube by means of cotton tape. After proper tube position is ascertained, it is helpful to place an indelible mark (arrow) on the tube for reference.

the tube, using the level of the external naris as the point of reference (Fig. 12-1). Meticulous attention to these details minimizes tracheal damage at points of contact and reduces the chances of inadvertent endobronchial intubation by preventing excessive endotracheal tube motion.

As a prophylaxis against nasal necrosis, excessive tension and angulation of the nasotracheal tube must be avoided (Zwillich and Pierson, 1973). This can be accomplished by securing the ventilatory tubing in such a fashion that patient movement does not produce undue tension on the tube. Use of a short length of flexible corrugated tube and a swivel-type connector interposed between the ventilator tubing and the endotracheal tube are helpful in this regard (Fig. 12-2). In addition, frequent inspection of the site of contact between tube and nose must be conducted; at the first sign of severe erythema, provisions for endotracheal intubation via alternative routes must be made and the nasotracheal tube removed.

Prevention of Tracheal Damage. Successful conduct of long-term mechanical ventilatory assistance requires the use of a cuffed tracheal tube to insure no-leak ventilation and to protect the respiratory tract from aspiration. This technique is now universally accepted and widely employed; however, there is the ever-present possibility of producing significant tracheal damage at the site of the inflatable balloon cuff. Such tracheal damage from prolonged intubation became a serious problem in the early years that followed the widespread use of mechanical ventilatory support techniques (Murphy et al., 1966; Cooper and Grillo, 1969b; Fishman et al., 1969; Shelly et

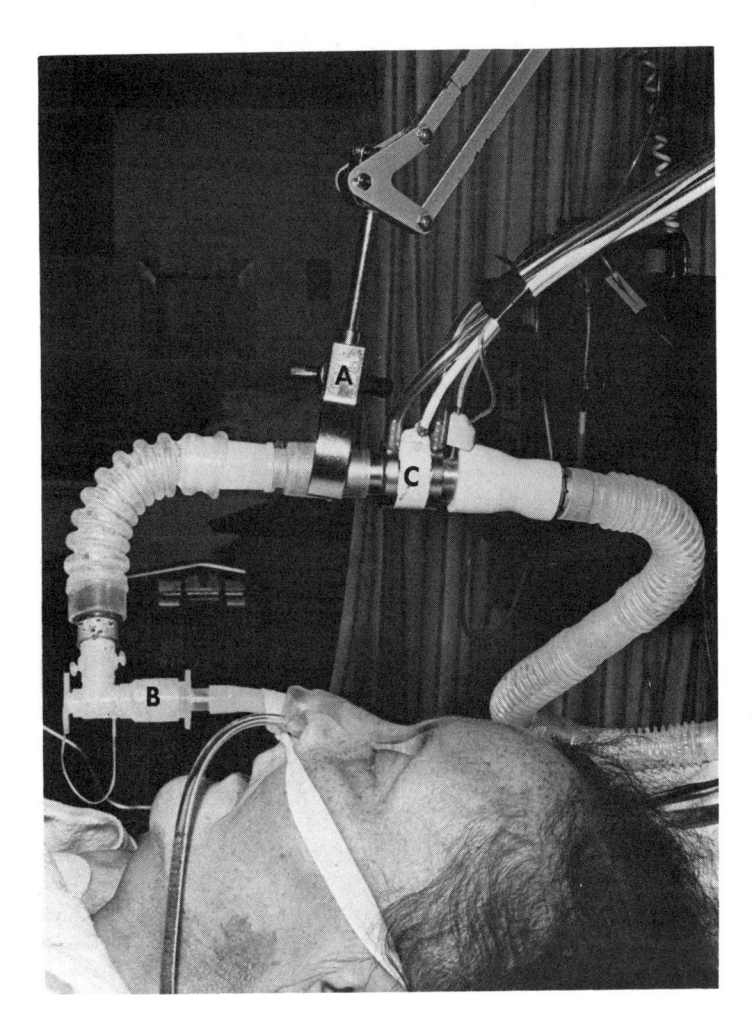

Figure 12-2. The use of a special holder (**A**) and a swivel connector (**B**) at the flex tube-to-tracheal tube junction helps relieve the pressure on the alae nasi while permitting sufficient patient mobility. A modified Fleisch pneumotachograph (**C**) is shown interposed in the patient's airway; the device permits automatic measurements of respiratory function.

al., 1969; Miller and Sethi, 1970; Andrews & Pearson, 1971; Geffin et al., 1971; Hedden et al., 1971; Tornvall et al., 1971). Indeed, it remains an important cause of morbidity despite advances in respiratory care techniques (Ching et al., 1974).

It has been established that the injury produced is ischemic in origin and that the pressure exerted on the tracheal wall by the inflated balloon cuff is the primary cause of the tracheal damage (Carroll et al., 1969; Cooper and Grillo, 1969a; Shelly et al., 1969; Miller and Sethi, 1970; Ching et al., 1971; Pearson and Andrews, 1971). A number of studies have clearly shown that ischemic injury with pressure necrosis is a virtual certainty if the transtracheal pressure (which is the difference between the intracuff pressure and airway pressure) is maintained in excess of the capillary and venous transmural pressures (Carroll et al., 1974; Dobrin et al., 1974), which normally are of the order of 20 to 25 mm Hg and 2 to 7 mm Hg, respectively (Guyton, 1965). Theoretically, sustained increases of transtracheal pressure over and above the 25 mm Hg level results in the cessation of all blood flow to the affected area, with ischemic pressure necrosis as the ultimate outcome. This was a common occurrence with the earlier types of balloon cuffs (i.e., the low-volume, high-pressure cuffs) (Cooper and Grillo, 1969a). Happily, use of the high-pressure balloon cuffs has largely been abandoned.

In recent years, substantial changes in cuff design and composition have been incorporated in the manufacture of tracheal tubes —the object being the prevention of tracheal damage achieved through the reduction of the resultant pressures exerted on the tracheal wall during cuff inflation (Grillo et al., 1971; Kamen and Wilkinson, 1971; Magovern et al., 1972). A most significant advance in tracheal tube design is the incorporation of a compliant, low-pressure balloon cuff with a large residual volume at atmospheric pressure (Carroll, 1973; Carroll et al., 1974). When air is injected, the cuff inflates symmetrically and conforms to the tracheal contour, minimizing transtracheal pressures. Moreover, cuff overinflation is accompanied with but a minimal increase in intracuff pressure.

Carroll et al. (1974) also showed that large-diameter, large-residual-volume cuffs possess the highly desirable property of automatically adjusting intracuff pressure to equal airway pressure, if the airway pressure rises above the resting cuff pressure during mechanical ventilation. When properly used, such a system ensures the maintenance of cuff and transtracheal pressures at the lowest levels possible, ranging from that which is necessary to prevent aspiration during expiration (generally achieved at resting cuff pressures of no greater than 15 mm Hg) to that which is required to provide an airtight seal during inflation of the lungs (highest possible pressure reached will be no greater than the airway pressure, as cuff pressure will rise above resting levels only if it is exceeded by the airway pressure). Certain tracheal tubes are equipped with a pressure-regulating device that prevents pressure in excess of 20 to 25 mm Hg on the tracheal wall (Magovern et al., 1972). An example of this type of tube is shown in Figure 12-3. In some models, no-leak ventilation can be achieved with the pressure-regulating device operating at 16 to 18 mm Hg (Carroll et al., 1974).

Routine care plans for patients requiring prolonged mechanical ventilation should include provisions for periodic cuff deflation and measurements of intracuff pressure and cuff volume. Cuff deflation allows removal of potentially contaminated secretions trapped in the cul-de-sac between the vocal cords and the balloon cuff; in addition, it provides an opportunity to measure intracuff pressure. Intracuff pressure measurements, in turn, permit estimations of transtracheal pressure to be made as long as the cuff is under no circumferential tension (Carroll et al., 1974). Moreover, when performed by properly trained personnel, such measurements prevent accidental overinflation. In practice, these maneuvers are performed once during each nursing shift (i.e., three times a day). Frequent (hourly) cuff deflation, which was originally thought to be essential in the prevention of tracheal injury, has largely been abandoned because it was found to be not only ineffective but also potentially harmful because it increased the chances of accidental overinflation (Bryant et al., 1971). Cuff pres-

Figure 12–3. An example of an endotracheal tube equipped with a large-volume, low-pressure, inflatable cuff and a regulating valve that precludes cuff inflation to pressures in excess of 20 to 25 mm Hg.

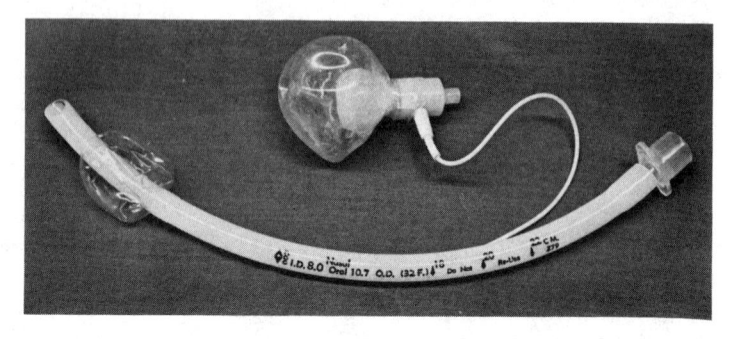

sure and volume measurements are performed easily with simple and readily available equipment (Fig. 12-4).

To summarize, use of the tracheal tubes equipped with large-volume, low-pressure inflatable cuffs and careful attention to the details of proper tube positioning and cuff inflation and deflation help reduce the likelihood of permanent tracheal damage in patients requiring prolonged mechanical ventilation.

Maintenance of Airway Patency. A properly functioning and patent airway can be ensured by assiduous care with meticulous attention to the techniques outlined below (see Care of the Patient Requiring Mechanical Ventilatory Assistance).

Guidelines for the Proper Conduct of Mechanical Ventilation

Successful application of mechanical ventilation to patient care requires understanding of respiratory and cardiovascular physiology and some of the basic principles of physics and chemistry. Of equal importance is a good working knowledge of the obligatory alterations in lung function that occur after cardiac surgery and the pathophysiologic mechanisms that underlie respiratory failure. In addition, knowledge of pulmonary disease and of currently available respiratory care methods and technology is most useful. For more detailed information about respiratory function, respiratory therapy, and mechanical ventilators, the reader is referred to the monographs and reports of Peters (1969), Pontoppidan et al. (1970), Egan (1973), and Lough et al. (1974).

Basic Physical Principles. One should remember that the patient's tracheobronchial tree and alveoli, as well as the devices used during mechanical ventilation, conform to the basic physical principles that govern gases and gas flows. The proper use of a mechanical ventilator requires attention to the following physical variables: (1) *volume;* (2) *pressure;* (3) *flow;* and (4) *time,* which is subdivided into *inspiratory* and *expiratory* periods. *Volume* and *pressure* are, of course, related directly to each

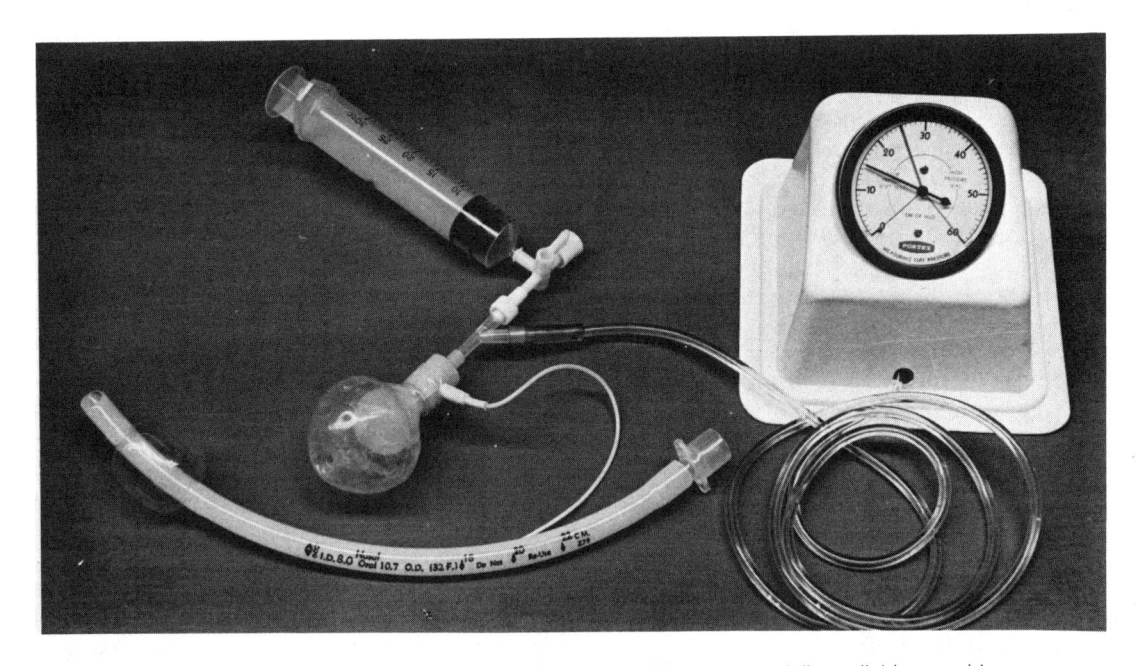

Figure 12–4. A simple method of monitoring intracuff pressure with a commercially available aneroid gauge.

other by *compliance*, defined as the change in volume divided by the change in pressure, or $\Delta V/\Delta P$. If a *time* base is added to the volume-pressure relationship, it becomes possible to calculate *flow rate;* additionally, inspiratory and expiratory times can then be determined with relative ease.

It is important to distinguish between two entirely different flow rates. The *minute volume* is defined as the tidal volume multiplied by the respiratory frequency. The *instantaneous flow rate* is the actual rate at which gas flows into and out of the respiratory system at any instant (dV/dt). Peak flow rates are the maximum flow rates during breathing and are usually at four to five times greater than the minute volume. It is appropriate to consider peak flow rates when assessing the effects of *resistance* to breathing.

Resistance, although not directly measurable, can be readily calculated. Using Ohm's law, resistance is defined as pressure divided by flow (R = P/F). It should be remembered that any change in airway resistance when a volume-limited mechanical ventilator is used will have its expressed consequence in the pressures being generated. Similarly, such a change in a pressure-limited device will be expressed as a change in the volume delivered. That is, an increased system resistance in a volume-limited machine will increase the pressure required to deliver the volume, and, where the pressure is fixed, the same increase in resistance will produce a fall in delivered volume. Of course, the opposite also holds true.

Choice of Ventilator. Fundamental to the care of patients who require assisted ventilation is a thorough understanding of one or more versatile ventilators. Since the optimal pattern for mechanical ventilation varies from patient to patient and frequently in the same patient from one moment to another, available equipment must be versatile enough to allow for such changes. A number of modern-day volume-cycled ventilators satisfy this requirement for flexibility.

In the selection of the proper ventilator, it is generally acceptable to use the pressure-cycled machines for short-term postoperative ventilation, especially in patients with minimal cardiorespiratory dysfunction, and for weaning from mechanical ventilation. On the other hand, the use of volume-cycled ventilators is mandatory for patients with impending or established respiratory failure with significantly deranged lung mechanics (with changing airway resistance or low compliance), for those in whom prolonged support is anticipated (as for patients with chronic valvular disease with severe pulmonary hypertension and pulmonary fibrosis), and for patients with impaired cardiac performance (reduced cardiac output). In comparison with the pressure-cycled types, volume-cycled ventilators possess the highly desirable property of ensuring predictable delivery of the predetermined inspiratory volume even in the face of rapidly changing airway resistance and lung compliance, while bringing about a greater reduction in the work of inspiration.

The Elema-Schonander servo-ventilator (Fig. 12-5) is an example of a unit that appears to be able to satisfy all reasonable technical and medical requirements in most, if not all, clinical situations (Ingelstedt et al., 1972). Full selectivity and control of ventilator performance has been made possible by a built-in electronic servo-system that provides continuous control of the airflow to and from the patient. In addition to a number of other desirable technical features, it is capable of being operated in both the pressure-cycle and volume-cycle modes.

Ventilation Patterns. In the selection of ventilator settings, consideration must be given to the effects of the ventilation pattern on pulmonary mechanics, arterial oxygenation, and circulation. One should remember that, as a general rule, those ventilatory patterns that are favorable to circulation usually are unfavorable to the efficiency of ventilation; the converse is equally true. Frequently a compromise will have to be reached between the type

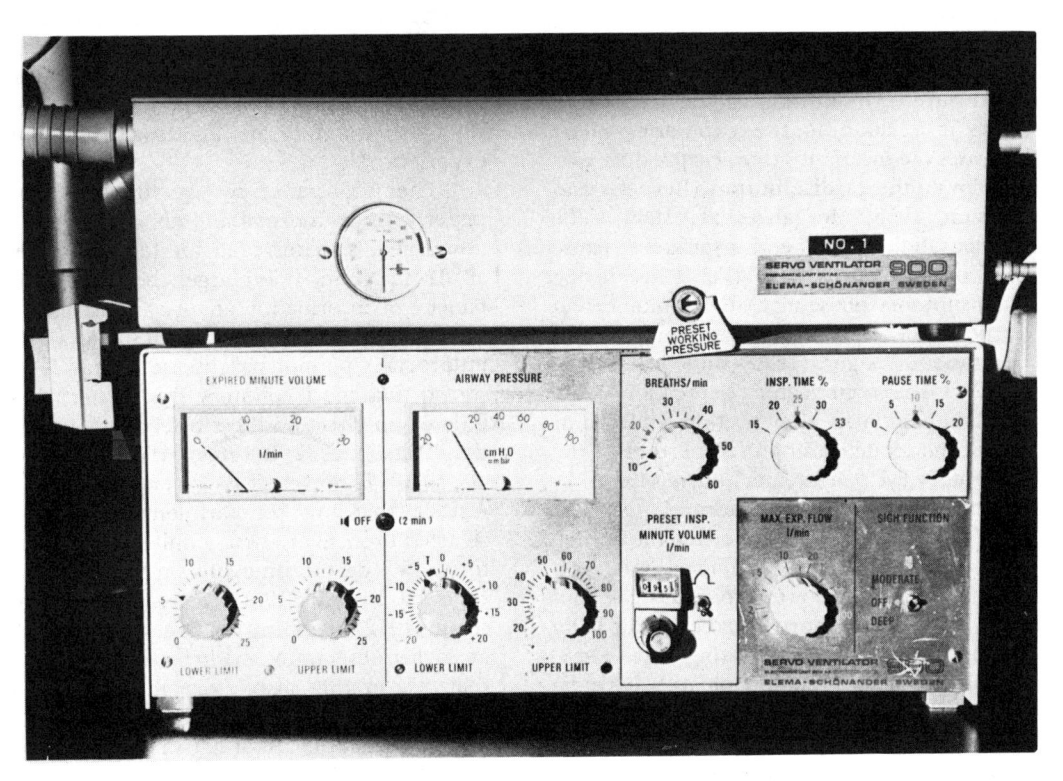

Figure 12-5. An example of a versatile ventilator that can operate either in the volume-limited or pressure-limited mode. The ventilator consists of a pneumatic unit (top compartment) and an electronic unit (bottom portion). An electronic servo-system provides continuous control of airflow to and from the patient. Full selectivity of inspiratory and expiratory patterns and intermittent mandatory capability are provided for. In addition, electrical signals representing airway pressure and inspiratory and expiratory flow are accessible via built-in output jacks and can be recorded on a bedside recorder.

of ventilatory pattern that is best suited for circulatory homeostasis and that which is best for gas exchange.

It is well-known that an increase in intrathoracic pressure produces circulatory depression by impeding venous return (Cournand et al., 1948; Morgan et al., 1966). Consequently, the general recommendation is to establish a ventilation pattern that minimizes increases in mean airway and intrathoracic pressures and optimizes gas exchange.

During mechanical ventilation, the level of airway pressure is determined by the interaction of several factors: (1) tidal volume; (2) the resistance (elastic and nonelastic) in the system; (3) the duration of inspiration (when the airway pressure is higher than atmospheric) relative to expiration (when the airway pressure is normally equal to atmospheric); (4) the inspiratory flow pattern, and (5) whether or not PEEP is used. Knowing that volume is the integral of flow (i.e., flow × time), the relationship between tidal volume, airway pressure, and resistance can best be described by Ohm's law. Thus, pressure is equal to the product of flow and resistance ($P = F \times R$), and any change in either flow or resistance or both will be reflected as a change in pressure, all other factors remaining constant.

Variations in the inspiratory phase also may bring about changes in mean intrathoracic pressure. Prolongation of the inspiratory phase in relation to the expiratory phase increases the mean intrathoracic pressure and may lower the cardiac output (Berneus and Carlsten, 1955; Morgan et al., 1966). The incorporation of an end-inspiratory pause (EIP) or "inspiratory hold" (Fig. 12-6) during the inspiratory phase may, for all intents and purposes, be regarded as a prolongation of inspiration. Lyager (1970) and Nordstrom (1972) observed circulatory depression in experimental animals after the introduction of EIP of moderate duration (20 percent of the respiratory cycle or greater) during intermittent positive-pressure ventilation.

Another important determinant of airway pressure is the pattern of inspiratory flow, of which three types are recognized: (1) constant (square wave) flow; (2) accelerating (sine wave) flow; and (3) decelerating flow. Theoretically, the decelerating pattern—where the greatest flow occurs during the early phases of inspiration—results in a somewhat higher mean intrathoracic pressure than if the greatest flow occurs toward the end of the inspiratory phase as seen in the accelerating pattern (Adams et al., 1970). The constant flow pattern results in even lower mean airway pressures (Ingelstedt et al., 1972), an observation we have found to be in accord with our experience.

The importance of the different flow patterns under normal and abnormal conditions remains an unsettled question (Adams et al., 1970; Nunn, 1970) largely because of the paucity of information about various disease states (Ingelstedt et al., 1972). In subjects with little or no pulmonary disease, it has been shown that the inspiratory flow pattern has little or no effect on the efficiency of ventilation (Watson, 1962; Bergman, 1967; Adams et al., 1970). However, it has been shown theoretically that lung compartments behind obstructed bronchi are best ventilated if inspiratory flow is decelerating, of long duration, and followed by an EIP (Lyager, 1968; Nordstrom, 1972), a finding that is at variance with an earlier observation made by Herzog (1964) that accelerating inspiratory flow produced even ventilation. Various workers have demonstrated that the use of EIP or the prolongation of inspiration improves alveolar ventilation in healthy subjects or dogs (Watson, 1962; Bergman, 1967; Knelson et al., 1970; Lyager,

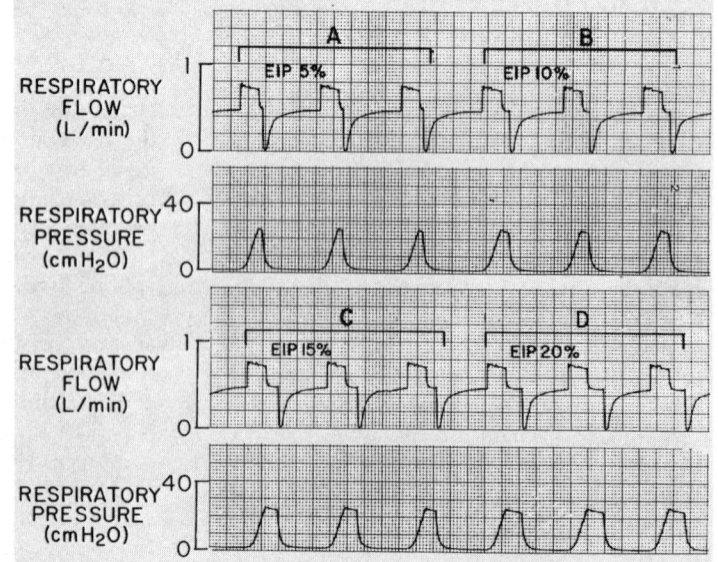

Figure 12–6. The effect of increasing the duration of end-inspiratory pauses (EIP), with an unchanging tidal volume and respiratory rate, on mean airway pressure. The increase in mean airway pressure is maximal when the EIP is increased to 20 percent of the respiratory cycle.

1970). Moreover, when an EIP is used the inspiratory flow pattern may be characterized as early lung filling decelerating flow pattern irrespective of the flow pattern during the insufflation time proper (Ingelstedt et al., 1972). Conversely, it has been shown that if the inspiratory phase is significantly shortened, gas mixing is impaired, resulting in reduced ventilatory efficiency (Horsfield and Cumming, 1968).

The expiratory pattern also exerts a great influence on the mean intrathoracic pressure. The use of PEEP and increased flow resistance (expiratory retard) both increase the pressure level. PEEP merely implies the use of positive pressure, with reference to atmospheric pressure, in the airway at the end of expiration. Under conditions of ordinary intermittent positive pressure ventilation (IPPV), the expiratory phase is unobstructed in the normal patient and pressures rapidly return to atmospheric levels, i.e., zero end-expiratory pressure (ZEEP). With PEEP, inspiration and the initial portion of the expiratory phase remain unchanged; however, when a preset exhalation pressure is reached, further exhalation is stopped by a valve attached to the exhalation port of the ventilator. With expiratory retard, a fixed resistance to flow is imposed at the beginning of expiration resulting in an expiratory phase that is slow and prolonged but with eventual return of airway pressure to zero. Both PEEP and expiratory retard are intended to prevent collapse of smaller airways, but the former is more effective than the latter in improving oxygen transport (Petty, 1974). The physiologic effects and clinical uses of PEEP will be discussed in a later section.

From the foregoing, it appears that a long inspiration, decelerating flow pattern, an EIP, and the use of PEEP exert a salutary effect on alveolar ventilation and gas exchange, but may be detrimental to circulatory homeostasis. On the other hand, an accelerating inspiratory flow pattern, absence of EIP, and a long expiration at zero-end expiratory pressure (ZEEP) would be favorable to circulatory function. The dictum is to use those ventilator settings that are favorable to the most seriously compromised function in the critically ill patient.

At present, it is our practice to start with a constant flow inspiratory pattern (with its relatively benign effect on mean airway pressure) in combination with an EIP of 10 percent of the respiratory cycle. This particular ventilatory pattern improves pulmonary gas exchange with minimal effects on circulatory function.

Tidal Volume. Use of large tidal volumes (10 to 15 ml/kg) has been shown to be effective in avoiding or minimizing postoperative atelectasis (Bendixen et al., 1963). Moreover, the evidence is persuasive that prolonged constant volume ventilation with small tidal volumes (less than 7 ml/kg) almost invariably leads to progressive atelectasis (Hedley-White et al., 1965). To prevent progressive alveolar closure and widening of the alveolar-arteriolar oxygen gradient (A-aDO_2), tidal volumes of 10 to 15 ml/kg are routinely employed, supplemented by periodic hyperinflations (sighs) to volumes 20 percent higher than the set tidal volume occurring six to eight times every hour. If, as often happens, hypocarbia (PaCO_2 <35 mm Hg) ensues, an appropriate length of tubing is added between the ventilator and the endotracheal tube to serve as additional mechanical dead space. This is the simplest method that can be employed to ensure maintenance of normocarbia (PaCO_2 between 38 and 42 mm Hg). In this regard, the formula for calculating the required additional mechanical dead space worked out by Suwa and Bendixen (1968) is extremely useful. In certain instances (e.g., patients with compensatory hyperventilation during assisted or "triggered" ventilation), the addition of 1 to 3 percent CO_2 to the inspired gas mixture via a CO_2 mixer may be a more predictable method of normalizing low arterial CO_2 tensions (Breivik et al., 1973).

The importance of avoiding hypocarbia during mechanical ventilation cannot be overemphasized. Hypocarbia causes a reduction in arterial oxygen tension (Michenfelder et al.,

1966; Suwa and Bendixen, 1968), cardiac output (Prys-Roberts et al., 1968), and cerebral blood flow (Sugioka and Davis, 1960), and shifts the oxyhemoglobin dissociation curve to the left, the so-called Bohr effect (Nunn, 1969), which impairs release of oxygen from hemoglobin to the tissues. Further, the combined presence of hypocarbia, alkalosis, and hypokalemia—the latter a common occurrence after cardiopulmonary bypass employing hemodilution—sets the stage for life-threatening ventricular arrhythmias and impaired myocardial performance. Breivik et al. (1973) have demonstrated the effectiveness of adding CO_2 (1 to 3 percent) to the inspired gas during prolonged mechanical ventilation to achieve normocarbia. In their study, significant increases in arterial Po_2, cardiac output, and arterial O_2 transport occurred as low arterial Pco_2 and high pH were normalized, while both systemic vascular resistance and oxygen use coefficient decreased.

In the rare instance when carbon dioxide retention and hypercarbia ensue despite the intentional hyperventilation, as occurs in patients with significantly increased physiologic dead space, the respiratory rate is increased to lower $Paco_2$ to the desired level (see below).

Respiratory Rate. Initially, a respiratory frequency of 10 to 15 breaths per minute generally is adequate for most adults, but occasionally this may have to be increased temporarily to prevent ventilator fighting in patients with a more rapid spontaneous rate. Moreover, in patients with circulatory embarrassment, it may be preferable to satisfy augmented ventilatory requirements by increasing the respiratory frequency rather than increase the tidal volume further in order to substantially decrease the mean intrathoracic pressure and minimize the interference with circulatory function (Nordstrom, 1972).

Inspiratory-to-Expiratory Time Ratio. During mechanical ventilation, prolongation of the inspiratory phase in relation to the expiratory phase increases the intrathoracic mean pressure and may lower cardiac output (Berneus and Carlsten, 1955; Morgan et al., 1966). While shortening of the inspiratory phase will theoretically have the opposite hemodynamic effect, gas mixing and ventilatory efficiency may be impaired if the inspiratory phase is significantly shortened (Horsfield and Cumming, 1968). To minimize the increase in mean intrathoracic pressure and to optimize venous return and gas mixing, an I:E ratio of 1:2 to 1:3 is recommended.

Fraction of Oxygen in the Inspired Gas. The required F_{IO_2} is a function of the indication for ventilator support and the necessity to maintain the Pao_2 as close to "normal" as possible. The objective is to be able to maintain satisfactory oxygenation (Pao_2 >70 mm Hg) at the lowest possible F_{IO_2}. Obviously, the ideal situation would be where ventilation with room air ($F_{IO_2} = 0.21$) achieves adequate oxygen exchange. However, the presence of ventilation-perfusion imbalance, reduced cardiac output, or perhaps a diffusion block and an increased venous admixture from shunting often results in hypoxemia and mandates the use of oxygen-enriched gas mixtures (F_{IO_2} >0.21) to insure adequate oxygenation.

There is no known advantage to using an F_{IO_2} greater than that which results in a Pao_2 of 95 to 100 mm Hg (Sao_2 of 95 to 98 percent at a pH of 7.40). On the other hand, there is experimental evidence that prolonged ventilation (two to five days) using high oxygen concentrations (i.e., $Pao_2 \geq 400$ mm Hg) can produce serious or fatal pulmonary injury (Spencer et al., 1966). Thus, to avoid the consequences of pulmonary oxygen toxicity, every effort should be made to satisfy the need for oxygen without exceeding an F_{IO_2} of 0.6. This also means careful attention to the other components of the oxygen transport system: maintenance of an adequate cardiac output and optimal levels of hemoglobin. In some cases, it may be necessary to modify therapeutic goals so that lower Pao_2 values and some degree of arterial desaturation are accepted.

Controlled vs. Assist Mode ("Triggered") Ventilation. Although the metabolic cost of breathing may be increased as much as twenty times normal in postoperative cardiac surgical patients (Thung et al., 1963), it has been shown that this can be reduced significantly during mechanical ventilation (Dammann et al., 1963). Wilson et al. (1973) observed a 20 percent increase in whole body oxygen consumption following initiation of spontaneous ventilation in patients who had initially been on controlled ventilation after mitral valve replacement.

Even in the absence of controlled studies comparing the metabolic costs of controlled versus patient-triggered (assist mode) ventilation, it would seem logical to think that the resultant savings in energy expenditure and reduction in oxygen consumption would be greater with the former, since the patient is totally relieved of respiratory muscle work. Thus, controlled ventilation would seem to be more appropriate for critically ill patients and for those in whom cardiac performance is impaired. On the other hand, assist mode ventilation can be safely employed in those who are in good condition otherwise and in those who are being weaned from mechanical ventilation; indeed, spontaneous breathing efforts should be encouraged in these patients.

Use of PEEP during Mechanical Ventilation. On the basis of available physiologic data, PEEP would seem to be most useful in clinical situations characterized by atelectasis, alveolar instability, pulmonary edema, reduced FRC, significant hypoxemia, high physiologic shunts, and significant A-aDo$_2$ (Asbaugh and Petty, 1973; Petty, 1974). The primary effect of PEEP is to increase the FRC (McIntrye et al., 1969; Kumar et al., 1970). Theoretically, with a larger FRC, more alveoli remain open and a better ventilation-perfusion relationship is maintained with a resultant improvement in oxygen exchange. Indeed, the use of PEEP results in a rise in Pao$_2$ and a fall in the amount of physiologic shunt ($\dot{Q}_s/\dot{Q}_T$) across the lung, the increment in Pao$_2$ being directly proportional to the decrease in the physiologic shunt, which, in turn, is inversely proportional to the FRC (Finley et al., 1960; Asbaugh, 1970; Kumar et al., 1970). Similarly, Falke et al. (1972) demonstrated a positive correlation between the level of PEEP and FRC, on one hand, and between FRC and Pao$_2$ on the other (Fig. 12-7). PEEP appears to be most beneficial when used to raise a low FRC to optimal values, but may be detrimental when used in the patient with optimal or high values (Asbaugh and Petty, 1973).

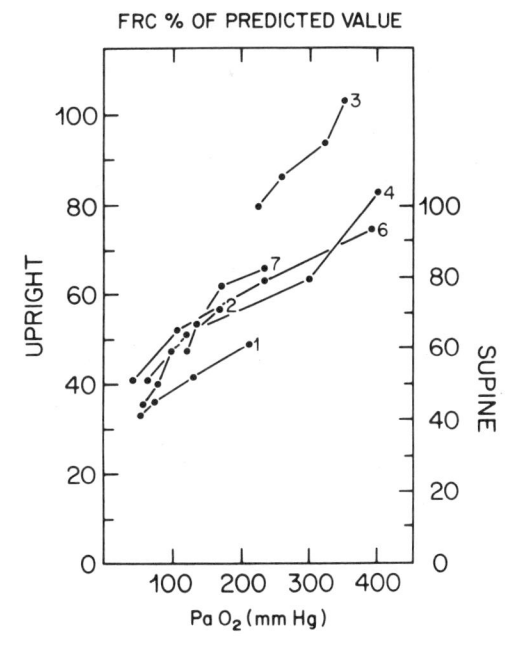

Figure 12-7. The effect of PEEP on FRC and Pao$_2$ (Fio$_2$ = 1.0). Data were obtained from patients with acute respiratory failure ventilated with end-expiratory pressures of 0, 5, 10, and 15 cm H$_2$O in random order. Each lowest point represents the relationship during ventilation with ZEEP, the next at PEEP of 5 cm H$_2$O, etc. There was correlation between FRC and Pao$_2$. *(Adapted from Falke et al., 1972.)*

The increase in mean intrathoracic pressure that accompanies the use of PEEP has been shown to raise venous pressure, decrease venous return to the heart, and decrease cardiac output in both experimental animals and humans (Barach et al., 1938; Cournand et al., 1948; Lenfant and Howell, 1965; Cheyney et al., 1967; Uzawa and Asbaugh, 1969). However, it is difficult to predict the net effect of PEEP on the circulation in the individual patient, presumably because of the multiplicity of factors that affect cardiac performance and the complexity of the mechanisms that regulate and control circulatory function. Such factors as the circulating blood volume, adequacy of cardiac performance, and underlying pulmonary pathology appear to be the more important determinants of response. PEEP may produce or accentuate circulatory embarrassment in the patient who is hypovolemic, in cardiac failure, or emphysematous. In reviewing three independent studies of patients with acute respiratory failure, Pontoppidan et al. (1973) noted a large variation in the hemodynamic response to different levels of PEEP; lower levels of PEEP (5 cm H_2O) were accompanied by only minor changes in cardiac output, whereas a mean decrease of approximately 15 to 20 percent (compared with intermittent positive pressure ventilation) occurred when higher levels (10 to 15 cm H_2O) of PEEP were employed (Fig. 12–8). From the foregoing, it is apparent that the net effect of PEEP on oxygen transport and available oxygen supply depends on the interplay of its frequently opposing effects on cardiac output and pulmonary gas exchange.

In the individual patient, the optimal level of PEEP is determined by careful titration of the responses to perturbation. Thus, starting from ZEEP, PEEP gradually is increased until the desired results are obtained. As the PEEP level is increased, the hemodynamic responses are carefully monitored, while serial measurements of arterial blood-gas tensions are performed. Suter et al. (1975) have demonstrated that, in normovolemic patients, measurements of total static compliance may provide a simple and reliable means of determining the optimal degree of lung distention, i.e., that which promotes the best gas exchange with the least risk of alveolar overdistention and rupture. Regardless of the method employed, the importance of cardiac output or arteriovenous oxygen difference measurements during PEEP titration cannot be overemphasized. Such measurements are essential for the proper interpretation of changes in Pao_2 and provide a rational basis for therapy. The relationship between arterial Po_2 and cardiac index or arteriovenous oxygen difference in the presence of varying degrees of right-to-left shunting is illustrated in Figure 12–9. A number of important facts emerge from examination of this relationship. First, reduced cardiac output is an important cause of hypoxemia, an effect that presumably is due to tissue hypoxia and decreased mixed venous oxygen tension. Second, in the presence of low to moderate levels of right-to-left shunting ($\dot{Q}_s/\dot{Q}_T$ of 5 to 10 percent), an in-

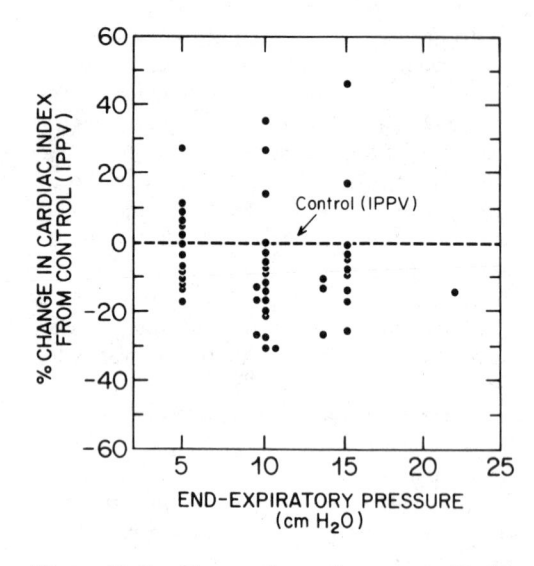

Figure 12–8. Changes in cardiac output with different levels of PEEP in patients with acute respiratory failure. Data obtained from three different studies reviewed by authors; different "controls" were employed. *(Modified from Pontoppidan et al., 1973.)*

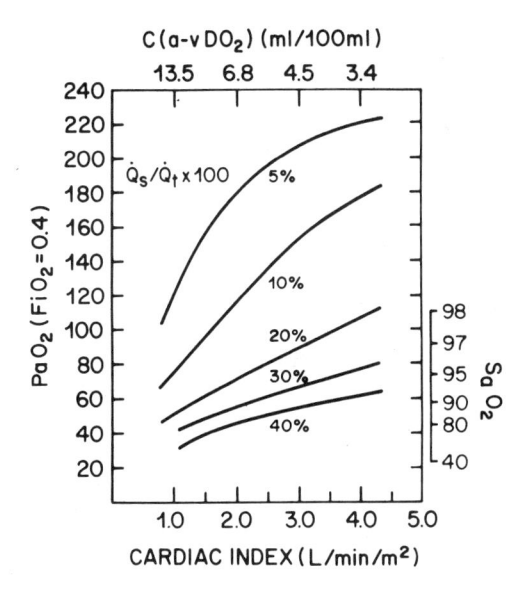

Figure 12-9 The relationship between Pa_{O_2} and cardiac index or arteriovenous oxygen difference $C(a\text{-}vD_{O_2})$ at various degrees of right-to-left shunts ($\dot{Q}_S/\dot{Q}_T$) calculated for a patient breathing 40 percent oxygen using the classic shunt and Fick equations. Sa_{O_2} = arterial oxygen saturation. Assumptions made: hemoglobin = 15 gm %; oxygen consumption = 135 ml/min/m²; normal oxyhemoglobin dissociation; pH = 7.40. *(Modified from Gray, 1977.)*

crease in cardiac output is accompanied by a sharp increase in arterial P_{O_2}. Third, an increase in arterial P_{O_2} brought about by a reduction in the magnitude of right-to-left shunting secondary to the use of PEEP may be accomplished at the expense of a reduced cardiac output, widened A-V O_2 difference, and decreased oxygen transport. The practical implications of the above are obvious.

When properly employed, PEEP is a useful therapeutic adjunct for patients with significant pulmonary dysfunction. In general, the use of PEEP is indicated when there is difficulty in maintaining a Pa_{O_2} above 70 mm Hg at an $F_{I_{O_2}}$ of 0.6 or greater and when gross pulmonary edema is evident. For postoperative cardiac surgical patients, it is rarely necessary to exceed a PEEP level of 15 cm H_2O.

Care of the Patient Requiring Mechanical Ventilatory Assistance

The fundamental elements of care include careful monitoring, adequate sedation, proper humidification, meticulous tracheobronchial toilette, and assiduous nursing care and chest physiotherapy. These measures will be discussed below.

Monitoring. Since cardiovascular and pulmonary subsystems dysfunction may be present in patients requiring mechanical ventilation, the margin for error is slim. Therefore, optimal patient management demands constant staff attendance and close surveillance. Maintenance of a 1:1 nurse-to-patient ratio is desirable. Periodic patient examinations are conducted routinely, with frequent examination of the chest to insure proper synchrony with ventilator cycling and satisfactory air entry and lung expansion. Chest roentgenograms are taken at least once daily and changes in the bacterial flora of the tracheobronchial tree carefully noted by periodic cultures. In addition, periodic checks of the various components of the patient's life-support systems, including the patient-to-ventilator interface, are carried out.

Close surveillance of vital subsystems functions—particularly cardiovascular, pulmonary, and renal—is mandatory. To a large degree, the same monitoring routine employed after open intracardiac operations will suffice (Chapter 6). These methods are reviewed here.

In situations in which the likelihood of postoperative cardiopulmonary dysfunction is great, it is mandatory to continuously monitor not only systemic arterial pressure via indwelling intravascular catheters, but right and left ventricular filling pressure as well. It is also essential to be able to measure cardiac output intermittently to gain better insight into the adequacy of cardiac performance and the oxygen transport system. Right ventricular filling pressure (right ventricular end-diastolic pressure) is reflected in measurements of central venous or right atrial pressure, assuming normal tricuspid valve function. On the other hand, left ventricular filling pressure (left ventricular end-diastolic pressure) is mirrored in measurements of left atrial or of pulmonary capillary wedge pressure, assuming mitral valvular function is normal.

Left atrial pressure measurements may be obtained through catheters positioned intraoperatively. Pulmonary capillary wedge pressure measurements are easily made with a properly positioned Swan-Ganz type balloon-tipped, flow-directed catheter. Specially designed thermistor-containing, balloon-tipped, flow-directed catheters permit: (1) mensuration of right atrial, pulmonary artery, and pulmonary capillary wedge pressures; (2) measurement of cardiac output using the indicator-dilution principle (thermodilution method); and (3) frequent sampling of pulmonary arterial blood (i.e., mixed venous blood) for serial determinations of the oxygen content of mixed venous blood ($C\bar{v}_{O_2}$), calculations of shunt fractions ($\dot{Q}_S/\dot{Q}_T$) and estimation of cardiac output by the direct Fick method (if measurements of arterial oxygen content (Ca_{O_2}) and oxygen consumption ($\dot{V}_{O_2}$) are simultaneously available.

Analysis of pulmonary subsystem performance requires careful assessment of oxygenation, ventilation, and estimation of ventilatory reserves. This is accomplished primarily through careful clinical observations, arterial blood-gas tension and acid-base measurements, and by serial chest x-rays. For the most part, these measures are sufficient for patients who come to the operation with normal cardiopulmonary function. When there is concern about the possibility of cardiopulmonary instability or acute respiratory failure, more intensive monitoring is indicated. For instance, measurements of mixed venous oxygen content ($C\bar{v}_{O_2}$), arteriovenous oxygen content difference, alveolar-arterial oxygen tension difference (A-aD_{O_2}), and estimations of the magnitude of right-to-left shunting ($\dot{Q}_S/\dot{Q}_T$) provide additional insight into the adequacy of oxygenation. Other methods used in the assessment of the adequacy of ventilation include measurements of end-tidal carbon dioxide tension (Pa_{CO_2}) and physiologic dead space-to-tidal volume ratio (V_D/V_T). Ventilatory reserve capacity may be assessed by measurements of inspiratory force, vital capacity (VC), forced expiratory volume (FEV_1), and functional residual capacity (FRC). Periodic sampling of the sputum for bacteriologic culture and sensitivity tests should also be carried out as necessary.

Careful monitoring of renal function, fluid balance, and daily weights are also of paramount importance.

Sedation. The conscious, cooperative, and adequately ventilated patient who tolerates the presence of the indwelling endotracheal tube may well require no more than reassurance and analgesic medication to remain comfortable. In general, these patients have satisfactory cardiorespiratory and cerebral functions and are otherwise ready for weaning or extubation. However, more often than not, the remainder of patients will require additional sedative medication to allay anxiety, prevent unnecessary struggling, and insure proper ventilator phasing and cycling. The importance of adequate sedation cannot be overemphasized; indeed, in patients with significant cardiorespiratory dysfunction, sedation is mandatory to reduce oxygen consumption and ensure satisfactory pulmonary gas exchange.

Morphine is perhaps the most effective drug for this purpose and it is used for both its analgesic and sedative actions. It frequently is employed alone but may be combined with tranquilizers such as diazepam. The appropriate dosage schedule is determined by careful titration to the individual patient's needs. In practice, small increments of the drug (i.e., 2 to 6 mg every three to four hours, intravenously) are administered rather than large "bolus" doses to avoid the occurrence of profound hypotension, which is rare and generally occurs in the hypovolemic patient. A mild and transient drop (5 to 10 mm Hg) in mean arterial pressure, presumably secondary to peripheral vasodilation, is the usual observed side effect with the smaller doses; this, by itself, is usually of no consequence, but may, on the other hand, be beneficial to cardiac dynamics because of afterload reduction.

The use of muscle relaxants such as pancuronium or curare and related drugs should be reserved only for special situations in which it is absolutely essential to achieve total muscular paralysis and other methods have been ineffective in bringing about proper synchronization with the ventilator (see Special Problems below). One should remember that muscle relaxants do not by themselves possess sedative properties. Therefore, sole reliance should not be placed on these agents to achieve controlled ventilation in otherwise conscious patients, because the absence of muscle tone and total inability to move could be a source of distress and anxiety to them, particularly if they are not properly forewarned and reassured.

Humidification. Proper humidification of inspired gas reduces the viscosity of secretions, prevents drying and encrustation, and helps maintain normal bronchial ciliary integrity and minimize postoperative atelectasis. The steps taken to accomplish this merely represent an attempt to reduplicate the state of affairs that obtain in a normal person during spontaneous respiration wherein inspired air is warmed and becomes fully saturated with water by the time it reaches the bronchi. During mechanical ventilation, efficient humidification is accomplished either with an ultrasonic nebulizer or by the passage of the inspiratory gas over a heated water bath so that it becomes saturated with water vapor. The ultrasonic nebulizer delivers a mist of particles of one micron or less (Herzog et al., 1964) and such nebulization is so efficient that one must guard against the possibility of overloading the patient with water (Sladen et al., 1968). When a hot water humidifier is used, it is essential to maintain the water bath temperature at 55C to prevent bacterial growth in the tank and deliver gas that is saturated at approximately body temperature at the end of the ventilator tubing. Because condensation of water in the ventilator tubing is a frequent occurrence with hot water humidifiers, provisions should be made for easy collection and emptying of the condensate with minimal interruption of mechanical ventilation.

Tracheobronchial Toilette. Secretions from within the respiratory tract are removed by periodic suction. This can be accomplished with relative ease with minimal interruption of ventilation. The patient is simply disconnected from the ventilator and manual ventilation is maintained by means of an Ambu bag, while suction removal of bronchopulmonary secretions is carried out via a sideport in the swivel connector attached to the end of the endotracheal or tracheostomy tube. Suction is performed once every two to three hours or as often as necessary. It is generally convenient to combine this perturbation with scheduled changes of position, physiotherapy, changes of ventilator tubing, and other maneuvers requiring temporary interruption of mechanical ventilation.

While suction removal of bronchopulmonary secretions is an essential element of respiratory care, the attendant staff should be cognizant of the hazards associated with suctioning. These include: (1) hypoxia resulting from improper and prolonged suction; (2) hypoxia-induced arrhythmias and even cardiac arrest; (3) introduction of pathogenic organisms into the tracheobronchial tree; and (4) repeated trauma to the tracheobronchial mucosa. These procedures should therefore be conducted with dispatch and with utmost precision and care, especially in patients with severely compromised cardiopulmonary function.

To reduce the possibility of significant hypoxia, certain measures are followed during suctioning. First, the patient is ventilated with 100 percent oxygen (F_{IO_2} = 1.0) for two to three minutes before disconnection from the ventilator. Second, during manual ventilation with the Ambu bag, the same high F_{IO_2} is delivered. Third, negative pressure is applied only during withdrawal of the suction catheter, and the duration of suction should be no more than 10 seconds for each attempt. Proper selective control of the suction (negative) pressure can be readily accomplished through the use of appropriate Y-connectors or of catheters designed with a thumb hole. Fourth, the patient is manually reinflated and allowed sufficient time for recovery after each application of suction.

Needless to say, meticulous asepsis is mandatory. To accomplish this, two persons are required to perform suctioning; one maintains manual ventilation while the other aspirates the secretions. A fresh, sterile catheter is used for each aspiration and the nurse or therapist must handle the catheter with either sterile glove or clamp, preferably the former (Fig. 12–10). The frequency of suctioning should be limited to the necessary minimum consistent with satisfactory tracheobronchial toilette to lessen mucosal trauma and the potential for infection. Use of certain suction catheters (e.g., Argyle, Aero-Flow) may also help reduce mucosal trauma; this is made possible by a special design feature that prevents attachment of mucosa to catheter as negative pressure is applied.

Where the tracheobronchial secretions are thick and viscid, aspiration is facilitated by prior loosening of the secretions accomplished by periodic instillation of and lavage with 2 to 3 ml of sterile saline. However, with efficient humidification, the need for frequent tracheal lavage with saline has decreased significantly.

Selective suctioning of the left bronchial tree may not be so readily accomplished with the classic maneuvers of shoulder positioning or head-turning to the right, but the success rate of catheter-entry into the left main bronchus is significantly increased when special angle-tipped catheters are used (Haberman et al., 1973).

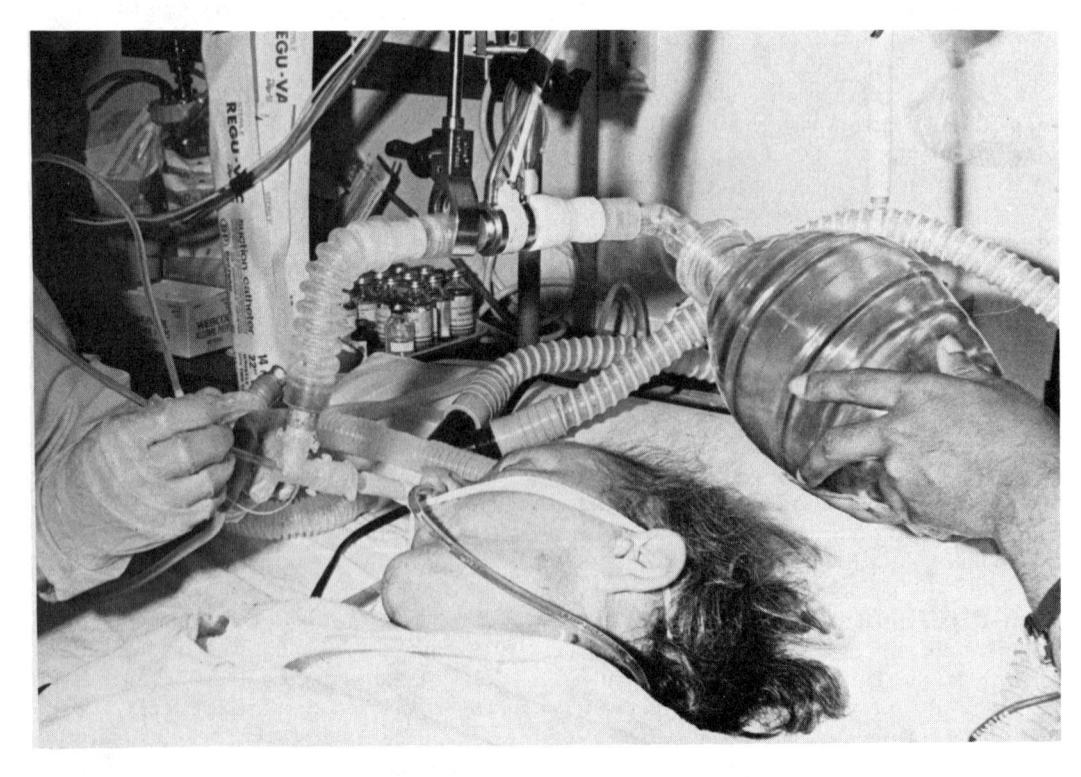

Figure 12–10. A method of endotracheal suctioning.

Chest Physiotherapy. Mobilization of secretions is facilitated by periodic chest phyiotherapy. Such maneuvers as manual hyperinflation combined with shaking and tapotage to the chest during expiration, chest wall percussion with cupped hands, and the use of electric vibrators have all been found to be effective. For optimal results, these procedures are best combined and coordinated with postural drainage sessions whenever the patient's condition permits.

Nursing Care. A patient on prolonged mechanical ventilatory assistance requires intensive nursing. In practical terms, this means careful attention to the basic physical, hygienic, and emotional needs of an intubated, often immobile, and otherwise totally helpless person who is unable to care for himself or herself. Above all, this demands round-the-clock coverage by a stable, well-motivated, competent, and compassionate nursing staff. The maintenance of close surveillance and meticulous attention to *all* subsystems are mandatory.

Constant reassurance of the conscious patient is essential, and particular care must be given to the eyes, mouth, bowels, urinary bladder, limbs, and skin—especially of the back and pressure areas. To reduce the incidence of respiratory complications, the principles outlined in previous sections of this chapter must be adhered to. Adequate nutrition should be maintained.

Special Problems

"Fighting" the Ventilator. A patient on the ventilator, when in proper condition, is quiet and relaxed. When the patient is restless and agitated or when he or she "fights" or is out of phase with ventilator cycling, the situation requires urgent attention. "Fighting," by itself, may result in impaired gas exchange, reduced cardiac performance, and increased whole body oxygen consumption. A careful systematic search for the cause must, therefore, be conducted expeditiously. The most common causes of ventilator fight are: (1) inadequate ventilation; (2) collection of tracheobronchial secretions; (3) acute pulmonary pathology, such as pneumothorax and atelectasis; (4) pain from any cause; (5) sudden deterioration of cardiac function; (6) gastrointestinal distension; and (7) neurologic damage.

Fighting usually can be suppressed and restlessness relieved by eliminating the cause. If fighting persists despite successful elimination of the presumed cause, certain maneuvers may be instituted provided ventilation is proven adequate and cardiac performance is deemed satisfactory. Adjustment of the rhythm of mechanical ventilation, sedation, or induction of total muscular paralysis by administration of muscle relaxants usually helps bring about proper synchronization of the patient's spontaneous respiratory efforts with ventilator cycling. Following the temporary disturbance of endotracheal suctioning, proper ventilator phasing usually can be reestablished by momentary hyperventilation (i.e., 25 to 30 breaths per minute). This maneuver almost always abolishes spontaneous inspiratory efforts and the respiratory rate can then be conveniently readjusted to the original setting. One must, however, guard against inducing marked hypocarbia.

If the patient is still restless or agitated despite readjustments of the ventilatory pattern, morphine is given intravenously for sedation (see Sedation). Larger than usual doses of morphine or concomitant use of other sedatives such as diazepam sometimes may be necessary to achieve the desired results.

If, in spite of these maneuvers, the patient remains intractably restless, the use of muscle relaxants is definitely indicated. These agents are capable of completely abolishing spontaneous respiratory efforts while all muscular activity is suppressed. Thus, total control of ventilation is facilitated while whole body oxygen consumption presumably is reduced —a most desirable action in patients with significantly reduced cardiac performance or impaired gas exchange. However, when induction of total muscular paralysis is contemplated, certain precautions have to be taken. First, muscle relaxants should never be used unless inadequate ventilation has been ruled out or corrected. Second, completely paralyzed patients should be watched more carefully, because the hazards of accidental interruption of mechanical ventilation are greater in the absence of spontaneous respiratory activity. Third, as indicated earlier, relaxants should always be combined with sedatives in awake and conscious patients. Fourth, one should remember that such functions as swallowing and coughing are lost while gastrointestinal peristalsis is impaired; further, some neurologic signs may be either obscured or abolished.

Tracheostomy. In recent years, there has been an increasing tendency to use nasotracheal or orotracheal intubation for a few days before the decision to perform tracheostomy is made. This appears to be sound policy in view of the temporary and reversible nature of some of the indications for tracheostomy. Moreover, it has been shown that a secure airway can be safely maintained with a loosely fitting nasotracheal tube for a period of seven to ten days without danger of permanent laryngeal or vocal cord damage (Lindholm, 1969).

In postoperative cardiac surgical patients requiring temporary mechanical support of ventilation, it may be possible to avoid tracheostomy if support is not required for more than seven to ten days. In these patients, a tracheostomy is electively performed after five to seven days when it seems likely that ventilatory assistance will be necessary for an additional week or more. In practice, the procedure is delayed (usually until after the seventh postoperative day) in patients with midsternal splitting incisions, the rationale being to prevent contamination of the surgical incision and the mediastinum.

A cuffed plastic tube (low pressure, large volume, soft cuff) commonly is used and the same principles of care outlined previously are followed (see Care of Airway).

Weaning from Mechanical Ventilation

Weaning from mechanical ventilatory assistance should be started as soon as the pathophysiologic condition for which ventilatory assistance was initiated has improved. This is a systematic process, culminating in extubation and discontinuance of ventilatory assistance. In general, one proceeds in reverse stepwise manner, starting from the maximum level of ventilatory assistance. Thus, from continuous positive-pressure ventilation (CPPV) the level of support is reduced to intermittent positive-pressure ventilation (IPPV) of which two stages are recognized, namely, IPPV (controlled mode) and IPPV (assisted or patient-cycled mode). Up to this point the patient generally is still on a volume-cycled ventilator; as his or her condition improves, a pressure-cycled ventilator may be substituted for the volume-cycled ventilator and IPPV maintained in the pressure-cycled mode. The patient then progresses to spontaneous ventilation; this is done through the tracheal tube connected to a T-piece adaptor and heated nebulizer. Initially, he or she is allowed *short periods* (less than 15 minutes) of spontaneous ventilation followed by trials of *longer periods* (longer than 15 minutes) of the same, with the F_{IO_2} set at a slightly higher level than the patient was receiving during controlled ventilation. The final step, of course, is extubation.

The different steps in the weaning process leading to the discontinuance of ventilatory assistance is schematically outlined in Figure 12–11. Generally one proceeds from Steps 1 through 10, allowing the patient to progress from one level to the next if certain established criteria are met and delaying progression when these requirements are not satisfied. Conversely, in patients who are doing extremely well, certain steps may be bypassed. In all cases, close surveillance and monitoring of vital functions are maintained throughout the entire process.

Criteria for Initiation of Weaning. In the broadest terms, weaning may be initiated if cardiac, respiratory, renal, and central nervous subsystems functions are adequate and if potentially life-threatening complications are not present.

As a general rule, the presence of circulatory instability is a contraindication to weaning; conversely, the maintenance of hemodynamic stability is essential to its success. For

CONCEPTS OF VENTILATORY AND RESPIRATORY CARE

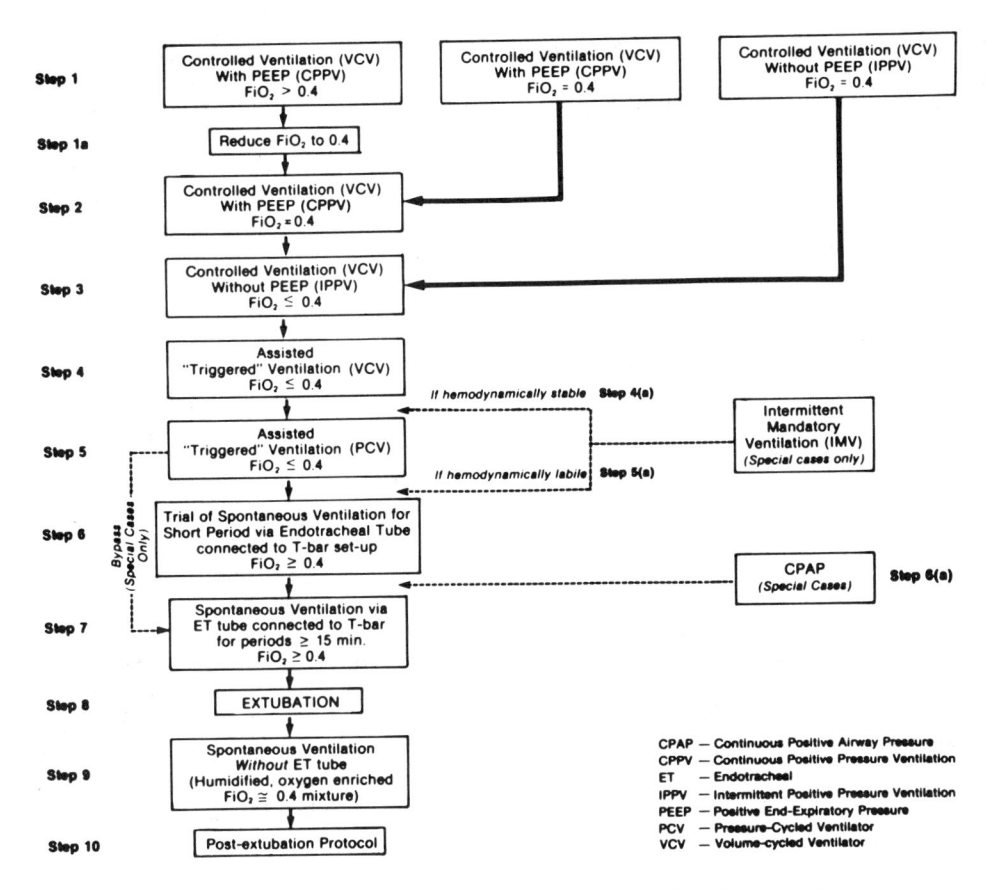

Figure 12-11. Schematic guide to weaning a patient from mechanical ventilatory assistance.

purposes of weaning, cardiac performance is said to be satisfactory if the following conditions obtain: (1) cardiac index is ≥ 2.5 liters/min/m^2; (2) mean systemic arterial pressure is ≥ 75 mm Hg; (3) mean left atrial pressure is ≤ 15 mm Hg; (4) mean right atrial pressure is ≤ 15 mm Hg; (5) circulatory assistance is no longer necessary or is being discontinued; (6) substantial inotropic support is not required; (7) urine output ≥ 15 ml/m^2/hr; and (8) significant acid-base deficit, life-threatening arrhythmias, and pulmonary edema are not present.

Another desideratum is the maintenance of a satisfactory overall pulmonary function. This generally means: (1) $Pa_{O_2} \geq 100$ mm Hg at $F_{I_{O_2}} \leq 0.4$; (2) A-a$D_{O_2}^{1.0} \leq 350$ mm Hg or $Pa_{O_2} \geq 300$ mm Hg at $F_{I_{O_2}} = 1.0$; (3) $V_D/V_T < 0.6$; (4) lung compliance >35 ml/cm H$_2$O; and (5) lung fields that are relatively clear by auscultatory and radiographic criteria.

While a fully reacted patient with good neuromuscular coordination and stable cardiopulmonary function is the ideal candidate for weaning, alterations in the state of consciousness should not greatly affect the decision to discontinue controlled ventilation provided the patient is able to "trigger" respirations and seizures are absent. Extubation, however, should await the return of consciousness as well as the return of an adequate cough and gag reflex.

In the presence of established acute renal failure, weaning may be delayed until there is a return of a satisfactory urinary output.

Likewise, weaning is delayed in the presence of life-threatening complications, such as continued mediastinal bleeding, until after the condition is treated or resolved.

As indicated earlier, progression from controlled to spontaneous ventilation is a deliberate step-by-step process. If cardiorespiratory stability is maintained after trials of short periods of spontaneous ventilation, longer periods of spontaneous ventilation are allowed if: (1) vital capacity exceeds 10 ml/kg; (2) arterial blood gases are satisfactory after 15 minutes of spontaneous ventilation; (3) respiratory rate is less than 35 breaths per minute; and (4) significant dyspnea, anxiety, restlessness, pallor, or cyanosis does not develop.

Criteria for Extubation. The criteria for extubation following step-by-step weaning are essentially the converse of those for the institution of mechanical ventilatory assistance. These criteria are outlined in Table 12–2.

Following extubation, the patient is monitored very closely, especially during the first hour. The patient is placed in the semi-Fowler position (15–30°) and breathes a humidified, oxygen-enriched mixture ($F_{IO_2} \geq 0.4$), usually through a face mask or face hood, and rarely through bipronged nasal cannulae. Children two to twelve years of age are best managed with an oxygen tent or canopy device. Intensive nursing care is continued, which should include a program of periodic patient turning, chest physiotherapy, deep breathing and coughing exercises, and other respiratory maneuvers designed to prevent atelectasis. Arterial blood-gas measurements are made one hour after extubation. If $Pa_{O_2} \geq 80$ mm Hg, $Pa_{CO_2} \leq 50$ mm Hg, respiratory rate <35, work of breathing not unduly increased, tussive force adequate, secretions able to be cleared effectively, and hemodynamic stability maintained, the patient's condition is considered satisfactory. Otherwise, reintubation and reinstitution of ventilatory assistance should be considered.

If a tracheostomy tube is in place during weaning, immediate decannulation is not aimed for. Instead, the tracheostomy site is allowed to remain patent for a few days in case it becomes necessary to reinstitute ventilatory assistance. The cuffed plastic tube is simply replaced with a fenestrated Jackson tube. The latter type of tube, when plugged, allows the patient to breathe through his or her own upper respiratory tract, talk, and cough secretions into the oropharynx. When it seems certain that the patient will not need reinstitution of ventilatory assistance, the fenestrated tube is gradually reduced in size and eventually removed.

Alternative Methods of Weaning. For patients who have required prolonged ventilatory support, the use of intermittent mandatory ventilation (IMV) may facilitate weaning from mechanical ventilation (Downs et al., 1973). IMV is a system of mechanical ventilation that allows the patient to breathe spontaneously, with or without PEEP, and delivers a mechanical hyperinflation at preset intervals. The mechanical hyperinflations are gradually reduced in frequency until weaning is complete.

Other patients may benefit from the use of PEEP during the weaning process. PEEP will find most successful application in patients with high closing volumes and those

TABLE 12–2 CRITERIA FOR EXTUBATION AFTER STEP-BY-STEP WEANING

Vital capacity exceeds 10 ml/kg

Maximum inspiratory force greater than -20 cm H$_2$O

Pa$_{O_2}$ ≥ 100 mm Hg at F$_{IO_2}$ = 0.4* (spontaneous ventilation through a T-piece connected to tracheal tube)

Pa$_{CO_2}$ stable at ≤ 50 mm Hg

Respiratory rate < 35 breaths/min

Absence of significant dyspnea, restlessness, pallor, cyanosis

Tussive force adequate

*Or an A-aD$_{O_2}^{1.0}$ of <300 to 350 mm Hg.

with prolonged respiratory failure. These patients tend to develop rapid alveolar collapse and hypoxemia upon discontinuance of mechanical ventilation, a process that is minimized or reversed by using 5 cm H_2O of PEEP. It has been shown that the use of PEEP during spontaneous ventilation favorably improves the relation between the closing volume and functional residual capacity, thereby improving arterial oxygenation (Craig and McCarthy, 1972).

For infants and children, we employ IMV and low PEEP; this technique is described in Chapter 19. Although continuous positive airway pressure (CPAP) with spontaneous breathing has been effectively employed in infants, it has been employed less frequently in the past few years.

REFERENCES

Adams AP, Economides AP, Finlay WE, Sykes MK: The effects of variations of inspiratory flow waveform on cardiorespiratory function during controlled ventilation in normo-, hypo- and hypervolemic dogs. Br J Anaesth 42:818, 1970.

Andrews MJ, Pearson FG: Incidence of tracheal injury following cuffed tube tracheostomy with assisted ventilation. Ann Surg 173:249, 1971.

Asbaugh DG: Effect of ventilatory methods and patterns on physiologic shunt. Surgery 68:99, 1970.

———, Petty TL: Positive end-expiratory pressure: physiology, indications, and contraindications. J Thorac Cardiovasc Surg 65:165, 1973.

Barach AL, Martin J, Eckman M: Positive pressure respiration and its application to the treatment of acute pulmonary edema. Ann Intern Med 12:754, 1938.

Bartlett RH, Gazzaniga AB, Geraghty TR: Respiratory maneuvers to prevent postoperative pulmonary complications. A critical review. JAMA 224:1017, 1973.

Bendixen HH, Hedley-Whyte JJ, Laver MB: Impaired oxygenation in surgical patients during general anesthesia with controlled ventilation. A concept of atelectasis. N Engl J Med 269:991, 1963.

Bergman NA: Effects of varying respiratory waveform on gas exchange. Anesthesiology 28:390, 1967.

Berneus B, Carlsten A: Effect of intermittent positive-pressure ventilation on cardiac output in poliomyelitis. Acta Med Scand 152:19, 1955.

Boyd AA, Tremblay RE, Spencer FC, Bahnson HT: Estimation of cardiac output soon after intracardiac surgery with cardiopulmonary bypass. Ann Surg 150:613, 1959.

Breivik H, Grenvik A, Miller E, Safar P: Normalizing low arterial CO_2 tension during mechanical ventilation. Chest 63:525, 1973.

Bryant LR, Trinkle JK, Dubilier L: Reappraisal of tracheal injury from cuffed tracheostomy tubes. JAMA 215:625, 1971.

Carlston A, Norlander O, Widman B: Observations on the postoperative circulation. Surg Gynecol Obstet 99:227, 1954.

Carroll R, Hedden M, Safar P: Intratracheal cuffs: performance characteristics. Anesthesiology 31:275, 1969.

Carroll RG: Evaluation of tracheal tube cuff designs. Crit Care Med 1:45, 1973.

———, McGinnis GE, Grenvik A: Performance characteristics of tracheal cuffs. Int Anesthesiol Clin 12 (3):111, 1974.

Cheyney FW, Hornkein HF, Crawford EW: The effects of expiratory resistance on the blood gas tensions of anesthetized patients. Anesthesiology 28:670, 1967.

Ching NP, Ayres SM, Paegle RP, Linden JM, Nealson TF Jr: The contribution of cuff volume and pressure in tracheostomy tube damage. J Thorac Cardiovasc Surg 62:402, 1971.

———, ———, Spina RC, Nealson TF Jr: Endotracheal damage during continuous ventilatory support. Ann Surg 179:123, 1974.

Cooper JD, Grillo HC: Experimental production and prevention of injury due to cuffed tracheal tubes. Surg Gynecol Obstet 139:1235, 1969a.

———, ———: The evolution of tracheal injury due to ventilatory assistance through cuffed tubes. A pathologic study. Ann Surg 169:334, 1969b.

Cournand A, Motley HL, Werko L, Richards DW: Physiological studies of the effect of intermittent positive pressure breathing on cardiac output in man. Am J Physiol 152:162, 1948.

Craig DB, McCarthy DS: Airway closure and lung volumes during breathing with maintained airway positive pressures. Anesthesiology 36:540, 1972.

Dammann JF Jr, Thung N, Christlieb II, Littlefield JB, Muller WH Jr: The management of the severely ill patient after open-heart surgery. J Thorac Cardiovasc Surg 45:80, 1963.

Dobrin PB, Goldberg EM, Lunfield TR: Endotracheal cuff: a comparative study. Anesth Analg 53:456, 1974.

Downs JB, Klein EF Jr, Desautels D, Modell JH, Kirby R: Intermittent mandatory ventilation: a new approach to weaning patients from mechanical ventilators. Chest 64:331, 1973.

Egan DF: Fundamentals of Respiratory Therapy. 2nd ed. St. Louis, C.V. Mosby, 1973.

Falke KJ, Pontoppidan H, Kumar A, Leith DE, Geffin B, Laver MB: Ventilation with end-expiratory pressure in acute lung disease. J Clin Invest 51:2315, 1972.

Finley TN, Lenfant C, Haab P, Riiper J, Rahn H: Venous admixture in pulmonary circulation of anesthetized dogs. J Appl Physiol 15:418, 1960.

Fishman NH, Dedo HH, Hamilton WK, Hinchcliffe WA, Roe BB: Postintubation tracheal stenosis. Ann Thorac Surg 8:47, 1969.

Geffin B, Grillo HC, Cooper JD, Pontopiddan H: Stenosis following tracheostomy for respiratory care. JAMA 216:1984, 1971.

———, Pontopiddan H: Reduction of tracheal damage by the prestretching of inflatable cuffs. Anesthesiology 31:462, 1969.

Gray BA: Clinical applications of mixed venous oxygen measurements. In Rogers RM (ed): Respiratory Intensive Care. Springfield, Ill, Thomas, 1977, pp 190–207.

Grillo HC, Cooper JD, Geffin B, Pontopiddan H: A low pressure cuff for tracheostomy tubes to minimize tracheal injury. J Thorac Cardiovasc Surg 62:898, 1971.

Guyton AC: Interstitial fluid pressure. II. Pressure-volume curves of interstitial space. Circ Res 16:452, 1965.

Haberman PB, Green JP, Archibald C, Dunn DL, Hurwitz SR, Ashburn WL, Moser KM: Determinants of successful selective tracheobronchial suctioning. N Engl J Med 289:1060, 1973.

Hedden MD, Ersoz CJ, Safar P: Tracheoesophageal fistulas following prolonged artificial ventilation via cuffed tracheostomy tubes. Anesthesiology 34:482, 1971.

Hedley-Whyte J, Pontoppidan H, Laver MB: Arterial oxygenation during hypothermia. Anesthesiology 26:595, 1965.

Herzog P: Advice and practical instructions for use of the Engstrom respirator. Opusc Med Stockh 9:280, 1964.

———, Norlander OP, Engstrom CG: Ultrasonic generation of aerosol for the humidification of inspired gas during volume-controlled ventilation. Acta Anaesthesiol Scand 8:79, 1964.

Horsfield K, Cumming G: Functional consequences of airway morphology. J Appl Physiol 24:384, 1968.

Ingelstedt S, Jonson B, Nordstrom L, Olsson SG: On automatic ventilation: a servo-controlled ventilator measuring expired minute volume, airway flow and pressure. Acta Anaesthesiol Scand (Suppl) 47:5, 1972.

Kamen JM, Wilkinson CJ: A new-low-pressure cuff for endotracheal tubes. Anesthesiology 34:482, 1971.

Kirklin JW, Theye RA: Cardiac performance after open intracardiac surgery. Circulation 28:1061, 1963.

Knelson JH, Howatt WF, DeMuth GR: Effect of respiratory pattern on alveolar gas exchange. J Appl Physiol 29:328, 1970.

Kuman A, Falke KJ, Geffin B, Aldridge CF, Laver MB, Lowenstein E, Pontoppidan H: Continuous positive-pressure ventilation in acute respiratory failure. N Engl J Med 283:1430, 1970.

Lenfant C, Howell BJ: Cardiovascular adjustments in dogs during continuous pressure breathing. J Appl Physiol 15:425, 1965.

Lindholm CE: Prolonged endotracheal intubation. Acta Anaesthesiol Scand (Suppl) 33:131, 1969.

Lomholt N: A new tracheostomy tube: cuff with controlled pressure of the tracheal mucuous membrane. Acta Anaesthesiol Scand 11:311, 1967.

Lough MD, Doershuk CF, Stern RC (eds): Pediatric Respiratory Therapy. Chicago, Year Book, 1974.

Lowenstein E, Bland JHL: Anesthesia in cardiac surgery. In Norman JC (ed): Cardiac Surgery, 2nd ed. New York, Appleton-Century-Crofts, 1972, pp 75–102.

Lyager S: Ventilation/perfusion ratio during intermittent positive-pressure ventilation. Acta Anaesthesiol Scand 14:211, 1970.

———: Influence of flow pattern on the distribution of respiratory air during intermittent positive pressure respiration. Acta Anaesthesiol Scand 12:191, 1968.

Magovern GJ, Shively JG, Fecht D, Theovitz F: The clinical and experimental evaluation of a controlled-pressure intratracheal cuff. J Thorac Cardiovasc Surg 64:747, 1972.

McGinnis GE, Shively JG, Patterson RL: An engineering analysis of intratracheal tube cuffs. Anesth Analg (Cleve) 50:557, 1971.

McIntyre BW, Laws AK, Ramachandran PR: Positive expiratory pressure plateau: improved gas exchange during mechanical ventilation. Can Anaesth Soc J 16:477, 1969.

Michenfelder JD, Fowler WS, Theye RA: CO_2 levels and pulmonary shunting in anesthetized man. J Appl Physiol 21:1471, 1966.

Miller DR, Sethi G: Tracheal stenosis following prolonged cuff intubation: cause and prevention. Ann Surg 171:283, 1970.

Morgan BC, Martin WE, Hornbein TF, Crawford EW, Guntheroth WG: Haemodynamic effects of intermittent positive pressure respiration. Anesthesiology 27:584, 1966.

Murphy DA, MacLean LD, Dobell ARC: Tracheal stenosis as a complication of tracheostomy. Ann Thorac Surg 2:44, 1966.

Nordstrom L: On automatic ventilation: haemodynamic effects of intermittent positive-pressure ventilation with and without an end-inspiratory pause. Acta Anaesthesiol Scand (Suppl) 47:29, 1972.

Nunn JF: Comment. Surv Anesth 14:333, 1970.

———: Applied Respiratory Physiology with Special Reference to Anaesthesia. London, Butterworths, 1969, p 313.

Pearson FG, Andres MJ: Detection and management of tracheal stenosis following cuffed tube tracheostomy. Ann Thorac Surg 12:359, 1971.

Peters RM: The Mechanical Basis of Respiration. Boston, Little, Brown, 1969.

Petty TL: Intensive and Rehabilitative Respiratory Care, 2nd ed. Philadelpha, Lea & Febiger, 1974.

Pontoppidan H, Geffin B, Lowenstein E: Acute Respiratory Failure in the Adult. Boston, Little, Brown, 1973.

———, Laver MB, Geffin B: Acute respiratory failure in the surgical patient. Adv Surg 4:163, 1970.

Prys-Roberts C, Kelman GR, Greenbaum R, Kain ML, Bay J: Hemodynamics and alveolar-arterial PO_2 differences at varying $Paco_2$ in anesthetized man. J Appl Physiol 25:80, 1968.

Shelly WM, Dawson RB, May IA: Cuffed tube as a cause of tracheal stenosis. J Thorac Cardiovasc Surg 57:623, 1969.

Sladen A, Laver MB, Pontoppidan H: Pulmonary complications associated with water retention during prolonged mechanical ventilation. N Engl J Med 279:448, 1968.

Spencer FC, Bosomworth PP, Richter W: Fatal pulmonary injury from prolonged inhalation of high concentrations of oxygen. Proc Third Int Conf Hyperbaric Med, 1966, p 189.

Sugioka K, Davis DA: Hyperventilation with oxygen —possible cause of cerebral hypoxia. Anesthesiology 21:135, 1960.

Suter PM, Fairley HB, Isenberg MD: Optimum end-expiratory airway pressure in patients with acute pulmonary failure. N Engl J Med 292:284, 1975.

Suwa K, Bendixen HH: Change in $Paco_2$ with mechanical dead space during artificial ventilation. J Appl Physiol 24:556, 1968.

Thung N, Herzog P, Christlieb II, Thompson WM Jr, Dammann JF Jr: Cost of respiratory effort in postoperative cardiac patients. Circulation 28:552, 1963.

Tornvall SS, Jackson KH, Oyanedel ET: Tracheal rupture, complication of cuffed endotracheal tube. Chest 59:237, 1971.

Uzawa T, Asbaugh DG: Continuous positive pressure breathing in acute hemorrhagic pulmonary edema. J Appl Physiol 26:427, 1969.

Watson WE: Observations on physiological dead space during intermittent positive pressure respiration. Br J Anaesth 34:502, 1962.

Wilson RS, Sullivan SF, Malm JR, Bowman FO Jr: The oxygen cost of breathing following anesthesia and cardiac surgery. Anesthesiology 39:387, 1973.

Zwillich C, Pierson DJ: Nasal necrosis: a complication of nasotracheal intubation. Chest 64:376, 1973.

13. Management of Ventilatory and Respiratory Complications

ROY A. JURADO   SIDNEY OWITZ
JOSEPH JAGUST

Respiratory problems constitute the most frequent complication after all types of thoracic and cardiac operations. While most of these conditions are self-limited processes, they remain an important cause of morbidity and sometimes mortality. Atelectasis, pneumonitis, pleural effusions, and acute respiratory failure are the most commonly encountered complications; discussions will, therefore, focus mainly on these problems. While the incidence of the classic "pump lung" syndrome has dramatically declined in recent years, cases of severe postoperative respiratory failure still are encountered from time to time. Occasionally, when pulmonary damage is severe, residual function in the native lung may no longer be adequate to sustain life, so that other modes of therapy and support measures, such as extracorporeal membrane oxygenation, may have to be availed of to forestall death from hypoxia and hypercarbia.

In the interest of brevity, discussions on the complications of assisted ventilation and intubation of the trachea and other iatrogenic complications will not be included in this chapter; the reader is referred to a selected list of monographs and articles that offer detailed information on these subjects (Sladen et al., 1968; Cooper and Grillo, 1969; Grillo, 1969, 1976, 1977; Lindholm, 1969; Winter and Smith, 1972; Wolfe et al., 1972; Zwillich et al., 1974).

The reported incidence of pulmonary complications after open heart surgery ranges from 61 to 84 percent, depending on the diagnostic criteria employed (Provan et al, 1966; Templeton et al., 1966; Gauert et al., 1971; Turnbull et al., 1974). The overwhelming majority of reported complications are atelectatic (Gauert et al., 1971). Operations for congenital lesions are followed by the lowest incidence of respiratory complications, while procedures for acquired valvular heart disease are accompanied by the highest respiratory complication rate (Provan et al., 1966). Although the *overall* incidence of pulmonary complications remains high, the incidence of *severe* dysfunction is lower and has been estimated to be between 18 and 20 percent (Provan et al., 1966; Gauert et al., 1971). However, Downes et al. (1970) reported a higher incidence (41 percent) of acute respiratory failure in infants less than two years of age undergoing either palliative or corrective surgery for various congenital cardiac and great vessel anomalies.

PATHOGENESIS OF POSTOPERATIVE PULMONARY DYSFUNCTION

The proposed mechanisms for the genesis of pulmonary dysfunction are multitudinous. A number of preoperative, intraoperative, and postoperative factors play a role, but more often than not, the interaction of these various factors is the important determinant.

Preoperative Factors

Severity of Cardiac Dysfunction. Of importance is the patient's overall cardiopulmonary status. Anderson and Ghia (1970) found that patients with class II, III, or IV cardiac disease (old New York Heart Association classification) invariably had disturbances of pulmonary perfusion and ventilation; in particular, Class III and IV patients had significant impairment of pulmonary function preoperatively. Measurements of their total flow resistance of the airway (TFR), total static compliance (TSC), and physiologic dead space-to-tidal volume ratio (V_D/V_T) were significantly different than those of patients with less severe cardiac disease (Class I) and in the control group of noncardiacs. Specifically, the mean values of TFR and V_D/V_T were higher, while TSC measurements were lower in Class III and IV cardiacs. The same investigators demonstrated further deterioration of pulmonary function after cardiopulmonary bypass in the same group of patients.

Similarly, Bates and Christie (1964), in a study of pulmonary function in patients with increasing severity of mitral stenosis, noted decreased maximum midexpiratory flow rate and dynamic compliance associated with progression of the severity of symptoms and rising airway resistance and mean pulmonary artery pressures. Moreover, patients with chronic mitral valve disease are known to have uneven distribution of ventilation and perfusion (Carroll et al., 1953; Curti et al., 1953; Dollery and West, 1960; Hallowell et al., 1965).

Pulmonary Venous Hypertension. The presence of chronic pulmonary venous hypertension or left ventricular failure is of equal importance. The hallmark of abnormal pulmonary function in heart disease is the clinical presence of dyspnea, which, in turn, is the direct result of acute or chronic vascular congestion (Marshall et al., 1954; Sharp et al., 1958; Daly et al., 1964; Gazetopoulos et al., 1966; Yu, 1969). A rise in pulmonary venous pressure increases the transmural hydrostatic force that favors translocation of water from the intravascular to the extravascular space (Levine et al., 1965). Indeed, in a study of patients with valvular heart disease, McCredie (1967) demonstrated that the degree of accumulation of pulmonary extravascular water was greater when the lesion was mitral stenosis, with its associated persistent rise in left atrial pressure. Patients with aortic valve disease also exhibited increased pulmonary extravascular water accumulation, but the changes were smaller in magnitude compared with those observed in the mitral valve disease group and were far more in keeping with the severity of their congestive failure (Fig. 13–1). Further, there was a positive correlation between the clinical severity of mitral and aortic valve disease and measured pulmonary extravascular water (Fig. 13–2). Finally, the increase in pulmonary extravascular water observed in the study groups was related to both pulmonary arterial and left atrial pressures, presumably reflecting increased transudation of fluid due to increased capillary hydrostatic pressure.

In addition to alterations in lung mechanics, abnormalities in gas exchange also are present in cardiac patients with or without heart failure (Carroll et al., 1953; Cosby et al., 1957; Saunders, 1965, 1966). It appears that the observed abnormalities in lung function stem from the increase in pulmonary blood volume and water content (Sharp et al., 1958; Daly et al., 1963, 1964; Forsberg, 1964; Gazeltopoulos, 1966; McCredie, 1967). Changes in pulmonary blood volume may, in turn, alter the physical characteristics of the pulmonary vasculature. Indeed, when pulmonary blood volume is elevated in either aortic or mitral valve disease, vascular compliance or distensibility is reduced (Giuntini et al., 1974; Yu et

Pulmonary Vascular Disease. Patients with pulmonary arteriolar hypertension and increased pulmonary vascular resistance are more likely to develop respiratory complications (Provan et al., 1966). These hemodynamic changes reflect morphologic alterations in pulmonary vascular anatomy, which, in turn, lead to uneven distribution of pulmonary blood flow and an abnormal $\dot{V}/\dot{Q}$ ratio. As an example, long-standing mitral valve disease is associated with regional changes in pulmonary vascular morphology that are preponderant in the lower lobes (Parker and Weiss, 1936). The ultimate result of these morphologic changes is an abnormal distribution of pulmonary blood flow (Friedman and Braunwald, 1966; Jebavy et al., 1970; Bjure et al., 1971). Other investigators (Dollery and West, 1960; Dawson et al., 1965) also have shown that an increase in pulmonary vascular

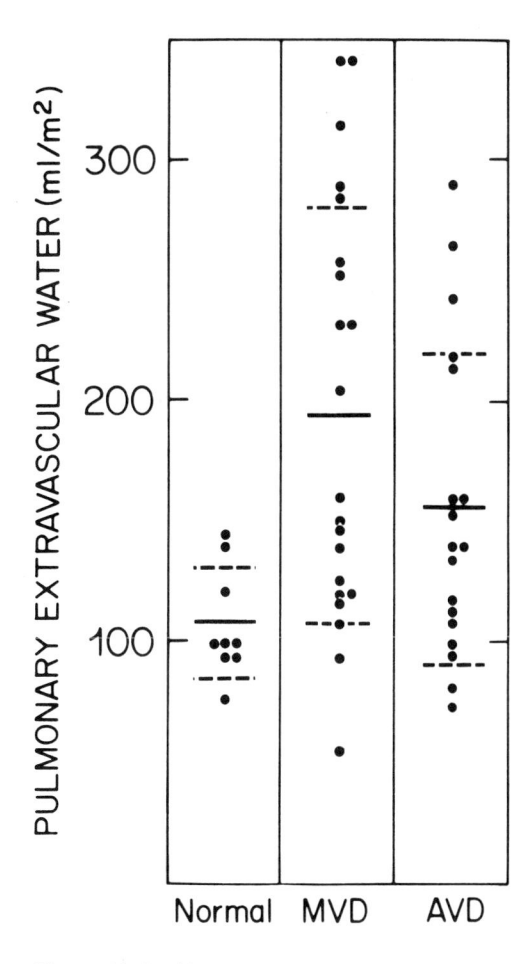

Figure 13-1. Measurements of pulmonary extravascular water showing higher values in patients with valvular heart disease than in normal subjects. Pulmonary extravascular water accumulation appears to be greatest in patients with mitral valve disease. Bars represent mean values; dashed lines represent ± 1 SD. MVD = mitral valve disease; AVD = aortic valve disease. *(Modified from McCredie, M. Measurement of pulmonary edema in valvular heart disease. Circulation 36:381–386, 1967.)*

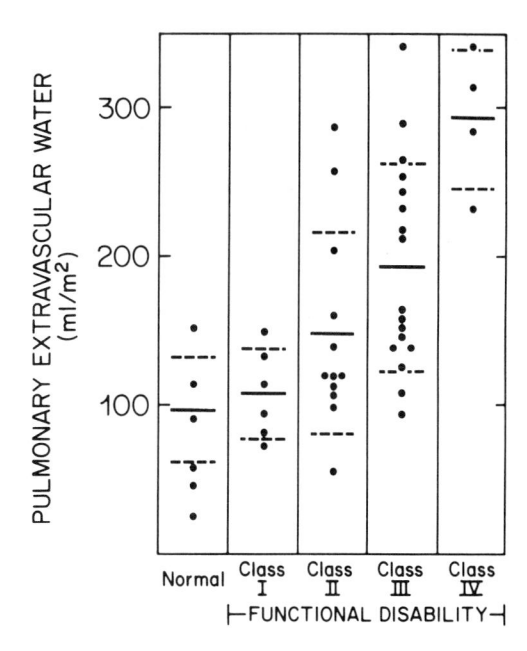

Figure 13-2. Relationship of measured pulmonary extravascular water and severity of dyspnea as reflected by functional classification. Measurements from normal subjects are shown for comparison. *(Modified from McCredie, M. Measurement of pulmonary edema in valvular heart disease. Circulation 36:381–386, 1967.)*

al., 1967). The practical implications are obvious. In the presence of severe pulmonary venous hypertension, only small increments in intravascular volume can be tolerated; injudicious administration of fluids or blood can readily result in pulmonary edema.

resistance in patients with chronic mitral valve disease is accompanied by increased blood flow to the upper lobes of the lung, resulting in a $\dot{V}/\dot{Q}$ maldistribution. Parenthetically, this may explain the different responses observed when positive end-expiratory pressure (PEEP) is added to the ventilatory pattern in patients with high (mitral valve disease) and those with normal (aortic valve disease) pulmonary vascular resistances (Trichet et al., 1975).

Patients with elevated pulmonary vascular resistance also have altered lung mechanics. Deal et al. (1968), in a study of patients with congenital heart disease, found that an elevated pulmonary vascular resistance was associated with a reduced pulmonary compliance. The obvious implication is that the energy cost of breathing may be increased in such patients.

Anatomic Factors. Mechanical compression of the large bronchi by enlarged cardiac chambers and great vessels may predispose to the development of atelectasis and secondary infection. The predilection of postoperative atelectasis to involve the left lower lobe in patients with significant left ventricular enlargement has been attributed to mechanical factors, i.e., compression of the left lower bronchus by the enlarged ventricular mass (Stanger et al., 1969). Conceivably, upward displacement of the left main stem bronchus by an enlarged left atrium may have the same effect by increasing the angle of the tracheal bifurcation.

It also has been demonstrated that extrinsic pressure by enlarged pulmonary arteries can produce bronchial obstruction, especially in infants (Stanger et al., 1969). The same investigators suggest that this anatomic lesion may explain certain symptoms of respiratory distress occurring in some infants with hypertensive pulmonary arteries and may be responsible for certain cases of infantile lobar emphysema occurring in association with congenital heart disease.

Preexisting or Intercurrent Lung Disease. The presence of parenchymal, airways, or chronic pleural disease heightens the possibility of postoperative respiratory complications. The two major areas of concern in these patients are the adequacy of pulmonary function and the presence of infection.

Ventilatory capacity and reserve are already both reduced in the patient with emphysema, who frequently exhibits an increased work of breathing, a prolonged expiratory phase, increased airway resistance, air trapping, and uneven pulmonary gas distribution. Maximum breathing capacity and timed vital capacity are also usually reduced in such patients. The chronic bronchitic will exhibit similar abnormalities in lung mechanics and, in addition, concomitant tracheobronchial infection may be present. The relationship between smoking and bronchitis is well-known and needs no further elaboration. Restriction of lung expansion by pleural fibrosis likewise reduces pulmonary reserve.

In the preoperative preparation of these patients, emphasis should be placed on eradication of infection, control of bronchospasm, and improvement of overall pulmonary function. These measures are discussed in Chapter 3.

Other Factors. Additional factors that are important include age, obesity, and enfeeblement that accompanies chronic heart failure. The physiologic handicaps imposed by the extremes of age, obesity, and cardiac cachexia have already been discussed in Chapter 3. Suffice it to say that the effects of these factors on respiratory subsystem performance increase the likelihood of postoperative problems.

Intraoperative Factors

Surgical Incision. It is generally accepted that midline sternal splitting incisions are associated with the lowest incidence of postoperative respiratory complications (Humphreys et al., 1964), presumably because pleural entry usually can be avoided (Sullivan et al., 1966; Ghia and Anderson, 1970) and less incisional pain results compared with the other types of incision. Additionally, since muscle cutting and dissection are minimal, substantially fewer alterations in chest wall mechanics occur. Indeed, Peters et al. (1969) observed that, while total compliance of the chest wall and lungs dropped significantly after both lateral thoracotomy and median sternotomy, far fewer changes resulted with the latter. It is felt that much of the apparent fall in total compliance is due to fixation of portions of the chest wall by local muscle spasm and pain (Peters et al., 1969).

However, regardless of the type of surgical incision employed, spirometric studies consistently have shown that tidal volume, vital capacity, and maximum breathing capacity are all reduced soon after open intracardiac operations (Howatt et al., 1962). Similar distortions in ventilatory function are seen in patients undergoing thoracotomies for various pulmonary diseases (Martin and Stead, 1953) and in patients with restriction of thoracic excursions because of a painful wound. Other postoperative changes observed include a decrease in functional residual capacity and an increase in residual volume. These changes appear to be maximal 24 hours postoperatively.

Left Heart Distention. The causal relationship between left heart distention (i.e., acute pulmonary venous hypertension) and postoperative pulmonary dysfunction is well-known (Kolff et al., 1958; Edmunds and Austen, 1966). For this and other reasons, provisions routinely are made for effective drainage and decompression of the left heart during cardiopulmonary bypass and mandatory when effective systolic contractions are not present.

Effects of Cardiopulmonary Bypass on Pulmonary Function. Certain changes in pulmonary function occur predictably after cardiopulmonary bypass. Impaired respiratory gas exchange almost invariably is present and most often is characterized by arterial hypoxemia caused by increased venous admixture (Fordham, 1965; Hedley-Whyte et al., 1965; McClenahan et al., 1965). While this is usually mild, arterial oxygen tensions may be at hypoxic levels 24 hours or more after cardiopulmonary bypass, if the patient is breathing room air (Turnbull et al., 1974). The time course of changes in Pao$_2$ is shown in Figure 13–3. These investigators observed that the duration of cardiopulmonary bypass was the only clinical factor significantly related to the Pao$_2$ 24 hours postoperatively; specifically, there was an inverse relationship between the two variables. Measurements of alveolar-arterial oxygen tension gradient (A-aDo$_2$) also revealed progressive widening, with the peak occurring between 24 and 72 hours after the operation, an observation similar to that made by Geha et al. (1966). These changes in A-aDo$_2$ are shown in Figure 13–4.

Moderate to marked reductions in diffusing capacity have been demonstrated (Howatt et al., 1962; Ellison et al., 1963). Turnbull et al. (1974) observed a marked reduction in the steady-state diffusion capacity for carbon monoxide (Dco$_{ss}$) postoperatively, which slowly improved with time (Fig. 13–5).

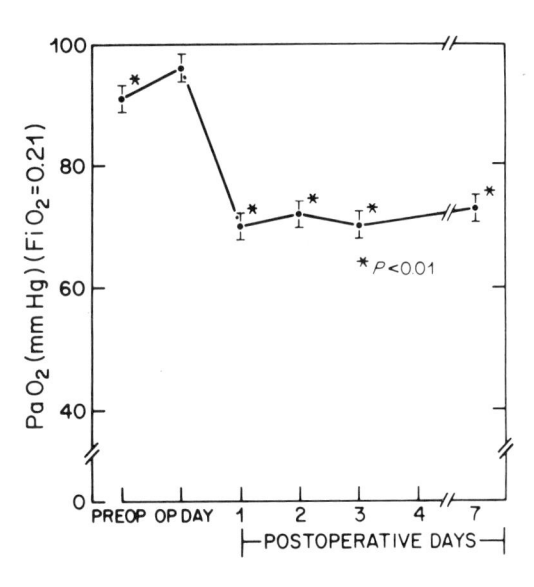

Figure 13–3. Changes in arterial oxygen tension (PaO$_2$) soon after open heart surgery with subjects breathing room air (FiO$_2$ = 0.21). PaO$_2$ levels remained significantly lower than preoperative values throughout the first postoperative week. *(Modified from Turnbull, KW, Miyagishima, RT, Gerein, AN. Pulmonary complications and cardiopulmonary bypass.* Can Anaesth Soc J *21:181–194, 1974.)*

Figure 13-4. Changes in arterial oxygen tension (PaO₂) and alveolar-arterial oxygen tension difference (A-aDO₂) soon after open heart surgery with subjects breathing 100 percent oxygen (FIO₂ = 1.0). A-aDO₂ appears to be highest 24 to 72 hours postoperatively. *(Modified from Turnbull, KW, Miyagishima, RT, Gerein, AN. Pulmonary complications and cardiopulmonary bypass. Can Anaesth Soc J 21:181–194, 1974.)*

Figure 13-5. Changes in lung diffusing capacity for carbon monoxide (Dco$_{ss}$) seen in patients soon after open heart surgery. Dco$_{ss}$ appears to be lowest on the first postoperative day. *(Modified from Turnbull, KW, Miyagishima, RT, Gerein, AN. Pulmonary complications and cardiopulmonary bypass. Can Anaesth Soc J 21:181–194, 1974.)*

A significant increase in a-ADco₂ has also been demonstrated; this occurs in the first postoperative day, with no significant changes observed beyond this time (Turnbull et al., 1974). Physiologic dead space-to-tidal volume ratios (V_D/V_T) remain apparently unchanged in the immediate and early postoperative intervals (Ghia and Andersen, 1970; Turnbull et al., 1974), but slowly begin to rise and remain significantly elevated from the third to the seventh postoperative days (Turnbull et al., 1974). The findings of reduced diffusing capacity, widened A-aDo₂, and increased V_D/V_T suggest the presence of $\dot{V}/\dot{Q}$ abnormalities that become significant three to seven days after surgery, presumably when collapsed or atelectatic lung segments are reexpanding.

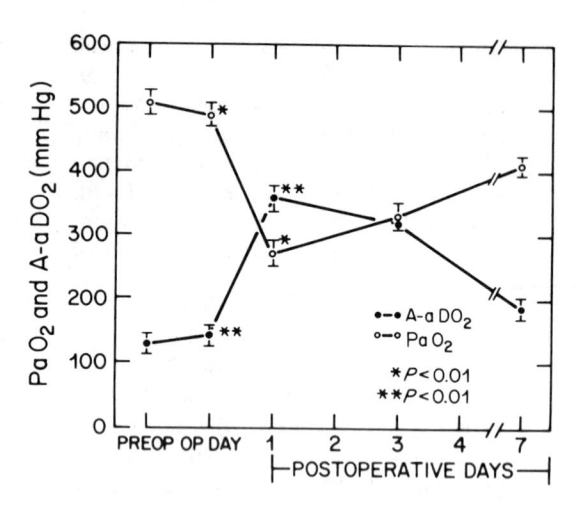

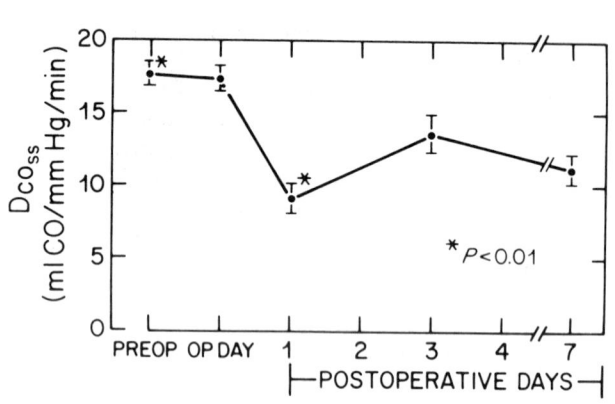

Rhodes et al. (1974) observed similar changes in puppies undergoing total cardiopulmonary bypass with bubble or membrane oxygenators. A decrease in alveolar ventilation, reduction in diffusing capacity, and a widening of the A-aDo₂ were seen in all animal groups. It was also noted that the distortions observed were directly related to the duration of cardiopulmonary bypass, but not to the type of oxygenator used.

Alterations in pulmonary mechanics likewise have been observed after open intracardiac operations. Pulmonary compliance has been shown to be decreased for a period of a few weeks after anesthesia and open heart operations (Garzon et al., 1966; Ellison et al., 1967; Hand et al., 1970). There is evidence that the decrease in compliance observed postoperatively represents a further change from the low preoperative values seen in patients with heart disease and pulmonary hypertension (Garzon et al., 1967; Andersen and Ghia, 1970). Work of breathing is markedly increased after open intracardiac operations (Garzon et al., 1966; Ellison et al., 1967; Peters et al., 1969; Hand et al., 1970), as is the total flow resistance of the airway (Andersen and Ghia, 1970). These alterations in lung mechanics appear to be maximal in the immediate postoperative period and gradually return toward preoperative control values over several postoperative weeks (Garzon et al., 1966; Ellison et al., 1967; Hand et al., 1970).

In a study of postcardiotomy patients, Hand et al. (1970) observed that pulmonary compliance and arterial oxygen tensions (F_{IO_2} of 0.21 and 1.0) decreased while total work of breathing increased in the immediate postoperative period and were significantly different than preoperative values. Pa_{O_2} values remained significantly lower than preoperative values during the first postoperative week. Total work of breathing was still significantly increased 6 to 10 days postoperatively. The time course of these changes is reproduced in Figure 13–6. In the same study, measurements of vital capacity and percentage of predicted vital capacity were the only values that still showed a significant change at 14 to 21 days.

While the nature of these alterations in pulmonary function after cardiopulmonary bypass is fairly well-defined, the exact pathogenetic mechanisms remain undetermined. The pathologic changes described are nonspecific and frequently include pulmonary atelectasis, congestion, and hemorrhage. Mechanical, chemical, embolic, hemodynamic, immunologic, physical, and other factors have been implicated in the genesis of postperfusion pulmonary dysfunction. This syndrome probably is the variable result of the interplay of a host of factors. A comprehensive discussion of these factors is beyond the scope of this chapter; the reader is, therefore, enjoined to refer to the reports and reviews of

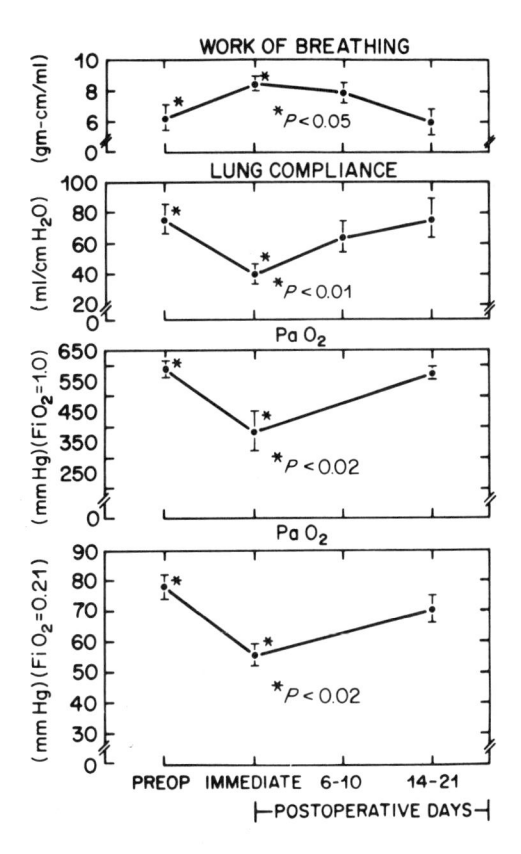

Figure 13–6. Changes in lung mechanics and arterial oxygen tension (Pa_{O_2}) seen in patients soon after open heart surgery. Lung compliance and arterial oxygen tension decreased, while work of breathing increased in the immediate postoperative period. *(Modifed from Hand, BR, Malm, JR, Bowman, FO, Jr, Sullivan, SF. The effects of anesthesia and cardiac bypass on pulmonary compliance in man. Bull N Y Acad Med 46:22–33, 1970.)*

Dodrill (1958), Lee et al., (1961), Hepps et al. (1963), Hollenberg et al. (1963), Litwak et al. (1963), Neville et al. (1963), Schramel et al. (1963), Nahas et al. (1965), Awad et al. (1966), Tilney and Hester (1967), Veith et al. (1968), Panossian et al. (1969), Sobonya et al. (1972), and Ratliff et al. (1973).

Postoperative Factors

Incisional pain produces muscle splinting and promotes hypoventilation. Moreover, it prevents effective coughing, thereby promoting retention of tracheobronchial secretions and obstructive atelectasis (Dammann et al., 1963). *Central depression* from neurologic damage or from the combined effects of residual anesthetic drugs and sedatives also promotes hypoventilation in patients who are not on mechanical ventilation. Likewise, the residual effects of muscle relaxant drugs may prevent effective spontaneous ventilation.

Pneumothoraces and hemothoraces, when not adequately drained, prevent full lung expansion, promote alveolar collapse, and impair respiratory gas exchange.

Myocardial dysfunction, when accompanied by a *low cardiac output,* adversely affects pulmonary function. Suwa et al. (1966) have demonstrated an inverse relationship between cardiac output and V_D/V_T in experimental animals with normal pulmonary function. Philbin et al. (1970), in a study of postcardiotomy patients, demonstrated that low cardiac output contributed significantly to arterial hypoxemia when venous admixture was already present. When the cardiac index fell below 2.5 liters/min/m^2, in patients with abnormally high values of venous admixture ($\dot{Q}_S/\dot{Q}_T$), the magnitude of arterial oxygen desaturation increased significantly during breathing of room air. Further, the same investigators, using derived data, reemphasized the point that increasing the F_{IO_2} will have a very minimal effect on arterial oxygenation when cardiac output is very low, assuming venous admixture, hemoglobin, and oxygen remain constant (see Fig. 12–9).

In the presence of *congestive heart failure,* secondary to myocardial dysfunction and other causes, an acute and sustained rise in pulmonary venous pressure may result in pulmonary edema, with its dire consequences on pulmonary mechanics and gas exchange.

After major operations, metabolic requirements are increased (Carlsten et al., 1954). In postcardiotomy patients, this is partially caused by the increased energy cost of breathing (Wilson et al., 1973). *Postoperative fever,* sepsis, and other conditions that cause whole body oxygen consumption to be augmented even further could impose additional demands on the body economy. If compensatory mechanisms fail to satisfy the need for increased alveolar ventilation or if proper therapy is not instituted promptly, ventilatory failure could supervene.

Miscellaneous factors considered important in the genesis of pulmonary dysfunction in the postcardiotomy patient include injudicious use of crystalloids, misuse of colloids, and multiple transfusions, especially when carried out without adequate filtration of donor blood. When sole reliance is placed on crystalloids for intravascular volume repletion, pulmonary interstitial edema could result. Similarly, the use of excessive amounts of concentrated albumin could result in the accumulation of albumin within the interstitial space, especially in patients with pulmonary edema or increased capillary permeability (Marty, 1974).

It is known that microaggregates of leukocytes, platelets, and fibrin accumulate in stored blood. If allowed to remain in transfused blood, these aggregates are filtered by the lung and cause pulmonary dysfunction (Hissen and Swank, 1965; Radegran, 1971; McNamara et al., 1972; Connell and Swank, 1973). It has been shown that, during the storage of blood in acid citrate dextrose (ACD) solution, microaggregate formation initially is minimal, as evidenced by a low screen filtration pressure. After five days, the mean screen filtration pressure increases markedly (indicating increased microaggregate formation) and continues to increase gradually from that point on (McNamara et al., 1971; Harp et al., 1974). While the reason for this sudden increase in microaggregate formation is not known, it has been suggested that fibrin formation may be responsible (Harp et al., 1974). It has been estimated that, after one week of ACD storage, there are over 140,000 microaggregates per milliliter of blood, ranging in size from 10 to 164 μ (Connell and Swank, 1973). Available experimental data show that infusion of stored blood with high screen filtration pressures results in increases in pulmonary vascular resistance, end-expiratory bronchial pressure, and lung water (Bennett et al., 1972; McNamara et al., 1972).

A rise in pulmonary arterial pressure and gross and microscopic evidence of pulmonary edema also have been observed (Hissen and Swank, 1965; Bennett et al., 1972), along with an increase in dead space-to-tidal volume ratio, suggesting an increase in alveolar dead space and microvascular occlusion. In a study of combat casualties, McNamara et al., (1970) observed a definite correlation between the amount of stored blood infused and the degree of shock and severity of trauma. Respiratory failure was noted in those casualties requiring massive transfusion, even in the absence of any known pulmonary injury. Moreover, significant amounts of microemboli were demonstrated in the pulmonary arterioles and capillaries of those casualties who eventually succumbed. Ultrapore filtration is perhaps the most effective method known to date of removing microaggregates during transfusion of banked blood (Swank, 1961; McNamara et al., 1972; Solis and Gibbs, 1972; Connell and Swank, 1973).

Pathogenesis of Postcardiotomy Acute Respiratory Failure

Despite advances in respiratory care techniques, the development of acute respiratory failure after cardiac surgery still carries serious prognostic implications, especially in patients who come to the operation with significantly compromised cardiopulmonary reserves. The pathogenesis of this complication is complex and involves the interaction of multiple preoperative, intraoperative, and postoperative factors, with the eventual development of life-threatening hypoxia or hypercarbia (Fig. 13–7). It is apparent that a significant number of factors believed to cause postcardiotomy respiratory failure are largely controllable, if not outright preventable. Therefore, the patient management program employed must stress the control, if not elimination, of those conditions known to predispose to the development of postoperative respiratory complications.

CLINICAL RECOGNITION OF PULMONARY COMPLICATIONS

Retention of Secretions, Atelectasis, and Pneumonitis

After major operations, an increase in tracheobronchial secretions is common. Frequently, the secretions remain mucoid and are easily cleared by coughing. The patient remains afebrile unless *acute bronchitis, atelectasis,* or *penumonitis* develops.

In patients with a history of heavy smoking or frequent upper respiratory tract infections the increase in tracheobronchial secretions is more marked. The sputum rapidly changes from mucoid to mucopurulent and even frankly purulent coincident with the appearance of signs of an acute tracheobronchial infection. The patient becomes febrile, a wheeze or a "rattle" becomes audible, and respirations may become labored. At this point, the chest roentgenogram is generally unremarkable.

Segmental atelectasis is more common than *lobar* collapse. Unless the atelectasis is massive, the classic signs of sudden onset of high fever, rapid pulse, tachypnea, cyanosis, mediastinal shift, and an inspiratory lag on the involved side are not seen. Segmental atelectasis is usually detected by the presence of diminished breath sounds with bronchial breathing over the involved segment of lung, or by the presence of moist rales, usually localized posteriorly or toward the lung bases. The patient is usually febrile, and his or her condition may deteriorate rapidly if lobar collapse is present. The roentgenographic picture of massive collapse is characteristic, but may be totally nonspecific in focal or patchy atelectasis.

Pneumonitis generally develops on a background of atelectasis, with infection being introduced from either the tracheobronchial tree or the blood stream (Shields, 1949) or both. The clinical signs are generally those of

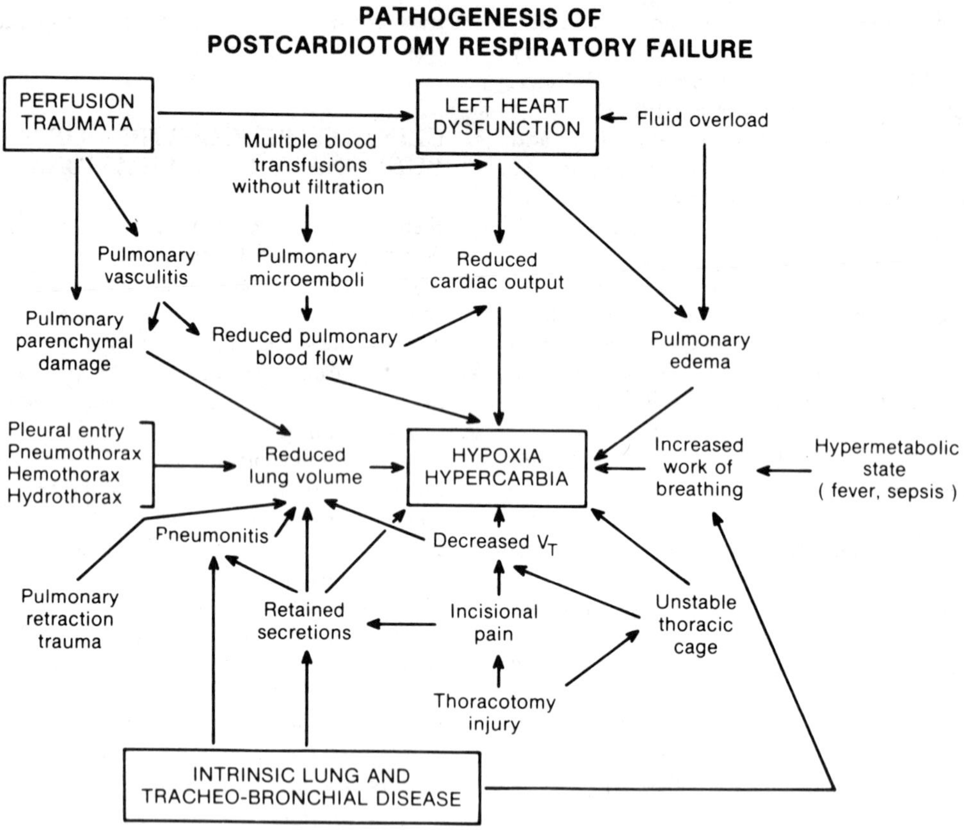

PATHOGENESIS OF POSTCARDIOTOMY RESPIRATORY FAILURE

Figure 13-7. Pathogenetic mechanisms in acute respiratory failure complicating cardiac surgery.

atelectasis. However, the patient remains febrile and may look septic despite efforts to remove secretions and reexpand atelectatic segments. If the infection spreads to surrounding lung parenchyma, the result is bronchopneumonia, which generally presents radiographically as confluent opacities scattered throughout the lung bases.

Pleural Effusion

Collections of fluid in the pleural space are generally due to either congestive heart failure or retained blood drainage from the operative site. The clinical signs are dullness to percussion and diminished to absent breath sounds over the lung bases. The patient may be dyspneic and tachypneic, and fever may also be present from secondary atelectasis. Unless the effusion is massive, shift of the mediastinal structures to the opposite side is not seen. The chest roentgenogram is usually diagnostic.

Pulmonary Vascular Overload

Strictly speaking, this is not a pulmonary complication per se but rather represents the inability of the left heart to handle its volume load. As a consequence, pulmonary edema develops and signs of respiratory distress appear. This condition can develop as a result of volume overloading or left ventricular failure, and, rarely, from mitral valve dysfunction.

Clinically, there is usually a marked tachypnea, which is accompanied by tachycardia, respiratory distress, and cyanosis. Frothy and bloody secretions may be expectorated. Concomitantly, signs of left ventricular overload are usually present. The left atrial or pulmonary capillary wedge pressure is elevated and a gallop may be present. There is usually a marked fall in lung compliance and in the arterial oxygen tension (Pa_{O_2}). The radiologic picture is characteristic, with pulmonary venous engorgement and pulmonary infiltrates.

Acute Respiratory Failure

For this and subsequent discussions in this chapter, the term "acute respiratory failure" is used liberally to include acute ventilatory failure and the so-called postperfusion lung or the pump-lung syndrome.

For patients allowed to breathe spontaneously soon after operative termination, the earliest signs of ventilatory insufficiency generally include tachypnea, mild dyspnea, and slight tachycardia. If pulmonary function tests are performed at this point, the tidal volume, vital capacity, and maximum breathing capacity are reduced. The Pa_{O_2} on room air ($F_{IO_2} = 0.21$) is borderline (i.e., 60 to 70 mm Hg) while hypocarbia is usually present, reflecting the hyperventilation. The A-a$D_{O_2}^{1.0}$ is increased and a rise in $\dot{Q}_S/\dot{Q}_T$ also is seen, indicating increased right-to-left shunting and venous admixture.

As the patient's condition worsens, signs of acute respiratory distress become manifest. Respirations become more labored with active use of the accessory muscles. The patient becomes diaphoretic. The heart rate increases even further and the patient becomes more dyspneic. Signs of progressive pulmonary insufficiency may now supervene. Hypocarbia persists as hypoxemia worsens despite intensive respiratory management. Signs of CO_2 retention (i.e., hypertension, tachycardia, and elevated left heart filling pressures) are rarely seen. Auscultation reveals increasing rales and rhonchi, and chest radiographs show spotty and diffuse infiltrates. At this point, endotracheal intubation generally is mandated and mechanical ventilatory assistance is instituted. Following this, the patient may show signs of improvement that may culminate in recovery or may only be transient, lasting for hours or at most a few days.

If recovery is not in store, the subsequent clinical course is characterized by a progressive deterioration in cardiorespiratory function. There is progression of the pulmonic process by clinical examination and by x-ray, with the appearance of widespread areas of consolidation. There is gradual failure of spontaneous ventilation. In addition, there is: (1) progressive drop in Pa_{O_2} despite rising F_{IO_2} and an augmented minute ventilation; (2) a progressive rise in maximum inspiratory and mean airway pressures; (3) a progressive decrease in lung compliance; (4) an increase in V_D/V_T and $\dot{Q}_S/\dot{Q}_T$. These soon are followed by loss of consciousness and the appearance of signs of circulatory instability, and death may ensue shortly thereafter.

For patients electively placed on mechanical ventilation at operative termination, the first signs of respiratory insufficiency may be hypoxemia (Pa_{O_2} <65 to 70 mm Hg) while breathing an oxygen-enriched gas mixture, a widened alveolar-arterial oxygen gradient (A-a$D_{O_2}^{1.0}$ >350 mm Hg), and an increased physiologic dead space (V_D/V_T>0.6). Confirmatory evidence is provided by the inability to wean off mechanical ventilatory assistance (See Chapter 12, Weaning from Mechanical Ventilation).

PREVENTION OF POSTOPERATIVE PULMONARY COMPLICATIONS

In the management of postoperative pulmonary complications, the emphasis should be on prophylaxis rather than actual treatment. This means meticulous attention to those factors considered important in the genesis of pulmonary dysfunction in general and of each specific complication in particular.

Prophylactic measures should be started early in patients undergoing elective operations if the risk of their developing postoperative pulmonary problems is high. This applies particularly to heavy smokers, chronic bronchitics, the elderly, and patients with chronic obstructive lung disease. Ideally, patients should stop smoking two weeks preoperatively. Bronchospasm should be cleared and tracheobronchial infection eradicated. A preoperative regimen of chest physiotherapy and respiratory exercises emphasizing deep abdominal diaphragmatic breathing and productive coughing should be instituted in all patients. This program has been shown to decrease significantly the incidence of postoperative pulmonary complications (Tarhan et al., 1973).

The patient's general condition should be improved as far as possible. Congestive heart failure should be treated and cardiac performance should be optimized. Ideally, overweight and obese patients should, if at all possible, be placed on a weight-reduction program preoperatively.

Some operative measures will help reduce the incidence of postoperative pulmonary problems. Whenever possible, transpleural procedures should be avoided by approaching the heart through a midline sternal incision with careful preservation of the intact pleural spaces (Sullivan et al., 1966; Ghia and Andersen, 1970). Adequate and effective venting of the left heart during cardiopulmonary bypass should be ensured to prevent left heart distention and acute pulmonary venous hypertension. The use of hemodilution (Hepps et al., 1963), minimizing hemolysis (Schramel et al., 1963), and periodic inflation of the lungs and avoidance of prolonged pulmonary collapse (Kirklin et al., 1958) have all been found helpful. Recently, the use of Dacron-wool filters during bypass has been found to be effective in preventing lung damage by removing leukocytes and damaged platelets from the circulation (Hill et al., 1975). Since the severity of postcardiotomy hypoxemia appears to be related to the duration of cardiopulmonary bypass (Turnbull et al., 1974), it stands to reason that the expeditious performance of the intracardiac repair with shortening of the bypass time may also be beneficial.

Postoperatively, the main object is to keep the lungs normally expanded and to maintain optimal volumes. It appears that functional impairment of a damaged lung can be minimized and its recovery facilitated if it can be kept at a normal FRC. This is accomplished by an aggressive general respiratory management program that emphasizes early mobilization, regular full turning, deep breathing, chest physiotherapy, and proper humidification, adequate tracheobronchial toilette, and careful fluid administration. To accomplish this, the patient should be adequately and properly medicated for pain at all times. Narcotic analgesics should be given in doses large enough to allay pain without producing central depression. If the pleural cavity had been entered, adequate pleural drainage should be maintained. If blood administration becomes necessary, transfusion filters should be used (see Postoperative Factors). Maintenance of optimal cardiac performance and elimination of factors conducive to hypermetabolism and increased oxygen consumption are essential. Close patient surveillance is mandatory to insure early detection and treatment of respiratory complications.

MANAGEMENT OF PULMONARY COMPLICATIONS

Retained Secretions, Atelectasis, and Pneumonitis

The fundamental elements of therapy are good nursing and assiduous respiratory care. Removal of viscid tracheobronchial secretions may sometimes be rendered difficult by enfeeblement or a lowered level of consciousness. More frequently, however, the failure to effectively clear secretions is due to chest wall splinting because of incisional pain. It is essential, therefore, that the patient be properly medicated for pain; for this purpose, reliance is placed on adequate doses of narcotics (see Chapter 12).

Deep breathing and coughing should be actively encouraged. Within the limits imposed by the patient's cardiorespiratory status and general condition, a carefully coordinated program of regular full turning, early mobilization, and periodic chest physiotherapy should be instituted. The maneuvers are best timed to follow the injections of the analgesic medication. Proper humidification of the inspired gas should also be ensured.

If atelectasis is already present or if the patient is unable to clear the secretions on his or her own, other methods of treatment should be employed. For instance, secretions may be removed by nasotracheal aspiration with a sterile catheter. Removal of thick, tenacious secretions is facilitated by prior instillation of 2 to 3 ml of normal saline solution into the tracheobronchial tree through the suction catheter.

When the secretions become so copious or viscid that clearance by nasotracheal aspirations fails, bronchoscopic aspiration is indicated. Bronchoscopy generally can be carried out at the bedside with topical anesthesia. When combined with saline instillation and manual hyperinflation with the Ambu bag, bronchoscopic aspiration can be a very effective method of clearing tenacious secretions and reexpanding atelectatic segments.

If bronchoscopic aspiration fails, or is required frequently, endotracheal intubation is indicated. After passage of the endotracheal tube, frequent aspiration of secretions can be performed and the patient usually is placed on mechanical ventilation for a few days. It is rarely necessary to perform a tracheostomy for the sole purpose of removing retained secretions. If tracheostomy is performed, there are usually more compelling reasons.

The hazard of improper tracheal suctioning are well-known and are discussed in Chapter 12 (see Tracheobronchial Toilette). The secretions obtained during tracheal aspiration can be collected aseptically in appropriate containers for microbiologic studies.

In the presence of known bronchitis or if atelectasis appears to be progressing to pneumonitis, appropriate antibiotics should be administered.

Pleural Effusion

Significant collections of fluid in one or both pleural spaces may impair ventilation and promote atelectasis. If the effusion simply represents retained bloody drainage, mechanical aspiration by thoracentesis usually suffices. When congestive heart failure is the cause, treatment should be directed toward the amelioration of the primary condition, although drainage by aspiration may be indicated if respiratory embarrassment is present.

Thoracentesis should be performed carefully and atraumatically in patients receiving anticoagulant drugs. In some cases, it may be preferable to taper the dose of the anticoagulant medication before thoracentesis is carried out. Likewise, patients with congestive heart failure and right-sided pleural effusions should be approached with caution. In these patients the likelihood of producing hepatic injury during thoracentesis is great because the liver is enlarged and encroaches into the chest. Moreover, liver function usually is deranged and coagulation abnormalities may be present.

Pulmonary Edema

Traditionally, primary reliance has been placed on digitalis, diuretics, morphine, and rotating tourniquets or phlebotomy in the treatment of this condition. However, if significant disturbances in ventilation or gas exchange are present, endotracheal intubation should be carried out and mechanical ventilatory assistance instituted, especially if cardiac output is reduced. Mechanical ventilation should be maintained as long as significant cardiopulmonary dysfunction persists. In weaning from mechanical ventilation, the same guidelines outlined in Chapter 12 are followed.

Acute Respiratory Failure

Acute respiratory insufficiency following cardiac surgery, though no longer a frequent problem, still occurs occasionally. Once pulmonary insufficiency is established, primary reliance is placed on mechanical ventilation to sustain life. Established principles and practices of respiratory therapy are meticulously adhered to, but the therapeutic program chosen should carefully balance the therapeutic goals against the potential for producing additional pulmonary damage as a result of the therapy. These principles and management techniques are discussed in Chapter 12.

In brief, the essential elements of intensive respiratory care include: (1) volume-cycled ventilation; (2) maintenance of optimal lung volumes; (3) oxygen-enriched inspiratory gas mixture using minimum F_{IO_2}'s; (4) judicious use of positive end-expiratory pressure; (5) proper humidification; (6) aseptic airway management; (7) good nursing care, which includes regular full turning and mobilization of the patient and chest physiotherapy; (8) stringent fluid management; (9) judicious use of diuretics and colloids; (10) use of antibiotics on indication only; and (11) careful patient monitoring.

When pulmonary dysfunction is severe and mechanical ventilatory assistance and other support measures are ineffective to support adequate gas exchange, resulting in life-threatening hypoxemia and hypercarbia, extracorporeal respiratory support with a membrane lung could be life-saving (Soeter et al., 1973). The rationale for the employment of extracorporeal membrane oxygenation (ECMO) is that it provides time and more favorable conditions for recovery of lung function, provided the underlying pulmonary pathology is still reversible (Hill et al., 1971, 1972a, 1972b). ECMO ensures maintenance of adequate gas exchange by artificial means; at the same time, it is an effective method of circulatory support (see Support of the Failing Right Heart, Chapter 21), an important consideration in patients who have severe cardiopulmonary failure. Discussion of procedural details of ECMO employment is beyond the scope of this chapter; for a comprehensive treatment of the subject, the reader is referred to the reports of Hill et al. (1971, 1972a, 1972b) and those of Zapol et al. (1972, 1976).

REFERENCES

Andersen N B, Ghia J: Pulmonary function, cardiac status, and postoperative course in relation to cardiopulmonary bypass. J Thorac Cardiovasc Surg 59:474, 1970.

Awad J A, Lemieux J M, Lou W: Pulmonary complications following perfusion of the lungs. J Thorac Cardiovasc Surg 51:767, 1966.

Barter W D, Levine R S: An evaluation of intermittent positive pressure breathing in the prevention of postoperative pulmonary complications. Arch Surg 98:795, 1969.

Bates D V, Christie R V: Respiratory Function in Disease. Philadelphia, Saunders, 1964.

Bennett S H, Geelhoed G W, Aaron R K, Solis R T, Hoye R C: Pulmonary injury resulting from perfusion with stored bank blood in the baboon and dog. J Surg Res 13:295, 1972.

Bjure J, Liander B, Widimsky J: Effect of exercise on distribution of pulmonary blood flow in patients with mitral stenosis. Br Heart J 33:438, 1971.

Carlsten A, Norlander O, Widman B: Observations on the postoperative circulation. Surg Gynecol Obstet 99:227, 1954.

Carroll D, Cohn J E, Riley R L: Pulmonary function in mitral valvular disease: distribution and diffusion characteristics in resting patients. J Clin Invest 32:510, 1953.

Clarke A D, Jackson P W: Postoperative care of patients undergoing cardiopulmonary bypass. Br J Anaesth 43:248, 1971.

Connell R S, Page U S, Bartley T D, Bigelow J C, Webb M C: The effect on pulmonary ultrastructure of dacron-wool filtration during cardiopulmonary bypass. Ann Thorac Surg 15:217, 1973.

———, Swank R L: Pulmonary microembolism after blood transfusion: an electron microscopic study. Ann Surg 177:40, 1973.

Cooper J D, Grillo H C: The evolution of tracheal injury due to ventilatory assistance through cuffed tubes. A pathologic study. Ann Surg 169:334, 1969.

Cosby R S, Stowell E C Jr, Hartwig W R, Mayo M: Pulmonary function in left ventricular failure,

including cardiac asthma. Circulation 15:492, 1957.
Curti P C, Cohen G, Castleman B, Scannell J G, Friedlich A L, Myers G S: Respiratory and circulatory studies of patients with mitral stenosis. Circulation 8:893, 1953.
Daly W J, Giammona S T, Ross J C, Feigenbaum H: Effects of pulmonary vascular congestion on postural changes in the perfusion and filling of the pulmonary vascular bed. J Clin Invest 43:68, 1964.
———, Ross J C, Behnke R H: The effect of changes in pulmonary vascular bed produced by atropine, pulmonary engorgement and positive-pressure breathing on diffusion and mechanical properties of the lung. J Clin Invest 42:1083, 1963.
Dammann J F Jr, Thung N, Christlieb I I, Littlefield J B, Muller W H Jr: The management of the severely ill patient after open-heart surgery. J Thorac Cardiovasc Surg 45:80, 1963.
Dawson A, Kaneko D, McGregor M: Regional lung function in patients with mitral stenosis studied with xenon during air and oxygen breathing. J Clin Invest 44:999, 1965.
Deal C, Osborn J J, Muller G E Jr, Gerbode F: Pulmonary compliance in congenital heart disease and its relation to cardiopulmonary bypass. J Thorac Cardiovasc Surg 55:320, 1968.
Dodrill F: Effects of total body perfusion upon the lungs. In Allen J G (ed): Extracorporeal Circulation. Springfield, Ill, Thomas, 1958, p 327.
Dollery C T, West J B: Regional uptake of radioactive oxygen, carbon monoxide and carbon dioxide in patients with mitral stenosis. Circ Res 8:765, 1960.
Downes J J, Nicodemus H F, Pierce W S, Waldhausen J A: Acute respiratory failure in infants following cardiovascular surgery. J Thorac Cardiovasc Surg 59:21, 1970.
Edmunds, L H Jr, Austen W G: Effect of cardiopulmonary bypass on pulmonary volume-pressure relationships and vascular resistance. J Appl Physiol 21:209, 1966.
Ellison, L T, Duke J F, Ellison R G: Pulmonary compliance following open heart surgery and its relationship to ventilation and gas exchange. Circulation 35(Suppl): 217, 1967.
———, Yeh T J, Moretz W H, Ellison R G: Pulmonary diffusion studies in patients undergoing nonthoracic, thoracic and cardiopulmonary bypass procedures. Ann Surg 157:327, 1963.
Fordham R M M: Hypoxaemia after aortic valve surgery under cardiopulmonary bypass. Thorax 20:505, 1965.
Forsberg S A: Pulmonary blood volume in man. Acta Med Scand (Suppl) 410: 1, 1964.
Friedman W F, Braunwald E: Alterations in regional pulmonary blood flow in mitral valve disease studied by radio-isotope scanning: a simple nontraumatic technique for estimation of left atrial pressure. Circulation 34:363, 1966.
Garzon A A, Seltzer B, Karlson K E: Respiratory mechanics following open heart surgery for acquired valvular heart disease. Circulation 33(Suppl 1):57, 1966.
———, ———, Lightenstein S, Karlson K E: Influence of open-heart surgery on respiratory work. Dis Chest 52:392, 1967.
Gauert W B, Anderson D S, Reed W A, Templeton A W: Pulmonary complications following extracorporeal circulation. South Med J 64:679, 1971.
Gazetopoulos N, Davies H, Oliver C, Deuchar D: Ventilation and hemodynamics in heart disease. Br Heart J 28:1, 1966.
Geha A S, Sessler A D, Kirklin J W: Alveolar-arterial oxygen gradients after open intracardiac surgery. J Thorac Cardiovasc Surg 51:609, 1966.
Ghia J, Andersen N B: Pulmonary function and cardiopulmonary bypass. J A M A 212:593, 1970.
Giuntini C, Mariani M, Barsotti A, Fazio F, Santolicandro A M: Factors affecting regional pulmonary blood flow in left heart valvular disease. Am J Med 57:421, 1974.
Grillo H C: Tracheostomy and its complications. In Sabiston D C Jr (ed): Davis-Christopher Textbook of Surgery, 11th ed. Philadelphia, Saunders, 1977, pp 2056–2063.
———: Congenital lesions, neoplasms, and injuries of the trachea. In Sabiston D C Jr, Spencer F C (eds): Gibbon's Surgery of the Chest, 3rd ed. Philadelphia, Saunders, 1976, pp 256–293.
———: The management of tracheal stenosis following assisted respiration. J Thorac Cardiovasc Surg 57:52, 1969.
Hallowell P, Hedley-Whyte J, Austen W G, Laver M B: Oxygenation during closed mitral valvulotomy. J Thorac Cardiovasc Surg 50:42, 1965.
Hand B R, Malm J R, Bowman F O Jr, Sullivan S F: The effects of anesthesia and cardiac bypass on pulmonary compliance in man. Bull N Y Acad Med 46:22, 1970.
Harp J R, Wyche W Q, Marshall B E, Wurzel H A:

Some factors determining microaggregate formation in stored blood. Anesthesiology 40:398, 1974.
Hedley-Whyte J, Corning H, Laver M B, Austen W G, Bendixen H H: Pulmonary ventilation-perfusion relations after heart valve replacement or repair in man. J Clin Invest 44:406, 1965.
———, Winter P M: Oxygen therapy. Clin Pharmacol Ther 8:696, 1967.
Hepps S A, Roe B B, Wright R R, Gardner R E: Amelioration of the pulmonary post-perfusion syndrome with hemodilution and low molecular weight dextran. Surgery 54:232, 1963.
Hill J D, de Lanerolle P, Heiden D, Aguilar M J, Gerbode F: Protection from lung damage by blood filtration during deep hypothermia in puppies. J Thorac Cardiovasc Surg 70:133, 1975.
———, de Laval M R, Fallat R J, Bramson M L, Eberhart R C, Schulte H D, Osborn J J, Barber, R, Gerbode F: Acute respiratory insufficiency. Treatment with prolonged extracorporeal oxygenation. J Thorac Cardiovasc Surg 64:55, 1972b.
———, Fallat R, Cohn K, Eberhart R, Dontigny L, Bramson M L, Osborn J J, Gerbode F: Clinical cardiopulmonary dynamics during prolonged extracorporeal circulation for acute respiratory failure. Trans Am Soc Artif Intern Organs 17:355, 1971.
———, O'Brien T G, Murray J J, Dontigny L, Bramson M L, Osborn J J, Gerbode F: Prolonged extracorporeal oxygenation for acute post-traumatic respiratory failure (shock-lung syndrome). N Engl J Med 286:629, 1972a.
Hissen W, Swank R L: Screen filtration pressure and pulmonary hypertension. Am J Physiol 209:715, 1965.
Hollenberg M, Pruetts R, Thal A: Vasoactive substances liberated by prolonged bubble oxygenation. J Thorac Cardiovasc Surg 45:402, 1963.
Howatt W F, Talner N S, Sloan H, DeMuth G R: Pulmonary function changes following repair of heart lesions with the aid of extracorporeal circulation. J Thorac Cardiovasc Surg 43:649, 1962.
Jebavy P, Runczik I, Opelt A, Tilsch J, Stanek V, Widimsky J: Regional pulmonary function in patients with mitral stenosis in relation to hemodynamic data. Br Heart J 32:330, 1970.
Kaplan S L, Sullivan S F, Malm J R, Bowman F O Jr, Papper E M: Effect of cardiac bypass on pulmonary diffusing capacity. J Thorac Cardiovasc Surg 57:738, 1969.

Kirklin J W, McGreen D C, Patrick R T, Theye R A: What is adequate perfusion? In Allen J G (ed): Extracorporeal Circulation. Springfield, Ill, Charles C Thomas, 1958, p 132.
Kolff W F, Effler D B, Graves L K, Hughes C R, McCormack L J: Pulmonary complications of open heart operations: their pathogenesis and avoidance. Cleve Clin Q 25:65, 1958.
Laver M B, Hallowell P, Goldblatt A: Pulmonary dysfunction secondary to heart disease. Anesthesiology 33:161, 1970.
Lee W H Jr, Krumharr D, Fonkalsrud E W, Schjeide O A, Maloney J V Jr: Denaturation of plasma proteins as a cause of morbidity and death after intracardiac operation. Surgery 29:50, 1961.
Levine O R, Mellins R B, Fishman A P: Quantitative assessment of pulmonary edema. Circ Res 17:414, 1965.
Lindholm C E: Prolonged endotracheal intubation. Acta Anaesth Scand (Suppl)33:131, 1969.
Litwak R S, Slonim R, Wisoff B G, Gadboys H L: Homologous blood syndrome during extracorporeal circulation. N Engl J Med 268:1377, 1963.
Lucier E R, Angel J J: Changes in oxygen consumption at weaning after thoracotomy and after respiratory failure. Anesth Analg (Cleve) 53:93, 1974.
Mandelbaum I, Giammona S T: Extracorporeal circulation, pulmonary compliance and pulmonary surfactant. J Thorac Cardiovasc Surg 48:881, 1964.
Marshall R, McIlroy M B, Christie R V: The work of breathing in mitral stenosis. Clin Sci 13:137, 1954.
Martin F E, Stead W W: Physiologic studies following thoracic surgery. III. Ventilatory studies in the immediate postoperative period. J Thorac Surg 25:417, 1953.
Marty A T: Hyperoncotic albumin therapy. Surg Gynecol Obstet 139:105, 1974.
McClenahan J B, Young W E, Sykes M K: Respiratory changes after open heart surgery. Thorax 20:545, 1965.
McCredie M: Measurement of pulmonary edema in valvular heart disease. Circulation 36:381, 1967.
McNamara J J, Boatright D, Burran E L, Molot M D, Summers E, Stremple E F: Changes in some physical properties of stored blood. Ann Surg 174:58, 1971.
———, Burran E L, Larson E, Omiya G, Seuhiro G, Yamase H: Effect of debris in stored blood on pulmonary microvasculature. Ann Thorac Surg

14:133, 1972a.

———, ———, Suehiro G: Effective filtration of banked blood. Surgery 71:594, 1972b.

———, Molot M D, Stremple J F: Screen filtration pressure in combat casualties. Ann Surg 172:334, 1970.

Nahas R A, Melrose D G, Sykes M K, Robinson B: Post-perfusion lung syndrome: role of circulatory exclusion. Lancet 2:251, 1965.

Neville W E, Kontaxis A, Gavin T, Clowes G H A Jr: Postperfusion pulmonary vasculitis: its relationship to blood trauma. Arch Surg 86:126, 1963.

Norden I, Norlander O, Rodriguez R: Ventilatory and circulatory effects of anesthesia and cardiopulmonary bypass. Acta Anaesth Scand 14:297, 1970.

Panossian A, Hagstrom J W C, Nehlsen S, Veith F J: Secondary nature of surfactant changes in postperfusion pulmonary damage. J Thorac Cardiovasc Surg 57:628, 1969.

Parker F, Weiss S: The nature and significance of the structural changes in the lungs in mitral stenosis. Am J Pathol 12:573, 1936.

Peters R M, Wellons H A Jr, Htwe T M: Total compliance and work of breathing after thoracotomy. J Thorac Cardiovasc Surg 57:348, 1969.

Philbin D M, Sullivan S F, Bowman F D Jr, Malm J R, Papper E M: Postoperative hypoxemia: contribution of the cardiac output. Anesthesiology 32:136, 1970.

Provan J L, Austen W G, Scannell J G: Respiratory complications after open-heart surgery. J Thorac Cardiovasc Surg 51:626, 1966.

Radegran K: Circulatory and respiratory effects of induced platelet aggregation. An experimental study in dogs. Acta Chir Scand (Suppl) 420:1, 1971.

Ratliff N B, Young W G Jr, Hackel D B, Mikat E, Wilson J W: Pulmonary injury secondary to extracorporeal circulation: an ultrastructural study. J Thorac Cardiovasc Surg 65:425, 1973.

Reul G J Jr, Greenberg S D, Lefrak E A, McCollum W B, Beall A C Jr, Jordan G L Jr: Prevention of post-traumatic pulmonary insufficiency. Fine screen filtration of blood. Arch Surg 106:386, 1973.

Rhodes E L, Kirsh M M, Howatt W, O'Rourke P T, Straker J, Sloan H: A comparison of pulmonary function in puppies undergoing total cardiopulmonary bypass with bubble or membrane oxygenators. J Thorac Cardiovasc Surg 68:658, 1974.

Saunders K B: Physiological dead space in left ventricular failure. Clin Sci 31:145, 1966.

———: Alveolar-arterial gradient for oxygen in heart failure. Lancet 2:160, 1965.

Schramel R, Schmidt F, Davis F, Palmisano D, Creech O Jr: Pulmonary lesions produced by prolonged partial perfusion. Surgery 54:224, 1963.

Sharp J T, Griffith G T, Bunnell I L, Greene D G: Ventilatory mechanics in pulmonary edema in man. J Clin Invest 37:111, 1958.

Shields R T Jr: Pathogenesis of postoperative pulmonary atelectasis. Experimental study. Arch Surg 58:489, 1949.

Sladen A, Laver M B, Pontoppidan H: Pulmonary complications and water retention in prolonged mechanical ventilation. N Engl J Med 279:448, 1968.

Sobonya R E, Kleinerman J, Primiano F, Chester E H: Pulmonary changes in cardiopulmonary bypass. Chest 61:154, 1972.

Soeter J R, Mamiya R T, Sprague A Y, McNamara J J: Prolonged extracorporeal oxygenation for cardiorespiratory failure after tetralogy correction. J Thorac Cardiovasc Surg 66:214, 1973.

Solis R T, Gibbs M B: Filtration of microaggregates in stored blood. Tranfusion 12:245, 1972.

Stanger P, Lucas R V Jr, Edwards J E: Anatomic factors causing respiratory distress in acyanotic congenital cardiac dieseas. Special reference to bronchial obstruction. Pediatrics 43:760, 1969.

Sullivan S F, Patterson R W, Malm J R, Bowman F O Jr, Papper E M: Effect of heart-lung bypass on the mechanics of breathing in man. J Thorac Cardiovasc Surg 51:205, 1966.

Suwa K, Hedley-Whyte J, Bendixen H H: Circulation and physiologic deadspace changes on controlling the ventilation of dogs. J Appl Physiol 21:1855, 1966.

Swank R L: Alteration of blood on storage: measurement of adhesiveness of "aging" platelets and leukocytes and their removal by filtration. N Engl J Med 265: 728, 1961.

Tarhan S, Moffitt E A, Sessler A D, Douglas W, Taylor W F: Risk of anesthesia and surgery in patients with chronic bronchitis and chronic obstructive lung disease. Surgery 74: 720, 1973.

Templeton A W, Almond C H, Seaber A, Simmons C, MacKenzie J: Postoperative pulmonary patterns following cardiopulmonary bypass. Am J Roentgen 96:1007, 1966.

Tilney N L, Hester W J: Physiologic and histologic changes in the lungs of patients dying after prolonged cardiopulmonary bypass: an inquiry into the nature of post-perfusion lung. Ann Surg 166:759, 1967.

Trichet B, Falke K, Togut A, Laver M B: The effect

of pre-existing pulmonary vascular disease on the response to mechanical ventilation with PEEP following open-heart surgery. Anesthesiology 42:56, 1975.

Turnbull K W, Miyagishima R T, Gerein A N: Pulmonary complications and cardiopulmonary bypass. Can Anaesth Soc J 21:181, 1974.

Veith F J, Hagstrom J W C, Panossian A, Nehlsen S L, Wilson J W: Pulmonary microcirculatory response to shock, transfusion, and pump-oxygenator procedures: a unified mechanism underlying pulmonary damage. Surgery 64:95, 1968.

Wilson R S, Sullivan S F, Malm J R, Bowman F O Jr: The oxygen cost of breathing following anesthesia and cardiac surgery. Anesthesiology 39:387, 1973.

Winter P M, Smith G: The toxicity of oxygen. Anesthesiology 29:210, 1972.

Wolfe W G, Ebert P A, Sabiston D C Jr: Effect of high oxygen tensions on mucociliary function. Surgery 72:246, 1972.

Yu P N: Pulmonary Blood Volume in Health and Disease. Philadelphia, Lea and Febiger, 1969.

———, Murphy G W, Schreiner B F Jr, James D H: Distensibility characteristics of the human pulmonary vascular bed. Study of the pressure-volume responses to exercise in patients with and without heart disease. Circulation 35:710, 1967.

Zapol W M, Pontoppidan H, McCullough N, Schmidt V, Bland J, Kitz K J: Clinical membrane lung support for acute respiratory insufficiency. Trans Am Soc Artif Intern Organs 18:553, 1972.

———, Schneider R, Snider M, Rie M: Partial bypass with membrane lungs for acute respiratory failure. Int Anesthesiol Clin 14 (1):119, 1976.

Zwillich C W, Pierson D J, Creagh C E, Sutton F D, Schatz E, Petty T L: Complications of assisted ventilation: a prospective study of 354 consecutive episodes. Am J Med 57:161, 1974.

14. Renal Failure In Cardiac Surgery

SHELDON GLABMAN   BEAT VON ALBERTINI
ROBERT S. LITWAK

Acute renal failure (ARF) after open intracardiac surgery is fortunately an infrequent complication. When it does occur the prognosis is poor, with 65 to 90 percent of the patients succumbing (Abel et al., 1974a, 1976; Bhat et al., 1976; Hilberman et al., 1979). Although many factors contribute to the development of ARF after open heart surgery, by far the single most important one is persistent low cardiac output and its accompanying reduction in renal blood flow.

Although life-threatening ARF is uncommon, evidence of transient renal dysfunction is not. A slight elevation of both blood urea nitrogen (BUN) and serum creatinine levels is not infrequently observed soon after open heart surgery (OHS) in patients who did not manifest any clinical signs of abnormal renal function before the operation. If cardiac output is adequate postoperatively, these alterations quickly return to normal levels.

It is beyond the scope of this discussion to explore the complex and still incompletely understood pathophysiologic mechanisms believed to be etiologic to the development of ARF. No single mechanism has as yet been able to convincingly account for the wide spectrum of clinical phenomena and biochemical alterations encountered in ARF. For a lucid review of these matters the reader is referred to Schrier (1981).

FACTORS CONTRIBUTING TO THE DEVELOPMENT OF ACUTE RENAL FAILURE (ARF) AFTER CARDIAC SURGERY

Preoperative Factors

There is a much higher incidence of ARF in patients coming to surgery with *advanced cardiac dysfunction* (Hilberman et al., 1979, 1980), since the probability of postoperative low cardiac output in this group is higher than for those with adequate preoperative performance. Moreover, those with advanced cardiac dysfunction frequently will have required vigorous and prolonged preoperative diuretic therapy resulting in extracellular fluid and salt depletion, factors that tend to further reduce renal blood flow.

It has long been established that *intrinsic renal disease* also is associated with an increased risk of worsening renal function. In one series, more than 90 percent of patients who succumbed from renal failure after major surgical procedures had postmortem evidence of preexisting renal disease (Sawyer et al., 1963). Because the situation is compounded by *advanced age*, it is not surprising that Abel et al. (1974b) observed a higher incidence of significant renal dysfunction after OHS in an older subgroup of patients and those who came to surgery with substantially higher preoperative serum values of both BUN and creatinine.

Operative and Postrepair Events

The Operation. Measurable alteration of renal function is an inescapable component of the surgical experience, which, after all, is controlled trauma. Fluid restriction, surgical dissection, and hypovolemia all compromise renal perfusion, thereby curtailing the kidney's ability to excrete a water load. Additionally, anesthetic induction may be accompanied by a significant fall in cardiac output (and therefore renal blood flow), particularly in patients with advanced cardiac dysfunction. These factors, which attend all major operations, are particularly important when cardiac patients are subjected to surgery and result in a reduced functional capacity of the kidney to effectively clear nitrogen and other metabolic byproducts.

Cardiopulmonary Bypass. Although present methods of *cardiopulmonary bypass* (CPBP) are remarkably safe, the evidence is incontrovertible that renal function is compromised to some degree by whole body perfusion. This is not surprising, since so many of the physiologic patterns of normal people are distorted by CPBP. Man, a homoiotherm, is accustomed to a temperature of 37.5C, a resting cardiac index of 3 liters/min/m^2, a mean arterial pressure approximating 100 mm Hg, and pulsatile blood flow. CPBP, as conducted in most centers, violates virtually every one of these biologic desiderata. Perfusion hypothermia commonly is induced and flow rates considered to be "high" (2.2 to 2.4 liters/min/m^2) are still lower than that in the normal resting person. Perfusion pressure is usually substantially lower and pulsatile flow is still not widely employed. Absence of pulsatile flow has been shown to adversely affect renal performance, primarily by increasing renal vascular resistance (Mandelbaum and Burns, 1965; Jacobs et al., 1969) and thus decreasing total renal function. Clinical and experimental evidence suggests that the reduction in renal blood flow tends to worsen with prolonged perfusion times and that this decrease is accompanied by intrarenal shunting of blood away from the cortex of the medulla (Porter et al., 1966; Engelman et al., 1974). During perfusion, glomerular filtration is reduced and the renal tubular concentrating mechanism altered (Porter et al., 1966; Kahn et al., 1968). Other adverse influences during perfusion include excessive hemolysis, persistent acidemia, and platelet-fibrin microemboli (Ashmore et al., 1968). Rarely, macroemboli consequent to removal of calcific valves lodge in the renal vasculature.

Low Cardiac Output. In most cases, the alterations in renal performance imposed by cardiopulmonary bypass tend to be reversible and are therefore clinically tolerable. The *added insult of other factors,* together with perfusion trauma, tips the balance toward the onset of life-threatening renal dysfunction. Despite optimal perfusion conduct and precise operative repair, patients coming to surgery with severe cardiac dysfunction almost invariably have lower postrepair levels of cardiac output than patients with less preoperative cardiac disability. At the very least, after completion of the repair a patient with poor or marginal cardiac performance almost always requires a prolonged supplemental period of circulatory support with the pump-oxygenator. Additionally, positive inotropic agents and other interventions often must be employed before some measure of acceptable hemodynamic stability is attained. Hence, it is not surprising that prolonged periods of perfusion, aortic cross-clamping, and the duration of the operation correlate well with the development of ARF (Abel et al., 1976, Hilberman et al., 1979). On the other hand, employment of hypothermia, low perfusion pressure, and reduced flow rates have not been found to be of major clinical importance in the development of ARF (Abel et al., 1976; Hilberman et al., 1979). These factors suggest the kidney's remarkable ability to adjust to alterations in blood flow, i.e., autoregulation.

PATTERNS OF RENAL FAILURE AFTER CARDIAC SURGERY

Previous discussion has stressed the dominant role of the postrepair hemodynamic state in determining the adequacy of renal performance after OHS. In the presence of low cardiac output and the resultant renal ischemia, two patterns of deranged renal function are identifiable, each with a different pathophysiologic course and prognosis (Table 14–1).

THREATENED ACUTE RENAL FAILURE

These are patients who, while exhibiting marked depression of cardiac performance soon after OHS, subsequently manifest significant and progressive hemodynamic improvement. At the height of dysfunction, glomerular filtration rate (GFR) is still sufficiently adequate to keep extracellular fluid composition approximately normal. Azotemia tends to be only moderate, with the BUN rising out of proportion to the serum creatinine. The former is generally less than 70 mg/dl while the creatinine usually does not exceed 2.5 mg/dl.

Tubular function, while compromised, is sufficiently intact to reabsorb an increased quantity of water and sodium. As a consequence, the urinary sodium (U_{Na}) is low (≤20 mEq/liter) and the urine osmolality (U_{osm}) remains higher than plasma (P_{osm}) with a $U_{osm}:P_{osm}$ ratio ≥ 1.5 and a specific gravity ≥ 1.015. Nitrogenous wastes are concentrated in the urine because of the increased tubular reabsorption. As a result, the urine:plasma ratio for both creatinine and urea is usually greater than 30:1.

In some instances values for U_{Na} and the $U_{osm}:P_{osm}$ ratio fall into an indefinite zone. Derived indices often are helpful in separating the threatened ARF group from those who are in frank ARF, particularly the *Renal Failure Index* (urine sodium ÷ urine:plasma creatinine ratio) and the *fractional excretion of sodium* (urine:plasma sodium ratio ÷ urine:plasma creatinine ratio × 100). Values less than 1.0 for both indices are indicative of ischemia with relatively intact tubular function. Values greater than 1 percent for both are suggestive of the development of life-threatening ARF.

Characteristically, in the threatened ARF group, improved cardiac performance is par-

TABLE 14–1 URINARY INDICES*

Measurement	Threatened ARF	Established ARF
Urinary Sodium (U_{Na})	≤ 20 mEq/liter	> 40 mEq/liter
Urine:Plasma Osmolality	$U_{osm} > P_{osm}$ (ratio ≥ 1.5)	$U_{osm} = P_{osm}$
Relationship between BUN and Creatinine Elevation	BUN rises out of proportion to creatinine (ratio usually > 10:1)	BUN rise proportionate to creatinine elevation (ratio 10:1)
Urine: Plasman Creatinine Ratio (U/P) Cr	≥ 30:1	< 20:1
Renal Failure Index (U_{Na} ÷ U/P Cr)	< 1	> 1
Fractional Excretion of Sodium	< 1	> 1

*Adapted from Schrier (1981).

alleled by a gradual return to preoperative levels of renal function within a few days. As would be anticipated, mortality is low.

ESTABLISHED ACUTE RENAL FAILURE

These patients characteristically fail to demonstrate any significant improvement in the sharply reduced postrepair cardiac output in the early days after the operation. Despite aggressive supportive therapy, ventricular filling pressures remain high and the cardiac index is consistently low ($\leq$ 1.9 liters/min/m^2). Hence, renal performance is severely compromised and mortality is high.

Oliguric and Nonoliguric ARF

While oliguria (< 15 ml/hr/m^2) is typically identified with frank ARF, it is important to appreciate that nonoliguric ARF (with urine volumes in adults reaching as high as 85 ml/hr) occurs more often than is generally appreciated. Nonoliguric ARF has a lower but still substantial mortality (26 percent) in comparison to oliguric ARF (65 percent) in surgical patients (Anderson et al., 1977).

Pathophysiology and Clinical Patterns. Tubular function is severely impaired and GFR reduced as well. The sharply reduced concentrating capacity of the damaged tubules results in an isosmolar relationship between plasma and urine. Additionally, the osmolality of the urine approximates that of plasma. The daily nitrogen load cannot be adequately eliminated (even in the nonoliguric cases) and a positive nitrogen balance with progressive azotemia is observed. Unlike the threatened ARF group, there is a commensurate elevation of BUN with creatinine (approximately 10:1). Typically, the urine:plasma creatinine ratio is less than 20:1 and the urinary concentration of sodium is high (tending to exceed 40 mEq/liter).

The magnitude of blood chemistry alterations is influenced by both the type of established ARF (i.e., whether oliguric or nonoliguric) and the postsurgical catabolic state. Oliguric patients generally excrete less water, electrolytes, and nitrogenous wastes in the urine and, as a rule, manifest more severe blood chemistry abnormalities than the nonoliguric cases. The postsurgical catabolic state further aggravates the renal problem, since the BUN and serum creatinine rise sharply, with daily increments as high as 50 mg/dl and 2 mg/dl, respectively, in oliguric patients. Frequently, hyponatremia can occur, the consequence of excessive administration of water in a patient no longer capable of handling such a fluid volume. Since the kidney can no longer eliminate the quantity of organic acid daily produced by the body (approximately 1 mEq/kg), the plasma bicarbonate falls and metabloic acidosis is observed. Inability of the kidney to excrete potassium adequately results in hyperkalemia, which adversely affects myocardial and striated muscle function when it exceeds 6.5 mEq/liter.

If the patient survives the oliguric phase, it may be followed by a polyuric or diuretic phase, which may occur as early as the seventh day or as late as six weeks after the onset of ARF. The characteristics of the urine remain as they were during the oliguric phase, i.e., with high sodium concentrations and isotonic to the serum, with the exception that more potassium appears in the urine. The polyuric phenomenon is best explained by the recruitment of more nephrons in the presence of a high osmotic load, but with damaged tubules still unable to properly reabsorb sodium. In well-dialyzed patients the polyuric phase may be minimal.

A characteristic of this type of ARF is that the onset of diuresis does not lead to immediate amelioration of the biochemical or clinical picture of uremia, since the BUN may continue to rise for several days. It is not until the urine output exceeds 2 to 3 liters a day that clinical and biochemical improvement occur. The diuretic stage is difficult to manage because of the magnitude of electrolyte and fluid losses. Many patients who succumb to uremia, sepsis, and bleeding do so in the diuretic phase.

Patients who survive ARF will ultimately experience restoration of renal function to precardiac surgical levels. However, polyuria and failure to conserve sodium appropriately may persist for many months following recovery.

Complications of ARF

The combination of continued low cardiac output and ARF adversely affects the functioning of virtually every subsystem. The prognosis is dismal despite dialysis, death almost always resulting from multiple subsystem failure.

In the postoperative cardiac surgical patient, *cardiovascular manifestations* commonly include hypotension and arrhythmias, the latter most often caused by the effects of hyperkalemia on a poorly contractile heart that is being supported by aggressive digitalis glycoside and other drug therapy. Electrocardiographic changes accompanying the development of significant hyperkalemia include the onset of tall, peaked T waves, widening QRS complexes and a variety of dysrhythmias (Fig. 14–1). *Pulmonary dysfunction* can be severe, in part due to elevated pulmonary venous pressures and generalized fluid retention. *Neurologic abnormalities* commonly are observed, including somnolence, muscle twitching, tetany (in part related to hyperphosphatemia and hypocalcemia), and even generalized seizures, which can be seen in advanced cases.

The *hematologic subsystem* is severely deranged. Anemia, an inevitable postperfusion event, is further exaggerated by ARF. Thrombocytopenia and qualitative defects in platelet function are observed. *Hepatic dysfunction,* often already present because of the cardiac dysfunction, worsens, and can be accompanied by measurable reduction in the level of various clotting factors. Hence, hemostatic conditions are highly abnormal and gastrointestinal bleeding is frequent in these patients. Finally, the *resistance to infection* is severely impaired. Lethal arrhythmias and infection are the two most common causes of death in postoperative cardiac patients suffering ARF.

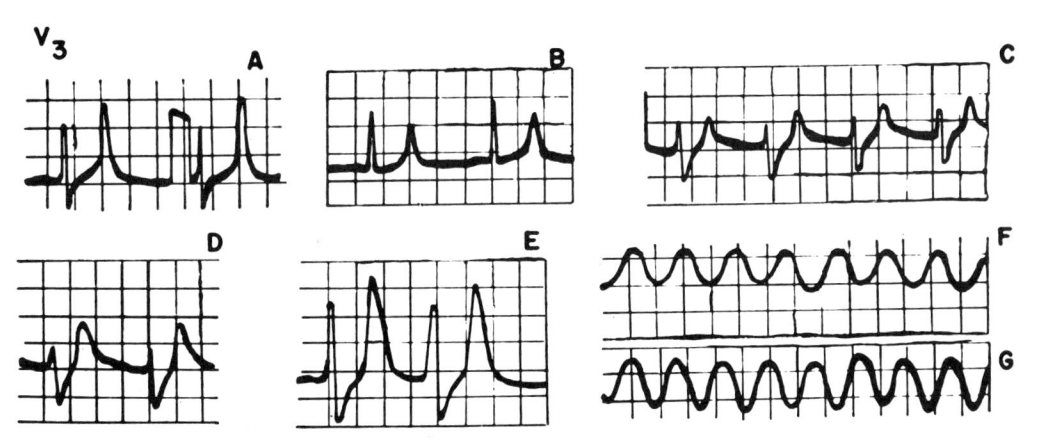

Figure 14–1. Representative electrocardiograms (ECG) in potassium intoxication. Early changes include the development of tall, peaked T waves while the P and R waves tend to decrease in height **(A** and **B).** As intoxication progresses, the P wave increases in duration while its amplitude decreases. The P-R interval becomes prolonged and the QRS complex begins to widen **(C).** Later, the Q-T interval lengthens and the P wave either disappears or becomes engulfed in the preceding T wave **(D).** With progressive worsening of intoxication, the QRS complex continues to widen **(E).** Terminally, the ECG is compatible with ventricular tachycardia **(F** and **G),** which usually proceeds to lethal ventricular fibrillation. *(Reproduced with permission from Merrill, J P, The Treatment of Renal Failure. 2nd ed. New York and London: Grune & Stratton, 1965.)*

MANAGEMENT OF THREATENED OR ESTABLISHED ACUTE RENAL FAILURE

Threatened Acute Renal Failure

The Cardiovascular Subsystem. Unless a satisfactory level of systemic blood flow is maintained after cardiac surgery, the onset of ARF is an absolute certainty. Hence, the sine qua non of management centers on measures employed to optimize performance of the cardiovascular subsystem. As detailed in Chapter 9, for patients with marginal or low cardiac output this requires a systematic approach involving not only the usual continuous monitoring of intracardiac and great vessel pressures but also sequential quantitation of systemic blood flow and appropriate supportive interventions.

When positive inotropic agents are employed, it is important that α-adrenergic drugs (which are systemic vasoconstrictors) should be avoided, since they decrease renal perfusion despite elevation of systemic arterial pressure. Of the currently available therapeutic agents, dopamine is probably the safest to use in threatened or established ARF. In addition to its positive inotropic effect, dopamine has a low dosage renal vasodilator effect (Goldberg, 1974). The drug may be administered in doses between 5 and 10 μg/kg/min without fear of worsening the renal failure.

Diuretics. The efficacy of mannitol and furosemide in preventing or ameliorating the severity of ARF is controversial. In part, these agents promote diuresis by decreasing tubular reabsorption of salt and water and thereby increase intratubular pressure. This may protect the tubules from collapse and obstruction with cellular debris. Additionally, both drugs dilate renal afferent arterioles and thus reduce vasoconstriction, an event believed to be of major importance in the development of ARF.* In this regard, it is noteworthy that studies of dogs have shown that furosemide significantly increases renal blood flow and reduces cortical ischemia after CPBP (Engleman et al., 1974).

A few clinical reports have suggested that both mannitol and furosemide can convert the highly lethal oliguric ARF to the more favorable nonoliguric form (Cantarovich et al., 1971). However, such a positive response has not been observed by others (Fries et al., 1971). Our own experience in a cardiac surgical setting suggests that the patients who do respond favorably to diuretics probably have had less renal impairment to begin with. Despite the experimental and occasional clinical reports suggesting beneficial effects, there is no convincing clinical information supporting the contention that diuretic agents can abort threatened ARF or reduce its severity in postoperative cardiac surgical patients (Abel et al., 1976).

Although the unresolved questions about the usefulness of diuretic therapy in ARF await clarification, there is general agreement that higher urine flows are certainly preferable in threatened ARF. When, despite optimized performance of the cardiovascular subsystem, oliguria and the urinary indices suggest threatened ARF, a trial of intravenous furosemide (2 mg/kg) is employed to promote a diuresis. This dosage may be repeated hourly for 4 to 6 doses. If effective, the urine output will increase and will be dilute and salt rich. It could be argued that such urinary findings are not necessarily diagnostic of tubular damage, since furosemide is a loop diuretic that interferes with tubular concentrating mechanisms. However, in a postoperative open heart surgical patient with threatened ARF, these observations must assume the presence of a tubular defect.

ESTABLISHED ACUTE RENAL FAILURE

Once a diagnosis has been made of established ARF, a detailed protocol involving surveillance and therapy is essential if there is to

---

See Patak et al. (1979), Burke et al. (1980), and Schrier (1981) for comprehensive discussions of the actions of mannitol and furosemide in ARF.

be any chance of recovery from this frequently lethal complication.

Optimizing Performance of Cardiovascular and Pulmonary Subsystems

Without adequate cardiorespiratory function, recovery from ARF will be impossible. Chapters 9 and 12 detail concepts and methods employed in seeking to optimize performance of these two vital subsystems. To achieve this it frequently will be necessary to employ prolonged ventilatory support as well as some type of mechanical circulatory support. These supportive interventions must be guided by sequential quantitation of systemic blood flow (in addition to the usual continuous determination of cardiac rate, rhythm, preload, and afterload) and assessment of hematocrit, acid-base, and blood-gas data every 6 to 8 hours.

Body Weight and Other Assessments

Because of the heightened potential for fluid overloading and pulmonary edema in ARF, intake and output of all fluids is recorded for each eight-hour shift. While accurate weighing can be difficult in a postoperative cardiac surgical patient because of the many tubes and other attachments, daily calculation of weight gain or loss is exceedingly helpful in guiding therapy. Body weight should decrease by 0.2 to 0.5 kg/day because of tissue catabolism.

Determination is made every 12 hours of serum electrolytes (sodium, potassium, chloride), BUN, creatinine, calcium, and phosphorus.

In addition to output, other urinary measurements of importance that should be obtained daily include osmolality, sodium, and creatinine. The data will allow derivation of the urinary indices (previously discussed) that provide insight into the nature and severity of the ARF.

Fluid and Cation Management

In the usual postoperative cardiac surgical patient in incipient or established ARF, the need to maximize cardiac preload presents a therapeutic dilemma. While it is essential to exploit the Frank-Starling relationship as much as possible and also to infuse cardiotonic and vasoactive drugs, these are precisely the interventions that acutely and dangerously expand all fluid compartments.

To the extent that it is possible, the daily crystalloid fluid intake is restricted to a volume equalling the urinary output, any extrarenal loss (such as from nasogastric suction), and insensible loss (estimated to be approximately 350 to 500 ml/day in the average euthermic adult). Fever, of course, significantly increases insensible loss. Additional volume (either blood or plasma) is given cautiously to replace blood loss or to increase preload.

In *oliguric ARF* it is satisfactory to initiate volume repletion with dilute salt solutions. The serum sodium concentration can be helpful in determining whether water and solute intake are appropriate (a decreased serum sodium would suggest an excess of water administration, and an elevated serum sodium a deficit in water intake).

Because of its diminished urinary excretion in oliguric ARF, potassium obviously is not administered unless a rare and specific indication clearly is apparent. When serious hyperkalemia exists (> 6.5 mEq/liter), the only efficient and predictable means of lowering this cation is prompt dialysis. Under different clinical circumstances (specifically in an ARF patient who can be given oral medication), the administration of a potassium binding resin such as sodium polystyrene sulfonate (Kayexalate) could be helpful. However, in a postoperative open heart surgery patient in ARF, the need to deliver the drug via the rectal route, its limited effectiveness, and the heightened potential for infection (i.e., the possible contact of loose stool material with intravascular lines) make the use of this agent inadvisable.

In circumstances where the electrocardiogram indicates a life-threatening situation due to hyperkalemia, cardiac toxicity can be transiently lessened with the administration of increments of 10 percent calcium chloride intravenously. While it can momentarily stabilize the clinical state, it is important to appreciate that the drug does nothing to lower the elevated serum potassium concentration.

Hypertonic glucose in combination with insulin temporarily shifts potassium from the extracellular to the intracellular space so that the serum level of potassium falls. In the adult, 50 grams of 50 percent glucose are administered with 15 units of regular insulin. This can be repeated every 15 to 30 minutes until other measures (i.e., dialysis) can be instituted. In acidotic patients, concomitant use of intravenous sodium bicarbonate (50 mEq) is also helpful in reducing serum potassium by causing it to shift intracellularly. The buffer must be used cautiously in oliguric postoperative cardiac surgical ARF because of its effect on volume loading. While these therapeutic measures are capable of transiently lowering the serum potassium concentration, they have no effect on total body potassium stores. This can only be accomplished by dialysis.

In *nonoliguric ARF*, primary concerns center on appropriate volume and cation repletion. Electrolyte losses can be considerable and it is important that frequent assessment be made of both serum and urinary cations so that proper replacement therapy can be designed. It must be borne in mind that inadquate volume or electrolyte repletion can convert nonoliguric ARF into oliguric ARF.

Dialysis

Replacement of renal excretory function by dialysis remains the most effective therapy for any form of advanced renal failure. Although the role of "prophylactic" dialysis is controversial, there is a growing consensus in support of this approach. The goal would be to avoid the complications of uremia with early dialysis rather than be forced to treat them (Schrier, 1981). In this regard, Gailiunas et al. (1980) specifically attribute the lowered mortality of ARF after cardiac operations to early institution of dialysis.

Immediate *indications for dialysis* are: (1) prevention of the manifestations of uremia (neurologic disturbances, gastrointestinal bleeding, etc.); (2) refractory hyperkalemia; (3) severe metabolic acidosis; and (4) fluid overload.

Peritoneal dialysis is best avoided in the postoperative open heart surgical patient because of the inherent risk of infection and the ventilatory compromise accompanying a fluid-filled distended abdominal cavity.

Hemodialysis is preferable because of its effectiveness, which allows reversal of acute complications of renal failure within a short time. In elective circumstances it is performed through an arteriovenous shunt in an extremity. In emergencies, blood can be drawn from a catheter in the femoral vein and returned to a peripheral vein.

Hemodialysis is not always well-tolerated, particularly in a patient with compromised cardiovascular function. The rapid lowering of plasma potassium levels can result in fatal arrhythmias. Effective fluid removal is often limited by the occurrence of hypotension and other symptoms of intravascular volume depletion. Rapid changes in plasma osmolality (mainly because of the rapid removal of urea) may result in a host of neurologic symptoms (Wakim, 1969). Hypoxemia often is noted during dialysis and may be related to ventilatory changes induced by rapid alterations in the acid-base status (von Albertini et al., 1976).

For the reasons just cited, hemodialysis must be carried out extremely carefully in postoperative cardiac surgical patients. We have found the following management details helpful. The dialysate is prepared with a potassium concentration no lower than 3.5 mEq/liter. The dialyzer (a noncompliant, low priming volume unit) can be filled with crystalloid or colloid, depending on the specific requirements of the patient. Immediately before the start of dialysis, a 50-mg bolus of lidocaine is given intravenously. During dialysis, lidocaine administration is continued at a rate of 1 to 2 mg/min and tapered off after dialysis over a three-hour period.

To minimize hypotension, blood flow rates to the dialyzer should not exceed 150 ml/min for the first 30 minutes. Additionally, ultrafiltration rates should be kept low, especially at the beginning of dialysis. Despite these precautions, it may be necessary to administer small increments of pressors (such as dopamine) to maintain hemodynamic stability. Hemodialysis is performed daily for 2 to 3 hours, with the goal of keeping the BUN below 100 mg/dl and the serum creatinine below 7 mg/dl. During the hemodialysis, cardiovascular variables are continuously observed. The acid-base state and blood chemistries are checked each hour.

In patients with severe volume overload, fluid removal can be carried out by ultrafiltration. It has been found that fluid removal is better tolerated if ultrafiltration is done separately from regular dialysis. (Bergström et al., 1976). During the ultrafiltration, the parallel flow dialyzer is disconnected from the dialysate delivery system and a negative pressure created inside the empty dialysate compartment of the dialyzer by connecting it to a vacuum source. With large enough transmembrane pressure gradients, high ultrafiltration rates can be achieved. Using this method, substantial volumes of fluid can be removed with relatively little evidence of intravascular volume depletion. Presumably, the increased oncontic pressure of the hemoconcentrated blood facilitates movement of interstitial fluid, thereby maintaining intravascular volume to a greater extent so that the hemodynamic status of the patient remains relatively stable. By contrast, the fall in plasma osmolality that occurs during regular hemodialysis (mainly because of the rapid diffusion of urea to the dialysate) may render patients more volume-depleted and hypotensive. The explanation, however, remains unsettled.

Current methodology of hemodialysis still requires administration of some heparin. Even when minimal amounts are used and protamine sulfate subsequently employed to neutralize the heparin, various reports indicate that a significant percentage of the patients (as high as 19 percent) have experienced hemorrhagic complications (Lazarus, 1981). Therefore, the recent report of uneventful hemodialysis without heparin (Zusman et al., 1981) may prove to be a major advance. These investigators used prostacyclin as the sole antithrombotic agent during hemodialysis. No hemorrhagic complications were experienced (despite the fact that one postoperative cardiac surgical patient in ARF had bled massively during prior hemodialyses with heparin) nor was clotting within the dialysis coils observed.

Additional Measures

Nutritional support with delivery of adequate calories (3,000 per day) is essential to minimize catabolic breakdown of proteins. Since oral intake is almost never feasible in the type of patient under consideration, nutrition must be provided by parenteral means. Faster recovery and improved survival have resulted from use of a specific renal failure hyperalimentation solution containing essential l-amino acids and hypertonic glucose (Abel et al., 1973, 1974a).

Modification of drug prescriptions is necessary. Agents that are nephrotoxic per se or those that are primarily excreted by the kidney (certain antibiotics, cardiac glycosides, etc.) should ideally be replaced with drugs that are excreted along other routes (not always possible) or have their dosage reduced and the intervals between their administration extended. Whenever feasible, serum levels of drugs should be performed at regular intervals. For detailed information about dosage and dialyzability of commonly used drugs in renal failure, the reader is referred to Bennett et al. (1974) and Anderson et al. (1976).

Since *infection* and *gastrointestinal hemorrhage* are common causes of death in ARF, measures must be taken to minimize the potential for these two dreaded complications to occur. Systemic antimicrobial agents are selected and administered in doses appropriate for ARF patients. Meticulous management of tracheobronchial aspiration combined with careful aseptic cleansing and redressing of all areas where drainage tubes exit or vascular lines are in place is essential. Although it has not been documented that cimetidine (given at half the usual dose) can prevent gastrointestinal bleeding, it would seem reasonable to empirically use this drug in these high risk patients.

OPEN HEART SURGERY IN A DIALYSIS-DEPENDENT PATIENT

The presence of nearly 50,000 chronic hemodialysis patients throughout the United States has necessitated resorting to cardiovascular surgery in some of them. They usually need such surgery because of either accelerated angina or severe congestive heart failure following infective endocarditis. Although it formerly had been thought that "anephric" patients could neither tolerate nor benefit from OHS, favorable experience in the past decade has documented that such pessimism is unwarranted (Lansing et al., 1968; Connors and Shaw, 1978;* Monson et al., 1980).

Preoperative Measures
Hemodialysis is performed within 12 hours of surgery to reduce total body and serum potassium levels and partially correct hemostatic derangements so commonly present in patients with chronic renal failure. Packed red cells are infused during dialysis if the hematocrit is less than 30.

The Operation
Fluid volumes (devoid of potassium) administered intravenously are kept to a minimum. The *priming perfusate* is designed with appreciation of the facts that (1) diuresis is not possible and (2) anemia commonly exists in these patients. Therefore, only limited hemodilution is employed. The prime is adjusted to achieve a desired mixed hematocrit† of 25 and consists of both fresh blood (to minimize the potassium load) and a crystalloid solution that does not contain potassium.

---

*Contains summary of worldwide published experience up to the date of publication.
†See Chapter 5 for details.

At the termination of perfusion, only limited infusion of perfusate volume is carried out to keep ventricular filling pressures as low as is consistent with satisfactory cardiovascular stability. Perfusate remaining in the heart-lung machine is centrifuged and the packed red cells slowly administered to the patient to ensure a hematocrit of 30.

Postoperative Measures
All of the procedures previously detailed in managing established ARF are employed. Although hemodialysis and ultrafiltration can be performed soon after the operation if volume overload or sharply elevated levels of BUN or potassium require it, delay of the procedure for 24 hours is usually possible and desirable to minimize the possibility of excessive bleeding. Regional rather than systemic heparinization is employed for the first postoperative week. Patients who are ordinarily dialyzed three times a week may require the procedure daily during the early postoperative period.

REFERENCES

Abel R M, Abbott W M, Beck C H Jr, Ryan J A, Fisher J E: Essential l-amino acids for hyperalimentation in patients with disordered nitrogen metabolism. Am J Surg 128:317, 1974a.

————, Beck C H Jr, Abbott W M, Ryan J A Jr, Barnett G O, Fischer J E: Improved survival from acute renal failure after treatment with intravenous essential l-amino acids and glucose: results of a prospective double-blind study. N Eng J Med 288:695, 1973.

————, Buckley M J, Austen W G, Barnett G O, Beck G H, Fischer J E: Etiology, incidence, and prognosis of renal failure following cardiac operations. J Thorac Cardiovasc Surg 71:323, 1976.

————, Wick J, Beck C H Jr, Buckley M J, Austen W G: Renal dysfunction following open heart operations. Arch Surg 108:175, 1974b.

Anderson R J, Gambertoglio J G, Schrier R W: Clinical Use of Drugs in Renal Failure. Springfield, Ill, Thomas, 1976.

————, Linas S L, Berns A S, Henrich W L, Miller T R, Gabow P A, Schrier R W: Nonoliguric acute renal failure. N Eng J Med 296:1134, 1977.

Ashmore P G, Svitek V, Ambrose D: The incidence

and effects of particulate aggregation and microembolism in pump oxygenator systems. J Thorac Cardiovasc Surg 55:691, 1968.

Bennett W M, Singer I, Coggins C J: A guide to drug therapy in renal failure JAMA 239:1544, 1974.

Bergström J, Asabatt S, Fürst P, Queles E: Dialysis, ultrafiltration and blood pressure. Proc Eur Dial Transplant Assoc 13:293, 1976.

Bhat J G, Bluck M C, Lowenstein J, Baldwin D S: Renal failure after open heart surgery. Ann Intern Med 84:677, 1976.

Burke T J, Cronin R E, Duchin K L, Peterson L N, Schrier R W: Ischemia and tubule obstruction during acute renal failure in dogs: mannitol in protection. Am J Physiol 238 (Renal, Fluid, Electrolyte Physiol 7) :F305, 1980.

Cantarovich F, Ferandez J D, Locatelli A, Perez-Loredo J: Furosemide in high doses in the treatment of acute renal failure. Postgrad Med J 47 (Suppl):13, 1971.

Connors J P, Shaw R C: Considerations in the management of open-heart surgery in uremic patients. J Thorac Cardiovasc Surg 75:400, 1978.

Engleman R M, Gouge T H, Smith S J, Stahl W M, Gombos E A, Boyd A D: The effect of diuretics on renal hemodynamics during cardiopulmonary bypass. J Surg Res 16:268, 1974.

Fries D, Pozet N, Dubois N, Traiger J: The use of large doses of furosemide in acute renal failure. Postgrad Med J 47 (Suppl): 18, 1971.

Gailiunas P Jr, Chawla R, Lazarus JM, Cohn L, Sanders J, Merrill J P: Acute renal failure following cardiac operations. J Thorac Cardiovasc Surg 79:241, 1980.

Goldberg LI: Dopamine—clinical uses of an endogenous catecholamine. N Eng J Med 291:707, 1974.

Hilberman M, Derby G C, Spencer R J, Stinson E B: Sequential pathophysiological changes characterizing the progression from renal dysfunction to acute renal failure following cardiac operation. J Thorac Cardiovasc Surg 79:838, 1980.

———, Myers B D, Carrie B J, Derby G, Jamison R L, Stinson E B: Acute renal failure following cardiac surgery. J Thorac Cardiovasc Surg 77:880, 1979.

Jacobs L A, Klopp E H, Seamone W, Topaz S R, Gott V L: Improved organ function during cardiac bypass with a roller pump modified to deliver pulsatile flow. J Thorac Cardiovasc Surg 58:703, 1969.

Kahn M, Goodman B, Litwak R S, Gadboys H L: High flow whole body hemodilution perfusion: acid base, renal, electrolyte and body fluid alterations. J Mount Sinai Hosp 35:111, 1968.

Lansing A M, Leb D E, Berman L B: Cardiovascular surgery in end-stage renal failure. JAMA 204:682, 1968.

Lazarus J M: Complications of hemodialysis. Kidney Int 18:783, 1981.

Mandelbaum I, Burns W H: Pulsatile and nonpulsatile blood flow. JAMA 191:121, 1965.

Monson B K, Wickstrom P H, Haglin J J, Francis G, Comty C M, Helseth H K: Cardiac operation and end-stage renal disease. Ann Thorac Surg 30:267, 1980.

Patak R V, Lifschitz M D, Stein J H: Acute renal failure: clinical aspects and pathophysiology. Cardiovasc Med 4:19, 1979.

Porter G A, Kloster F E, Herr R J, Starr A, Griswold H E, Kimsey J, Lenertz H: Relationship between alterations in renal hemodynamics during cardiopulmonary bypass and postoperative renal function. Circulation 34:1005, 1966.

Sawyer K C, Sawyer R B, Robb W C: Postoperative renal failure. Am J Surg 106:668, 1963.

Schrier R W: Acute renal failure: pathogenesis, diagnosis, and management. Hosp Pract 16:93, 1981.

von Albertini B, Kirpalani A, Goldstein M, Glabman S, Bosch J: Changes in Pco_2 during and after hemodialysis. Proc Clin Dial Transplant Forum 6:199, 1976.

Wakim K G: The pathophysiology of the dialysis dysequilibrium syndrome. Mayo Clin Proc 44:406, 1969.

Zusman R M, Rubin R H, Cato A E, Cocchetto D M, Crow J W, Tolkin-Rubin N: Hemodialysis using prostacyclin instead of heparin as the sole antithrombotic agent. N Eng J Med 304:934, 1981.

15. Bleeding And Hemorrhagic Complications

J. Donald Hill   Robert Rodvien
C. Harold Mielke, Jr.

The coagulation disturbances observed during open heart surgery are best understood by first comprehending the nature of the body's response to hemorrhage, and then by considering how the components of open heart surgery may alter this response.

COMPONENTS OF THE HEMOSTATIC RESPONSE

Vasoconstriction

Hemostasis is achieved through interaction of the vessel wall and the various components of the blood. First, it is important to realize the profound effect vasoconstriction has on bleeding at the site of a transsected arterial vessel. If, through vasoconstriction, the diameter of a vessel is narrowed by one half, the flow through that vessel is reduced by a factor of 16. Mathematically, this is expressed by the Hagen-Poiseuille formula:

$$F = \frac{\pi d^4 \Delta P}{128 \eta L}$$

Where: F = flow rate
d = internal diameter of vessel
P = pressure drop along length of vessel
L = length of vessel
η = viscosity of blood

For example, if the length of the vessel and the pressure gradient in the vessel are constant, a flow of 100 ml/min through a vessel is reduced to 6.25 ml/min if the diameter is halved.

The Hemostatic Mechanism

Blood remains liquid as long as its only exposure is to the normal blood vessel wall. Blood exposed to any other surface—biologic or otherwise—will be altered to promote vasoconstriction, platelet adhesion, release, and aggregation, and fibrinogen conversion to an insoluble latticework of fibrin. This invariant sequence of events can be qualitatively modified by the ability of an altered vessel to constrict, the quality and quantity of blood flow, the lipids of the platelet membrane and of the plasma, the degree of tissue damage, the capabilities of fixed or mobile histiocytic cells to remove activated coagulation factors, and the diet and drugs of the person in whom hemostasis is challenged. The initial events occur in seconds to minutes and will favor platelet participation when the flow is high or turbulent. Sluggish or laminar flow tends to exclude the platelets; the fibrin deposition then consists of entrapped leucocytes and erythrocytes without a bridge of platelets between the altered vessel wall and the bulk of the thrombus.

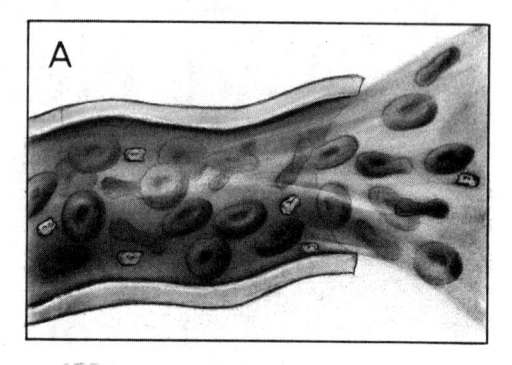

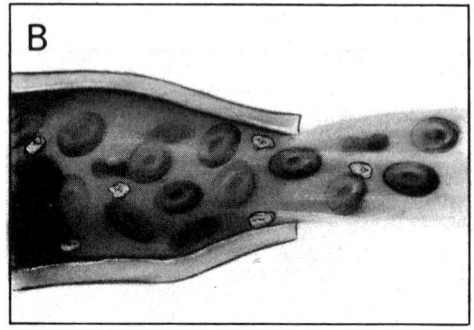

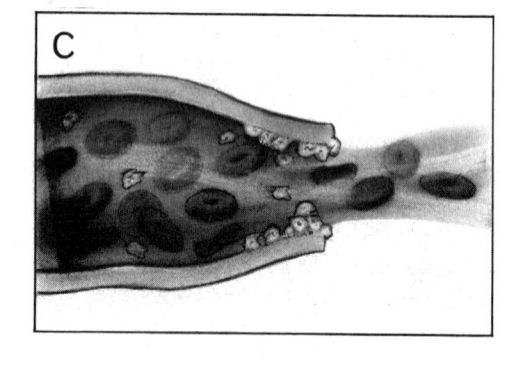

Figure 15–1. High or disordered blood flow that may be caused by either biochemical or physical alterations in the vessel wall causes change in the blood, resulting in early platelet adhesion and aggregation. Low or laminar flow states tend to exclude the platelet, but contact activation of clotting factors still leads to fibrin deposition. Not shown are the complex interactions of platelets and coagulation factors involving so-called platelet factor 3 activity to amplify thrombin's production, thrombin's effect on platelet aggregation and release, and the role of platelet surface lipids to allow the concerted biochemical reactions of the coagulation proteins to proceed. Ultimately, thrombus dissolution occurs and new intima forms to restore blood flow.

First, initial vasoconstriction reduces the flow of blood (Fig. 15-1A and B). Next, platelets adhere to the exposed subintimal tissue, particularly collagen fibers, and the platelet aggregates form (Fig. 15-1C). As the platelets contact one another and the foreign surface, they swell, degranulate, and release a vasoactive substance, adenosine diphosphate (ADP), potentiating the adherence of platelets to one another at the site of the injury (Fig. 15-1D) and creating a reversible hemostatic plug. Within minutes, the plug enlarges (Fig. 15-1E) and trace amounts of thrombin are generated via the extrinsic coagulation pathway. The hemostatic plug becomes impermeable, blood flow ceases (Fig. 15-1F), platelet Factor 3 becomes available, and the intrinsic mechanism of the coagulation system is activated. Thrombin is then formed in large quantities and fibrin is laid down (Fig. 15-1G). Formation of a stable hemostatic plug follows (Fig. 15-1H) as Factor XIII cross-links the fibrin strands. Through the action of the platelet contractile protein thrombosthenin, the clot retracts (Fig. 15-1I). Thrombus dissolution normally occurs in days, although this time scale may be compressed to hours if the enzymes of fibrinolysis are markedly activated.

The Platelet

Platelets are small, complex, cellular elements that lack a nucleus and contain a large concentration of highly active materials (Rodvien and Mielke, 1976). The peripheral platelet count varies from 150,000 to 350,000 per microliter. Apparently, production is under the control of a plasma factor, thrombopoietin. It is estimated that each megakaryocyte can produce approximately 2,000 to 3,000 platelets as evaginations of megakaryocytic cytoplasm. The younger platelets are believed to be large and heavy compared with the older ones; the younger the platelet, the more its hemostatic capability. Platelet life span varies from nine to eleven days in the circulation.

BLEEDING AND HEMORRHAGIC COMPLICATIONS

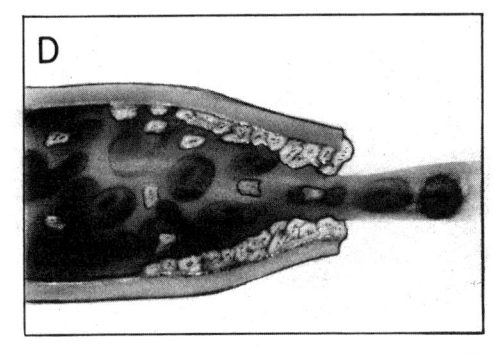

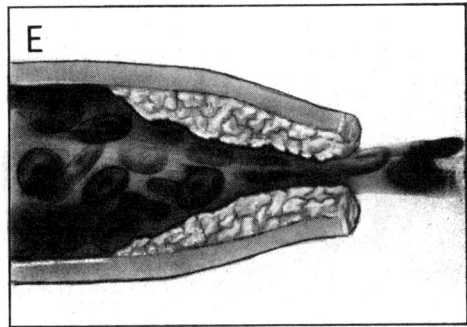

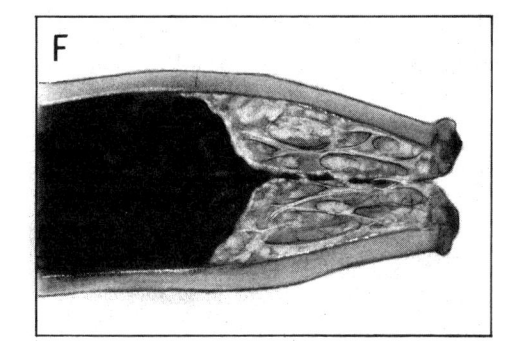

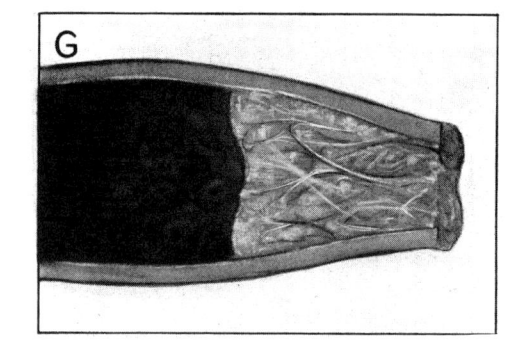

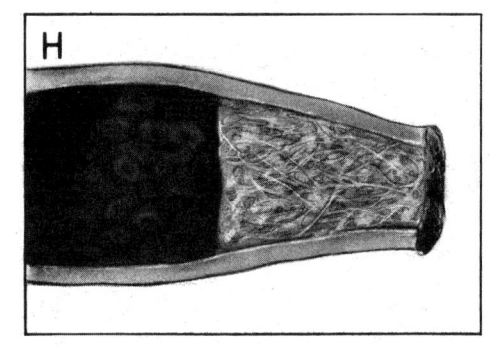

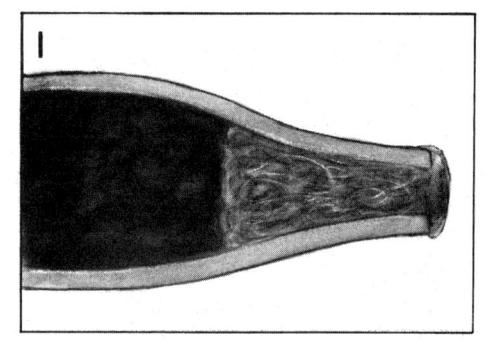

When a blood vessel is injured and subendothelial tissue is exposed, plasma proteins adhere extremely rapidly. The critical proteins in this process may or may not be among those included as part of the coagulation cascade. These proteins then serve as "bridge proteins" between the surface of platelets. If platelets are exposed to stimuli as diverse as collagen, thrombin, adenosine diphosphate (ADP), polyvinyl chloride (PVC) tubing, gas bubbles, or silicone rubber, they will adhere to the "new" surface and spew out vasoconstrictors, structural proteins, enzymes, cations, and ADP, which prompt more platelets to adhere and undergo the so-called release reaction. Therefore, the platelet reaction consists of the physical events of adherence to foreign materials, change in shape and aggregation to each other, and the biochemical events of "release" (Fig. 15–2). These biochemical reactions are mediated, at least in part, by the "second messengers" common to most cells: the cyclic nucleotides, the intermediates of prostaglandin (PG) synthesis, and the

Figure 15-2. Several plasma proteins are altered when they are exposed to an abnormal surface. The protein may be changed in shape, or it may be retained on the surface and proteolytically cleaved with or without return of fragments to the blood. Of the contact-activated proteins, factor XII (Hageman factor) may be central to the activation of other proteins in different cascades of enzymes. Consequently, contact activation may lead to thrombus production and ultimately dissolution; vasodilatation or constriction (mediated by kinins and metabolites of arachidonic acid); chemotaxis (mediated by complement components); or a host of other biologic events.

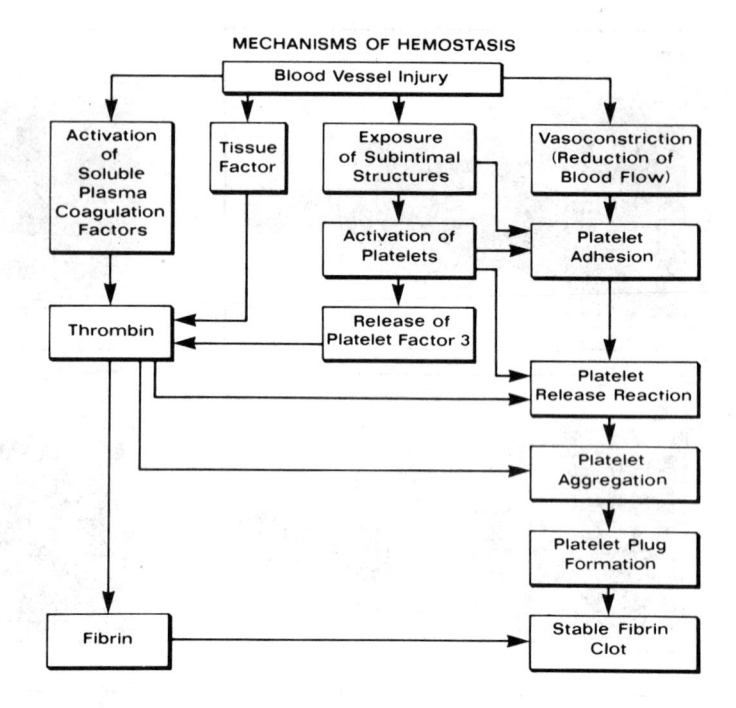

divalent cations. The exact interactions between PGs, cyclic AMP and GMP, and calcium are still not clear despite intensive investigations (Salzman et al, 1976; Glass et al., 1977; Minkes et al., 1977). It recently has been shown that platelet-biomaterial interaction causes synthesis of specific PGs and their intermediates (Addonizio et al., 1979). It is also clear that the pharmacologic use of endothelial PGs (specifically PGI_2) can prevent platelet consumption by foreign surfaces. It may be that phosphorylation-dephosphorylation reactions involving the enzymes of synthesis and degradation of these second messengers also control platelet reactivity (Assaf, 1976).

Part of the platelet's response involves membrane alterations that make the cell adhere to the rent in the endothelium as well as accelerate the production of thrombin and ultimately fibrin. Platelets may adhere only transiently but long enough to gather other platelets into an amorphous mass with or without fibrin. Physical blockade of vessels by released circulating platelet aggregates can then lead to tissue ischemia of varying degrees. The best tests of platelet adequacy are the platelet count and the bleeding time. New tests of platelet activation, such as measurement of platelet Factor 4, beta thromboglobulin, or circulating platelet aggregates, though important for other reasons, do not help in the evaluation of hemorrhage.

Blood Clotting

The blood coagulation mechanism consists of fibrinogen and nine trace plasma proteins, one tissue protein, and calcium. Their interaction results in a complex physiologic mechanism providing normal hemostasis. The usual normal levels of these coagulation factors, where they are produced, how they are found, and their biologic half-life is outlined in Table 15-1.

Any abnormal surface will cause contact-sensitive proteins in the blood to be retained by the surface, then to be fragmented and activated to cause another protein in greater amounts to be fragmented and activated. At present we recognize at lease three different

TABLE 15-1 PLASMA COAGULATION FACTORS

Factor	Synonyms	Site of Origin	Approximate Biologic Half-Life	Minimum Hemostatic Level	Blood Product Availability	Laboratory Tests
I	Fibrinogen (N = 200–400 mg%)	Liver, exact cell unclear	3–4 days	80–100 mg%	Stored blood or plasma cryoprecipitates	Specific assay, thrombin time, clot observation
II	Prothrombin (N = 50–150 activity)	Hepatocyte	2–3 days	20–40%	Plasma, stored blood concentrates	Protime, PTT, specific assay
V	Labile factor (N = 50–150 activity)	Hepatocyte	15–36 hours	5–25%	Fresh frozen plasma or fresh whole blood	Protime, PTT, specific assay
VII	Stable factor (N = 70–130% activity)	Hepatocyte	5 hours	10–25%	Stored blood or plasma concentrates	Protime, specific assay
VIII	Antihemophilic factor (AHF) (N = 50–200% activity)	Multiple sites of production, liver not primary	10–12 hours	20–30%	Fresh frozen plasma or fresh whole blood, concentrates, cryoprecipitates	PTT, specific assay
IX	Plasma thromboplastin component (PTC) (N = 60–160% activity)	Hepatocyte	20–40 hours	25–30%	Stored blood, frozen plasma, concentrates	PTT, specific assay
X	Stuart-Prower factor (N = 50–150% activity)	Hepatocyte	48–60 hours	10–20%	Stored blood, frozen plasma, concentrates	Protime, PTT, specific assay
XI	Plasma thromboplastin antecedent (PTA) (N = 50–185% activity)	Probably liver, unproven	2–4 days	15–25%	Stored blood, frozen plasma, concentrates	PTT, specific assay
XII	Hageman factor (N = 30–225% activity)	Probably liver, unproven	2–3 days	—	Stored blood or frozen plasma	PTT, specific assay
XIII	Fibrin stabilizing factor (FSF)	Probably liver, unproven	10–12 days	<5%	Stored blood or frozen plasma cryoprecipitates	Clot solubility, specific assay

plasma proteins that are contact-activated by any abnormal surface—Factors XII and XI as well as Fitzgerald Factor (Schiffman and Lee, 1974; Stormorken, 1975). With each different protein's activation, the amount of the next protein to be activated is increased and the time taken to be activated diminished; hence the terms "cascade" and "waterfall." By-products of this activation may modify thrombus formation or have other effects on the blood. For example, when fibrinogen is changed to fibrin, chemotactic and permeability factors (Malofiejew, 1971) as well as platelet inhibitory substances are produced (Niewiarowski et al., 1973; Stormorken, 1975).

Fibrinogen, when it is converted to fibrin and its several fragments, does not activate other proteins but forms an insoluble plug against the abnormal endothelium, silicone rubber, or gas bubble. Thrombin and therefore thrombus production can occur independent of the platelet's presence; but the catalytic process of coagulation factor activation occurs much more rapidly on the platelet's surface (Walsh, 1974).

One of the first proteins that interacts with the abnormal tissue or surface, Factor XII, undergoes adherence and proteolysis, after which fragments are returned to the circulation. As shown in Figure 15–3, Factor XII exists in multiple forms—the holoprotein prior to surface contact and fragments that can be retained or released. Which of these forms is physiologically the enzymatically active moiety that activates the other systems is not completely determined (Cochrane and Griffin, 1979). Figure 15–3 also hints at the complexities of the coagulation system. Factor XII may, by pathways alternative to the classic ones, promote thrombin generation by alteration of Factor VII (Nemerson, 1976). Other investigations also are blurring the traditional concepts of "intrinsic" and "extrinsic" pathways to thrombin generation. Factor VII may activate Factor X to a form that can activate Factor IX and therefore amplify the production of more Factor X (Nemerson, 1976). The more historically accepted reactions are that Factor XII can activate Factor XI or be enzymatically active in other "cascade" systems;

Figure 15–3. Activation of the coagulation proteins first involved (factor XII, factor XI) is slow to occur and few molecules are activated. With each succeeding step in the process, less time is required to activate more and more molecules. Heparin acts stoichiometrically to alter a plasma protein, antithrombin III, to enhance the rate of destruction of several activated clotting factors. Not shown is the belief that heparin's effect may be overwhelmed if fewer heparin molecules are circulating than there are activated factors. Conversely, few heparin molecules (unmeasurable by routine clotting studies) could prevent the cascade from getting beyond the initial contact-activated proteins.

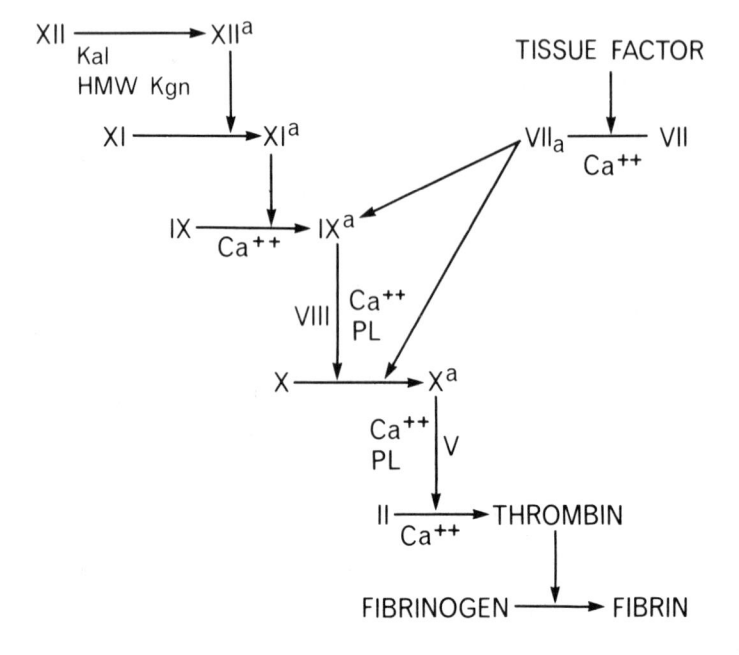

i.e., the kinin, complement, and fibrinolytic systems (see Fig. 15-3) (Stormorken, 1975). Excessive fibrinolysis is said to occur frequently during cardiopulmonary bypass (Ekert et al., 1970). When activated, the complement and kinin systems also result in potentially active fragments. Their creation during cardiopulmonary bypass surgery has not been identified nor have their effects been measured.

Lipids are in numerous compartments of the blood: the red cell membrane, leucocytes and platelets, and the cell-free plasma. There is probably slow equilibration between each of these pools. Within the plasma itself, the lipids are solubilized within the physical structure of the lipoprotein particles and their ghosts (Havel, 1974). For the platelet, the membrane lipids are crucial determinants of the response to various stimuli, since the intermediates of PG synthesis, endoperoxides and thromboxanes, are determined by the availability of arachidonate (Blackwell et al., 1977). Determinants of the fractions within each lipid pool are multiple: genetic factors, diet, drugs, and liver disease, to name a few. Rapid alterations in pool content can be achieved by activation or release of hepatic and extrahepatic lipases and other enzymes from nonblood pools (Glueck, 1975). These alterations in enzymatic activity occur in the presence of heparin and contribute to alterations in lipid metabolism that occur with open heart surgery.

Blood Lysis

A complete understanding of the normal coagulation system is not possible without consideration of the fibrinolytic system, since the body is in delicate balance between coagulation and fibrinolysis (Pechet, 1965; Sherry, 1968). The latter refers to the physiologic mechanism by which the body dissolves established thrombi. Plasminogen is the inactive precursor to plasmin in the fibrinolytic system. It is found in all body fluids but is especially high in the globulin fraction of the plasma (Fig. 15-4). The protein can be adsorbed to polymerizing fibrin and activated by thrombin so that as the thrombus forms, conditions are created within the thrombus for its eventual lysis. Other activators of the plasmin system are enzymes found in the body tissues, particularly in the vascular endothelium. Indirect activators include streptokinase and tissue kinases, which act as proactivators converting the activators into the active form, which in turn influences plasminogen to form plasmin. Direct activators also are found in the plasma. They are usually labile and soluble. It should be noted that endothelial cells have been shown to exercise a local fibrinolytic activity, underscoring the premise that the coagulation mechanism is continually being activated, producing fibrin in certain areas. Patency of a vessel is normally maintained as a result of the action of local fibrinolysis.

PREOPERATIVE FACTORS AFFECTING BLEEDING

Inherited Coagulation Disorders

Among the inherited disorders, hemophilias A and B and Von Willebrand's syndrome account for most cases. The other inherited coagulation disorders and the clinically significant inherited thrombocytopenias and thrombocytopathias will not be discussed because of their rarity. The combined incidence of the three disorders is about one in 10,000 live births.

Hemophilia A (Factor VIII deficiency) is the best known of the inherited coagulopathies. It is sex-linked: males have the disease; females are carriers except in the rare instance when an affected male and a female carrier have offspring. Bleeding usually is apparent in early childhood, though milder cases may go undiagnosed until surgery is done as an adult. The degree of the bleeding correlates fairly well with the level of Factor VIII, and the severity tends to remain constant in both the patient and the afflicted family members. Patients with less than 1 percent Factor VIII activity have severe disease while those with 5 percent or more are only mildly afflicted and rarely bleed spontaneously.

Figure 15–4. When blood contacts a foreign surface, or when factors are released from damaged tissue, two highly active proteolytic enzymes (thrombin and plasmin) are transformed from inert blood precursors. Whenever thrombin forms, fibrinogen's conversion to fibrin produces an insolubilized compartment in the blood stream. Plasminogen adheres to the fibrinogen-fibrin in the thrombus and is converted by thrombin to plasmin. Both enzymes then act on fibrinogen—one to produce more thrombus, and one to produce competitive inhibitors of fibrin production. Platelet participation in the thrombus is enhanced by thrombin and is unaffected by plasmin. Alternatively, foreign surface contact alone can activate the platelets, causing retention on the surface with release of aggregates from the surface to lodge downstream. Several of the coagulation reactions initiated by blood-foreign surface contact may be heparin-sensitive, but the platelet reactions are not.

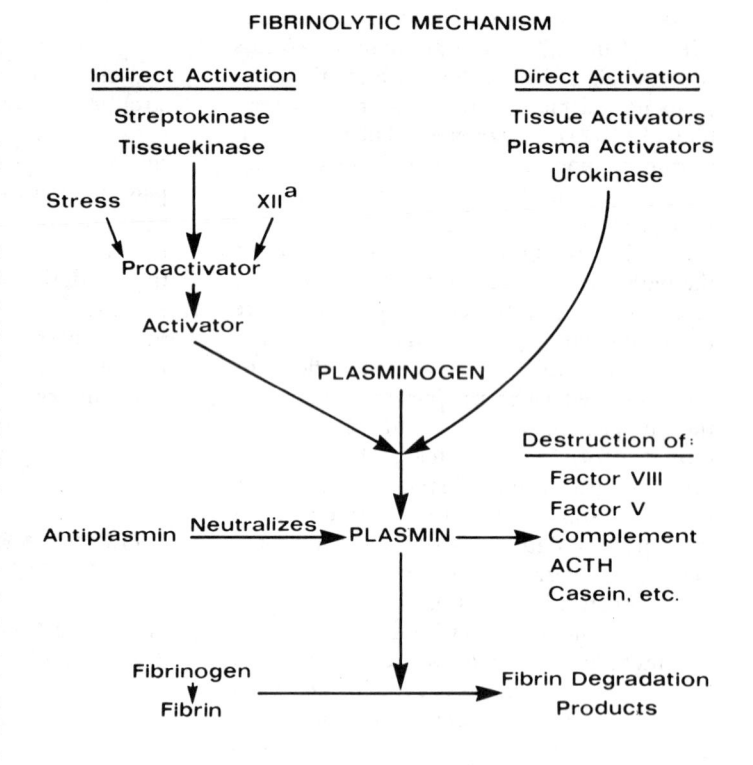

FIBRINOLYTIC MECHANISM

Indirect Activation: Streptokinase, Tissuekinase, Stress, XII^a → Proactivator → Activator

Direct Activation: Tissue Activators, Plasma Activators, Urokinase

PLASMINOGEN

Antiplasmin —Neutralizes→ PLASMIN

Destruction of: Factor VIII, Factor V, Complement, ACTH, Casein, etc.

Fibrinogen → Fibrin

Fibrin Degradation Products

In hemophilia, platelet function is normal unless certain drugs are ingested. Bleeding in people with hemophilia tends to affect deeper structures (muscles, retroperitoneal areas, and joints) and does cause petechiae or oozing from mucous membranes. The diagnosis of severe hemophilia usually is evident from the history and physical examination. Coagulation tests show a prolonged whole blood clotting time and partial thromboplastin time, and a normal platelet count, bleeding time, thrombin time, and prothrombin time. Thus the defect is confined to the *intrinsic* mechanism. The discovery of cryoprecipitate (Pool et al., 1964) and the commercial production of Factor VIII concentrates have revolutionized the care of the hemophiliac. Major surgery is now possible and open heart surgery has been performed. As a rule, the patient should receive enough Factor VIII to approach normal levels before surgery, and should be transfused every 12 hours thereafter to keep his Factor VIII levels above 30 percent. This level should be maintained until the surgical wound has healed (approximately 14 days).

Hemophilia B (Factor IX deficiency) is clinically indistinguishable from hemophilia A, but it appears to result in a larger proportion of milder cases. The screening tests are similar to those for Factor VIII deficiency. Differentiation of the two hemophilias must be done with specific factor assays. Factor concentrates for replacement therapy (Proplex, Konyne) are available (Hoag et al., 1969). They contain vitamin K-dependent clotting factors (II, III, IX, and X) but not Factor VIII. Caution must be exercised in using these materials, since the risk of hepatitis is high (Kasper, 1973; Blatt et al., 1974), and in some instances several preparations may contain activated factors which may inappropriately produce undesired thrombosis.

Von Willebrand's disease is characterized by both a defect in Factor VIII and a qualitative defect in platelet function. Therefore, bleeding from and into the skin and mucous membranes along with menorrhagia and bruising is a major clinical finding. In the classical picture of von Willebrand's disease, the patient has a prolonged bleeding time and a normal clotting time. Factor VIII is decreased, varying from 5 to 40 percent; it is rarely undetectable as is the case in severe hemophilia. The levels of Factor VIII vary; in fact, laboratory evidence of the disease may be obscured by pregnancy or the use of birth control pills. Patients with von Willebrand's disease have impaired platelet adhesiveness, both in vivo and in vitro (Salzman, 1963), and platelet aggregation studies are normal except for the impaired response to Ristocetin (Weiss and Moyer, 1973). Recent work has shown that this syndrome occurs when there is a decreased amount of plasma von Willebrand Factor (VWF), a large molecular weight protein that occurs in normal plasma and can correct the lack of aggregation of von Willebrand platelets to Ristocetin. Classic von Willebrand's syndrome is characterized by an equivalent decrease in circulating Factor VIII activity and antigen, unlike hemophilia A. Cryoprecipitate, which contains VWF and its subunit Factor VIII, is the treatment of choice in von Willebrand's disease, with levels of Factor VIII approaching 30 percent for up to 14 days desired for most major surgical procedures. It is not clear if correction of Factor VIII levels or correction of the bleeding time is more important to achieve hemostasis in this disorder.

Acquired Coagulation Disorders

Several acquired disorders can promote bleeding during cardiac surgery.

Vitamin K Deficiency. Coagulation Factors II, VII, IX, and X (also termed the vitamin K-dependent factors) cannot be synthesized in the liver without adequate supply of vitamin K. Lack of vitamin K results in a characteristic laboratory abnormality of the coagulation mechanism. Only when the deficiency is pronounced does bleeding occur. Conditions that interfere with the body's access to vitamin K include parenteral feeding (intravenous fluids), the use of broad spectrum antibiotics that sterilize the gut, and impaired fat absorption (from biliary tract obstruction or malabsorption syndromes). Any member of the coumarin family of anticoagulants can mimic vitamin K deficiency because they prevent the proper synthesis of this same group of coagulation proteins. Without vitamin K the four coagulation factors disappear from the blood stream in the following order: VII, IX, X, II. Disappearance correlates with their biologic half-lives. When vitamin K is supplied, the coagulation factors return in the reverse order. Because of this pattern of response, the prothrombin time may return to normal by 12 hours, though the hemostatic mechanism still may be impaired. If vitamin K is given and the abnormality is caused by liver disease, the prothrombin time will not correct.

Liver Disease (Hepatocellular Damage). Liver disease, the most common acquired coagulation defect, may produce a complex disturbance in the coagulation mechanism. Since the liver is responsible for production of all of the factors except Factor VIII, all but Factor VIII will be depressed in severe disease. The degree of depression correlates roughly with the extent of hepatocellular damage. Prothrombin and Factor V are the first and most severely depressed. At times, cirrhosis is associated with splenomegaly and a deficiency of circulating platelets is seen (Finkbiner et al., 1959). Trapping in the liver or spleen can be readily demonstrated by employing isotopic labeling and scanning techniques with ^{51}Cr labeled platelets. Patients with liver disease may also have increased fibrinolytic activity, perhaps because the liver cannot remove plasminogen activators from the circulation. Hepatic dysfunction is especially common in severe, intractable right heart failure and tricuspid disease. Systemic bleeding associated with liver disease is most often seen in patients with Factor V levels less than 20 percent or markedly reduced plasminogen levels. Treatment of the coagulopathy of liver disease is best undertaken with fresh blood or plasma to provide Factor V and with platelet concentrates if thrombocytopenia is present. Prothrombin concentrates are not advocated because of the high risk of hepatitis.

Circulating Anticoagulants. A number of disease states produce specific circulating factor inhibition. The most commonly seen are the Factor VIII inhibitors. They can appear spontaneously, usually in previously healthy elderly people or in women after childbirth. The Factor VIII inhibitors are most common in severe hemophilia and develop after multiple transfusions of plasma (Strauss, 1969). The antibody is stimulated by transfusion and the titer rises accordingly; however, if transfusions are withheld the titers subside and may spontaneously disappear. Transfusions in patients with inhibitors are contraindicated except for life-threatening situations. Surgery is contraindicated because of the high risk of hemorrhage and difficulty in controlling it. In an emergency the use of high potency Factor VIII concentrates of either bovine or porcine Factor VIII may provide temporary neutralization of the inhibitor. If this is achieved, hemostasis will take place.

In addition to the Factor VIII inhibitors, inhibitors to Factors IX, V, and XIII have been reported. Therapy is similar to that for the Factor VIII inhibitors. Inhibitors have been described in other diseases suspected of having an immunologic basis; e.g., lupus erythematosis, rheumatoid arthritis, ulcerative colitis, penicillin reaction, and regional enteritis (Green, 1968; Shapiro and Holburn, 1970).

Cyanotic Heart Disease (CHD). The problems posed by CCHD deserve special attention. Some investigators have found that the fibrinolytic mechanism is activated (Ekert et al., 1970). This coagulation disturbance does not explain the low platelet count or abnormal platelet function that is frequently observed (Ekert et al., 1970). In addition, these patients have a long partial thromboplastin time that can be explained only partially by technical difficulties in determining the proper amount of anticoagulant to use in the test (Naiman, 1970). People with CCHD frequently have elevated venous pressure that persists postoperatively and may cause "anatomic" bleeding independent of a coagulopathy. These same people also are often poorly nourished, frequently need a second or third operation, and have diffuse collateral pulmonary circulation. Reoperation for any reason is frequently associated with increased postoperative bleeding, which in part reflects the need for dissection through fibrous adhesive tissue.

Drugs. Deliberate administration of heparin or warfarin by the patient or physician is the most common cause of an acquired circulating anticoagulant and should be considered first for any workup. The aminoglycosides also can cause a circulating anticoagulant, in this instance Factor V. Drugs also can be "platelet suppressive." Drugs such as indomethacin and sulfinpyrazone appear to reversibly affect platelet cyclooxygenase. Other drugs, such as Keflin (Cazenave et al., 1976), atropine (White, 1969), and propranolol (Bygdeman and Johnsen, 1969), also should be stopped at least one day before the operation. Aspirin should be avoided for the week before surgery because of its prolonged irreversible effect on the circulating platelet. A good screen for some of these drug effects is the TBT (Mielke et al., 1969).

INTRAOPERATIVE EVENTS DURING OPEN HEART SURGERY

Thrombocytopenia and Thrombopathy

Thrombocytopenia and a decrease in fibrinogen concentration are essentially universal after cardiopulmonary bypass (CPB) (Parker-Williams, 1972; Umlas, 1976). Platelets will adhere to any foreign surface, be it solid or gaseous. In bubble oxygenators the constantly forming new bubbles continue to alter platelets so that in routine CPB, the longer the bypass, the worse the thrombopenia. Those platelets that do circulate may not be maximally competent: they do not perform normally in the glass bead retention test and aggregate poorly (McKenzie et al., 1969). Transient platelet retention and its consequences (intermittent microembolization with endarteriolar occlusion) may be one of the coagulation disturbances induced by CPB that has been difficult to define and yet may have profound long-range effects on each patient's overall health.

Filters have been used to prevent the direct consequences of circulating platelet aggregates (Swank et al., 1974). When these filters are used the thrombocytopenia may be more severe. The introduction of depth (Dacron wool) and microporous grid (less than 200 microns pore size) filters into the coronary suction circuit or the arterial perfusion lines theoretically could lead to a permanent reduction in the available platelets and excess bleeding in the intraoperative and postoperative period. The author's records do not corroborate this. Our early experience indicated that there was no difference in the amount of bleeding when Dacron wool filters were used in the coronary suction line. Subsequently, Dacron wool filters also were placed in the arterial perfusion line. Again, the amount of postoperative bleeding was not increased. The platelet count did decrease during perfusion but it did not appear to matter. However, the added surface of the filter can activate platelets leading to plasma substances that are vasoactive if not toxic to the endothelium. A blocked filter reintroduced into the circulation can cause transient hypotension, presumably because of released vasoactive substances from the platelet.

The decrease in platelet numbers (thrombopenia) and the impaired function of the platelets that circulate (thrombopathy) are probably the most common cause of nonsurgical bleeding during open heart surgery. In individuals with cyanotic congenital heart disease (CCHD), the thrombopenia and thrombopathy may precede surgery (Ekert et al., 1970). The platelet problems are exaggerated by the hemodilution of the prime and usually are made worse by the preoperative condition of the patient; specifically the presence of liver disease or the use of drugs such as aspirin (Bick, 1976).

Heparin Excess

None of the just discussed effects of CPB on the platelet are heparin-sensitive. Heparin is necessary for CPB because it accelerates the destruction of activated coagulation factors and therefore prevents thrombin production (Rosenberg, 1975) (see Fig. 15–3). Without heparin, the surface-induced activation of the coagulation cascade would clot the blood. In our hospital we give 300 units/kg heparin IV bolus and will not give any more unless the CPB lasts more than two hours and the activated clotting time is less than 400 to 500 seconds. At that time, 100 units/kg heparin are given. The only other heparin is in the blood transfusions given during CPB.

Excess heparin is an unusual cause of bleeding; it has been observed to occur after hypothermia is reversed and heparin is released from fat stores. This event is well-known and rarely results in unexpected bleeding (Ellison et al., 1974). However, heparin may contribute to bleeding through effects on lipoprotein lipase that modify both plasma and platelet lipids. We have shown that in both these lipid compartments lysolecithin and proteolipids increase and the phosphatidyl inositols are altered. This latter lipid is the major source of arachidonic acid for the platelet to convert into thromboxanes and prostaglandins. Heparin can cause loss of platelet function when given in smaller doses than those given in most CPB procedures (Heiden et al., 1977). The template bleeding time (TBT) currently is the most sensitive indicator of in vivo platelet dysfunction available. As shown in Table 15–2, 100 U/kg IV heparin prolongs the TBT in approximately one third of a population of normal human volunteers, in some instances markedly. In this short period of time platelet counts do not change. In those normal people in whom heparin does not prolong the TBT, aspirin's ability to prolong the TBT can be exaggerated by heparin (Heidin et al., 1977). We have no explanation for why heparin alters lipids in all people and the TBT in only some. It may be that there are multiple parallel pathways for platelet activation and that heparin's capacity to modify platelet function exists only in those in whom the prostaglandin pathway is dominant. This effect of heparin may be an important part of the "thrombopathy" of open heart surgery.

Protamine Excess

Protamine is used to reverse heparin, but it too has "anticoagulant" properties (Egerton and Robinson, 1961). Furthermore, it may exaggerate the thombopenia, especially when used in conjunction with heparin (Radegran et al., 1971). Protamine excess can be a cause of nonsurgical bleeding after CPB by forming a complex with fibrinogen that acts as an anticoagulant. We recently have lowered our dose of protamine to 3 mg/kg followed by an optional 0.5 mg/kg protamine one-half hour later if the ACT has not returned to a normal range. This regimen has diminished the extent of chest tube and wound bleeding seen in the postoperative period.

Plasmin Excess

Some workers have found that primary fibrinolysis occurs frequently with CPB and advocate that this phenomenon is a major contributor to postoperative bleeding (Bick et al., 1976). However, mild reductions in plasminogen with the apparent production of plasmin occurs very commonly in CPB, while unacceptable bleeding is unusual. In addition, prevention of fibrinolysis with the routine use of Amicar has not decreased the bleeding seen

TABLE 15-2 DIFFERENCES IN IN VIVO RESPONSE OF TBT TO TWO DIFFERENT HEPARINS IN HUMANS

SUBJECT	Beef Lung Heparin BASELINE	Beef Lung Heparin 15 MIN	Pork Gut Heparin BASELINE	Pork Gut Heparin 15 MIN
1	6' 00"	7' 00"	5' 00"	9' 00"
2	6' 00"	9' 30"	7' 00"	9' 00"
3	4' 30"	5' 00"	5' 00"	15' 30"
4	4' 30"	5' 00"	6' 00"	12' 00"
5	5' 00"	10' 30"	5' 30"	4' 00"
6	7' 00"	7' 30"	6' 30"	20' 00"
7	8' 00"	15' 00"	5' 30"	20' 00"
8	3' 00"	4' 00"	6' 30"	9' 30"
9	5' 30"	6' 00"	3' 00"	5' 00"
mean	5' 30"	7' 51"	5' 30"	11' 30"
s.d.	1' 23"	3' 28"	1' 10"	5' 32"

Each individual was given 100 U/kg IV bolus heparin of each type from coded vials. Administrations were one week apart. TBTs were done before and 15 minutes after heparin administration. As shown here, the TBT was prolonged by two minutes or more in three of the nine persons receiving beef lung heparin, whereas the pork gut heparin prolonged eight of the nine TBTs for two minutes or more.

with CPB (Rice and Worth, 1968; Verska et al., 1972). Changes in the fibrinolytic mechanism may be epiphenomena, akin to the elevation of the sedimentation rate with infection, and explain little of the bleeding seen with CPB.

Thrombin Excess (Disseminated Intravascular Coagulation, or DIC)

Thrombin excess in CPB is the most feared of the forms of nonsurgical bleeding. Any thrombin generation not only insolubilizes fibrinogen as thrombus but also consumes platelets and coagulation factors and generates plasmin (see Fig. 15–4). In this situation, bleeding and clotting can occur simultaneously. A working laboratory definition of DIC is the documentation of a fall in circulating fibrinogen concentration and platelet numbers associated with a rise in fibrin(ogen) split products. "Thrombin excess" (DIC) and "plasmin excess" (primary fibrinolysis) therefore should be distinguishable because platelets are spared in hyperplasminemia (see Fig. 15–4). In CPB where thrombopenia occurs independent of "thrombin excess," this rule is not helpful. During CPB the distinction between heparin and thrombin excess also is made by laboratory tests alone, since the clinical bleeding patterns of too little and too much heparin may be virtually indistinguishable. The pattern of an infinite thrombin time (TT) and normal reptilase time is virtually pathognomonic of heparin's presence.

Thrombin may not be the only way to consume coagulation proteins and therefore place the individual at risk to bleed. Gas-liquid interfaces caused by the bubble oxygenator and exaggerated by coronary suction may denature the coagulation proteins, producing impaired hemostasis (Wright et al., 1962; Pruitt et al., 1971). Platelet dysfunction from continuous blood-material interaction also occurs. These changes are probably the major cause of bleeding associated with prolonged CPB. Once bypass has lasted 6 to 8 hours, hemostasis may be difficult to accomplish with protamine administration alone. A combination of DIC and gross depletion or destruction of coagulation factors may be occurring to cause bleeding, but no one has used heparin successfully at this point in the operation to combat DIC and control the bleeding. Heparin administration at this point would seem to be the sensible thing to do if DIC could be documented. Once intraoperative DIC begins after the initial use of heparin, the only treatment consists of support with fresh blood, fresh frozen plasma, and platelets.

Laboratory Diagnosis and Treatment

Diagnosis of the cause of bleeding in the operating room requires preoperative laboratory evaluation. These baseline data identify the patient who is at risk to bleed and allow for interpretation of changes during CPB. Before surgery, a platelet count, TBT, partial thromboplastin time, and fibrinogen level serve both these purposes. If nonsurgical excessive bleeding is suspected *during* surgery after protamine should have restored normal hemostasis, one can collect specimens for a platelet count (plt), prothrombin time (PT), partial thromboplastin time (PTT), thrombin time (TT), protamine sulfate corrected thrombin time, fibrin split products (FSP), fibrin monomer (FM), fibrinogen, and activated clotting time (ACT).

Hattersley's (1966) method of ACT provides an accurate control of heparin administration (deLeval et al., 1972; Hill et al., 1974). The technique is automated and minimizes the logistics of monitoring heparin in the operating room. It has excellent repeatability and reliability, and is easy to perform. Traditionally, the whole blood clotting time has been used to monitor heparin. This test is time-consuming and poorly reproducible.

We have a standard response to bleeding that occurs after the first dose of protamine. If the ACT is normal there is no heparin excess and probably no coagulation disorder. We then give platelet transfusions (12 to 16 units in the adult). If the ACT is prolonged a small additive dose of protamine may be given (0.5 mg/kg). If protamine does not correct the ACT, we give fresh frozen plasma and watch for signs of improved clotting in the wound. Amicar rarely is needed and certainly should not be used first. With the first signs of excess bleeding, we establish good quick contact with the laboratory.

The aim of these tests is to diagnose the cause of bleeding. Therapy has been mentioned first because therapy precedes the definitive diagnosis of bleeding in the open heart suite. Interpretations of the tests can be made only in the context of how much heparin and protamine have been given. The PT is relatively unaffected by either drug but is sensitive to thrombin excess. The PTT is more sensitive and the TT most sensitive to heparin. If protamine corrects the TT, there is heparin excess. If not, give more fresh frozen plasma. We have not found that rapid lysis of the clot observed when doing the TT is a good measure of clinically important fibrinolysis. If clot lysis can be demonstrated in a test tube, give Amicar. The presence of fibrin monomers or FSP occurs most frequently with DIC; i.e., thrombin excess. Repeat the platelet counts and coagulation test to see if a trend can be established. Continue to support the patient with platelet transfusions and fresh frozen plasma. If gross coagulation defects are not improving, pooled plasma concentrates may be given (e.g., Konyne), but their administration runs a considerable risk of hepatitis. Local methods of controlling "general ooze" with Gelfoam, Surgicel, and Avitene are often very effective. Their action in arresting bleeding is both mechanical and biochemical.

The investigation and management of postoperative nonsurgical bleeding is handled in a similar fashion. One also has the additional advantage of being able to do a TBT to assess platelet function.

Postoperative DIC

In the immediate postoperative period, the causes of DIC are sepsis and trauma. Prolongation of the period of DIC can occur because of hypotension, liver disease, and inability to control the precipitating events. DIC can cause multiple thrombi but activation of the fibrinolytic system not only makes these thrombi morphologically difficult to find but also makes them unimportant pathophysiologically. The only clinically important consequence of DIC is if consumption of platelets and coagulation factors occurs to such an extent that exaggeration of other causes for bleeding occurs. In general, because both CPB and DIC are associated with hypofibrinogenemia and thrombocytopenia and bleeding may be treated in part by transfusion, it is extremely difficult to be sure that DIC is occurring. The differentiation of true DIC from the immediate post-CPB state becomes more difficult if transient acute respiratory failure (ARF) also occurs. ARF itself may be associated with third-spacing of fibrinogen and trapping of platelets *or* may cause true consumption of these blood elements as thrombi are formed and dissolved. The ambiguities of diagnosis diminish as the postoperative period is prolonged. In general, these ambiguities, along with the chest tube and other bleeding, have led us to treat suspected DIC by treating the underlying cause (such as sepsis), correcting the hypotension and gas exchange, giving platelets and plasma as necessary, but not using heparin.

Surgical Bleeding

Surgical bleeding is continuous bleeding that occurs from any surgical wound in the presence of a relatively normal hemostatic mechanism. Despite most surgeons' earnest statements to the contrary, most bleeding associated with surgery is of surgical origin. Differentiation of bleeding is based on the knowledge of the details of the surgical procedure as it was performed and the systematic exclusion of hematologic causes. Bleeding from multiple incisions into the wound dressings is often an indication of a coagulation disorder. In the absence of a demonstrable hematologic explanation, one must treat the patient as though there were one or more areas of specific mechanical leaks from the venous, arterial, or cardiac portion of the circulation. Most of these leaks self-seal, but some will persist. Early persistent general ooze sometimes can be arrested by the mechanical effects of 5 to 10 cm of PEEP.

The treatment of continuous surgical bleeding is prompt surgical intervention. The reoperation rate for bleeding should be less than 5 percent. The time for surgery is early rather than late. A patient continuing to bleed more than 2 ml/kg/hr (140 ml per hour in a 70-kg man) six hours after surgery should be reexplored. The overall effect of waiting too long is to prolong recovery time, and increase morbidity and sometimes mortality. The consequences of procrastination outweigh the momentary benefits of waiting except in exceptional circumstances. An unstable cardiovascular state will persist as long as bleeding continues. The borderline cardiac output results in a compensatory peripheral vasoconstriction and subsequent inadequate renal perfusion. Accumulated blood in the mediastinum and pleural space diminishes venous return and impairs the ventilatory mechanism. Finally, the continuous administration of transfused blood carries with it hematologic, metabolic, and infectious dangers as well as subjecting the patient to antibody development. Transfused blood should be warmed. Following the work of Swank (1968) and Solis and Gibbs, (1972) the development of depth and microporous blood transfusion filters has reduced the adverse effects resulting from transfusing large amounts of particulate matter into the patient's lungs. In addition to the filters, better blood banking procedures as well as availability of blood component therapy also has reduced the risks of blood transfusion therapy.

Occasionally, bleeding will persist and then stop, leaving a large volume of blood in the mediastinum or pleural space. This blood clot should be removed. A large volume of blood in the pleural space will hamper breathing for several weeks. An attempt should be made to remove it by thoracentesis, but if this is unsuccessful, as it usually is, early reexploration can be performed through a small lateral thoracotomy incision or through the original sternotomy incision. Large amounts of retained blood in the mediastinum liquify and, under pressure, seep through the mediastinal wound. This seepage will protect the patient from developing late mediastinal tamponade but can lead to a more serious complication: an infected sternum and mediastinum with complete breakdown of the wound and sternal separation.

The risks of early reoperation are small. Forty-eight hours later the patients who have been reexplored are at the same stage of recovery as patients who did not bleed. Reoperation can be performed quickly and easily without danger of infection. Caution must be used during induction of anesthesia. The patient may have pronounced compensatory peripheral vasoconstriction that precipitously decreases during the induction of anesthesia. This condition results in a dangerous level of hypotension. This anticipated problem can be prevented by giving the patient an adequate blood volume before the induction of anesthesia and by the liberal use of transfusion in the operating room. We continue to give calcium when large volumes of blood are transfused to enable the myocardium to contract vigorously. Pharmacologically administered ionized calcium has little or no practical effect on the coagulation values during bleeding.

Acute Pericardial or Mediastinal Tamponade

Acute tamponade is the rapid accumulation of blood or fluid in a confined space in the pericardium or mediastinum, compressing the heart and preventing diastolic filling of the cardiac chambers. The cardiac output is sharply decreased, producing the signs of hypovolemic shock. Tamponade can occur in the first 2 to 18 hours after cardiac surgery; a mediastinal or pleural chest tube does not guarantee that tamponade will not occur. A chest tube can be plugged with clot and the opened mediastinal pleura, which allows drainage into the pleural space, can seal very quickly once the chest is closed. The routine closure of the pericardium will further reduce the leeway one has in postoperative bleeding before tamponade can occur.

The diagnosis of tamponade is made on physical signs, hemodynamic values, and sometimes the chest x-ray. Generally, an unusual amount of bleeding has occurred. The patient is peripherally vasoconstricted, cool, and oliguric. Mental confusion may be present because of both the postoperative state and inadequate cerebral perfusion. Pulsus parodoxicus, combined with distended neck veins, indicative of a high central venous pressure, is almost pathognomonic of tamponade. In this situation, transfusing the patient with increased blood volume produces a slight increase in blood pressure and a marked increase in central venous pressure. Intracardiac pressure catheters or a Swan-Ganz catheter will show that the right atrial, left atrial, left ventricular end-diastolic, right ventricular end-diastolic, and pulmonary artery diastolic pressures are all slightly elevated and the same. Shoemaker et al. (1973) measured and described the hemodynamic effects of acute tamponade in clinical trauma patients. The same physiologic effects are observed in acute tamponade after cardiac surgery. There is a rapid heart rate and a small stroke volume, reflecting the small volume of blood that the cardiac chamber can accept during diastole. The systemic peripheral resistance is at first increased, but with the onset of acidosis it will fall, resulting in a dangerously low central aortic pressure. The chest x-ray may show mediastinal or pericardial widening. Once again all the symptoms and signs need not be present and a strong index of suspicion in a hypotensive patient is reason to explore.

The treatment is prompt surgery to relieve tamponade, remove blood clot, and arrest hemorrhage. In an emergency, substernal exploration can be performed with a sucker (see Fig. 15–5). This can also serve as a definitive procedure if the tamponade is anterior. Another emergency procedure to consider is to elevate the sternum one or two centimeters with the use of a finger or retractor under the xyphoid. A larger mediastinal space will occur and allow more diastolic cardiac filling. Relief of tamponade will produce a sharp increase in the systemic blood pressure. If a large volume of blood has been transfused before surgery and there is a very high central venous pressure, relief of the tamponade may be followed by prompt improvement, or acute left heart failure may then occur. The latter must be recognized and the heart supported pharmacologically for a short time or the blood removed by phlebotomy.

Late Bleeding Complications

Late bleeding complications are unusual in cardiac surgery. The early administration of various pharmacologic anticoagulants is responsible for most of the mishaps. The development of less thrombogenic prosthetic valves has reduced the urgency and aggressiveness in obtaining maximal anticoagulation effects; hence, fewer late bleeding problems have occurred as well.

Hematomas

Postoperative hematomas are best classified as minor and major. The minor hematomas are self-limited and account for little increase in morbidity or mortality. Common examples are bleeding into wounds, into catheterization sites, and into sites of deep intravenous injections, especially in patients taking anticoagulants. Two major hematomas merit special attention. A large, spontaneous, retroperitoneal hematoma is a highly morbid and even fatal complication in the postoperative period. Anticoagulants should be discontinued. A spontaneous retroperitoneal hematoma is difficult to evacuate satisfactorily, and unless its size is causing respiratory, cardiac, or gastrointenstial symptoms, it should be allowed to absorb. Subdural or subarachnoid hemorrhage and hematoma are serious and often produce fatal postoperative bleeding complications. Infection is a late complication of hematoma. It is most serious when it occurs in the mediastinal incision or within the mediastinum. It is more completely discussed in the chapter on infections.

Late Mediastinal or Pericardial Tamponade

A patient can accumulate clinically significant quantities of blood in the closed pericardial or

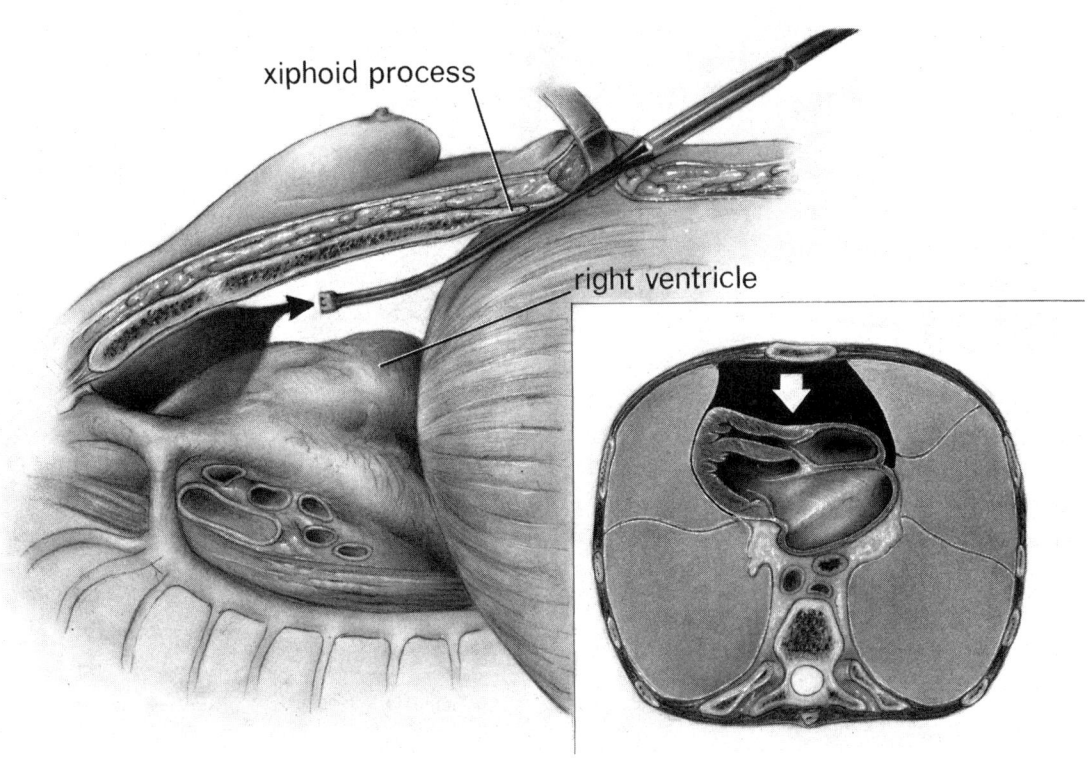

Figure 15–5. Retrosternal collection of blood causing a mediastinal tamponade to the heart. It can be effectively and rapidly treated by the substernal insertion of a sucker.

mediastinal space 4 to 40 days following cardiac surgery. As in acute tamponade, having had the right or left pleural space open is not protection against development of late tamponade. Almost always, the patients are receiving anticoagulants. Nelson et al. (1969) emphasize that these patients have had excessive postoperative bleeding.

In a group of patients we have evaluated, we (Hill et al., 1969) found the symptoms are vague; all patients have malaise that is difficult to distinguish from postpericardiotomy syndrome. They very often complain of back, neck, or chest pain. The most important findings are an elevated central venous pressure and a pulsus paradoxicus. Mild fever is often present.

The pathology is illustrated in Figures 15–5 and 15–6. Most commonly, liquified blood has collected in the retrosternal position (Fig. 15–5). Less often, it is behind or along the diaphragmatic surface of the heart (Fig. 15–6). Pulmonary embolus, postpericardiotomy syndrome, and congestive heart failure are the principal differential diagnoses. Chest x-rays are not usually helpful, but they may show a mediastinal widening. The symptoms progress to shortness of breath and oliguria. If the diagnosis is not clear, cardiac catheterization and angiography should be performed to establish the diagnosis. The presence of equal left ventricular end-diastolic, right ventricular end-diastolic, left atrial, and right atrial pressures are diagnostic. In addition, the patient will have a low cardiac output, rapid pulse, and low stroke volume due to inadequate cardiac filling. Superior vena cava angiography may reveal a filling defect on the right side of the heart. Increasingly sophisticated echocardiography

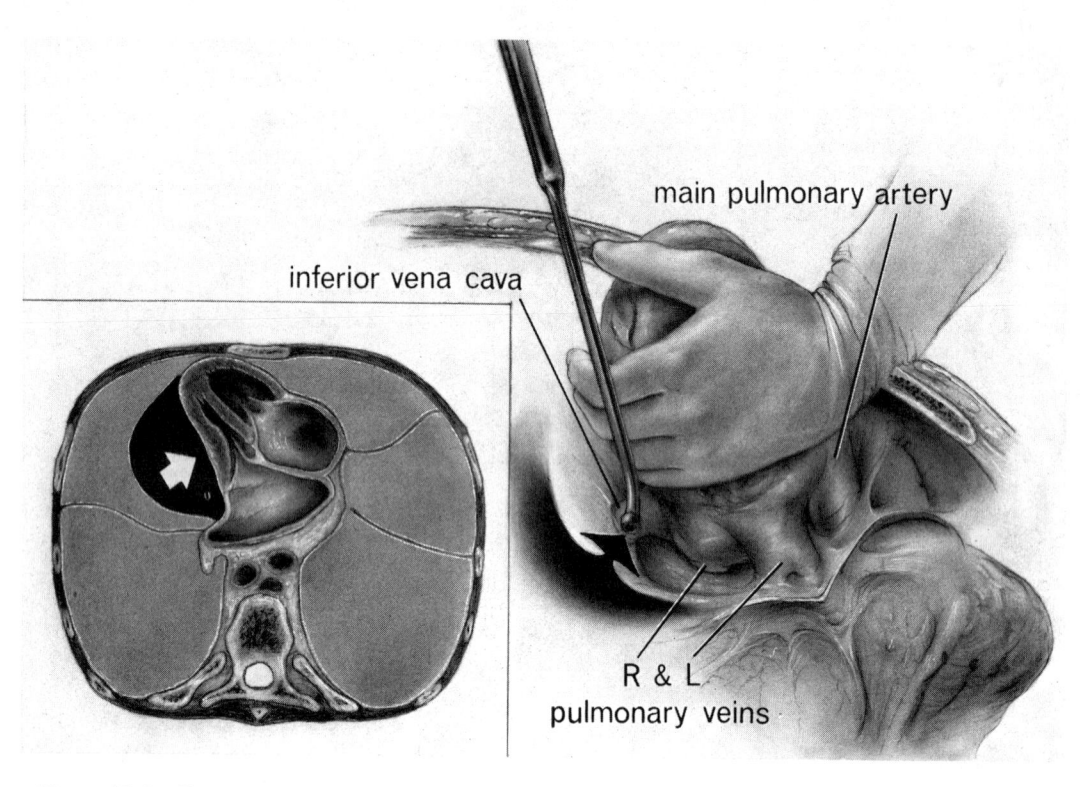

Figure 15–6. Retrocardiac pericardial tamponade. It can only be relieved by exploratory median sternotomy with elevation of the heart and removal of the clot and liquid blood under direct vision.

can be expected to displace cardiac catheterization as the diagnostic method of choice.

The treatment is pericardiocentesis, substernal exploration, or median sternotomy, with exploration of the mediastinum. Pericardiocentesis often is not successful because of adhesions and loculated fluid. Ellison and Kirsh (1974) and Englemann et al. (1970) also have reported dissatisfaction with the mediastinocentesis as a definitive form of therapy. The patient should be transferred to the operating room and prepared for exploration of the mediastinum. A retrosternal and superdiaphragmatic exploration is performed first through the subxyphoid area with a finger and suction (Fig. 15–5). If successful, when the blood under pressure is released there is an immediate increase in the systemic blood pressure. Tamponade behind the heart requires reopening the sternotomy incision to evacuate the blood (Fig. 15–6). Immediately after the operation, there should be a dramatic improvement of the patient's well-being.

REFERENCES

Addonizio VP, Strauss JF, Colman RW, Edmunds LH: Effects of prostaglandin E$_1$ on platelet loss during *in vivo* and *in vitro* extracorporeal circulation with a bubble oxygenator. J Thorac Cardiovasc Surg 77:119, 1979.

Assaf SA: Cyclic AMP-mediated phosphorylation reactions in the regulation of blood platelet aggregation. Int J Biochem 7:535, 1976.

Bick RL: Alterations of hemostasis associated with cardiopulmonary bypass: pathophysiology, prevention, diagnosis and management. In Mammen EF (ed): Seminars in Thrombosis and

Hemostasis. New York, Stratton Intercontinental, 1976, pp 59–82.
_____, Schmalhorst WR, Arbegast NR: Alterations of hemostasis associated with cardiopulmonary bypass. Thrombus Res 8:285, 1976.
Blackwell GJ, Duncombe WG, Flower RJ, et al: The distribution and metabolism of arachidonic acid in rabbit platelets during aggregation and its modification by drugs. Br J Pharmacol 59:353, 1977.
Blatt PM, Lundblad RL, Kingdon HS, McLean G, Roberst HR: Thrombogenic materials in prothrombin complex concentrates. Ann Intern Med 81:766, 1974.
Bygdeman S, Johnsen O: Studies on the effect of adrenergic blocking drugs on catecholamine-induced platelet aggregation and uptake of noradrenaline and 5-hydroxytryptamine. Acta Physiol Scand 75:129, 1969.
Cazenave JP, Reimers HJ, Senyi AF, et al: Effects of penicillin g. and Cephalothin on platelet function in vivo. Proc Soc Exp Biol Med 152:641, 1976.
Cochrane CG, Griffin JH: Molecular assembly in the contact phase of the Hageman factor system. Am J Med 67:657, 1979.
deLeval M, Hill JD, Mielke CH, Bramson ML, Smith C, Gerbode F: Platelet kinetics during extracorporeal circulation. Trans Am Soc Artif Intern Organs 18:355, 1972.
Egerton WF, Robinson CLN: The anti-heparin, anticoagulant and hypotensive properties of hexadimethrine and protamine. Lancet 2:635, 1961.
Ekert H, Gilchrist GS, Stanton R, Hammond D: Hemostasis in cyanotic congenital heart disease. J Pediatr 76:221, 1970.
Ellison LH, Kirsh MM: Delayed mediastinal tamponade after open heart surgery. Chest 65:64, 1974.
Ellison N, Beatty CP, Blake Dr, Wurzel HA, MacVaugh H: Heparin rebound. J Thorac Cardiovasc Surg 67:723, 1974.
Engleman RM, Spencer RC, Reed GE, Tice DA: Cardiac tamponade following open heart surgery. Circulation 41, 42 (Suppl 2): 165, 1970.
Finkbiner RB, McGovern JJ, Goldstein R, Bunker JP: Coagulation defects in liver disease and response to transfusions during surgery. Am J Med 26:199, 1959.
Glass DB, Frey W, Carr DW, et al: Stimulation of human platelet guanylate cyclase by fatty acids. J Biol Chem 252:1279, 1977.
Glueck CJ: Postheparin lipoprotein lipases. N Engl J Med 292:1347, 1975.
Green D: Spontaneous inhibitors of factor VIII. Brit J Haematol 15:57, 1968.
Hattersley PG: Activated coagulation time of whole blood. JAMA 196:436, 1966.
Havel RJ: Lipoproteins and lipid transport. In Kritchevsky D, Paoletti R, Holmes WL (eds): Lipids, Lipoproteins and Drugs. New York, Plenum, 1974, pp 37–59.
Heiden D, Mielke CH, Rodvien R: Impairment by heparin of primary haemostasis. Br J Haematol 36:427, 1977.
Hill JD, Dontigny L, deLeval MR, Mielke CH: A simple method of heparin management during prolonged extracorporeal circulation. Ann Thorac Surg 17:129, 1974.
_____, Johnson DC, Mill GE, Kerth WJ, Gerbode F: Latent mediastinal tamponade after open-heart surgery. Arch Surg 99:808, 1969.
Hoag MS, Johnson FF, Robinson JA, Aggeler PM: Treatment of hemophilia B with a new clotting factor concentrate. N Engl J Med 280:581, 1969.
Kasper CK: Postoperative thrombosis in Hemophilia B. N Engl J Med 289:160, 1973.
Malofiejew M: The biological and pharmacological properties of some fibrinogen degradation products. Scand J Haematol 13(Suppl 8):303, 1971.
McKenzie FN, Dhall DP, Arfors KE, et al: Blood platelet behavior during and after open-heart surgery. Br Med J 2:795, 1969.
Mielke CH, Kanoshiro MM, Maher IA, Weiner JM, Rapaport SI: The standardized normal Ivy bleeding time and its prolongation by aspirin. Blood 34:205, 1969.
Minkes M, Stanford N, Chi MM, et al: Cyclic adenosine 3', 5'-monophosphate inhibits the availability of arachidonate to prostaglandin synthetase in human platelet suspensions. J Clin Invest 59:449, 1977.
Naiman JL: Clotting and bleeding in cyanotic congenital heart disease. J Pediatr 76:333, 1970.
Nelson RM, Jenson CB, Smoot WM: Pericardial tamponade following open heart surgery. J Thorac Cardiovasc Surg 58:510, 1969.
Nemerson Y: Biological control of factor VII. Thromb Haemost 35:96, 1976.
Niewiarowski S, Senyi AF, Gillies P: Plasmin-induced platelet aggregation and platelet release reaction. J Clin Invest 52:1647, 1973.
Parker-Williams EJ: Platelets in prostheses and pumps. In O'Brien JR (ed): Clinics in Haematology. Philadelphia, Saunders, 1972, pp 413–423.
Pechet L: Fibrinolysis. N Engl J Med 273:966, 1965.

Pool JG, Hershgold EJ, Pappenhagen AR: High-potency antihemophilic factor concentrate prepared from cryoglobulin precipitate. Nature 203:312, 1964.

Pruitt KM, Stroud RM, Scott JW: Blood damage in the heart-lung machine. Proc Soc Exp Biol Med 137:714, 1971.

Radegran K, Taylor GA, Olsson P: Mode of action of protamine in regard to its circulatory and respiratory side effects. Eur Surg Res 3:139, 1971.

Rice DA, Worth MH: Recognition and treatment of postoperative bleeding associated with open heart surgery. Ann NY Acad Sci 146:745, 1968.

Rodvien R, Mielke CH: Role of platelets in hemostasis and thrombosis. West J Med 125:181, 1976.

Rosenberg RD: Actions and interactions of antithrombin and heparin. N Engl J Med 292:146, 1975.

Salzman EW: Measurement of platelet adhesiveness: a simple in vitro technique demonstrating an abnormality in von Willebrand's disease. J Lab Clin Med 63:724, 1963.

———, Lindon JN, Rodvien R: Cyclic AMP in human blood platelets: relation to platelet prostaglandin synthesis induced by centrifugation or surface contact. J Cyclic Nucleotide Res 2:25, 1976.

Schiffman S, Lee P: Preparation, characterization and activation of a highly purified factor XI: evidence that a hitherto unrecognized plasma activity participates in the interaction of factors XI and XII. Br J Haematol 27:101, 1974.

Shapiro SS, Holburn RR: Pathophysiology of anticoagulants in hemophilia A and B. In Brinkhous K (ed): The Hemophilias. International Symposium (1968). Chapel Hill, University of North Carolina Press, 1970, p 141.

Sherry S: Fibrinolysis. Ann Rev Med 19:247, 1968.

Shoemaker WC, Carey JS, Yao ST, Morh PA, Printen KJ, Kark AE: Hemodynamic monitoring for physiologic evaluation, diagnosis and therapy of acute hemopericardial tamponade from penetrating wounds. J Trauma 13:36, 1973.

Solis RT, Gibbs MB: Filtration of microaggregates in stored blood. Transfusion 12:245, 1972.

Stormorken H: Relation of the fibrinolytic to other biological systems. Thromb Diathes Haemorrh 34:378, 1975.

Strauss HS: Acquired circulating anticoagulants in hemophilia A. N Engl J Med 281:866, 1969.

Swank RL, Connell RS, Webb MC: Dacron wool filtration and hypotensive shock: an electron microscopic study. Ann Surg 179: 427, 1974.

———, Edwards M: Microvascular occlusion by platelet emboli after transfusion and shock. Microvasc Res 1:15, 1968.

Umlas J: Fibrinolysis and disseminated intravascular coagulation in open heart surgery. Transfusion 16:460, 1976.

Verska JJ, Lonser ER, Brewer LA: Predisposing factors and management of hemorrhage following open-heart surgery. J Cardiovasc Surg (Torino) 13:361, 1972.

Walsh PN: Platelet coagulant activities and hemostasis: a hypothesis. Blood 43: 597, 1974.

Weiss HJ, Moyer LW: Von Willebrand factor: dissociation from antihemophilic factor procoagulant activity. Science 182:1149, 1973.

White JG: Effects of atropine on platelet structure and function. Scand J Haematol 6:236, 1969.

Wright ES, Sarkozy E, Harpur ER, et al: Plasma protein denaturation in extracorporeal circulation. J Thorac Cardiovasc Surg 44:550, 1962.

16. Neurologic Complications of Cardiac Surgery

Murray Budabin

Signs and symptoms of central nervous system dysfunction may be observed as untoward sequelae of almost any type of major surgery. However, the potential for and the incidence of such complications following intracardiac procedures performed with the assistance of extracorporeal circulation clearly occurs more frequently.

Both survival and the quality of the clinical result after open cardiac surgery with cardiopulmonary bypass depend on delivery of oxygen to the brain. More than any other organ, the brain epitomizes Haldane's dictum: "Anoxia does not only stop the machine, it wrecks it." With an obligatory aerobic metabolic requirement, the brain consumes 3 to 5 ml of oxygen/100 gm/min, or more than 20 percent of the total body oxygen consumption. Approximately 15 percent of the cardiac output is needed to deliver this oxygen requirement, although the brain accounts for only 2.5 percent of body weight.

Studies performed in the past 15 years indicated that postoperative neurologic complications had been encountered in 19 to more than 50 percent of cardiac surgical patients (Gilman, 1965; Tufo et al., 1970; Branthwaite, 1972; Gotze et al., 1980).* However, recent technical modifications in cardiopulmonary bypass (specifically, methods that reduce particulate and gaseous emboli) appear to have resulted in a significant decline in neurologic morbidity (Branthwaite, 1974, 1975; Bjork and Ivert, 1980).

ETIOLOGIC CONSIDERATIONS

Although present understanding is incomplete, a number of factors can be identified that contribute to cerebral dysfunction after cardiac surgery. Events that alter cerebral perfusion and metabolism by adversely affecting (1) regional distribution of blood flow, (2) pressure-volume relationships; and (3) blood characteristics (viscosity, gas-hemoglobin affinity, gas tensions, hematocrit, and pH) may be etiologic to either neurologic or behavioral abnormalities. The latter alterations, as will be discussed later, also may become manifest in the absence of any clearly defined neurologic dysfunction.

A number of predisposing factors frequently are present in cardiac patients that may contribute to reduced cerebral blood flow. Significant reduction of blood flow to the brain, apparently unrelated to intrinsic cerebral vascular disease, has been observed in patients with severe congestive heart failure, and it is not surprising that a higher frequency of postcardiotomy delirium has been related to severe preoperative cardiac disability

---

While the incidence of these complications in the various reported series would seem to be inordinately high, it must be appreciated that these data were derived by means of prospective attempts to evaluate systematically postperfusion nervous system dysfunction.

and reduced postoperative cardiac output (Blachly and Starr, 1964; Blachly and Kloster, 1966). It would also appear that older patients are particularly at risk, since there is evidence that the frequency of cerebral dysfunction after cardiac surgery is higher for them (Heller et al., 1970), particularly those over 50 years of age, and those with a history of a previous neurologic lesion even when there are no residual stigmata (Javid et al., 1969; Tufo et al., 1970; Branthwaite, 1972). The higher incidence of such abnormalities with advancing years suggests that coexisting cerebral arterial occlusive disease probably plays a significant role in reducing perfusion of the brain during cardiac surgery, particularly since it has been observed that general anesthesia itself (before sternotomy) may impose a 20 to 25 percent reduction of systemic blood flow in adult cardiac surgical patients (Litwak et al., 1972).

Precisely how preoperative neurologic damage increases the probability of postoperative cerebral dysfunction is unclear, although the frequent history of antecedent emboli in patients with chronic heart disease suggests the hypothesis that an established embolic cerebral vascular occlusive lesion sets the stage for a major intraoperative reduction in blood flow to that area of the brain supplied by the involved vessel. Recently, an attempt has been made to identify patients who have significant extracranial occlusive vascular lesions before open heart surgery and to perform carotid endarterectomy in patients considered at risk in selected cases (Budabin, 1980).

Specific operative factors of major importance in cerebral dysfunction states discerned after open intracardiac surgery are primarily related to either use of a pump-oxygenator or technical problems accompanying the surgical procedure. The direct exposure of blood to gas in nonmembrane oxygenators (particularly the commonly used bubble oxygenators) produces protein denaturation and fat globulinemia (Lee et al., 1971; Wright et al., 1963). Additional sources of fat globules derive from intrapericardial blood (that has pericardial fat floating on it), which is aspirated, returned to the pump-oxygenator, and thence to the patient (Caguin and Carter, 1963). It is noteworthy that trauma, including the operation per se, is also a common source of fat emboli (Peltier, 1968). Eighty percent of patients who die after open heart surgery have cerebral fat emboli (Hill et al., 1969).

A variety of nonfat emboli also may be generated by the pump-oxygenator. Aggregates of fibrin, platelets, and leukocytes (Allardyce et al., 1966; Ashmore et al., 1968; Osborn et al., 1970) or occasionally silicone emboli (Helmsworth et al., 1963) have been described. Recent evidence suggests that the use of prostacycline during the operation preserves platelets and platelet function, thereby decreasing the risk of embolization due to platelet aggregation (Longmore, 1980; Pokar et al., 1980). The incidence of nonfat emboli has been correlated directly with perfusion times of 90 minutes or longer (Hill et al., 1969), and it is noteworthy that use of Dacron wool filters in the bypass system has effectively prevented fibrin, platelet, and foreign body microemboli, although fat emboli still occur (Aguilar et al., 1971). Gas emboli originating from the perfusion system have been shown to occur, and a clear relationship of even minute amounts of air and subsequent brain damage has been well-documented (Fries et al., 1957).

A higher incidence of cerebral dysfunction (over half of the patients) has been noted when mean arterial blood pressures remained low during whole body perfusion (Javid et al., 1969; Tufo et al., 1970). When mean systemic arterial pressures remained below 40 mm Hg, clinically apparent cerebral dysfunction was three times that seen when the mean pressure level remained over 60 mm Hg, especially in older patients (over age 40). In these patients, even transient periods of hypotension (longer than 10 minutes) resulted in a cerebral damage rate four times that of an identical age group in which systemic pressures were maintained above 50 mm Hg. It is of interest that Kolka and Hilberman (1980) were unable to discern a significant difference between patients who did and did not manifest neurologic dysfunction when mean arterial pressures approximated 50 mm Hg in both groups. It is apparent that unless major deviations from normal perfusion pressure exist for a significant period of time, the incidence of neurologic complications is unlikely to be influenced by pressure per se.

Apart from the deleterious influence of whole body perfusion per se, certain intraoperative technical problems may occasionally contribute to cerebral dysfunction. These include problems of cannulation, such as obstruction of cerebral venous return with a poorly placed superior vena caval cannula or malposition of an aortic arch perfusion cannula. Intracardiac left heart pathology, such as dislodged fragments of either calcium from a valve or thrombotic material, continue to be occasional sources of brain damage. Finally, small quantities of air may remain trapped in the pulmonary veins or left heart at the termination of the operative procedure and be a source of cerebral dysfunction despite deliberate attempts to evacuate the air (Peirce, 1980; Stoney et al., 1980).

It may be concluded that most instances of neurologic dysfunction after open heart surgery result from a combination of predisposing and operative factors, the latter largely having to do with current methods of cardiopulmonary bypass. Superimposed intraoperative technical problems appear to influence significantly both the frequency and severity of such problems.

CLINICAL AND PATHOLOGIC CONSIDERATIONS

Mortality in those patients clinically identified as having sustained cerebral damage as a result of their cardiac surgical procedure is approximately 25 percent. In such cases, postmortem examination may demonstrate gross hemorrhages and infarcts scattered throughout the brain. Diffuse bilateral changes as well as areas of cortical infarction may be present on microscopic examination (Javid et al., 1969).

Paradoxically, equally symptomatic patients may fail to show any significant pathologic changes on routine microscopic examination. On the other hand, detailed neuropathologic study of the brains of cardiac surgical patients dying in the course of intracardiac surgery and bypass has demonstrated microscopic changes consisting of emboli, acute hemorrhages, and diffuse and focal neuronal necrosis in up to 85 percent of the entire postmortem population (Aguilar et al., 1971). It has thus been postulated that most patients undergoing intracardiac surgery and bypass have varying degrees of fat emboli in their brains (Hill et al., 1969).

Since the clinical incidence of organic brain syndromes does not correlate accurately with the plethora of neuropathologic findings, a considerable variability must exist between the presence of such structural lesions and their mode of clinical expression. In addition, the contribution of purely psychologic factors in the genesis of postcardiotomy behavioral disorders cannot be overlooked, although organic involvement of the central nervous system undoubtedly plays the major role.

DIAGNOSIS OF NEUROLOGIC COMPLICATIONS IN THE CARDIAC SURGICAL INTENSIVE CARE UNIT

Approximately 80 percent of neurologic complications occurring in cardiac surgical patients are evident at the time the patient is returned from the operating suite and are directly related to events in the surgical period. The remainder of the complications evolve in the postoperative unit as a consequence of primary cardiac, pulmonary, or renal dysfunction.

The importance of early diagnosis of neurologic complications in cardiac surgical patients is underlined by the frequency of convulsions that occur in the postoperative period. Approximately one out of every three noncomatose patients with neurologic lesions will have a seizure. For a small number of patients, seizure will be their sole initial sign that the central nervous system is involved. Grand mal, focal, or Jacksonian types of seizure activity present no problem in identification. However, focal or generalized muscle twitching in an otherwise alert patient may be confused with metabolic or electrolytic disturbances. Electroencephalography may be helpful in differentiating between these two classes of disorder.

Coma, stupor, and frank motor deficits are readily apparent and do not escape attention. However, more subtle signs of neurologic dysfunction, such as visual or sensory impairment and brainstem syndromes, may easily escape initial detection. In particular, confusional states and difficulty with communication may be overlooked. Agitation may be a mask for disorientation, and what is considered to be unwillingness to respond and to follow commands may be, in reality, an aphasic state. These patients and others who require a prolonged period to fully react after surgery should be carefully examined for neurologic deficits, because such symptoms may be signs of underlying cerebral dysfunction and may be harbingers of generalized seizures.

A few simple questions directed at ascertaining the postoperative patient's ability to understand commands and follow them, in addition to gauging the general level of his or her orientation, will serve to distinguish the presence of an organic mental syndrome from ordinary drowsiness or reaction to pain.

Coma is the most serious neurologic problem seen in cardiac surgical patients. Failure to awaken following the conclusion of the operative procedure carries a grave prognosis. More than likely, irreversible central nervous system damage has occurred. Because of the possibility that an occasional patient may have been hypersensitive to induction of anesthetic agents or that the condition is self-limited and reversible, it is wise to delay offering a prognosis for at least 24 hours. During that period, further examination (including the performance of laboratory tests at the bedside) may shed some light on the etiology of the coma. If the possibility of drug intoxication is seriously considered, the use of antagonist agents is advised.

DIAGNOSTIC EXAMINATIONS

Diagnostic examinations available at the bedside that may assist in establishing both neurologic diagnosis and prognosis in cardiac surgical patients include electroencephalography, lumbar puncture, and caloric testing. Tests such as radioisotope brain scanning and computerized transaxial tomography of the brain are not initially indicated or possible in the postoperative unit. This is true as well for contrast studies such as carotid or brachial angiography, which may be performed at a later period during the patient's course should such a need arise. Since the majority of the neurologic syndromes seen in cardiac surgical patients are the result of diffuse involvement of the brain on the microscopic or submicroscopic level, these latter examinations would be performed only if a mass lesion such as an abscess or a bleeding lesion such as an aneurysm is suspected. Angiography remains the only means of providing definitive information about the concurrent presence of intra- and extracranial vascular occlusive disease.

ELECTROENCEPHALOGRAPHY

This noninvasive laboratory test is probably the single most useful tool available for neurologic diagnosis in the cardiac surgical unit. All patients suspected of having sustained neurologic damage (in particular, those who exhibit lethargy or inappropriate behavior) should be so examined.

An abnormal electroencephalographic tracing is a compelling indication to initiate anticonvulsant therapy regardless of how innocuous the patient's symptoms may appear. Evidence of focal or diffuse cerebral dysfunction may be seen on such tracings. At times spike and wave patterns ordinarily seen in patients with seizure disorders may be demonstrated.

The electroencephalogram also may be useful in ascertaining the prognosis of comatose patients. So called "flat" tracings seen on two occasions 24 hours apart suggest "brain death."

LUMBAR PUNCTURE

Lumbar puncture need be performed only on selected patients where intercurrent hemorrhage or infection of the brain is suspected postoperatively. In view of the possibility of exciting traumatic bleeding in postperfusion patients or in those who are already anticoagulated, this procedure should be performed only by experienced persons. This caveat in no way should inhibit the performance of lumbar puncture where improvement fails to occur within a reasonable amount of time and the diagnosis of the nature of the neurologic dysfunction remains in doubt. Evidence of increased intracranial pressure obtained by this method may be an indication for the initiation of therapy (osmotically active agents such as mannitol, steroids, etc.) in cases of severe reactive cerebral edema.

CALORIC EXAMINATION

Caloric testing consists of introducing ice water into the external auditory canal of cardiac patients with neurologic problems to study the response of the oculomotor system. This is particularly valuable in the unresponsive patient in whom perverted responses suggest brainstem dysfunction. Absent response usually indicates that the prognosis will be unfavorable. The intact patient will respond by developing horizontal nystagmus of the eyes in the direction contralateral to the side stimulated. If the level of consciousness is reduced, the quick phases may be absent and replaced by a slow tonic deviation of the ipsilateral side.

MANAGEMENT

Apart from the use of hyperbaria in air embolism (Peirce, 1980), management of the neurologic complications of intracardiac surgery is both prophylactic and symptomatic. The goals are twofold: prevention of further sequelae as a result of seizures and restoration of neurologic functions secondary to central nervous system insult. The course of the majority of cardiac surgical patients who manifest neurologic complications is relatively benign, except those patients received in coma. However, the presence of postoperative low cardiac output or pulmonary or renal subsystem dysfunction may influence neurologic prognosis unfavorably. In most uncomplicated cases recovery may be a matter of days. An occasional patient with a hemiplegia may require a more extended period to recover. Permanent disability is more likely to occur when neurologic deficits have existed before cardiac surgery.

Seizure prophylaxis should begin immediately upon determination that neurologic damage has occurred. An initial dose of 200 mg of Dilantin should be administered intramuscularly and followed by 100 mg every eight hours during the patient's postoperative period. Phenobarbital and other sedative medications should be used cautiously until parameters of the level of consciousness are established.

Control of seizuring patients may be effected with intravenous Valium used in 10-mg intravenous doses or, in the case of status epilepticus, with a sodium amytal drip infusion. Curariform drugs must be immediately available. Additionally, endotracheal intubation and controlled mechanical ventilation should be continued until convulsions have been predictably eliminated and the patient is alert and cooperative.

An occasional refractory seizure disorder may require the additional use of Mysoline, which is available in oral and suppository form.

It has been suggested that steroids may be helpful in acute cases where widespread cerebral damage is suspected, particularly when prolonged unresponsiveness is encountered.

Physiotherapy should be started as soon as is practicable to forestall contractures and help mobilize the inert patient's extremities.

PSYCHIATRIC COMPLICATIONS*

Of all the psychiatric manifestations seen in the postoperative unit, the "postcardiotomy delirium" is the most striking. The psychotic state is characterized by illusions, hallucinations, and paranoid elaborations and usually appears after a two- to five-day lucid interval (Blachly and Starr, 1964). As originally described, its incidence ranged from 1 to 19 percent of patients (Heller et al., 1970). Since the occurrence of this postoperative psychosis was more often associated with improving cardiac function, environmental factors (as well as organic ones) were implicated in its etiology (Blachly and Kloster, 1966; Layne and Yudofsky, 1971). Sleep deprivation, the stress of postoperative intensive care, and failure to elicit the repressed anxiety of the cardiac surgical patients before their procedures were thought to contribute to this behavioral disorder. More recent studies have demonstrated a reduced incidence of postcardiotomy delirium that cannot be ascribed to psychologic or environmental manipulation (Heller et al., 1970). The most affected patients are those in older age groups, those more seriously ill, and those who have had previous neurologic insults. Controlled studies suggest that a likely primary cause of this psychiatric syndrome is a microvascular perfusion defect generated by factors inherent in the extracorporeal circulation system (Lee et al., 1969, 1971). Fortunately, most psychiatric manifestations observed in patients after cardiac surgery tend to be both subtle and transient.

Data on the effect of the traumata of open heart surgery employing extracorporeal circulation on intellectual function are inconclusive at this time. Several studies suggest that proper and uncomplicated operative conduct does not appear to significantly alter intellectual performance (Frank et al., 1972; Whitman et al., 1973). On the other hand, Åberg (1974) concluded that certain patients without clinically apparent cerebral complications exhibit impairment of intellectual function, particularly if perfusion time was prolonged. The possible influence of lengthy periods of cardiopulmonary bypass in diminishing *intellectual gains* after open heart surgery has been suggested by Frank et al. (1972). Åberg (1974) noted that the inclusion of a micropore filter in the arterial line (which presumably reduced the volume of microemboli to the brain) reduced the intellectual impairment of subjects studied postoperatively. Additional studies are required before definitive conclusions can be drawn about these matters.

REFERENCES

Åberg T: Effect of open heart surgery on intellectual function. Scand J Thorac Cardiovasc Surg 8:1, 1974.

Aguilar MJ, Gerbode F, Hill D: Neuropathological complications of cardiac surgery. J Thorac Cardiovasc Surg 61:676, 1971.

Allardyce DB, Yoshida SH, Ashmore PG: The importance of microembolism in the pathogenesis of organ dysfunction caused by prolonged use of the pump oxygenator. J Thorac Cardiovasc Surg 52:706, 1966.

Ashmore PG, Svitek V, Ambrose P: The incidence and effects of particulate aggregation and microembolism in pump oxygenator systems. J Thorac Cardiovasc Surg 55:691, 1968.

Bjork VO, Ivert T: Early and late neurological complications after prosthetic heart valve replacement. Second International Symposium on Psychopathological and Neurological Dysfunctions Following Open Heart Surgery, Milwaukee, March 1980.

Blachly PH, Kloster FE: Relation of cardiac output to postcardiotomy delirium. J Thorac Cardiovasc Surg 52:422, 1966.

Blachly PH, Starr A: Post-cardiotomy delirum. Am J Psychiatry 121:371, 1964.

Branthwaite MA: Prevention of neurological damage during open-heart surgery. Thorax 30:258, 1975.

⸺: Cerebral blood flow and metabolism during open-heart surgery. Thorax 29:633, 1974.

⸺: Neurological damage related to open-heart surgery. Thorax 27:748, 1972.

---

*An expanded discussion of these complications will be found in the next chapter.

Budabin M: Diagnosis and prevention of neurological complications in patients undergoing open heart surgery. Second International Symposium on Psychopathological and Neurological Dysfunctions Following Open Heart Surgery, Milwaukee, March 1980.

Caguin F, Carter NG: Fat embolization with cardiotomy with the use of cardiopulmonary bypass. J Thorac Cardiovasc Surg 46:665, 1963.

Frank KA, Heller SS, Kornfeld DS, Malm JR: Long-term effects of open-heart surgery on intellectual functioning. J Thorac Cardiovasc Surg 64:811, 1972.

Fries CC, Levowitz B, Adler S, Cook AW, Karlson KE, Dennis C: Experimental cerebral gas embolism. Ann Surg 145:461, 1957.

Gilman S: Cerebral disorders after open-heart operations. N Engl J Med 272:489, 1965.

Gotze P, Huse-Kleinstoll G, Speidel H: Psychopathological and neurological dysfunctions following open heart surgery: a review of the present state of research. In Psychic and Neurological Dysfunctions after Open-Heart-Surgery. Stuttgart, George Thieme Verlag, 1980.

Heller SS, Frank KA, Malm JR, Bowman FO Jr, Harris PD, Charlton MH, Kornfeld DS: Psychiatric complications of open-heart surgery. N Engl J Med 283:1015, 1970.

Helmsworth JA, Gall EA, Perrin EZ, Braley SA, Flege JB Jr, Kaplan S, Keirle AM: Occurrence of emboli during perfusion with an oxygenator pump. Surgery 53:177, 1963.

Hill JD, Aguilar MJ, Baranco A, Lanerolle P, Gerbode F: Neuropathological manifestations of cardiac surgery. Ann Thorac Surg 7:409, 1969.

Javid H, Tufo H, Najafi H, Dye WS, Hunter TA, Julian OC: Neurological abnormalities following open-heart surgery. J Thorac Cardiovasc Surg 58:502, 1969.

Kaplan S, Achtel RA, Callison CB: Psychiatric complications following open-heart surgery. Heart Lung 3:423, 1974.

Kolka R, Hilberman M: Neurological dysfunction following cardiac operation with low-flow, low-pressure cardiopulmonary bypass. J Thorac Cardiovasc Surg 79:432, 1980.

Kornfeld DS, Zimberg S, Malm JR: Psychiatric complications of open-heart surgery. N Engl J Med 273:287, 1965.

Layne OL Jr, Yudofsky SC: Postoperative psychosis in cardiotomy patients. The role of organic and psychiatric factors. N Engl J Med 284:518, 1971.

Lee WH, Brady MP, Rowe JM, Miller WC: Effect of extracorporeal circulation upon behavior, personality, and brain function: Part II, hemodynamic, metabolic, and psychometric correlations. Ann Surg 173:1013, 1971.

———, Miller W Jr, Rowe J, Hariston P, Brady MP: Effects of extracorporeal circulation on personality and cerebration. Ann Thorac Surg 7:569, 1969.

Litwak RS, Jurado RA, Lukban SB, Mitchell BA, Kahn M, Berger S, Estioko MR, Aledort L: Perfusion without donor blood. J Thorac Cardiovasc Surg 64:714, 1972.

Longmore D: The effects of prostacyclin on reducing cerebral damage following open heart surgery. Second International Symposium on Psychopathological and Neurological Dysfunctions Following Open Heart Surgery, Milwaukee, March 1980.

Osborn JJ, Swank RL, Hill JD, Aguilar MJ, Gerbode F: Clinical use of Dacron wool filter during perfusion for open heart surgery. J Thorac Cardiovasc Surg 60:575, 1970.

Peirce EC: Specific therapy for arterial air embolism. Ann Thorac Surg 29:300, 1980.

Peltier LF: A few remarks on fat embolism. J Trauma 8:812, 1968.

Pokar H, Bleese H, Fisher-Dusterhoff H, Gotze P, Huse-Kleinstoll G, Koedijk J, Prussman K, Tilsner V: Prevention of postoperative neurological disturbances after open heart surgery using prostacyclin—a clinical study. Second International Symposium on Psychopathological and Neurological Dysfunctions Following Open Heart Surgery, Milwaukee, March 1980.

Stoney WS, Alford WC, Burrus GR, Glassford DM, Thomas CS: Air embolism and other accidents using pump oxygenators. Ann Thorac Surg 29:336, 1980.

Tufo HM, Ostfeld AM, Shekelle R: Central nervous system dysfunction following open-heart surgery. JAMA 212:1933, 1970.

Whitman V, Drotar D, Lambert S, Van Heeckeren D, Borkat G, Ankeney J, Liebman J: Effects of cardiac surgery with extracorporeal circulation on intellectual function in children. Circulation 48:160, 1973.

Wright ES, Sarkozy E, Dobell ARC, Murphy DR: Fat globulinemia in extracorporeal circulation. Surgery 53:500, 1963.

17. Psychiatric Complications of Cardiac Surgery

Stuart H. Bartle

Despite improved perfusion techniques, psychiatric syndromes still occur with greater frequency in patients undergoing open heart surgery than is observed in those having general surgical procedures. One study made some years ago estimated the incidence of these syndromes to be less than 0.1 percent after general surgery, 15 percent after closed heart surgery, and 57 percent after open heart procedures (Abram, 1971). These data suggest an incidence far higher than that experienced by most cardiac surgical centers. However, it is essential to appreciate that major advances in heart-lung bypass methods (such as hemodilution, microfilters, etc.)* as well as better perioperative support of the cardiovascular system undoubtedly have been instrumental in sharply reducing the incidence of postcardiac surgical psychiatric syndromes in recent years.

If these syndromes are properly understood, preventive measures, diagnosis, and treatment can mitigate them and help in recovery and rehabilitation. The most dramatic and best known of these syndromes is *postoperative delirium*. Other names that have been used include postoperative psychosis, postcardiotomy syndrome or delirum, and ICU syndrome (Fox et al., 1954; Lazarus and Hagens, 1968; Dubin et al., 1979). Almost any psychiatric syndrome can occur under the nonspecific stress of surgery. *Depression, persistent postoperative pain,* and *anxiety,* however, are most characteristic of the recovery period following cardiac surgery and also will be discussed.

POSTOPERATIVE DELIRIUM

General Description and Etiology

Postoperative delirium is an acute psychotic state, almost always reversible (Lee et al., 1971), caused primarily by organic impairment of brain function. It is characterized by impairment of: (1) orientation; (2) short-term memory; (3) judgment; (4) all intellectual functions such as comprehension, learning, knowledge, and calculation; and, in addition, one sees (5) lability and shallowness of affect (Engel and Romano, 1959). Patients found to have increased susceptibility are those over 55 (Tufo et al., 1970); those with multiple valvular defects (Tufo et al., 1970); those whose mean pressure falls below 60 mm Hg for more than a brief period during cardiopulmonary bypass (Tufo et al., 1970); those with a history or the presence of organic brain syndrome (Morse and Litin, 1969; Tufo et al., 1970). Psychiatric factors associated with increased susceptibility include emergency surgery, a family history of psychosis, alcoholism, past or present depression, a history of functional gastrointestinal disorders, or a clinical

---

*Comprehensive discussion of these methodologic advances will be found in Chapter 5.

psychiatric description approximating a diagnosis of paranoid personality (Morse and Litin, 1969).

The initial insult appears to be neurologic, usually occurring during cardiopulmonary bypass, most likely secondary to microembolic phenomena (Blachly and Starr, 1966; Tufo et al., 1970).* In these cases, careful neurologic examination in the immediate postoperative period frequently will show a deficit, often a gross one (Tufo et al., 1970) not routinely detected because the patient's immobilization and endotracheal tube present obstacles to neurologic assessment. The minimal deficit is a cognitive one. People usually are ashamed of any defective thinking, however, and do not spontaneously disclose it. Conscious of a defect in their thought processes but feeling the need to hide this from the staff, their sense of isolation increases. They try to be hyperalert (to compensate for defective perceptual ability), causing further physiologic stress. They lose sleep and become more anxious, with increasing fears of losing control. If everything else goes well, they eventually may recover. They may succeed in hiding the defect from the staff and may even forget it themselves, although a high percentage of patients will recall some aberrant thinking before discharge (Blacher, 1971).

If, however, greater stresses are placed on people with certain preexisting psychologic sets, the process may go on to produce last-ditch psychologic defenses; i.e., paranoid delusions, hallucinations, and escape into a full-blown psychosis. Additional psychologic stress would result from: (1) drugs causing drowsiness and thus threatening alertness; (2) any complication that delays recovery and that can be misinterpreted as further evidence of imminent death or permanent disability; (3) an ICU environment preventing rest, with the resultant tremendous sensory overload (Kornfeld et al., 1965); (4) any perception or misperception of something occurring or heard on the ward, for example a patient's death, a misunderstood remark; (5) difficult communication because of a tracheostomy or aphasia, which prevents patients from getting their needs met, threatens their sense of control, and increases their sense of isolation; and (6) poor postoperative relationships with members of their family. The major preexisting psychologic factor that increases the stress on their defenses is the expectation of a bad outcome; this often results from identification with a relative or friend who has died after an operation, frequently based on unconscious fantasies of guilt and punishment.

Initially this syndrome was thought to follow a "lucid interval" of two to four days (Kornfeld et al., 1965), and emphasis was placed on events occurring in the ICU environment. Subsequently it has emerged that there is a high incidence of neurologic insult in these patients, and early postoperative mentation often is grossly disturbed (Blachly and Starr, 1966; Kimball, 1969; Tufo et al., 1970) but hidden from the staff. The pendulum, then, swung toward an organic explanation for the findings (Editorial, 1970). In all probability, however, delirium is a final common pathway for a heterogeneous mixture of organic, social-environmental, psychologic, and possibly even hereditary factors (Engel and Romano, 1959).

Treatment

Once delirium becomes obvious, treatment is considerably more difficult than if initiated at an early stage—or, even better, anticipated. The basic principle of treatment is to relieve the overwhelming anxiety that has conquered the patient's normal psychologic coping defenses.

1. A major tranquilizer is indispensible. The drug of choice is chlorpromazine because of its sedating qualities (important to the staff as well as to the patient), its ease of administration (IM is readily given) as well as its familiarity to the staff. Twenty-five mg, orally or intramuscularly, is given as an initial dose, which can be repeated in an hour if there is no

---

For more complete analysis of etiology, see the preceding chapter.

effect. Twenty-five to 50 mg every six to eight hours is an average dose, but this must be individualized. Orthostatic hypotension, the chief cardiovascular side effect, is usually transient, especially in these amounts (Nadelson, 1976). If the patient is too sedated, haloperidol, 1 to 2 mg, can be given every eight hours; this is a butyrophene and has less action on the cardiovascular system. Barbiturates should not be used. The minor tranquilizers such as diazepam and chlordiazepoxide usually do not help and may increase agitation. A psychiatrist familiar with postoperative delirium should be called at this point to help plan treatment.

2. The most effective treatment is based on understanding what patients are experiencing; since they fear that they are "crazy" and are going to die, they need repeated explanations that their experience is common, that problems can be handled and, most important, are transient (true, even though some may still have nocturnal confusion and decreased intellectual function at time of discharge).

3. The staff should try to remain calm and react with flexibility to the patient's unusual behavior. Patients easily perceive an attitude of fear, which intensifies their own fears of losing control. One of the hazards is that the staff may be oversensitized to *cardiac* patients who are agitated and seek stronger measures to quiet them. Restraints should only be a last resort.

4. Efforts should be made constantly to remind patients of every bit of progress they have made, to remind them of events that have happened or are about to (short-term memory is very poor).

5. Keep a clock and calendar in sight at all times to help maintain orientation.

6. Allow as much privacy as feasible.

7. Arrange for understanding family members to spend prolonged periods of time with patients, if they are comfortable with this.

8. Say nothing in or out of earshot that could be misinterpreted (medical terms such as heart failure or heart block can be terrifying to a layperson) (Blacher, 1972).

9. Be sure that they are treated as knowledgeable adults able to share details of their present condition and expectations with the staff. Even though they may appear grossly incompetent, at some level they will appreciate and respond to this with increased trust.

10. Inform the family of the problem, either directly or through the nurse-clinician or social worker assigned to the ward, so that they can understand and help rather than aggravate the problem.

It is not fully appreciated that delirium is truly terrifying to patients and can interfere with treatment and recovery (Cook, 1974). Patients who have progressed to or near psychosis have sustained a serious injury to their ego; they are humiliated, isolated, fearful that there is something terribly wrong with their mind, afraid that they have lost the ability to control themselves. They are afraid even to ask questions that might indeed even bring reassuring answers. They desperately need understanding help.

DEPRESSION

Etiology
Mild depression and withdrawal from staff and family is common, perhaps even normal, following transfer from the ICU and after discharge (Kimball, 1969). In the intense drama of the operation and the ICU all attention is focused on the patient, who, like an infant, seems to be the center of the universe. Suddenly all this support and attention seem to be taken away, losses that can create the setting for a depression. If now other factors are added, a more serious depression can result.

The most important stress contributing to this is the patients' perception that they are going to be far more limited postoperatively, physically, sexually, or economically than they had (rightly or wrongly) anticipated. It is important to note again the role of preoperative *denial* in this regard. For most people, denial is absolutely necessary to diminish anxiety and allow themselves to submit to the possibility of death or mutilation as a result of surgery. Thus, fantasies of a rapid and complete cure, though often held secretly, are common, and having to give them up can be a severe loss.

Serious depression is also particularly often found in patients who have formed an unconscious dependency on their illness and must now give it up; this is especially common if there is long-standing disease and consequent limitation of function, and a personality colored by having *used* the disease to relate to or control people in the environment. Severe financial load as a result of hospitalization can also provoke strong feelings of guilt and depression.

Treatment
Antidepressants are of little value and may complicate the clinical picture in a patient who may already be taking a good share of the pharmacopoeia. A discussion with a successfully rehabilitated patient often will relieve some doubts or fears. It is also helpful for a staff worker familiar with postoperative psychologic events to speak to the patient. A chair-at-the-bedside talk with the surgeon can clear up many misconceptions and also establish that the doctor is not afraid to talk to the patient. One extremely common fantasy is that the reason for the surgeon's often very brief bedside rounds is that he or she does not want to face the patient and is in fact trying to conceal a bad result. Another type helped by this bedside approach is the narcissistic patient (VIP's tend to fall into this category), who does not believe anything unelss it comes from the "top."

If these measures are not successful, the patient should be referred for consultation to a psychiatrist familiar with postoperative depression. Optimally a liaison psychiatrist making regular rounds on the ward would know and be known to the patient and be in an excellent position to help. Referral should be made in a nonjudgmental way, with the explanation that emotional reactions are part of the overall reaction to cardiac surgery, profound-

ly affect physiology, and, if understood, can help the staff and patient deal with the physiologic processes more constructively. Depression often can be detected preoperatively—sometimes it is obvious. If questioned, patients will state that they feel hopeless and that they are being pushed into surgery. A "giving up" syndrome (Engel and Schmale, 1967) is associated with an extremely high mortality in all phases of the recovery period; even survivors show either no improvement or a deterioration of function (Kimball, 1969). Postponement of the operation is essential in seriously depressed patients, many of whom may be acting out unconscious suicidal feelings.

PROLONGED POSTOPERATIVE PAIN

General Description
Continued pain out of proportion to any apparent physical cause occurs often and is extremely difficult for the staff to deal with because of the subjective nature of pain as well as the great number of possible sources after cardiac surgery. An angry, guilt-laden nontherapeutic relationship between staff and patient often results, in which the staff can come to hate the patient who threatens their identity as "healers." Under these conditions the staff often make minor "mistakes" resulting in inconvenience to the patient; increasing rigidity in interpreting rules or allowing the patient to ignore them are further reactions as the staff become more defensive. Medical staffs may be too afraid of the addiction potential in narcotic, pleasure-giving drugs over a short time. They will then either give inadequate doses or withhold them for too long a time. Conversely, some physicians feel that their patients should feel no pain at all and will err on the side of creating unrealistic expectations. Both positions lead to conflict when pain is prolonged.

Etiology
There are several common types of pain-prone people (Engel, 1959): (1) those who

become addicted to narcotics; (2) those who retain or develop a compensation neurosis; (3) those with pain as part of a posttraumatic neurosis or as a somatic expression of anxiety, anger, or depression; (4) those who get secondary gain from the perpetuation of psychoneurotic pain, i.e., more attention or more control of their environment.

The last three types overlap a good deal in personality and etiology; they are much more commonly seen in patients with long-standing heart disease, rheumatic or congenital in etiology, than in coronary artery disease, which has usually not been mainfest for many years before surgery is contemplated. The many years of days and nights spent fearing death, feeling dependent on others to alleviate suffering, perhaps even to preserve life, can solidify a dependent character structure; anxiety may then be easily provoked by the need to become independent. Compensation neurosis is an escape from independence, though patients are unconscious of this, as they are of their use of pain to control the environment. Posttraumatic neurosis pain is an expression via the sensorimotor system of the unconscious hurt that patients feel was done to them; the pain may thus express *anger* at the surgeon (on another level displaced from a parent), *anxiety* about what was done to them, or can represent a *depressive* equivalent.

Treatment

A common mistake is to give a placebo. This offers no help in differential diagnosis; because of the powerful effect of suggestion, a placebo almost always works, no matter what the underlying reason for the pain. But, if exposed, it represents a breach of trust that alienates the patient and is difficult to reverse because of the humiliation felt by the patient. The staff's fear that the patient is manipulating them and does not really need medication to cure the pain is valid only in the case of the previously addicted person; this can be detected, though it should rarely be necessary to do it, by the intravenous injection of a narcotic antagonist to produce classic withdrawal signs in minutes.

The cardinal principle, however, is to recognize that, whatever the reason for the pain, it is real to the patients and they are not aware of the psychologic mechanism causing them to perceive increased amounts of pain above that suffered by others with equal (or more) apparent organic cause. If the staff understand this, it is possible to avoid the customary contretemps mentioned above. This can be accomplished by staff conferences allowing open ventilation of feelings and attended preferably by a psychiatrist or other persons trained in postoperative medical psychologic problems. It may be necessary, if the problem persists, to get direct psychiatric consultation; individual, group, or family therapy may be indicated, depending on the etiology.

ANXIETY

Anxiety is a psychobiologic reaction to any threat to the self (Cannon, 1915), to a physical threat, as in surgery or combat, or to a psychologic one, as seen in stage fright, for example. The *heart* is the center of our self (Meyer et al., 1961; Blacher, 1972). Imagery abounds to document this: "broken" hearts, hearts "stopping" from either fear or love, a vice president is "one heartbeat" from the presidency, heart "strain" has long been thought to lead to death. Thus, heart surgery, especially when the heart is actually stopped and opened, is enormously frightening in a profound, even unconscious, way (Abram, 1965). No amount of technical explanation can completely allay this fear.

For a person to function adequately under the threat of death, it is necessary to *deny* this threat by some psychologic mechanism (Becker, 1973). The most effective denial is achieved by action; the combat soldier and the astronaut who face unknown terrors keep physically and mentally active in preparing for their ordeal. Surgical patients cannot be physically active; they are sick (or at least are in the "sick" role) and must remain passive, trusting others to care for them and cure them.

Thus, cardiac surgery patients are unique in their (1) enormous anxiety because of fear of death; (2) inability to take action themselves and, therefore, need to submit themselves to others; and, further, (3) realization that their operated-on heart has to function immediately to sustain life, contrary to the entrenched lay belief in the need for *rest* after any stress; cardiac patients often are afraid to do anything that would put a "strain" on their heart.

These three factors need special attention from the staff. (1) Fear of death is constantly present and patients need reassurance even if they do not verbalize it, especially in the preoperative period and postoperatively if complications occur. (2) Any patient who has problems in trusting others is especially vulnerable in the postoperative period to psychologic problems. For example, many hard-driving executives need to feel they can control their environment themselves and are threatened by having to rely on nurses and others. They should be informed as much as possible about what is happening or about to happen in an effort to give them a sense of control. They are apt to be especially threatened in the early postoperative period because of the necessity to submit to multiple, urgent procedures. (3) "Strain" anxiety will appear particularly when medical care is decreased suddenly, as in transfer from the ICU or upon news of imminent discharge. Most patients err on the side of not doing enough because of the "strain" factor. Many have fantasies that their chest or heart sutures will come apart if they exert themselves. Again, these fantasies can be handled by encouraging communication, by helping patients bring out questions they may be ashamed to ask.

DISCUSSION

The most effective way to reduce the incidence of postoperative psychologic problems is to anticipate them. Preoperative discussions should take advantage of the fact that well-informed patients require less narcotics and are discharged earlier than others (Egbert, 1964). The preoperative discussion should aim at giving the patient ways to actively help in the recovery process. Also important, they need to confront a realistic view of the probable postoperative course and of the ultimate benefit from the operation. They should not be permitted to keep a blanket denial that everything is going to be quick and easy, tempting as this may be for the surgeon. Rebounds from total denial are far worse than if the patient is psychologically prepared.

Janis has referred to the "work of worrying" as important emotionally in psychologic coping (1958, 1974). Specific reassurances are more effective after patients have expressed their anxieties. Blanket reassurances act as a cutoff to further discussion and may increase anxiety, particularly postoperatively, when followed by the surgeon or staff member walking away from the worried patient; often a specific, open answer (but not one exposing previously unknown dangers to the patient) would allow anxiety to subside, by clearing up a misapprehension.

REFERENCES

Abram HS: Psychiatric reactions after cardiac surgery—a critical review. Semin Psychiatry 3:70, 1971.

⸻: Adaptation to open heart surgery: a psychiatric study of response to the threat of death. Am J Psychiatry 122:659, 1965.

Becker E: The Denial of Death. New York, Free Press, 1973.

Blacher RS: The hidden psychosis of heart surgery. JAMA 222:305, 1972.

⸻: Open-heart surgery: the patient's point of view. Mount Sinai J Med 38:74, 1971.

Blachly PH, Starr A: Treatment of delirium with phenothiazine drugs following open heart surgery. Dis Nerv Syst 27:107, 1966.

⸻, ⸻: Post-cardiotomy delirium. Am J Psychiatry 121:371, 1964.

Cannon WB: Bodily Change in Pain and Rage. New York, Appleton-Century-Crofts, 1915.

Cook F: The operation was a success but the patient died. NY Magazine, Nov. 18, 1974.

Dubin WR, Field HL, Gastfriend DR: Postcardiotomy delirium: a critical review. J Thorac Cardiovasc Surg 77:586, 1979.

Editorial: Open Heart surgery and the psyche. JAMA 212:1370, 1970.

Egbert LD, Batit GE, Welch CE, Bartlett MK: Reduction of postoperative pain by encouragement and instruction to patient. N Engl J Med 270:825, 1964.

Engel G L: Psychogenic pain and the pain-prone patient. Am J Med 26:899, 1959.

———, Romano J: Delirium, a syndrome of cerebral insufficiency. J Chronic Dis 9:260, 1959.

———, Schmale AH Jr: Psychoanalytic theory of somatic disorder: conversion, specificity, and the disease onset situation. J Am Psychoanal Assoc 15:344, 1967.

Fox JM, Rizzo NO, Clifford S: Psychological observations of patients undergoing mitral surgery. Psychosom Med 16:186, 1954.

Janis IL: Psychological Stress. New York, Wiley, 1958. Reprinted, New York, Academic Press, 1974.

Kimball CP: The experience of open heart surgery. III. Toward a definition and understanding of postcardiotomy delirium. Arch Gen Psychiatry 27:57, 1972.

———: Psychological response to the experience of open heart surgery: I. Am J Psychiatry 126:348, 1969.

Kornfeld DS, Zimberg S, Malm JR: Psychiatric complications of open-heart surgery. N Engl J Med 273:287, 1965.

Lazarus HR, Hagens JH: Prevention of psychosis following open heart surgery. Am J Psychiatry 124:1190, 1968.

Lee WH, Brady MP, Rowe JM, Miller WC Jr: Effects of extracorporeal circulation upon behavior, personality, and brain function. Part II: Hemodynamic, metabolic, and psychometric correlations. Ann Surg 173:1013, 1971.

Meyer BC, Blacher RS, Brown F: A clinical study of psychiatric and psychological aspects of mitral surgery. Psychosom Med 23:194, 1961.

Morse RM, Litin EM: Postoperative delirium: a study of etiological factors. Am J Psychiatry 126:388, 1969.

Nadelson T: The psychiatrist in the surgical intensive care unit. I. Postoperative delirium. Arch Surg 111:113, 1976.

Tufo HM, Ostfeld AM, Shekelle R: Central nervous system dysfunction following open heart surgery. JAMA 212:1933, 1970.

18. Infections Associated with Open Heart Surgery

Burt R. Meyers   Roy A. Jurado

The incidence of infections after operations on the heart and great vessels has diminished steadily through the years (Amoury, 1972; Conte et al., 1972; Dismukes et al., 1973; Clark et al., 1976). However, infection, particularly prosthetic valve endocarditis, remains one of the most dreaded complications because of its frequently devastating sequelae. Specifically, the morbidity and mortality associated with such complications remain high (Peirce et al., 1970; Slaughter et al., 1973; Dismukes et al., 1973; Wilson et al., 1975; Karchmer et al., 1978; Rossiter et al., 1978; Richardson et al., 1978; Masur and Johnson, 1980).

Infections associated with cardiac surgery are caused by a variety of bacterial, fungal, viral, and protozoal organisms (Table 18–1). It has been estimated that, after cardiac surgery, the total wound infection rate (superficial and deep) is approximately 7 percent and the total nosocomial infection rate varies between 15 and 50 percent (reviewed by Clark et al., 1976). The incidence of prosthetic valve endocarditis has been estimated to be 2 to 3 percent (reviewed by Clark et al., and Watanakunakorn, 1979) with a mortality of 73 and 45 percent for early (infections occurring within two months of the operation) and late (infections occurring two months or longer after operation) endocarditis, respectively (Watanakunakorn).

This chapter will confine itself to discussions of the pathogenesis, diagnosis, and management of *major* infective complications of open heart surgery. In the interest of brevity, discussions of superficial wound infections and infections accompanying closed cardiac operations will not be included.

PATHOGENETIC MECHANISMS IN CARDIAC SURGICAL INFECTIONS

In simple terms, a surgical infection is the result of a disturbance of the exquisite balance that normally exists between a host (patient), his or her local and systemic defense mechanisms, and the environment, which is laden with a wide variety of microorganisms, all with infection-producing potential. This delicate balance may be disturbed if the systemic host resistance is decreased or, more commonly, if the local host defense mechanisms are depressed, as occurs in operative and traumatic wounding. Surgical infections may result

TABLE 18–1 INFECTIONS ASSOCIATED WITH OPEN HEART SURGERY

I. Prosthetic Valve Endocarditis
   A. Bacterial
   B. Fungal
II. Intravascular—Mycotic Aneurysm
III. Local
   A. Wound Infections
   B. Sternal Osteomyelitis, Sternal Dehiscense
   C. Mediastinitis
IV. Viral
   A. Hepatitis A, B, "non-A-non-B"
   B. Cytomegalovirus Infection
   C. Epstein-Barr Virus Infection
V. Pulmonary Infections
   A. Aspiration Pneumonia
   B. Bacterial Pneumonia; Empyema
   C. Tracheitis, Bronchitis
VI. Urinary Tract Infections
VII. Vascular Catheter Induced Infection (Bacterial or Fungal)
VIII. Protozoal: Transfusion-Induced Malaria

from the introduction of the offending organisms from without (exogenous) or from invasion by organisms normally harbored by the host (endogenous) when the latter's defense mechanisms are depressed or overwhelmed. Environmental control measures—which include, among other things, asepsis, antisepsis, air filtration, and use of antimicrobial agents—are designed to help maintain the balance in the host's favor so that no infection develops.

Environmental Factors

Using the classification devised by the National Academy of Sciences—National Research Council cooperative study on postoperative wound infections (Report of NAS—NRC, 1964), most cardiac operations can be categorized as "refined-clean" (i.e., elective, primary closure, no entry into the gastrointestinal or respiratory tract, no break in technique). As originally proposed, the classification was based on estimation of the amount of bacterial contamination occurring at the time of operation—accepting the premise that bacterial contamination is a prerequisite for wound infection. According to established criteria, "refined-clean" operations have the lowest degree of bacterial contamination. In the National Research Council cooperative study, there was a definite correlation between the degree of bacterial contamination occurring at the operation and the infection rate. The infection rate was *lowest* in "refined-clean" operations and highest in "dirty" operations.

Although most cardiac operations are "refined-clean," published reports indicate that operations entailing the use of cardiopulmonary bypass generally result in infection rates higher than the rate reported for surgical procedures in general (Altemeier, 1970). Several factors unique to open intracardiac operations may explain this difference. For instance, it is known that the larger number of personnel necessary for the conduct of such procedures and the increased intensity of personnel activity and traffic within the operating room contribute significantly to the amount of air-borne contamination (Blakemore et al., 1971). The conduct of cardiopulmonary bypass itself provides multiple avenues for microbial inoculation as blood circulates in the extracorporeal circuit. Repeated exposure of pump-oxygenator blood, banked donor blood, and intravascular catheters (Kluge et al., 1974) all have been identified as definite exogenous sources of contamination. In addition, the use of coronary suction units for recovery of blood shed on the operative field permits entry of ambient air, with its potential contamination, into the extracorporeal circuit (Blakemore et al., 1971).

The duration of the operation also appears to be of primary importance. A striking relationship has been noted between increasing duration of surgery and increasing infection rate that appears to be independent of other factors known to influence wound infection rate (Report of NAS—NRC, 1964). This is obviously of relevance, since most operations requiring the use of cardiopulmonary bypass entail a comparatively longer period of time for completion. While other factors related to the duration of the operation might be at play, it is known that airborne bacteria constitute a large inoculum in an open wound. It has been shown that as many as 30,000 to 40,000 organisms could fall into a three to four square meter sterile field of a major operation every hour (Sompolinsky et al., 1957), although stringent operating room environmental control measures could substantially reduce the amount of airborne contamination (Laufman, 1973a, 1973b, 1975; Clark et al., 1976).

Impairment of Host Defense Mechanisms

There is evidence that the use of extracorporeal circulation may impair host defense mechanisms. Cardiopulmonary bypass has been noted to cause leukopenia and produce certain morphologic, metabolic, and functional alterations in leukocytes (Kusserow and Larrow, 1968; Kusserow et al., 1969). Kusserow et al. have observed leukocyte morphologic changes ranging from total cellular disintegration and frank loss of cytoplasm to sublethal damage, including distortion and confluence of the lobes of the granulocytes, hyaloid transformation, homogenization of the nuclear substance, and vacuolization of the nucleus. The same group of investigators (Kusserow and Larrow; Kusserow et al., 1971) also observed decreased oxygen uptake and glucose utilization in leukocytes after perfusion. Since both oxygen and glucose play important roles in intracellular energy-producing processes, it has been suggested that derangements in oxygen and glucose utilization may be responsible for the impairment of leukocyte phagocytic capability observed by Kusserow et al. (1969).

It is also known that extracorporeal circulation produces denaturation of globulins and other serum proteins (Lee et al., 1961; Pruitt et al., 1971). Hairston et al. (1968) reported a significant depression in bactericidal capacity for *S. aureus* and *E. Coli* of the sera of eight patients after pump-oyxgenator perfusion, and the degree of depression was proportional to the duration of perfusion. The same investigators (Hairston et al., 1969) observed depletion of complement (total complement and complement fraction) and decrease in immunoglobulins with concomitant reduction in serum bactericidal capacity in 35 patients undergoing cardiopulmonary bypass. It is believed that the depletion of complement and immunoglobulins may be the direct consequence of plasma protein denaturation occurring during perfusion (Hairston et al., 1969).

In addition, Subramanian et al. (1968) reported defective clearance of bacteria by the reticuloendothelial system after perfusion in experimental animals. More recently, Silva et al. (1974) observed transient defects in phagocytic function in patients undergoing cardiopulmonary bypass.

From the foregoing, it appears that there is strong support for the belief that the use of cardiopulmonary bypass may compromise host resistance and increase susceptibility to microbial invasion.

Use of Intracardiac or Intravascular Prostheses

Operations requiring the use of prosthetic materials for intracardiac repair are associated with a higher incidence of infection (Denton et al., 1957; Lord et al., 1961; Barney et al., 1962; Geraci et al., 1963; Herr et al., 1965; Amoury et al., 1966; Peirce et al., 1970) than those procedures in which no foreign body is implanted (Engelman et al., 1973a). These observations are in complete accord with a body of experimental data showing that host resistance is decreased while susceptibility to infection is increased when foreign bodies are present (summarized by Alexander et al., 1967; Everett, 1970).

Intrinsic contamination of the implanted prosthesis is a potential source of endocarditic infection. Implantation of porcine xenograft prostheses contaminated by *Mycobacterium chelonei* has been reported to produce *M.*

chelonei infection in at least two patients (Laskowski et al., 1977; Levy et al., 1977).

General Factors

Advanced age (over 65 years), severe malnutrition, extreme obesity, the presence of infection remote from the operative site, and chronic steroid therapy have each been shown to be associated with higher infection rates, independent of other known adverse factors (Report of NAS—NRC, 1964).

The cardiac surgical patient is also constantly exposed to the infection hazards of anesthesia equipment (Duncalf, 1973), ventilators (Dreyden, 1968), blood and pooled blood products, and the intensive care unit (Northey et al., 1974; Rosendorf et al., 1974).

Many patients with native valve endocarditis now undergo valve replacement even in the presence of active infection, when the offending organisms may still be present in valvular vegetations or annular tissue. Although the overall incidence of infection of the newly implanted prosthesis by the original infecting organism is low (estimated to be 5 percent), certain infections (e.g., *Pseudomonas aeroginosa, Serratia marcescens,* and various *Candida* species) may be extremely difficult to eradicate (Sarot et al., 1970; English and Ross, 1972; Arbulu et al., 1972; Turnier et al., 1975; Mills and Drew, 1976; Stinson et al., 1976). Thus, valve replacement carried out in the presence of an active infectious process caused by one of these organisms imposes an added risk, albeit small, of prosthetic valve infection.

A number of devices used in the perioperative period, including arterial lines, atrial and central venous catheters, peripheral venous catheters, pulmonary artery catheters, cardiac pacemaker electrodes, endotracheal tubes, ventilators, and Foley catheters, may be sources of contamination and bacteremia (Stein et al., 1966; Conte et al., 1972; Sande et al., 1972; Dismukes et al., 1973; Kluge et al., 1974). A newly implanted intracardiac prosthesis may then become infected, although postoperative bacteremia does not always result in endocarditis (Sande et al., 1972).

In summary, patients undergoing open intracardiac operations are a subgroup at high risk of developing postoperative infection. In these patients, the natural host defense mechanisms are frequently impaired as a result of both underlying disease and the operative procedure. Further, the required surgical procedure, because of its duration and complexity, may involve the hazard of significant exogenous bacterial contamination. Moreover, intracardiac repair may entail the use of significant amounts of foreign prosthetic material.

PREVENTION OF INFECTIVE COMPLICATIONS

Maintenance of Microbiologic Cleanliness

In essence, maintenance of microbiologic cleanliness in the operating room is the cornerstone to surgical infection control. This is especially true in operations requiring the use of cardiopulmonary bypass where, for the reasons just discussed, the host resistance may be severely compromised. Attainment of this goal requires strict adherence to the elements of a multifaceted program designed to minimize the degree of exogenous and endogenous contamination during the intraoperative period. The basic components of the program are: (1) proper operating room design; (2) reliable air-filtration and air-handling systems; (3) proper operating room sterilization and cleaning procedures; (4) stringent traffic control and containment measures; (5) use of impervious, waterproof gowns and drapes; (6) identification of carriers; and (7) maintenance of a high level of staff discipline. For a more comprehensive treatment of the subject, the reader is referred to the published reports of Laufman (1973a, 1973b, 1975, 1979), Scannell et al. (1975), Clark (1976), and the American College of Surgeons (1976).

While the patient appears to be most vulnerable during the intraoperative interval, it must be remembered that the intensive care unit and its personnel are also important sources of nosocomial infection. Thus, maintenance of the same level of discipline and bacteriologic awareness in the intensive care unit as in the operating room is an essential component of infection control.

Supplementing Host Resistance: The Concept of Preventive Antibiotic Action

A number of investigators have reported a reduction in the incidence of clinical infections after open intracardiac operations if antibiotic therapy was initiated preoperatively and continued into the postoperative period (Slonim et al., 1963; Reed, 1965; Nelson et al., 1965; Amoury et al., 1966). Slonim et al., in a prospective randomized study, observed a significant increase in the incidence of infection after open heart surgery if antibiotic therapy was not employed. Of significance was the observation that the infection rate was lowest in those patients in whom antibiotic therapy was initiated in the preoperative period and continued postoperatively, but remained high in those in whom antibiotic administration was not started until after the operation. Unfortunately, the study had to be aborted before a large cohort could be enrolled because of a dramatic rise in postoperative infection rate. When the code was broken, it was noted that most infective complications occurred in patients who received no antibiotics.

Parallels can be drawn between the above clinical observations and the experimental studies of Miles (1956); Miles et al. (1957), Burke and Miles (1958), and Burke (1961). Miles et al. observed that the development of an experimental bacterial lesion is determined by the effectiveness of the host's nonspecific antibacterial defense mechanisms in the tissue at or shortly after the time of inoculation. Burke and Miles demonstrated that the host defense mechanisms began to act the instant the bacterial inoculum arrived and that there was a period of intense, effective antibacterial activity beginning at the moment of contamination and ending three to four hours after the arrival of bacteria, even though the anatomic bacterial lesion continued to develop in the sense of classic inflammation for 20 hours or longer. This early interval of intense activity on the part of the host had been termed by Miles the "decisive period in defense against bacterial invasion."

Subsequent studies by Burke (1961) demonstrated that administration of antibiotics, shortly before or after bacterial inoculation, suppressed experimental infections. The antimicrobial agents provided maximal protection when administered before the bacteria gained access to the tissue, but provided no protective effect when begun beyond three hours after bacterial inoculation. These experimental observations suggested the distinct possibility that certain interventions, when properly timed, may effectively supplement the host's natural defense mechanisms to bacterial inoculation so that no infection develops.

In a later report, Burke (1973) established certain principles based on the above experiments that are applicable to the prevention of infection in clinical surgery. First, the prevention of bacterial infection is, in large measure, dependent on the effectiveness of the natural defense mechanisms of the host. Second, host resistance is reduced by the stress and traumata of anesthesia and the operative procedure itself. Third, the risk of developing infection can be reduced and, in certain instances, infection prevented if the host's antibacterial resistance is supplemented before bacterial contamination of the tissue occurs. Fourth, if delivered beyond three hours after the end of the period of active bacterial contamination, interventions designed to supplement host resistance serve no useful purpose.

Thus, the concept of *preventive antibiotic management* in surgery can once more be stated, in Burke's (1973) own words, as follows:

> Preoperative preventive antibiotics are indicated if there is a high probability that the patient's natural resistance to bacterial invasion will not overcome the combined bacterial and physiologic challenge posed by a surgical procedure. Further, the antibiotic substance used

to supplement host resistance must be circulating at high concentrations in the patient's tissue before contaminating bacteria arrive.

The Question of Prophylactic Antibiotics.
Although the controversy remains unresolved, the practice of prophylactic antibiotic therapy has become commonplace in cardiac surgery. Proponents consider the large body of experimental data and clinical observations reviewed in the preceding sections as supportive of their view. On the other hand, those who argue against prophylactic antibiotics contend that its efficacy has never been conclusively demonstrated in a prospective randomized study involving a large number of patients and, further, that most reports frequently cited in support of prophylactic antibiotics involved retrospective analyses of data and had serious shortcomings (reviewed by Goldmann et al., 1977). The prospective randomized studies of Slonim et al. (1963) and Goodman et al. (1968) were both aborted before large cohorts could be enrolled, preventing any firm conclusions from being drawn.

It has also been pointed out by opponents that the use of prophylactic antibiotics may alter normal bacterial flora and promote the growth of antibiotic-resistant organisms that could then overwhelm the host. This is certainly a distinct possibility with prolonged, injudicious administration of antibiotics; however, there is evidence that a short course of prophylactic antibiotics is both effective (in preventing endocarditis) and safe (Goldmann et al., 1977). While conceding that incontrovertible statistical proof of the efficacy of prophylactic antibiotic therapy is still lacking, proponents consider the significant morbidity and high mortality associated with prosthetic valve endocarditis sufficient justification to continue the practice (Geraci et al., 1963; Nelson et al., 1965; Reed, 1965; Amoury et al., 1966; Stein et al., 1966; Yeh et al., 1967; Firor, 1967; Goodman et al., 1968; Carey and Hughes, 1970; Baffes et al., 1970; Shafer and Hall, 1970; Okies et al., 1971; Conte et al., 1972; Slaughter et al., 1973; Wilson et al., 1975). It is possible that the controversy may never be fully resolved to the satisfaction of most because of the complex ethical and moral issues involved in conducting a carefully designed, controlled prospective randomized study involving a large number of patients.

At present, the controversy on prophylaxis notwithstanding, the Cardiothoracic Surgical Service at our institution places patients undergoing intracardiac operations on a program of prophylactic antibiotics (preventive antibiotic management may be a more appropriate term to use). Adults are given cefazolin, while a combination of penicillin and gentamicin is employed in infants. When penicillin or cephalosporin hypersensitivity is present or suspected, a combination of vancomycin and gentamicin is preferred. Following Burke's concepts (1961, 1973), antibiotic administration is begun the night of surgery, continued the morning of the operation and immediately after it, and then maintained for five days postoperatively.

In a study comparing cefamandole and cephalothin prophylaxis in patients undergoing prosthetic valve replacement, Archer et al. (1978) demonstrated higher antibiotic levels in right atrial tissue obtained with the former. On a priori grounds, cefamandole would seem to be the "better" antibiotic; however, whether higher tissue levels translate into better protection remains to be seen.

IMPORTANT INFECTIVE COMPLICATIONS OF OPEN INTRACARDIAC OPERATIONS

Prosthetic Valve Endocarditis
General Considerations. Infection of a prosthetic valve remains one of the most dreaded complications of cardiac valve replacement because of its frequently devastating sequelae. It has been estimated that it occurs in approximately 2 percent of patients in whom prosthetic replacement of cardiac valves is performed (Watanakunakorn, 1979). Important differences in pathogenesis, microbiolo-

gy, and prognosis make it useful to classify prosthetic valve infections according to the time period in which the disease occurs (Block et al., 1970; Dismukes et al., 1973). Prosthetic valve infections occurring within two months of surgery are classified as "early," while infections occurring two months or longer after valve implantation are classified as "late." There is some evidence that the incidence of early prosthetic valve endocarditis has decreased significantly in recent years, but that of late prosthetic valve endocarditis has not. The overall mortality of prosthetic valve endocarditis remains high, with the prognosis for early prosthetic valve endocarditis significantly worse than that for the late infections. Early prosthetic valve endocarditis is associated with a mortality of approximately 73 percent, while late endocarditis has a mortality of 45 percent (reviewed by Watanakunakorn, 1979).

Infections involving the prosthetic aortic valve also have decreased in recent years and now occur about as often as infections of the prosthetic mitral valve; this was not the case in the early years of heart valve replacement when aortic involvement was more common. The risk of developing infective endocarditis appears to be higher after multiple valve replacement than after single valve implantation (Watanakunakorn, 1979).

Pathogenesis. The potential sources of infection accompanying open intracardiac operations have been discussed extensively in preceding sections of this chapter and need not be repeated here. It is believed that early prosthetic valve endocarditis results from contamination occurring during the perioperative period. Early endocarditis may also be associated with other infective complications occurring postoperatively, such as sternal wound infections, pneumonia, or urinary tract infection. The organisms involved in early prosthetic valve endocarditis tend to be more virulent (see Microbiology).

In contrast, the pathogenetic mechanism in late prosthetic valve endocarditis is frequently difficult to determine. While most cases of late prosthetic valve endocarditis caused by *Streptococcus* species may be attributable to dental and genitourinary procedures (Dismukes et al., 1973; Wilson et al., 1975; Quenzer et al., 1976), the source may not be readily apparent in certain cases of *Staphylococcus aureus* endocarditis and in infections caused by organisms of normally low virulence (i.e. *Staphylococcus epidermidis,* diphtheroids, certain *Candida* species).

Microbiology. Compared to native valve endocarditis, the microbiologic spectrum in prosthetic valve endocarditis is significantly different (Watanakunakorn, 1977). In native valve endocarditis, streptococci (predominantly *S. viridans*) are the offending organisms in approximately 50 percent of cases, while staphylococci (mostly *S. aureus*) account for approximately 20 percent of infections. In contrast, staphylococcal organisms (predominantly *S. epidermidis*) are the infecting agents in approximately 40 percent of all cases of early and late prosthetic valve endocarditis, while streptococci are responsible for approximately 22 percent of cases. Gram-negative bacteria and fungi together account for approximately 24 percent of early and late prosthetic valve infections (reviewed by Watanakunakorn, 1979). These organisms rarely are found in cases of native valve endocarditis, except in patient populations with a high rate of intravenous drug abuse (Ramsey et al., 1970; Linde and Rao, 1973; Stimmel et al., 1973).

S. epidermidis emerges as the single most important organism, accounting for more than 24 percent of *all* cases of early and late prosthetic valve infections (reviewed by Watanakunakorn, 1979). Approximately one half of the cases of early prosthetic valve endocarditis are caused by virulent organisms (*S. aureus,* gram-negative bacilli and fungi). In contrast, organisms with relatively low pathogenic potential *(Streptococcus* species and *S. epidermidis)* account for 60 percent of cases of late prosthetic valve endocarditis. In a more recent report, summarizing the experience at one university hospital, *S. epidermidis* was the infecting agent in 48 percent of patients and was the most common cause of early and late prosthetic valve endocarditis (Masur and Johnson, 1980).

Pathology. The annular tissue on which the prosthetic valve is seated is usually the primary site of the infectious process with involvement of the overlying endocardium and adjacent tissues. An annular abscess is frequently present (Madison et al., 1975; Arnett and Roberts, 1976), which may extend to adjacent tissues, including the conduction system. Partial detachment of the prosthetic valve sewing ring from the infected annular tissue with paravalvular leakage occurs much more commonly with the aortic valve, while formation of vegetations with obstruction tends to occur more frequently with the mitral valve (Colvin et al., 1965; Cheng et al., 1970; Suri et al., 1971; Arnett and Roberts, 1976; Anderson et al., 1977). Mycotic aneurysms may also form (Madison et al., 1975; Arnett and Roberts, 1976) and occasionally the aortotomy site may be involved in the infective process (Ostermiller et al., 1971).

Clinical Picture. The clinical manifestations of early and late prosthetic valve endocarditis are similar (reviewed by Watanakunakorn, 1979): *fever* and the presence of *new regurgitant or changing murmurs* are the two most common clinical findings. Almost all patients have fever, but new or changing murmurs are heard in only half of the patients (Amoury et al., 1966; Stein et al., 1966; Dismukes et al., 1973; Wilson et al., 1975). When present, the classical signs of subacute bacterial endocarditis (petecchiae, Osler's nodes, Janeway's lesion, and Roth's spots) are helpful in establishing the diagnosis, but they are often absent. *Splenomegaly,* which is found in approximately 35 percent of all patients, is more commonly seen in late than early prosthetic valve endocarditis. Approximately 10 percent of patients have evidence of systemic *embolization:* surgical removal of emboli from easily accessible peripheral arteries frequently allows a precise microbiologic diagnosis to be established. The diagnosis of fungal endocarditis has been made in this manner in a number of cases (Lawrence et al., 1971; Harford, 1974; Kammer and Utz, 1974, Upshaw, 1974).

Approximately half of the patients with prosthetic valve endocarditis show *leukocytosis* (Amoury et al., 1966; Stein et al., 1966; Dismukes et al., 1973; Wilson et al., 1975). The leukocyte count tends to be elevated in infections caused by pyogenic organisms such as *S. aureus* (Watanakunakorn and Baird, 1977), but may be normal in endocarditic infections caused by less virulent organisms such as *S. viridans* (Tan et al., 1973). Anemia in the early postoperative period can be due to a number of noninfective causes; as such, the significance of its presence is often difficult to interpret.

Signs and symptoms of heart failure may predominate the clinical picture. When present, a regurgitation murmur around prosthetic valves may provide the only diagnostic clue. The patient may also present with signs of prosthetic valve obstruction (Anderson et al., 1977).

The clinical diagnosis is based primarily on the presence of the triad of fever, new regurgitant or changing murmurs, and leukocytosis. Microbiologic confirmation is obtained when the offending organism is isolated from the blood stream. In cases of untreated prosthetic valve endocarditis, the blood cultures are, with a few exceptions, usually persistently positive. Not infrequently, bacteremia or fungemia may be the only finding in a febrile patient. It should be remembered, however, that sustained bacteremia occurring in the early postoperative period does not necessarily signify endocarditis, especially if a definite noncardiac focus of infection is identifiable, no murmur is heard, and the bacteremia is due to a gram-negative bacillus (Sande et al., 1972). Moreover, gram-negative bacteremia due to contaminated intravenous infusions has been reported (Dumas et al., 1971) and *Erwinia* species has been isolated from unused intravenous infusion bottles (Meyers et al., 1972). On the other hand, blood cultures are often negative in cases of prosthetic valve endocarditis caused by fungal organisms, especially *Aspergillus* species (Ostermiller et al., 1971; Hall, 1974; Kammer and Utz, 1974; Seelig et al., 1974), and certain fastidious organisms such as diphtheroids, *Serratia,* and *Hemophilus* species may take a few days to grow in standard culture media. Thus, in patients with fungal endocarditis and negative blood cultures, the definitive diagnosis may be established only after histologic and microbiologic examination of peripheral emboli or excised heart valve.

Although angiography may be required to provide radiographic documentation of a paravalvular leak, fluoroscopy and cinefluoroscopy have been found to be helpful in detecting prosthetic valve malfunction and abnormal valve motion (i.e., rocking) suggesting dehiscence (Stinson et al., 1968; Ellis et al., 1973; Masur and Johnson, 1980). In addition, echocardiography and combined echophonocardiography may help to demonstrate obstruction or paraprosthetic leak (Brodie et al., 1976; Strunk et al., 1977). However, echocardiography may be of limited value in detecting vegetations in prosthetic valve endocarditis (Dillon, 1977).

Management. The identification and isolation of the offending organism is essential to therapeutic success. The management program is determined by the type of infecting organism and its antimicrobial susceptibility and by the knowledge of the natural history of infections caused by the organism. Not infrequently, however, the clinical situation dictates that antimicrobial therapy be begun before a precise microbiologic diagnosis is on hand. Thus it is helpful for the staff to be familiar with the clinical characteristics of commonly encountered infections and to have a working knowledge of the antimicrobial susceptibilities of common pathogens (Table 18–2) and the therapeutic doses of available antimicrobial agents (Table 18–3).

Following isolation of the offending organism, appropriate in vitro antibiotic sensitivity tests are carried out. A *bactericidal antibiotic* is then chosen according to the results of the in vitro antibiotic sensitivity test against cultures of the offending organism. It is mandatory to perform these sensitivity tests, since an organism may show unexpected resistance to a particular antibiotic.

High doses of the specific bactericidal antibiotic are administered and the intravenous route is recommended to insure reliable drug absorption and reproducible serum levels of the antibiotic. Once antibiotic therapy has begun, it is essential to have insight into *serum bactericidal activity* so that the actual amount of antibiotic to be administered can be determined with a greater degree of precision. A sample of the patient's serum, obtained approximately 30 minutes after the last dose and before the next scheduled dose, is tested for bactericidal activity against the isolated organism. The organism is inoculated into serially diluted samples of the patient's serum, and the bactericidal level is determined from the highest serum dilution (i.e., lowest concentration of antibiotic) required to kill the organism. In practice, the antibiotic dosage schedule is adjusted to achieve a serum antibiotic concentration that is at least four times greater than that required to kill the organism in vitro or peak serum bactericidal titer (drawn 45 to 90 minutes after antibiotic administration) of at least 1:16. Determinations of serum bactericidal titers are of great importance because in vitro bactericidal levels do not faithfully mirror serum bactericidal activity.

The management of patients with prosthetic valve endocarditis is most difficult. The mortality remains high with a significantly worse outlook for early infections, presumably because patients tend to be in a poorer general state of health soon after cardiac surgery. Some patients (up to 25 percent) are cured with antibiotic therapy alone (Amoury et al., 1966; Block et al., 1970; Wehr and McCall, 1972), and there is suggestive, albeit not firm, evidence that xenograft valve endocarditis may be more easily sterilized—with medical therapy alone—than mechanical prosthetic valve endocarditis (Rossiter et al., 1978). However, most patients require a com-

TABLE 18–2 COMMON PATHOGENS AND ANTIBIOTIC SENSITIVITIES

Gram-Positive Bacteria	Antibiotics
Staphylococcus aureus: penicillin-resistant	Semisynthetic penicillins (Oxacillin, Nafcillin), Cephalothin, Cefamandole, Vancomycin, Clindamycin
Staphylococcus epidermidis	Any of the above if strains are sensitive. Rifampin in combination with above.
Streptococcus species	
1. B-hemolytic Group A	Penicillin, Erythromycin, Clindamycin
2. Group D (*Enterococcus* sp.)	Penicillin or Ampicillin + Aminoglycoside, Vancomycin + aminoglycoside, Piperacillin
3. Other groups and anaerobic species	Penicillin, Cephalosporin, Cephamycins, Erythromycin, Clindamycin, Vancomycin
Diplococcus pneumoniae	Penicillin, Cefamandole, Cefazolin, Cefoxitin, Erythromycin, Clindamycin
Diphtheroid species	Penicillin or Penicillin + aminoclycoside, Rifampin, Cephalothin, Cefamandole
Clostridial species	Penicillin, Tetracycline, Clindamycin, Chloramphenicol, Cefoxitin, Cefamandole
Gram-Negative Microorganisms	**Antibiotics**
Escherichia coli	Ampicillin, Cefamandole, Cefazolin, Cefoxitin, Piperacillin, Gentamicin, Tobramycin
Klebsiella species	Cefamandole, Cefoxitin, Gentamicin, Tobramycin, Chloramphenicol, Tetracycline, Piperacillin
Enterobacter species	Tobramycin, Gentamicin, Cefamandole, Piperacillin, Chloramphenicol
Proteus species—indole positive	Carbenicillin, Ticarcillin, Cefamandole, Cefoxitin, Gentamicin, Aminoglycoside, Chloramphenicol, Piperacillin
Serratia species	Tobramycin, Gentamicin, Aminoglycoside
Pseudomonas species	Gentamicin, Aminoglycoside, Piperacillin, Carbenicillin, Ticarcillin
Other aerobic gram-negative species	
1. *Acinetobacter*	Tobramycin, Gentamicin
Bacteriodes: other gram-negative anaerobic rods	Clindamycin, Cefoxitin, Cefamandole, Chloramphenicol, Tetracycline
Candida species, *Aspergillus* species	Amphotericin-B, 5-Fluorocytosine, Miconazole, Ketaconazole

bined approach: antibiotic therapy *plus* surgical removal of the infected prosthesis, with correction of the accompanying hemodynamic defect. Indeed, it has been suggested by many that all patients with prosthetic valve endocarditis should be candidates for early removal and replacement of the infected prosthesis except those with uncomplicated streptococcal infections (Arnett and Roberts, 1976; Saffle et al., 1977; Karchmer et al., 1978; Rossiter et al., 1979; Masur and Johnson, 1980).

The optimal duration of antimicrobial therapy remains a controversial issue. In the absence of incontrovertible evidence demonstrating superiority of one regimen over others, all current practices can only be considered empirical. In practice, antibiotics are given for six to eight weeks, regardless of whether they are being managed with antimicrobials alone or with combined therapy. Whenever possible, operations for removal of infected prostheses are deferred to a time when the patient has attained an optimally

TABLE 18–3 USUAL DAILY DOSE OF ANTIBIOTICS IN PATIENTS WITH NORMAL RENAL FUNCTION

Antibiotic	Total Dose	Route
Penicillin (Pen Vee) (V-cillin K)	2 to 24 million units in 4 to 8 divided doses 600,000 units Pro Pen q 12 h	IV IM
Cephalothin, cephalosporin (Keflin)	8 to 12 grams in 4 to 8 divided doses	IV
Cefazolin (Kefzol; Ancef)	4 to 8 grams in 6 to 8 divided doses	IV or IM
Cefamandole (Mandol)	4 to 12 grams in 4 to 6 divided doses	IV IM
Cefoxitin (Mefoxitin)	4 to 12 grams in 4 to 6 divided doses	IV IM
Cephalexin (Keflex)	2 to 4 grams in 4 divided doses	PO
Clindamycin phosphate (Cleocin)	1,200 to 3,000 mg in 4 to 6 divided doses	IV or IM
Ampicillin (Polycillin) (Principen) (Omnipen) (Penbritin)	4 to 12 grams, in 4 divided doses 4 grams, in 4 divided doses	IV PO
Erythromycin (Erythocin Lactobionate) (Ilotycin Gluceptate)	2 to 4 grams in 4 divided doses	IV
Oxacillin (Prostaphlin) (Nafcillin) (Unipen)	8 to 12 grams in 4 to 8 divided doses 2 to 4 grams	IV or IM PO
Piperacillin (Avocin)	8 to 24 grams in 4 to 6 divided doses	IV (Continued)

TABLE 18–3 USUAL DAILY DOSE OF ANTIBIOTICS IN PATIENTS WITH NORMAL RENAL FUNCTION (Cont.)

Antibiotic	Total Dose	Route
Vancomycin (Vancocin)	2 grams in 4 divided doses	IV
Tetracycline	2 grams in 4 divided doses	IV or PO*
Amikacin (Amikin)	15 mg/kg q 8 or 12 h	IV
Streptomycin	1 to 2 grams q 12 h	IM
Tobramycin	5 mg/kg in 3 divided doses	IM or IV
Gentamicin (Garamycin)	5 mg/kg in 3 divided doses	IM or IV
Chloramphenicol (Chloromycetin)	4 grams in 4 divided doses	IV†
Kanamycin	1 gram in 2 divided doses	IM
Carbenicillin (Geopen) (Geocillin)	40 to 60 grams in divided doses or continuously 4 to 8 grams in divided doses	IV PO
Ticarcillin (Ticar)	20 to 40 grams in 6 divided doses	IV
Trimethoprim-sulfamethoxazole (Bactrim) (Septra)	80/400 mg bid	PO
Amphotericin-B (Fungizone)	1 mg/kg qod	IV‡
5-Flurocytosine (Ancobon)	50 to 150 mg/kg	PO
Miconazole	50 to 150 mg/kg	IV

*Use with caution at the upper dose level.
†Fatal aplastic anemia (presumed to be idiosyncratic) has been caused by this compound. Its use should be restricted to life-threatening situations when other antibiotics are not useful.
‡Patient should be tested with 1 mg initially and final dose achieved in stages.

stable condition (e.g., cardiac failure and sepsis under control). Usually, these operations can be conveniently performed during the second or third week of antibiotic therapy, following which antibiotic therapy is continued and maintained until the prescribed six- to eight-week course has been completed.

Apart from other considerations, early operative intervention in prosthetic valve endocarditis is deemed prudent under the following conditions: (1) moderate to severe heart failure secondary to paravalvular leakage or prosthetic valve malfunction; (2) persistent bacteremia under adequate appropriate antibiotic therapy; (3) endocarditis caused by organisms resistant to available antibiotics; (4) evidence of invasive infection with involvement of the conduction system and aortic root structures (mycotic aneurysm formation); (5) repeated major embolization; (6) fungal or yeast infection; and (7) relapse of prosthetic valve endocarditis. There is accumulating evidence that prompt removal and replacement of infected prostheses may offer the best chance for survival and cure in most patients (Arnett and Roberts, 1976; Saffle et al., 1977; Karchmer et al., 1978; Rossiter et al., 1978), except those with uncomplicated streptococcal infections (Masur and Johnson, 1980).

Prophylaxis. Compared to the general population, patients with prosthetic valves are at a greater risk of developing endocarditic infections. In this sense, they may be likened to patients who have an abnormal endocardium. Patients with prosthetic valves appear to be particularly vulnerable during periods of bacteremia when the prosthesis may be colonized. Certain procedures are known to be accompanied by transient bacteremia (Everett and Hirschmann, 1977) and prosthetic valve endocarditis has been reported to occur after dental and genitourinary manipulations (Dismukes et al., 1973; Wilson et al., 1975; Quenzer et al., 1976), procedures known to produce bacteremia.

There is evidence that administration of antibiotics immediately before induction of bacteremia prevents the development of endocarditis in experimental animals (Durack and Petersdorf, 1973; Pelletier et al., 1975). Thus, it is recommended that patients with a prosthetic valve should receive appropriate antibiotic prophylaxis shortly before undergoing procedures associated with a significant risk of bacteremia (e.g., dental procedures, tonsillectomy, genitourinary operations or instrumentations, gastrointestinal operations) and in the presence of a remote infection. Certain guidelines for prophylaxis have been suggested and the reader is referred to the report of the Committee on Prevention of Rheumatic Fever and Endocarditis of the American Heart Association for details (Kaplan et al., 1977).

Postoperative Mediastinal Infection

General Considerations. Median sternotomy has been widely used for intracardiac surgery for more than two decades. Without doubt, it is the most commonly used incision in cardiac surgery and it is not surprising that it has gained universal acceptance. The incision affords the surgeon rapid access to and excellent exposure of the heart and great vessels, facilitates institution of cardiopulmonary bypass, and permits the performance of most cardiac procedures. Moreover, it allows for expeditious closure and its complication rate does not differ from that of other thoracic incisions (Nelson and Nelson, 1967).

With the steady increase in the number of cardiac operations (and, therefore, of median sternotomy incisions) performed, it is remarkable that the incidence of postoperative sternal and mediastinal infections has remained low. It has been reported to be between 0.5 and 5 percent (Nelson and Nelson, 1967; Jimenez-Martinez et al, 1970; Ochsner et al., 1972; Engelman et al., 1973a; Thurer et al., 1974; Grmoljez et al., 1975). When it occurs, however, postoperative mediastinal infection must be viewed as a serious complication and should be treated aggressively. It is potentially life-threatening because of the possibility of extension to cardiotomy and aortotomy suture lines (Bryant et al., 1969), prosthetic grafts, patch materials, and the increased likelihood of prosthetic endocarditis associated with it (Amoury, 1972).

Pathogenesis. Analysis of reports in the literature (Brown et al., 1969; Ochsner et al., 1972; Sanfelippo and Danielson, 1972a, 1972b; Thurer et al., 1974; Grmoljez et al., 1975) reveals that certain perioperative factors play a role in the development of major sternotomy complications (i.e., mediastinitis or sternal dehiscence). Brown et al. found a higher incidence of major sternotomy complications in patients in whom the sternum was improperly divided, reoperation was mandated by postoperative bleeding, external cardiac massage was performed postoperatively, prolonged assisted ventilation with tracheostomy was necessary, and postoperative cardiac output was low. The authors emphasized the importance of making a "clean cut" of the sternum, as this contributes to a firm and stable closure.

Sanfelippo and Danielson (1972a, 1972b) reported similar findings. They found that reoperation for postoperative bleeding, resuscitative external cardiac massage, prolonged mechanical ventilation, and the presence of a tracheostomy were all associated with an increased incidence of incisional complications. In addition, they reported that the use of nylon bands for sternal closure was accompanied by a threefold, fourfold, and eightfold increase in wound complication, dehiscence, and major infection rates, respectively (1972b). In their series, postoperative low cardiac output was not accompanied by a significant increase in wound complications.

Ochsner et al. (1972) alluded to the adverse effects of external cardiac massage, mechanical ventilatory assistance, and reoperation for bleeding, while emphasizing the importance of technical precision in making the incision and wound closure.

Engelman et al. (1973a) identified prolonged operative and perfusion times, along with low postoperative cardiac output, as important etiologic factors. Other conditions found to predispose to sternal and mediastinal infection were reoperation for bleeding, postoperative closed chest massage, and pneumonitis. It was also noted that the incidence of postoperative mediastinitis in patients undergoing myocardial revascularization procedures was three times higher than those having procedures not involving coronary artery bypass grafting. Eleven of 17 patients (65 percent) with mediastinitis had had myocardial revascularization. A possible explanation for this difference may have been that nearly all 11 patients had severely impaired myocardial function preoperatively, with 8 of 11 patients developing low cardiac output for a protracted period postoperatively. The prolonged operative and perfusion times were brought about primarily by poor cardiac reserve and the need for circulatory assistance postrepair. It is also pertinent to mention that almost half (8 of 17) of their patients required a tracheostomy in the early postoperative interval, perhaps reflecting further the advanced state of cardiac dysfunction present in their patients before surgery.

To summarize, the conditions known to predispose to the development of postoperative mediastinal sepsis can be broadly categorized as follows: (1) those that increase the likelihood of intraoperative mediastinal contamination (prolonged operation, reoperation, bleeding, tracheostomy); (2) those that promote sternal instability (technical imprecision, external cardiac massage, prolonged mechanical ventilatory assistance); and (3) those that impair host defense mechanisms and reduce resistance to infection (prolonged operation, prolonged cardiopulmonary bypass).

A wide variety of gram-positive and gram-negative bacteria and fungi can cause postoperative mediastinal sepsis. While the initial involvement may be primarily soft tissue, the infectious process could eventually involve sternal bone or costal cartilage.

Clinical Features. The presence of infection is usually heralded by persistent fever and leukocytosis, which are followed by the appearance of wound drainage or sternal instability or separation. Rarely, the signs of septic shock may predominate. The chest roentgenogram is frequently nonspecific, but may confirm the presence of sternal separation.

The clinical diagnosis usually can be made without difficulty. The offending organism is isolated from cultures of the wound drainage or mediastinal exudate.

Therapy. The therapeutic mainstays are the prompt institution of systemic bactericidal or fungicidal therapy, mediastinal drainage, sternal stabilization, and continuous mediastinal lavage with a nontoxic antimicrobial solution. Choice of the systemic antimicrobial agent is dictated by the cultures, and the dosage schedule is determined according to the guidelines described earlier (see Prosthetic Valve Endocarditis, Management).

The mediastinum is promptly explored to carry out sternal debridement, evacuate detritus and necrotic debris, place irrigating and drainage catheters, and restore sternal stability (Bryant et al, 1969). The sternum is debrided to bleeding, healthy bone. All exudate and necrotic material is evacuated and the subcutaneous tissue and skin are debrided as well. Regular mediastinal and pleural drainage tubes are positioned in appropriate locations and brought out through the skin via separate stab incisions. Irrigating catheters are positioned in the superior mediastinum and similarly brought out through the skin. The sternum is securely reapproximated with No. 5 monofilament wire suture. The subcutaneous tissue and skin are usually closed as a single layer employing heavy gauge nonreactive material.

Continuous irrigation is begun immediately after mediastinal exploration. A number of antimicrobial solutions have been used for mediastinal lavage (Bryant et al., 1969; Ochsner et al., 1972; Engelman et al., 1973a), but the method described by Thurer et al. (1974) appears to produce the best results. Thurer et al. used 0.5 percent povidone-iodine solution for continuous irrigation. Povidone-iodine appears to have the desirable properties of being bactericidal and fungicidal and nontoxic in the concentration recommended. In contrast, there have been reports of serious toxic reactions (Gruhl, 1971) and emergence of resistant fungal and bacterial infections following use of antibiotics for irrigation (Wray et al., 1973).

In summary, there is evidence that continuous mediastinal irrigation with povidone-iodine is a safe and effective method of therapy for postoperative mediastinal sepsis. The best results are obtained when this is combined with systemic antimicrobial therapy, mediastinal drainage and debridement, and restoration of thoracic cage integrity.

Postpericardiotomy Syndrome

General Considerations. The *postpericardiotomy syndrome* is a benign, self-limited, febrile illness, of still uncertain etiology, commonly complicating operations involving pericardial entry. In its classical form, it is characterized by *fever* and *signs of pericardial* and sometimes *pleural involvement* during the second or third postoperative week, with the illness lasting from one to four weeks. The syndrome does not specifically affect surgical outcome and is not in itself responsible for increased mortality. It is an important cause of postoperative morbidity, but its clinical significance stems primarily from the fact that it could render the differential diagnosis of more life-threatening conditions causing postoperative fever—such as endocarditis, mediastinitis, pneumonia, and septicemia—more difficult.

The incidence of this postoperative complication has been reported to be between 1 and 60 percent (Elster et al., 1954; Ito et al., 1958; Engle and Ito, 1961; Uricchio, 1963; Drusin et al., 1965; Engle and Marx, 1965; Engle et al., 1975; Livelli et al., 1978). This wide variability in the reported incidence reflects the nonspecific nature of the signs and symptoms of the disease and the lack of uniform criteria for diagnosis.

Pathogenesis. The exact pathogenetic mechanism remains unresolved. A number of the earlier theories have been discarded because of lack of supporting evidence. In the original description by Soloff et al. (1953), it was suggested that reactivation of rheumatic fever was responsible for the febrile illness seen after mitral commissurotomy *(postcommissurotomy syndrome)*. However, this theory largely has been debunked due to lack of supportive bacteriologic, serologic, and histologic evidence for an active rheumatic process (Elster et al., 1954; Epstein, 1957; Larson, 1957; Uricchio, 1963) and because of the occurrence of the syndrome in patients who never had rheumatic heart disease (Ito et al., 1958).

Inflammatory reaction to blood in the pericardial space also has been suggested as a possible causative factor (Ehrenhaft and Taber, 1952; Tabatznik and Isaacs, 1961). An intensive inflammatory response has been observed after the injection of autogenous blood and lipids into the pericardial cavity of dogs (Ehrenhaft and Taber). While this may explain the initial febrile response following the extravasation of blood into the pericardium, it does not account for the recurrent nature of the syndrome.

Dressler (1956) described a recurrent pericarditic illness developing in some patients after myocardial infarction. The clinical manifestations of postmyocardial infarction (Dressler's) syndrome are similar to those seen in the postpericardiotomy syndrome. The postpericardiotomy syndrome also has been reported following penetrating stab wounds of the chest (Segal and Tabatznik, 1960), nonpenetrating chest trauma (Goodkind et al., 1960), and percutaneous left ventricular puncture for measurement of intracardiac pressure (Peter et al., 1966). It is interesting to note that a feature common to these conditions and cardiac surgery is the presence of myocardial tissue damage.

An autoimmune mechanism was originally proposed by Ito et al. (Ito et al., 1958; Engle and Ito, 1961). These investigators suggested the possibility that the inflammatory response might be triggered by an immunologic reaction to damaged autologous tissue in the pericardial cavity. Subsequently, Robinson and Brigden (1963) and Van der Geld (1964) demonstrated the presence of antiheart antibodies in some patients with postpericardiotomy syndrome, lending some credence to the autoimmune theory. However, these findings are at variance with those of Gery et al. (1960) and Heine et al. (1966). Gery et al. found heart antibodies in the sera of patients with different forms of heart disease who did not develop the postpericardiotomy syndrome. In addition, Heine et al., in a study of 71 patients with recent myocardial infarction, found circulating antibodies to be increased in all patients, but only one patient exhibited the clinical manifestations of postpericardiectomy syndrome.

Meanwhile, Engle et al. (1974), in a prospective double-blind study, demonstrated high titers of heart-reactive antibody, using an indirect immunofluorescent technique, in the serum of patients in whom the postpericardiotomy syndrome developed after intraperi-cardial surgery. They noted a close correlation between the presence of high antibody titers and the clinical syndrome, and suggested that the demonstration of the antiheart antibody in high titer may provide a laboratory confirmation of the syndrome.

More recently, the same group of investigators (Engle et al., 1975) reported the results of a prospective triple-blind study that was designed to determine whether an autoimmune response or a viral infection or both were involved in the pathogenesis of the postpericardiotomy syndrome. Of 257 patients, heart-reactive antibody in high titer appeared in 62 (24 percent), all of whom had the clinical manifestations of the syndrome. None of the 102 patients with no heart-reactive antibody had the syndrome. Among 137 patients tested for titers to one or more viral agents (adenovirus, Coxsackie B, and cytomegalovirus), a significant rise and then a drop in titer occurred in 31. Twenty-one of 31 patients (68 percent) who exhibited a rise and fall in viral titer had positive antiheart antibody and the postpericardiotomy syndrome. The results of the study raised the possibility that an immunologic response and viral illness may be related to the postpericardiotomy syndrome. Years earlier, Kahn et al. (1967) had suggested the possibility of a viral etiology after they were able to isolate parainfluenza virus from a group of patients with the postpericardiotomy syndrome.

None of the theories advanced so far has gained widespread acceptance. The exact roles of the heart-reactive antibody and viral infection remain to be determined. These and other issues related to the pathogenesis of postpericardiotomy syndrome require further study.

Clinical Features. Signs of pleuropericardial inflammation dominate the clinical picture. In its classic form, fever, with diaphoresis but without chills, appears suddenly during the second or third postoperative week after a seemingly normal postoperative course. Sometimes the febrile illness merges with the temperature elevation normally seen in the early postoperative period, so that the patient appears to have a prolonged febrile course.

Pericardial involvement is indicated by retrosternal or precordial chest pain that frequently radiates to the neck, shoulders, and interscapular area and is made worse by recumbency or deep inspiration. Dyspnea, nonproductive cough, or arthralgia may also be present.

A pericardial friction rub is frequently audible. Signs of pericardial or pleural effusion also may be present. During the febrile period, moderate leukocytosis and neutrophilia are common findings. The electrocardiogram may show changes consistent with pericarditis or pericardial effusion. The chest roentgenogram may show an enlarged cardiac silhouette, consistent with the presence of pericardial effusion, and evidence of pleural effusion. Echocardiography confirms the presence of pericardial fluid.

The diagnosis is suggested by the clinical picture and is established by exclusion of other postoperative febrile illnesses. The absence of hepatosplenomegaly, atypical lymphocytosis, and rising viral titers rule out the *postperfusion syndrome*. The diagnosis of infective endocarditis is not likely in the absence of positive blood cultures.

Managment. Therapy is nonspecific and purely symptomatic and supportive. Antiinflammatory-antipyretic-analgesic agents are the therapeutic mainstays. Acetysalicylic acid and its congeners are usually effective in bringing about symptomatic relief. Thoracentesis or pericardiocentesis may be required to drain significant accumulations of fluids.

Where symptoms are severe or fail to be controlled by salicylates, the use of corticosteroids may bring about dramatic relief, with relief of pain and disappearance of fever (Engle and Ito, 1961).

Postperfusion Syndrome

General Considerations. The *postperfusion syndrome* is a postoperative febrile illness that is sometimes confused with the postpericardiotomy syndrome, though pericarditis is not featured. It is less common than the postpericardiotomy syndrome and is known to be caused by a viral infection transmitted by homologous blood transfusions (discussed later). It has been reported to occur in 3 to 11 percent of patients undergoing open heart surgery (Seaman and Starr, 1962; Wheller et al., 1962; Smith, 1964; Reyman, 1966; Paloheimo et al., 1968). The occurrence of the triad of *fever, splenomegaly,* and *lymphocytosis,* with many atypical forms, is characteristic of the syndrome; hepatomegaly is sometimes present. Chest pain, arthralgia, and neutrophilia are absent.

In the classic form, the postperfusion syndrome appears two to six weeks after cardiopulmonary bypass. Like the postpericardiotomy syndrome, it is a self-limited illness that runs a benign course.

Pathogenesis. There is evidence that the syndrome is caused by infection by a number of antigenically similar herpes viruses—specifically cytomegalovirus and the Epstein-Barr (EB) virus. Several investigators have provided serologic and virologic evidence of cytomegalovirus infection associated with the syndrome (Kääriäinen et al., 1966; Embil et al., 1968; Lang et al., 1968; Paloheimo et al., 1968; Lang and Henshaw, 1969). Gerber et al. (1969) provided serologic and virologic evidence of primary EB virus infection associated with the postperfusion syndrome in patients undergoing open heart surgery. Infection by CMV appears to be more common than EB virus infections (Henle et al., 1970).

There is ample evidence that both the cytomegalovirus and the EB virus can be transmitted through the transfusion of blood harboring the infective agents (Embil et al., 1968; Lang et al., 1968; Paloheimo et al., 1968; Foster and Jack, 1969; Lang and Henshaw, 1969; Henle et al., 1970; Prince et al., 1971). Moreover, CMV has been isolated from healthy blood donors (Diosi et al., 1969). Contrary to earlier beliefs, the infection can develop in patients undergoing cardiac operations in which extracorporeal circulation is *not* employed (Henle et al.) and also after noncardiac operations (Armstrong et al., 1969). Blood transfusion appears to be the only common factor in all these series describing a comparable syndrome. Also contrary to earlier belief, disease transmission is not confined to the use of fresh blood (Prince et al.); rather the risk of infection is related to the number of units of blood transfused (Armstrong et al.; Henle et al.; Prince et al.). Thus, strictly speaking, the term *postperfusion syndrome* is applicable only to patients who develop the infection after operations employing cardiopulmonary bypass.

Clinical Features. *Fever* is always present and is the predominant feature (Kreel et al., 1960; Seaman and Starr, 1962; Wheller et al., 1962; Smith, 1964; Reyman, 1966; Embil et al., 1968). The temperature elevation is usually low-grade (101 to 102F) and occurs two to six weeks postoperatively. Occasionally, the temperature may go up as high as 104F (Seaman and Starr; Wheller et al.; Smith; Reyman; Embil et al.). A striking feature is the absence of systemic toxic symptoms. The patient feels well otherwise and maintains a good appetite. Another distinguishing characteristic is the absence of chest pain and arthralgia.

Minimal *splenic enlargement* becomes appreciable with the appearance of the fever and may persist for many months and even as long as a year (Seaman and Starr, 1962; Wheller et al., 1962; Smith, 1964; Riemenschneider and Moss, 1966). Sometimes hepatic enlargement may be present as well. Rarely, a generalized maculopapular eruption may appear transiently (Smith; Riemenschneider and Moss). Anterior cervical node enlargement may also be present (Smith; Riemenschneider and Moss).

The total leukocyte count is usually normal, but sometimes may be slightly elevated. The characteristic hematologic picture is the presence of *lympocytosis* (as high as 85 percent of the total), with appearance of *atypical forms* (as high as 20 percent). Atypical lymphocytes appear in the peripheral blood with the onset of the febrile illness, reaching a peak count over a period of one to three weeks and slowly disappearing in one to three months (Seaman and Starr, 1962; Wheller et al., 1962; Smith, 1964; Reyman, 1966; Embil et al., 1968). The atypical lymphocytes are identical to the Downey Type I and II cells seen in infectious mononucleosis (Battle and Hewlett, 1958). Eosinophilia (Perillie and Glenn, 1962) and nonthrombocytopenic purpura (Behrendt et al., 1968) also have been reported.

Apart from the hematologic changes just described, no other abnormal laboratory findings are present. Bacteriologic cultures of blood, urine, and throat specimens are negative. The chest roentgenogram and electrocardiogram are unrevealing.

Heterophil agglutinins are usually negative (Seaman and Starr, 1962). Cytomegalovirus infection may elicit a rise in titer of complement-fixing antibody to the virus and may be accompanied by excretion of the virus in the sputum and urine from whence it might be cultured (Caul et al., 1971). Similarly, EB virus infection provokes a rise in anti-EBV antibody, and EBV antigens may be isolated from the leukocytes of patients if the infection remains active (Gerber et al., 1969).

Management. Like the postpericardiotomy syndrome, the illness is self-limited and runs a benign course. The therapy is mainly symptomatic and consists of the administration of salicylates for their antipyretic action. More serious causes of postoperative fever must be ruled out.

Viral Hepatitis
General Considerations. It is now known that viral hepatitis, characterized primarily by an inflammatory injury to the liver, results from infection with one of several viruses. Hepatitis results *most commonly* from infection with one of two viruses, namely *hepatitis A virus* (HAV) and *hepatitis B virus* (HBV). Recent studies suggest that other yet unidentified viruses *(hepatitis C virus,* also known as *hepatitis "non-A-non-B" virus)* may be important causes of posttransfusion hepatitis (Prince et al., 1974; Feinstone et al., 1975). Less frequently, hepa-

titis may be caused by cytomegalovirus or Epstein-Barr virus infections (Hersey and Shaw, 1968; Stern, 1972).

Hepatitis A (short incubation period or epidemic hepatitis) is usually transmitted by the fecal-oral route, although infusion of infected blood obtained from viremic donors may cause sporadic infection. The incubation period is usually between two and six weeks. Hepatitis A usually runs a benign, self-limited course and resolves without progression to a chronic hepatic disease. Since there is no evidence of a chronic hepatitis A carrier state in humans, infection results from exposure to virus from an acutely infected subject. It is known that the use of standard pooled immune serum prevents or attenuates the disease when given before infection or early in the incubation period.

Hepatitis B (homologous serum hepatitis or posttransfusion hepatitis or long incubation period hepatitis) is usually transmitted by direct parenteral inoculation, although there is ample evidence that nonparenteral modes of transmission may be just as important (reviewed by Deinhardt, 1976). The incubation period is usually six weeks to six months. Hepatitis B is a more serious disease with a fatality rate ranging between 1 and 2 percent. It could also lead to such chronic disabling conditions as chronic active hepatitis or postnecrotic cirrhosis. Standard pooled immune serum globulin has little or no effect on hepatitis B prevention, but specially prepared hyperimmune globulins with high antibody titers against HBV surface antigens offer some degree of protection when administered at the time of suspected inoculation (Ginsberg et al., 1972; Grady, 1975).

Hepatitis C (hepatitis "non-A-non-B") occurs after transfusions of infected blood and may account for more cases of posttransfusion hepatitis than HAV and HBV together. It is not known whether hepatitis C is also transmissible by other means. It is differentiated from hepatitis A and hepatitis B by failure to develop antibodies to the HAV and HBV and by a median incubation period (generally between four and nine weeks). Tests for the presence of HBV antigens during the acute stage of the disease will also help in the differential diagnosis.

Pathogenesis of Posttransfusion Hepatitis. In the setting of cardiac surgery, the major mode of disease transmission is the transfusion of infected blood and pooled blood products. The primary agents are the HBV and hepatitis C virus. It has been estimated that the overall incidence of symptomatic posttransfusion hepatitis after major cardiovascular surgery in the United States is approximately 2.8 percent (National Transfusion Hepatitis Study, 1972). In the same study, patients receiving fibrinogen and blood had a 19 percent incidence of hepatitis. Further, there was a strong correlation between the risk of hepatitis and the incidence of hepatitis B antigen in donor blood, the proportion of commercial donors, and the transfusion volume.

Since patients undergoing open intracardiac operations may use more blood, the risk of hepatitis is increased under these conditions. This is especially true in geographic areas where heavy reliance is placed on commercial sources for donor blood. Transmission of the infective agents by blood transfusion can be prevented in part by reducing blood usage during cardiopulmonary bypass and by testing donors for the presence of HBV antigens and by using voluntary rather than paid donors (Szmuness et al., 1975). However, testing for HBV antigens alone may not substantially reduce the total number of posttransfusion hepatitis because as many as 80 percent of cases of posttransfusion hepatitis currently reported in the United States are caused neither by HAV or HBV but probably by the largely yet unknown agents of hepatitis C (Prince et al., 1974; Feinstone et al., 1975).

Since little is known about the hepatitis C virus(es), the succeeding sections will be devoted to discussion of HBV infection.

Immunologic Considerations. The development of sophisticated immunologic methods for the detection of HBV and its components has led to major advances in the understanding of hepatitis B infection and in developing methods of prevention, particularly among recipients of transfused blood.

Hepatitis B virus antigen was first discovered in the serum of an Australian aborigine, and was initially called Australia antigen (Blumberg et al., 1965). Subsequently, the virus was identified by electron microscopy in the serum of patients with HBV infection. The virus particle (also known as the Dane particle) has been described as being 42 nm in diameter, with a central core and surface capsid. The virus core contains DNA and exhibits DNA polymerase activity, and has been designated the hepatitis B_{core} antigen (HB_cAg). The capsid, or surface antigen, on the other hand, has been designated $HB_{surface}$ antigen (HB_sAg). Both particles have distinct antigenic characteristics and provoke the formation of their corresponding antibodies, namely, anti-HB_c and anti-HB_s.

The advent of immunofluorescent and immunoelectron microscopic methods have made it possible to identify HB_cAg and HB_sAg in the nuclei and cytoplasm, respectively, of hepatic cells from patients who are chronic HB_sAg carriers. HB_sAg also has been identified as 20 nm filaments or spheres with the central virus core in peripheral blood of carriers using immunodiffusion, complement-fixation, and radioimmunoassay techniques (Koretz et al., 1973; Szmuness et al., 1975).

Clinical Features. The infection may manifest itself in a number of ways. In many subjects there is evidence of hepatitis without jaundice *(anicteric hepatitis)*. Infection is followed by a mild illness without clinical evidence of hepatitis; a transiently positive test for HB_sAg or a rise in viral antibody titer may be the only evidence of infection.

Other patients develop jaundice *(icteric hepatitis)*, which usually runs a short uncomplicated course, but sometimes has a prolonged course *(chronic active hepatitis)*. It is not uncommon to see acute exacerbations of the disease after partial recovery or for a seemingly complete recovery to be followed by a recurrence *(recurrent hepatitis)*. Sometimes, cholestasis is the predominant feature *(cholestatic hepatitis)* and, rarely, massive necrosis *(fulminant hepatitis)* may follow.

The symptoms of anicteric hepatitis are nonspecific and mimic those of other viral infections of the respiratory and gastrointestinal tracts. Fever may be present and is usually most pronounced at the onset. Frequently, the patient complains of anorexia, weakness, myalgia, and headaches. Occasionally, right upper abdominal quadrant pain may be present and hepatic enlargement may become discernible, but physical signs may be strikingly absent.

Icteric hepatitis, on the other hand, is generally ushered in by an initial *preicteric phase* wherein the symptoms are similar to those seen in anicteric hepatitis. As the disease progresses, fever continues and gastrointestinal symptoms generally become more pronounced, with increasing anorexia, nausea, vomiting, and right upper quadrant pain and tenderness. At times, the latter may simulate an acute surgical abdomen. The urine becomes discolored and clinical jaundice becomes apparent as the liver becomes more enlarged. Fever usually subsides after the onset of jaundice. Within a few days, there is generally a subsidence of nausea and appetite may improve slightly. Typically, the jaundice reaches its peak intensity within 10 to 14 days from onset and gradually subsides over four to six weeks. Hepatic enlargement also subsides and symptomatic improvement continues. Convalescence may take several weeks and even months. During this period the patient may complain of variable malaise and fatigue. Complete recovery is the usual outcome (Sherlock, 1972).

The cholestatic, chronic persistent, and fulminant forms of the disease are atypical and will not be discussed here.

During the preicteric and early icteric periods of the illness, the leukocyte count may be normal or slightly elevated and atypical mononuclear cells may appear. In the early icteric period, the urine contains increased amounts of urobilinogen and bilirubin. Increasing bilirubinemia reflects deepening clinical icterus, but urinary urobilinogen decreases to minimal levels as the jaundice reaches its peak. The serum transaminase (glutamic-oxalacetic and glutamic-pyruvic) levels rise, usually reaching maximum during the early icteric period and generally tending to return to normal during the remainder of the icteric phase. Mild elevations of the serum alkaline phosphatase frequently occur. Mild abnormalities in serum proteins are frequently seen, including a slight decrease in albumin and a late increase in gamma globulin.

In hepatitis B infection, tests for HBV antigens (HB_cAg and HB_sAg) usually become positive during the preicteric and early icteric phases of the illness, with HB_cAg disappearing from the blood earlier than HB_sAg. Anti-HB_s antibody titers begin to rise during the early recovery phase as most patients become HB_sAg negative. A small minority of patients remain HB_sAg positive and anti-HB_s negative. They could ultimately become carriers with or without manifestations of chronic residual liver disease.

Viral hepatitis must be differentiated from other causes of postoperative icterus, including drug-induced hepatitis, congestive heart failure, and hemolytic jaundice, especially in patients who have had valve replacement procedures. The diagnosis of viral hepatitis is suggested by the clinical and biochemical picture and confirmed by immunologic tests. Sometimes a liver biopsy might be helpful when the clinical course is atypical or the diagnosis remains uncertain. Special precautions are obviously necessary when liver biopsy is performed in patients who are taking anticoagulant or platelet deaggregating drugs and in those who might have some degree of heart failure.

Management. No specific therapy is available for hepatitis B infection; therefore management is mainly supportive. Hospitalization is advisable if symptoms are severe. Although the therapeutic value of rest has been questioned (Chalmers et al., 1955), it is common practice to impose a program of complete bedrest during the acute phase of the viral illness, especially in the elderly or chronically ill patient recovering from open heart surgery. The not infrequent occurrence of relapses after increased physical activity and of remissions after imposition of bed rest have been the reasons for this recommendation.

An adequate caloric intake must be ensured. Supplemental intravenous feeding may be indicated in patients who have marked anorexia and severe gastrointestinal symptoms.

Extreme caution must be exercised in administering drugs that require microsomal enzyme activity for metabolic degradation, since acute hepatic inflammation impairs microsomal enzyme function. Prime examples of such drugs are coumarin derivatives, barbiturates, and opiates and other sedatives.

Respiratory Tract Infections
General Considerations and Pathogenesis.
Lower respiratory tract infections seen in cardiac surgical patients are mostly nosocomial. Although by no means unique to the cardiac surgical experience, a number of factors are known to predispose to respiratory tract infections: poor oral hygiene, general debility, congestive heart failure, general anesthesia, endotracheal intubation, prolonged mechanical ventilation, tracheostomy, endotracheal suctioning, and injudicious use of antibiotics. The use of general anesthesia, endotracheal intubation, and tracheostomy impair natural local barriers to infection, and infectious material is either aspirated or introduced by the contaminated hands of hospital personnel and through use of contaminated ventilatory support equipment. Rarely, lower respiratory infection may develop as a direct result of the patient's inability to bring up secretions, leading to atelectasis and secondary infection.

The most important clinical infection encountered in the cardiac surgical patient postoperatively is *bacterial pneumonia*. Atelectasis, a more frequent cause of postoperative fever, is usually not accompanied by infection.

Clinical Picture. Fever and cough are the most common manifestations. The fever is low grade (101 to 102F) and generally merges with the normal postoperative temperature elevation. In the absence of congestive heart failure, the onset of productive cough suggests respiratory infection. The sputum may be purulent and sometimes foul-smelling. The presence of foul-smelling sputum suggests infection with anaerobic microorganisms (anaerobic streptococci or *Bacteroides* species). In the patient maintained on assisted ventilation, a change in the character of the tracheal aspirate may be the first sign.

Physical examination is frequently unrevealing except when frank lobar consolidation is present. Rales and rhonchi may be audible, but these could be confused with signs of heart failure.

The leukocyte count is usually elevated with neutrophilia. The chest roentgenogram usually shows some infiltrates and, rarely, some evidence of consolidation. Gram stains of the sputum or aspirate will usually reveal a mixed flora of gram-positive cocci and gram-negative rods; the presence of polymorphonuclears in large numbers suggests infection. Sputum cultures usually grow the bacteria and, occasionally, blood cultures will be positive. When infection by anaerobes is suspected, the proper anaerobic culture media (e.g., fluid thyoglycollate) should be used to enhance the chances of isolating the offending organism.

It must be remembered that microorganisms can rapidly colonize the upper respiratory tract after endotracheal intubation or tracheostomy without producing actual infection (Glover and Jolly, 1971), and it is difficult to differentiate colonization from infection, since similar microorganisms may be recovered in both settings. Thus, the results of the sputum smears and culture should always be correlated with the clinical picture.

Management. Specific therapy is dictated by the results of the microbiologic studies on the sputum or aspirate, including antibiotic sensitivity testing on the isolated organism. Assiduous tracheobronchial toilette is an important component of therapy. Measures to prevent cross-contamination of other patients should be strictly adhered to by the staff.

Urinary Tract Infection

General Considerations and Pathogenesis. In the setting of cardiac surgery, urinary (urethral) catheters serve as valuable adjuncts in monitoring critically ill patients (see Chapters 6 and 9). However, one should always be aware of the risks of such a procedure, particularly infection.

It has been estimated that the risk of urinary tract infection after a single in-and-out urethral catheterization carried out with careful aseptic technique is approximately 1 to 2 percent (Stamm, 1975). On the other hand, the risk of infection is higher with indwelling catheters and increases with time. It has been shown that almost all patients with urinary catheters will develop bacteriuria within ten days (Kass and Sossen, 1959); the use of systemic prophylactic antimicrobial agents may delay but not prevent this (Martin and Bookrajian, 1962). Use of an open drainage system with an indwelling urinary catheter will result in infection in almost all patients in four to six days. In contrast, use of a carefully maintained closed drainage system may delay development of bacteriuria, with substantial reduction in the risk of infection during the first week or two; however, if the catheter is left in place beyond two weeks infection is a virtual certainty (Thornton and Andriole, 1970; Stamm, 1975).

Most catheter-related infections are caused by bacteria that normally reside in the patient's perineum. Most of these organisms originate from the large bowel and may be deposited on the urethral catheter during the course of catheter manipulations by the hands of hospital personnel. The bacteria may gain entrance into the lower urinary tract by migrating up the exterior of the catheter. Occasionally—usually through a momentary break in the continuity of the closed drainage system—bacteria may gain access to the drainage system and migrate retrogradely inside the catheter lumen, up into the lower urinary passages. Mechanical trauma of both urethra and urinary bladder caused by frequent catheter motion may lower local host resistance further and set the stage for an invasive infection. Gram-negative septicemia is a serious complication.

Clinical Picture. Urinary burning (dysuria) is the most common symptom. Unless an invasive infection is developing, fever is not a prominent feature. Urinary frequency is usually present in patients in whom the urinary catheter has been removed. A purulent meatal drainage may be present, especially after an indwelling catheter has been in place for a long time. The urine may be cloudy.

Urinalysis shows a significant pyuria and bacteriuria (more than 100,000 colonies per ml). Urine cultures will reveal the offending organism.

Management. Prophylaxis is the most important aspect of management. There is evidence that the most effective means of reducing the risk of catheter-related infections are proper catheter insertion technique and the meticulous maintenance of a sterile, closed drainage system (Stamm, 1975). Urinary catheters should be removed promptly when no longer necessary.

Patients with significant bacteriuria should be given specific antimicrobial therapy with agents that achieve high urinary bactericidal levels. Examples of these agents are ampicillin, nitrofurantoin, trimethoprim, trimethoprim-sulfamethoxazole, and cephalexin. If *Pseudomonas* species are cultured, oral carbenicillin may be the drug of choice.

Fortunately, gram-negative septicemia originating from the urinary tract is rarely seen in cardiac surgery. When it occurs, therapy is directed to reversal of the shock state, control of septicemia, and eradication of the feeding focus whenever possible.

Infections Related to the Use of Intravascular Catheters

General Considerations and Pathogenesis.
Indwelling intravenous and intraarterial catheters are important adjuncts in the care of the cardiac surgical patient. Yet there is evidence that the presence of such catheters is an important source of potential bacterial and fungal infection (Smits and Freedman, 1967). The risk of infection appears to be related to the length of time the catheters are in place. In addition, septicemia can occur from contaminated intravenous infusions (Dumas et al., 1971).

Contamination occurs most commonly at the site where the cannula penetrates the skin, either during initial cannula insertion or following subsequent manipulations. The infusion set and the infusion fluid itself represent potential sites for introduction of microorganisms during therapy. It has been suggested that steel needles (e.g., "butterfly" needles) carry a lower risk of septic complications than plastic catheters. Use of indwelling long plastic cannulae for the administration of high osmolality intravenous hyperalimentation solutions has been associated with a high incidence of systemic fungal infections (Curry and Quie, 1971).

Clinical Picture. The presence of spiking fever, with shaking chills, is the predominant feature. Frequently, there is an accompanying bacteremia. The feeding focus may be easily discernible. For instance, signs of suppurative thrombophlebitis may be present.

Management. The importance of meticulous attention to the technical details of aseptic, atraumatic cannular insertion cannot be overemphasized. Cannulae should also be securely anchored to prevent excessive to-and-fro motion and possible introduction of bacteria into the vessel along the catheter tract. In addition, the cannular insertion site should be treated aseptically and protected with a sterile dressing. Finally, intravascular cannulae should be removed promptly when no longer necessary. There is evidence that the risk of bacterial endocarditis, particularly from *S. aureus*, is reduced if intravascular catheters are removed within 24 hours of insertion.

The onset of signs and symptoms of septicemia mandates prompt removal of the offending cannulae. Occasionally, surgical removal of an infected venous channel may be necessary in certain cases of suppurative thrombophlebitis.

Specific bactericidal or fungicidal therapy should be started promptly, especially in the presence of intracardiac prostheses. When *Staphylococcus aureus* is isolated from blood cultures, the presence of prosthetic valve infection should be seriously considered. In such an event, it seems prudent to institute therapy for endocarditis (i.e., intravenous antibiotics for at least two weeks) and then determine serum techoic acid and antibody levels. The demonstration of high techoic acid and antibody levels suggests *tissue infection*, and further therapy (i.e., four weeks) with antibiotics is indicated.

REFERENCES

Alexander J W, Kaplan J Z, Altemeier W A: Role of suture materials in the development of wound infections. Ann Surg 165: 192, 1967.

Altemeier W A: Current infection problems: surgical. Presented at International Conference on Nosocomial Infections, Atlanta, Aug. 3–6, 1970.

American College of Surgeons; Committee on Operating Room Environment: Definition of microbiologic clean air. Bull Am Coll Surg 61:19, 1976.

Amoury R A: Infections following cardiopulmonary bypass. Sternal infection. In Norman J C (ed): Cardiac Surgery, 2nd ed. New York, Appleton-Century-Crofts, 1979, pp 575–577.

――――: Infection following cardiopulmonary bypass. In Norman J C (ed): Cardiac Surgery. New York, Appleton-Century-Crofts, 1972, pp 555–597.

――――, Bowman F O, Malm J R: Endocarditis associated with intracardiac prostheses. Diagnosis, management and prophylaxis. J Thorac Cardiovasc Surg 51:36, 1966.

Anderson D J, Bulkley B H, Hutchins G M: A clinicopathologic study of prosthetic valve endocarditis in 22 patients: morphologic basis for diagnosis and therapy. Am Heart J 94:325, 1977.

Arbulu A, Thomas N W, Wilson R F: Valvulectomy without prosthetic replacement. J Thorac Cardiovasc Surg 64:103, 1972.

Archer G L, Polk R E, Duma R J, Lower R: Comparison of cephalothin and cefamandole prophylaxis during insertion of prosthetic heart valves. Antimicrob Agents Chemother 13:924, 1978.

Armstrong D, Balakrishnan S L, Steger L: A spectrum of cytomegalovirus infections during renal transplantation. J Clin Invest 48:3a, 1969.

Arnett E N, Roberts W C: Prosthetic valve endocarditis. Clinicopathologic analysis of 22 necropsy patients with comparison of observations in 74 necropsy patients with active infective endocarditis involving natural left-sided cardiac valves. Am J Cardiol 38: 281, 1976.

Baffes T G, Blazek W V, Fridman J L, Agustsson M H, Van Elk, J: Postoperative infections in 1136 consecutive cardiac operations. Surgery 68:791, 1970.

Barney J D, Williams G R, Cayler G G, Bracken E C: Influence of intracardiac prosthetic materials on susceptibility of bacterial endocarditis. Circulation 26:684, 1962.

Battle J D Jr, Hewlett J S: Hematologic changes observed after extracorporeal circulation during open-heart operations. Cleve Clin Q 25:112, 1958.

Behrendt D M, Epstein S E, Morrow A G: Postperfusion nonthrombocytopenic purpura. An uncommon sequel of open heart surgery. Am J Cardiol 22:631, 1968.

Blakemore W S, McGarrity G J, Thurer R J, Wallace H W, Mac Vough H III, Coriell L L: Infection by air-borne bacteria with cardiopulmonary bypass. Surgery 70:830, 1971.

Block P C, DeSanctis R W, Weinberg A N: Prosthetic valve endocarditis. J Thorac Cardiovasc Surg 60:540, 1970.

Blumberg B S, Alter H J, Visnich S: A "new" antigen in leukemia sera. J A M A 191:541, 1965.

Brodie B R, Grossman W, McLaurin L: Diagnosis of prosthetic mitral valve malfunction with combined echo-phonocardiography. Circulation 53:93, 1976.

Brown A H, Braimbridge M V, Panagopoulos P, Sabar E F: The complications of median sternotomy. J Thorac Cardiovasc Surg 58:189, 1969.

Bryant L R, Spencer F C, Trinkle J K: Treatment of median sternotomy infection by mediastinal irrigation with an antibiotic solution. Ann Surg 169:914, 1969.

Burke J F: Preventive antibiotic management in surgery. Ann Rev Med 24:289, 1973.

――――: The effective period of preventive antibiotic action in experimental incisions and dermal lesions. Surgery 50:161, 1961.

———, Miles A A: The sequence of bacterial events in early infective inflammation. J Pathol Bacteriol 76:1, 1958.
Carey J S, Hughes R K: Control of infection after thoracic and cardiovascular surgery. Ann Surg 172:916, 1970.
Caul E O, Clarke S K R, Mott M G, Perham T G M, Wilson R S E: Cytomegalovirus infections after open heart surgery. A prospective study. Lancet 1:777, 1971.
Chalmers T C, Eckhardt R D, Reynolds W E, Cigarros J G Jr, Deane N, Reinfenstein R W, Smith C W, Davidson C S: The treatment of acute infectious hepatitis. Controlled studies of the effect of diet, rest, and physical reconditioning on the acute course of the disease and on the incidence of relapses and residual abnormalities. J Clin Invest 34:1136, 1955.
Cheng T O, Kinhas V, Tice D A: Fatal thrombosis of the Starr-Edwards mitral valve prosthesis associated with bacterial endocarditis. Chest 57:151, 1970.
Clark R E, Amos W C, Higgins V, Bomberg K F, Weldon C S: Infection control in cardiac surgery. Surgery 79:89, 1976.
Colvin O M, Waldman R H, Lee S: Staphylococcal infection of a Starr-Edwards prosthesis with fatal obstruction of the mitral valve. N Engl J Med 273:1380, 1965.
Conte J E Jr, Cohen S N, Roe B B, Elashoff R M: Antibiotic prophylaxis and cardiac surgery: a prospective double-blind comparison of single-dose versus multiple-dose regimens. Ann Intern Med 76:943, 1972.
Curry C R, Quie P G: Fungal septicemia in patients receiving parenteral hyperalimentation. N Engl J Med 255:1221, 1971.
Deinhardt F: Epidemiology and mode of transmission of viral hepatitis A and B. Am J Clin Path 65:890, 1976.
Denton C, Pappas E G, Uricchio J F, Goldberg H, Likoff W: Bacterial endocarditis following cardiac surgery. Circulation 15:525, 1957.
Dillon J C: Echocardiography in valvular vegetations. Am J Med 62:856, 1977.
Diosi P, Moldovan E, Tomescu N: Latent cytomegalovirus infection in blood donors. Br J Med 4:600, 1969.
Dismukes W E, Karchmer A W, Buckley M J, Austen W G, Swartz M N: Prosthetic valve endocarditis. Analysis of 38 cases. Circulation 48:365, 1973.
Dressler W: Postmyocardial infarction syndrome: preliminary report of complications resembling idiopathic, recurrent, benign pericarditis. J A M A 160:1379, 1956.
Drusin L M, Engle M A, Hagstrom J W C, Schwartz M S: The pericardiotomy syndrome. A six-year epidermiologic study. N Engl J Med 272:597, 1965.
Dryden G E: Questionnaire study of anesthesia equipment sterility. J A M A 206:2524, 1968.
Dumas R J, Warner J F, Dalton H P: Septicemia from intravenous infusions. N Engl J Med 284:257, 1971.
Duncalf D: Care of anesthetic equipment and other devices. Arch Surg 107:600, 1973.
Durack D T, Petersdorf R G: Chemotherapy of experimental streptococcal endocarditis. I. Comparison of commonly recommended regimens. J Clin Invest 52:592, 1973.
Ehrenhaft J L, Taber R E: Hemopericardium and constrictive pericarditis. J Thorac Surg 24:355, 1952.
Ellis K, Jaffe C, Malm J R, Bowman F O Jr: Infective endocarditis roentgenographic considerations. Radiol Clin North Am 11:415, 1973.
Elster S K, Wood H F, Seely R D: Clinical and laboratory manifestations of the postcommisurotomy syndrome. Am J Med 17:826, 1954.
Embil J A, Folkins D F, Haldane E V, van Rooyen C E: Cytomegalovirus infection following extracorporeal circulation in children: a prospective study. Lancet 2:1151, 1968.
Engelman R M, Chase R M Jr, Boyd A D, Reed G E: Lethal postoperative infections following cardiac surgery: review of four years' experience. Circulation 47, 48 (Suppl III):31, 1973.
———, Williams C O, Gouge T H, Chase R M, Falk E A, Boyd A D, Reed G E: Mediastinitis following open heart surgery. Arch Surg 107:772, 1973.
Engle M A, Ito T: The postpericardiotomy syndrome. Am J Cardiol 7:73, 1961.
———, Marx N R: The postpericardiotomy and postperfusion syndromes. Heart Bull 14:33, 1965.
———, McCabe J C, Ebert P A, Zabriskie J: The postpericardiotomy syndrome and antiheart antibodies. Circulation 49:401, 1974.
———, Zabriskie J B, Senterfit L, Tay D J, Ebert P A: Immunologic and virologic studies in the postpericardiotomy syndrome. J Pediatr 87:1103, 1975.
English T A H, Ross J K: Surgical aspects of bacterial endocarditis. Br Med J 4:598, 1972.
Epstein S: Is the postcommissurotomy syndrome of

rheumatic origin? A M A Arch Intern Med 99:253, 1957.
Everett E D, Hirschmann J V: Transient bacteremia and endocarditis prophylaxis. Medicine 56:61, 1977.
Everett W G: Suture materials in general surgery. Prog Surg 8:14, 1970.
Feinstone S M, Kapikian A Z, Purcell R H, Alter H J, Holland P V: Transfusion-associated hepatitis not due to viral hepatitis A or B. N Engl J Med 292:767, 1975.
Firor W B: Infection following open-heart surgery with special reference to the role of prophylactic antibiotics. J Thorac Cardiovasc Surg 53:371, 1967.
Foster K M, Jack I: A prospective study of the role of cytomegalovirus in post-transfusion mononucleosis. N Engl J Med 280:1311, 1969.
Galleti P: Laboratory experience with 24 hour partial heart-lung bypass. J Surg Res 5:97, 1965.
Geraci J E, Dale A J D, McGoon D C: Bacterial endocarditis following cardiac operations. Wis Med J 62:302, 1963.
Gerber P, Walsh J H, Rosenblum E N, Purcell R H: Association of EB-virus infection with the post-perfusion syndrome. Lancet 1:593, 1969.
Gery I, Davies A M, Ehrenfeld E N: Heart-specific autoantibodies. Lancet 1:471, 1960.
Ginsberg A L, Conrad M E, Bancroft W H, Ling C M, Overby L R: Prevention of endemic HAA-positive hepatitis with gamma globulin. N Engl J Med 286:562, 1972.
Glover J L, Jolly L: Gram-negative colonization of the respiratory tract in postoperative patients. Am J Med Sci 261:24, 1971.
Goldmann D A, Hopkins C C, Karchmer A W, Abel R M, McEnary T, Akins C, Buckley M J, Moellering R C Jr: Cephalothin prophylaxis in cardiac valve surgery. J Thorac Cardiovasc Surg 73:470, 1977.
Goodkind M J, Bloomer W E, Goodyer V N: Recurrent pericardial effusion after non-penetrating chest trauma. Report of two cases treated with adreno-cortical steroids. N Engl J Med 263:874, 1960.
Goodman J S, Schaffner W, Collins H A, Battersby E J, Koenig M G: Infection after cardiovascular surgery: clinical study including examination of antimicrobial prophylaxis. N Engl J Med 278:117, 1968.
Grady G F: Post-transfusion hepatitis: passive immunization. Am J Med Sci 270:369, 1975.
Grmoljez P F, Barner H H, William V L, Kaiser G C: Major complications of median sternotomy. Am J Surg 130:679, 1975.
Gruhl V R: Renal failure, deafness, brain lesions following irrigation of the mediastinum with neomycin. Ann Thorac Surg 11:376, 1971.
Hairston P, Manos J P, Graber C D, Lee W H Jr: Depression of immunologic surveillance by pump-oxygenation perfusion. J Surg Res 9:587, 1969.
———, ———, ———, ———: Alteration of intrinsic bactericidial potential of blood by pump-oxygenator perfusion. Symposium— Organ Perfusion and Preservation. New York, Appleton-Century-Crofts, 1968, pp 911–928.
Hall W J III: *Pencillium* endocarditis following open heart surgery and prosthetic valve insertion. Am Heart J 87:501, 1974.
Harford C G: Postoperative fungal endocarditis. Arch Intern Med 134:116, 1974.
Heine W I, Friedman H, Mandell M S, Goldberg H: Antibodies to cardiac tissue in acute ischemic heart disease. Am J Cardiol 17:798, 1966.
Henle W, Henle G, Scriba M, Joyner C R, Harrison F S, von Essen R, Paloheimo J, Klemola E: Antibody responses to the Epstein-Barr virus and cytomegalovirus after open-heart and other surgery. N Engl J Med 282:1068, 1970.
Herr R, Starr A, McCord C W, Wood J A: Special problems following valve replacement: embolus, leak, infection, red cell damage. Ann Thorac Surg 1:403, 1965.
Hersey D F, Shaw E D: Viral agents in hepatitis: a review. Lab Invest 19:558, 1968.
Ito T, Engle M A, Goldberg H P: Postpericardiotomy syndrome following surgery for non-rheumatic heart disease. Circulation 17:549, 1958.
Jimenez-Martinez M, Arguero-Sanchez R, Perez-Alvarez J J, MinaCastaneda P: Anterior mediastinitis as a complication of median sternotomy. Diagnostic and surgical considerations. Surgery 67:929, 1970.
Kääriäinen L, Klemela E, Paloheimo J: Rise of cytomegalovirus antibodies in an infectious-mononucleosis-like syndrome after transfusion. Br Med J 1:1270, 1966.
Kahn D R, Ertrel P Y, Murphy W H, Kirsh M M, Vathayanon S, Stern A M, Sloan H: Pathogenesis of the post-pericardiotomy syndrome. J Thorac Cardiovasc Surg 54:682, 1967.
Kammer R B, Utz J P: *Aspergillus* species endocarditis. Am J Med 56:506, 1974.

Kaplan E L, Anthony B F, Bismo A, Durack D, Houser H, Millard D, Sanford J, Shulman S T, Stillerman M, Taranta A, Wenger N: Prevention of bacterial endocarditis (AHA Committee Report). Circulation 56:139 A, 1977.

Karchmer A W, Dismukes W E, Buckley M J, Austen W G: Late prosthetic valve endocarditis. Clinical features influencing therapy. Am J Med 64:199, 1978.

Kass E H, Sossen H S: Prevention of infection of urinary tract in presence of indwelling catheters: disruption of electromechanical valve to provide intermittent drainage of the bladder. J A M A 169:1181, 1959.

Kluge R M, Calia F M, McLaughlin J S, Hovnick R B: Sources of contamination in open heart surgery. J A M A 230:1415, 1974.

Koretz R L, Klahs D R, Ritman S, Damus K, Gitnick G L: Post-transfusion hepatitis in recipients of blood screened by newer assays. Lancet 2:694, 1973.

Kreel I, Zaroff L I, Frankel A, Canter J W, Baronofsky ID: A syndrome following total body perfusion. Surg Gynecol Obstet 111:317, 1960.

Kusserow B K, Larrow R: Studies of leukocyte responses to prolonged pumping-effects upon phagocytic capability and total white cell count. Trans Am Soc Artif Intern Organs 14:261, 1968.

———, ———, Nichols J: Metabolic and morphologoical alterations in leukocytes following prolonged blood pumping. Trans Am Soc Artif Intern Organs 15:40, 1969.

———, ———, ———: Perfusion and surface induced injury in leukocytes. Fed Proc 30:1516, 1971.

Lang D J, Henshaw J B: Cytomegalovirus infection and the postperfusion syndrome: recognition of primary infection in four patients. N Engl J Med 280:1145, 1969.

———, Scolnick E M, Willerson J T: Association of cytomegalovirus infection with postperfusion syndrome. N Engl J Med 278:1147, 1968.

Larson D L: Relation of the postcommissurotomy syndrome to the rheumatic state. Circulation 15:203, 1957.

Laskowski L F, Marr J, Spernoga J F, Frank N J, Barner H B, Kaiser G, Tyras D H: Fastidious mycobacteria growth from porcine prosthetic-heart-valve cultures. N Engl J Med 297:101, 1977.

Laufman H: Nosocomial infection complicating intrathoracic surgery, In Cordell A R, Ellison R G (eds): Complications of Intrathoracic Surgery. Boston, Little, Brown, 1979, pp 267–277.

———: The role of discipline in infection control in the operating room. Excerpta Medica International Congress Series No. 137. General Surgery, Orthopedics, Plastic Surgery: Controversial Opinions. Amsterdam, July 1975.

———: Current status of special air-handling systems in operating rooms. Med Instrum 7:7, 1973b.

———: Surgical hazard control. Effect of architecture and engineering. Arch Surg 107:552, 1973b.

Lawrence T, Shockman A T, MacVaugh H III: *Aspergillus* infection of prosthetic aortic valves. Chest 60:406, 1971.

Lee W H Jr, Kromhaar D, Fonkalsrud E W, Schjeide O A, Maloney J V Jr: Denaturation of plasma proteins as a cause of morbidity and death after intracardiac operations. Surgery 50:29, 1961.

Levy C, Cutin J A, Watkins A, Marsh B, Garcia J, Mispireta L: *Mycobacterium chelonei* infection of porcine heart valves. N Engl J Med 297:667, 1977.

Linde L M, Rao P S: A modern view of infective endocarditis. Cardiovasc Clin 5:15, 1973.

Livelli F D, Johnson R A, McEnany M T, Sherman E, Lewell J, Block P C, DeSanctis R W: Unexplained in-hospital fever following cardiac surgery. Natural history, relationship to postpericardiotomy syndrome, and a prospective study of therapy of indomethacin versus placebo. Circulation 57:968, 1978.

Lord J W, Imparato A M, Hackel A, Boyle E F: Endocarditis complicating open heart surgery. Circulation 23:489, 1961.

Madison J, Wang K, Gobel F L, Edwards J E: Prosthetic aortic valvular endocarditis. Circulation 51:940, 1975.

Martin C M, Bookrajian E N: Bacteriuria prevention after indwelling urinary catheterization. A controlled study. Arch Intern Med 110:703, 1962.

Massur H, Johnson W D Jr: Prosthetic valve endocarditis. J Thorac Cardiovasc Surg 80:31, 1980.

Meyers B R, Bottone R, Hirschman S Z, Schneierson S S: Infections caused by microorganisms of the Genus Erwinia. Ann Intern Med 76:9, 1972.

Miles A A: Nonspecific reactions in bacterial infections. Ann Acad Sci 66:356, 1956.

———, Miles E M, Burke J F: The value and

duration of defence reactions of the skin to the primary lodgement of bacteria. Br J Exp Pathol 38:79, 1957.

Mills J, Drew D: *Serratia marcescens* endocarditis, a regional illness associated with intravenous drug abuse. Ann Intern Med 84:29, 1976.

Mortensen J P, Hurd G, Hill G: Bacterial contamination of oxygen used clinically—importance and one method of control. Dis Chest 42:567, 1962.

National Transfusion Hepatitis Study: Risk of post-transfusion hepatitis in the United States—a prospective cooperative study. J A M A 220:692, 1972.

Nelson J C, Nelson R B: The incidence of hospital wound infections in thoracotomies. J Thorac Cardiovasc Surg 54:586, 1967.

Nelson R M, Jensen C B, Peterson C A, Sanders B C: Effective use of prophylactic antibiotics in open-heart surgery. Arch Surg 90:731, 1965.

Northey D, Adess M L, Hartsuck J M, Rhoades E R: Microbial surveillance in a surgical intensive care unit. Surg Gynecol Obstet 139:321, 1974.

Ochsner J L, Mills N L, Woolverton W C: Disruption and infection of the median sternotomy incision. J Cardiovasc Surg 13:394, 1972.

Okies J E, Viroslav J, Williams T W Jr: Endocarditis after cardiac valve replacement. Chest 59:198, 1971.

Ostermiller W E, Dye W S, Weinberg M: Fungal endocarditis following cardiovascular surgery. J Thorac Cardiovasc Surg 61:670, 1971.

Paloheimo A, von Essen R, Klemola E, Kääriäinen L, Siltanen P: Subclinical cytomegalovirus infections and cytomegalovirus mononucleosis after open-heart surgery. Am J Cardiol 22:624, 1968.

Peirce W S, Peckham G J, Johnson J, Waldhausen J A: Gram-negative sepsis following operations for congenital heart disease. Diagnosis, management and results. Arch Surg 101:698, 1970.

Pelletier L L Jr, Durack D T, Petersdorf R G: Chemotherapy of experimental streptococcal endocarditis. IV. Further observation on prophylaxis. J Clin Invest 56:319, 1975.

Perillie P E, Glenn W L: Fever, splenomegaly, lymphocytosis, and eosinophilia. A new postcardiotomy syndrome. Yale J Biol Med 34:675, 1962.

Peter R H, Whalen R E, Orgain E S, McIntosh H D: Postpericardiotomy syndrome as a complication of percutaneous left ventricular puncture. Am J Cardiol 17:718, 1966.

Prince A M, Bortman B, Grady G F, Huhns W J, Hazzi C, Levine R W, Millian S J: Long-incubation post-transfusion hepatitis without serological evidence of exposure to hepatitis B. virus. Lancet 2:241, 1974.

———, Szmuness W, Millian S J, David D S: A serologic study of cytomegalovirus infections associated with blood transfusion. N Engl J Med 284:1125, 1971.

Pruitt K M, Strood R M, Scott J W, McKibbin J M: Blood damage in the heart-lung machine. Proc Soc Exp Biol Med 137:714, 1971.

Quenzer R W, Edwards L D, Levin S: A comparative study of 48 host valves and 24 prosthetic valve endocarditis cases. Am Heart J 92:15, 1976.

Ramsey R G, Gunnar R M, Tobin J R Jr: Endocarditis in the drug addict. Am J Cardiol 25:608, 1970.

Reed W A: Antibiotics and cardiac surgery. J Thorac Cardiovasc Surg 50:888, 1965.

Report of an Ad Hoc Committee of the Committee on Trauma, Division of Medical Sciences, National Academy of Sciences—National Research Council: Postoperative wound infections. The influence of ultraviolet radiation of the operating room and of various factors. Ann Surg 160 (Suppl):1, 1964.

Reyman T A: Postperfusion syndrome: a review and report of 21 cases. Am Heart J 72:116, 1966.

Riemenschneider T A, Moss A J: Postperfusion syndrome. Report of four cases and review of the literature. J Pediatr 69:546, 1966.

Robinson J F, Brigden W: Immunological studies in the postcardiotomy syndrome. Br Med J 2:706, 1963.

Rosendorf L L, Daicoff G, Baer H: Sources of gram-negative infection after open-heart surgery. J Thorac Cardiovasc Surg 67:195, 1974.

Rossiter S G, Stinson E B, Oyer P R, Miller D C, Schapira J N, Martin R P, Shumway N E: Prosthetic valve endocarditis. Comparison of heterograft tissue valves and mechanical valves. J Thorac Cardiovasc Surg 76:795, 1978.

Richardson J V, Karp R B, Kirklin J W, Dismukes W E: Treatment of infective endocarditis. A 10 year comparative analysis. Circulation 58:589, 1978.

Saffle J R, Gardner P, Schoenbaum S C, Wild W: Prosthetic valve endocarditis. The case for prompt valve replacement. J Thorac Cardiovasc Surg 73:416, 1977.

Sande M, Johnson W, Hook E, Kaye D: Sustained

bacteremia in patients with prosthetic valves. N Engl J Med 286:1967, 1972.

Sanfelippo PM, Danielson G K: Complications associated with median sternotomy. J Thorac Cardiovasc Surg 63:419, 1972a.

———, ———: Nylon bands for closure of median sternotomy incisions. An unacceptable method. Ann Thorac Surg 13:404, 1972b.

Sarot I A, Weber D W, Schechter D C: Cardiac surgery in active primary infective endocarditis. Chest 57:58, 1970.

Scannell J G, Brown G E, Buckley M J, Ebert P A, Haufman H, Rackley C E, Sabiston D C Jr, Sloan H E: Optimal resources for cardiac surgery: Guidelines for program planning and evaluation I C H D Resources Report. Circulation 52 (Suppl): A-23, 1975.

Seaman A J, Starr A: Febrile postcardiotomy lymphocytic splenomegaly: a new entity. Ann Surg 156:956, 1962.

Seelig M S, Speth C P, Kozinn P J, Taschdjian C L, Toni E F, Goldberg P: Patterns of *Candida* endocarditis following cardiac surgery: importance of early diagnosis and therapy (an analysis of 91 cases). Prog Cardiovasc Dis 17:125, 1974.

Segal F, Tabatznik B: Postpericardiotomy syndrome following penetrating stab wounds in the chest: comparison with the postcommissurotomy syndrome. Am Heart J 59:175, 1960.

Shafer R B, Hall W H: Bacterial endocarditis following open-heart surgery. Am J Cardiol 25:602, 1970.

Sherlock S: The course of long-incubation (virus B) hepatitis. Br Med Bull 28:109, 1972.

Silva J Jr, Hoeksema H, Fekety F R Jr: Transient defects in phagocytic functions during cardiopulmonary bypass. J Thorac Cardiovasc Surg 67:175, 1974.

Slaughter L, Morris J E, Starr A: Prosthetic valve endocarditis. A 12 year review. Circulation 47:1319, 1973.

Slonim R, Litwak R S, Gadboys H L, Ehrenkranz N J: Antibiotic prophylaxis of infection complicating open-heart operation. In Proceedings of the Third Interscience Conference on Antimicrobial Agents and Chemotherapy. Sylvester J C (ed): Washington, D.C., 1963, pp 731-735.

Smith D R: A syndrome resembling infectious mononucleosis after open-heart surgery. Br Med J 1:945, 1964.

Smits H, Freedman L R: Prolonged venous catheterization as a cause of sepsis. N Engl J Med 276:1229, 1967.

Soloff L A, Zatuchni J, Janton H, O'Neil T J, Glover R P: Reactivation of rheumatic fever following mitral commissurotomy. Circulation 8:481, 1953.

Sompolinsky D, Hermann A, Oeding P, Rippon J E: A series of postoperative infections. J Infect Dis 100:1, 1957.

Stamm W E: Guidelines for prevention and management of catheter-associated urinary tract infections. Ann Intern Med 82:386, 1975.

Stein P D, Harken D E, Dexter L: The nature and prevention of prosthetic valve endocarditis. Am Heart J 71:393, 1966.

Stern H: Cytomegalovirus and EB virus infections of the liver. Br Med Bull 28:180, 1972.

Stimmel B, Donoso E, Dack S: Comparison of infective endocarditis in drug addicts and non-drug users. Am J Cardiol 32:924, 1973.

Stinson E B, Castellino R A, Shumway N E: Radiologic signs in endocarditis following prosthetic valve replacement. J Thorac Cardiovasc Surg 56:554, 1968.

———, Griepp R B, Vosti K, Copeland J G, Shumway N E: Operative treatment of active endocarditis. J Thorac Cardiovasc Surg 71:659, 1976.

Strunk B L, London E J, Fitzgerald J, Popp R L, Barry W H: The assessment of mitral stenosis and prosthetic valve obstruction, using the posterior aortic wall echocardiogram. Circulation 55:885, 1977.

Subramanian V, Lowman J T, Gans S: Effect of extracorporeal circulation on reticuloendothelial function. Arch Surg 97:330, 1968.

Suri R K, Selby D A, Hawks G H, Baker C B: *Serratia marcescens* endocarditis: a report of a case involving Cross-Jones mitral valve prosthesis with a review of the literature. Can Med Assoc J 104:1013, 1971.

Szmuness W, Hirsch R L, Prince A M, Levine R W, Harley E J, Ikram H: Hepatitis B surface antigen in blood donors: further observations. J Infect Dis 131:111, 1975.

Tabatznik B, Isaacs J P: Postpericardiotomy syndrome following traumatic pericardium. Am J Cardiol 7:83, 1961.

Tan J S, Watanakunakorn C, Terhune C A Jr: *Streptococcus viridans* endocarditis: favorable prognosis in geriatric patients. Geriatrics 28:68, 1973.

Thornton G F, Andriole V J: Bacteriuria during indwelling catheter drainage. J A M A 214:339, 1970.

Thurer R J, Bagnolo D, Vargas A, Isch J H, Kaiser

G A: The management of mediastinal infection following cardiac surgery. An experience utilizing continuous irrigation with povidone-iodine. J Thorac Cardiovasc Surg 68:962, 1974.

Turnier E, Kay J H, Bernstein S, Mendez A M, Zubiate P: Surgical treatment of *Candida* endocarditis. Chest 67:262, 1975.

Upshaw C B Jr: *Penicillium* endocarditis of aortic valve prostheses. J Thorac Cardiovasc Surg 68:428, 1974.

Uricchio J F: The postcommissurotomy (postpericardiotomy) syndrome. Am J Cardiol 12:436, 1963.

Van der Geld H: Anti-heart antibodies in the postpericardiotomy and the postmyocardial-infarction syndromes. Lancet 2:617, 1964.

Watanakunakorn C: Prosthetic valve infective endocarditis. Prog Cardiovasc Dis 22:181, 1979.

———: Changing epidemiology and newer aspects of infective endocarditis. Adv Intern Med 22:21, 1977.

———, Baird I M: Prognostic factors in *Staphylococcus aureus* endocarditis with a penicillin and gentamicin. Am J Med Sci 273:133, 1977.

Wehr K, McCall C: Infection of prosthetic valves. Successful therapy with antibiotics. South Med J 65:1224, 1972.

Wheller E Q, Turner J D, Scannell J G: Fever, splenomegaly, and atypical lymphocytes: syndrome observed after cardiac surgery utilizing pump oxygenator. N Engl J Med 266:454, 1962.

Wilson W R, Jaumin P M, Danielson G K, Giulianai E R, Washington J A, Geraci J E: Prosthetic valve endocarditis. Ann Intern Med 82:751, 1975.

Wray T M, Bryant R E, Killen D A: Sternal osteomyelitis and costochondritis after median sternotomy. J Thorac Cardiovasc Surg 65:227, 1973.

Yeh T H, Anabtawi I N, Cornett V E, White A, Stern W H, Ellison R G: Bacterial endocarditis following open-heart surgery. Ann Thorac Surg. 3:29, 1967.

Zinner S H, Denney-Brown B C, Braun P: Risk of infection with intravenous indwelling catheters: effect of application with an antibiotic ointment. J Infect Dis 120:616, 1969.

19. Operative and Postoperative Care of the Neonate and Pediatric Cardiac Surgical Patient

ROBERT S. LITWAK   EDWIN G. BROWN

Over the past two decades enormous strides have been made in the efficacy and safety of operations for an ever expanding list of congenital cardiac defects. Indeed, there are few cardiac lesions for which effective operative palliation or primary repair is not possible.

Despite the low risk and excellent results of "corrective"* procedures achieved over the years in older children, it was not until the past several years that the same operations performed in the first weeks or months of life could be performed with reasonable probability of early and late survival. Many factors have contributed to the lowered risk: precise diagnostic delineation of the cardiovascular pathophysiology, more effective preoperative supportive care of the infant, significant improvements in both perfusion conduct and technical quality of the repairs, and, finally, major advances in postoperative care. Failure to optimize any one of these components will sharply reduce the probability of a successful outcome. Gersony and Hayes (1972) have eloquently stated the case: "The modern 'perioperative' care of a newborn infant with a severe heart defect must be considered as a unique commitment.... In our experience, *unremitting attention to detail* is the single most important principle in the treatment of these seriously ill babies."

Obviously, in a single chapter it is not possible to deal comprehensively with the entire spectrum of care of infants and children requiring cardiac surgery. Rather, the discussion will be selective and focus primarily on those management techniques that are believed to have had major impact on the improved safety of surgery in the first few weeks or months of life.

CARDIOVASCULAR OPERATIONS WITHOUT CARDIOPULMONARY BYPASS

In theory, cardiovascular operations not requiring cardiopulmonary bypass should be associated with minimal risk, results that in-

---

*Until the late results of many intracardiac operations are better established, the term "corrective" would probably best be applied with due appreciation of deficiencies in our current information (Macartney et al., 1980).

deed are consistently achieved in infants and children beyond the age of three months having *elective* operations. On the other hand, the risk is significantly higher in babies who require urgent or emergent operations in the first days or weeks of life.

On occasion, emergency ductal ligation is required in premature infants after failure of a prostaglandin synthetase inhibitor (indomethacin) to induce ductal closure (Neal et al., 1977; Merritt et al., 1978). On the other hand, use of prostaglandin E_1 or E_2 to maintain ductal patency in severe cardiac lesions with diminished pulmonary blood flow (Olley et al., 1976; Neutze et al., 1977), interrupted aortic arch, or juxtaductal coarctation of the aorta (Heymann et al., 1979) frequently has made it possible to delay operations until the babies are in a more stable condition. However, despite these and other supportive measures, surgery is almost invariably superimposed on an already severely compromised clinical state. Hence, there is always great potential for sudden life-threatening intraoperative or postoperative deterioration in these babies.

Surgical Palliation Versus Primary Definitive ("Corrective") Repair

A number of cardiac lesions previously palliated during the early days or months of life can now be definitively repaired primarily, at a risk not substantially different from the palliative procedure. Thus, timing and selection of the appropriate procedure has become a complex matter and requires careful assessment of a number of considerations discussed below.

Palliation is obviously advisable if, in the experience of a particular surgical group, the alternative primary definitive repair carries an unacceptably higher risk. Second, despite the initial technical and clinical success of certain anatomic or physiologic "corrective" procedures performed in infancy, palliation might better be considered if there is great probability that a second open operation ultimately will be required (for example, the need for subsequent replacement of a small diameter pulmonary artery conduit that had been in-

serted in the first year of life). On the other hand, weighing the comparative risks of palliation versus primary repair must also include the possible heightened morbidity and occasional mortality of a corrective operation complicated by a previous palliative procedure (for example, the reconstructive problems imposed by extensive cicatrical scarring of the pulmonary artery trunk and adjacent structures by a previously placed pulmonary artery band, or bleeding accompanying mobilization of a previously constructed systemic-pulmonary artery shunt).

In summary, selection of the proper operation at the proper time is difficult. That a definitive repair *can* be done in the first few months of life does not necessarily imply that it *should* be done in all cases. Properly conducted palliative operations still have a major role to play. Central to the decision is the responsible surgeon's careful analysis of his or her own early and late results (Kirklin et al., 1979; Arcinieagas et al., 1980).

Management of Closed Procedures. Infants have a large surface area relative to their mass and a thin subcutaneous fat layer. Placed in a cold environment, they rapidly lose body heat, which is why the operating room temperature must be maintained at 29 to 30C (approximately 85F), a level approaching thermoneutrality (discussed later) in these tiny subjects.

Both the preliminary preparation of the patient and the operative procedure should proceed with all deliberate speed and require an experienced staff to carry out a coordinated plan in which, as much as practicable, preparatory measures are *performed simultaneously* rather than in sequence.

Electrocardiogram leads are positioned, the baby anesthetized, and a central venous line (generally the basilic or internal jugular vein) is inserted for delivery of fluids and drugs. With the exception of blood (administered by syringe), all fluids are delivered with infusion pumps equipped to operate on either line or battery power. This insures that postoperative transfer to the intensive care unit is simplified. All infusion lines must have been meticulously cleared of even the smallest air bubble since as little as 0.1 ml of air delivered to the brain or heart can cause severe damage. The anesthesiologist can now administer muscle relaxants and other agents through the line, thereby facilitating endotracheal tube (uncuffed) insertion. If systemic arterial access has not been previously obtained (umbilical artery of a newborn), an upper extremity artery is cannulated (either radial or brachial) percutaneously or, if necessary, by cutdown to monitor systemic pressure, blood gases, pH, hematocrit, electrolytes, and glucose levels. If attempts to enter the artery percutaneously are not promptly successful, the surgeon should approach the artery directly by cutdown.

An esophageal thermistor probe is inserted and urine is collected for measurement either with a plastic bag taped to the perineum or an indwelling bladder catheter.

Most palliative procedures are performed through a lateral thoracotomy, thereby requiring that one lung be compressed. Mediastinal movement (consequent to inflation of the contralateral lung or ventilatory efforts of the infant) must be controlled by the anesthesiologist to enable the surgeon to accurately carry out all technical manipulations without any delay. The operation must be planned to allow for periodic reexpansion of the compressed lung. Hence, the anesthesiologist must be able to see the operative field and *work with* the surgeon to ensure that ventilation is adequate, controlled, and coordinated with the surgical maneuvers.

When a systemic-pulmonary artery shunt is performed, one pulmonary artery is necessarily occluded, increasing sharply the probability of life-threatening hypoxia and acidosis. A sign of impending serious trouble is the onset of bradycardia (often before there is a noticeable change in blood pressure). Surgical maneuvers must cease, if at all possible; the lung is reexpanded and ventilatory exchange maximized. Although there is no blood flow from the heart to the lungs through the occluded pulmonary artery, reexpansion of the lung allows increased transit to the left atrium of aortopulmonary collateral blood contained within that lung. Reexpansion is frequently followed by an improvement in heart rate and blood pressure. If improvement does not occur promptly, it is helpful to begin a slow infusion of a dilute solution of epinephrine (1 mg in 250 ml of D5W) at a rate that will achieve an adequate hemodynamic response. Indeed, it has been the practice of one of us (R.S.L.) to electively institute administration of the drug slowly (0.1 µg/kg/min) in all neonates having palliative procedures, beginning at the time of lung compression for exposure and continuing until thoracic closure has begun.

OPEN INTRACARDIAC SURGERY IN NEONATES AND INFANTS

It is remarkable that precariously ill babies can now undergo primary definitive repair with an acceptably low mortality, particularly since neonates requiring emergency operations invariably manifest preoperative multiple subsystem dysfunction as a consequence of severe hypoxemia or congestive heart failure. Extraordinary as these contemporary accomplishments are, it is all the more impressive to recall that two decades ago Kirklin and DuShane (1961) and Sloan et al. (1962) demonstrated the efficacy of intracardiac correction employing cardiopulmonary bypass (CPBP) in infants. Indeed, it was Sloan (1962) who first combined surface cooling, circulatory arrest, and limited CPBP, a technique subsequently widely employed by Hikasa (1967) and further refined by Barratt-Boyes et al. (1971).

The following discussion will deal solely with perfusion methods used in neonates and infants, since perfusion conduct in larger children does not differ significantly from that employed in adults.*

Equipment and Priming Perfusate

Although hard evidence is still largely lacking,

A comprehensive discussion of the physiologic concepts, equipment, and procedures employed in open heart surgery will be found in Chapter 5.

there is general agreement that the perfusion equipment should be miniaturized as much as is safely possible to minimize the discrepancy between the infant's blood volume and the priming volume of the extracorporeal circuit. Currently available equipment still requires a *minimal* priming volume of 600 to 800 ml, an amount equal to the blood volume of a 6- to 8-kg infant. This represents a significant improvement over circumstances in earlier years, when priming-blood volume ratios of 5 and even 10 to 1 were common.

Both bubble and membrane oxygenators are in current use for infant perfusions; priming volumes for the *entire circuit* (oxygenator, tubing, etc.) approximate 600 to 800 ml. Improvements in bubble oxygenator design now permit reduced gas-blood flow ratios as low as 0.75/1.0. Hence, despite the theoretical physiologic advantages of membrane oxygenators, the simplicity and excellent clinical results associated with modern low prime bubble oxygenators continues to make them the device of choice in most pediatric cardiac surgical centers. All of the modern disposable bubble oxygenators have reasonably efficient integral heat exchangers, which are sufficient to conduct moderate hypothermic perfusions and subsequent rewarming. However, when profound levels of hypothermia are to be used, an additional heat exchanger is incorporated in either the venous or arterial line.

Ultrapore filtration of the cardiotomy return blood is essential. Whether filtration of the blood returning to the child via the arterial line is also essential (albeit desirable) remains less clear at present.

Although pulsatile perfusion is used in several centers, we and most groups continue to use nonpulsatile roller pumps. There simply is no convincing information that there are major advantages with pulsatile flow in the usual clinical circumstances. Indeed, there are several practical disadvantages (see Chapter 5). Adequate control of arterial flow and cardiotomy return requires that the pump housing be adjusted to accept 6.4 mm (one-fourth inch) I D tubing.

Hemodilute perfusate is routinely employed. Neonate and infant perfusions almost always require addition of blood to a heparinized, buffered, isosmolar crystalloidal diluent to achieve proper levels of hemodilution. The *desired mixed hematocrit* (i.e., the hematocrit achieved when the pump prime and the patient's blood volume are thoroughly mixed) is 30 if a short normothermic or mild hypothermic perfusion is anticipated, 25 for moderate hypothermia, and 20 for deep hypothermia.*
The importance of using a hemodilute perfusate when profound levels of hypothermia are used is now well recognized (Bove and Behrendt, 1980). In earlier years, when hypothermic circulatory arrest was carried out without hemodilution in patients with normal or high hematocrits, severe brain and kidney damage were often encountered. Undoubtedly, major factors etiologic to the damage included the viscous character of the cold blood, formed element sludging within the microvasculature, and a "no reflow phenomenon" at the time of circulatory restoration (Bjork and Hultquist, 1962; Brunberg et al., 1974).

Preliminaries

All of the preliminary procedures discussed earlier (see Management of Closed Procedures) are expeditiously carried out. Additionally, because perfusion hypothermia is almost invariably employed and since various areas of the body cool and rewarm at different rates, three temperature probes are inserted: in the esophagus (fastest rate of thermal change observed), the rectum (slowest rate of change), and either the nasopharynx or tympanic membrane (intermediate rate of change; approximate brain temperature).

Perfusion Conduct

After sternotomy and exposure of the heart and great vessels, a 000 polyester purse-string suture is placed in the ascending aortic wall and the adventitia in the circumscribed area is

---

The reader is referred to Chapter 5 for details of perfusate design, including buffering and the formula used to calculate the amount of blood needed to adjust the priming perfusate to achieve the desired mixed hematocrit *after the start of perfusion.*

cleared. Although this seems to be a small detail, it is important to do it before heparinization so that any small amount of bleeding that might occur at one of the aortic wall suture interstices will have a chance to clot. In the usual surgical situation, two purse-strings are placed in the right atrial wall, the first around the right atrial appendage and the second close to the inferior vena cava. Heparin (200 μ/kg) is injected directly into the right atrium and the activated coagulation time checked and adjusted as required (see Chapter 5).

Cannulation. Aortic cannulation is performed with a thin walled plastic cannula that is fitted with a snug but adjustable collar near its tip, permitting only a short cannula length to lie within the aortic lumen. A properly sized cannula must not be so large that it significantly impedes systemic ventricular ejection, while at the same time it must have a large enough orifice to prevent an unacceptably large pressure gradient across the cannula (> 100 mm Hg) from occurring at the predicted flow rate (see Table 5–1 of Chapter 5 for detailed data relating to cannula size).

Unless necessitated by either anomalies of systemic venous return or anticipation of total circulatory arrest, separate vena caval cannulation is performed with the largest cannula that can be *readily* accepted by each vena cava. If circulatory arrest is to be used, single cannula drainage from the right atrium is generally employed. After appropriately connecting the cannulae to the extracorporeal tubing lines, partial CPBP is initiated, usually at 32C. The entire system is checked for performance adequacy before total bypass is established and the intracardiac repair begun.

Perfusion Rates and Temperature. At normothermia or mild hypothermia, flow rates of 2.4 liters/min/m^2 are employed. It is more convenient and just as accurate to calculate the flow rate for tiny infants in relation to weight (kg) rather than surface area. Flow rates of 125 ml/kg/min are used if perfusion temperatures at or above 30C are elected. If deeper levels of perfusion hypothermia are to be used, it follows that proportionally lower flow rates can be employed, as will be discussed later.

If high flow rates were to be used in infants undergoing correction of complex defects, exposure of intracardiac structures could be obscured by coronary venous and aortopulmonary collateral blood returning to the heart. Thus, perfusion hypothermia with reduced flow is routinely employed in all but the simplest intracardiac repairs. Indeed, there are circumstances (discussed below) in which a period of *no flow* is desirable during the intracardiac repair.

Despite more than a quarter century of experience with perfusion hypothermia in humans, it is important to appreciate that the *permissible* levels of reduced flow relative to perfusion temperature reduction are derived largely from gross survival data and clinical assessment of cerebral function. The presently used methods are not always able to define subtle derangements that could become manifest years later. Moreover, the issue is further complicated by the fact that behavioral, intellectual, and motor abnormalities may have been caused by factors unrelated to the cardiac surgery. We must accept that the effects of current methods of cooling and rewarming of homoiotherms are still poorly understood. Norwood et al. (1979) pointedly remind us of our incomplete understanding with their observation that the "protective effect of hypothermia is not solely a result of reduced metabolic rate."

With these limitations, experience has suggested it is safe to reduce flow to 50 percent of the calculated normothermic flow rate for as long as 90 minutes at 28C (nasopharyngeal). At 20C, reduction of flow to 25 percent is readily tolerated for 60 minutes. Regardless of the final body hypothermic temperature that has been selected, it is essential that a period of high flow cooling be maintained for 8 to 15 minutes (depending on the child's mass) before reducing the perfusion rate to achieve even and adequate cooling of the muscle mass and vital organs. Organ cooling (particularly the brain) is facilitated by maintenance of normal to high carbon dioxide tensions (Payne et al., 1963). Accordingly, a 95/5 percent oxygen-carbon dioxide gas mixture is delivered to the oxygenator during the hypothermic perfusion.

A period of *circulatory arrest* is often desirable in infants under three months or those weighing less than 6 kg who are undergoing repair of complex intracardiac anomalies. During the arrest interval, the need is eliminated for space-occupying intracardiac suckers, vents, and vena caval cannulae; all of these compromise exposure and tend to distort delicate intracardiac structural relationships. Safe hypothermic circulatory arrest conditions can be induced by either external (surface) cooling or reduction of the perfusate temperature during CPBP (core cooling) or both.

Combined Surface and Core Cooling with Circulatory Arrest. Originally employed two decades ago, this method offers the advantage of preliminary cooling of the skin and skeletal muscle mass so that the subsequent period of perfusion cooling is relatively short, a major consideration in earlier years when perfusion techniques were certainly more crude than those of today. The procedure involves initial surface cooling with either plastic bags filled with crushed ice or a "hypothermic chamber" (Vidne and Subramanian, 1976) (Fig. 19–1). External cooling is continued until the core temperature (best reflected by the esophageal probe) has fallen to 25C, at which point sternotomy, cardiac exposure, and cannulation are carried out. A brief period of perfusion cooling (7 to 10 minutes) is employed to lower the nasopharyngeal or tympanic membrane temperature to 16 to 17C.*

Circulatory Arrest with Perfusion Cooling Alone. In recent years, as a result of improvement in perfusion equipment and methodology (see earlier discussion), many groups have tended to rely exclusively on perfusion cooling to achieve circulatory arrest conditions. The infant is brought into a cold operating room and anesthetized. Once asleep, the baby is stripped while the cutdowns and other preliminaries are carried out. In this cold environment the body temperature falls to approximately 34C by the time the skin incision is made. The aorta is cannulated, single cannula drainage of the right atrium is performed, and high flow CPBP instituted with the perfusate temperature lowered to 12C. Core cooling is continued until the rectal temperature† has fallen below 20C and the nasopharyngeal or tympanic membrane temperature has fallen to 16C. At this point the ascending aorta is cross-clamped, perfusion discontinued, and the venous blood allowed to drain into the oxygenator. The vena cavae are occluded, the right atrial cannula is removed, and the intracardiac repair begun.

Although limited data are available concerning the "safe" period of circulatory arrest in infants, sufficient experience has accumulated indicating that up to 60 minutes is well-tolerated at the above temperatures (Clarkson et al., 1980). However, if the surgical correction has not been completed by 45 minutes it seems prudent to reinstitute perfusion at 12C at a rate of 50 ml/kg/min for a 5- to 10-minute period. Cardiotomy suckers are used to recover the venous return, a technique first suggested by Ebert and colleagues (Smith et al., 1978).

Resumption of Perfusion and Discontinuance Measures. After completion of the intracardiac repair, the venous cannula is reinserted into the right atrium (the functional left atrium after the Mustard or Senning procedure),

---

Various surgical groups have specified slightly different temperature levels that are to be attained by both the initial (external cooling) and subsequent core cooling procedures. For these and other important procedural details, the reader is referred to Castaneda et al. (1974), Barrett-Boyes (1976), Vidne and Subramanian (1976), and Sade et al. (1977).

†*When perfusion cooling is employed (wthout prior surface cooling), the rectal temperature tends to lag behind other temperature measurements. Hence, once it has fallen below 20C one can be reasonably confident that adequate cooling of the other regions of the body has occurred. Nevertheless, confirmation by esophageal and nasopharyngeal (or tympanic membrane) temperatures is essential.*

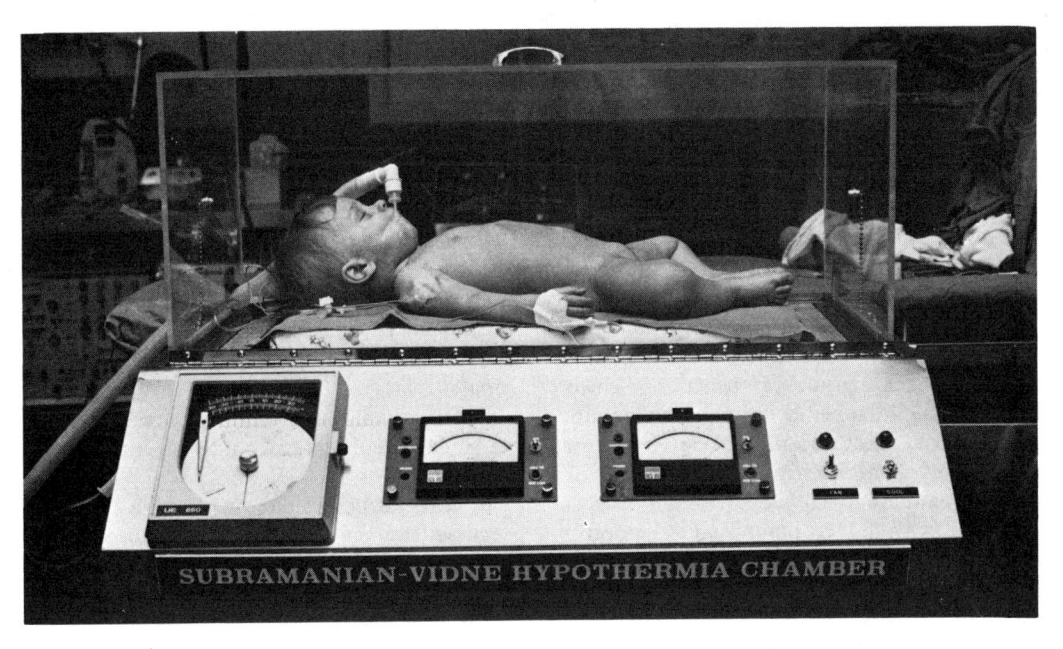

Figure 19–1. An infant in the hypothermia chamber. The plastic cooling box allows convenient access to the infant. *(Photograph courtesy of Dr. S. Subramanian).*

perfusion reinstituted at high flow rate, and the aortic crossclamp removed. Evacuation of air from the heart through an aortic root vent must be meticulous and perfusion rewarming precisely carried out with a blood-nasopharyngeal temperature gradient not to exceed 10C (see Chapter 5). The heart is massaged regularly to avoid overdistention until organized contractions occur. Electrical defibrillation, if required, is delayed until the esophageal temperature is 32C. Perfusion rewarming is continued until the *rectal* temperature is 34C. Core rewarming is supplemented by surface warming with a thermal blanket and raising the operating room temperature. During perfusion rewarming, small polyvinyl catheters are positioned in both atria and temporary atrial and ventricular pacing wires are sutured into place. Additionally, availability of a pediatric size (no. 2-2.5 Fr.) thermistor catheter now permits frequent and reliable thermodilution cardiac output measurements to be performed postoperatively in infants (Moodie et al., 1979). The catheter is passed into the pulmonary artery from the right ventricular outflow tract during the CPBP support period. Unless dictated by specific information requirements, a pulmonary artery line for pressure and blood gas sampling is not routinely inserted.

With completion of rewarming and apparently satisfactory performance of the cardiovascular and pulmonary subsystems, CPBP is gradually terminated. The aortic cannula is removed, as is one atrial cannula (assuming that two were used). The arterial pump line is connected to the one atrial cannula remaining within the heart and any desired volume increment from the pump-oxygenator is delivered by this route. As is customary, additional volume filling is guided initially by atrial and systemic arterial pressures.

Levels and relationships between left atrial (LA) and right atrial (RA) pressures are influenced by many factors after open intracardiac operation (see Chapter 9). In particular, the nature of the cardiac pathology and the repair as well as derangements imposed by the perfusion and the imperfections of myocardial protection importantly influence ventricular filling pressures and their management immediately after discontinuance of CPBP. For example, after repair of severe tetralogy of Fallot, right ventricular compliance is suboptimal, with the result that the RA pressure often will be higher than the LA pressure. Additionally, hemodilution perfusion and use of hypothermic cardioplegia tend to produce some transient myocardial edema and reduce ventricular compliance. These events may become apparent immediately after CPBP termination or, as a consequence of reperfusion dysfunction (which may take some time to become maximally manifest), 20 to 30 minutes later. Hence, in the *immediate postperfusion period* it seems prudent to maintain atrial pressures as low as is consistent with an acceptably stable hemodynamic state in anticipation of a possibly delayed rise in filling pressures consequent to altered ventricular compliance.

When the preload volume has been properly adjusted, the one remaining atrial cannula is withdrawn from the heart. If a substantial volume of perfusate is still in the heart-lung machine, it is centrifuged and the packed cells administered subsequently as required.

Even in the presence of adequate cardiac output, the use of perfusion hypothermia is frequently attended by significant elevation of mean arterial pressure and systemic vascular resistance in the early postperfusion period (Benzing et al., 1970). Management of afterload elevation and the other measures taken to optimize cardiac performance in infants will be discussed later.

Operative Completion

After decannulation, the heparinized state is reversed with protamine sulfate. Although the elegant dose-response curve of Bull et al. (1975) is ideal, we have found it simple and effective to calculate the total dosage of heparin used (the amount placed in the prime plus the amount administered to the baby throughout the procedure) and deliver a milligram-for-milligram dose of protamine.

Although it is a truism that hemostasis must be carefully secured, experience has documented the increased tendency in infants for even the smallest oozing point to stubbornly persist. Presumably, this is related in part to reduced tensile strength of the infants's tissues due to the immature character of collagen (Bove and Behrendt, 1980) and the fact that infants coming to surgery with severe polycythemia accompanying cyanotic heart disease tend to bleed more. Hence, it is essential that all suture lines be absolutely dry before closure is begun. Two intrapericardial drainage tubes are inserted and, whenever feasible, the pericardium is loosely approximated. Sternal and wound closure is now carried out, the skin being approximated with a slowly absorbable running subcuticular suture.

Unless specific circumstances dictate otherwise, the originally inserted orotracheal tube is not replaced. Because of the invariable occurrence of some degree of gastric dilatation, a nasogastric tube is inserted by the anesthesiologist. When all subsystems are stable, the infant is transferred to the Intensive Care Unit (ICU).

Transfer to the Intensive Care Unit

This is potentially an exceedingly treacherous period, since cardiorespiratory functional assessment and facility of management are limited. A portable open-care unit such as an Ohio Neonatal Intensive Care Center* is brought into the operating room and the baby gently moved to it from the operating table. This seemingly simple undertaking is fraught with many hazards, the most important of which is endotracheal tube dislocation. The anesthesiologist, having previously "unitized" the endotracheal tube and the head with a stabilizing gauze turban (Fig. 19–2), coordinates the move from the operating table.

It has been our practice to *first* move the baby to the open-care bed while all intraoperative monitoring systems are still completely functional, to ensure continued stability of the baby. Once the move to the open-care bed has been accomplished, the ECG leads that will be used in the ICU are attached and connected to

---

Ohio Medical Products, Madison, Wis. 53707.

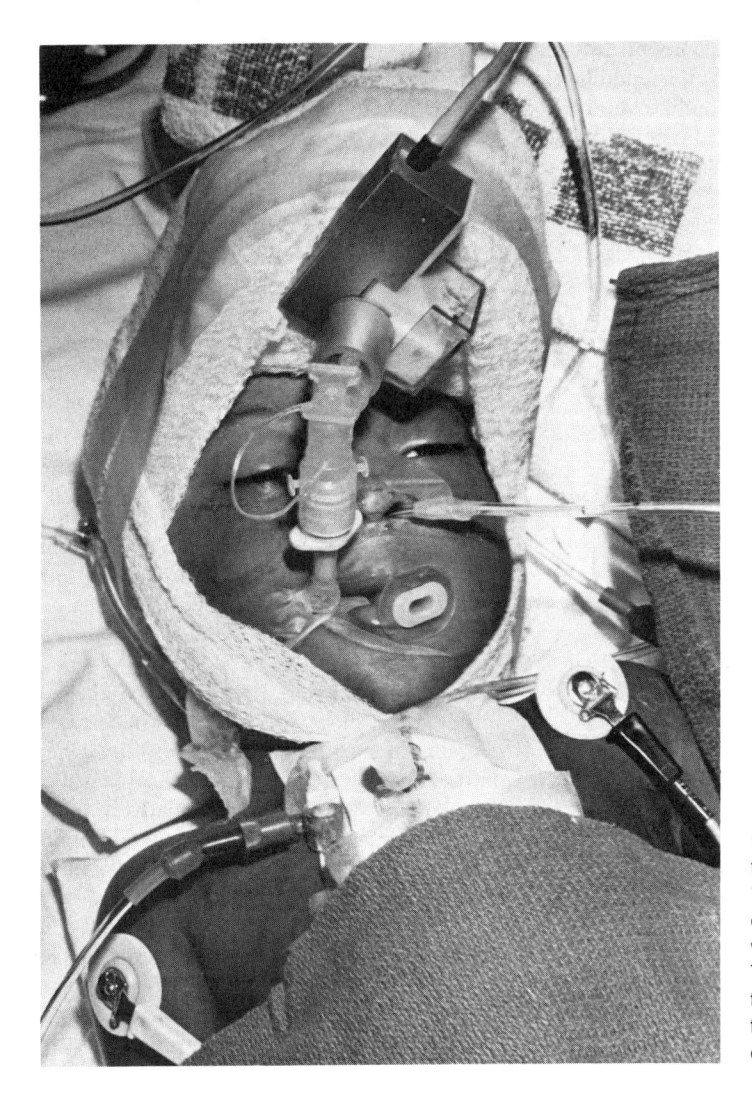

Figure 19-2. The endotracheal tube is immobilized with a gauze "turban" to avoid kinking or dislocation of the endotracheal tube when the baby's head is turned. The rectangular instrument (distal to the endotracheal tube connector) is the sensor for the carbon dioxide analyzer.

a battery-operated vital sign monitor* and all fluid filled pressure lines are capped to permit direct connections to transducers in the ICU immediately on arrival. However, if the ICU is some distance from the operating room or if vasoactive drugs are being administered, the systemic arterial pressure is continuously monitored during the transfer either with a battery-operated unit (ideal but cumbersome) or with a simple aneroid system connected to the arterial line through a three-way stopcock. All mechanical infusion pumps are now switched to battery power to permit uninterrupted delivery of fluid and drugs during the trip to the ICU; once in the ICU the pumps will be returned to line power, thereby obviating the delay and potential instability inherent in switching to ICU pumps.

Transfer to the ICU is now effected with the anesthesiologist ventilating the baby with simple hand compression of an oxygen-rich

---

*Tektronix, Inc., Beaverton, Ore. 97005.

reservoir bag system. While it is elemental that hypoventilation must be avoided, it is equally important that the baby not be made severely hypocarbic (with its potential dangers) by overly aggressive ventilation—a common error.

POSTOPERATIVE CARE

Postoperative supportive care of infants and children after cardiac surgery demands the efforts of a staff that has a specific commitment to and experience in the care of these tiny patients. There must be *constant attendance* of physicians and knowledgeable pediatric ICU nurses for the first 24 hours (longer if the baby has not been extubated or manifests any subsystem instability).

An orderly plan that, as much as possible, seeks to use quantitative indices of functional performance is the key to successful clinical assessment and management. The goal is to *prevent complications* and is facilitated by Kirklin's systems analysis approach (1970), in which the patient is considered to be a complex *system* composed of multiple functionally *integrated subsystems,* a concept that has been repeatedly stressed in this text. Hence, although the discussions that follow deal with each subsystem separately, it must be appreciated that the separation is one of literary convenience; the continued performance failure of one subsystem ultimately will adversely affect all of the others.

In the delivery of postoperative care, a conscious effort must be made to cluster and integrate assessment and management procedures so that adequate periods of rest are ensured. It should never be forgotten that rest is one of the indispensable components of convalescence for all seriously ill patients, particularly infants and children.

Admission Measures

Reception Procedures. Admission of the infant to the ICU requires the coordinated activity of a reception team of nurses, technicians, and other supporting staff. A well-organized and disciplined effort entails concurrent performance of assigned tasks by each member of the reception team: one assists the anesthesiologist in establishing controlled ventilation; another connects the pressure monitoring lines to transducers and clears the lines of any air; another switches the ECG to the ICU monitoring system and the battery driven infusion pumps to line power; another connects the nasogastric tube to a vented receptacle, checks the urine drainage system, and inserts a rectal thermistor, while someone else connects the open-care unit to ICU electrical power and reestablishes continuity of the pericardial drainage system. All efforts, properly concerted, can be carried out in several minutes. In these endeavors, a senior staff nurse stands by to coordinate all maneuvers, although few, if any, instructions will be required if the reception team is experienced.

Temperature Control. Regardless of age, all subjects must increase their metabolic activity to maintain normal body temperature when exposed to cold. Infants are at a particular disadvantage because of a relatively small amount of insulating subcutaneous fat and a large surface area relative to body mass. Hence, heat loss by both radiation and evaporation is increased. The heat production in response to even minimal cold stress can lead to serious depletion of energy stores causing hypoglycemia, hypoxia, and acidosis.

Obligatory increases in postoperative metabolic activity of the infant can be reduced by maintenance of ambient thermal neutrality (that temperature at which energy expenditure to generate heat is at a basal level). This temperature varies with the infant's age and size (Hey and Katz, 1970). For example, the thermoneutral ambient temperature (TNAT) of a five-day-old 1-kg baby is 34.7C, and 33.4C for a 3-kg baby of the same age. With increasing age, the infant's TNAT requirement falls slightly. At 30 days of age, the TNAT of the 1-kg infant falls to 33.3C, and 32.5C for the 3-kg baby (Rowe, 1979). In the ICU, close attention is paid to attaining proper environmental conditions by radiant heating of the open-care unit. The amount of radiant heat is servocontrolled by a skin temperature probe. For a comprehensive review of the subject, the reader is referred to Sinclair (1978).

Laboratory Studies. As soon as the reception procedures just described have been completed, an arterial sample is drawn for micromethod measurement of blood gases, pH, hematocrit, serum osmolality, electrolytes, urea nitrogen, and glucose. These latter two moieties sharply affect serum osmolality and sudden changes can have serious consequences (see later discussion). In addition to hourly measurement of urinary output, determinations are made of urinary sodium and potassium concomitantly with the other laboratory studies.

Even if the infant appears to be satisfactorily stable, the potential for adverse biochemical changes to occur insidiously and rapidly necessitates repetition of all determinations every two hours for the first eight postoperative hours and thereafter every four to six hours for the first 24 hours. Evidence of any instability obviously requires more frequent performance of appropriate studies and absolutely mandates prompt and sequential measurements of cardiac output, either by thermodilution or indocyanine green.

A portable chest film is obtained promptly on admission to the ICU, eight hours postoperatively, and daily thereafter for the first two to three days postoperatively. The films not only permit evaluation of the status of the lungs, pleura, and cardiac silhouette but also reveal the position of both the nasogastric and endotracheal tubes. It must be remembered that a newborn's trachea may be only 4 cm long; therefore, slight positional change can cause the endotracheal tube to enter the right main bronchus and completely obstruct the left main and right upper lobe bronchi.

The location and proper function of the nasogastric tube is all too frequently ignored. Improper positioning or kinking of the tube can result in acute gastric dilatation with compromise of cardiopulmonary function.

Subsystem Assessment and Management

The Pulmonary Subsystem. Despite major advances in postoperative ventilatory management, respiratory failure remains a major cause of morbidity and mortality in infants after cardiac surgery. These problems are particularly liable to occur in those infants with severe preoperative pulmonary dysfunction who require emergency operations. It is our current practice to continue mechanical ventilation in the early postoperative period of all infants and children, regardless of age, who have undergone open intracardiac operations.

It is recognized that extubation in the operating room can be carried out safely in infants, provided that they meet appropriate criteria (Barash et al., 1979). However, it is our view that the *routine* maintenance of intubated ventilatory control until the continued stability of all subsystems in the ICU is ensured offers advantages that outweigh the small incidence of potential complications associated with such a routine. Once satisfactory performance of all subsystems has been documented, our extubation protocol (discussed later) is promptly initiated. In most cases, extubation is carried out within several hours after the patient's arrival in the ICU.

MECHANICAL VENTILATION. A volume-controlled time-cycled ventilator is employed. Our experience is with the Siemens-Elema Model 900 B servoventilator with an in-line model 930 carbon dioxide analyzer.* In normal lungs, end-tidal P_{CO_2} accurately reflects systemic arterial P_{CO_2}. By providing breath-

---

*A principal feature of this analyzer is that the infrared cell is in series with the airway and requires no withdrawal of gas for the analysis. The level of peak expired CO_2 (E_{CO_2}) is read as a percentage of the concentration of the gas. For example, assuming an atmospheric pressure of 760 mm Hg, a vapor pressure 47 mm Hg, and a normal systemic arterial P_{CO_2} (Pa_{CO_2}) of 40 mm Hg, the CO_2 analyzer would read out 5.61 percent. A rising Pa_{CO_2} would be accompanied by an increased percent E_{CO_2}, while a falling Pa_{CO_2} would be reflected by a lower E_{CO_2} percentage.

by-breath assessment of the level of peak Eco_2, the analyzer permits convenient ventilator adjustments to optimize $Paco_2$ without necessarily resorting to multiple blood gas measurements. This is feasible since, once established, the relationship between Eco_2 and $Paco_2$ in a baby convalescing satisfactorily is relatively stable. Hence, by comparing the percent of Eco_2 with the initial $Paco_2$ measurement, it is possible to predict what the $Paco_2$ would be after a ventilator adjustment has been made by simply observing the directional change and percent Eco_2.

A cascade type of heated humidifier is used to maintain an inspiratory gas temperature no lower than 32C so that the humidity of the gas approximates or exceeds 85 percent.

The initial oxygen concentration (F_{IO_2}) is set at 0.4 in the absence of specific gas exchange problems that might have been experienced in the operating room and provided that the initial postoperative blood gas study reveals a Pao_2 of at least 60 mm Hg. Obviously, a higher F_{IO_2} is selected in more compromised circumstances, but this should be reduced as quickly as clinical conditions permit. It is important to appreciate that hyperoxia offers no physiologic advantage and, indeed, imposes the real dangers of pulmonary damage in all neonates and retrolental fibroplasia in preterm infants. Accordingly, the F_{IO_2} should be adjusted to ensure that the Pao_2 will not exceed 100 mm Hg. Intravascular catheters containing sensors to continuously measure oxygen saturation or Po_2 are useful for this purpose (Brown et al., 1980).

Tidal Volume (TV) is calculated at 10 ml/kg *plus* the measured compliance volume of the ventilator circuit.* Practical considerations such as inadequate thoracic expansion or poorly heard breath sounds may dictate the use of a slightly higher TV. Peak *inflation pressure* should be kept below 25 cm H_2O unless lung compliance is poor; this circumstance requires higher pressures for adequate ventilation.

Ventilatory rate is set between 20 and 30 per minute, depending on the size of the infant (older and larger infants are ventilated at the lower end of this range). It has been shown that relatively slow cycling rates are associated with higher Pao_2 (Smith et al., 1969). Slow ventilatory rates allow both a relatively long inspiratory phase—shown to be important in raising Pao_2 (Reynolds, 1971)—while also permitting an adequately lengthy expiratory phase, ensuring that cardiac output is not compromised. It has been our experience that an *inspiratory:expiratory* ratio of 1:2 is satisfactory in most cases.

Further adjustment of the ventilator settings of F_{IO_2}, TV, and rate are made after the first arterial blood gas report is received. As discussed previously, this information is correlated with the peak Eco_2 (from the CO_2 analyzer) to allow additional "fine tuning" of the ventilator. Optimally, the Pao_2 should be maintained between 70 and 100 mm Hg, the $Paco_2$ between 30 and 40 mm Hg, and the pH between 7.35 and 7.45.

When the infant's $Paco_2$ is observed to be abnormal, in theory three ventilator adjustments can be made: change (1) the dead space, (2) the ventilator rate, or (3) the TV. For example, if hypocarbia is present, dead space could be added, the ventilator rate reduced, or TV lowered. Since reduction of TV can increase the possibility of significant atelectasis, we believe that only the first two of the three approaches should be exploited. Similarly, in a hypercarbic state it seems advisable to either reduce the dead space or increase the ventilator rate. In both circumstances, the first option (changing the dead space) is preferable, if convenient.

POSITIVE END-EXPIRATORY PRESSURE (PEEP). There are certain potential problems with the use of high levels of PEEP (reduction of cardiac output and pneumothorax). Hence, employment of PEEP is restricted to those situations in which there is radiologic evidence of significant atelectasis or blood gas evidence of substantial intrapulmonary shunting ($Pao_2 < 60$ mm Hg with $F_{IO_2} > 0.8$ and normal or low $Paco_2$). It is also used briefly

---

Each ventilator manufacturer details a procedure to obtain this measurement.

during the weaning process (see page 446, Weaning from the Ventilator).

When PEEP is required, it is initially set at 2.5 cm H_2O at an FI_{O_2} of 0.5. The level of PEEP is raised only after clear evidence of no clinical improvement. Because of the potential dangers (see above), PEEP should not exceed 15 cm H_2O in these babies. If the Pa_{O_2} remains < 60 mm Hg despite increasing PEEP, the FI_{O_2} is then progressively raised above 0.5 with full recognition that a life-threatening respiratory problem exists.

Although *continuous positive airway pressure* (CPAP) in combination with spontaneous breathing (Gregory et al., 1971) has been effectively employed in infants after open heart surgery (Stewart et al, 1973), it has been used less frequently in the past several years, almost certainly because of the availability of more sophisticated ventilators and improved management techniques.

TRACHEAL TOILET. This procedure must be done with great care and with full appreciation that reduced Pa_{O_2} invariably accompanies the procedure and can persist for many minutes after termination of tracheobronchial suction (Fig. 19–3). The potential for the development of life-threatening hypoxemia as a consequence of protracted suctioning is apparent. Moreover, in a postperfusion child emerging from anesthesia, tracheobronchial suction may be accompanied by bucking and a consequent sharp increase in intracranial pressure, conditions that could precipitate serious neurologic sequelae, particularly if there still happens to be some residual circulating anticoagulant effect.

For these reasons, we do not consider that routine suctioning "by the clock" is desirable. Rather, the procedure is performed only if a secretion buildup is detected. From a practical standpoint, this usually requires that suctioning will be performed every two to three hours (and occasionally more frequently).

Sterile technique is employed (gloves, new sterile catheter each time, etc.). After a one- to two-minute period of modest hyperventilation (Pa_{CO_2} reduced to 25 to 30 mm Hg) with an Ambu bag and oxygen, a catheter (with a side vent hole or a Y-connector) is gently passed into the endotracheal tube as far as it will go conveniently *without suction being applied*. Suction is used *only* during withdrawal of the aspirating tube to minimize the hypoxia caused by sucking out the oxygen-rich tracheobronchial air. Moreover, since the endotracheal tube is all but occluded during this time, the entire residence period of the aspirating tube (in and out) should not exceed 10 seconds.

Gentle turning of the head from one side to the other facilitates entry of the catheter into each main stem bronchus. Each brief aspiration period should be preceded by a one- to two-minute Ambu ventilatory interval. If the secretions are tenaciously thick, 0.5 to

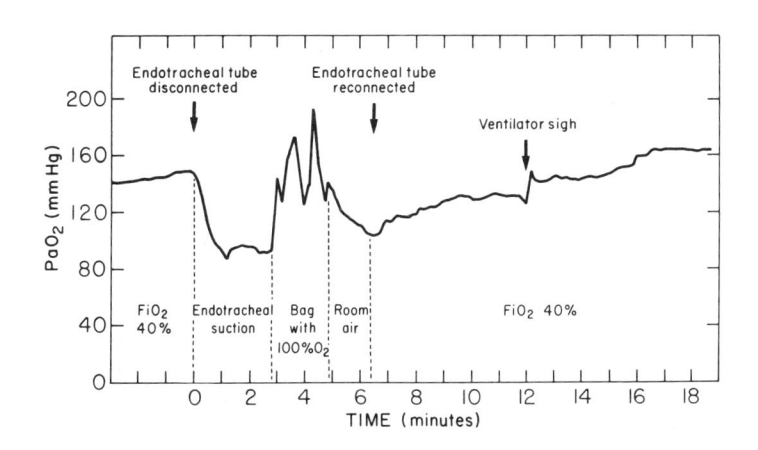

Figure 19–3. The effect of endotracheal suction and other interventions on systemic arterial oxygen tension (Pa_{O_2}). The sharp fall in Pa_{O_2} associated with the suction episode is noteworthy. Moreover, after discontinuance of suctioning, more than 11 minutes passed before the Pa_{O_2} stabilized at the level present before the aspiration. *(Redrawn after Brown et al., 1980).*

1.0 ml of physiologic saline solution is instilled before aspiration.

When tracheobronchial aspiration is required in a baby with elevated right atrial or superior vena caval pressures or those suspected of having cerebral edema, bucking must be avoided at all costs. In these circumstances a muscle relaxant such as pancuronium (0.05 mg/kg) is administered prior to the procedure.

VENTILATORY CONTROL. It is essential that the baby not "fight" the ventilator. If this does occur, one must immediately rule out ventilator malfunction, mechanical occlusion of the endotracheal tube, occlusive secretions in the distal tracheobronchial tree, or derangement of blood-gas levels and the acid-base state. If all appears to be well and the baby is simply awakening, increments of morphine (0.05 to 0.2 mg/kg) or diazepam (same dosage) will sedate the infant sufficiently to again permit unimpeded ventilatory control. Rarely it may be necessary to resort to use of pancuronium (0.05 mg/kg) to control the infant's uncoordinated ventilatory efforts.

Infants recovering uneventfully with adequate performance of all subsystems require minimal or no analgesia. Despite being awake and alert, they readily accommodate to the ventilator rate.

WEANING FROM THE VENTILATOR. An attempt is made to wean the infant as soon as he or she is alert, appears ready to breathe spontaneously, has minimal bleeding, and all subsystems are performing satisfactorily. The decision to extubate requires that a weaning protocol be followed that, on one hand, is "aggressive" enough to ensure that unnecessarily prolonged intubation does not occur but, on the other hand, is "conservative" enough to obviate all of the problems associated with urgent reintubation of an infant who has been extubated prematurely. All current extubation protocols include, in addition to quantitative data, *subjective* assessment of the infant. As conceptually undesirable as this is, the current limitation of purely quantitative criteria makes subjective assessment an essential component of the extubation decision.

Almost every currently used weaning protocol is keyed to the capability of the modern generation of mechanical ventilators to progressively reduce the ventilatory support of the infant through the use of intermittent mandatory ventilation (IMV). The approach allows the ICU staff to test the baby's ability to assume the increased work of breathing. IMV is a method in which the ventilator is set to deliver a known number of cycles per minute while the patient spontaneously breathes between these cycles. The frequency of ventilator cycling is gradually reduced as the infant demonstrates increased capacity to easily and effectively breathe spontaneously at an adequate rate and depth.

Our weaning protocol involves the use of both IMV and low PEEP. The decision to wean the infant assumes that any higher levels of PEEP that may have been used earlier are no longer required. If the baby is not on PEEP it is set at 2.5 cm H_2O and kept there until extubation. IMV rate is set at two breaths per minute below the previously set controlled rate. If this initial step elicits no spontaneous breathing, another stepwise reduction in mandatory rate is made (in decrements of two) until spontaneous breathing is observed. However, under no circumstances should the IMV rate be reduced below 50 percent of the controlled rate in the initial attempt to elicit spontaneous breathing. Rather, given these circumstances, controlled ventilation should be resumed and weaning attempts deferred for the moment.

The infant's hemodynamics, independent ventilatory rate, TV, minute volume (MV), and ECO_2 are carefully monitored to assess the baby's initial response to this challenge. In the system we employ, the latter three variables are automatically displayed.* The response to the initial challenge is considered to be satisfactory when, after a 5 to 10 minute period of IMV reduction: (1) the total ventilation rate (i.e. the sum of the spontaneous and IMV breaths), TV, and MV are ±10 percent of the previously controlled ventilator conditions; (2) an ECO_2 that, having risen transiently as a consequence of IMV reduction, does not increase more than 20 percent and thereafter begins to fall toward the level observed during controlled ventilator conditions; (3) thoracic wall movement is adequate without retraction or use of accessory muscles of ventilation; and (4) there are adequate breath sounds bilaterally. If an inappropriate trend is apparent in any of these variables or clinical observations, the baby is returned to controlled ventilation.

Satisfactorily stable conditions allow further progressive lowering (in decrements of two) of the IMV rate, provided that the assessment criteria have been fulfilled each time. If at any time the criteria are not satisfied, the IMV rate is promptly increased (by two) to the previous setting. A *fifth* assessment criterion (arterial blood-gas and acid-base check) is required when the IMV has been reduced to 50 percent of the initial controlled ventilator rate and again when the IMV is at five per minute. Arterial blood-gas data are deemed to be adequate if the Pco_2 is < 50 mm Hg, the Po_2 > 70 mm Hg, and the pH between 7.35 and 7.40. If, at the lowest IMV settings, all previously described criteria remain satisfactory, the baby has not tired after approximately one hour of spontaneous breathing, and all other subsystems are satisfactory, extubation is carried out.

EXTUBATION TECHNIQUE. Before initiating the extubation procedure, the stomach must have been adequately decompressed of air and fluid. The airway and oropharynx are carefully suctioned to minimize aspiration of any residual detritus after endotracheal tube removal. If the trachea of the child was large enough to have permitted use of a cuffed endotracheal tube, the cuff is not deflated until after these measures have been accomplished. The child is ventilated for 5 to 10 deep breaths at an unchanged FIO_2 and the tube is quickly removed at the peak of inspiration. This usually induces a cough (or a gag in an infant), which facilitates the expelling of any residual secretions in the airway. The child is then placed in an FIO_2 environment 5 to 10 percent higher than the ventilator FIO_2 setting. This is accomplished with a headhood for infants and a nonrestrictive face device (Fig. 19–4) for children.

POSTEXTUBATION CARE. The infants are maintained in a headbox, the air kept fully humidified with an FIO_2 of 0.5 to 0.7. Guided by arterial blood-gas measurements, the FIO_2 is gradually reduced to 0.3 to 0.4 over the next 24 hours. Chest films are obtained immediately after extubation and periodically thereafter.

Vigorous physiotherapy and stimulation of the baby to cry are carried out by the nursing staff every two to four hours, care being taken to permit an uninterrupted sleep period between these efforts. Periodic aspiration of the oropharnyx offers an effective means of clearing tenacious secretions that could block the pharynx or be aspirated into the tracheobronchial tree.

Although a glucocorticoid (either methylprednisolone or dexamethasone) has been used to reduce tracheal edema and postextubation stridor, we have not been impressed with its effectiveness and no longer use the drug routinely.

The Cardiovascular Subsystem. Inadequate cardiac performance remains the leading cause of death in infants and small children after open intracardiac operations. Parr et al. (1975) documented that when the cardiac index (CI) is less than 2.0 liters/min/m² and mixed venous oxygen tension (a reflection of adequacy of blood flow) is less than 30 mm Hg (normal approximately 40 mm Hg), the prob-

---

*Other systems may not provide such on-line information. In such circumstances, a Wright Respirometer can be used to obtain TV and MV. However, the instrument may prove to be relatively insensitive in small infants. Barash et al. (1979) recommend use of a minispirometer (Boehringer model No. 8805), which is more sensitive and also provides a measure of inspiratory force (which should exceed −20 cm H_2O in babies deemed ready for extubation). Additionally, in the absence of on-line TV, MV, and ECO_2 data, it is apparent that from the inception of the initial lowering of IMV, sequential determinations of arterial blood gases and pH will be necessary as IMV is progressively reduced.

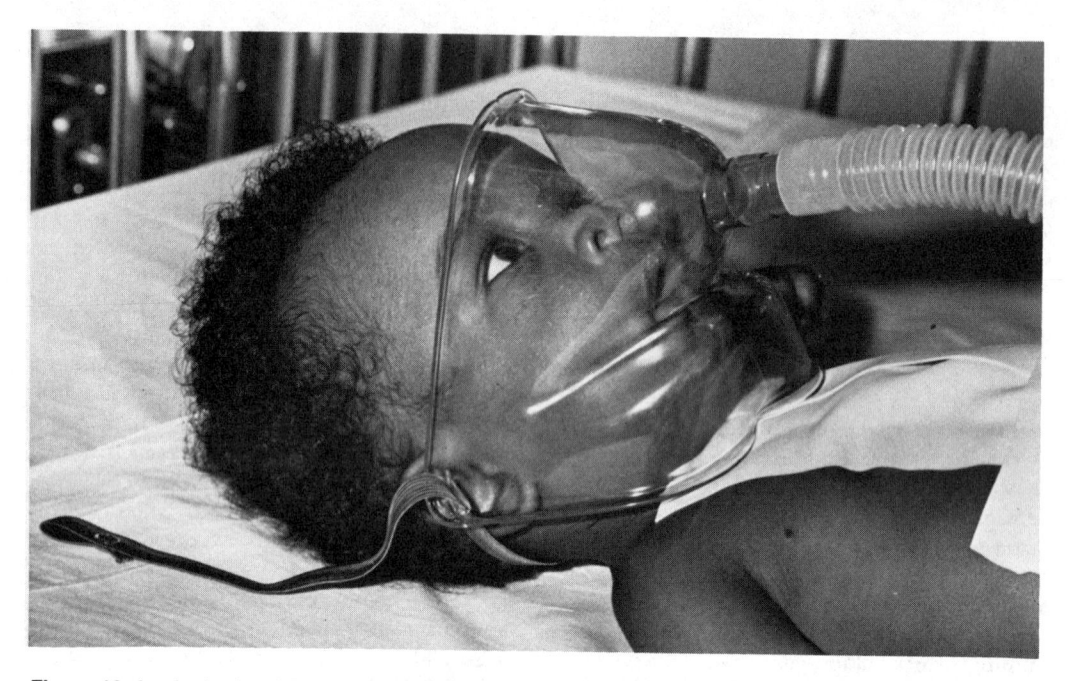

Figure 19–4. A plastic adult "face tent" is simply inverted and conforms nicely to an infant's face.

ability of acute cardiac death is sharply heightened (Fig. 19–5). Age per se is not a factor in maintenance of adequate levels of cardiac output after surgery. On the other hand, both the nature of the cardiac pathology and events in the operating room (length and conduct of perfusion, adequacy of myocardial protection, and the degree to which the repair establishes normal cardiovascular function) do influence the probability of postrepair low cardiac output.

For example, one would not expect problems after uncomplicated transatrial repair of a ventricular septal defect, because both atrial reservoir and ventricular pumping functions are not compromised. Contrarily, despite optimal management of the perfusion and myocardial protection, failure to satisfactorily "correct" a complete atrioventricular canal in which significant mitral incompetence persists would almost certainly be accompanied by low cardiac output. Similarly, after repair of total anomalous pulmonary venous connection, postoperatively low cardiac output may occur

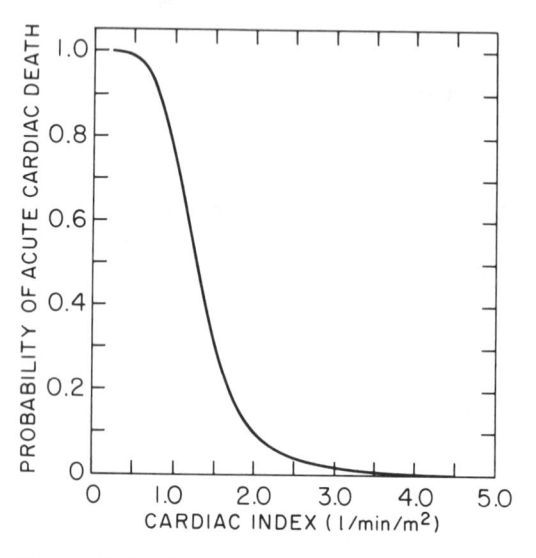

Figure 19–5. Prediction of acute cardiac death based on the mean cardiac index of patients during the first 72 hours after open intracardiac operations. The heightened probability of mortality is apparent in those patients whose mean cardiac index was less than 2.0 liters/min/m^2. (After Parr et al., 1975).

on occasion because the LA is small (low reservoir function), thereby limiting stroke volume (Parr et al., 1974). These are but several examples of the fact that well-described derangements of cardiac function after specific intracardiac repairs must be understood, anticipated, and properly managed to optimize cardiac function.

MANAGEMENT CONCEPTS. When the heart is viewed as a volume displacement pump, it is apparent that for its function to be optimized both rate and the factors affecting stroke volume must be manipulated to approach ideal performance characteristics. A broad discussion dealing with analysis, maintenance, and support of cardiac function after open intracardiac operation will be found in Chapter 9. The following comments are intended to emphasize those cardiovascular management procedures that are of particular pertinence to infants and small children.

In infants one to two years of age, the cardiac rate should be maintained between 120 and 130 beats per minute. The availability of temporary bipolar atrial and ventricular pacing wires not only allows low rates to be effectively managed but, equally important, facilitates diagnosis of complex arrhythmias (see Chapter 10 for expanded discussion of the recognition and management of arrhythmias).

In the absence of abnormal atrioventricular conduction and electrolyte problems, most infants are *electively digitalized,* particularly those who required ventriculotomy. Apart from the positive inotropic effect, another advantage of digitalis glycoside administration is the efficacy in reducing the incidence of troublesome postoperative atrial tachyarrhythmias. Certainly the severity of these abnormalities is far less and they are more readily controlled if digitalization is promptly begun as soon as the infant reaches the ICU. The drug (Lanoxin) is given either intramuscularly or intravenously. The initial dose varies from .03 to .04 mg/kg, with a daily maintenance dosage of .01 mg/kg.

Montioring of LA, RA, and systemic arterial pressures has long been a routine after open cardiac surgery in all but the simplest cases. The availability of convenient and reliable methods to measure cardiac output in even the smallest infant now makes it possible to analyze and more effectively manipulate the three factors directly influencing stroke volume: *preload, afterload,* and—by deductive reasoning—the *inotropic state.* Routine performance of sequential cardiac output measurements in infants after repair of complex intracardiac lesions would seem to be the most effective means of avoiding the onset of severe low cardiac output. At the very least, the method permits early detection of an adverse trend and is a critical guide to appropriate therapy.

During the first 18 hours after surgery, *preload* of the least compliant ventricle is electively maintained between 10 and 15 mm Hg in uncomplicated circumstances. Higher levels may be necessary upon quantitation of marginal cardiac output (see later discussion).

It has long been established that increased *afterload* is commonly observed after perfusion hypothermia (Benzing et al., 1970), particularly in infants who are in low cardiac output (Parr et al, 1975). An elegant study by Applebaum et al. (1977) documented in infants the effectiveness of sodium nitroprusside in concomitantly lowering both mean systemic and pulmonary arterial pressures, increasing CI, and reducing LA and RA pressures. In addition to the augmented venous capacity caused by the venodilating effect of nitroprusside, it must be assumed that the LA and RA pressure reduction in the presence of increased cardiac output (at an unchanged heart rate) is a direct consequence of drug-induced decreased afterload and improved ventricular performance.

IMPAIRED CARDIAC PERFORMANCE. A systematic approach to the management of suboptimal cardiac performance after surgery has been detailed in Chapter 9. Briefly, if cardiac rate and rhythm are satisfactory (a first step), the Frank-Starling mechanism is then exploited by preload augmentation. Since the pressure is highest in the atrium that provides filling of the ventricle with the most severe intrinsic or surgically induced pathology, maximal preload augmentation is dictated by the pressure in that atrium. For example, after extensive repair of severe tetralogy of Fallot, RA pressure often will exceed LA pressure, while the converse would be expected in an infant undergoing emergency intracardiac surgery for an obstructive lesion of the left ventricular outflow tract. Except in unusual circumstances, it is not advisable to add volume that will make mean LA or RA pressures exceed 20 mm Hg.

If, after having optimized rate and maximized preload, CI remains below 2 liters/min/m^2 and calculated resistances in either the pulmonary or systemic circuit are high, sodium nitroprusside is administered in a continuous drip (with a concentration of 100 μg/ml in 5 percent dextrose in water) until there is an appropriate reduction in arterial pressure. The required dosage tends to vary from 1.5 to 12 μg/kg/min. During the nitroprusside infusion, a fall in atrial pressures must be anticipated (see above) and preparations for volume filling must be made before starting the drug.

If the CI continues to be below 2 liters/min/m^2 despite the interventions just described, a positive inotropic agent to enhance myocardial contractility is infused concomitantly with both sodium nitroprusside administration and appropriate volume loading. Dopamine (2 to 10 μg/kg/min) or epinephrine (0.15 to 0.5 μg/kg/min) are equally effective, the latter having been used electively by Benzing et al. (1978) with impressive results.

The positive feedback nature of persistent and severe low cardiac output (CI < 2 liters/min/m^2) will inexorably be characterized by the onset of progressive metabolic acidosis and its lethal consequences. A buffer can transiently improve the clinical state while other therapeutic measures are being carried out to eliminate the cause of the acidosis (almost invariably impaired cardiac performance). We consider a significant metabolic acidosis to be present if the pH is < 7.30 or the buffer base deficit of the extracellular fluid (calculated from the Siggaard-Andersen nomogram) is > 5 mEq/liter. In such circumstances, either sodium bicarbonate (available in a 50-ml ampoule; concentration 1 mEq/ml) or a nonsodium-containing buffer, THAM (0.3 molar solution), is administered. The buffer should be administered through a central line, the *total dose* for either agent being calculated from the formula:

$$\text{Buffer (ml)} = \text{Base deficit (mEq/liter)} \times \text{weight (kg)} \times 0.3$$

One half of the total dose is administered slowly over a five-minute period and the other half delivered over the next hour. Blood pH must be followed carefully every 15 minutes to avoid creation of alkalosis, with its attendant danger of cardiac arrhythmias. It is particularly important that the sodium bicarbonate be given slowly and with an appreciation of the potential problems it can cause. In the limited amount of diluent usually permissible in infants, the agent is markedly hypertonic (at the concentration mentioned above, each ml = 1,648 mOsm/kg H$_2$O), and rapid administration can result in intracranial hemorrhage because of the sudden rise in serum osmolality. Tris (hydroxymethyl) amino-methane (THAM) offers several advantages as a buffer. Although still hypertonic as a 0.3 molar solution, it is far less so than the 1 mEq/liter sodium bicarbonate solution. Additionally, the agent has the capacity to cross the cell membrane and act as an intracellular buffer. Finally, THAM does not contribute a sodium load to an already compromised circulation.

A complicating component of low cardiac output is the oliguria and accompanying hyperkalemia associated with reduced renal perfusion. Apart from the primary goal of improving cardiac performance, concomitant adjustments are made in the volume and constituents of intravenous fluids. These details of management are discussed later.

The Renal Subsystem. Rowe (1979) has observed that "the kidneys [of the infant] are not fully mature until about one year of age, but the control mechanisms for maintaining homeostasis are perfectly adequate. . . . Perhaps the regulatory mechanisms are not as finely tuned as in the older individuals and, as a result, may not effectively handle conditions brought on by extreme stress." Characteristically, the infant kidney performs its diluting function satisfactorily although its concentrating capability is reduced. Thus, infants cannot conserve sodium as completely as adults (even in the presence of hyponatremia). Normal postoperative urinary sodium loss is 20 to 40 mEq/liter. Hence, infants usually require some sodium in the postoperative fluid and electrolyte prescription.

What constitutes *adequate urinary output*? In a full-term infant, 1 ml/kg/hr is satisfactory. This volume is relatively higher than that anticipated in older children (15 ml/m^2/hr), but is necessary because the infant kidney's limited concentrating capacity creates conditions requiring a larger urine volume to excrete the solute load (the maximal urine osmolality in an infant rarely exceeds 400 mOsm/kg H$_2$O, whereas almost twice that level can be observed in an older child).

Despite the immaturity of the infant kidney, perfusion trauma, and the often attendant problem of congestive heart failure, oliguria after cardiac surgery rarely is due to dehydration or intrinsic renal dysfunction. Rather, the most common cause is prerenal: low cardiac output. Therefore, in the presence of oliguria, first efforts should be directed toward quantitative assessment and optimizing of cardiac performance (see previous discussion). Concomitantly, sequential measurement of serum and urine sodium and osmolality should be initiated. Renal failure must be considered to be present if the oliguria persists, the urinary sodium exceeds 60 mEq/liter, and the urine and plasma are essentially isosmolar. A diagnosis of renal failure is reinforced if furosemide (1 mg/kg and repeated once after 20 minutes) fails to induce a prompt diuresis.

FLUID REQUIREMENTS. It is not possible to rigidly prescribe a specific fluid volume that will be appropriate for all babies after cardiac surgery. Age, preoperative condition (nature of the lesion, preoperative need for diuretics), the type of procedure (closed or open), and the postoperative hemodynamic and metabolic state all play major roles in determining fluid requirements of a particular baby. After open intracardiac operations, infants tend to have a substantial water load, primarily (but not solely) because of the perfusate they were exposed to during the operative procedure. Therefore, the calculated fluid volume is kept on the low side. Planned maintenance for babies of 10 kg or less after open operations approximates 60 to 70 ml/kg/24 hr and 100 ml/kg/24 hr after closed procedures. It is important that all fluids (including the anticipated volume necessary to maintain patency of all monitoring lines) be included in the calculations. The fluid volume originally projected requires periodic modification, guided by careful assessment of all fluid losses and sequential measurements of urinary output and osmolality.

INFUSATE COMPOSITION. Urinary cation losses in infants after cardiac surgical operations are similar (but not identical) to those observed in older patients, i.e., a brisk kaliuresis and modest sodium excretion (recall previous discussion of the limited ability of the infant kidney to conserve sodium). Because of the substantial amount of *sodium* usually delivered to the baby by the sodium bicarbonate buffer in the pump perfusate, repletion of this cation rarely is required in the early postoperative period. Similarly, there is usually no need to routinely administer calcium or magnesium in the postoperative period unless untoward events (elevated serum citrate levels from stored blood administration or excessive hemodilution) have occurred. However, the large *potassium* loss must be carefully replaced.

Blood *glucose* levels can vary significantly in either direction after open intracardiac operations. Hyperglycemia commonly is observed, generally as a consequence of a large glucose load from the pump and a transient decrease in insulin release (Mandelbaum and Morgan, 1968; Stremmel et al., 1972). In the usual circumstances, elevated glucose levels correct themselves in the first few postoperative hours without specific therapy and are not hazardous. On the other hand, for reasons still unclear, hypoglycemia can also be seen (particularly after hypothermic circulatory arrest), which, if severe, can cause both lethargy and seizures.

Because of the anticipated alterations discussed above, it seems prudent to initiate postoperative fluid therapy as a 5 to 10 percent dextrose solution in water. In the rare event of significant hyponatremia (serum sodium below 125 mEq/liter), the basic fluid should be 0.25 sodium chloride in 5 percent D/W. In the presence of hypoglycemia, the infusion rate or concentration of the glucose solution should be increased to deliver 6 to 8 mg/kg/min (one can give as high as 24 mg/kg/min) until the blood glucose concentration is at a normal or slightly higher level for 6 to 12 hours. Thereafter, the rate and concentration of the glucose infusion may be reduced slowly until the basal infusion rate of 4 to 6 mg/kg/min maintains the blood glucose at normal concentrations. Under such conditions, blood glucose levels must be checked every 30 minutes until a satisfactorily stable level has been attained.

Potassium repletion is most safely accomplished in the first 18 hours postoperatively by administering increments of potassium chloride to maintain a serum potassium level of 4 to 4.5 mEq/liter. Repletion usually begins with 1 to 2 mEq administered over 60 minutes, additional doses being guided by subsequent blood studies. It is essential to appreciate how rapidly the levels of serum potassium can change, and the importance of frequent measurements cannot be overstressed.

As suggested earlier, the most common cause of life-threatening hyperkalemia (serum potassium ≥ 7 mEq/liter) is low cardiac output with reduced renal perfusion. Apart from therapy of the primary etiology, treatment of the hyperkalemia is initiated immediately by injecting intravenously 0.5 ml/kg of 10 percent calcium gluconate over two to four minutes. The effect of the calcium is rapid but transient, and it should be followed by the injection of 1 ml.kg of 50 percent glucose over 30 to 60 minutes. Subsequently, an infusion of glucose (1.5 gm/kg) with one unit of regular insulin for each three grams of glucose is administered at a rate equal to the calculated fluid requirements. In conjunction with these measures, sodium polystyrene sulfonate (Kayexalate), a sodium-potassium exchange resin (1 gm/kg), is given rectally (1 gm dissolved in 2 to 4 ml of 10 percent dextrose).

It is necessary that this substance be retained for 30 to 60 minutes to reduce the serum potassium by 1 mEq/liter within two to four hours. It should be remembered that Kayexalate exchanges sodium for potassium with a consequent gain in body sodium. If these measures fail to reduce and maintain the serum potassium below 6.0 mEq/liter, dialysis must be initiated.

Host Defenses and Antibiotic Therapy. It is generally agreed that, regardless of age, host defenses are reduced after CPBP (Subramanian et al., 1968; Silva et al., 1974). Additionally, the phagocytic capability of polymorphonuclear cells of stressed babies is known to be diminished (data summarized by Rowe, 1979). Moreover, there is evidence that the incidence of clinical infection is significantly higher after open intracardiac surgery with CPBP if antimicrobial therapy is not employed. In a study by Slonim et al. (1963), infection was lowest when antibiotic administration was begun preoperatively and continued postoperatively. These clinical observations are in accord with several elegant experimental studies. Miles et al. (1957) demonstrated that the size of an experimental infectious lesion is largely determined by the presence or absence of bacterial defense mechanisms in the tissue at or shortly after the time of inoculation, and Burke (1961) showed that experimental infections could be suppressed by antibiotics if administered shortly before or after bacterial inoculation. Maximal suppression was observed if the antimicrobial agents were administered before the bacteria gained access to the tissue. No protective effect of the antibiotics was observed if begun beyond three hours after the experimental bacterial implantation.

A variety of antibiotic programs have been employed with equal success. At our institution, administration of penicillin and gentamicin is begun one day preoperatively and continued postoperatively for five days.

REFERENCES

Applebaum A, Blackstone E, Kouchoukos N T, Kirklin J W: Afterload reduction and cardiac output in infants early after intracardiac surgery. Am J Cardiol 39:445, 1977.

Arciniegas E, Farooki Z Q, Hakimi M, Green E W: Results of two-stage surgical treatment of tetralogy of Fallot. J Thorac Cardiovasc Surg 79:876, 1980.

Barash P G, Lescovich F, Katz J D, Talner N S, Stansel H C, Jr: Early extubation following pediatric cardiothoracic operation: a viable alternative. Ann Thorac Surg 29:228, 1979.

Barratt-Boyes B G: The technique of intracardiac repair in infancy using deep hypothermia with circulatory arrest and limited cardiopulmonary bypass. In Current Techniques in Extracorporeal Circulation. London, Butterworths, 1976, pp 197–228.

———, Simpson M J, Neutze J M: Intracardiac surgery in neonates and infants using deep hypothermia with surface cooling and limited cardiopulmonary bypass. Circulation 43, 44 (Suppl I): I-25, 1971.

Behrendt D M, Austen W G: Management of infants undergoing cardiac surgery. In Patient Care in Cardiac Surgery, (2nd ed.) Boston, Little, Brown, 1976, pp 53–65.

Benzing G III, Helmsworth J A, Schreiber J T, Kaplan S: Nitroprusside and epinephrine for treatment of low output in children after open-heart surgery. Ann Thorac Surg 27:523, 1978.

———, Stockert J E, Kaplan S: Human myocardial performance during surgical treatment of cardiac defects. J Thorac Cardiovasc Surg 59:809, 1970.

Bjork V O, Hultquist G: Contraindications to profound hypothermia in open heart surgery. J Thorac Cardiovasc Surg 44:1, 1962.

Bove E L, Behrendt D M: Open-heart surgery in the first week of life. Ann Thorac Surg 29:130, 1980.

Brown E G, McDonnell F E, Cabatu E E, Jurado R A, Maier S L, Wynn R J: Clinical evaluation of three types of continuously measuring oxygen sensors—their potential use for computer control of blood oxygenation. In Nair, S (ed.): Computers in Critical Care and Pulmonary Medicine. New York, Plenum, 1980, pp 103.

Brunberg J, Reilly E, Doty D: Central nervous system consequences in infants of cardiac surgery using deep hypothermia and circulatory arrest. Circulation 49, 50 (Suppl II): II-60, 1974.

Bull B S, Huse W M, Brauer F S, Korpman R A: Heparin therapy during extracorporeal circulation. II. The use of a dose-response curve to individualize heparin and protamine. J Thorac Cardiovasc Surg 69:685, 1975.

Burke J F: The effective period of preventive antibiotic action in experimental incisions and dermal lesions. Surgery 50:161, 1961.

Castaneda A R, Lamberti J, Sade R M, Williams R G, Nadas A S: Open heart surgery during the first three months of life. J Thorac Cardiovasc Surg 68:719, 1974.

Clarkson P M, MacArthur B A, Barratt-Boyes B G, Whitlock R M, Neutze J M: Developmental progress after cardiac surgery in infancy using hypothermia and circulatory arrest. Circulation 62:855, 1980.

Gersony W, Hayes C J: Perioperative management of the infant with congenital heart disease. Prog Cardiovasc Dis 15:213, 1972.

Gregory G A, Kitterman J A, Phibbs R H, Tooley W H, Hamilton W: Treatment of the idiopathic respiratory-distress syndrome with continuous positive airway pressure. N Engl J Med 284:1333, 1971.

Haller J A Jr, Talbert J L: The physiologic challenge. In Surgical Emergencies in the Newborn. Philadelphia, Lea & Febiger, 1972, pp 1–3.

Hey E N, Katz G: The optimum thermal environment for naked babies. Arch Dis Child 45:328, 1970.

Heymann M A, Berman W Jr, Rudolph A M, Whitman V: Dilatation of the ductus arteriosus by prostaglandin E_1 in aortic arch abnormalities. Circulation 59:169, 1979.

Hikasa Y, Shirotani H, Satomura K: Open-heart surgery in infants with the aid of hypothermic anesthesia. Arch Jpn Chir 36:495, 1967.

Kirklin J W: Systems Analysis in Surgical Patients with Particular Attention to the Cardiac and Pulmonary Subsystems (Macewen Memorial Lecture). Glasgow, University of Glasgow Press, 1970.

———, Blackstone E H, Pacifico A D, Brown R N, Bargeron L M Jr: Routine primary repair vs two-stage repair of tetralogy of Fallot. Circulation 60:373, 1979.

———, DuShane J H: Repair of ventricular septal defect in infancy. Pediatrics 27:961, 1961.

Macartney F J, Taylor J F N, Graham G R, DeLaval M, Stark J: The fate of survivors of cardiac surgery in infancy. Circulation 62:80, 1980.

Mandelbaum I, Morgan C R: Effect of extracorporeal circulation upon insulin. J Thorac Cardiovasc Surg 55:526, 1968.

Merritt T A, DiSessa T G, Feldman B H, Kirkpatrick S E, Gluck L, Friedman W F: Closure of the patent ductus arteriosus with ligation and indomethacin: a consecutive experience. J Pediatr 93:639, 1978.

Miles A A, Miles E E, Burke J F: The value and duration of defence reactions of the skin to the primary lodgement of bacteria. Br J Exp Pathol 38:79, 1957.

Moodie D S, Feldt R H, Kaye M P, Danielson G K, Pluth J, O'Fallon M: Measurement of postoperative cardiac output by thermodilution in pediatric and adult patients. J Thorac Cardiovasc Surg 78:796, 1979.

Neal W A, Kyle J M, Mullett M D: Failure of indomethacin therapy to induce closure of patent ductus arteriosus in premature infants with respiratory distress syndrome. J Pediatr 91:621, 1977.

Neutze J M, Starling M B, Elliott R B, Barratt-Boyes B G: Palliation of cyanotic congenital heart disease in infancy with E-type prostaglandins. Circulation 55:238, 1977.

Norwood W I, Norwood C R, Ingwall J S, Castaneda A R, Fossel E T: Hypothermic circulatory arrest: 31-phosphorus nuclear magnetic resonance of isolated perfused neonatal rat brain. J Thorac Cardiovasc Surg 78:823, 1979.

Olley P M, Coceani F, Bodach E: E-type prostaglandins: a new emergency therapy for certain cyanotic congenital heart malformations. Circulation 53:728, 1976.

Parr G V S, Blackstone E H, Kirklin J W: Cardiac performance and mortality early after intracardiac surgery in infants and young children. Circulation 51:867, 1975.

———, Kirklin J W, Pacifico A D, Blackstone E H, Lauridsen P: Cardiac performance in infants after repair of total anomalous pulmonary venous connection. Ann Thorc Surg 17:561, 1974.

Payne W S, Theye R A, Kirklin J W: Effect of carbon dioxide on rate of brain cooling during induction of hypothermia by direct blood cooling. J Surg Res 3:54, 1963.

Reynolds E O R: Effect of alterations in mechanical ventilator settings on pulmonary gas exchange in hyaline membrane disease. Arch Dis Child 46:152, 1971.

Rowe M I: Preoperative and postoperative management: the physiologic approach. In Ravitch M et al. (eds): Pediatric Surgery, 3rd ed. Chicago, Year Book, 1979, Vol I, pp 39–53.

Silva J Jr, Hoeksma H, Fekety F R: Transient defects in phagocytic functions during cardiopulmonary bypass. J Thorac Cardiovasc Surg 67:175, 1974.

Sloan H, McKenzie J, Morris J D, Stern A, Sigmann J: Open heart surgery in infancy. J Thorac Cardiovasc Surg 44:459, 1962.

Slonim R, Litwak R S, Gadboys H L, Ehrenkranz N J: Antibiotic prophylaxis of infection complicating open-heart operations. Antimicrob Agents Chemother 731, 1963.

Smith D L, Wilson J M, Ebert P A: Cardiac surgery in infants up to one year old. Cardiovasc Med 3:925, 1978.

Smith P C, Daily W J R, Fletcher G, Meyer H B P, Taylor G: Mechanical ventilation of newborn infants. I. The effect of rate and pressure on arterial oxygenation of infants with respiratory distress syndrome. Pediatr Res 3:244, 1969.

Stewart S III, Edmunds L H Jr, Kirklin J W, Allarde R R: Spontaneous breathing with continuous positive airway pressure after open intracardiac operations in infants. J Thorac Cardiovasc Surg 65:37, 1973.

Stremmel W, Schlosser V, Koehnlein H E: Effect of open-heart surgery with hemodilution perfusion upon insulin secretion. J Thorac Cardiovasc Surg 64:263, 1972.

Subramanian S, Vlad P, Fischer L, Cohen M: Sequelae of profound hypothermia and cardiocirculatory arrest in infants and small children. In Kidd B S L, Rowe R D (eds): The Child with Congenital Heart Disease After Surgery. New York, Futura, 1976, p 421.

Subramanian V, Lowman J, Gans H: Effect of extracorporeal circulation on reticuloendothelial function. Arch Surg 97:330, 1968.

Vidne B A, Subramanian S: Surface induced profound hypothermia in infant cardiac surgery: a new system. Ann Thorac Surg 22:572, 1976.

RECOMMENDED READING

Sade R M, Cosgrove D M, Castaneda A R: Infant and Child Care in Heart Surgery. Chicago, Year Book, 1977.

Sinclair J C (ed): Temperature Regulation and Energy Metabolism in the Newborn. New York, Grune & Stratton, 1978.

20. Permanent Cardiac Pacemakers: Management And Problems[*]

ALVIN J. GORDON MANUEL R. ESTIOKO

Although many of the principles of electrical stimulation of the heart were enunciated by McWilliam in 1889 and by others even earlier, Hyman (1932) ushered in the modern era by developing and employing an electrical generator that he called an artificial pacemaker. Zoll (1952) applied an external pacemaker for the treatment of patients with complete heart block. The first fully implantable pacemaker was used by Elmqvist and Senning in 1959, and, in the same year, a practical method for endocardial stimulation in humans was described by Furman and Schwedel.

Current methods for long-term or so-called permanent pacing is the subject of this chapter, which will include a summary of indications for pacing; the pathophysiology of heart block and pacing; the etiology of heart block; classification of pacemakers; preoperative management; surgical technique and complications; instructions for patients; and follow-up. Techniques of temporary pacing will be omitted.

INDICATIONS FOR PERMANENT PACING

The prime indication for long-term pacing is the presence of a slow heart rate with consequent low cardiac output, which leads to serious compromise of one or more organ systems. When the brain is affected (and this is the most common indication for pacing), there can be Stokes-Adams seizures or an organic mental syndrome. When the heart is affected, serious cardiac arrhythmias, congestive heart failure, or angina pectoris may occur. The latter is a rare complication of bradycardia. Azotemia may supervene and, rarely, intermittent claudication.

The indications for pacing are usually unequivocal, except in a small group of patients who present with occasional syncopal episodes and an abnormal electrocardiogram, often with partial atrioventricular block or intraventricular block. Unless the etiology of the fainting spells can be established by continuous monitoring in the hospital or by taped electrocardiograms, a decision about the implantation of a pacemaker may be extremely difficult.

Some patients with second- or third-degree block, on the other hand, may be asymptomatic, and it may be equally difficult to decide at what point pacing should be

---

[*]Dr. Salvador B. Lukban, a former member of the Cardiothoracic Surgical Attending Staff of The Mount Sinai Hospital, collaborated in the early drafts of this chapter.

instituted. Catheter recording of His bundle potentials has been advocated in these cases (Rosen, 1973), and pacing recommended when the block is localized in or distal to the His bundle.

In the past, the majority of patients requiring permanent pacing suffered from complete atrioventricular heart block. In recent years the emphasis has shifted to affections of the sinoatrial node, "sick sinus" or "diseased sinus" syndrome (Ferrer, 1973), as a more common cause of bradycardia. Many of these patients are susceptible to paroxysmal tachycardia and may also have a sensitive carotid sinus. In general, symptoms in this group of patients are less severe, and pacing often may be withheld for long periods.

Permanent pacing is sometimes undertaken to prevent or terminate arrhythmias, such as paroxysmal supraventricular tachycardia and ventricular tachycardia. In situations such as these, a demand pacemaker may be required as insurance against toxic effects of certain indicated drugs—particularly propranolol and digitalis. For the control of supraventricular tachycardia, such as may occur in the Wolff-Parkinson-White syndrome, a permanent atrial pacemaker may be implanted, which can then be activated when necessary by radio frequency control or a magnetic switch (Preston and Kirsh, 1970). Patient-activated ventricular pacemakers may be used to terminate ventricular tachycardia as well. Also undergoing clinical evaluation are pacemakers that respond to ventricular tachycardia by a short run ("burst") of rapid ventricular pacing (Kim et al., 1979) and other units that revert to fixed rate pacing at a normal rate (underdrive pacing).

ETIOLOGY OF HEART BLOCK AND SINUS NODE DYSFUNCTION

Congenital heart block is uncommon, is accompanied in a majority of cases by additional congenital lesions, and usually does not require pacing. Most cases of heart block are acquired. Some follow acute myocardial infarction. Diaphragmatic wall infarction may lead to sequential heart block (first-degree, second-degree, including Wenckebach, and often complete block), but the lesion is in the atrioventricular node or the bundle of His, the ventricular focus is high, the QRS is narrow, and the heart rate often is between 50 and 60. If such a patient survives, the block regresses, and the patient rarely, if ever, requires permanent pacing.

With anterior wall or combined myocardial infarction, complete heart block is often preceded by QRS widening (such as bundle branch block). Complete block may occur suddenly, with low ventricular focus and very slow rate. The block may be trifascicular (right bundle and both main branches of the left bundle) and may also involve the bundle of His. Many of these patients will succumb despite temporary pacing. If they survive, the complete heart block usually regresses. However, since these patients have a high incidence of sudden death in the year following the acute infarct (Atkins et al., 1973), a permanent demand pacemaker may be indicated.

In most patients with complete heart block, there is no history or later anatomic evidence of infarction. The lesion is thought to be fibrosis of the conduction system (Lev, 1964). These patients' hearts may otherwise be structurally sound and their prognosis excellent once the heart block is controlled. Rarely, heart block may be noted during episodes of variant angina and may be grave enough to require permanent pacing.

Other less common causes of heart block are:

1. Trauma—such as cardiac surgery
2. Sarcoidosis
3. Infections, particularly Chagas' disease
4. Valvular heart disease, particularly involving the aortic valve, with calcification and fibrosis spreading to the atrioventricular node and bundle of His
5. Metastatic tumors.

Physiologic derangement of the sinoatrial node (particularly sinus bradycardia) occurs in about 5 percent of patients with acute myocardial infarction (Rokseth and Hatle, 1971). Most of these are diaphragmatic infarcts. Such disturbances are usually transient and rarely require pacing in the acute stage. Few anatomic studies of patients with the "sick sinus" syndrome are available (Ferrer, 1973), nor is the etiolgy in most cases clinically evident (James, 1979). This is primarily, but not exclusively, a disease of advanced age.

ELECTROPHYSIOLOGY OF PACING

The heart is exquisitely sensitive to electricity. When bipolar or unipolar catheter electrodes stimulate the right ventricular endocardium, the minimum amount of energy required for depolarization is 0.5 microjoules. This may be delivered by a one-volt, one-milliampere stimulus acting for 0.05 milliseconds (msec). This quantity of energy is equivalent to one two-millionth of a watt-second and would light a 100-watt bulb for 0.05 msec. When applied to the tongue (a convenient method of testing battery-powered external pacemakers), this electrical stimulus is barely perceptible.

The minimum quantity of energy required by a pacemaker to initiate a propagated impulse is called the *threshold*. Threshold values are influenced by the type of electricity (usually direct current), the duration as well as the voltage and quantity of current, the polarity of the impulse (i.e., whether cathodal or anodal), its shape, and the current density at the site of stimulation.

Electrical threshold rises for the first few weeks after implantation, reaches a maximum in two to four weeks, and then may either fall somewhat or remain stationary (Siddons and Sowton, 1967). Knowledge of this fact is important for the proper use of pacemakers in which output or pulse width can be changed after implantation.

Strength-duration curves (Davies and Sowton, 1966) indicate that the human heart can be paced by impulses as short as 0.1 msec, although more power is required than at longer durations. Although formerly most manufacturers preferred a 1-msec impulse, the trend has been toward shorter stimuli, resulting in considerable saving of battery power.

Cardiac factors are also of great importance. Of particular concern is the state of the underlying myocardium, as influenced by ischemia, infection, fibrosis, drugs, and electrolytes. In order of decreasing sensitivity the heart responds to endocardial, intramural, and epicardial stimulation. The ventricle may be slightly more sensitive than the atrium. The stimulating electrode must be in contact with viable heart muscle to ensure stable pacing.

The heart responds in an all-or-none fashion to pacemaker stimuli, which are then spread through the myocardium, presumably via the Purkinje system.

If more than one pacemaker fires simultaneously (i.e., a spontaneous and an artificial one), depolarization may begin at different sites and give rise to a *fusion beat*, which electrocardiographically usually contains elements of both parent beats. Retrograde conduction through the His bundle usually does not occur when the heart block is complete but may be a factor when sinus node dysfunction is treated by ventricular pacing. Then the atria may be stimulated and contract against closed atrioventricular valves, giving rise to cannon waves in the venous pulse and reducing cardiac output.

Phases of Excitability

The ventricular contraction cycle (Castellanos and Lemberg, 1969; Hoffman and Cranefield, 1960) is divided into an *absolute refractory period* from the onset of the QRS to the peak of the T wave, a short *relative refractory period* close to the peak and early downslope of the T wave, and a supernormal period, toward the end of the T wave, when the ventricle may be 10 to 15 percent more sensitive to electrical stimulation. The latter may only be observed clinically during the phase of battery failure of an implanted pacemaker, when the power is just at threshold.

A *vulnerable* period of the ventricle is present during the upstroke of the T wave, during which single stimuli may produce repetitive responses (ventricular tachycardia or fibrillation). The importance of the vulnerable period in clinical cardiac pacing is a matter of controversy, insofar as competition between a spontaneous and an artificial pacemaker is concerned. On the basis of the authors' experience it appears that competition may be dangerous only when the heart is ischemic or irritable.

Phases of excitability exist in the atria, similar to those in the ventricles, although they have not been the subject of as much study.

CLASSIFICATION OF PACEMAKERS

Pacemakers may be classified according to the chamber that is stimulated; whether endocardial or epicardial; unipolar or bipolar; fixed rate (asynchronous), demand, atrial-triggered, or sequential; programmable or designed for treating tachyarrhythmias. The nature of the power supply may vary and special features may be incorporated.

Endocardial versus Epicardial Pacing

The epicardial approach has been almost entirely replaced by intracavitary electrodes. Thoracotomy introduces unnecessary risks and a significant mortality. The heart has also been approached by median sternotomy (Guilmet et al., 1964), subxiphoid (Stewart et al., 1975), parasternal transmediastinal (Dixon et al., 1972), and mediastinoscopy (Carlens et al., 1965). Routes other than endocardial are only justified in infants or when an atrial electrode is required for sensing or stimulation or when transvenous pacing has failed, or in conjunction with open heart surgery.

Atrial Pacing

Permanent atrial pacing and its variations may be clearly indicated in certain cases of the "sick sinus" syndrome and in some recurrent tachycardias. It has enjoyed little vogue because of the difficulty in maintaining a stable catheter position in the atrium. Of the various methods that have been reported, that of Moss and Rivers (1978) is often effective. The electrode tip is passed into the great cardiac vein through the coronary sinus, which serves to keep it in place, and in contact with atrial musculature. J-shaped catheter electrodes have been used by Smyth et al. (1971), De Sanctis et al. (1968), and by Zucker et al. (1973). The latter authors have reported stable long-term pacing from the right atrial appendage.

Even if stable atrial pacing could be regularly achieved, its use would be inadvisable in many cases because of the possibility of later development of atrial fibrillation of atrioventricular block. In a given patient, if there is no history of atrial fibrillation, if the P-R interval is not prolonged, and if rapid atrial pacing (at least up to 120 bpm) at the time of implantation produces no A-V block, permanent atrial pacing is justified.

Ventricular Pacing

Unipolar versus Bipolar Pacing. At this time endocardial pacing from the apex of the right ventricle is the method of choice. This can be done by means of a bipolar electrode, in which the poles are approximately one centimeter apart, or by a "unipolar" configuration in which the metal casing of the generator is the indifferent electrode. Each variant has its proponents, but there is little to choose between them. The pacemaker stimulus of the unipolar pacemaker, as measured from the body surface, has five to ten times the voltage of the bipolar. This may deceive a cardiac alarm, which may interpret the artefact as a cardiac depolarization. The recharge pulse of the unipolar pacemaker artefact, which is opposite in phase and returns very slowly to the baseline, grossly distorts the electrocardiogram. This has been eliminated in the "Spectrax,"* in which the repolarization current

---

*Medtronic, Inc.

completes its cycle before the inscription of the QRS. By the same token, the Spectrax artefact in the routine electrocardiogram is biphasic. The larger artefact generated by unipolar pacing may facilitate impulse analysis ("spike analysis") by oscilloscopic means (Furman and Norman, 1972), although the authors' wide-band amplifier (discussed later) displays the bipolar pacemaker impulse with equal accuracy. With unipolar pacing, local muscle twitching may occur in proximity to the indifferent electrode at the base of the generator. Skeletal muscle potential may inhibit a unipolar pacemaker.

Inadequate sensing in the demand mode may be more common with bipolar electrodes. The inhibiting signal sensed by the pacemaker is the difference in potential between the two poles. In the case of a bipolar unit, the endocardial electrogram from each of the two poles may be similar, and the difference in voltage too small (i.e., less than 2 mv) to be sensed. This may be recognized by recording endocardial electrograms at the time of implantation and changing the electrode position if indicated.

The dispersion of the electrical field in the unipolar configuration makes this pacemaker more sensitive to electrical interference from outside the body. However, bipolar pacemakers, by the same token, must provide more amplification of the incoming signal, so that the net result is little practical difference in susceptibility to outside interference (Tarjan, 1973).

Pacing Modes

Asynchronous (Fixed Rate). The pacemaker fires at a regular rate independent of cardiac activity. This mode is indicated when there is little or no spontaneous ventricular activity. It has the advantage of simpler electronics and may last longer than equivalent demand models. It introduces the possibility of competition should spontaneous cardiac activity occur, with the attendant danger of provoking arrhythmias by firing in the vulnerable phase of the cardiac cycle (the upstroke of the T wave). In the authors' experience, this danger has been exaggerated (also see Siddons, 1974). This mode of pacing is now rarely used although it can be programmed in certain units.

Ventricular Inhibited (Demand). A spontaneous depolarization resets the pacemaker, which then does not fire until the preset interval has elapsed (860 msec when the rate has been set at 70 beats per min). A refractory period (varying from 75 to 400 msec in different models) prevents the pacemaker from being inhibited by the trailing edge of the paced beat or a prominent T wave. Spontaneous beats that fall in the refractory period of paced or other spontaneous beats are not sensed and do not inhibit the subsequent paced ventricular contraction.

Ventricular Synchronous (Ventricular Triggered or Standby). Each spontaneous depolarization provokes an immediate pacing impulse that produces no response. In the event of no spontaneous cardiac activity for the preset interval, an impulse occurs, and the heart follows. There is a set maximum rate (150 in Cordis Ectocor and twice the programmed rate in Omni-Ectocor) above which the pacemaker cannot be triggered. This mode of pacing is losing its popularity and today would be useful chiefly in a patient who is frequently exposed to electrical interference, such as an electrician.

Atrial Triggered. Atrial contraction is sensed by an endocardial or epicardial atrial lead, and after a suitable delay (0.16 sec) a second (ventricular) electrode fires and depolarizes the ventricle. If a P wave is not detected, the ventricles are stimulated at a fixed rate (70). Maximum rate here is also fixed. Variations of this mode include ventricular sensing as well, so that a ventricular premature beat recycles the unit.

This form of pacing has two theoretical advantages: (1) it preserves the normal sequence of atrial and ventricular contraction, which has been shown to increase cardiac output and eliminate phasic variations thereof; (2) it allows the heart to respond to physiologic stimuli as triggered by variations in atrial rate. From the practical standpoint, atrial triggered pacing is chiefly of value in the treatment of children and young adults.

Variants of this form of pacing are: (1) sequential pacing, in which the atrium and ventricle are stimulated in proper sequence by two catheters. (2) "bifocal" demand pacing, in which A-V sequential pacing on demand is accomplished by catheter electrodes in both atrium and ventricle. Ventricular electrical activity alone is monitored, which programs both atrial and ventricular stimulation (Castillo et al., 1971). Advanced function pacemakers which are under investigation have both atrial and ventricular sensing and pacing (DDD mode). They are potentially advantageous in the attempt to simulate physiologic functions (Sutton et al., 1980).

A three-letter identification code, proposed by a commission sponsored by the U.S. Department of Health, Education and Welfare, (Parsonnet et al., 1974), is now in common use. The first letter indicates the chamber pace (V, A, or D–dual), the second, the chamber sensed (O–fixed rate, V, A, or D), and the third, the mode of response (O, I–inhibited, T–triggered, or D). The common ventricular-inhibited demand pacemaker, for example, would be coded VVI. Because of the increasing complexity of pacing, this code has recently been revised to include a fourth letter to indicate programmable functions (P–programmable [rate and/or output]; M–multiprogrammable; O–none). A fifth letter includes special tachyarrhythmia functions (B–bursts; N–normal rate competition; S–scanning; and E–external) (Furman et al., 1981).

Power Sources

Mercury-Zinc Cells. For many years the standard cell for pacemakers throughout the world, the Mallory RM 1 cell has a long shelf life and small size for its voltage (1.35 v per cell). Output is constant over long periods of time until the end of its life, when it usually fails rapidly (days or weeks). For economic reasons this cell is still being used frequently outside of the United States.

Lithium Iodine Cells and Other Lithium Cells. This nonrechargeable cell lasts longer than the mercury-zinc battery, has a long shelf life, and can be hermetically sealed. It fails slowly. It has gained popularity rapidly and is used exclusively by most American manufacturers (Greatbatch, 1973; Lillehei et al., 1974).

Rechargeable Cells. Pacemakers with nickel-cadmium cells, which could be recharged through the skin, were available for several years but recently have been withdrawn from the market (Pacesetter Systems, Inc.). The latest model required 60 minutes of charging time per week or four hours per month. Experience with this unit was good (Lewis et al., 1974; Hauser and Giuffre, 1976) but the inconvenience of recharging, coupled with the failure of some patients to adhere to the recharging schedule, led to its abandonment (Stertzer et al., 1978).

Radio Frequency and Inductive Coupling. In both these systems, current is transmitted through the intact skin to an implanted receiver. The latter may be sutured directly to the heart (Cammilli, 1967) or connected to the heart by epicardial (Glenn et al., 1959; Abrams et al., 1960) or cavity leads (Glenn et al., 1966).

Radioisotope Sources. The first implantation of an isotope-powered pacemaker was performed in Paris in April 1970. Although long life is possible for the power source, attributes of other components vitiate its usefulness. Furthermore, disposal problems after the patient's death and political difficulties crossing national boundaries have contrived to limit its popularity.

^{238}Pu (plutonium 238) with a half-life of 87.5 years provides the power for some units by thermopile conversion from heat to electric current. ^{147}Pm (prometheum 147) (half-life = 2.6 years) has been used for its beta-voltaic (photo) effect. Although ^{238}Pu-powered units have performed very well, the experience with the ^{147}Pm has been poor, with early failure in a high proportion of one series (Williams et al., 1979).

Pacemaker Electronics

Improvements in pacemaker longevity resulting from newer power sources have been matched by component miniaturization, leading to striking decreases in generator volume and weight. This has resulted chiefly from the so-called integrated circuit, in which many microscopic electronic components are contained in a "chip" whose actual size may be 2 × 2 mm. A "hybrid" circuit contains both chips and discrete components. Microcomputers are employed for noninvasive programming. Despite their small size these circuits are proving their reliability.

Special Feature Pacemakers

The keen commercial competition among pacemaker manufacturers (Greene, 1976) has fostered numerous improvements, of which the most important is programmability (the option of changing one or more variables after implantation). This is not a new concept, a unit having become available in the early 1960s that allowed the patient to change the rate from 65 to 85 by applying a magnet. Two manufacturers had external radio-frequency rate controls for some models. In a later development, the rate, output, or both could be varied by a special needle passed through the skin into a projecting nipple.

Programmability now encompasses noninvasive changes in mode, rate, output, pulse width, refractory period, sensitivity, hysteresis, and, in an A-V sequential model, A-V delay and atrial unit shutdown. Complete temporary inhibition of ventricular pacemakers is possible, and one unit permits conversion from bipolar to unipolar pacing. These changes are accomplished by magnetic or radio-frequency means (Figs. 20-1 and 20-2).

Other special features permit threshold analysis by various means as well as telemetry, which may include all programmed variables and battery voltage, lead impedance, battery impedance, and battery current drain. It is also possible in some recent pacemakers to record an endocardial electrogram.

Some of the advantages of programmable units are apparent. Spontaneous rhythm may be promoted by rate decrease.

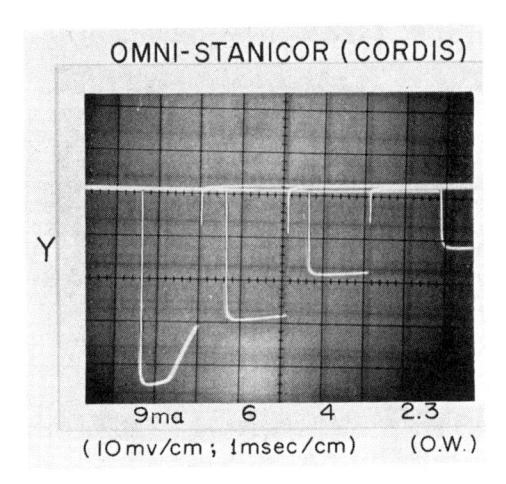

Figure 20-1. Oscillograms of stimulus artefact in Y component lead of the Frank system at four successive mA settings (9, 6, 4, and 2.3 mA) of the Omni-stanicor. The programmer was used after skin closure, while the patient was still in the operating room. Sensitivity: 10 mV/cm; speed: 1 msec/cm. The traces have been retouched.

Battery longevity is enhanced by slowing the rate, dropping the output, and narrowing the pulse width. Undesirable skeletal muscle and diaphragmatic stimulation may sometimes be eliminated by decreasing the output or pulse width, while rising threshold may be counteracted by the reverse maneuver. Angina may be ameliorated by rate decrease, and changes in rate or hysteresis may lead to a more stable pulse in the presence of some rhythm disturbances. Mode and rate change may be of value in the early postoperative management of patients with sinus node dysfunction and retrograde atrial conduction, and in the determination of pacemaker dependence and the diagnosis of acute myocardial infarction. Sensitivity change may prevent pacemaker inhibition by skeletal muscle potentials. These maneuvers should make it possible to prevent reoperations that might otherwise be needed.

Programmability, however, is not without its drawbacks. Of particular concern is the occasional occurrence of unwanted or unexpected programming by false signals (Sinnaeve et al., 1980) and potentially dangerous errors made by faulty programmers or gen-

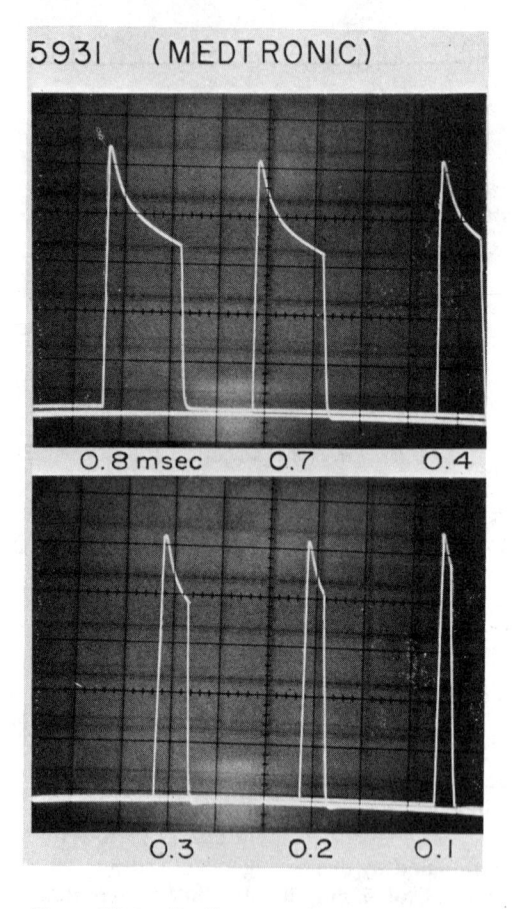

Figure 20-2. Oscillograms of stimulus artefact in X component lead of the Frank system at six successive settings of pulse width in a patient with a Medtronic Model 5931 pacemaker with epicardial leads. The pulse width was adjusted by external application of the magnetic controller. Sensitivity: 10 mV/cm; speed: 0.5 msec/cm. The traces have been retouched.

erators (Fieldman and Dobrow, 1978) or by those of the wrong manufacturers.

PREOPERATIVE MANAGEMENT

Many of the patients requiring pacemaker implantation are admitted electively after cardiologic evaluation. The others are in-hospital patients referred by internists or cardiologists. The average patient in our experience is 72 years of age and often has associated medical illnesses. Some patients require temporary pacemaker insertion because of their unstable condition (severe bradycardia with symptoms). Recurrent and recent Stokes-Adams attacks are particularly dangerous. Subsequent permanent pacemaker implantation can be done more safely on an elective basis. On the other hand, the additional procedure of a temporary pacemaker should be avoided if the patient is not jeopardized. The cardiologists and implanting surgeons should individualize the indication for temporary pacing according to the clinical course of the patient.

Foci of infection should be carefully excluded during the preoperative evaluation to prevent serious complication. Special care is exercised in preparing the skin at the operative site. Antibiotics usually are given before surgery and for a few days afterwards. They are particularly indicated in the presence of associated valvular lesions. Bacterial endocarditis has been reported in association with implantation of temporary and permanent pacemakers. Siddons et al. (1979), on the other hand, advocate using antibiotics only when the patient has special risks of infection.

Drugs that are not necessary or may interfere with the surgical procedure should be discontinued. For example, aspirin and anticoagulants should be discontinued to prevent bleeding. If coagulopathy is suspected the appropriate studies should be performed. Correction of electrolyte imbalance, especially of the serum potassium, is necessary. Drugs such as propranolol and digitalis may further aggravate the bradycardia and should be avoided. The use of atropine and isoproterenol to increase the heart rate is unnecessary in stable patients.

Legal consent is obtained from the patient or from the next of kin (if the patient is not able). The function of the pacemaker implantation procedure, as well as possible complications, should be explained to the patient and to the responsible member of his or her family. Adequate premedication is useful, but too much sedation, especially with barbiturates, must be avoided. Respiratory depression can easily occur in elderly patients.

SURGICAL TECHNIQUE OF PERMANENT PACEMAKER IMPLANTATION

Our experience with pacemakers covers 17 years and more than 5,000 operations. The results of pacemaker implantation today are predictably favorable with a minimum of complications. Advances in pacemaker technology and improved surgical techniques are primarily responsible for the good results.

Transvenous Pacemaker Implantation

Transvenous or endocardial pacemaker implantation is the procedure of choice and is simpler than other approaches. It is performed under local infiltration anesthesia (Furman et al., 1966, 1969). This technique is used in about 92 percent of all pacemaker implantations in the United States (Goldman and Parsonnet, 1979). We prefer the sterile environment in the operating room rather than the special procedures room in the x-ray department or the cardiac catheterization laboratory. The equipment needed in the cardiac operating room includes a special table to allow fluoroscopy, a fluoroscopy machine with a C-arm, a TV screen, and an oscilloscope for the electrocardiogram. The surgeon's assistants should include a surgical assistant, a scrub nurse, a circulating nurse, and an x-ray technician. An anesthesiologist should be standing by for seriously ill patients or when there is a possibility of epicardial pacemaker implantation.

An oblique incision over the deltopectoral groove or a transverse incision below the clavicle is made and the cephalic vein is dissected. The electrode, inserted through the *left* cephalic vein, usually takes a smooth curve, which facilitates insertion. In left-handed patients, implantation in the right side may be preferable. If the cephalic vein is small, more proximal dissection down to the junction with the axillary vein may be necessary (Gadboys et al., 1968). The side of the axillary vein may be used with a purse-string suture without occluding the main venous channel. Alternatively, the external jugular vein and sometimes the side of the internal jugular vein on either side may be used. The various venous accesses are shown in Figure 20–3. The jugular approach requires another small incision, with tunneling of the electrode to the main incision. Prior to insertion into the cephalic vein, the electrode with the stylet(s) in place is molded into a gentle curve of about 90°, four centimeters proximal to its tip. The electrode is then advanced gently under fluoroscopic control to the right atrium and then to the right ventricle, traversing the tricuspid valve. Proper positioning of the electrode in the right ventricle (RV) is facilitated by the following maneuvers:

1. With the electrode advanced into the pulmonary artery, slowly pulling down and replacing the curved stylet with a straight one will point the electrode downward toward the apex of the RV. Without the stylet, the electrode in the main cavity of the RV will have wide up-and-down swings with the contraction of the heart, indicating that the electrode is free in the cavity of the RV.

2. After placement of the electrode tip in the apex of the right ventricle, fluoroscopy in the oblique and lateral views demonstrates the electrode pointing anteriorly and downward.

3. The electrode is probably in the coronary sinus if it repeatedly returns to the same transverse position during manipulation. Fluoroscopy in the lateral projection shows the electrode pointing posteriorly. Atrial pacing may be observed during testing when the electrode is in the coronary sinus, or the endocardial electrogram may contain characteristic tall P waves.

Under no circumstances should force be applied to the electrode, especially when the stylet is in place, as perforation or myocardial penetration may occur. This complication can also be avoided by partially withdrawing the stylet during the final stage of manipulation, making the tip of the electrode soft and yeilding. Our experience with the use of tined electrodes is excellent (Estioko et al., 1979). The snagging feel on slight pulling of the electrode is a very important test indicating that the tines are securely engaged in the

Figure 20-3. Veins used for transvenous pacemaker implantation. The most commonly used vein is the cephalic (1), followed by the external jugular (2). The others are: axillary (3), internal jugular (4), and subclavian (5) veins. The procedure may be performed either on the left or right side.

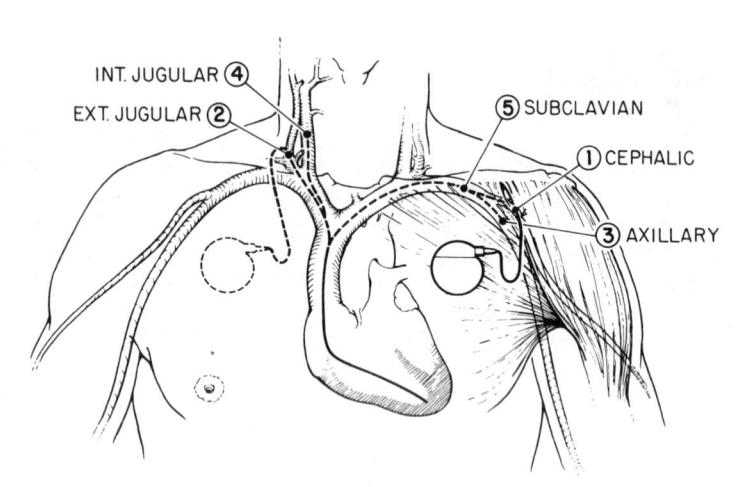

trabeculae of the endocardium. Once a satisfactory position is achieved, the stylet is removed, allowing a slight redundancy at the level of the right atrium. Fluoroscopy (and overpenetrated postoperative chest x-ray) in the PA and lateral projections will demonstrate the correct electrode position. Figure 20-4 shows the ideal electrode position in the frontal and lateral views.

Threshold measurements are done as the next step. A pacemaker system analyzer is used to measure the pacing thresholds, R-wave sensing, and the electrical characteristics of the generator to be implanted. Several pacemaker system analyzers are available, and the surgeon must be completely familiar with the one he or she chooses. Before testing thresholds, the analyzer should be adjusted to the pulse width of the generator the surgeon is planning to use. Sterile cables attach the electrode to the analyzer. The lowest voltage (V) and current flow (in milliamperes) that stimulate the heart are referred to as pacing threshold. The aim is to obtain thresholds below one volt, or even 0.5 V or lower and less than 2.5 milliamperes (mA) (Furman et al., 1968). The testing is accomplished by gradually decreasing the voltage (or current) until there is loss of pacing capture. The electrical resistance can be calculated or directly measured in ohms by some analyzers. The electrode and cardiac factors determine the resistance.

The measurement of sensing function is imperative and another indication of proper electrode position. The sensing circuit of the pacemaker system analyzer detects the amplitude of the endocardial R wave and generates a digital readout in millivolts (mV). The sensing circuits in most pacemaker generators can detect cardiac signals of 1.5 to 2.5 mV. However, R-wave amplitudes of about twice that figure (5 mV or higher) are desirable. Satisfactory sensing is obtained with small tip electrodes with a surface area of 8 millimeters square. This favors low current drain and longer battery life. The electrode surface must be small enough to pace efficiently but large enough to sense effectively.

The determination of sensing function may be difficult in some patients. A patient may be pacemaker-dependent during the R-wave measurement and develop asystole. It is advisable in this situation to gradually decrease the pacing rate and wait for the patient's intrinsic rhythm to manifest itself, which usually will occur eventually. As soon as the patient has some of his or her own beats (after pacing about 40 per minute), a brief test of the R-wave button of the analyzer determines whether the patient has adequate intrinsic cardiac activity. The test button must be released immediately (and pacing resumed) if he or she becomes symptomatic or asystolic. The surface electrocardiogram is watched carefully. A similar maneuver is per-

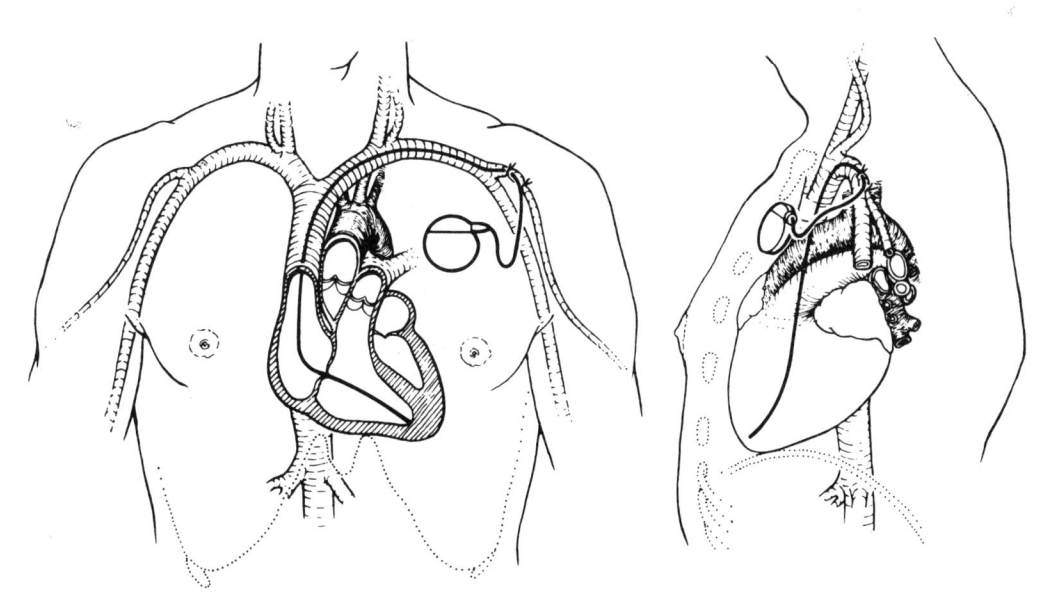

Figure 20–4. Correct Electrode Position. The transvenous electrode is shown in its proper position with the tip at the apex of the right ventricle. It is pointing downward in the frontal view and anteriorly in the lateral view. (See also Fig. 20–10 A, B.)

formed in the patient with a temporary pacemaker. There are some who cannot tolerate even brief discontinuation of temporary pacing. Windmann et al. (1979) warned of the pitfalls in measuring R waves in pacemaker-dependent patients, emphasizing that the pacemaker analyzer may record the temporary pacemaker spike instead of the R wave.

It is useful to measure the threshold of both the tip and proximal poles of the bipolar electrode separately and in bipolar arrangement. It is important that all of these thresholds are satisfactory, otherwise repositioning should be done. If a satisfactory threshold of the proximal electrode cannot be achieved despite repositioning, the system should be unipolarized (using the tip electrode). The practice of changing to a new unipolar electrode is unnecessary and wasteful. During the electrical testing, the electrode movement and stability are rechecked periodically with fluoroscopy. Physiologic functions such as deep breathing and coughing should not interfere with pacemaker function. These provocative tests are done and the possibility of diaphragmatic pacing is explored by increasing the voltage of the analyzer. If diaphragmatic pacing is not provoked with the voltage about twice that of the permanent pacemaker (for example, 10 V) this complication is highly unlikely.

Endocardial electrograms are also helpful in determining proper electrode position (Gordon et al., 1968). They can indicate the following: (1) that the electrode is in the RV, as indicated by tall R waves; (2) that ST elevation (contact current) is present, indicating good endocardial contact (but if the ST elevation is excessive, perforation may follow); (3) that the electrode is in an aberrant position, such as right atrium or coronary sinus; (4) that there is sufficient amplitude for proper sensing.

As soon as the position and the threshold are satisfactory, the vein is tied around the electrode and the latter anchored to the edge of the pectoralis major muscle with a suture ligature. The subcutaneous pocket is developed by sharp dissection. The proper plane of the pocket is anterior to the pectoralis major muscle, leaving the fascia of the muscle intact. There is minimal bleeding with correct dissection. The subcutaneous pocket should be located downward and medially, so that the generator will be away from the clavicle, the shoulder, and the axilla. The use of a drainage system (for example, closed vacuum) is recommended, although with the newer small generators some surgeons find it unnecessary. There is no substitute for good hemostasis with or without a drain.

The generator can now be selected by the surgeon and tested for proper function. The electrical properties of the pacemaker generator (amplitude, pulse interval, pulse rate, pulse width, and sensing) are tested with the analyzer. The results are compared with the specifications furnished by the manufacturer. It is considered sound practice to test the pacemaker prior to implantation to avoid the possibility of using a faulty generator. The rate of the generator at room temperature may be a few beats lower than postimplantation body temperature. The generator is then connected to the electrode and the connections are sealed. Many models require the use of sealing glue (silastic glue) and a nonabsorbable tie on the connecting sleeve. The generator is placed in the subcutaneous pocket with the redundant portion of the electrode behind the generator. This avoids the prominent protrusion of the electrode beneath the skin in thin people. The wound is closed in layers with absorbable sutures. These usually give a good cosmetic result without the necessity of removing sutures. The pocket should be adequate in size without tension on the suture line. When a unipolar generator is used, if the indifferent electrode is a window in the metallic capsule, it should be directed toward the skin and away from the pectoralis muscle. This orientation avoids two possible complications: (1) pectoral muscle stimulation and (2) myopotential inhibition of the pacemaker.

The electrocardiogram is continuously monitored on the oscilloscope during the implantation. Maintaining a conversation with the patient is a practical way of checking his or her condition. Supplemental intravenous sedation may be given when necessary.

The permanent pacemaker function is rechecked at the end of the procedure. If the patient's intrinsic rhythm is constantly inhibiting the pacemaker, a magnet is used to determine the pacing function. At this time, reprogramming may be done. The final reprogrammed variables are recorded in the patient's chart and card. Postoperative monitoring in the cardiac intensive care unit for about 24 hours is ideal. Early failure may be detected by a bedside ECG oscilloscope, telemetry, serial ECGs, or Holter monitor.

Epicardial Implantation

Epicardial pacemaker implantation is the other method of electrode placement. The indications for epicardial pacemaker implantation are:

1. Failure of transvenous or endocardial method
2. Conditions that contraindicate the transvenous method; for example, the presence of a tricuspid valve prosthesis, severe tricuspid valve disease, or bacterial endocarditis
3. When the heart is already exposed during open heart surgery
4. When the patient is an infant or child.

A small anterolateral thoracotomy with placement of a sutureless screw electrode on the left ventricle is the preferred approach. In elderly patients with associated medical problems, careful evaluation should be done in preparation for general anesthesia. After general endotracheal anesthesia, the patient is placed in the supine position with the left side of the chest slightly elevated about 30°. The skin of the operative field is sterilized. Anterolateral thoracotomy is performed in the fifth or fourth intercostal space. The lung is retracted laterally and the pericardium is opened vertically, anterior to the phrenic nerve. An area of exposed myocardium away from the coronary vessels is selected for the placement of the electrode. Areas with abundant epicardial fat or scarring should be avoided.

The myocardial test electrode is used to determine the best site for implantation (Varriale et al., 1977). The test electrode has a metal pin with surface area that approximates the permanent electrode. The threshold obtained by the test electrode closely approximates the threshold of the permanent lead. The sutureless myocardial screw electrode is then implanted at the selected site and threshold testing is performed similar to that described for transvenous pacemaker implantation. It is recommended that a second and even a third spare electrode be used, especially if a bipolar system is contemplated. If reoperation ever becomes necessary because of some lead problem, the spare electrode can be used without the need for another thoracotomy. The pericardium is partially closed to allow drainage. Some redundancy of the electrode in the pericardium and in the chest is recommended. The electrodes are then tunneled subcutaneously to the pocket, preferably in the left pectoral area, although the left upper abdomen is sometimes chosen. The generator is connected to the electrode and the spare electrode is capped and sealed. The thoracotomy incision is closed after a chest tube has been inserted for underwater drainage.

Other Methods of Epicardial Pacemaker Implantation. Subxiphoid pacemaker implantation has enjoyed popularity during the past several years. The procedure is generally done under general anesthesia but can be done under local. A five- to seven-centimeter vertical incision is made in the midline at the level of the xiphoid process. The xiphoid is excised and the abdominal fascia incised at the midline. A substernal dissection is carried out with the diaphragm retracted. The lower anterior aspect of the pericardium is exposed bluntly, with both plurae pushed away laterally. The pericardium is grasped by a forceps and a vertical incision is made, exposing the heart. A transverse incision is added inferiorly for wider exposure of the right ventricle. A suitable area of the RV (anterior or diaphragmatic) is exposed and selected for the electrode implantation. It is important to avoid the atrioventricular groove and epicardial fat. The myocardial sutureless screw electrode is then implanted. Exposure is facilitated by applying a retractor downward on the pericardium with the underlying diaphragm and lifting the lower sternum. The testing of the electrode, subcutaneous tunneling at the site of the pacemaker pocket, and connections to the generator are similar to those described for the transvenous pacemaker. It is not necessary to close the pericardium. A pericardial tube is placed for drainage.

Problems have been encountered with the subxiphoid placement of the electrodes in the right ventricle (Brenner et al., 1974; Naclerio and Variale, 1979). Electrode contact also may be lost because of the thinness of the RV wall. Some patients lose sensing and capture because of rising thresholds weeks or months after implantation. In a few such patients we elected to implant new epicardial electrodes in the left ventricle by a left thoracotomy. There are clinical as well as laboratory studies (Tyers et al., 1975) indicating better thresholds in the left ventricle.

The surgical approaches for epicardial electrode implantation are shown in Figure 20–5. Other illustrated techniques are: left subcostal (Lawrie et al., 1976; Frazier et al., 1979); left parasternal transmediastinal (Kostiainen and Appelqvist, 1977); right parasternal (Carney and Anderson, 1979); and median sternotomy.

Atrial Electrode Implantation

A reliable atrial electrode is the common factor in the application of modes of pacing other than the commonly used ventricular demand mode (VVI). In atrial demand pacing (AAI), good pacing as well as sensing are required. Sensing function is all that is necessary in atrial triggered pacing (VAT) or its variant, atrial syncrhronous, ventricular in-

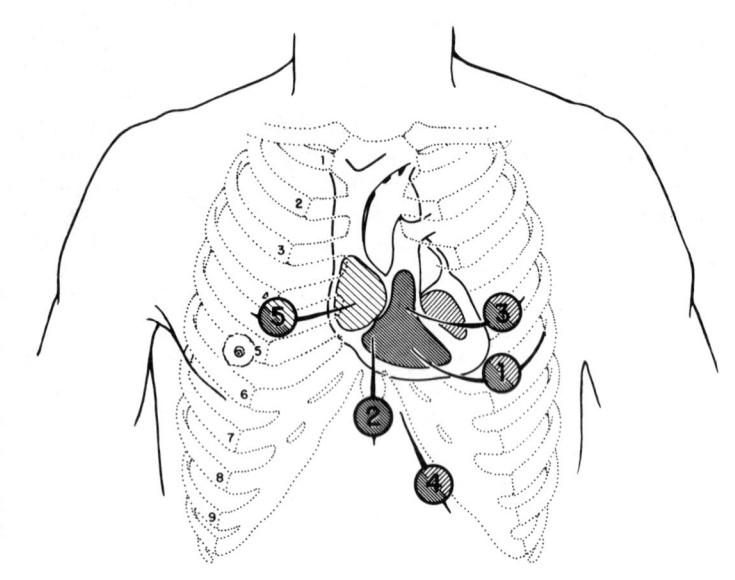

Figure 20–5. Surgical approaches for epicardial implantation. The incisions are illustrated, and the different shaded areas correspond to the cardiac chambers that can be approached. 1 = left antero-lateral thoracotomy (left ventricle, LV, or right ventricle, RV). 2 = subxiphoid (RV). 3 = left parasternal (RV or LV). 4 = left subcostal (RV or LV). 5 = right parasternal (right atrium or RV).

hibited (VDD). In AV sequential bifocal pacing (DVI), only the pacing function is necessary because the sensing is accomplished by the ventricular electrode. There are different ways of implanting atrial electrodes: (1) transvenous in the coronary sinus; (2) transvenous in the atrial appendage; (3) atrial epicardial; (4) endocardial screw electrode.

Coronary Sinus Approach. Various coronary sinus electrodes are available, the most common of which has an electrode ring placed proximally away from the tip for better contact and stability. The electrode is inserted into the cephalic vein or other suitable vein. Before passage, a 60° bend is placed about six centimeters from the tip and another gentler curve close to the tip. Under fluoroscopy the electrode is passed to the coronary sinus (Moss and Rivers, 1978). The electrode in the coronary vein points posteriorly in the oblique and lateral projections on fluoroscopy. The vein is explored to obtain the greatest amplitude of endocardial P waves, which must be greater than 2 mV for proper sensing. The ventricular complex should be smaller than the atrial, lest it recycle the pacemaker (Fig. 20–6). Pacemakers with long refractory periods (about 400 msec) and rate programmability are advantageous in insuring against recycling by the R wave.

Transvenous Electrode in the Right Atrial Appendage. Another transvenous method employs a J-shaped electrode. Different types of J-shaped electrodes are commercially available, with or without silicone rubber tines. The electrode is straightened for passage, using a stylette that is removed after the tip reaches the lower atrium. The electrode then assumes its natural J configuration with the tip pointing cephalad. The electrode is pulled upward, with the tip pointing posteriorly and to the left (medially) until it lodges in the atrial appendage. When in good position, in the atrial appendage, the tip does not move when slight clockwise and counterclockwise rotation is applied to the electrode. On fluoroscopy the tip sways from side to side with each atrial contraction (Zucker et al., 1973). Good contact of the electrode is confirmed by satisfactory thresholds. Postoperative chest x-ray of posterior anterior and lateral views document the position of the J electrode.

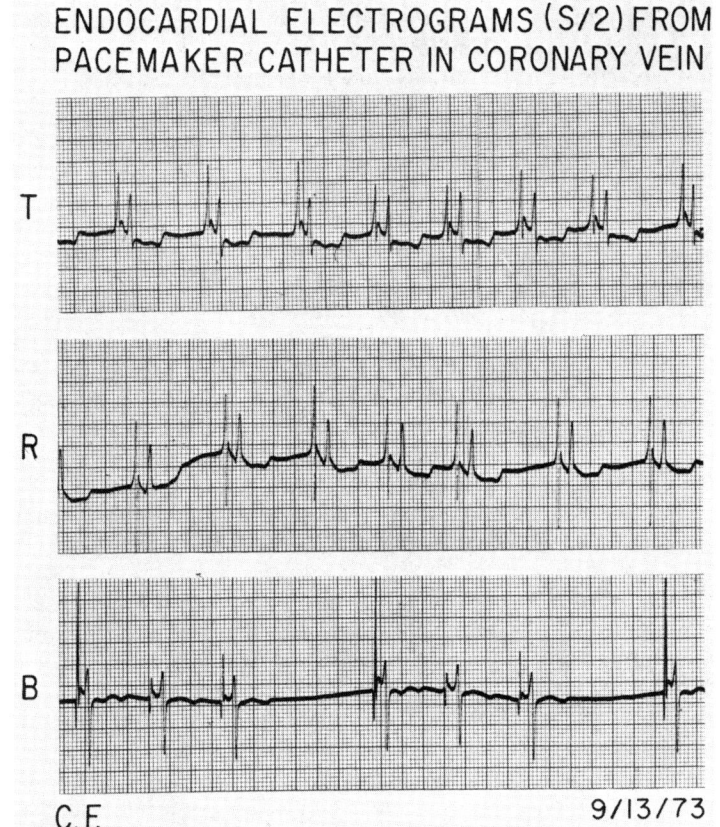

ENDOCARDIAL ELECTROGRAMS (S/2) FROM
PACEMAKER CATHETER IN CORONARY VEIN

Atrial Pacer Spikes

Figure 20–6. Endocardial electrograms from pacemaker catheter in coronary vein. T=tip; R=ring; B=bipolar. The atrial complex is mainly positive in T and biphasic in R and B. Variations in amplitude in B are probably the result of catheter movement during ventricular contraction. The three tall atrial complexes in B have been retouched. (1/2 standardization.)

Epicardial Placement of Atrial Electrode. Direct implantation of a right atrial electrode may be accomplished by right anterolateral thoracotomy, right parasternal extrapleural (transmediastinal) approach, median sternotomy, or left thoracotomy. The ability to gain adequate exposure and the need to place an additional ventricular electrode are the two factors that determine the choice of the surgical approach. Gentle handling of the right atrium is necessary because the wall is usually thin. The epicardial atrial electrode may be sutured or a sutureless screw electrode may be used. The sutureless electrode is much more convenient and requires less surgical exposure. The electrode tip should be short to avoid loss of contact from overpenetration of the wall. The ventricle is not usually accessible with the right parasternal approach. Another incision is necessary if a ventricular wire is also required. With only a right parasternal incision, a transatrial right ventricular endocardial electrode was passed in a few cases (Carney and Anderson, 1979). This was accomplished by inserting the endocardial electrode through the wall of the right atrium into the right ventricle. A purse-string suture avoids bleeding and secures the electrode. The positioning of the electrode is facilitated by fluoroscopy.

Endocardial Screw Electrode. Active fixation transvenous electrode (endocardial screw) has been used successfully to correct or prevent ventricular electrode displacement. The principle is finding its application in the atrial position (Kreuzer and Bisping, 1980). The technique involves localizing a suitable area in the right atrium by endocardial electrogram and threshold measurements. Once this is accomplished, the screw mechanism is activated. A certain model that uses a modified stylette as the screwdriver works very well. Repeat testings are done after the fixation to be certain that the thresholds are good. The actual motion of the screw as it is activated is also readily observed under fluoroscopy. The active fixation in the endocardium can be verified by applying gentle traction on the electrode and observing the tip of the electrode.

Epicardial Pacemaker Implantation During Open Heart Surgery

In some patients undergoing an open heart procedure, there are specific indications for permanent pacemaker implantations. Examples of these conditions are: (1) sick sinus syndrome with severe bradycardia; (2) severe calcific aortic stenosis with significant A-V block (second or third degree); and (3) atrial fibrillation with a very slow ventricular response, not caused by digitalis.

A sutureless myocardial screw electrode is placed in the left ventricle at the end of the open heart procedure. The pacing thresholds and R-wave sensing are tested as usual. The electrodes are connected to the generator in the subcutaneous pocket as described previously. We recommend the use of a drain in the pocket because of oozing secondary to the systemic heparinization during cardiopulmonary bypass. The use of a programmable pacemaker has the advantage of noninvasive manipulation in the immediate postoperative period. Nevertheless, for most patients undergoing open heart surgery who require a permanent ventricular pacemaker, we recommend additional temporary atrial and ventricular epicardial wires for possible use during the immediate postoperative period. Rate augmentation by atrial pacing optimizes cardiac output. Overdrive pacing (Cooper et al., 1978), diagnostic testing with atrial electrograms, and A-V sequential pacing may be used postoperatively as indicated. When temporary pacing is used, the rate should be set higher to suppress the permanent pacemaker generator, or the latter should be programmed to a lower rate.

In the presence of bradycardia or intermittent complete heart block, when the indication for permanent pacing has not been definitely established, permanent epicardial electrodes are advised. The terminals are capped and placed in the subcutaneous pocket. If permanent pacing later becomes necessary, a generator can be connected under local anesthesia. The permanent epicardial electrode can also be used in a temporary system by connecting a temporary lead extension, which is brought out through the skin for pacing. The temporary extension is removed later by applying traction, leaving the permanent lead capped in the subcutaneous pocket (Fig. 20-7).

When patients with permanent pacemakers undergo heart surgery, there are concerns about the deleterious effect of electrocautery and defibrillators on the pacemaker and the heart. These potential problems (which are not well-documented in the literature) include: (1) ventricular fibrillation or other arrhythmias caused by electrocautery; (2) electrocautery-induced myocardial injury at the electrode tip, resulting in a rise in threshold; and (3) damage to the pacemaker generator by defibrillatory currents (Aubry-Frize et al., 1979; Aylward et al., 1979; Hauser et al., 1979, Shepard et al., 1979). One approach to these problems is the temporary removal of the generator at the beginning of the open heart procedure. The generator is saved in a sterile field to be reimplanted later. If the patient required temporary pacing, the electrode is connected to a temporary pacemaker. There is usually extensive use of the electrocautery and occasional use of the defibrillator. The temporary removal of the generator avoids its possible injury.

Cold potassium cardioplegia is now the established method of myocardial protection during open intracardiac surgery. Myocardial oxygen consumption is remarkably decreased during deep hypothermia and with the heart asystolic. Electrical stimulation by the perma-

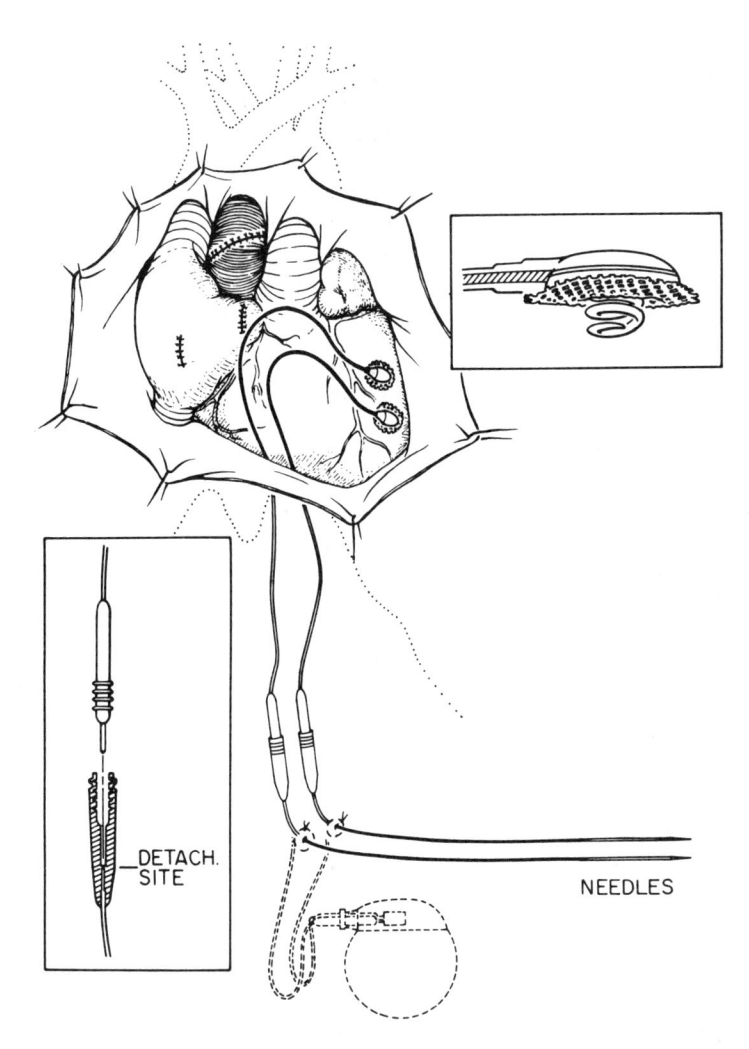

Figure 20-7. Permanent epicardial electrode implantation at the time of open heart surgery. Two permanent sutureless screw electrodes are implanted in the left ventricle (after an aortic valve replacement). They are brought out subcutaneously and attached to the *temporary* lead extensions. The inset at the top right is the closeup of the sutureless electrode. The details of the temporary lead extension and the site of detachment are shown in the left lower inset. In dotted lines, the permanent generator is connected.

nent pacemaker at this time is not desirable. However, open heart operations have been performed without temporarily disconnecting the generator. Most pacemakers are now well enough protected from electromagnetic interference and we have not seen any problems so far. If a transvenous electrode has been in place a long time, cannulation of the superior and inferior vena cavae does not usually interfere with it. On the other hand, intraoperative manipulations during open heart surgery will most likely dislodge a recently implanted transvenous electrode. It is desirable to retest the electrode and generator at the completion of the intracardiac procedure. A spare permanent epicardial electrode is recommended with a temporary lead extension for temporary pacing.

TECHNIQUE OF PACEMAKER GENERATOR REPLACEMENT

Elective and prophylactic pacemaker generator replacement was customary when mercury-zinc batteries were widely used. The newer power sources are more reliable and generator replacement is only necessary in the presence of pacemaker failure or with the appearance of end-of-life indications. In the follow-up of 422 lithium generators over 12,500 patient months, we found no power failure and only one random circuit failure (Estioko et al., 1980). Although the lithium-powered pacemakers are performing well, there have been some advisories (recalls), which required closer monitoring of some units and generator replacement in others. The failures commonly were rate decrease, but some had rate increase and others no output (Bilitch, 1981). Random circuit failures have also been observed. Reoperations are more commonly related to electrode problems. With any contemplated generator change, the surgical team should be prepared for possible complete system replacement. The fluoroscopy setup should always be available for electrode change. The patient is also made aware of this possibility preoperatively.

The operative field is prepared to include both neck and upper chest areas. Under local infiltration anesthesia, an incision is made into the subcutaneous pocket, following the previous incision. An unsightly scar may be excised. If there is much downward migration of the generator, the incision may be made over the upper part of the generator. The incision is carefully carried downward to the generator, avoiding damage to the electrode. The placement of the redundant part of the electrode behind the generator at the initial implantation protects the electrode during dissection at reoperation. The generator is exteriorized and disconnected from the electrode. Temporary pacing must be established promptly in patients who are pacemaker-dependent. When the system is bipolar, temporary unipolar pacing is maintained while the electrodes are disconnected one at a time. With a unipolar electrode, quick disconnection and temporary pacing must be undertaken. This can be accomplished by inserting a 25-gauge needle through the electrode insulation and parallel to the electrode, thus making temporary contact for pacing while the pin is disconnected.

As soon as the generator is removed, the temporary cable can be switched from the 25-gauge needle to the terminal pin. The temporary pacemaker cable can be switched back to the needle after the thresholds are tested. The new generator can now be connected safely while temporary pacing is continued without interruption. The needle is removed and the tiny puncture in the insulation is sealed with silastic glue.

Pacing thresholds, R-wave sensing, and the new generator should be checked with a pacemaker system analyzer. The subcutaneous pocket is usually adequate in size for the currently used generators, which are quite small. Revision of the pocket may be required if it is too large, in a poor location, or if the generator has migrated excessively.

ELECTRODE REPOSITIONING AND REPLACEMENT

In transvenous implantation, pacemaker failure is often electrode-related. This may occur in the first few days, weeks, or months because of electrode displacement, instability, or rise in thresholds. This problem may be corrected as follows:

1. The same electrode is repositioned to obtain good stability and thresholds. A third failure could occur but this is unusual.
2. The electrode may be changed to one with an active fixation mechanism. The most promising in our experience is the endocardial screw electrode. Figure 20–8 illustrates the various electrodes classified into passive, semi-active, and active.
3. The transvenous approach is abandoned and epicardiac electrode implantation is carried out. Some centers will proceed with epicardial pacemaker implantation without attempting repositioning or electrode change. With the availability of reliable active fixation transvenous electrodes, at least one reoperation is justified prior to epicardial implantation.

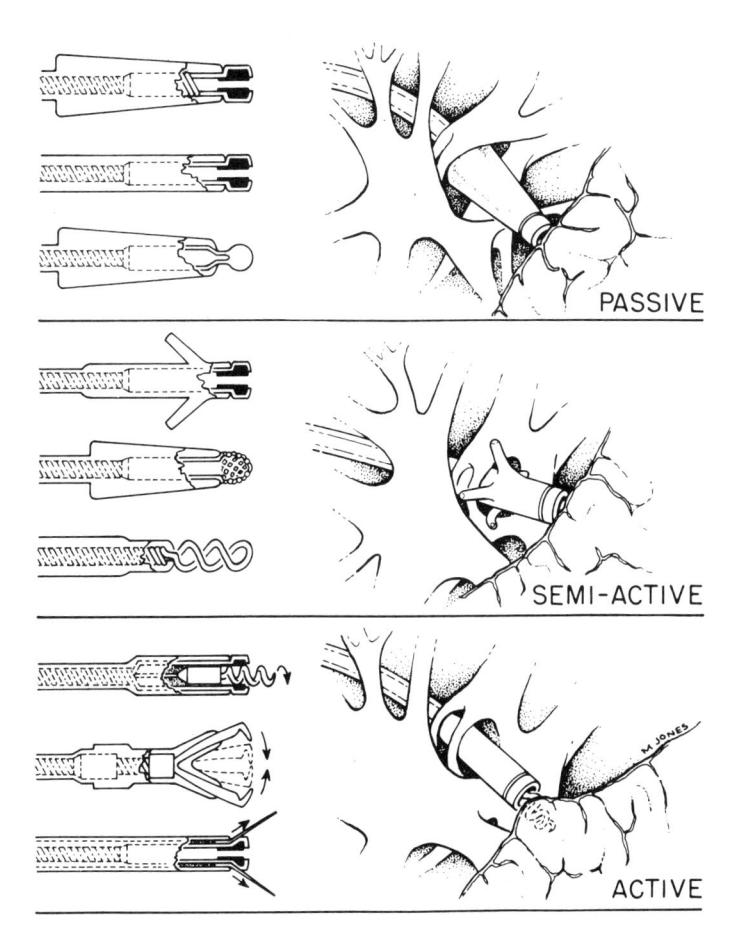

Figure 20-8. Common Types of Transvenous electrodes. The electrodes may be classified into passive, semiactive, or active types. Representatives of each type are shown at left (from top to bottom). *Passive:* flanged tip, straight, flanged with ball tip. *Semiactive:* tined with ring tip, flanged with porous tip, helically coiled tip. *Active:* endocardial screw, pinching or grasping type, pronged type. Note the relationship of the three types to the endocardium and trabeculations as shown by the illustrations on the right.

Electrode replacement is also indicated in the presence of high thresholds during elective generator replacement. Reusing an old electrode with high threshold causes excessive drain on the battery and may lead to premature pacemaker failure. The electrodes used several years ago had large surface areas with higher current drain. The old electrode is dissected down to its entrance into the vein and it can be withdrawn. The same vein may be used to insert the new electrode. If the same vein is not suitable or the old electrode cannot be withdrawn, a new venous access would be used, as described earlier. Again, provisions should be made for the patient to be continuously paced if he or she is pacemaker-dependent. Alternatively, if there is limitation of venous access because of previous multiple operations, subclavian puncture can be done (Littleford et al., 1979; Neihus et al., 1979). In our opinion, this technique should not be used routinely because of possible complications (notably pneumothorax and bleeding).

COMPLICATIONS OF PACING

Complications may be divided into early and late. The early complications are related to those immediately postimplantation in the hospital or shortly after discharge. Late complications refers to those that occur after one month.

Early Complications

Electrode Displacement. Displacement or dislocation of the electrode is usually manifested by intermittent or sustained loss of pacing or sensing. Displacement of the electrode may be detectable in the chest x-ray. Figure 20-9 illustrates various displaced positions in the frontal and lateral views. The incidence of this complication is high if there is improper positioning and testing of the electrode at the initial implantation. Ideally, the incidence should be below 5 percent with meticulous technique and an experienced team (Parsonnet et al., 1979). Our experience has been favorable with the use of the tined electrode. A review of 300 recent consecutive primary implantations with the tined electrode revealed only two displacements (0.67 percent). Electrode repositioning, electrode change, or epicardial implantation as previously described are undertaken to correct this complication.

Pacemaker Failure Due to "Exit Block". The term "exit block" has been used to describe early pacemaker failure caused by rise in threshold. Sometimes it is difficult to distinguish rising threshold from minor change in transvenous electrode position, which cannot be detected by chest x-ray. "Exit block" has also been observed in epicardial pacemaker implantation, with a higher incidence in the right ventricle. Reprogramming of certain variables of the pacemaker (increasing pulse width or output) may correct this problem. In a transvenous pacemaker, repositioning the electrode or electrode change may be necessary.

Generator Pocket Hematoma. When there is adequate hemostasis, pocket hematoma is uncommon. A drain is useful but ineffective if excessive oozing is present. A small hematoma usually does not require treatment. Needle aspiration is not recommended because of the possibility of contamination. If there is a large hematoma of the pocket, reoperation with evacuation of the hematoma and control of bleeding should be done early. A review of 1,000 initial implantations in our institution revealed only two patients requiring reoperation because of bleeding, or a complication rate of 0.2 percent.

Diaphragmatic Stimulation. This complication is rare if it is specifically excluded at the time of operation (see previous discussion). It is manifested by intermittent or rhythmic contraction of the left hemidiaphragm (visible by fluoroscopy) and possibly of the abdominal wall. The patient may complain of palpitations or thumping sensations. Reoperation and repositioning of the electrode usually corrects the problem, or it may disappear spontaneously. It can sometimes be solved by using the features of a programmable pacemaker (for example, decreasing the output or pulse width).

Pectoral Muscle Stimulation. Occasionally, pectoral muscle stimulation occurs secondary to a break in the insulation or the seal of the electrode connection to the generator. The unipolar generator may be improperly oriented and produce muscle twitchings. Reoperation is necessary to correct this problem. Pectoral muscle stimulation may still occur with a properly oriented unipolar generator. A change to a bipolar pacemaker is the treatment of choice. Subpectoral placement of a unipolar generator only invites this complication.

Myocardial Perforation and Penetration. With increasing experience there has been a significant reduction in the incidence of myocardial perforation or penetration. This complication is often, but not always, associated with loss of pacemaker function. The simultaneous loss of pacemaker function and diaphragmatic stimulation often indicates myocardial penetration or perforation. This is usually a benign complication that can be corrected by withdrawing and repositioning the electrode. It is confirmed by recording a continuous electrocardiogram from the cathe-

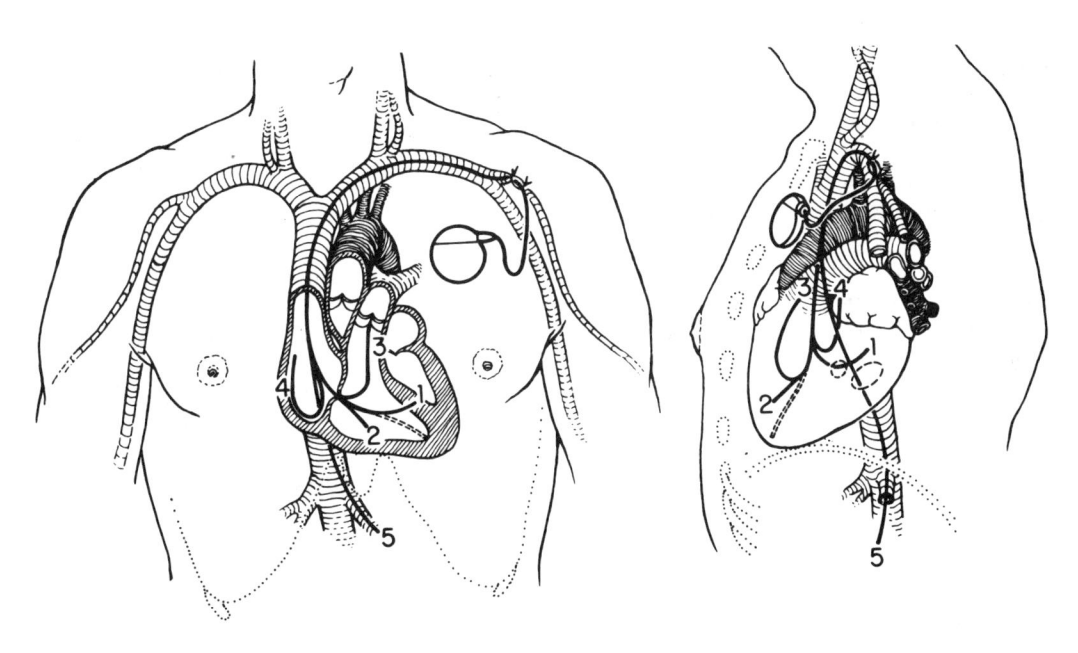

Figure 20-9. Electrode displacements. The various displacement positions are illustrated in the frontal and lateral views. 1 = coronary sinus. 2 = midcavity of the RV. 3 = outflow tract of the RV, close to the pulmonary artery. 4 = right atrium. 5 = inferior vena cava and hepatic vein.

ter tip during its withdrawal. As the electrode traverses the myocardium, the amplitude of the tracings will suddenly increase and there is a transient ST elevation (current of injury). Cardiac tamponade may result, especially if the patient is receiving anticoagulants. Central venous pressure measurement and echocardiogram may be helpful in the diagnosis. Left thoracotomy is the treatment of choice to decompress the pericardium and withdraw the transvenous electrode. Often it is not necessary to suture the site of perforation. The pacemaker should then be converted to an epicardial implantation. Pericardiocentesis is performed only for diagnosis and for emergency decompression. Creation of a pericardial window by the subxiphoid approach is the other alternative.

Wound Infection. Infection of the pacemaker generator pocket is fortunately rare (0.2 percent in our experience). The presence of a foreign body makes it highly resistant to treatment with antibiotics. It is usually necessary to completely remove the infected pacemaker and implant a new system at another location. When this is done it is extremely important to isolate the sterile field of the new implantation site. The new pacemaker implantation should be finished and the incision closed before removal of the infected pacemaker. Culture and sensitivity tests from the pocket are obtained so that treatment with appropriate antibiotics can be instituted. The infected wound is debrided. The wound is closed per primum and a closed suction drain inserted. Continuous irrigation with saline for a few days has been used. Single layer closure of the wound with fine wire or monofilament material is recommended. Leaving an open wound without closure creates a risk of cross-contamination of the new pacemaker incision.

Arrhythmia. Catheter-induced arrhythmia can occur at the time of electrode manipulation. It is unusual for a stable electrode to cause arrhythmias. They are mainly related to intrinsic disease of the heart and require the usual pharmacologic treatment. Temporary increase of the pacemaker rate by reprogramming may abolish some of the rhythm disturbances, but this is rarely necessary.

Late Complications

Electrode Displacement. Electrode displacement may still occur after several months. Fibrosis and psuedoendothelial formation secure the electrode, making late displacement unusual. The management of this complication has been described.

Skin Erosion and Wound Infection. Skin erosion over the pacemaker generator has been observed in very thin patients with large and heavy generators. Pressure necrosis of the overlying skin occurs at the areas corresponding to the edges of the generator. Reoperation should be considered before complete erosion of the skin and secondary infection supervene. The operation is designed to excise this area of necrosis and to prevent its recurrence. The generator may be relocated at another site, located deeper behind the pectoralis muscle, or changed to a thinner and lighter one. If there is a break in the integrity of the skin, the pacemaker is considered infected. In the presence of infection, a new pacemaker system should be placed on the opposite side and the infected pacemaker removed as previously described.

Septicemia and Bacterial Endocarditis. This is an uncommon complication. Infection of the pacemaker electrode should be suspected in the presence of persistently positive blood cultures. The electrode may have vegetations or any of the cardiac valves may be involved. A new murmur of valvular insufficiency may appear. Appropriate intravenous antibiotic treatment should be administered aggressively. If infection cannot be controlled, removal of the infected pacemaker electrode is the next step. The electrode is completely removed and an epicardial pacemaker electrode should be implanted. There is a risk of reinfection if a new transvenous electrode is used, even at a different vein site. It may be difficult to remove an old electrode that has been trapped by fibrosis. In one case we were successful by using an intravascular grasping forceps under fluoroscopy. Urologic or bronchoscopic instruments can be used for this purpose by introducing them through the right internal jugular vein. If all else fails, the infected electrode must be removed by median sternotomy or right thoracotomy. It can be extracted through the right atrium, superior vena cava, or innominate vein. Exposure and access to the different structures is excellent with median sternotomy. The operating team should also be prepared to use cardiopulmonary bypass (this is rarely necessary).

The need for prophylactic measures against endocarditis in pacemaker patients is uncertain.

Venous Thrombosis. Upper deep-vein thrombosis is a rare complication in transvenous pacemaker implantation. Stoney et al (1976), however, demonstrated that the incidence of abnormal findings on routine venous angiogram is not low. We encountered four symptomatic cases in 1,000 primary implants. The treatment is anticoagulation with heparin. The swelling of the upper extremity usually quickly disappears. There are a few reports of an even rarer complication—superior vena caval obstruction associated with a transvenous pacemaker (Williams and Demos, 1974). We had one patient with massive and fatal pulmonary embolism three weeks after transvenous implantation in another hospital. There are few reports in the literature of this complication (Kaulbach and Krukonis, 1970).

Electrode Fracture. Electrode fracture was one of the leading complications in the past, but improvement in electrode design has diminished its incidence. It may occur at any point of stress within or outside the heart and usually leads to loss of pacing and sensing function. Fracture without insulation break may cause intermittent loss of pacemaker artefact. Insulation break located in the subcutaneous tissue may produce muscle twitchings of the pectoralis. It may also lead to a change in the vector of the pacemaker artefact and pacing may continue. Electrode change is required. Splicing and other kinds of repairs are not recommended.

"Twiddler's Syndrome" and Wandering Generator. "Twiddler's syndrome" refers to an interesting complication that results when patients manipulate their generator by turning it in the subcutaneous pocket (Bayliss et al., 1968). The electrode is pulled away from its contact with the endocardium, causing pacemaker failure. Proper fixation of the electrode at the time of implantation and instruction of patients not to manipulate their pacemaker will prevent this complication. When it occurs, reoperation is necessary.

The generator may gravitate excessively in elderly patients with loose subcutaneous tissue. This usually does not present a problem because there is enough redundancy of the electrode in the subcutaneous pocket. Some patients, however, complained of pain at the pacemaker pocket. Large generators that were improperly located laterally tended to migrate to the axilla. This causes discomfort, especially with arm motions. Revision of the pocket or relocation of the generator is the treatment in symptomatic patients.

Tricuspid Regurgitation. Post-mortem examinations have established that there may be adhesion of the electrode to the tricuspid valve. On occasion this may interfere with valve function and lead to severe regurgitation.

Premature Generator Failure. The generator may fail earlier than anticipated because of electronic circuit or power source problems. Circuit failures are usually random and can appear as loss of pacemaker function or abnormal function (Chirife et al., 1976). A faulty magnetic reed switch may result in asynchronous pacing. Battery failures are uncommon in the present state of the art. Lithium batteries have significantly improved the reliability and longevity of pacemakers (Burr, 1977).

ELECTRICAL INTERFERENCE

Any pacemaker designed to modify its function by electrical or magnetic signals may, by the same token, be subject to undesirable effects by outside influences that mimic these signals. Demand pacemakers vary in their susceptibility to such "interference," which may inhibit ventricular-inhibited pacers, accelerate synchronous units, or convert them into asynchronous operation. Short-wave diathermy and electrocoagulation current will interfere with most pacemakers, while proximity to microwave ovens, radar, and radio transmitters, gasoline engine distributors, and electric razors should probably be avoided. Weapons' detectors (magnetometers) used at airports (Keshishian et al., 1972) are not a significant hazard, but magnets used for testing pacemakers will be detected. Certain anti-theft devices used in libraries may interfere with demand pacemakers (Cueni, et al., 1979).

Skeletal muscle potentials frequently interfere with function of unipolar pacemakers (Wirtzfeld et al., 1972), but this is not often severe enough to cause symptoms.

PATIENT EDUCATION

Patients with implanted pacemakers are understandably anxious and should be instructed in detail about the conduct of their lives and the necessity for careful follow-up. Most manufacturers publish illustrated pamphlets for patients. These will include warnings about the type of outside interference that is most likely to affect their particular brand of pacemaker.

It is generally agreed (Sowton, 1972) that most patients be permitted to drive automobiles, with the possible exception of those who are known to have either no or very slow idioventricular rhythm, or those in whom there is doubt about the effectiveness of the pacemaker. Pacemaker patients, like diabetics and people taking anticoagulants, should carry identification cards or tags.

FOLLOW-UP OF PATIENTS WITH PACEMAKERS

The surgeon's responsibility does not cease when the patient leaves the hospital. A followup system must be instituted that will probably include the patient's primary physician and perhaps a cardiologist as well. The patient must be seen at intervals of a few months. With the mercury-zinc batteries, which tend to fail suddenly, a decision has to be made whether to replace the generator at a fixed interval or to attempt to obtain as long a life as possible for the generator by close observation for change in rate and pulse width or by electronic analysis. The latter course requires special equipment, including a calibrated high-speed oscilloscope and electronic counter. Some of the newer threshold testing pacemakers (discussed previously) may be analyzed by simpler methods. Hand-held analyzers of rate and pulse width (Instromedix) may eventually obviate the need for oscilloscopic analysis. One pacemaker, by telemetry, is capable of transmitting values for electrode-tissue interface impedance, loaded battery impedance, and average current drain. These figures can be used in the determination of time for replacement (Programalith).

The newer lithium-powered units last longer and generally lose their power much more slowly, so that follow-up need not be as frequent.

The most exacting follow-up program will not eliminate the occasional pacemaker failure caused by catheter displacement, electronic fault, or premature battery depletion. The great majority of failures, however, may be anticipated in time. Fortunately, very few patients are so dependent on their pacemaker that they would not survive without it. The surgeon will be aware which patients fall into this category and will be particularly cautious in these cases.

Office Analysis

A great deal of information about the pacemaker may be gleaned by history, physical examination, roentgenography, and a twelve-lead electrocardiogram. If the heart is usually completely captured, the patient or a companion should be taught to take the pulse once a day and keep a record of it. If the pulse is often irregular, counting it does more harm than good. Symptoms such as dizziness or syncope should be sought. Dizziness is a common complaint among older patients and may be labyrinthine in origin. If so, it often occurs with change in position. Muscle contractions, often described by patients as "palpitations" or "twitching," when in certain positions, may be troublesome but are usually tolerable.

In the office, the pulse should be taken for a full minute. In most pacemakers, application of an ordinary transistor radio over the generator (see below) elicits a click each time the pacemaker fires. This click may be used to time the pacemaker rate and to determine (by simultaneous auscultation or palpation of the pulse) whether the heart is following the pacemaker. The location of the pacemaker generator should be noted in relation to the nipple. Contractions of the abdominal muscles might indicate stimulation of the diaphragm. Pericardial friction rubs are common during the first few weeks after implantation. Both of these events are of little significance, unless accompanying loss of capture.

It is well-known that sizable phasic variations in blood pressure may occur in paced patients and the intensity of the first sound may vary. An extraneous sound preceding the first heart sound and often called a pacemaker "knock" may be heard in certain phases of respiration or in some positions. This sound may indicate a perforation of the heart wall, but in most instances it is benign and presumably the result of intercostal muscle contractions caused by excessive current.

In seeking to establish the site of pacemaker electrodes in the heart by roentgenograms, the film should be overexposed. Lateral projections must be taken as well as postero-anterior (Fig. 20-10 A, B). Image intensification fluoroscopy, if available, will yield even more information about the location and behavior of the electrode.

A standard twelve-lead electrocardiogram should be obtained. It can easily be determined from this whether the pacemaker is functioning normally. Even a single pacemaker artefact occurring outside the refractory period that does not capture the heart indicates malfunction. The location of the electrodes will determine the configuration of the surface electrocardiogram, and the direction of current flow in the pacemaker electrodes will be indicated by the vector of the pacemaker stimulus.

With bipolar right ventricular apical cavity pacing, the standard leads invariably show abnormal left axis deviation and the precordial leads a left bundle branch block pattern or a variant thereof (Figs. 20-11 and 20-12). When a right bundle branch block pattern appears in the precordial leads, one must suspect pacing from the left ventricle, although a pacing site high on the right ventricular side of the septum is also possible (Fig. 20–13). The routine recording of V_1 on the operating table is important in this regard.

When P waves cannot be identified in the paced electrocardiogram, several possibilities exist: (1) atrial fibrillation is present; (2) the P waves are small and not visible because of a low gain setting of the EGG; (3) retrograde P waves are buried in the QRS-T complexes. In the latter case they can sometimes be identi-

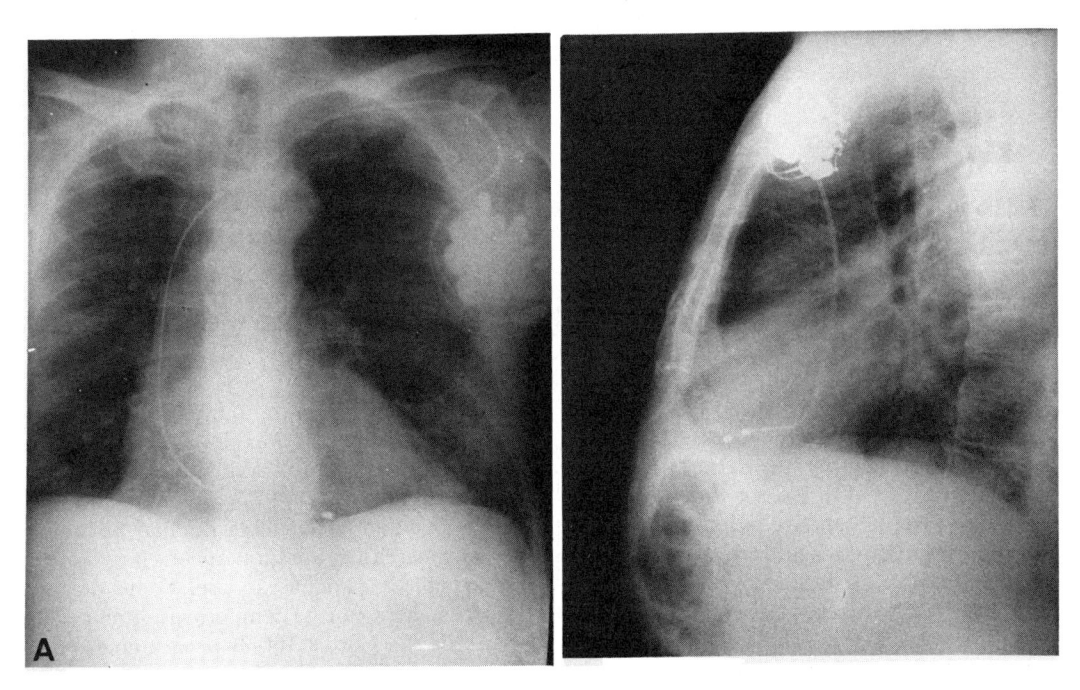

Figure 20–10. Antero-posterior **(A)** and left lateral roentgenograms **(B)** showing the preferred location of a pacemaker catheter in the apex of the right ventricle.

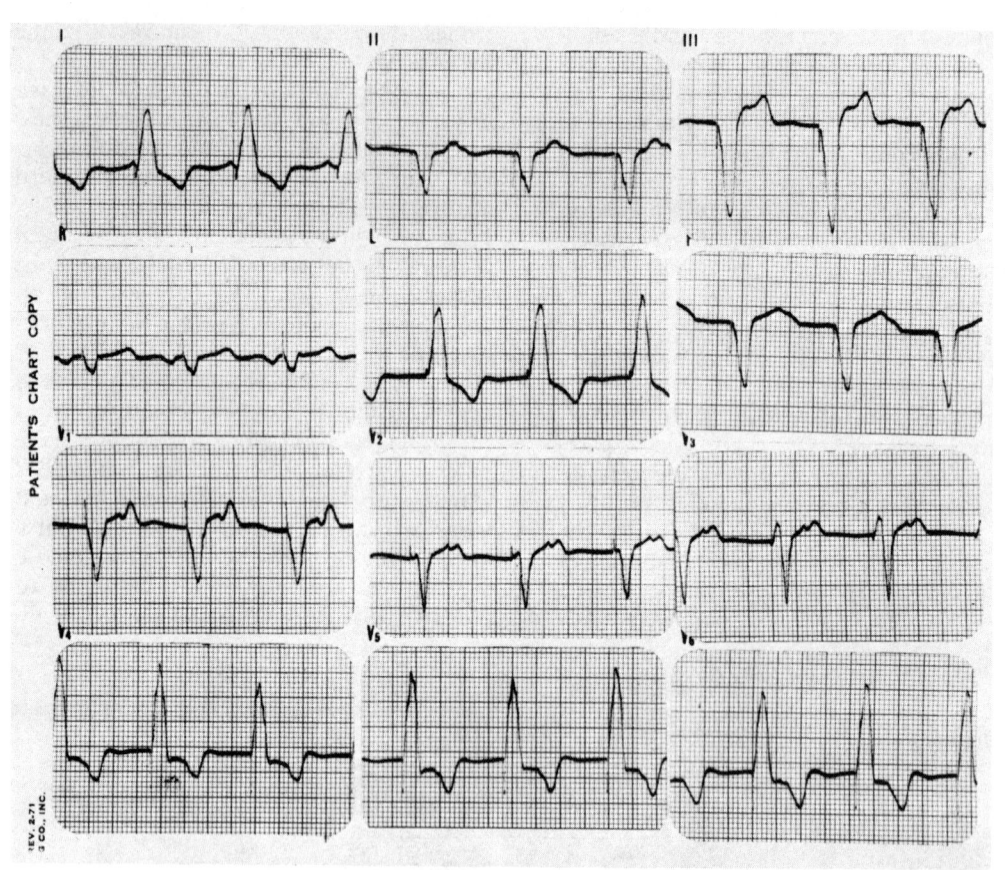

Figure 20–11. Twelve-lead electrocardiogram showing characteristic left bundle branch block configuration in a patient with endocardial bipolar pacing from apex of right ventricle.

fied in some leads or suspected by the finding of "cannon" waves in the venous pulse. Retrograde P waves are much more common in sinus node dysfunction than in heart block.

In unipolar pacing the electrocardiogram is often distorted by the large pacemaker artefact (Fig. 20–14). Except for minor QRS shift in AVR, the standard paced electrocardiogram does not change during the life of a given electrode, unless it moves or perforates the heart. In patients with demand pacemakers, however, T-wave changes may occur in the unpaced electrocardiogram, which may be reversible and may not indicate myocardial damage (Chatterjee et al., 1969).

Demand pacemakers may be inhibited by chest wall stimulation (Barold et al., 1970; Gordon et al., 1970) to permit the spontaneous electrocardiogram to be studied or to test inhibitory function. Pin electrodes usually require less current for inhibition than standard ones (Mattes et al., 1977).

Demand pacemakers also may be inhibited by increasing the spontaneous heart rate by having the patient exercise. Some demand pacemakers can be temporarily inhibited by use of the Cordis 166-B programmer (Latif and Ewy, 1977). Cordis Stanicor can be shut off by turning the horseshoe magnet in 180° arcs (Voukydis et al., 1975). The Medtronic

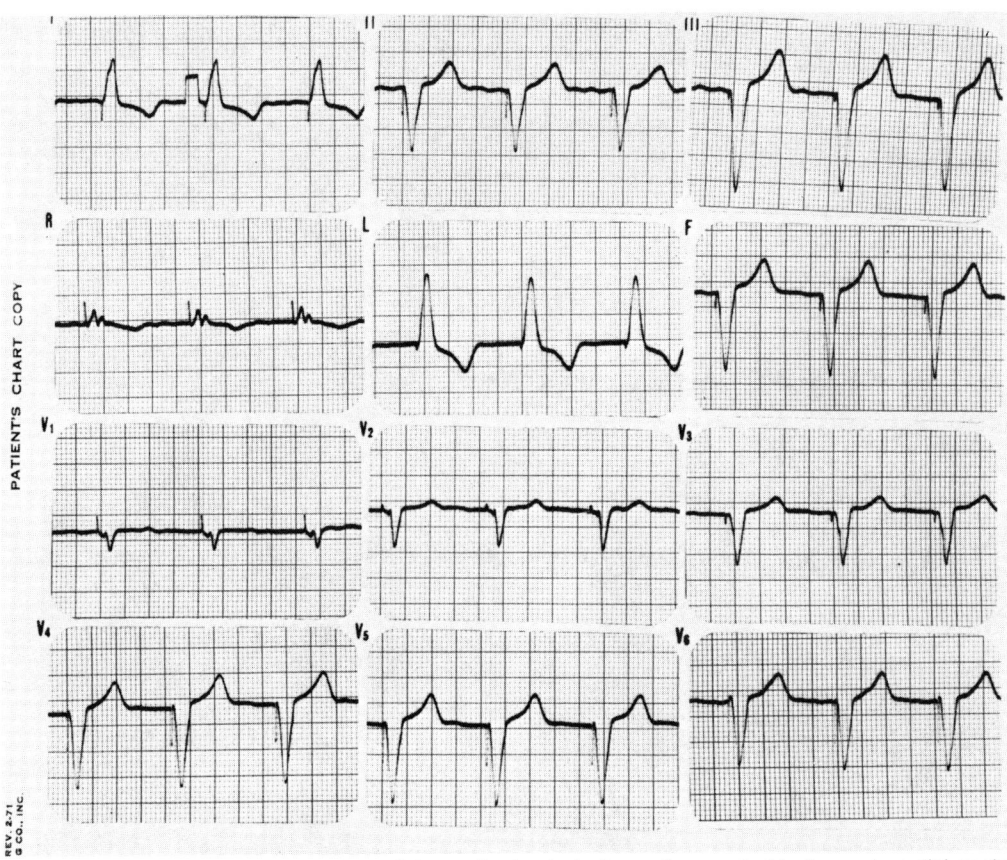

PERMANENT CARDIAC PACEMAKERS: MANAGEMENT AND PROBLEMS 481

Figure 20–12. A more common variant of the twelve-lead electrocardiogram in bipolar endocardial pacing from apex of right ventricle. In contrast to Figure 20-11, the precordial QRS complexes are all negative.

Spectrax programmer has an inhibitor mode. In some other units it may be possible to program the demand pacemaker slow enough to permit the underlying rhythm to manifest itself.

Conversely, most pacemakers may be made to fire in asynchronous mode by application of a magnet to the generator. It is dangerous to apply pressure over the carotid sinus to slow the heart and activate a demand pacemaker. A careful Valsalva maneuver may accomplish the same purpose and with less risk. The authors have successfully used this method in a patient whose magnetic switch was inoperative.

ELECTRONIC ANALYSIS

First described by Knuckey et al. (1965), oscilloscopic analysis of the pacemaker impulse forms the backbone of most pacemaker follow-up clinics. This is usually performed on one or more standard extremity leads, but one of the authors (AJG) has employed a custom-built, wide-band amplifier to display X, Y, and Z component leads and frontal, transverse, and left sagittal vectors of the inpulse in the Frank system (Fig. 20–15, p. 484). Information can thus be obtained not only about the voltage, duration, and time constant of the pacemaker impulse, but also about the

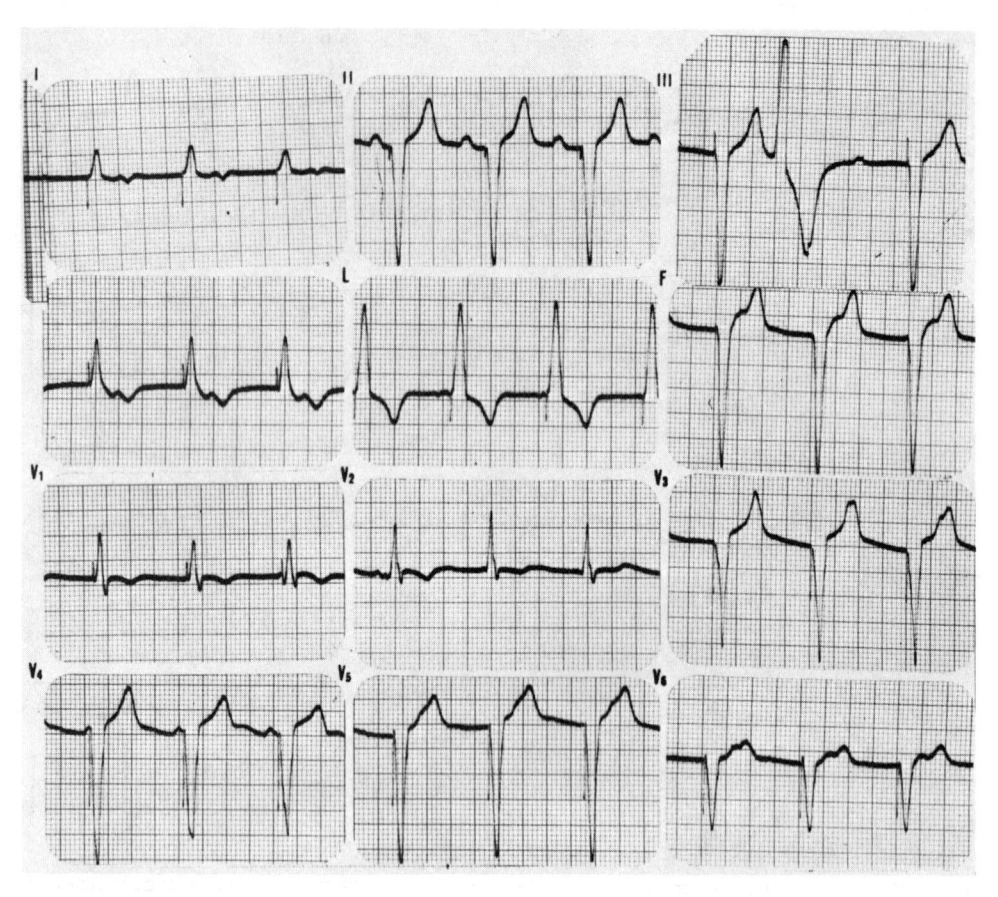

Figure 20-13. Right bundle branch block configuration caused by bipolar endocardial catheter pacing from high on right ventricular side of interventricular septum.

orientation of the electrode (Gordon, 1971). Impending battery failure, lead fracture, insulation break, and electrode displacement may be diagnosed. An electronic counter also may be used for accurate determination of pacemaker interval. Recently, instruments have become available (Vitatron, Gutmann) that display this type of information in digital form. Follow-up clinics have been computerized for more efficient operation for large numbers of patients (Parsonnet et al., 1970).

Remote Monitoring

Some patients, because of their age or infirmities, are not able to visit the doctor's office or pacemaker clinic regularly. For this group and for patients who are approaching the end of the life of their pacemaker generators, it is helpful to have a complementary system, which the patient or a companion may use at home at frequent intervals or transmit over the telephone. Many such systems are available, ranging in complexity from the simple determination of the patient's pulse rate by palpation to the transmission of the electrocardiogram containing the pacemaker artefact over the telephone.

The pulse rate alone is probably the least accurate of these methods, but it is also the simplest. Almost all pacemakers manufactured today are designed to slow when the batteries begin to fail. If the heart is complete-

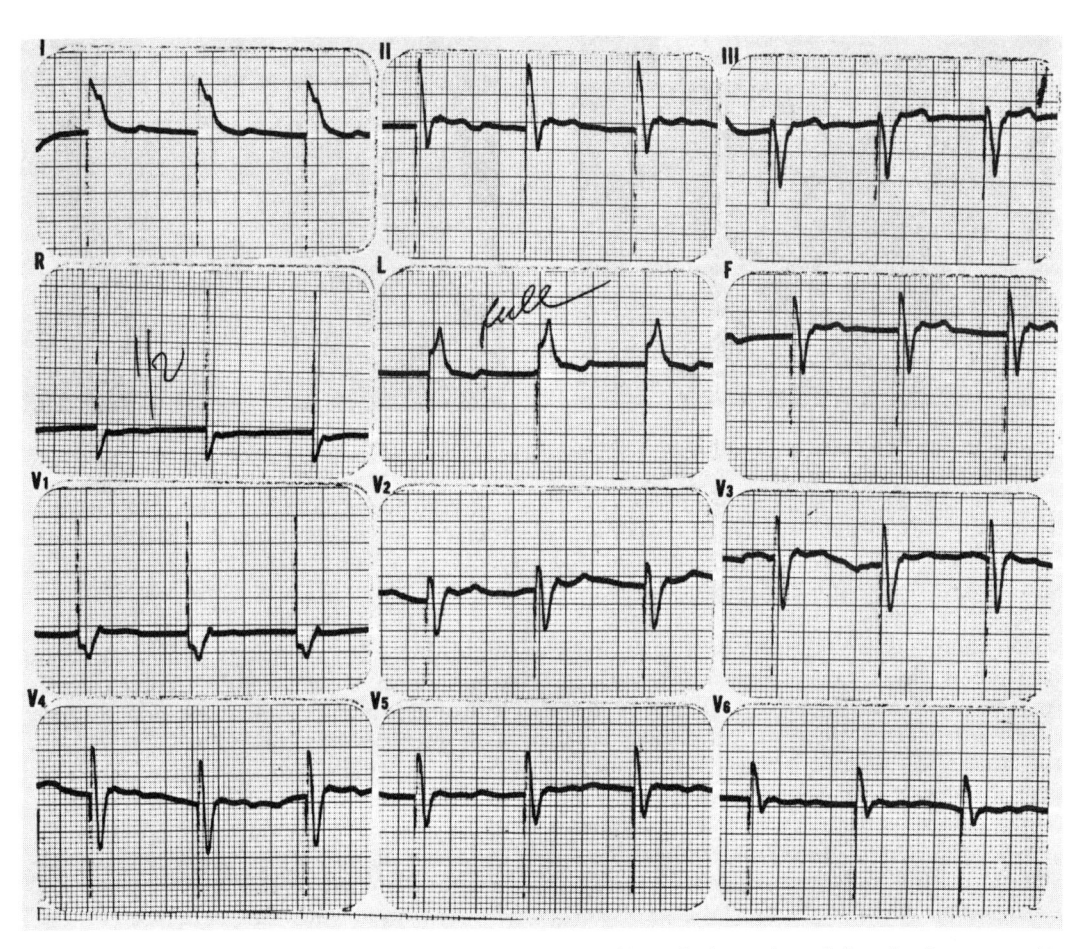

Figure 20-14. Distortion of surface electrocardiogram caused by unipolar endocardial pacing from apex of right ventricle. On another occasion, when the heart was paced by a bipolar catheter at approximately the same location, the twelve-lead electrocardiogram was essentially the same as that in Figure 20-12.

ly captured by either an asynchronous or demand pacemaker, the pulse rate, taken once a day for a full minute, often alerts the patient to a failing unit. If the heart is not completely captured, this method may be confusing.

Better surveillance is possible by telephone transmission. Systems are available that transmit the pacemaker rate alone with or without the application of a magnet that converts the pacemaker to an asynchronous mode. Temporary application of the magnet in this context is associated with little risk (Parsonnet, 1973), although one case of ventricular fibrillation has occurred after use of a magnet in a patient with no additional factors (such as acute myocardial infarction) causing increased cardiac irritability (Seipel et al., 1975). Accurate pacemaker interval may be established when the system employs an electronic counter at the receiving end.

A simple yet effective method the authors use (Gordon, 1974) consists of holding an ordinary transistor radio over the implanted generator (Furman and Escher, 1970) and timing the resulting clicks by a stopwatch. The

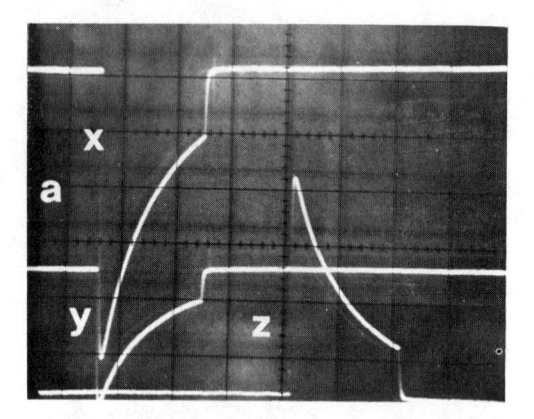

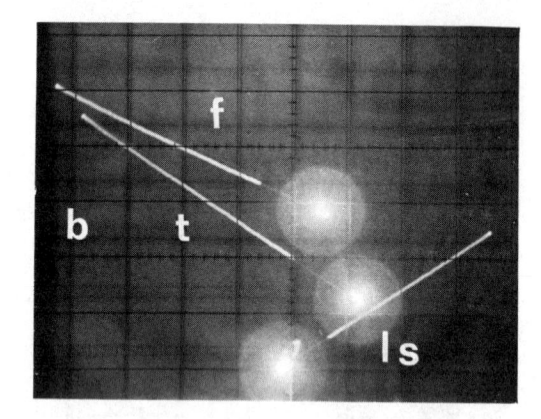

Figure 20–15. The Frank X, Y, and Z component leads **(a)** and frontal, transverse, and left sagittal vectors **(b)** of the stimulus artefact in the patient whose roentgenograms are shown in Figure 20–10. In **(a)**, sweep speed is 1 msec/cm; sensitivity: 2 mV/cm. In **(b)**, sensitivity is 2 mV/cm. (Figs. 20–10 and 20–15 reproduced by permission of North Holland Publishing Company, from *Vectorcardiography 2*, Proceedings of the XI International Symposium on Vectorcardiography, Amsterdam and London, 1971.)

radio volume is turned up to maximum and the station selector turned to the lowest setting on the AM band (540 kHz). The axis of the radio antenna relative to the pacemaker may be critical, so the radio is slowly turned until the maximum volume is obtained. With a stopwatch calibrated to tenths of a second, the elapsed time for 100 beats is determined. This figure, multiplied by ten, gives the average pacemaker interval to the nearest msec. Pacemakers fire with such regularity that great accuracy may be achieved by this method, which is easily adapted to telephone transmission.

If capture is not complete, a magnet must first be applied. The magnet will inactivate the radio if it is too close to the speaker. In that case various positions of the radio, adjacent to the generator, should be tried. Several relatively inexpensive transmission devices are available that contain a magnet as well as a radio or inductive instrument.

Any system based on the rate at which a pacemaker fires, without indicating whether the heart is following, has obvious drawbacks. Combined transmission of pacemaker impulse and pulse from a finger plethysmograph (Cardiac Data Corp.) is one method of improving telephone surveillance. We favor transmission of electrocardiographic tracings with and without application of a magnet. This provides data to evaluate pacing and sensing functions of the pacemaker. The electronic counter gives readout of the rate, pulse interval, and pulse width. The use of the magnet is important because some pacemakers are designed so that the magnetic rate decreases as an early sign of failure.

REFERENCES

Abrams LD, Hudson WA, Lightwood R: A surgical approach to the management of heart block using an inductive coupled artificial cardiac pacemaker. Lancet 1:1372, 1960.

Atkins JJ, Leshin SJ, Blomqvist G, Mullins CB: Ventricular conduction blocks and sudden death in acute myocardial infarction. N Engl J Med 288:281, 1973.

Aubry-Frize M, Gagnon RM, Beaudet R, Poirier N, Lemire J: Measurement of electrosurgical leakage current in pacemaker leads. In Meere C (ed): Cardiac Pacing, Proceedings of the VI World Symposium on Cardiac Pacing, Montreal, 1979, Chap 35–1.

Aylward P, Blood R, Tonkin A: Complications of defibrillation with permanent pacemaker *in situ*.

PACE 2: 462,1979.

Barold SS, Keller JW: Sensing problems with demand pacemakers. In Samet P (ed): Cardiac Pacing. New York, Grune & Stratton, 1973, p 407.

———, Pupillo GA, Gaidula JJ, Linhart JW: Chest wall stimulation in evaluation of patients with implanted ventricular-inhibited demand pacemakers. Br Heart J 32: 783, 1970.

Bayliss CE, Beanlands DS, Baird RJ: The pacemaker twiddlers syndrome. Can Med Assoc J 99: 371, 1968.

Bilitch M: Performance of cardiac pacemaker pulse generators. PACE 4:124, 1981.

———, Hauser RG, MacGregor DC, Furman S, Parsonnet V: Performance of cardiac pacemaker pulse generator. PACE 4:254, 1981.

Brenner AS, Wagner GS, Anderson ST, Rosati RA, Morris JJ Jr: Transvenous, transmediastinal, and transthoracic ventricular pacing. Circulation 49:407, 1974.

Burr LH: The lithium iodide-powered cardiac pacemaker. Clinical experience with 250 implantations. J Thorac Cardiovasc Surg 73:421, 1977.

Cammilli L, Pozzi R, DeSaint Pierre G, Gallenga GC, Buttini C, Grassi G: An implantable micropacemaker without wire electrodes for continuous control of heart block. Isr J Med Sci 3: 236, 1967.

Carlens R, Johansson L, Karloff I, Lagergren H: New method for atrial-triggered pacemaker treatment without thoracotomy. J Thorac Cardiovasc Surg 50:229, 1965.

Carney AL, Anderson EM: The system concept of physiologic pacing: right parasternal approach to atrial and ventricular pacing, atrial mapping, EEG, and staging. In Meere C (ed): Cardiac Pacing, Proceedings of the VI World Symposium on Cardiac Pacing, Montreal, 1979, Chap 14–4.

Castellanos A Jr, Lemberg L: Electrophysiology of Pacing and Cardioversion. New York, Appleton-Century-Crofts, 1969.

Castillo CA, Berkovits BV, Castellanos A Jr, Lemberg L, Callard G, Jude JR: Bifocal demand pacing. Chest 59:360, 1971.

Chatterjee K, Harris A, Davies G, Leatham A: Electrocardiographic changes subsequent to artificial ventricular depolarization. Br Heart J 31:770, 1969.

Chirife R, Frankl WS, Mendizabal R, Estioko MR: Ventricular fibrillation induced by a defective demand pacemaker. Chest 69:247, 1976.

Cooper TB, MacLean WAH, Waldo AL: Overdrive pacing for supraventricular tachycardia: a review of theoretical implications and therapeutic techniques. PACE 1:196, 1978.

Cueni T, Shenasa M, Kappenberger L, Sowton E: The effect of electromagnetic interference (EMI) from anti-theft devices upon demand pacemakers. In Meere C (ed): Cardiac Pacing, Proceedings of the VI World Symposium on Cardiac Pacing, Montreal, 1979, Chap. 35–10.

Davies JG, Sowton E: Electrical threshold of the human heart. Br Heart J 28:231, 1966.

DeSanctis RW, Kastor JA, Leinbach RC, Harthorne JW: Long-term pervenous atrial pacing. Circulation 38 (Suppl VI) 65, 1968.

Dixon SH, Perryman RA, Morris JJ, Young WG Jr: Transmediastinal permanent ventricular pacing. Ann Thorac Surg 14:206, 1972.

Elmqvist R, Senning A: Implantable pacemaker for the heart. In Smyth CN (ed): Proceedings of the 2nd International Conference on Medical Electronics, Paris, June 1959. London, p 253.

Estioko MR, Gomez E, Camuñas J, Estioko RM, Mindich BP, Jurado RA: Early clinical experience with a new transvenous tined electrode without displacement. In Meere C (ed): Cardiac Pacing, Proceedings of the VI World Symposium on Cardiac Pacing, Montreal, 1979, Chap 31–34.

———, ———, Jurado RA, Mindich BP, Fitzkee H, Blust J, Litwak RS: Clinical experience with 422 lithium pacemakers (abstr). PACE 3:369, 1980.

Ferrer MI: The sick sinus syndrome. Circulation 47:635, 1973.

Fieldman A, Dobrow RJ: Phantom pacemaker programming. PACE 1:166, 1978.

Fields J, Berkovits BV, Matloff J: Permanent transvenous atrioventricular sequential demand (bifocal) pacing in atrial bradycardias and "sick sinus syndrome" (abstr). Am J Cardiol 31:131, 1973.

Frazier OH, Ostarhild K, Cooley DA: Consecutive experience with 310 epicardial pacemaker patients: evolving implantation techniques and results. In Meere C (ed): Cardiac Pacing, Proceedings of the VI World Symposium on cardiac pacing, Montreal, 1979, Chap 14–9.

Furman RW, Hiller AJ, Playforth RH, Bryant LR, Trinkle JK: Infected permanent cardiac pacemaker: management without removal. Ann Thorac Surg 14:54, 1972.

Furman S, Escher DJW: Principles and Techniques of Cardiac Pacing. New York, Harper Row, 1970.

———, ———, Solomon N: Experiences with myocardial and transvenous implanted pacemakers. Am J Cardiol 23:66, 1969.

———, ———, ———, Schwedel JB: Implanted transvenous pacemakers: equipment, techniques and clinical experience. Ann Surg 164: 465, 1966.

———, Parker B, Escher DJW, Solomon N: Endocardial threshold of cardiac response as function of electrode surface area. J Surg Res 8:161, 1968.

———, Schwedel JB: An intracardiac pacemaker for Stokes-Adams seizures. N Engl J Med 261: 943, 1959.

Gadboys HL, Lukban SB, Litwak RS: Long-term follow-up of patients with cardiac pacemakers. Am J Cardiol 21:55, 1968.

Glenn WWL, Furman S, Gordon AJ, et al.: Radio frequency-controlled catheter pacemaker. N Engl J Med 275: 137, 1966.

———, Mauro A, Longo E, Lavietes PH, McKay FJ: Remote stimulation of the heart by radio frequency transmission: clinical application to a patient with Stokes-Adams Syndrome. N Engl J Med 261: 948, 1959.

Goldman BS, Parsonnet V: World survey on cardiac pacing. PACE 2: W–1 1979.

Gordon AJ: Vector analysis of the stimulus artefact in patients with endocardial pacemakers. J Electrocardiol 4:91, 1971.

———: Pacemaker follow-up with transistor radio and stopwatch. Chest 66:557, 1974.

———, Klein L, Rosenstock N: Functional analysis of implanted pacemakers (abstr). Circulation 42 (Suppl III): 159, 1970.

———, Vagueiro MC, Barold SS: Endocardial electrograms from pacemaker catheters. Circulation 38:82, 1968.

Greatbatch W: Chemical power sources for implanted cardiac pacemakers. In Cardiac Pacing, Proceedings of the IV International Symposium on Cardiac Pacing, Assen, The Netherlands, Van Gorcum, 1973.

Greene J: Ya gotta have heart to survive in the competitive field of cardiac pacemakers. Barrons, Dec. 27, 1976, p11.

Guilmet D, Piwnica A, Pedeferri G: Implantation d'un stimulateur cardiaque intern par sternotomie mediane verticale. Ann Chir Thorac Cardiovasc 3: 443, 1964.

Hauser RG, Giuffre VW: Newer developments in pacemakers. Med Clin North Am 60:369, 1976.

———, McKeever WP, Sweeney MB, Giuffre VW: Clinical pulse generator malfunction after DC countershock. In Meere C (ed): Cardiac Pacing, Proceedings of the VI World Symposium on Cardiac Pacing, Montreal, 1979, Chap 35–5.

Hoffman BF, Cranefield PF: Electrophysiology of the Heart. New York, McGraw-Hill, 1960.

Hyman AS: Resuscitation of the stopped heart by intracardiac therapy. Arch Intern Med 50:283, 1932.

James TN: Anatomy and pathology of the conduction system of the human heart. In Thalen HJ Th, Meere C (eds): Fundamentals of Cardiac Pacing. The Hague, Martinus Nijhoff, 1979, p 23.

Kastor JA, Leinbach RC: Pacemakers and their arrhythmias. Prog Cardiovasc Dis 13:240, 1970.

Kaulbach MG, Krukonis EE: Pacemaker electrode-induced thrombosis in the superior vena cava with pulmonary embolization. Am J Cardiol 26:205, 1970.

Keshishian J, Smyth NPD, Hood OC, Hoffman AA, Baker NR, Podolak E, Basu AP: The behavior of triggered unipolar pacemakers in active magnetic fields. J Thorac Cardiovasc Surg 64:772, 1972.

Kim SG, Fisher JD, Furman S, Escher DJW: Implantable ventricular burst pacemakers for termination of ventricular tachycardia. In Meere C (ed): Cardiac Pacing, Proceedings of the VI World Symposium on Cardiac Pacing, Montreal, 1979, Chap 6–12.

Knuckey L, McDonald R, Sloman G: A method of testing implanted cardiac pacemakers. Br Heart J 27:483, 1965.

Kosowsky B, Barr I: Complications and malfunctions of electrical cardiac pacemakers. Prog Cardiovasc Dis 14:501, 1972.

Kostianinen S, Appelqvist P: Parasternal mediastinomy for implantation of a myocardial electrode. Scand J Thorac Cardiovasc Surg 11:233, 1977.

Kramer DH, Moss AJ: Permanent pervenous atrial pacing from coronary vein. Circulation 42:427, 1970.

Kreuzer J, Bisping HJ: Four years experience treating outpatients with transvenous screw-in leads in atrial and ventricular position (abstr). PACE 3:365, 1980.

Latif P, Ewy GA: Temporary inhibition of permanently implanted demand pacemakers. Circulation 55:27, 1977.

Lawrie GM, Morris GC Jr, Howell JF, DeBakey ME: Left subcostal insertion of the sutureless myocardial electrode. Ann Thorac Surg 21:350, 1976.

Lev M: The pathology of complete atrioventricular block. Prog Cardiovasc Dis 6:317, 1964.

Lewis KB, Love JW, O'Neal Humphries J, Voigt GC, Ross RS: Current status of the Hopkins rechargeable cardiac pacemaker (abstr). Circulation 50 (Suppl III):95, 1974.

Lillehei RC, Romero LH, Beckman CB, Burroughs J, Friedburg HD: A new solid-state, long-life, lithium-powered pulse generator. Ann Thorac Surg 18:479, 1974.

Littleford PO, Parsonnet V, Spector DS: A subclavian introducer for endocardial electrodes. In Meere C (ed): Cardiac Pacing, Proceedings of the VI World Symposium on Cardiac Pacing, Montreal, 1979, Chap 14–12.

Mascarenhas E, Center S: Results of permanent pacemaker therapy. In Samet P (ed): Cardiac Pacing. New York, Grune & Stratton, 1973, p 184.

Mattes LM, Elster SK, Gordon AJ: Chest wall stimulation by pin electrodes in patients with implanted pacemakers. J Electrocardiol 10:411, 1977.

McWilliam JA: Electrical stimulation of the heart in man. Br Med J (Fed. 16):348, 1889.

Moss AJ, Rivers RJ Jr: Atrial pacing from the coronary vein. Circulation 57:103, 1978.

———, ———, Griffith LS, Carmel JA, Millard EB Jr: Transvenous left atrial pacing for control of recurrent ventricular fibrillation. N Engl J Med 278:928, 1968.

———, ———, Kramer DH, Resnicoff S: Permanent pervenous atrial synchronized ventricular pacing. Circulation 48:37, 1973.

Naclerio EA, Varriale P: Anterior axillary minithoracotomy: the optimal approach for left ventricular sutureless electrode implantation. In Meere C (ed): Cardiac Pacing, Proceedings of the VI World Symposium on Cardiac Pacing, Montreal, 1979, Chap 14–3.

Niehus B, Behrenbeck DW, Tauchert M, Hilger HH: Puncture of the subclavian vein for permanent pacemaker implantation. In Meere C (ed): Cardiac Pacing, Proceedings of the VI World Symposium on Cardiac Pacing, Montreal, 1979, Chap 14–1.

Parsonnet V: Magnet pacemaker reversion. JAMA 224:1428, 1973.

———, Bilitch M, Furman S, Fisher J, Escher DJW, Myers G, Cassidy E: Early malfunction of transvenous pacemaker electrodes. Circulation 60:590, 1979.

———, Furman S, Smyth NPD: Implantable cardiac pacemakers: status report and resource guideline. Am J Cardiol 34:487, 1974.

———, ———, ———: A revised code for pacemaker identification. PACE 4:400, 1981.

———, Gilbert L, Zucker IR, Assefi I: Subcostal transdiaphragmatic insertion of a cardiac pacemaker. J Thorac Cardiovasc Surg 49:739, 1965.

———, Myers GH, Gilbert L, Zucker IR: Prediction of impending pacemaker failure in a pacemaker clinic. Am J Cardiol 25:311, 1970.

———, ———, ———, ———, Rockland R: A clinic for long-term pulse generator surveillance. In Samet P (ed): Cardiac Pacing. New York, Grune & Stratton, 1973, p 216.

Preston TA, Kirsch MM: Permanent pacing of the left atrium for treatment of WPW tachycardia. Circulation 42:1073, 1970.

Rokseth R, Hatle L: Sinus arrest in acute myocardial infarction. Br Heart J 33:639, 1971.

Rosen KM: Catheter recording of His bundle electrograms. Mod Concepts Cardiovasc Dis 42:23, 1973.

Seipel L, Bub E, Driwas S: Kammerflimmern bei funktions-prüfung eines demand-shritt machers. Dtsch Med Wochenschr 100:2439, 1975.

Shepard RB, Russo AG, Breland VC: Radio frequency electrocoagulator hemostasis, and chronically elevated pacing thresholds in cardiopulmonary bypass procedure patients. In Meere C (ed): Cardiac Pacing, Proceedings of the VI World Symposium on Cardiac Pacing, Montreal, 1979, Chap 35–2.

Siddons H: Deaths in long-term paced patients. Br Heart J 36:1201, 1974.

———, Nowak K: Surgical complications of implanting pacemakers. Br J Surg 62:929, 1979.

———, Sowton R: Cardiac Pacemakers. Springfield, Ill, Thomas, 1967, p 86.

Sinnaeve A, Piret J, Stroobandt R: Potential causes of spurious programming: report of a case. PACE 3:541, 1980.

Smyth NPD, Keshishian JM, Basu AP, Bacos JM, Massumi RA, Fletcher RD, Baker NR: Permanent transvenous atrial pacing. Ann Thorac Surg 11:360, 1971.

Sowton E: Driving licenses for patients with cardiac pacemakers. (Editorial). Br Heart J 34:977, 1972.

Stertzer SH, DePasquale NP, Cohn LJ, Bruno MS: Evaluation of a rechargeable pacemaker system. PACE 1:186, 1978.

Stewart S, Cohen J, Murphy G: Sutureless epicardial pacemaker lead: a satisfactory preliminary experience. Chest 67:564, 1975.

Stoney WS, Addlestone RB, Alford WC Jr, Burrus GR, Frist RA, Thomas CS Jr: The incidence of venous thrombosis following long-term transvenous pacing. Ann Thorac Surg 22:166, 1976.

Sutton R, Citron P: Electrophysiological and haemodynamic basis for application of new pacemaker technology in sick sinus syndrome and atrioventricular block. Br Heart J 41:600, 1979.

———, Perrins J, Citron P: Physiological cardiac pacing. PACE 2:207, 1980.

Tarjan PP: Engineering aspects of implantable cardiac pacemakers. In Samet P (ed): Cardiac Pacing. New York, Grune & Stratton, 1973, p 60.

Tyers GF, Hughes HC Jr, Torman HA, Waldhausen JD: The advantages of transthoracic placement of permanent cardiac pacemaker electrodes. J Thorac Cardiovasc Surg 69:8, 1975.

Varriale P, Naclerio EA, Niznik J: Selection of site for permanent epicardial pacing using myocardial test electrode. NY J Med 77:1272, 1977.

Voukydis PC, Shulman AN, Cohen SI: Unmasking of slow intrinsic ventricular excitation by magnetic inhibition of R-wave inhibited demand pacemakers. Chest 67:304, 1975.

Waugh RA, Wagner GS, Haney TL, Rosati RA, Morris JJ Jr: Immediate and remote prognostic significance of fascicular block during acute myocardial infarction. Circulation 47:765, 1973.

Williams DR, Demos NJ: Thrombosis of superior vena cava caused by pacemaker wire and managed with streptokinase. J Thorac Cardiovasc Surg 68:134, 1974.

Williams WG, Goldman BS, Izukawa T, MacGregor DC, Trusler GA, Smith JM: The failure of nuclear pacing. In Meere C (ed): Cardiac Pacing, Proceedings of the VI World Symposium on Cardiac Pacing, Montreal, 1979, Chap 22–4.

Windman WD, Edoga JK, Thomas L, Trotta JJ, Muccione S: Pitfalls in measuring R-waves in pacemaker-dependent patients. PACE 2:186, 1979.

Wirtzfeld A, Lampadius M, Ruprecht ED: Unterdrückung von demandschrittmachern durch muskel potentiale. Dtsch Med Wochenschr 97:61, 1972.

Zoll PM: Resuscitation of the heart in ventricular standstill by external electric stimulation. N Engl J Med 247:768, 1952.

Zucker RI, Parsonnet V, Gilbert L: A method of permanent transvenous implantation of an atrial electrode. Am Heart J 85:195, 1973.

RECOMMENDED READING

Furman S, Norman JC: Cardiac pacing and pacemakers. In Norman JC (ed): Cardiac Surgery, 2nd ed. New York, Appleton-Century-Crofts, 1972.

Thalen HJ Th, Van den Berg JW, Homan Van der Heide JN, Nieveen J. The Artificial Cardiac Pacemaker. Assen, The Netherlands, Royal Van Gorcum, Ltd., 1970.

Varriale P, Naclerio EA (eds): Cardiac Pacing. Philadelphia: Lea & Febiger, 1979.

21. Special Techniques of Care Employed in the Cardiac Surgical Intensive Care Unit

Roy A. Jurado

The overall mortality and morbidity soon after open intracardiac operations have declined steadily through the years. The improved surgical results can be ascribed largely to advances in preoperative, intraoperative, and postoperative care techniques. However, the operative risk remains high for those patients who come to the operation with advanced cardiac dysfunction. In general, they require more assiduous care after intracardiac repair.

This chapter will confine itself to discussions of certain surveillance and management techniques that have been found to be extremely helpful, especially in the care of seriously ill cardiac surgical patients. The discussions that follow will be limited to considerations of: (1) pulmonary arterial catheterization; (2) measurement of cardiac output; and (3) mechanical circulatory support techniques. Computer-assisted surveillance and therapy—another special technique of care—has already been discussed in Chapter 6.

PULMONARY ARTERY CATHETERIZATION

Rationale

A significant disparity between right and left ventricular function has been clearly demonstrated in severely ill patients with or without obvious heart disease (Cohn et al., 1969; Civetta et al., 1971; Forrester et al., 1970, 1971). In such patients, the use of right atrial (central venous) pressure to estimate left-heart filling pressure has serious limitations. In practice, we routinely monitor left atrial pressure (LAP) after open intracardiac operations and, in rare instances, make direct measurements of left ventricular pressure. When it is not feasible to measure either left atrial or left ventricular pressure, indirect estimations of left-heart filling pressure offer valuable clinical information. Measurements of the pulmonary capillary wedge (PCW) or end-diastolic pressure (PAD) allow such estimations to be made.

The development of a safe, reliable, and simple technique of pulmonary arterial catheterization has undoubtedly been one of the important advances in critical care medicine in recent years. An indwelling pulmonary artery catheter permits frequent, if not moment-to-moment, measurements of pulmonary artery and pulmonary capillary wedge pressures and provides an easy avenue for periodic sampling of pulmonary mixed venous blood in the critically ill patient. The introduction of a flow-directed balloon-tipped catheter has greatly simplified the technique of pulmonary artery catheterization (Swan et al., 1970).

Reliability of Methods Used for Estimation of Left Ventricular Filling Pressures

The measurement of pulmonary capillary wedge pressure appears to be a reliable index of left atrial pressure (Fitzpatrick et al., 1972; Lappas et al., 1973). Lappas et al. found a very high correlation between pulmonary capillary wedge pressure and left atrial pressure in a group of patients undergoing open heart surgery. In contrast, although overall correlation was close, the pulmonary artery diastolic pressure was a less reliable indicator of changes in left atrial pressure.

Certain interventions may cause changes in the relationship between PCW and LAP, on one hand, and PCW and PAD, on the other. Lozman et al. (1974) observed that, during the application of positive end-expiratory pressure (PEEP) in patients requiring prolonged ventilatory support, PCW sometimes may reflect a pressure other than LAP. Rahimtoola et al. (1972) have reported an average gradient of 6.7 mm Hg between PAD pressure and mean PCW pressure in patients with acute myocardial infarction who had slightly to moderately increased pulmonary vascular resistance. These conditions should be borne in mind when such indirect measures of left-heart filling pressures are used to assess left-heart performance.

The Balloon-Tipped, Flow-Directed Catheter

For bedside pulmonary artery catheterization, the Swan-Ganz model* is perhaps the most commonly used catheter. Other commercially available models are functionally similar but are not as popular.

In its simplest form, the Swan-Ganz catheter consists of a double lumen, polyvinylchloride catheter measuring 100 cm in length, with an outside diameter of 1.6 mm. A balloon is attached at the tip of the catheter and may be inflated through the smaller of the two lumens in the shaft of the catheter. The minor lumen connected to the inflatable balloon terminates in a one-way stopcock for the inflating syringe. The balloon at the catheter tip has a bursting volume of approximately 3 ml, but the manufacturer recommends that, for a 5 French catheter (Fig. 21-1), the inflation volume should not exceed 0.8 ml. For a 7 French catheter, the recommended inflation volume is 1.0 ml.

The smaller lumen connected to the inflatable balloon is generally filled with air, and balloon inflation, during catheter passage and measurements of PCW, is maintained by means of a one-way stopcock attached to an air-filled tuberculin syringe. The other lumen is saline filled before passage of the catheter and is connected to an appropriate pressure-recording device; lumen size is adequate for the recording of intracardiac and great vessel pressures, with a frequency response uniform to approximately 10 Hz with the most commonly used electromanometers.

Different lengths and sizes of the catheter are now available for specific applications. For instance, a 7 French quadruple lumen thermistor catheter (Fig. 21-2) permits repeated measurements of cardiac output by the thermodilution method and monitoring of right atrial, pulmonary arterial, and pulmonary capillary wedge pressures. Other right heart catheters designed along the balloon flotation concept are also available (discussed later).

Technique of Pulmonary Artery Catheterization

In practice, catheter passage is performed at the patient's bedside under sterile conditions. Local infiltration anesthesia is used and, depending on personal experience and preference and availability of suitable veins, the catheter is advanced either by percutaneous puncture of an appropriate vein in the brachial, subclavian, or femoral region or by a cutdown in the antecubital fossa or in the deltopectoral groove. In most instances, fluoroscopy is not necessary for successful catheter passage. However, it is mandatory that catheter travel inside the vascular tree be monitored by continuous recordings of cavity

---

*Edwards Laboratories, Santa Ana, Calif.

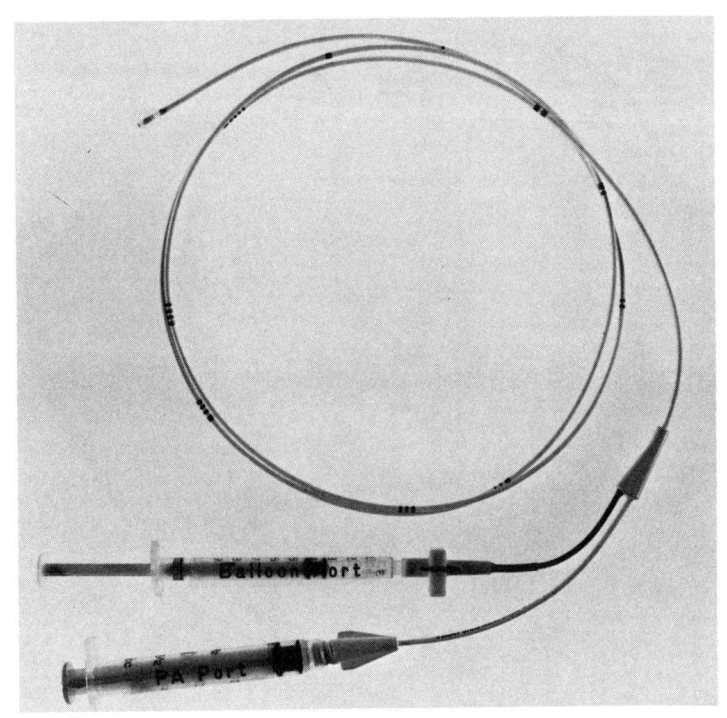

Figure 21-1. Double lumen (French 5), balloon-tipped, flow-directed catheter.

pressures with oscilloscopic display of the pressure waveforms to gauge the location of the catheter tip (Fig. 21-3). Easy-to-read markings on the shaft of the catheter also help the operator to determine at all times the approximate length of the catheter that already has been introduced.

As soon as the catheter is passed centrally (approximately 40 cm from an antecubital or brachial insertion site as guided by the markings on the catheter shaft), it is gently flushed with saline to ensure an undamped pressure tracing. The patient may be requested to cough or take deep breaths, and oscillations of pressure indicate that the catheter is in a large systemic vein—generally the superior vena cava at this point. The balloon is inflated (generally with 0.8 ml of air) and the catheter is advanced slowly and gently. The catheter is flexible enough to permit the inflated balloon at its tip to be guided by the stream of blood flowing through the tricuspid valve and then slowly propelled into the right ventricle and out into the pulmonary artery.

Balloon inflation should be maintained at all times to facilitate catheter travel and prevent entrapment of the catheter tip in the ventricular wall trabeculations. Also, with the balloon inflated, the relationship of the balloon to the catheter tip possibly prevents subendocardial injury or irritation. The operator should also guard against overanxious and overenthusiastic pushing of the catheter at this point, for this could lead into looping in the right ventricle and, perhaps, subsequent knotting of the catheter. Once the catheter tip gets into the right venticle, the trick is to wait for a few cardiac contractions and allow the flowing blood to catch and drag the inflated balloon into the outflow tract and out into the pulmonary artery.

With balloon inflation still maintained, the flowing blood will continue to direct the catheters more distally into the pulmonary arterial tree. Further catheter advance is halted as soon as the balloon-tipped catheter enters a vessel that approximates the size of the inflated balloon. The catheter is now said

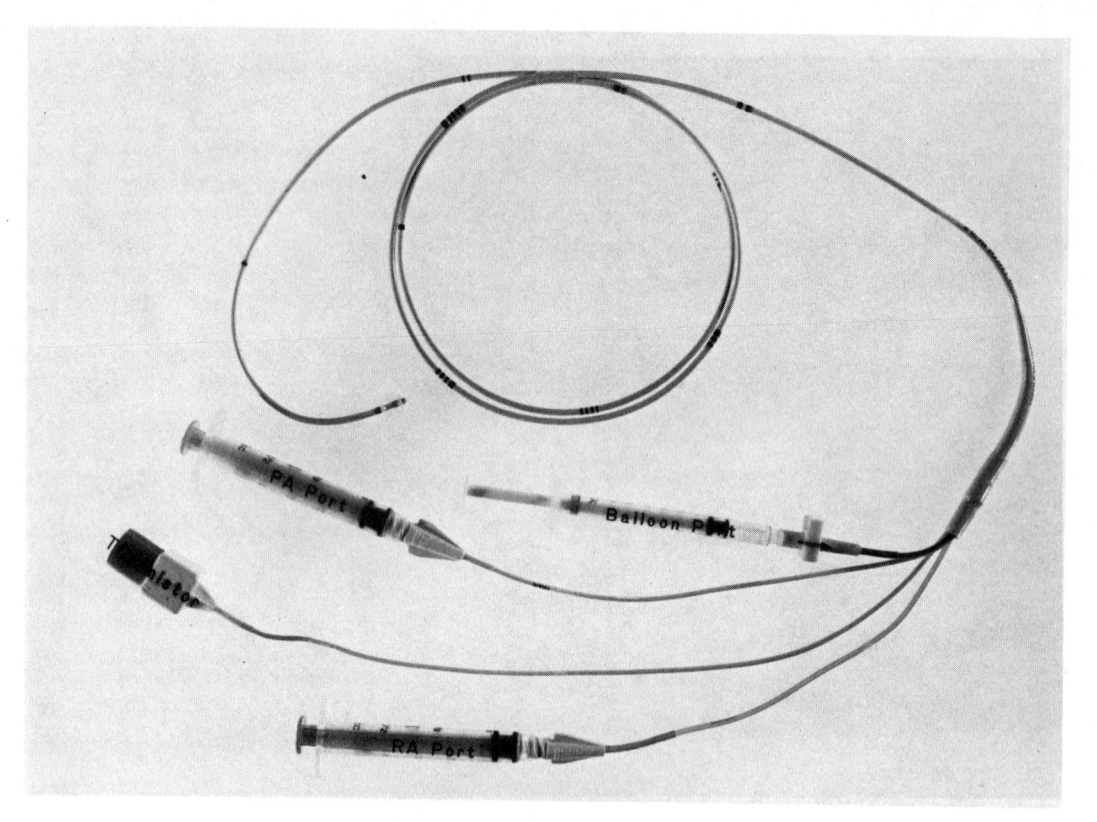

Figure 21-2. Quadruple lumen (French 7), thermistor-bearing, balloon-tipped, flow-directed catheter used for bedside measurements of right atrial, pulmonary artery and pulmonary capillary wedge pressures, and cardiac output. When properly positioned, it provides a convenient means of sampling true mixed venous blood.

to be "wedged." There is a static, nonflowing column of blood in the pulmonary arterioles, capillaries, and veins of that pulmonary segment, the vessel that is occluded by the balloon. This fluid column allows transmission of the pressure wave in the dynamic vascular system immediately downstream from the position, namely, the pulmonary veins and the left atrium. This is what is ordinarily known as the PCW pressure and is a phase-delayed and amplitude-damped version of the left atrial pressure. As indicated earlier, the mean values for PCW pressure and LAP are practically identical. The operator verifies a true wedge position by the characteristic pressure waveform, the presence of respiratory variation, a mean pressure lower than mean pulmonary arterial pressure, and the ability to withdraw arterialized blood (Yu, 1969).

To reduce the possibility of subsequent permanent catheter wedging, and, therefore, permanent obstruction of the vessel, the catheter tip is carefully placed in the most proximal position from which a satisfactory wedge pressure recording could be obtained when the balloon is inflated. The operator should also see to it that a redundant loop is not present in the right ventricle; this can be easily verified by simply withdrawing the catheter slowly while maintaining a wedge position for the catheter tip. The catheter is then carefully transfixed as soon as the optimal position is achieved. The transfixation suture should be securely tied but should avoid pinching the catheter lumina.

To maintain patency and to ensure an undamped pressure tracing, the catheter-transducer system is connected to a constant

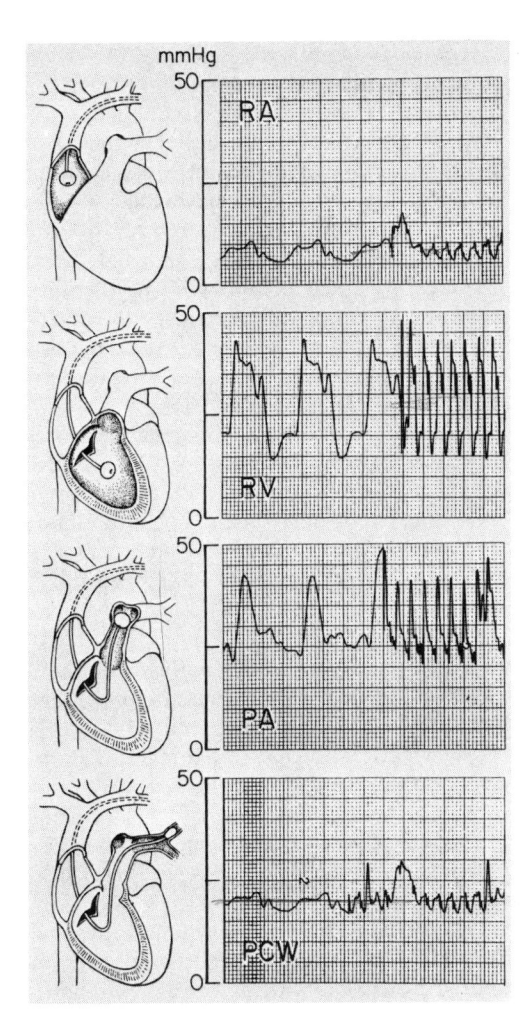

Figure 21–3. Continuous visual display of intracavitary pressure waveforms allows the operator to monitor catheter passage and gauge catheter tip location with relative precision. Fluoroscopic guidance is rarely necessary. (RA = right atrium; RV = right ventricle; PA = pulmonary artery; PCW = pulmonary capillary wedge)

infusion setup containing heparinized saline solution.

Complications of Pulmonary Artery Catheterization

The complications that have been reported are similar to those that accompany right heart catheterization and the use of indwelling intravascular catheters. These range from balloon rupture (Cerra et al., 1973) and transient minor atrial and ventricular arrhythmias (Swan et al., 1970) to rupture or perforation of a pulmonary artery (Chun and Ellestad, 1971; Lapin and Murray, 1972; Golden et al., 1973; Lemen et al., 1975), pulmonary valve injury (O'Toole et al., 1979), pulmonary infarction (Scott et al., 1972; Foote et al., 1974), persistent atrial arrhythmias (Geha et al., 1973), and complete heart block (Abernathy, 1974). Other reported complications include intracatheter thrombosis (Scott et al.), axillary, subclavian, and peripheral vein thrombosis (Foote et al.), local wound infection (Cerra et al.), catheter coiling in the right ventricle (Cerra et al.), intracardiac knotting of the catheter (Lipp et al., 1971), the formation of aseptic thrombotic endocardial vegetations (Greene and Cummings, 1973; Pace and Horton, 1975), and septic endocarditis (Greene et al., 1975).

The majority of these complications are largely preventable if meticulous attention is paid to the technique of catheter insertion and to the maintenance and aftercare once the catheter is in place. In most cases, balloon rupture can be avoided by careful attention to the details of inflation and deflation. Perforative complications and major arrhythmias can best be prevented by gentle handling of the catheter during insertion and by making sure that the balloon is maximally inflated during passage from the superior vena cava out the pulmonary artery.

Other measures that reduce the likelihood of perforative complications include careful attention to the details of catheter positioning and fixation and, possibly, the use of fluoroscopy during technically difficult insertions. Gentle catheter handling may also help reduce intimal trauma and minimize thrombotic complications. The use of a heparinized continuous infusion system prevents intracatheter thrombosis. While pulmonary ischemic lesions may result from emboli propagated from thrombi within the catheter lumen or attached to the shaft of the catheter, pulmonary infarctions are most commonly caused by direct arterial occlusion by the catheter itself (Foote et al., 1974). It has been observed that the catheter tip tends to advance and move peripherally within the first 24 hours after insertion (Scott et al., 1972; Foote et al.). This appears to be due to the rhythmic contractions of the heart and the pulsatile propelling force of the blood flow. A certain allowance should be given for this occurrence before final catheter positioning to avoid not only permanent wedging but perforative complications as well.

Frequent, if not continuous, monitoring of the pressure wave form, careful adherence to balloon inflation and deflation protocols, and frequent chest roentgenograms to check catheter tip position and for trapped air in the inflatable balloon may help prevent unintentional catheter wedging and pulmonary infarction. Meticulous asepsis, assiduous local wound and catheter care, and prompt catheter removal as soon as circumstances permit are the most effective prophylactic measures against infective complications.

Fortunately, the incidence of serious and fatal complications is low and, in certain critically ill patients, the benefits of pulmonary artery catheterization far outweigh the risks associated with the procedure.

MEASUREMENT OF CARDIAC OUTPUT

Rationale

Traditionally, heavy reliance has been placed on blood pressure measurements in the clinical assessment of cardiovascular subsystem performance. The ease and rapidity with which such measurements can be made has helped establish the method as a standard monitoring technique. Unfortunately, the concept of equating seemingly normal blood pressure measurements with satisfactory cardiovascular subsystem performance is grossly erroneous. The error becomes even more apparent when one considers the classic relationship described by Ohm's law, which states that *pressure* (P) is the product of *flow* (F) and *resistance* (R); thus: $P = F \times R$.

Cardiac output (the volume of blood pumped by the heart per minute) represents *flow* when the above equation is applied to the intact organism. It is obvious that measurements of *pressure* (blood pressure) *alone* cannot properly characterize cardiovascular subsystem performance; more importantly, the maintenance of a seemingly normal blood pressure alone may not be sufficient to ensure adequate perfusion. Moreover, the third variable in the equation, *resistance* (vascular resistance), is *not* directly measurable, but is derived from the relationship: $R = P/F$.

Therefore, it is mandatory that measurements of *both* blood pressure and cardiac output be made to properly assess cardiovascular subsystem performance. The methods employed in the evaluation of such performance have been discussed in Chapters 6 and 9.

Methods

A number of invasive and noninvasive techniques of cardiac output measurement have been devised (Tables 21–1 and 21–2). The invasive methods include the direct Fick, indicator dilution, pressure-pulse contour, pressure gradient, electromagnetic flowmeter techniques, and x-ray cardiometry. The noninvasive methods include the indirect Fick, photoelectric colorimetric oxygen detection, ballistocardiography, echocardiography, and impedance plethysmography. For a comprehensive discussion of these different methods, the reader is enjoined to review the publications of Guyton et al. (1973), Rushmer (1976), and Schenk and Race (1966).

In practice, cardiac output is measured by either the direct Fick method or by indicator-dilution techniques (dye dilution and thermodilution). A brief review of these methods is given in the sections that follow. Other methods of cardiac output estimation that have been tried in the clinical setting and hold some promise include the pulse contour (Jurado et al., 1973), echocardiographic (Steingart et al., 1980), and the electromagnetic flowmeter techniques (Williams et al., 1971). For a variety of reasons, the latter methods have not yet found widespread clinical application.

TABLE 21-1 INVASIVE METHODS OF CARDIAC OUTPUT MEASUREMENT

Application of the Fick Principle
   Direct Fick method
Indicator Dilution Methods
   Dye dilution
   Thermodilution
   Radioisotopic
Pressure-Pulse Contour Methods
Pressure Gradient Technique
Electromagnetic Flowmeter Technique
X-ray Cardiometry

TABLE 21-2 NONINVASIVE METHODS OF CARDIAC OUTPUT MEASUREMENT

Application of the Fick Principle
   Indirect Fick method
Photoelectric Colorimetric Oxygen Detector Technique
Ballistocardiography
Echocardiography
Impedance Plethysmography

Measurement of Cardiac Output by the Direct Fick Method

The Fick Principle. In simple terms, the Fick principle states that flow in a given period of time is equal to the amount of substance entering the stream of flow in the same period of time divided by the difference between the concentrations of the substance upstream and downstream of the point of entry. This principle is applicable to any flowing stream of fluid when a substance either enters or leaves the stream, provided the rate of entry or exit of the substance and its concentrations on the two sides of entry or exit can all be measured. Another requirement that must be satisfied is that the indicator substance must be thoroughly mixed with the flowing fluid at each point of sampling.

Oxygen satisfies the above requirements for an indicator and has traditionally been the indicator of choice in clinical applications of the direct Fick principle. To calculate cardiac output by the direct Fick method, using oxygen as the indicator, measurements of oxygen consumption and of arterial and mixed venous oxygen contents are required (Fig. 21–4). Cardiac output is calculated as follows:

$$\dot{Q} = \frac{\dot{V}_{O_2}}{(Ca_{O_2} - C\bar{v}_{O_2}) \times 10}$$

where,

$\dot{Q}$ = Cardiac output in liters/min
$\dot{V}_{O_2}$ = Oxygen consumption in ml O_2/min
Ca_{O_2} = Arterial oxygen content in ml O_2/100 ml blood (or vol%)
$C\bar{v}_{O_2}$ = Mixed venous oxygen content in ml O_2/100 ml blood (or vol%)
10 = Factor to convert units to liters/min.

The oxygen-Fick equation may be rewritten thus:

$$CO = \frac{O_2 \text{ consumption}}{av_{O_2} \text{ difference} \times 10}$$

where,

CO = Cardiac output (liters/min)
av_{O_2} difference = Ca_{O_2} minus $C\bar{v}_{O_2}$ (vol%).

Measurements of O_2 consumption and av_{O_2} difference are performed simultaneously while the subject is in a steady state, since the Fick principle depends on the condition that the tissue uptake of oxygen is *equal* to the oxygen uptake of the lungs. The accuracy of the oxygen-Fick method is affected by changes in cardiac output and respiration (Nahas et al., 1953; Visscher and Johnson, 1953).

Determination of Oxygen Consumption. For the calculation of O_2 consumption, the volume of the expired air is measured (or collected) over a given period of time (usually three to five minutes) by a variety of methods, and the O_2 concentration of the ambient and expired air is measured with a gas analyzer. The total oxygen consumed during the given period of

$$Q = \frac{\dot{V}O_2}{(C_aO_2 - C_{\bar{v}}O_2) \times 10}$$

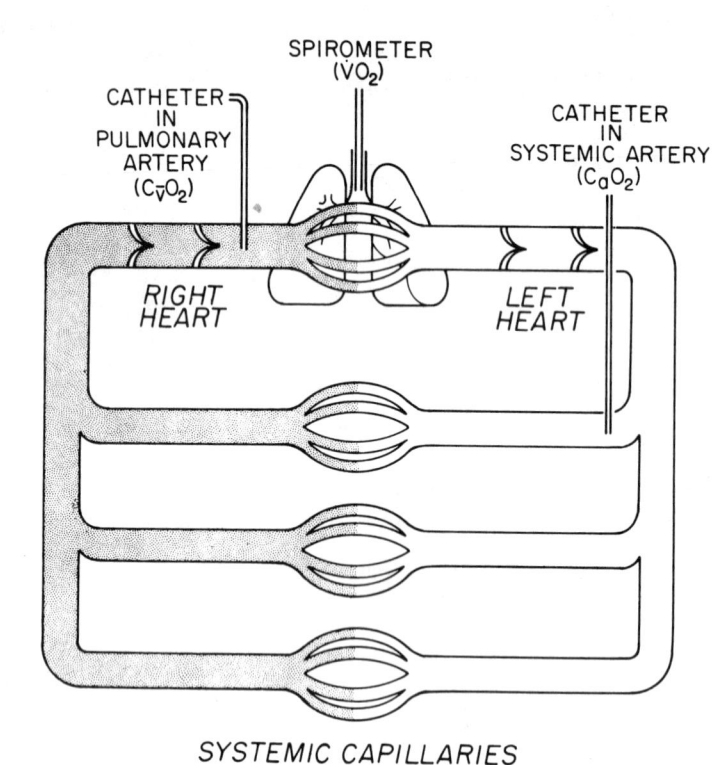

Figure 21–4. Schematic representation of oxygen-Fick methodology. To estimate cardiac output with this method, measurements of total body oxygen consumption ($\dot{V}O_2$) and the arterial-venous oxygen content difference (C_aO_2 minus $C\bar{v}O_2$) are required. Ideally, *true* mixed venous blood should be sampled from the pulmonary artery.

time is the product of the total volume of expired air measured (or collected) and the O_2 concentration difference between the ambient and expired airs. In the spontaneously breathing subject, the volume of expired air is usually measured with the aid of a specially designed hood, a Douglas bag, or a calibrated spirometer with either a special mask or a mouth piece and a nose clip. The latter contraptions may not be well-tolerated by the acutely ill patient who may already be dyspneic or tachypneic. In the disoriented or extremely uncooperative patient, tracheal intubation after adequate sedation may provide the only effective and reliable means of gas sampling and analysis. In clinical practice, reliable measurements of oxygen consumption have been made with a computer-assisted measurement system that incorporates a modified Fleisch pneumotachograph and an oxygen analyzer (Osborn et al., 1968; also see Chapter 6).

Determination of Arteriovenous Oxygen Content Difference. To determine avo_2 difference, representative samples of *mixed arterial* and *mixed venous* blood are required. For this purpose, any systemic artery may be used for arterial blood sampling, since the O_2 content of arterial blood (downstream of the left ventricle) is fairly uniform throughout. On the other hand, true mixed venous blood can be obtained only from the pulmonary artery. Sampling from chambers proximal to the pulmonary artery may introduce errors because of incomplete mixing (Shore et al., 1945; Warren et al., 1946; Warren et al., 1948). The introduction of balloon-tipped, flow-directed pulmonary artery catheters for clinical use (see previous section) has made mixed venous blood sampling relatively simple. Sampling of arterial and mixed venous blood must be carried out simultaneously with the measurement of O_2 consumption. In addition, blood withdrawal must be done slowly at a steady rate over a period of 10 to 15 seconds to obtain a representative average sample rather than an instantaneous sample.

The oxygen content of arterial and mixed venous blood may be determined by direct or indirect methods. Direct determination of blood oxygen content is performed using the Van Slyke manometric apparatus (Peters and Van Slyke, 1932), which permits the measurement of *all* the O_2 contained in the sample (O_2 bound to hemoglobin and O_2 dissolved in the plasma).

The indirect method requires separate determinations of blood hemoglobin content (usually by colorimetric methods), the hemoglobin saturation (by spectrophotometric methods), and the partial pressure of O_2 with blood (Po_2) with the Clark electrode. With the indirect method, the amount of O_2 bound to hemoglobin is calculated as follows:

O_2 bound to Hb (ml O_2/100 ml blood) = (Hb × 1.36) × S

where,
Hb = Hemoglobin content (gm %)
1.36 = Amount of O_2 (ml) that binds with 1 gm Hb at full saturation
S = Oxygen saturation of blood sample (%).

The amount of O_2 dissolved in the plasma is also determined thus:

O_2 dissolved in plasma (ml O_2/100 ml plasma) = Po_2 × 0.003026

where,

Po_2 = Partial pressure of O_2 in the blood sample (mm Hg)
0.003026 = Coefficient of solubility of O_2 in plasma at physiologic (36 to 38C) temperature ranges (0.003026 ml of O_2 enter in physical solution in 100 ml of blood for every mm Hg rise in Po_2).

From the foregoing, it becomes a simple matter to calculate the total O_2 content in the arterial and mixed venous blood samples, which are analyzed simultaneously. The O_2 content in a blood sample is the sum of the O_2 bound to Hb and the O_2 dissolved in plasma.

Clinical Utility of the Oxygen-Fick Method.
The impeccability of the Fick principle remains unchallenged. In addition, numerous studies have shown that the direct Fick method—when carefully and meticulously carried out under absolutely steady-state conditions—gives an accurate measure of *true* cardiac output. For instance, it has been shown that there is fairly good agreement between Fick and direct rotameter measurements of cardiac output in the experimental animal (Huggins et al., 1950; Seely et al., 1950). Comparisons made both in humans and in animals have also demonstrated that cardiac output measurements by the oxygen-Fick method agree favorably with output measurements obtained by indicator-dilution methods (Hamilton et al., 1948; Eliasch et al., 1955; Cross et al., 1957). Furthermore, repetitive measurements of cardiac output in the same subject under constant study conditions have given reproducible results (Wood et al., 1955; Howell and Horvath, 1959). It is not surprising, therefore, that the direct Fick method became established as the standard reference for measurement of cardiac output. It also became apparent early on that O_2 would be an ideal indicator because of the relative ease by which O_2 uptake (amount of O_2 entering the blood through the lungs per unit time) and the arteriovenous oxygen difference (O_2 content of blood leaving the lungs

minus O_2 content of blood entering the lungs) could be measured in the laboratory.

However, the methodology is as complex as the principle is sound. It is undoubtedly for this reason that the method has not gained widespread clinical application. The facility with which bedside pulmonary artery catheterizations (hence, mixed venous blood sampling) can now be carried out has done little to stimulate enthusiasm for the oxygen-Fick method as a monitoring tool. The lack of a rapid and simple—yet reliable—technique of measuring O_2 consumption (especially in the spontaneously breathing, critically ill patient) remains the single most important impediment. Moreover, compared with other techniques (see subsequent sections), the oxygen-Fick method is both cumbersome and time-consuming and may, therefore, not be suited for use in clinical situations where rapid, sequential determinations of cardiac output are required. The opportunities for measurement error are numerous and the clinician must be familiar with them (Guyton et al., 1973).

In clinical practice, application of the oxygen-Fick method in the intensive care unit has been restricted largely to the diagnosis and localization of intracardiac shunts by simple bedside oximetric techniques. The same intravascular catheters employed for hemodynamic monitoring provide ready access for blood sampling from the great veins and arteries and the cardiac chambers. The presence of a left-to-right shunt (e.g., postinfarctional ventricular septal defect, incomplete repair of congenital or acquired ventricular septal defect) is suggested by the demonstration of an oxygen-saturation step-up at the level of the intracardiac shunt and downstream to it. In contrast, the presence of a right-to-left shunt (e.g., unrecognized interatrial communication in a patient who develops right heart hypertension following intracardiac repair) is suggested by the demonstration of a decreased oxygen saturation in the peripheral arterial blood, while normal saturation is maintained in *true* pulmonary venous blood.

Quantification of the magnitude of the intracardiac shunt requires measurement of O_2 consumption in addition to oximetry. The following formulas apply:

$$Q_T \text{ (liters/min)} = \frac{\dot{V}_{O_2} \text{ (ml/min)}}{(C_aO_2 - C_{mv}O_2) \times 10}$$

$$Q_P \text{ (liters/min)} = \frac{\dot{V}_{O_2} \text{ (ml/min)}}{(C_{pv}O_2 - C_{pa}O_2) \times 10}$$

$$Q_{EP} \text{ (liters/min)} = \frac{\dot{V}_{O_2} \text{ (ml/min)}}{(C_{pv}O_2 - C_{mv}O_2) \times 10}$$

where,

Q_T = Total systemic blood flow (liters/min)
Q_P = Total pulmonary blood flow (liters/min)
Q_{EP} = Effective pulmonary blood flow (liters/min)
C_aO_2 = Oxygen content of systemic arterial blood (vol%)
$C_{mv}O_2$ = Oxygen content of mixed venous return to right atrium (vol%)
$C_{pv}O_2$ = Oxygen content of pulmonary venous blood (vol%)
$C_{pa}O_2$ = Oxygen content of pulmonary artery blood (vol%).

If a direct pulmonary venous sample is not available, it is permissible to calculate $C_{pv}O_2$ on the basis of an assumed O_2 saturation of 95 percent.

For practical purposes, pulmonary blood flow is equal to systemic blood flow ($Q_P \cong Q_T$); that is, if the relatively small amount of physiologic right-to-left shunting into the left ventricle, left atrium, and pulmonary veins is ignored. In the presence of intracardiac shunts, this normal relationship is disturbed. For instance, if a left-to-right shunt is present, the pulmonary blood flow is greater than total systemic blood flow ($Q_P > Q_T$). In contrast, the total systemic blood flow is greater than pulmonary blood flow ($Q_T > Q_P$) in the presence of a right-to-left shunt. To determine the magnitude of left-to-right and right-to-left shunting in the presence of a bidirectional shunt, it is essential to calculate "effective pulmonary blood flow" (Q_{EP}) first, using the appropriate formula above. Q_{EP} is defined as the volume of mixed blood that, after returning to the right atrium, is presented for gas exchange in the pulmonary capillaries. After Q_{EP} has been calculated, the amount of left-to-right shunting can be estimated as follows:

$$Q_{l\text{-}r} = Q_P - Q_{EP}$$

where,

$Q_{l\text{-}r}$ = left-to-right shunt (liters/min). Similarly, the magnitude of right-to-left shunting can be determined as follows:

$$Q_{r\text{-}l} = Q_T - Q_{EP}$$

where,

$Q_{r\text{-}l}$ = right-to-left shunt (liters/min).

Where measurements of $\dot{V}O_2$ are not available, a rough index of the magnitude of the left-to-right shunt may be expressed by the ratio of Q_P to Q_T, which is normally unity (i.e., $Q_P/Q_T \cong 1$). In the presence of a left-to-right shunt, $Q_P/Q_T > 1$. The pulmonary-to-systemic blood flow ratio may also be rewritten as follows:

$$\frac{Q_P}{Q_T} = \frac{\dfrac{\dot{V}O_2}{(C_{pv}O_2 - C_{pa}O_2) \times 10}}{\dfrac{\dot{V}O_2}{C_aO_2 - C_{mv}O_2 \times 10}} = \frac{(C_aO_2 - C_{mv}O_2)}{(C_{pv}O_2 - C_{pa}O_2)}$$

Since the $\dot{V}O_2$ expressions in the above equations are equal and therefore cancel each other out, it is not always necessary to have direct measurements of $\dot{V}O_2$. Moreover, since the amount of O_2 normally dissolved in plasma is negligible, it is permissible to rewrite the Q_P/Q_T relationship as follows:

$$\frac{Q_P}{Q_T} = \frac{S_aO_2 - S_{mv}O_2}{S_{pv}O_2 - S_{pa}O_2}$$

where,

S_aO_2 = Systemic arterial oxygen saturation (%)
$S_{mv}O_2$ = Mixed venous return (to right atrium) oxygen saturation (%)
$S_{pv}O_2$ = Pulmonary venous oxygen saturation (%)
$S_{pa}O_2$ = Pulmonary arterial oxygen saturation (%).

The above relationship assumes that the hemoglobin content of systemic arterial, mixed venous return, pulmonary venous, and pulmonary arterial blood are equal. In practice, it is also frequently assumed that $S_{pv}O_2$ is the same as S_aO_2.

In the analysis of oximetric data, one should remember that desaturation of arterial blood can be secondary to pulmonary causes (i.e., ventilation-perfusion mismatch, hypoventilation, and impaired diffusion) and does not necessarily indicate the presence of a right-to-left intracardiac shunt. It should also be recognized that in left-to-right shunts less than 20 percent of the pulmonary blood flow ($Q_{l\text{-}r}/Q_P < 0.20$) may not be detectable by conventional blood oximetry.

Measurement of Cardiac Output by Indicator-Dilution Methods

The Indicator-Dilution Principle. Estimation of cardiac output by indicator-dilution methods is based on the principle that injection of a substance (the indicator) into the circulation produces a time-concentration curve that can be recorded and analyzed as blood is sampled at a constant rate at some point downstream of the injection site. The resultant curve consists of an initial rapid upslope (rising concentration of indicator) that, after reaching a peak, is followed by a slower descending limb that falls off exponentially if no recirculation of the indicator has taken place. If recirculation has occurred, a secondary rise (recirculation curve) is inscribed at some point on the downslope of the primary curve before the first circulation ends. The passage time for the indicator is recorded and its average concentration is calculated from the time-concentration curve.

The flow is deduced from the total amount of indicator injected, its time of passage, and the average indicator concentration during this time. In the analysis of the time-concentration curve, certain difficulties are introduced by the presence of recirculation; these will be dealt with in the section that follows (Measurement of Cardiac Output by Dye-Dilution Method).

For accurate measurements of cardiac output, the method requires passage of the indicator through some portion of the central circulation to allow complete mixing before the sampling site is reached. It is also required that *no* loss of indicator from the blood take place during the measurement.

A number of substances (various dyes, radioactive substances, hypertonic saline, warm or cool saline) have been used as indicators. These substances appear to be well-suited for this purpose because they mix with blood instantaneously and completely and are amenable to rapid and accurate quantitative analysis. In addition, when used judiciously, they are generally nontoxic and produce no significant perturbation of the steady state.

In clinical practice, the indicator substances employed most commonly have been tricarbocyanine (dye-dilution) and room-temperature or cold saline (thermodilution).

Measurement of Cardiac Output by the Dye-Dilution Method.

THE DYE-DILUTION PRINCIPLE. The commonest method involves the sudden injection (single injection bolus or slug method) of a known amount of tricarbocyanine (more popularly known as indocyanine green) into the central circulation, usually the right heart, following which the indicator concentration is measured or recorded at a point downstream (usually a peripheral artery) as change in the optical density of the blood-indicator mixture over time. A concentration-versus-time curve is thus produced.

Following indicator bolus injection, the concentration rapidly rises to a peak, followed by a slower downslope and a recirculation curve (Fig. 21–5). The recirculation curve begins before the first circulation ends. To calculate cardiac output, it is necessary to estimate the mean indicator concentration during its first circulation through the vascular tree. This estimation would be more accurate if most of the indicator has passed the sampling site after the first circulation. In the absence of recirculation or if the first circulation ends before recirculation, the mean indicator concentration can be easily estimated by integrating the area under the first circulation curve employing planimetric methods, and dividing it by the base (representing the total duration of the curve).

In reality, however, the presence of the recirculation curve (before the first circulation ends) makes it difficult to determine with precision the end of the disappearance time, so that an accurate estimation of the mean indicator concentration during the first circulation may seem impossible. Once recirculation occurs, the mathematics of the function relating flow to indicator concentration becomes difficult to manage. However, it has been found that if the time-concentration curve is replotted on semilogarithmic paper (with the indicator concentration on the logarithmic axis), the descending limb (i.e., the disappearance slope) of the replot after the initial curved portion becomes a straight line, followed by a recirculation curve. The disappearance slope does, in fact, follow an exponential law (presumably because the indicator concentration declines exponentially in the absence of recirculation). Because of this property, the downslope can be extrapolated past the point of recirculation to the theoretical zero concentration. If the extrapolated line is replotted onto the original coordinates, the area under the curve, ignoring recirculation, can be measured. It then becomes a simple matter to estimate the mean indicator concentration.

CALCULATION OF CARDIAC OUTPUT. To perform the calculation of cardiac output, the amount of indicator injected, the passage time of the indicator, and the mean

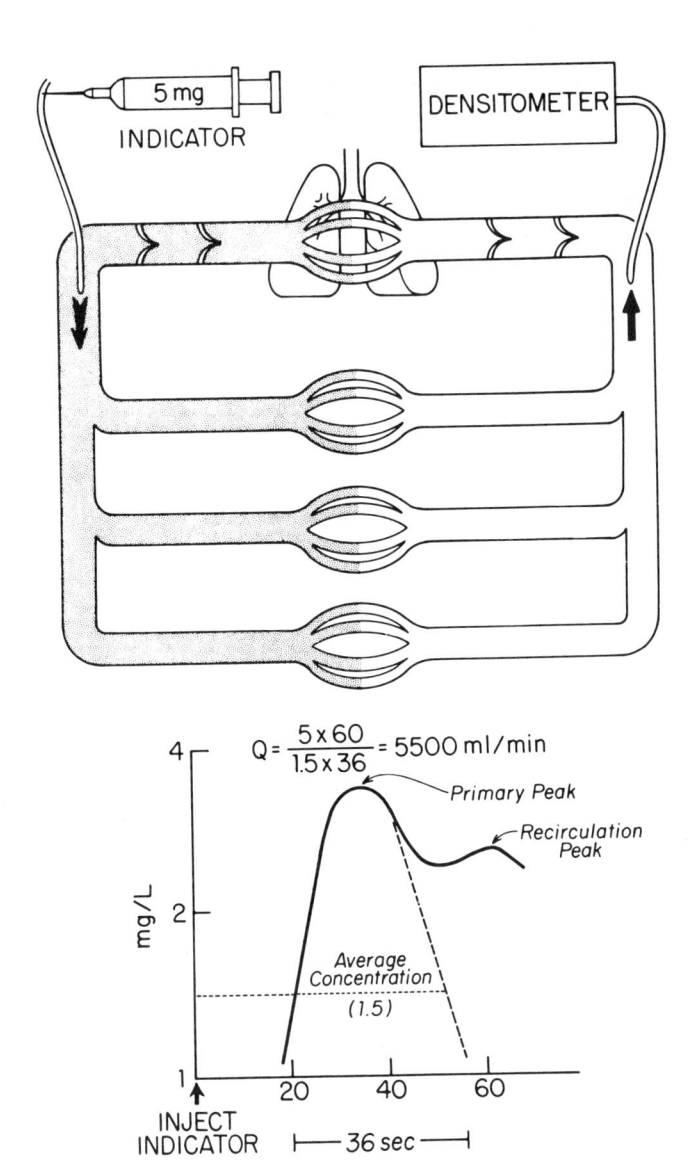

Figure 21-5. Schematic representation of the dye-dilution cardiac output measurement methodology. An idealized dye concentration-versus-time curve is shown.

indicator concentration during the first circulation must be known. The inscribed concentration-versus-time curve provides these data. Cardiac output may then be calculated with the basic Hamilton equation (Hamilton et al., 1932) as follows:

$$CO = \frac{I \times 60}{Cm \times t}$$

where,

CO = Cardiac Output (liters/min)
I = Amount of indicator injected (mg)
Cm = Mean indicator concentration (mg/liter)
t = Total curve duration (sec)
60 = 60 sec/min.

In practice, the mean concentration of the indicator substance (dye) is measured with the aid of an optical densitometer. Blood is drawn at a steady rate through a cuvette that allows light of constant intensity to pass and be detected by a photoelectric cell on the other side. The amount of light that passes is modified by the density of the blood and the amount of indicator in the blood. If the density of the blood remains constant during passage of the sample through the cuvette, the recorded changes in optical density reflect changes in indicator concentration (i.e., optical density is proportional to the indicator concentration). Since the electrical output from the photocell (reflecting changes in optical density) is recorded as galvanometer deflection expressed in millimeters, it is necessary to convert it to actual indicator concentration (mg/liters). This is done by calibrating the densitometer to known serial dilutions of the indicator and a blood sample without indicator. A calibration curve is thus constructed by plotting indicator concentration against the corresponding densitometer deflections. The calibration factor (K) is obtained by dividing the indicator concentration (mg/liters) by the corresponding densitometer deflection on the calibration curve (i.e., the slope of the calibration line is K). Cardiac output can then be more accurately calculated with the rewritten Hamilton equation, thus:

$$CO = \frac{I \times 60}{Cm \times K \times t}$$

where,

CO = Cardiac Output (liters/min)
I = Amount of indicator injected (mg)
Cm = Mean indicator concentration (mg/liter)
K = Calibration factor (mg/liter/mm)
t = Total curve duration or indicator passage time (sec)
60 = 60 sec/min.

The mean indicator concentration, Cm, is obtained by dividing the area under the complete curve (mm^2) by the base of the complete curve (mm), the complete curve being the primary curve that has been corrected for recirculation by downslope extrapolation.

An alternate method uses the sum of the concentration-time values read at one-second intervals from the start to the finish of the complete curve or from a semilogarithmic plot. The following formula is used:

$$CO = \frac{I \times 60}{C \times K}$$

where,

CO = Cardiac output (liters/min)
I = Amount of indicator injected (mg)
C = Sum of concentration-time values (mm sec) read at one-second intervals
K = Calibration factor (mg/liter).

The equation may also be rewritten as follows:

$$CO = \frac{I \times 60}{\int_0^\infty C\, dt}$$

where,

CO = Cardiac output (liters/min)
I = Amount of indicator injected (mg)
C = Concentration of the indicator (mg/liters)
t = Time (sec).

PROCEDURE FOR DYE-DILUTION CARDIAC OUTPUT MEASUREMENT. The procedure for measurement of cardiac output by the dye-dilution method is fairly straightforward.

The cuvette densitometer to be used is calibrated in a sterile fashion with four indicator-blood solutions (containing known indicator concentrations, usually 8.0, 4.0, 2.0, and 1.0 mg/liter) and whole blood without indicator. A calibration curve is constructed and the calibration factor (K) determined. The hematocrit is also determined for reference purposes since the density of blood is hematocrit-dependent. Any significant change in hematocrit mandates recalibration of the densitometer. The indicator must also be freshly prepared each day since it becomes unstable with time and exposure to light.

Both the injection and sampling catheters are positioned in the appropriate loci so that the requirements for having the indicator traverse a portion of the central circulation and for complete indicator-blood mixing are satisfied. The usual injection site is the right atrium, while downstream sampling is conveniently done via a radial artery catheter. A special syringe assembly allows reproducible withdrawal and injection of a precisely known amount of indicator solution. The dye is injected as a single slug or bolus as rapidly as possible. Ideally, injections should be of constant volume (usually 5 mg in 1 ml for adults, 2.5 mg in 1 ml for children, and 1.25 mg in 1 ml for infants). After dye injection, the catheter system is immediately cleared of residual dye by a rapid injection of saline solution from a flushing syringe. Alternatively, the connector/adaptor-catheter dead space may be primed with indicator (drawn from the same vial as the injection dose) prior to the actual bolus injection. With the latter method, the necessity to rapidly clear the catheter system of indicator after the slug injection is obviated; however, one must make sure that there is no loss of indicator from the catheter dead space before injection of the bolus dose. Regardless of what injection method is used, the object is to rapidly administer an accurately known amount of indicator.

Meanwhile blood is withdrawn at a constant rate (10 to 30 ml/min) through a catheter from a selected site downstream in the vascular system. For this purpose, a withdrawal pump is used. Sampling is begun before actual dye injection, to ensure a stable baseline for recording, and this is continued until a time-concentration curve is inscribed. A suitable speed for the chart recorder used to display in real time the output signal from the densitometer would be 5 mm per second. The sampling catheter or cannula is usually connected to a sterile three-way tap that allows ready access for either sampling, flushing and pressure recording, or reinfusing sampled blood. It has been our practice to employ a totally sterile withdrawal-densitometer system; this has allowed us to reinfuse sampled blood and perform repetitive measurements without unnecessary loss of blood.

The inscribed concentration-versus-time curve is carefully examined for basic morphology, distortions, artefacts, or abnormal contours. If the measurement is deemed valid, the primary curve is reconstructed by extrapolating the downslope beyond the point of recirculation down to the horizontal time axis. The area under the extrapolated curve and the total duration of the curve are used to obtain the mean indicator concentration during the first circulation, employing one of the methods described above.

CARDIAC OUTPUT COMPUTERS. Manual methods of curve analysis are notoriously tedious and time-consuming and may not be suitable for use in intensive care situations where frequent measurements of cardiac output are necessary. Bedside analog computers with built-in integrators are now being used with increasing frequency for dye curve analysis (Leighton and Czekajewski, 1971). These computers may be specially programmed to analyze the output from the densitometer, reconstruct the curve, and carry out an almost instantaneous calculation of cardiac output if the other known variables of the Hamilton equation (see p. 501) have been entered beforehand.

ACCURACY OF DYE-DILUTION CARDIAC OUTPUT ESTIMATES. Cardiac output estimates obtained by the dye-dilution method correlate very closely with measurements made using the Fick method; careful technique results in estimates with a ± 5 percent error (Alpert and Dexter, 1974). While accuracy suffers under low flow states, it improves in the higher ranges of cardiac output. In contrast, Fick estimates are more accurate under low output conditions.

In the presence of intracardiac shunts, the time-concentration curve becomes distorted, leading to inaccurate cardiac output estimates. Nevertheless, the indicator-dilution method (primarily the dye-dilution method) has been used to detect the presence and quantitate the magnitude of cardiovascular shunts. This is based on the principle that the passage of the indicator through the anatomic defect causes variable distortion of the resultant indicator-dilution curve. The exact morphology of the distorted curve is determined by the arrangement of the injection and sampling sites. For a comprehensive discussion of the various qualitative and quantitative methods of evaluating cardiovascular shunts using the indicator-dilution principle, the reader is referred to standard textbooks of cardiac catheterization methodology.

LIMITATIONS OF THE DYE-DILUTION METHOD. The dye-dilution method has several disadvantages that limit its routine use in clinical settings. First, preparation of the indicator can be a tedious process, and an intricate calibration procedure is required. Second, tricarbocyanine itself is a relatively unstable substance, especially after it has been dissolved in diluent. Third, the method requires blood withdrawal, which not only makes the technique complex and cumbersome, but also renders rapid, sequential measurements extremely difficult. Fourth, recirculation of indicator distorts the primary concentration-versus-time curve, necessitating extrapolation of the downslope; this complicates calculations and may introduce inaccuracies in both the high and low ranges of cardiac output encountered clinically. Finally, the slow dissipation of tricarbocyanine limits the total number of measurements that can be performed over a short period of time because of buildup of high background concentration of the indicator.

Measurement of Cardiac Output by the Thermodilution Method

THE THERMODILUTION PRINCIPLE. This method also uses the indicator-dilution principle and depends on the induction of a change in the heat content of the blood stream. Theoretically, this change can either be positive (addition of heat, with a resultant increase in blood stream temperature) or negative (abstraction of heat from the blood stream, resulting in a decrease in temperature). In simple terms, the heat content of the blood stream may be altered by the addition of either heat or cold.

In clinical practice, the technique requiring addition of heat to the blood stream is almost never used. Rather, the desired change in the heat content is achieved by the bolus injection of a substance that is readily and completely miscible with blood and at a lower temperature (the injectate that is commonly used is either saline solution or 5 percent dextrose in water). In reality, it is *cold* (or the temperature change induced by the addition of cold) that is the indicator—the injectate merely serves as the vehicle for the introduction of the indicator into the circulation.

In principle, thermodilution is identical with other indicator-dilution methods for the measurement of blood flow. The same assumptions are made, namely: (1) that there is no, or at least only negligible, loss of indicator between the point of injection and the point of temperature measurement; and (2) that complete indicator and blood commixture has taken place before the point of detection is reached. It is performed in the following manner. A measured amount of liquid (which had been kept at a temperature lower than that of the blood stream) is injected into some portion of the central circulation (usually the right atrium) in such a way as to produce rapid and complete injectate-blood mixing, following which the resultant change in blood temperature over time is detected at a suitable point downstream (usually by a thermistor positioned in the pulmonary artery). A temperature-time curve is inscribed and analyzed. The cardiac output is inversely proportional to the fall in temperature.

The change in bloodstream temperature brought about by the bolus injection of indicator is sensed by a detection thermistor. The latter forms one arm of a Wheatstone bridge, the output of which is taken via a DC amplifier to a chart recorder whose speed is known. When cold is the indicator used, as is customarily done, the bloodstream temperature will initially fall, causing a "negative" galvanometer deflection (i.e., deflection below baseline), followed by an exponential return to baseline. The actual temperature-time curve will have a configuration resembling a mirror image of a dye-dilution curve, except that there is no secondary (recirculation) curve in the former, although, in practice, its "polarity" is reversed so that the final curve is also upright. The presence of an intracardiac shunt invalidates the temperature-time curve.

CALCULATION OF CARDIAC OUTPUT.

The thermodilution principle involves the application of the calorimetric "method of mixtures" to the dynamic situation existing in the circulation (i.e., system of a flowing stream of fluid). Analysis of the temperature-time curve and knowledge of the magnitude of the change in the heat content produced by the injectate allow the estimation of blood flow in a manner analogous to that used for other indicator-dilution methods. Hosie (1962) gave a detailed explanation of the derivation of the thermodilution analog of the basic Stewart-Hamilton equation. The cardiac output measured by thermodilution is given by:

$$CO = \frac{V \times (T_B - T_I) \times S_I \times C_I \times 60 \times 0.82}{A \times K \times S_B \times C_B}$$

where,
CO = Cardiac output (ml/min)
V = Volume of injectate (ml)
A = Area under the deflections-time curve (mm/sec)
K = Calibration factor for the thermistor (°C/mm deflection)
T_B = Initial blood temperature (°C)
T_I = Initial injectate temperature (°C)
S_B = Specific gravity of blood
S_I = Specific gravity of injectate
C_B = Specific heat of blood
C_I = Specific heat of injectate
60 = 60 sec/min
0.82 = Empirical correction factor for injectate temperature rise between injection port and tip of catheter (Forrester et al., 1972).

The area under the deflections-time curve (i.e., A, expressed in mm sec) is calculated as follows. The area under the curve (mm²) is first determined by planimetry and the value obtained is divided by the recorder paper speed mm/sec). Since galvanometer deflections are recorded in millimeters, the deflections-time curve (A) is converted into a temperature-time curve. This conversion is accomplished by multiplying A (mm sec) by a calibration factor, K (°C/mm). The latter describes the temperature-resistance relationship of the thermistor, and its value has usually been determined prior to thermistor passage.

When 5 percent dextrose is used as the injectate, $(S_I \times C_I)/(S_B \times C_B) = 1.08$, so that the thermodilution equation can be rewritten as:

$$CO = \frac{V (T_B - T_I) \times 1.08 \times 60 \times 0.82}{_0\!\int^\infty \Delta T_B (t) \, dt}$$

where,
$_0\!\int^\infty \Delta T_B (t) \, dt$ = integral of blood temperature change (°C sec).
[This is equal to A × K (see previous equation).]

For calculation of cardiac output, only four variables need be known: the volume of the injectate (V), the initial temperature of the injectate (T_I), the initial temperature of the blood (T_B), and the thermistor calibration factor (K) appropriate for the blood temperature. The patient's body temperature (usually measured rectally) may be conveniently used as an indicator of initial blood temperature (T_B) as there is usually no significant difference between the two, except where there is severe peripheral vasoconstriction (hypothermia with slow peripheral rewarming, low cardiac output states), when rectal temperature may be lower than true central circulation temperature. More modern monitoring hardware has eliminated this potential source of error by allowing direct measurement of pulmonary artery blood temperature by the indwelling detection thermistor. The integration of the temperature-time curve is usually performed electronically with direct online computer techniques. The computation itself is made considerably simpler, as an extrapolation of the exponential curve (downslope) is unnecessary because of the virtual absence of the recirculation phenomenon.

One important practical point revolves around the question of what the ideal injectate temperature should be. Both iced (0°C) and room temperature saline or 5 percent dextrose in water are used clinically. When iced injectate is used, warming of the injectate (with consequent loss of indicator) invariably occurs as the fluid traverses the length of the injection catheter. The cold injectate mixes with the warmer residual fluid in the catheter injection lumen, with additional heat transfer occurring from the catheter walls to the injectate. Indeed, it has been shown that saline at a temperature of 4C injected through a catheter 48 cm long will warm up to 12C (Meisner et al., 1973). A satisfactory solution to this problem would seem to be the use of a two-thermistor setup, in which one thermistor head measures injectate temperature at the latter's entry point into the central circulation, with the other element serving as the downstream detection thermistor (Ganz et al., 1971). Such an arrangement, however, would complicate bedside hardware and other equipment requirements.

Another ingenious method has been devised to balance this loss of indicator in a single thermistor setup where iced injectate was used. Goodyer et al. (1959) and Forrester et al. (1972) have been able to quantitate the magnitude of indicator loss in in vitro studies, making it possible to compensate for this loss of indicator by introducing a correction factor in the thermodilution cardiac output formula. It has been suggested that for most clinical applications, the value of the correction factor should be 0.825 (Forrester et al., 1972).

It should be remembered, however, that the empirical correction factor does not take into account any additional loss of "negative heat" that can occur as a result of any delay in or improper handling of the injection syringe after its removal from the ice water bath. The latter probably may be eliminated by injecting the indicator at room temperature, since any portion of the injection catheter that was exposed to room air would be at the same temperature as the injectate. (Evonuk et al., 1961). Moreover, the method provides for a more accurate determination of the temperature of the delivered injectate. However, use of room temperature injectate may decrease the sensitivity of the method by two to three times (Wessel et al., 1971), presumably because the change in blood temperature induced by the injectate ("signal") may not be large enough to be significantly different from the normal cyclic variations in pulmonary artery temperature ("physiologic noise"). The "signal-to-noise" ratio can be increased by using iced injectate or by increasing the volume of room temperature injectate (Wessel et al., 1971; Ganz and Swan, 1972). The use of analog computers that employ electronic averaging of baseline pulmonary artery temperatures has also minimized the influence of these periodic fluctuations (Berger et al., 1976; Woods et al., 1976).

ADVANTAGES OF THE THERMODILUTION METHOD. The accuracy and reproducibility of the thermodilution method have been established (Fegler, 1954; Goodyer et al., 1959; Evonuk et al., 1961; Sanmarco et al., 1971; Berger et al., 1976). Since its clinical application in 1971 (Ganz et al., 1971), the thermodilution method has become the most commonly employed technique of cardiac output measurement. The thermodilution method permits rapid, accurate, and repetitive cardiac output measurements, which can be readily performed at the bedside. Preparation of the indicator is simple and the injectate is stable. Since thermistor catheters are now commercially available and come precalibrated, virtually no operator intervention is required for complex calibration procedures. Blood withdrawal is not required, allowing rapid, sequential measurements to be performed with ease. With the exception of patients requiring strict fluid restriction (e.g., acute oliguric renal failure), numerous indicator injections can be made with relative safety. Moreover, since dissipation of the thermal indicator is rapid and complete, there is no buildup of background indicator concentration. Presumably because the systemic circuit acts as an excellent heat sink, the recirculation phenomenon is either absent or, if present, is late and minimal (Goodyer et al., 1959). Extrapolation of the downslope is not required, rendering analog computation simple.

Currently available instrumentation has the capability of directly measuring both blood and injectate temperature and allows manual entry of the injectate volume, catheter calibration, and catheter correction factors. It also can average baseline pulmonary artery temperature fluctuations, integrate the temperature-time curve, introduce a calibration signal, solve the thermodilution cardiac output equation, and display the result (cardiac output in liters per minute) in less than 60 seconds after the indicator injection. The relatively simple methodology and the rapidity by which meaningful physiologic information can now be obtained have enhanced widespread acceptance of the thermodilution method.

Derived Hemodynamic Parameters. Measurements of blood flow (i.e., cardiac output) and of great vessel and intracardiac pressures provide the quantitative basis for the clinical assessment of cardiovascular subsystem performance and for evaluating the effect of therapy. From these basic measurements of flow and pressure, a number of clinically useful values can be obtained. These derived values, which provide alternative methods of characterizing cardiovascular subsystem performance, will be reviewed in brief.

CARDIAC INDEX AND STROKE INDEX. Cardiac output (CO) is defined as the amount of blood ejected by the heart per unit time. By convention, CO is expressed in liters per minute. Based on the premise that the cardiac output is proportional to the body mass, an established practice in physiology is to relate cardiac output to the body surface area (BSA). Although the validity of this concept can be challenged (Kleiber, 1947), it remains the only method, albeit imperfect, of accounting for variability in cardiac output due to individual differences in body size. *Cardiac index* (CI) is the customary method of expressing *normalized* cardiac output values; thus CI (liters/min/m^2) = CO (liters/min)/BSA (m^2). The BSA normally is obtained from the original Dubois and Dubois (1916) height-weight equation.

Stroke volume is the amount of blood ejected per heartbeat, expressed in milliliters per beat. Stroke volume (SV) is obtained by dividing cardiac output by the heart rate (HR) recorded at the time of measurement; thus, SV (ml/beat) = CO (ml/min)/HR (beats/min). It is also customary to normalize SV to body mass, so that *stroke volume index* or, simply, stroke index (SI), is obtained by dividing SV by the BSA. Thus, SI (ml/beat/m^2) = SV (ml/beat)/BSA (m^2). Both cardiac index and stroke index decrease progressively with age (Brandfonbrener et al., 1955). In the adult, the normal stroke index at rest is approximately 43.0 ± 9.5 ml/beat/m^2.

STROKE WORK INDEX. Cardiac performance is sometimes measured in terms of the external work performed by the ventricle with each systolic ejection. External work per beat is commonly referred to as *stroke work.* Stroke work is the product of the pressure generated by the ventricle during a heartbeat and the volume of blood ejected during that heartbeat. The commonly employed parameter, stroke work index (SWI), is usually calculated by the formula:

$$SWI = (VP_{sm} - VP_{ed}) \times SI \times 0.0136$$

where,

SWI = Stroke work index (gm m/m^2 BSA/beat)

VP_{sm} = Mean ventricular systolic pressure (mm Hg)

VP_{ed} = Ventricular end-diastolic pressure (mm Hg)

SI = Stroke index (cm^3/m^2 BSA/beat)
0.0136 = Conversion factor from mm Hg cm^3 to gm m (gm m/mm Hg cm^3).

This equation assumes a constant rate of ventricular ejection and ignores the kinetic energy developed. By and large, these assumptions may be acceptable, since normally the kinetic factor is only of trivial importance in considering ventricular work done per beat in the resting person. However, they may not hold true when cardioactive drugs are used or when conditions are other than basal and resting. Since the formula also requires direct measurements of ventricular pressure and planimetry to calculate VP$_{sm}$, its application in critical care settings has been limited.

An alternative method of calculating SWI conveniently employs the following formula:

$$SWI = (\overline{AP} - VFP) \times SI \times 0.0136$$

where,

- $\overline{AP}$ = mean arterial pressure (mm Hg), using mean aortic (mean systemic arterial) pressure or mean pulmonary arterial pressure for calculation of left (SWI$_{LV}$) or right (SWI$_{RV}$) ventricular stroke work index, respectively.*
- VFP = ventricular filling pressure (mm Hg), using mean left atrial pressure (pulmonary capillary wedge pressure) or mean right atrial pressure for calculation of left (SWI$_{LV}$) or right (SWI$_{RV}$) ventricular stroke work index, respectively.

Other designations as in the previous equation.

Since mean pulmonary arterial pressure is one fifth to one fourth of that in the aorta, the right heart, under ordinary circumstances, does less work per beat than the left.

VASCULAR RESISTANCE. The terms *afterload* (impedance to blood flow) and *vascular resistance* frequently are used interchangeably. Conceptually, this is not totally accurate, since impedance to blood flow is determined by a variety of factors. While it is true that impedance to blood flow is determined largely by arterial/arteriolar resistance, other factors are at play. Thus, ventricular chamber geometry (myocardial wall tension), the physical characteristics of the arteries, and the mass and viscosity of blood are the other important determinants of afterload.

The inverse relationship between stroke volume and afterload are well-documented, both experimentally (Sonnenblick, 1966; Ross et al., 1966) and clinically (Ross and Braunwald, 1964). Thus, the therapeutic implications are obvious.† In clinical practice, the closest approximations of afterload may be gleaned from calculations of vascular resistance.

Vascular resistance, or simply resistance (R), can be calculated, from pressure and flow measurements, through simple application of Ohm's law and the Hagen-Poiseuille equation: Resistance = Pressure Gradient/Flow.
This can be rewritten as:

$$R = \frac{P_1 - P_2}{Q}$$

where,

R = Resistance (mm Hg)/(liters/min)
$P_1 - P_2$ = Pressure gradient across a segment of the circulation (mm Hg)
Q = Flow (liters/min).

By convention, resistance is expressed in absolute units of force. To accomplish this, a

---

*SWI may be calculated with more precision if mean systolic arterial pressures are used, a method that would require time-consuming and often cumbersome planimetric techniques.

†See Chapter 9: Analysis, Maintenance, and Support of Cardiac Function after Cardiac Surgery.

number of conversions are necessary. Since

$$\frac{1 \text{ mm Hg}}{1 \text{ liters/min}} = \frac{1{,}332 \text{ dynes/cm}^2}{1{,}000 \text{ cm}^3/60 \text{ sec}}$$

$$= \frac{1{,}333 \times 60 \text{ dynes sec}}{1{,}000 \text{ cm}^5} = 80 \text{ dynes sec cm}^{-5}$$

then,

$$R = \frac{P_1 - P_2 \times 80}{Q}$$

where,
R = Resistance (dynes sec cm^{-5})
$P_1 - P_2$ = Pressure gradient (mm Hg)
Q = Blood flow (liters/min)
80 = Conversion factor.

Applied to the systemic circulation, the equation can be rewritten as follows:

$$\text{SVR} = \frac{(\text{MAP} - \text{RAP}) \times 80}{Q_T}$$

where,
SVR = Systemic vascular resistance (dynes sec cm^{-5})
MAP = Mean systemic arterial pressure (mm Hg)
RAP = Mean right atrial pressure (mm Hg)
Q_T = Total systemic blood flow (liters/min).

Similarly, pulmonary vascular or arteriolar resistance may be calculated as follows:

$$\text{PVR} = \frac{(\text{MPAP} - \text{LAP}) \times 80}{Q_P}$$

where,
PVR = Pulmonary vascular (arteriolar) resistance (dynes sec cm^{-5})
MPAP = Mean pulmonary artery pressure (mm Hg)
LAP = Mean left atrial pressure or equivalent (mm Hg)
Q_P = Total pulmonary blood flow (liters/min).

In the absence of intracardiac shunts, Q_T and Q_P are equal and equivalent to the clinically measured cardiac output. To make comparisons of measurements obtained from infants, children, and adults, resistance calculations should be related to flow normalized to body mass (i.e., liters/min/m^2 BSA).

Based on measurements made on healthy subjects, the systemic vascular resistance is normally around 1130 ± 178 dynes sec cm^{-5}, while the pulmonary vascular resistance is approximately 67 ± 23 dynes sec cm^{-5} (Barratt-Boyes and Wood, 1958).

MECHANICAL CIRCULATORY ASSISTANCE

A variety of ingenious methods of circulatory support have been devised, but only a few have found more than sporadic clinical application. For an overview of these various methods, the reader is referred to published reviews on the subject (National Academy of Sciences—National Research Council, 1966; Sugg et al., 1967; Soroff et al., 1969; Kolff and Lawson, 1975; Bregman, 1976; Mundth, 1976).

This section will confine itself to discussion of *three* methods of mechanical circulatory support that, in the editors' experience, have been clinically helpful. Left heart support methods currently employed at our institution include *intra-aortic balloon counterpulsation* and *partial left ventricular (left atrium-to-aortal bypass)*. On the other hand, mechanical support of the right heart has been successfully accomplished with *femoro-femoral venoarterial bypass* techniques. These methods will be discussed subsequently.

Intraaortic Balloon Counterpulsation
The Counterpulsation Principle. The concept of physically reducing left ventricular afterload (through properly timed, rapid withdrawal of arterial blood during ventricular systole) and augmenting aortic diastolic pressure (through pulsatile return of the same

quantity of blood into the arterial system during ventricular diastole) was first suggested by Clauss et al. (1961). The method required systemic arterial cannulation, use of a proportioning pump (the arterial counterpulsator), and electrocardiographic gating for proper synchronization of blood withdrawal and return with cardiac events. When properly phased, arterial counterpulsation has been accompanied by a reduction in left ventricular work and myocardial oxygen consumption (Lefemine et al., 1962; Soroff et al., 1963; Rosensweig and Chatterjee, 1968). It has also been shown that, when instituted soon after acute coronary occlusion, counterpulsation significantly lowers mortality from cardiogenic shock in experimental animals (Jacoby et al., 1963), presumably by limiting the extent of myocardial infarction (Nachlas and Siedband, 1967; Sugg et al., 1969).

However, despite the apparent effectiveness of arterial counterpulsation in experimental animals, it never gained widespread clinical application. For one, deployment of the system in patients with cardiogenic shock did not improve survival (Sugg et al., 1970). Second, it has been shown that rapid withdrawal of the requisite volume of arterial blood during systole was frequently not possible to accomplish, especially in the presence of severe hypotension and tachycardia, since the arterial walls almost invariably collapsed around the cannula under these conditions. Hence, effective afterload reduction may not always be possible. Finally, rapid withdrawal and forceful pulsatile return of arterial blood induced significant formed element trauma.

In 1962, Moulopoulos and co-workers demonstrated that effective counterpulsation could be achieved through phasic mechanical displacement of blood within the arterial system, made possible by the use of a catheter-mounted cylindrical balloon positioned in the descending thoracic aorta. The balloon-containing catheter was connected to a carbon dioxide driving console and rhythmic balloon inflation and deflation were accomplished in this fashion. The driving system was gated to the electrocardiogram and both left ventricular and systemic arterial pressures were continuously monitored, permitting proper synchronization of balloon inflation and deflation with cardiac electromechanical events. The hemodynamic effects achieved with intraaortic balloon counterpulsation (IABC) were similar to those obtained with the more classic methods of arterial counterpulsation described earlier. A distinct advantage of the IABC technique over earlier methods of counterpulsation is that blood withdrawal is not required.

Successful clinical application of IABC was reported by Kantrowitz et al. (1968). These investigators demonstrated the effectiveness of IABC in improving the hemodynamic state of patients with postinfarctional cardiogenic shock, particularly when circulatory assistance was instituted early in the course of shock. Subsequent reports (Buckley et al., 1970; Mundth et al., 1970; Bregman et al., 1971; Mueller et al., 1971; Dunkman et al., 1972; Buckley et al., 1973b; Gold et al., 1973) reaffirmed the efficacy, simplicity, and safety of the measure and helped establish IABC as a valuable adjunctive tool in the management and support of the failing or ischemic left ventricle.

Physiologic Considerations. The intraaortic balloon (IAB) normally is positioned in the descending thoracic aorta by insertion of the balloon catheter through another site in the arterial tree. The preferred IAB insertion site is the common femoral artery. In its proper position, the IAB tip lies at least 4 cm below the upper part of the aortic knob (see Technical Considerations below).

Counterpulsation is achieved through alternate inflation and deflation of the IAB, controlled by an electrocardiographically regulated console. IAB inflation is timed to occur at the beginning of ventricular diastole (aortic valve closure), while deflation is set to take place during the period of isovolumetric contraction just before left ventricular ejection of the succeeding cycle. Thus, counterpulsation operates by raising aortic pressure during diastole and lowering it before left ventricular ejection of the succeeding cycle. The physiology of IABC is best understood by relating balloon inflation and deflation to cardiac electromechanical events (Fig. 21-6). In practice, the electrocardiographic signal is used primarily for triggering the intraaortic balloon pump (IABP), while the arterial pressure waveform is a necessary reference for optimal timing of IAB inflation and deflation.

When the IAB inflates, as a result of entry of gas into the balloon, it takes up a volume of space in the aorta and causes blood displacement in proportion to the inflated balloon volume. In addition, the peak aortic diastolic pressure rises, with a resultant increase in coronary perfusion pressure. Since approximately 90 percent of coronary perfusion takes place during diastole, it is logical to expect an increase in coronary blood flow when the aortic diastolic pressure is augmented. However, changes in coronary blood flow in response to IABC have been variable and have not necessarily paralleled directional changes in aortic diastolic pressure. For instance, Mueller et al. (1971) reported significant increases in coronary blood flow in patients with postinfarctional cardiogenic shock. On the other hand, Leinbach et al. (1971) observed either a reduction or no significant change in coronary blood flow during IABC support in the majority of patients studied.

Earlier observations made in dogs with or without myocardial infarction showed similar variable effects of IABC on coronary blood

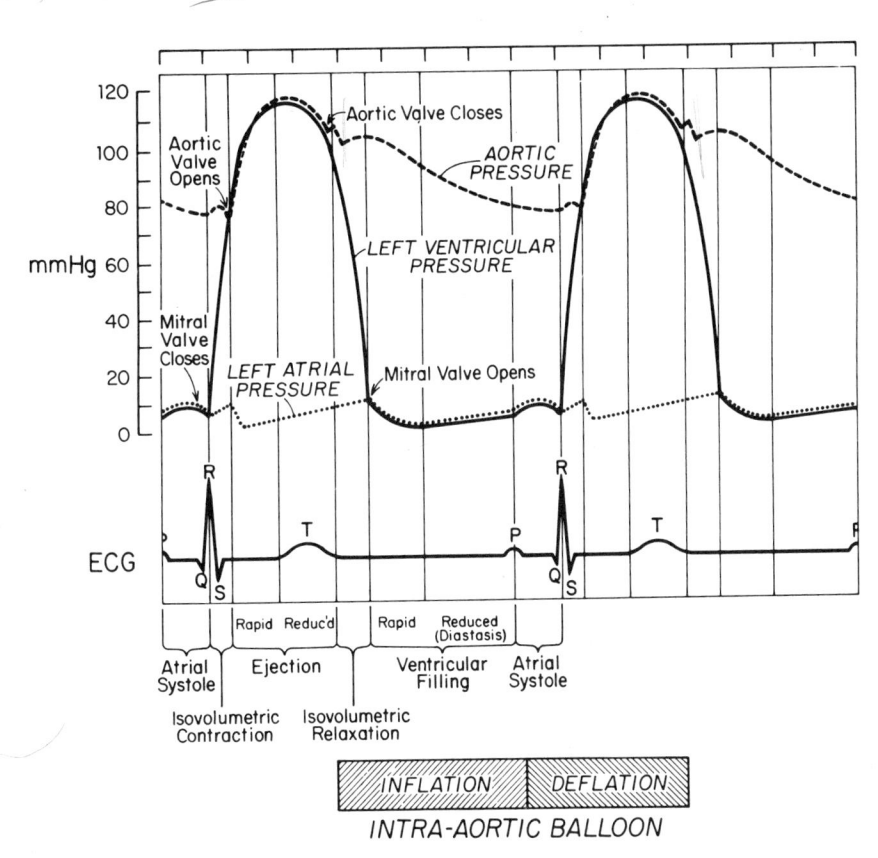

Figure 21-6. Schematic representation of the temporal relationships of the electromechanical events of the cardiac cycle and IAB inflation and deflation.

flow (Brown et al., 1967; Yahr et al., 1968; Powell et al., 1970). It has been postulated that the net effect of IABC in coronary flow is determined largely by the interplay between increased blood flow to ischemic areas brought about by the augmented diastolic perfusion pressure and diminution of blood flow to normal myocardium in which the oxygen requirements are reduced by decreased afterload (Leinbach et al.). It is possible that local autoregulatory mechanisms play a dominant role in determining regional distribution of coronary flow, as suggested by Powell et al.

Balloon deflation, which is brought about by the rapid escape of the inflating gas from the balloon, is timed to be completed during the peroiod of isovolumetric contraction, which is the interval between the peak of the R wave of the electrocardiogram and the earliest rise in ventricular pressure after atrial contraction to the opening of the aortic valve. This means that IAB deflation should be timed to actually begin in late ventricular diastole a few milliseconds before the inscription of the QRS complex (Fig. 21–7). IAB deflation has the effect of lowering aortic end-diastolic pressure. Since the aortic valve normally opens the instant developed pressure in the left ventricle (during isovolumetric contraction) exceeds aortic pressure, lowering the aortic end-diastolic pressure (by IAB deflation) *shortens the* duration of isovolumetric contraction by allowing the aortic valve to

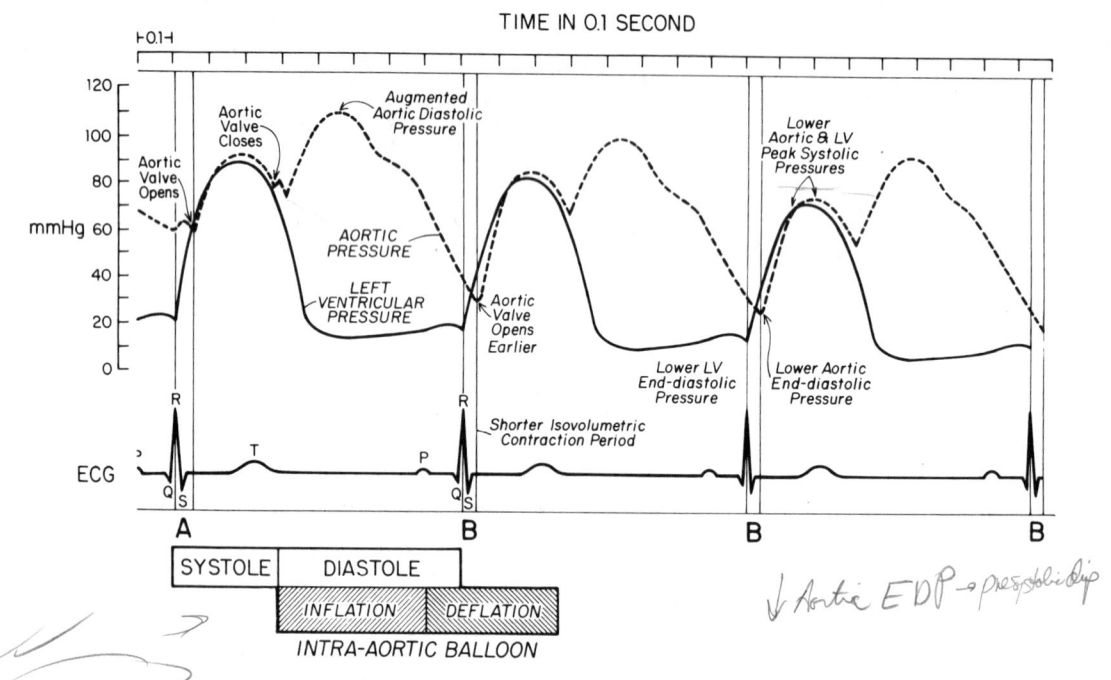

Figure 21–7. Schematic representation of the relationships of the electrical and mechanical events of the cardiac cycle during intraaortic balloon counterpulsation. IAB inflation early in diastole augments aortic diastolic and coronary perfusion pressure, while IAB deflation in late diastole lowers aortic diastolic pressure and shortens the duration of isovolumetric contraction by allowing the aortic valve to open earlier (B vs. A) and at a lower level of developed left ventricular pressure. Properly synchronized IAB counterpulsation eventually results in lower left ventricular and aortic peak systolic and end-diastolic pressures. (IAB inflation and deflation indicators shown in only one cardiac cycle.)

open earlier and at a lower level of developed ventricular pressure. Consequently, impedance to left ventricular ejection is reduced and both left ventricular and aortic peak systolic pressures fall. Reduction of impedance to emptying of the left ventricle results in a corresponding decrease in energy expenditure (Braunwald et al., 1970). From a mechanical standpoint, it can be said that part of the energy supplied for inflation and deflation of the balloon is ultimately used for the propulsion of blood. The net result is a further reduction in myocardial oxygen requirements.

Other hemodynamic and associated metabolic changes observed during IABC appear to be related to precounterpulsation cardiovascular subsystem performance (Powell et al., 1970; Mueller et al., 1971; Berger et al., 1973; Buckley et al., 1973b; Mueller, 1977). In the presence of cardiogenic shock, IABC support of the failing left ventricle is accompanied by the following desirable changes: (1) a fall in heart rate and left ventricular filling pressure; (2) an increase in cardiac output; (3) an increase in coronary blood flow with a concomitant fall in myocardial oxygen consumption; (4) a decrease in myocardial lactate production (or a shift from lactate production to lactate extraction), accompanied by a fall in arterial lactate content; and (5) a decrease in arterial-coronary sinus oxygen content difference. The important hemodynamic and metabolic effects of IABC on the failing, ischemic left ventricle are summarized in Table 21-3.

Available data indicate that the salutary effects of IABC are related primarily to the reduction in cardiac work (afterload) and augmentation of aortic diastolic pressure (i.e., coronary perfusion pressure) that it brings about. While the net effect on coronary blood flow may be variable, myocardial oxygen con-

TABLE 21-3 HEMODYNAMIC AND METABOLIC EFFECTS OF INTRAAORTIC BALLOON COUNTERPULSATION ON THE FAILING, ISCHEMIC LEFT VENTRICLE

Measurement	Effect
Arterial Pressure	
End-diastolic	Decreased
Mean diastolic (or coronary perfusion pressure)	Increased
Peak systolic	Decreased
Mean arterial	Variable
Heart Rate	Deceased
Cardiac Output	Increased
Left Ventricular Ejection resistance	Decreased
Left Ventricular Filling pressure	Decreased
Coronary Blood Flow	Increased
Myocardial Oxygen Consumption	Decreased
Arterial-Coronary Sinus Oxygen Content Difference	Decreased
Myocardial Lactate Extraction	Increased
Arterial Lactate Content	Decreased

Information derived from the reports of Powell et al., 1970; Leinbach et al., 1971; Mueller et al., 1971; Berger et al., 1973; Buckley et al., 1973a; and Mueller, 1977.

sumption also invariably falls as a result of the shortening of the isovolumetric phase of ventricular contraction and the reduction in left ventricular ejection resistance. The secondary fall in heart rate and left ventricular filling pressures frequently observed during IABC also lead to further reductions in myocardial oxygen consumption. The result is a more favorable myocardial oxygen supply and demand relationship. The latter, in turn, frequently results in an improved myocardial metabolic performance (Summers et al., 1969; Maroko et al., 1972; Mueller et al., 1972). In addition, cardiac output rises modestly (500 to 900 ml/min) during IABC support (Berger et al., 1973; Buckley et al., 1973b; Mueller et al., 1977).

Clinical Indications. IABC has been employed primarily as an adjunctive tool in the management of patients with low cardiac output accompanying two major clinical disorders: (1) acute myocardial infarction shock due to either myocardial injury or dysfunction, ventricular septal perforation, papillary muscle rupture, or a combination of these conditions (Kantrowitz et al., 1968; Buckley et al., 1970; Mundth et al., 1970; Bregman et al., 1971; Mueller et al., 1971, 1972, 1977; Dunkman et al., 1972; Buckley et al., 1973b); and (2) left ventricular power failure following open intracardiac surgery, often characterized by the inability to wean the patient from cardiopulmonary bypass support (Buckley et al., 1973a; Berger et al., 1973; Bregman et al., 1975). IABC also has been used in the management of patients with myocardial ischemic syndromes (unstable or preinfarction angina), specifically those in whom pharmacologic measures have been ineffective in controlling ischemic pain or those requiring emergency cardiac catheterization, angiography, and surgery (Gold et al., 1973; Mundth et al., 1975). In addition, the intraaortic balloon and a modification of the technique (the "pulsatile assist device") have been employed to create pulsatile flow during clinical cardiopulmonary bypass and to initiate counterpulsation support during weaning from bypass (Pappas, 1974; Bregman et al., 1977).

IABC is contraindicated in the presence of aortic regurgitation, since aortic diastolic pressure augmentation increases the amount of reflux of aortic blood into the left ventricle. IABC also is contraindicated in the presence of an aortic dissection or aneurysm because of the increased likelihood of aortic rupture, both during IAB insertion and counterpulsation.

Technical Considerations

EQUIPMENT AND PERSONNEL REQUIREMENTS. For IABC support, an intraaortic balloon pump (IABP), a supply of intraaortic balloons, and equipment for ECG and hemodynamic monitoring—with the capability for direct display and/or write-out of the systemic arterial pressure waveform—are the basic essentials.

A discussion of the IABP systems in current use will be given in the section that follows (The IABP System).

IAB insertion and removal are performed under the same conditions of sterility that obtain in a regular operating room. An operating team (consisting of a surgeon, an assistant, a scrub nurse, and a circulating nurse) and a technician skilled in the use of the IABP device should be in attendance. Since most of these procedures are carried out at the bedside in intensive care unit settings, it is desirable to have specially constituted surgical packs and trays that can be transported with relative ease. Instruments and devices (vascular grafts, embolectomy catheters) required for basic vascular operations should be available. Adequate lighting to illuminate the surgical field is required; mobile operating room type lighting fixtures are most helpful.

A portable x-ray apparatus operated by a trained technician must be available on a standby basis, especially during IAB insertion. It is mandatory that the IAB position be checked before the balloon catheter is anchored and the insertion site closed. This ensures that proper IAB position is achieved promptly and optimal counterpulsation support established without delay. Alternatively, image intensification fluoroscopy may be used. However, this method has several drawbacks. First, it requires that additional space-taking equipment (i.e., TV monitor, C-arm, and collimator) be moved to the frequently cramped bedside area. Second, the patient will have to be placed on a suitable radiolucent bed or platform. Third, the necessary radiation protection measures required are an encumbrance to the scrubbed members of the operating team. When IAB insertion is performed in the course of cardiac surgery, x-ray or fluoroscopic control is usually not required since the chest is generally open and the thoracic aorta is usually either directly visible or palpable.

THE IABP SYSTEM. A number of IABP systems are now commercially available, but the Avco-Roche* and the Datascope† systems have found the widest clinical acceptance. While both systems employ the same principle, there are important differences in systems design and operation.

The Avco-Roche IABP system uses a cylindrically shaped, triple-segmented, polyurethane balloon that has been designed to be nonocclusive. IAB inflation brings about both cranial and caudal displacement of intraaortic blood and propagation of the augmented aortic diastolic pressure pulse wave. Thus, the term *omnidirectional* has sometimes been used to characterize the Avco-Roche balloon. In the trisegmented balloon, inflation begins in the middle segment, followed by inflation of the two end segments. As presently designed, each of the three segments is of equal length and is separated by baffles affixed to a perforated catheter. The catheter perforations in the middle segment are larger than those in the proximal and distal segments to allow inflation to begin in this segment. It is believed that inflation of a tricompartmental balloon in this sequence avoids entrapment of blood between the two end segments. This IAB design concept evolved from the observations made by Laird et al. (1968) on the effects of balloon configuration on diastolic pressure augmentation. These investigators demonstrated that single-segment cylindrical or sausage-shaped balloons are susceptible to high lateral wall pressure. The latter would lead to preferential inflation of the balloon ends, trapping of blood between the preferentially inflated balloon ends, and ineffective volume displacement and pressure augmentation (the so-called bubble blowing phenomenon).

The Datascope IABP system, on the other hand, employs mainly a dual-chambered polyurethane balloon. It has a spherical distal chamber that inflates early in diastole and occludes the aorta. This is sequentially followed by the inflation of a narrower cylindrical proximal pumping chamber, in the same diastolic interval, that reportedly produces displacement of intraaortic blood entirely (unidirectionally) toward the aortic root. This particular IAB design concept evolved from the original work of Talpins et al. (1968). These investigators studied the hemodynamic effects of IABC in experimental cardiogenic shock using both a single-chambered cylindrical balloon and a two-chambered balloon. A substantially greater increment in coronary blood flow was observed when IABC was carried out with a two-chambered balloon. Subsequent work by Bregman et al. (1970) confirmed these observations.

The Avco-Roche system uses helium as the driving gas for balloon inflation while the Datascope system uses carbon dioxide. The choice of driving gas has been based on considerations of response time and safety. Helium, being lightweight, has rapid transport and inflation capabilities and offers a greater advantage when short inflation and deflation times are required under conditions of tachycardia (i.e., heart rates in excess of 120 beats per minute). Carbon dioxide is heavier with a

---

*Roche Medical Electronics Inc., Cranbury, N.J.
†Datascope Corp, Paramus, N.J.

slower response time; however, because of its greater solubility, it may have a lesser risk of gas embolism in the event of catastrophic balloon rupture or leakage. It is gratifying to note that gas embolism is an exceedingly rare complication of IABC. The primary reasons for the low incidence of gas embolism are the rigid quality control measures employed during balloon manufacture and the fail-safe mechanisms built into the pump system.

The present generation Avco-Roche (Model 10) and Datascope (System 80) IABP control consoles exemplify the most advanced and sophisticated technology. Both systems have been found to be effective, reliable, safe, and easy to use. It is not our intention to recommend any particular IABP system. However, since most of our experience has been with the Avco-Roche system, it is understandable that the discussions that follow pertain to it.

THE AVCO IABP SYSTEM. The basic components of the system are the catheter-mounted trisegmented balloon and the pump itself. The trisegment balloon is available in three adult and two pediatric sizes attached to catheters of various sizes (Table 21–4).

The pump essentially consists of two parts: the pneumatics part and the electronics part. The pneumatics part contains the compressor system and the helium supply and is connected to the IAB by the catheter. The balloon is inflated with helium and is deflated at every cardiac cycle. IAB inflation and deflation are accomplished by means of an isolating piston that moves back and forth under the influence of alternating low and high air pressures. The piston connects to a high and low pressure chamber by means of a pulse valve. Two pumps operating continuously permit maintenance of high and low pressures in separate chambers. Appropriate signals supplied from the electronics part of the pump alternately switches the pulse valve to high and then to low pressure.

The electronic part of the pump consists essentially of an R-wave detector triggered by the patient's electrocardiogram; the pulse of the detector in turn triggers an inflation and a deflation signal that can be applied on the pulse valve with a variable delay. In its most basic configuration, the pump console provides an oscilloscopic screen that continuously displays the patient's electrocardiogram and the pressure in the helium compartment. The inflation and deflation signals are displayed as flags superimposed on the patient's ECG. In addition, there are also a number of control buttons and a screen where malfunction messages appear when necessary.

PATIENT PREPARATION. Patients requiring IABC support should be closely monitored and cared for in a unit staffed by personnel skilled in the use of the IABP device.

A good quality ECG signal is required to accurately *trigger* balloon inflation and deflation. This signal may be obtained either from a bedside monitor or directly from the patient via a separate set of ECG paste-on electrodes

TABLE 21–4 DIMENSIONS OF CURRENTLY AVAILABLE TRISEGMENTED INTRA-AORTIC BALLOONS

Application	Balloon Volume (ml)	Outside Diameter (mm) of Inflated Balloon	Catheter Size (Fr)
Adult	40	18	14 & 12
	30	16	14
	20	14	12
Pediatric	12	11	9
	4	8.6	7

Data furnished by Roche Medical Electronics, Cranbury, N.J. 08512.

and fed to the balloon console computer. Regardless of the method employed, it is essential to insure that the signal acquired gives the tallest possible R wave and is both stable and interference-free. Proper ECG electrode position is essential to the acquisition of a good electrical signal. For IAB triggering, the ideal ECG signal is one with a large QRS deflection with a relatively small T wave. In the majority of cases, a modified Lead 2 is satisfactory; in certain instances, however, the technician must determine the mean electrical axis in the frontal and horizontal planes and position the electrodes accordingly. When attempts to obtain an adequate QRS signal have failed (fortunately rare), artificial cardiac pacing—whenever appropriate—may provide an alternate method of IAB triggering.

To accurately *time* balloon inflation and deflation an undamped systemic arterial waveform is necessary. This means that systemic arterial pressure must be continuously monitored via an indwelling intravascular catheter and the waveform displayed in real time. For precise balloon timing, a central aortic pressure pulse would be the ideal reference, since it provides the closest temporal approximation of cardiac electromechanical events. In practice, however, systemic arterial pressure is continuously monitored via a catheter positioned in the radial artery for reasons of ready accessibility, ease of cannulation, and adequacy of collateral circulation. Sometimes it is measured by a brachial artery catheter. Whenever systemic arterial pressure is measured from either the radial or brachial artery (or, for that matter, from any peripheral artery), allowances must be made for pulse wave propagation delays when setting the timing of IAB inflation and deflation.

Continuous monitoring of left ventricular filling pressures and periodic measurements of cardiac output are indicated in patients undergoing IABC for left ventricular power failure, cardiogenic shock, or low cardiac output, but generally not in those requiring support purely because of myocardial ischemic pain poorly controlled by pharmacologic measures.

Preparatory to IAB insertion, the lower abdomen, pubic area, and both thighs are shaved and scrubbed (most IAB insertions are done through the common femoral artery). These areas are generally included in the routine surgical "prep" for most, if not all, open intracardiac operations, so that the common femoral vessels are almost always readily accessible.

TECHNIQUE OF IAB INSERTION. The IAB is inserted through a longitudinal arteriotomy, most commonly in the common femoral artery. Other vessels (including iliac artery, lower abdominal aorta, ascending aorta, and subclavian artery) have been used as IAB insertion sites, but only when access through the common femoral artery is not feasible. Regardless of the vessel used, the balloon catheter is secured in place with the aid of a sidearm graft to allow maintenance of perfusion distal to the insertion site (see below).

The description that follows applies to IAB insertion through the common femoral artery, performed without fluoroscopic control.

It is recommended that both groins be encompassed in the sterile field to allow easy access to either common femoral artery. Not infrequently, IAB passage up one side may be prevented by the presence of previously unsuspected arteriosclerotic obstructive disease; in this event, IAB passage could then be attempted up the contralateral side. It must be remembered that there is approximately a 10 percent chance that IAB passage up both common femoral arteries will not be successful because of the presence of iliofemoral arteriosclerotic obstructive disease bilaterally. While the quality of the femoral arterial pulse largely dictates which vessel to use, it is helpful to establish—at least on clinical grounds—the presence or absence of significant arteriosclerotic obstructive disease before attempting IAB insertion in order to reduce the likelihood of complications.

Once the insertion site has been selected, the operative site is infiltrated with 0.5 percent lidocaine solution. Of course, this step is omitted if the patient is already under general anesthesia (as is the case when IAB insertion is done in the course of open intracardiac operations). The preferred skin incision is a vertical one made over the femoral triangle from a point just above the inguinal crease to 6 to 8 cm below, along the course of the artery. The incision is carried down to the femoral sheath. The femoral sheath is opened and the common femoral artery is isolated between the level of the inguinal ligament and the origin of the profunda femoris artery. If there is a high origin of the profunda femoris artery, it is sometimes necessary to incise the inguinal ligament and carry the common femoral artery exposure to the origin of the deep inferior epigastric artery. To facilitate vascular control during balloon catheter passage, pull-up tourniquets (Dacron tapes passed through short segments of 16 Fr. or 18 Fr. red rubber catheters) are placed around the proximal and distal portions of the exposed common femoral artery.

At this point, heparin (75 to 100 IU/kg) is administered intravenously, unless systemic heparinization had been established previously (e.g., heparinization during the conduct of cardiopulmonary bypass). Appropriate IAB size is determined. It must be remembered that IAB performance characteristics are determined in large measure by balloon volume. That is, all other variables being equal, the larger the balloon volume, the greater the efficacy of diastolic pressure augmentation and impedance reduction (Weber et al., 1972). The anatomic studies performed by Weikel et al. (1971) showed that the diameter of the midthoracic aorta is greater than 19 mm in 90 percent of subjects. Since the largest available balloon (40 ml) has an outside diameter of less than 19 mm (i.e., 18 mm) when fully inflated, it appears that it will be possible to use a 40-ml balloon in most instances without exceeding optimal inflated IAB-to-aortic diameter ratio (i.e., occlusivity). Whereas the greatest augmentation in aortic diastolic pressure (at any level of aortic pressure and aortic size) is seen with complete occlusion on IAB inflation, the possibility of aortic wall and formed element damage at 100 percent occlusion suggests that perhaps 90 to 95 percent occlusivity might be optimal (Weber et al., 1972). In selecting optimal IAB size, a good rule of thumb to follow is to use the largest IAB that one can pass through the common femoral and iliac arteries. In children, the options are fewer because of the small size of the femoral arteries.

It has been our experience that an IAB that passes up the femoroiliac system with relative ease is almost never completely occlusive to the aorta at full balloon inflation. The recent introduction of the 40-ml balloon mounted on a 12 Fr. catheter will undoubtedly expand the usage of this large volume IAB. However, it must be borne in mind that use of such a balloon catheter system will make it readily possible to pass an IAB that will turn out to be completely occlusive during balloon inflation. Fortunately, complete occlusivity is readily recognizable from the character of the balloon pressure waveform and the magnitude of the aortic-diastolic pressure augmentation.

The balloon catheter that has been selected is brought onto the operative field with the balloon carefully protected from damage by minimizing handling and keeping the protective sheath in place until just before actual insertion. The length of the catheter to be inserted intravascularly (to achieve the desired IAB position) is determined. This is accomplished by laying the balloon catheter straight and flat against the patient's body along the approximate course of the femoroiliac vessels and the abdominal and descending thoracic aorta. With the catheter tip positioned at the level of the angle of Louis, a nonabsorbable ligature is tied snugly around the catheter to mark the anticipated point of exit of the balloon catheter at the lower angle of the groin incision. With this method, the surgeon is assured that the catheter tip will almost invariably come to be within 2 to 4 cm distal to the takeoff of the left subclavian artery if, following insertion, the catheter marker is aligned with the lower angle of the skin incision. This, of course, constitutes satisfactory IAB position in most instances.

The sidearm graft is selected and prepared. A 10- to 12-mm synthetic tubular vascular graft is perhaps the most widely used material for this purpose, but we prefer to use formalin-preserved iliac vein or inferior vena caval allografts (Ortiz et al., 1975). Vein allografts offer the advantages of handling and suturing ease and of being more hemostatic in the face of systemic heparinization. Moreover, subsequent repair, especially of a significantly sclerotic femoral artery, is easier because of the greater pliability of vein allografts.

The sidearm graft is trimmed to the appropriate length, beveled to allow a catheter exit angle of approximately 45°, and slid over the balloon catheters. The balloon is kept constantly deflated, which is readily accomplished by attaching a three-way stopcock and a 50-ml syringe to the connector end of the balloon catheter. The balloon is deflated by application of negative pressure at the end of the catheter; this state of complete deflation is maintained during IAB catheter passage with the aid of the three-way stopcock arrangement.

The balloon is thoroughly washed with heparinized normal saline solution to remove all loose foreign material. The common femoral artery is isolated between two atraumatic vascular clamps and a 12- to 14-cm longitudinal arteriotomy is made on the anterior wall of the excluded arterial segment. The balloon catheter is introduced into the arterial lumen as the vascular clamps are slowly removed and proximal and distal vascular control established by snaring down on the artery with the previously applied pull-up tourniquets. The balloon catheter is gently advanced into the iliac system. Often it is helpful to gently rotate the catheter along its long axis, as it is advanced, so that the collapsed balloon neatly wraps around it—thereby effectively reducing the bulk of the balloon-catheter complex. Use of vigorous force should be avoided to reduce the dangers of arterial perforation, dissection, and dislodgement of intimal plaques.

When significant resistance to catheter passage is encountered, a number of technical maneuvers may be helpful. First, the balloon catheter may be removed and the tip bent gently to allow passage beyond any tortuosity in the aortoiliac vessels. Second, hyperextension of the body to the opposite side (especially with the left femoral artery approach) may help straighten the aorto-ilio-femoral system and allow easier passage. Third, whenever feasible, the contralateral common femoral artery should be used and catheter passage attempted up this vessel. Fourth, if none of these maneuvers succeeds, passage of a smaller size balloon may be attempted or the technique of progressive arterial dilatation with regular silastic rubber or Fogarty catheters may be tried. It must be remembered that serious arterial injury may result from very vigorous attempts at dilatation.

If balloon catheter passage still cannot be accomplished after all of these maneuvers, catheter insertion through one of several alternative insertion sites may be tried (see below) after the groin incisions are repaired.

In most patients (approximately 90 percent), balloon catheter passage can be carried out successfully with the common femoral artery approach. After negotiating the femoroiliac system, the balloon catheter is advanced into the aorta until the previously applied tie marker on the catheter is at the level of the lower angle of the skin incision. This generally ensures proper IAB position in the descending thoracic aorta with the catheter tip situated 2 to 4 cm distal to the takeoff of the left subclavian artery (Fig. 21-8). Attempts at further catheter passage beyond this point may be met with resistance as the catheter tip abuts against the transverse aortic arch, or the operator may observe either a reduction or obliteration of the systemic arterial pressure pulse—that is, if the arterial pressure is being monitored via one of the distal radicles of the left subclavian artery, as is frequently the case. When one or both of the latter phenomena are observed, the balloon catheter is pulled back 2 to 4 cm.

The balloon catheter is temporarily secured to the surgical drapes or to the skin and the distal end is handed over to the IABP technician, who proceeds to connect the cath-

Figure 21-8. *Left Panel.* Diagram illustrating IAB insertion through the common femoral artery. Optimal IAB tip position relative to the aortic knob and the take-off of the left subclavian artery is shown. *Right Panel.* Technical details of IAB catheter insertion showing use of an anchoring sidearm graft sutured to the common femoral artery in an end-to-side fashion (**A, B, C**). For this purpose, an autogenous vein graft or a formalin-preserved vein allograft is preferred over synthetic material. When prompt institution of counterpulsation is required, the graft may be slid over the IAB catheter as the latter is passed and counterpulsation initiated while the graft-to-femoral artery anastomosis is fashioned out. Use of a vein graft facilitates arterial repair (**D**).

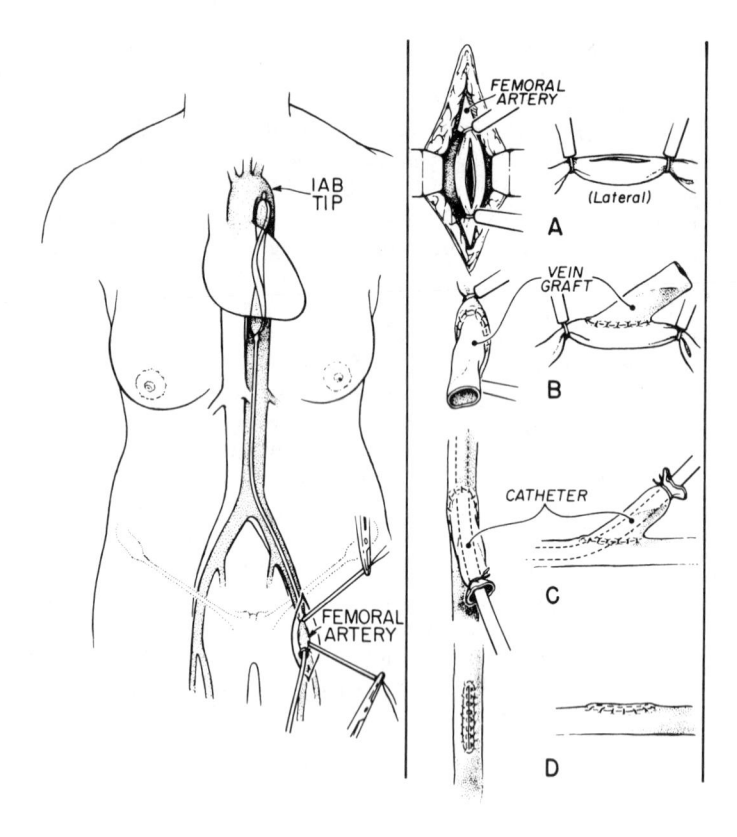

eter to the ready-to-operate IABP console. If so desired, IABC can promptly begin after the usual catheter vent-and-purge procedures. Meanwhile, the sidearm graft is slid down the catheter and anastomosed to the femoral artery end-to-side with 5-0 or 6-0 monofilament vascular sutures, generally polypropylene. A pull-up tourniquet is applied around the sidearm graft and the exiting catheter, while the tourniquets (first the distal, then the proximal) around the common femoral artery are slowly released. The graft-to-artery suture line is carefully inspected and hemostasis ensured.

A bedside chest x-ray is taken at this point to confirm optimal balloon position (this is a step that can safely be dispensed with when the chest is open). The occasions when major IAB repositioning is required after the radiographic check are rare, if careful attention has been paid to the technical details just described. As pointed out in an earlier section, we have not found it necessary to routinely use bedside fluoroscopy. Once optimal IAB position has been confirmed, the sidearm graft is doubly ligated with heavy (#0) nonabsorbable ligatures around itself and the balloon catheter. The proximal ligature should be applied close to the anastomotic line (without producing distortion) to avoid the creation of a blind cul-de-sac where a thrombus could form and propagate. It is also important to ensure that balloon position not be disturbed while the catheter is secured.

The catheter is sutured to the inferior point of the skin incision with a heavy, nonabsorbable suture that is wrapped several times around the catheter and tied. The deep and superficial fascial layers and the subcutaneous tissue are closed with interrupted absorbable sutures with the balloon catheter exiting inferiorly. The skin is closed with interrupted nonabsorbable sutures. The area of catheter exit is cleaned and covered with a bactericidal ointment.

A sterile occlusive dressing is applied to cover the incision and a few inches of catheter. This dressing maintains sterility of the area and further secures catheter fixation.

ALTERNATE IAB INSERTION SITES. If balloon catheter passage cannot be accomplished through the common femoral artery route as described, alternate IAB insertion sites should be considered.

If arteriosclerotic obstructive disease involves the femoral or external iliac systems, catheter passage may be attempted through the common iliac artery or distal abdominal aorta by a retroperitoneal approach. Regional or general anesthesia is required and the procedure should be carried out in a regular operating room. A muscle-splitting incision is made in the iliac or lower lumbar region and deepened to the retroperitoneum. The iliac vessels and the aortic bifurcation are exposed. If a suitable common iliac vessel is found, pull-up tourniquets are placed around the artery for proximal and distal control and the balloon catheter is inserted with the same techniques described under the common femoral artery approach. However, if IAB insertion has to be done through the distal aorta, a partially occluding clamp is used. A longitudinal aortotomy (12 to 14 cm) is made over the excluded portion of the vessel and a vascular graft is sutured onto the aorta with 4-0 or 5-0 vascular sutures. The vascular graft should be long enough to reach to a readily accessible subcutaneous location where it can easily be exposed with minimal dissection at the time of IAB removal. The balloon catheter is inserted through this graft and advanced to the proper anatomic location in the thoracic aorta. Once proper IAB position is achieved, the sidearm graft is doubly ligated with heavy, nonabsorbable ligatures around itself and the balloon catheter. Catheter position is secured by the same anchoring techniques described above.

Occasionally, antegrade insertion of the balloon catheter may become necessary in patients with severe aorto-ilio-femoral arteriosclerotic disease who manifest such severe, life-threatening, left ventricular dysfunction during the conduct of cardiac surgery that they cannot be separated from cardiopulmonary bypass. This can be accomplished by suturing a vascular graft to the ascending aorta (Krause et al., 1976; Roe and Chatterjee, 1976) and is possible only under open chest conditions. The balloon catheter is introduced through a small separate intercostal or subcostal incision. A partially occluding vascular clamp is applied tangentially on the ascending aorta. A longitudinal aortotomy is made and the graft-to-aorta anastomosis is fashioned out using 4-0 vascular sutures. The balloon catheter is inserted through the graft and the balloon is advanced to and positioned in the descending thoracic aorta distal to the left subclavian artery takeoff. The graft is doubly ligated in a subcutaneous location and anchored to the skin. Access to the graft at the time of IAB removal can be accomplished easily under local infiltration anesthesia without thoracic reentry. After balloon catheter removal, the graft is transected, oversewn, and allowed to retract into the chest.

INITIATION OF IABC SUPPORT. It is desirable to have in attendance a skilled technician who has a working knowledge of cardiovascular and counterpulsation physiology and who has been well-schooled in the proper mechanical operation of the IABP system. By the time optimal IAB position has been attained, all other preparations necessary for initiating counterpulsation support will have been completed. The IABP technician will have conducted a thorough systems check of the pump console and of all ancillary equipment. He or she ensures the acquisition of a high-quality, interference-free ECG signal, which is fed to the IABP computer console. The technician also sees to it that an undamped systemic arterial pressure waveform is conveniently displayed in real time and that the helium tank contains an ample amount of driving gas.

As soon as a satisfactory ECG signal is obtained, preliminary adjustments of the inflate-deflate timing controls are made. The start of inflation is made to coincide with the peak of the T wave and the start of deflation with the interval between the P wave and the R wave. Some of the late model IABP pump consoles have the capability of having inflation-deflation timing triggered by the arterial pressure waveform. This feature makes it possible to maintain uninterrupted IABC support when the patient is IABP-dependent yet effective ECG triggering is not possible because of a small R wave (as in massive myocardial infarction) or when 60-cycle interference is present or electrocautery has to be used. Ideally, however, ECG triggering is employed whenever possible because optimal timing is more predictably achieved in this operational mode.

The helium supply is turned on and the volume adjust control is set to read one half the balloon volume (for adult size balloon) or the full balloon volume (for pediatric size balloons). The IABP console is now ready to pump.

The balloon catheter is connected to the IABP console. The catheter vent is opened and the IABP console pneumatic system is turned on to deliver helium gas to purge and displace all the air contained in the balloon catheter. The usual purge time is approximately 45 to 60 seconds, after which the vent hole is closed. The pneumatic system is temporarily turned off and the balloon is inflated to its full volume. Balloon pumping can then begin.

The reader is encouraged to consult the appropriate operator's manual for additional IABP technical information.

TIMING OF IAB INFLATION AND DEFLATION. While phasic triggering of balloon inflation and deflation is ECG regulated, the finer adjustments necessary to achieve optimal IAB synchrony with cardiac electromechanical events require careful study of the morphology of an undamped systemic arterial pressure waveform in its balloon-assisted and unassisted forms. During IAB assistance, the arterial pressure waveform characteristically exhibits two peaks per cardiac cycle. The earlier of the two is produced by left ventricular ejection, the second by balloon inflation.

On the other hand, balloon deflation produces a pressure drop immediately before the opening of the aortic valve, which marks the beginning of the succeeding cardiac cycle (see Fig. 21-7).

Balloon inflation is timed to occur after aortic valve closure, which marks the beginning of ventricular diastole. Aortic valve closure, in turn, is marked by the dicrotic notch on the arterial pressure waveform. IAB deflation is set to occur just before the aortic valve opens. Aortic valve opening is marked by the earliest rise in systolic arterial pressure.

In making the necessary adjustments in the inflation-deflation controls, one should remember that there are inherent time delays in the propagation of the arterial pressure pulse; the magnitude of the delay is a function of the distance between the left ventricle and the recording site. For instance, the inscription of the dicrotic notch will take place later, in terms of real time, when the recording site is the radial artery rather than the ascending aorta. If the femoral artery is the pressure recording site, the time delay is even greater.

For maximal therapeutic benefit, IAB inflation and deflation should be carefully *timed to cardiac rather than peripheral arterial events.* A central aortic pressure pulse, when available, would be the ideal reference for timing, since it provides the closest temporal approximation of cardiac events. If arterial pressure is recorded from other than the ascending aorta, the operator must allow for pulse wave propagation delays in setting the inflation-deflation controls.

If a central aortic pulse is available, IAB inflation and deflation can be done with ease and dispatch. With the IABP off, the dicrotic notch is identified; with the IABP on, inflation is adjusted to coincide with the dicrotic notch. IAB deflation timing is set to ensure that the pressure dip in late diastole reaches its lowest point before the succeeding ventricular ejection. Too early deflation will produce a significant flat at the bottom of the valley before ventricular ejection. On the other hand, too late deflation will decrease the duration and magnitude of the pressure drop before the next systole.

SPECIAL TECHNIQUES EMPLOYED IN THE INTENSIVE CARE UNIT

Systemic arterial pressure is most commonly monitored from the radial artery. To set balloon inflation timing, the dicrotic notch is located with the IABP off. Inflation is then timed to occur approximately 50 msec (2.5 mm at a recording paper speed of 50 mm/sec) before the estimated dicrotic notch (Fig. 21-9). Since left ventricular generated pressure pulses appear earlier at the aortic root than at the radial artery and pressure pulses originating from the IAB appear later at the aortic root than at the origin of the brachiocephalic artery (approximate location of the IAB tip), IAB-generated pressure pulses should occur earlier by *twice* the time required for a pressure wave to travel from the IAB to the aortic root (i.e., 25 msec × 2 = 50 msec). Balloon deflation timing is set to ensure that the pressure drop preceding ventricular ejection has a 50-msec wide flat bottom (see Fig. 21-9). In theory, this all looks nice and neat; in actual practice, however, it is difficult to precisely discern timing changes of the order of magnitude of 50 msec on a normal oscilloscopic sweep or conventional recording paper speed. Moreover, the actual pulse wave propagation delay varies from one patient to another and even in the same patient with time, depending on changes in the inotropic state. While it may seem convenient to remember a guide number (i.e., 50 msec), it is more informative to carefully examine the morphology of the balloon-assisted arterial waveform.

With experience, the operator can set optimal IAB inflation and deflation without difficulty in most patients.

The femoral artery pressure pulse is an undesirable timing reference signal because of the inherent pulse wave propagation delays and the waveform distortion past the IAB, which could be very significant. The time delays vary from one person to another (influenced by the length of the patient's torso, presence or absence of significant aortoiliac atherosclerotic disease) and in the same person with changes in the inotropic state of the myocardium. Therefore, use of the femoral arterial pulse as a timing reference signal should be reserved only for situations in which the arterial pressure could not be monitored from a more suitable site. In this case, IAB inflation is timed to occur approximately 120 msec (roughly equal to the total delay time to the aortic root) before the estimated dicrotic notch, and the duration of the pressure drop between the end of deflation and the onset of ventricular ejection should also be approximately 120 msec (6.0 mm at a recording paper speed of 50 mm/sec).

Examples of improper IAB inflation and deflation are shown in Figure 21-10.

Once optimal timing of IAB inflation-deflation is achieved, IABC is maintained at the 1:1 assist level. The management of a patient maintained on IABC support is described in the section that follows.

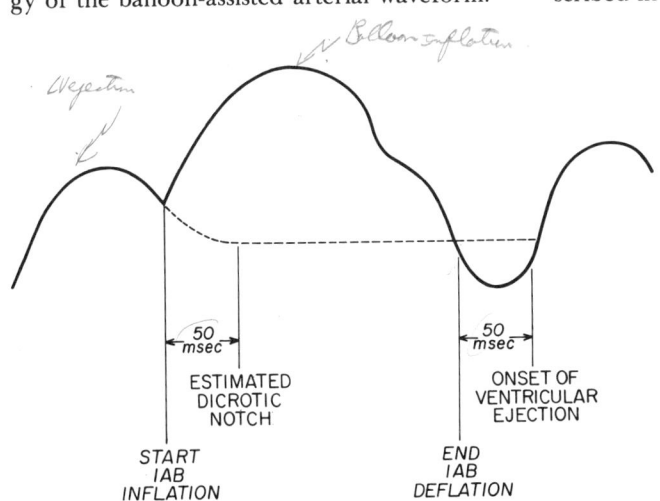

Figure 21-9. Diagram illustrating proper adjustment of IAB inflation and deflation when a radial artery pressure waveform is used as timing reference.

PROPER INFLATION/DEFLATION TIMING

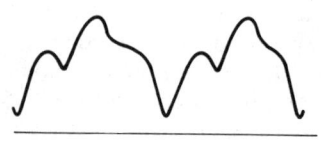

Figure 21-10. The central aortic pressure pulse is the ideal reference for timing IAB inflation and deflation. Actual central aortic pressure tracings are reproduced showing the morphologic characteristics of the aortic pressure pulse when inflation and deflation are properly and improperly timed. For comparison, "normal" or "typical" tracings are superimposed (dashed lines).

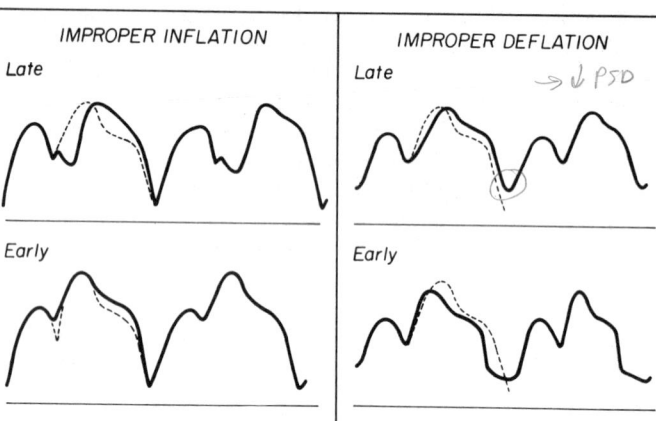

Management of the Patient on IABC Support.

Patients on IABC support require either close surveillance or other therapeutic modalities designed to support a failing or ischemic left heart or both. For a comprehensive discussion of these management measures, the reader is referred to Chapter 9.

This section will be devoted to a discussion of certain management measures that apply specifically to the care of a patient maintained on IABC support.

MAINTENANCE OF A STABLE CARDIAC RHYTHM. Maximal hemodynamic benefits from IABC are obtained under conditions of a regular rhythm and a cardiac rate maintained within "physiologic" limits (heart rate between 60 and 120 bpm). The IABP operates most effectively under these conditions. Therefore, prompt control of cardiac dysrhythmias or arrhythmias, employing pharmacologic or electrophysiologic techniques or both, is a prerequisite to effective counterpulsation support.

Proper lead placement is essential to the maintenance of a stable high-quality, interference-free ECG signal, which, in turn, insures proper IABP triggering.

PATIENT ACTIVITY. Physiologic and safety considerations dictate that the patient on IABC support be confined to bed. For patients who are awake and who are in a position to cooperate with the nursing personnel, physical activity must be restricted. Regular full turning in bed and other bedside nursing activities are permissible, but must be done under supervision or with assistance. Hip motions that may induce motion at the IAB insertion site and possibly produce vascular damage must be avoided. Similarly, extreme elevation of the patient's head and upper torso (>45°) must not be permitted, as this tends to produce excessive balloon catheter flexing at the level of the insertion site and predisposes to catheter fracture; in addition, it can force the balloon tip proximally into the aortic arch and produce brachiocephalic obstruction or intimal trauma (O'Rourke and Shepherd, 1973). Excessive leg movements, which may cause separation of the catheter-tygon tubing connection, must also be forbidden.

ANTICOAGULATION. As a prophylactic measure against IAB-induced thrombogenesis, patients are maintained on an intravenous infusion drip of heparin (3 to 10 IU/kg/hr) to keep the activated coagulation time (ACT) between 110 and 140 seconds (particulate-activated method) as determined by a modified Hattersley method (1966).* In our experience, this level of heparinization provides adequate protection against clinically significant thrombogenesis, at least during the interval that balloon assistance is maintained at the 1:1 level. It is possible that, as the level of assistance is reduced during weaning from support, the likelihood of thrombotic complications may increase. For this reason, the amount of heparin given is increased to attain higher ACT level (approximately 160 to 180 seconds).

In general, the ACT is determined hourly until a stable therapeutic level is attained, after which it is sufficient to determine the ACT once every three to four hours.

MONITORING LIMB VIABILITY. The balloon catheter is a space-taking device that, when introduced through a limb artery, will almost invariably bring about a reduction in blood flow distal to the site of insertion. This alteration in regional blood flow can be significant if the artery used is anatomically small, peripheral vascular disease is present, or cardiac output is reduced, more so if compensatory vasoconstriction is marked.

It is, therefore, mandatory that the vascular integrity of the ipsilateral limb be assessed periodically. The staff should be on the lookout for signs and symptoms of limb ischemia. A careful record is maintained of changes in skin color and temperature, capillary refill time, venous filling, the quality and character of the distal arterial pulses, the consistency of the different muscle compartments, and petechiae. Where no distal pulses are present, use of Doppler ultrasound techniques to assess distal blood flow may be helpful.

At the earliest sign of limb compromise the IAB is removed and alternate insertion sites considered if counterpulsation support is still needed.

LOCAL WOUND CARE. The balloon catheter must be securely anchored to minimize local tissue trauma, which, in conjunction with the presence of a foreign body, could enhance the chances of a potentially serious wound infection. The catheter exit site is treated with a topical antibiotic ointment and an occlusive dressing is used.

The dressings are carefully changed every other day with strict aseptic technique. Systemic antibiotics also are used routinely for prophylaxis.

WEANING FROM THE IABC SUPPORT. Simply stated, the criteria for weaning from IABC support are the exact opposite of the criteria for IABC deployment. In general, weaning from IABC is begun when it is apparent that satisfactory cardiac performance (CI≥2.5 liters/min/m^2; left ventricular filling pressures ≤15 mm Hg; heart rate within "physiologic" limits) can be maintained by nonmechanical forms of therapy (pacing, cardioactive and vasoactive drugs, preload optimization, pharmacologic afterload reduction) or when myocardial ischemic pain can be controlled by other means (pharmacologic agents, revascularization).

The weaning procedure consists of progressively decreasing the frequency of balloon assistance. Whereas full assistance means that every heart beat (1:1) is mechanically assisted, 1:2 assistance means that only every other beat is assisted. Present-generation IABP consoles permit progressive reduction in assistance in steps from 1:2 to 1:4 to 1:8. The actual duration of each step varies widely and is largely dictated by the patient's response to the reduction in the level of assistance. Close surveillance and careful hemodynamic assessment must be maintained during each step of the weaning process.

At the 1:8 level of assistance, the magnitude of cardiac support afforded is nil. This means that, if hemodynamic stability had been maintained at the 1:4 assistance for at least one to two hours, it is safe to discontinue IABC and remove the IAB.

---

*ACT is measured with the aid of a blood coagulation timer (Hemochron Model 400, International Technique Corp., Edison, N.J.).

IAB REMOVAL. Balloon removal is performed under the same conditions described in an earlier section (Technical Considerations), with the exception that a portable x-ray apparatus would, ordinarily, not be required.

After a careful preparation, sterile drapes are applied and the IAB insertion site exposed. Local infiltration anesthesia is adequate in most cases. The incision is opened and the common femoral artery is exposed. Pull-up tourniquets are applied around the artery proximally and distally. The pull-up tourniquets are tightened to establish proximal and distal control.

The anchoring ligatures are removed, including those around the sidearm graft. The sidearm graft is opened and clots, if any, are removed. Meanwhile, the IABP console is turned off as the balloon catheter is disconnected from the console. A three-way stopcock and a 50-ml syringe are connected to the balloon catheter and the balloon is kept partially inflated (approximately 15 to 20 percent). The partially inflated balloon will conveniently act as an embolectomy catheter as it is gently withdrawn. During catheter withdrawal the air volume can be easily adjusted to maintain a snug passage.

Following catheter withdrawal, the proximal pull-up tourniquet slowly is released to flush out any retained clots while proximal flow is checked. Back bleeding is then checked by releasing the distal tourniquet. A Fogarty catheter is routinely passed distally to insure that no clots are left behind.

After it is established that satisfactory forward and backward flow are present, both tourniquets are tightened once more. Much of the vein allograft is excised, leaving just a narrow rim for repair purposes. Arterial repair is accomplished with 4-0 or 5-0 vascular sutures. It has been our practice to use the vein allograft remnant as a patch graft. This method facilitates repair, especially of a sclerotic artery (see Fig. 21-8).

The tourniquets are removed after completion of the arterial repair. If the distal circulation is deemed satisfactory, after reestablishment of forward flow the wound is thoroughly irrigated with antibiotic-containing solution and then closed in anatomic order.

Support of the Failing Left Ventricle with a Left Heart Assist Device

Although IABC has been effective in improving the hemodynamic status of some patients (see section on Intraaortic Balloon Counterpulsation: Clinical Indications), others will not survive unless increases in blood flow substantially greater than can be achieved with IABC are provided. A number of other ingenious methods of left ventricular support have been devised and employed in humans (Dennis et al., 1962; Baird et al., 1963: Cappelletti and Reynold, 1967; Trinkle and Bryant, 1970; Zwart et al., 1970; DeBakey, 1971; Litwak et al., 1974; Glassman et al., 1975; Norman, 1976; Radvany et al., 1977). An impediment to the use of many of these techniques is the need to reenter the thoracic cage for subsequent device removal, since patients requiring circulatory support are precisely those in whom reoperation under general anesthesia would almost certainly impose significant added risk.

The editors and their colleagues have developed a simple left heart assist device (LHAD) that can be conveniently deployed in patients with severe postcardiotomy left ventricular dysfunction, unresponsive to conventional support measures including IABC, and who could not be separated from cardiopulmonary bypass. The device permits rapid establishment of partial left ventricular (left atrium-ascending aorta) bypass by means of specially designed cannulae positioned in the left atrium and ascending aorta and an extracorporeal roller pump system. With improved cardiac performance, separation from the device and termination of left ventricular support can be readily accomplished without need for thoracic reentry. This is made possible by the use of precisely fitting obturators that obliterate the cannular lumina and allow the tubes to remain permanently implanted. Design, development, and early clinical use of the LHAD have been described previously

(Litwak et al., 1973, 1974, 1976).

The physiologic basis and criteria for LHAD deployment are discussed in Chapter 9. Procedural details concerning deployment of the device and subsequent management will be summarized in this section.

Deployment of the LHAD. The decision to institute partial left ventricular bypass support is based on objective evidence of such inadequate cardiac performance after intracardiac operation that conventional cardiopulmonary bypass cannot be discontinued despite maximal supportive therapy. Once this decision is reached, total cardiopulmonary bypass is reestablished. If the left atrial pressure remains elevated (≥15 mm Hg), left ventricular sump drainage is resumed and regulated to maintain left atrial pressure of 10 to 15 mm Hg.

INSERTION OF LHAD CANNULAE. Each cannula is prepared for insertion by circumferential placement of 8 to 10 horizontal double-armed mattress sutures of 3-0 polyester in the proximal sewing skirt. The atrial cannula is inserted through a 1.8 cm left atrial incision adjacent to the interatrial sulcus. In most instances, this can be accomplished through the usual left ventricular sump insertion site, which can readily be enlarged. The sutures are passed through the full thickness of the atrial wall and the cannula is positioned so that the proximal skirt lies on the endocardial surface of the atrium. The sutures are then passed through the distal skirt and tied, thereby sandwiching the atrial wall between the sewing skirts.

A similar technique is followed in the insertion of the aortic cannula, which must be positioned on the *right lateral* wall of the ascending aorta to avoid possible compression when the sternum is closed. Aortic cannula insertion is accomplished either by partial exclusion of the aortic wall or by temporarily occluding the aorta. The latter method is less desirable and must be avoided whenever possible. However, if multiple coronary artery bypass grafts, aortic valve replacement, or both have been performed, it may be necessary to occlude the ascending aorta briefly so that cannula insertion can be precisely accomplished without traumatizing adjacent suture lines.

PREPARATION OF EXTRACORPOREAL CIRCUIT AND CONNECTIONS TO CANNULA. The extracorporeal pump and tubing components of the LHAD are readied for use and primed with perfusate withdrawn from the cardiopulmonary bypass circuit, while the atrial and aortic cannulae are being implanted. Perfusate is slowly recirculated through the extracorporeal loop enough times to remove all microbubbles from the system.

The cannular connections to the extracorporeal circuit must be situated so that both cannulae and their respective metal connectors remain wholly intracorporeal; none of these components should traverse the skin. This is accomplished by connecting both cannulae to short lengths of polyvinyl chloride (PVC) tubing using 6.4 × 6.4 cm straight stainless steel connectors. The firm gripping quality of the PVC tubing allows two thirds the length of each connector to be occupied by more slippery LHAD (silicone elastomer) cannulae, while only one third of the connector length is needed for the PVC attachment. The connections are secured with No. 5 Tevdek ligatures.

The two PVC tubing lengths are passed through the full thickness of the rectus abdominis muscle in the right upper abdomen and made to traverse a subcutaneous tunnel before the skin is crossed at their respective points of exit. The subcutaneous tunnel must be long enough to permit an intracorporeal location of at least the distal 7.5 cm of the cannular tips, the metal connectors, and at least 8 to 10 cm of the PVC tubing. This is facilitated by using a 32F trocar catheter* to traverse the entire thickness of the rectus muscle and a varying distance of the subcutaneous fat. After the rectus is traversed, subcutaneous tunneling is continued for an addi-

---

*Argyle trochar catheter, Sherwood Medical Industries, St. Louis, M.

tional 6 to 8 cm. The skin is then punctured, a portion of the trocar catheter is delivered across the skin, and the trocar is withdrawn. The proximal fluted end of the catheter (still within the mediastinum) allows "press-fit" insertion of the PVC tubing, which is now drawn to the tunnel.

This procedure is followed for both cannula connections. Separate exit tunnels are made for each of the two PVC tubing lengths and securely anchored to the skin. When properly positioned, both LHAD cannulae remain intracorporeal with their distal tips under the skin in the right upper abdomen.

The cannulae and PVC tubing lengths are allowed to fill up with blood. The PVC tubing lengths are connected to the appropriate segments of the previously primed extracorporeal circuit with stainless steel connectors with stopcocks. Air bubbles remaining in the LHAD circuit are meticulously removed and the system is ready to operate.

LHAD Management in the Operating Room

ESTABLISHMENT OF SUPPORT. Before partial left ventricular bypass support with the LHAD is initiated, a number of vital technical maneuvers must be executed to prevent air embolism. Since air bubbles can be sucked into the system at the left atrial cannulation site as the LHAD flow rate is increased and the left atrial pressure falls, the pericardial sac must be flooded with physiologic irrigating solution to constantly maintain a fluid level over the left atrial cannulation site. It is also helpful to tilt the operating table so that the patient's left side is slightly elevated, thereby insuring constant "flooding" of the atrial cannulation site. The intravascular volume is adjusted to maintain a left atrial pressure of around 15 mm Hg before LHAD support is begun.

The LHAD flow rate is slowly increased while the conventional cardiopulmonary bypass flow rate is correspondingly reduced. Initially, adjustments in flow rates of the two systems are guided solely by measurements of arterial pressure and ventricular filling pressures. As the LHAD flow rate is increased, the left atrial pressure may tend to fall rapidly. At this point, it is convenient to volume load the patient from the regular pump-oxygenator circuit. It is advisable to maintain the left atrial pressure above 10 mm Hg to avoid the potential of aspirating air should an adequate fluid level at the left atrial cannulation site fail to be properly maintained.

Once hemodynamic stability has been maintained, conventional cardiopulmonary bypass is discontinued and the regular cannulae are removed. The heparin effect is partially reversed with protamine sulfate (1 mg/kg). This generally allows hemostasis to be established while the LHAD continues to function.

ADDITIONAL OPERATING ROOM MEASURES. After termination of cardiopulmonary bypass, one would normally aim for complete or near-complete reversal of the heparin effect to restore satisfactory hemostatic capability. However, in patients requiring LHAD support, it is necessary to maintain modest levels of heparin to avoid thromboembolic complications. Measurements of the whole-blood activated coagulation time (ACT) allow rapid repetitive estimations of residual heparin activity. An ACT between 110 and 140 seconds (particulate-activated method) is satisfactory. After prolonged periods of cardiopulmonary bypass, it is frequently necessary to administer additional doses of protamine (0.25 to 0.5 mg/kg) to reduce heparin activity to desired levels.

If a hemostatic check of a deeply situated anatomic structure or suture line becomes necessary, it is advisable to momentarily turn the LHAD *completely* off and clear the pericardial sac of irrigating fluid and blood before examining the area in question. The pericardial sac may then be promptly refilled with irrigating solution, and only then is LHAD assistance reinstituted. The thoracic drainage catheters should remain clamped until sternal closure is completed. Again, prevention of air embolism is one of the major concerns.

At operative termination, antibiotic ointment (bacitracin or povidone-iodine) is applied around the skin exit sites of the LHAD tubing followed by an occlusive dressing. The patient is moved to the intensive care unit with the LHAD operating on battery power.

Thus, manipulation of left ventricular filling pressures and the LHAD flow rate permit maintenance of adequate levels of systemic blood flow. Not infrequently, however, concomitant right ventricular dysfunction may limit one's ability to make these manipulations.

LHAD Management in the Intensive Care Unit

HEPARIN ADMINISTRATION. It is necessary to maintain modest levels of anticoagulation (ACT between 110 and 140 seconds). This is accomplished by continuous administration of heparin (3 to 10 IU/kg/hr) by intravenous infusion drip.

ADJUSTMENT OF LHAD FLOW RATE. Logical decisions regarding adjustment of the LHAD flow rate are made possible by knowledge of total systemic blood flow, which is equivalent to pulmonary blood flow ($\dot{Q}_T = \dot{Q}_P$). Pulmonary blood flow is readily measured by the thermodilution method using a thermistor catheter positioned in the pulmonary artery and an analog computer. Since total systemic blood flow is the *sum of LV output and LHAD flow,* regulation of the LHAD flow rate becomes a simple matter. Manipulations of volume filling and LHAD flow rate allow easy maintenance of total systemic blood flow at or above 2.5 liters/min/m² and mean left atrial pressure below 20 mm Hg. Satisfactory urine output and hyperosmolality (relative to plasma) as well as absence of metabolic acidosis provide clinical evidence of adequate systemic blood flow.

MONITORING HEMATOLOGIC FUNCTION. Close surveillance of hematologic function is essential, especially if high bypass flow rates and prolonged support are required. A complete blood count and coagulation profile (prothrombin time, partial thromboplastin time, platelet count, fibrinogen, fibrin-split products) are obtained daily. Tests to estimate hemolytic rates (bilirubin, plasma hemoglobin, serum haptoglobins) are likewise necessary.

CARE OF THE EXTRACORPOREAL COMPONENTS OF THE LHAD. As soon as hemodynamic stability is achieved, partial side-to-side turning of the patient is permissible. The perfusionist in attendance must see to it that no kinking of the extracorporeal tubing components occurs. To minimize wear and possible tubing rupture, the pump head tubing is periodically lubricated with mineral oil. Use of a 1.20-m tubing length also allows shifting of the segment in the pump head every 72 to 96 hours.

CRITERIA FOR LHAD DISCONTINUANCE. The decision to wean the patient from LHAD support is based on objective evidence of a: (1) stable and adequate cardiac performance—total systemic blood flow at or above 2.5 liters/min/m² at left atrial pressures below 20 mm Hg; and (2) steadily increasing left ventricular contribution to total systemic blood flow. Left ventricular contribution to total systemic blood flow can easily be calculated using the formula:

$$\text{Percent LV contribution to TSBF} = \frac{\text{TSBF} - \text{LHAD flow}}{\text{TSBF}} \times 100$$

where,
LV = left ventricular
TSBF = total systemic blood flow.

As the left ventricular contribution to total systemic blood flow rises (in the presence of adequate systemic blood flow and satisfactory levels of left atrial pressure), the LHAD flow rate is gradually reduced. When cardiac performance has improved so that left ventricular contribution to total systemic blood flow is 90 percent or more, LHAD support is terminated, provided that total systemic blood flow is adequate and the left atrial pressure is stabilized at satisfactory levels. During weaning from LHAD assistance, it is advisable to continue all other supportive measures, unless dramatic improvements in cardiac performance occur that allow discontinuance of other therapy.

DISCONTINUANCE MEASURES. As the LHAD flow rate is brought to low levels (i.e., below 1,000 ml/mm), the potential for thromboembolic complications is heightened due to reduced blood flow velocity and prolonged residence time within the circuit. Under these conditions, it is advisable to administer additional heparin so that the ACT rises to between 160 and 200 seconds.

Separation from the LHAD is carried out at the bedside under strict aseptic conditions. The patient is lightly sedated and all chest and abdominal dressings are removed. The afferent and efferent limbs of the LHAD circuit are exposed. The chest and abdomen, including the adjacent tubing, are thoroughly scrubbed with an iodophor-detergent compound, and the area is dried and finally prepared with iodophor alone. After the patient is draped, the distal cannula tips are exposed through a small right upper quadrant incision (4 to 6 cm inferior and oblique to the costal margin) under local infiltration anesthesia. The location of the incision is determined by palpation of the two cannula-to-PVC connectors that are situated subcutaneously.

Once both cannula tips are exposed, the LHAD is turned off and the cannulae are clamped and disconnected from the PVC tubing. The extracorporeal components can now be withdrawn from the operative field by the pump technician. Each cannula is filled with saline and the obturators are inserted, care being taken to avoid entrapment of air. With the aortic obturator, this hazard is minimal because of the systemic arterial pressure. On the other hand, the relatively low left atrial pressure presents a greater potential for entrapping or sucking in air when the atrial obturator is inserted. It is helpful to momentarily maintain a positive intrabronchial pressure during insertion of the atrial obturator. The obturators are inserted in such a way that the bias-cut hub of each one is accurately fitted against the distal angulated edge of the cannula. Each mated obturator and cannula is secured with two ligatures of No. 5 Tevdek, and the junction is sealed by overlaying medical-grade silicone adhesive.* Both obturated cannulae are then replaced in the subcutaneous position.

The operative area is irrigated with bacitracin-neomycin solution† and a Hemovac drain‡ is inserted (to be removed after 24 hours). The incision is closed. The skin edges where the PVC tubing entered and exited are then debrided and sutured.

If IABC has been employed in conjunction with the LHAD, it is generally continued as a supportive measure after LHAD discontinuance.

Mechanical Support of the Failing Right Ventricle

Because life-threatening low cardiac output secondary to acute right ventricular failure is relatively rare, as a primary clinical entity it has not aroused a great deal of interest. Clinical recognition of the condition is often difficult and its presence is frequently masked by signs of left ventricular failure. When it develops, the prognosis is generally poor because available supportive measures are either insufficient or inefficient. Moreover, application of appropriate therapy is frequently delayed.

The conditions most commonly associated with acute right ventricular failure include: (1) massive pulmonary embolism; (2) right ventricular infarction; and (3) postcardiotomy right ventricular dysfunction (in the absence of infarction), frequently superimposed on a background of significant pulmonary vascular disease with severe resistive pulmonary hypertension. As with acute left ventricular power failure, the principal pathogenetic mechanisms responsible for the development of acute right ventricular failure are impaired myocardial contractility (with or without loss of contractile mass), marked increase in right

---

*Dow Corning Corp, Midland, Mich.

†Upjohn Co., Kalamazoo, Mich.
‡Zimmer, Warsaw, Ind.

ventricular afterload, or both. However, the prognostic implications may be graver since conventional therapeutic measures are generally not effective in reducing impedance to right ventricular ejection and most circulatory assist devices have been designed for the systemic circulation.

Rationale. The use of mechanical circulatory assistance in acute right ventricular failure devolves from a number of experimental and clinical observations suggesting that venoarterial bypass over a few hours or days is an effective means of circulatory support in this setting. Connolly et al. (1958) reported that venoarterial bypass (without an oxygenator in the circuit) was effective in relieving right ventricular failure and improving cardiac output in experimental animals in whom acute right ventricular failure was produced by pulmonary artery constriction. In the early 1970s, a number of investigators reported the efficacy of extracorporeal membrane oxygenation (ECMO) as a method of providing *both* respiratory and circulatory support in patients with cardiopulmonary failure (Lande et al., 1970; Hill et al., 1972; Zapol et al., 1972; Bartlett et al., 1974). More recently, Jardin et al. (1978) reported survival after venoarterial bypass support (with membrane lung oxygenation) in a patient with massive pulmonary embolism, acute pulmonary hypertension, and shock. After 60 hours of bypass support the patient was successfully weaned from circulatory assistance; no surgical embolectomy was necessary, as the embolus lysed.

Our own experience (Jurado et al., 1979) provides further corroboration of these observations. Two patients with advanced rheumatic mitral valvular disease and severe resistive pulmonary hypertension who developed life-threatening low cardiac output after mitral valve replacement were successfully managed with venoarterial bypass support (60 and 84 hours). In both instances, conventional therapeutic measures had failed to bring about hemodynamic and metabolic stability before employment of mechanical circulatory assistance.

From the foregoing, it would appear that there is ample evidence that venoarterial (usually femorofemoral) bypass is indeed an effective—yet relatively simple—means of providing temporary mechanical support to a failing right ventricle. The employment of this technique of support is based on the hypothesis that partial right ventricular bypass over a period of hours to days would allow a functionally depressed myocardium time to recover while providing sufficient systemic blood flow to satisfy metabolic requirements.

In acute right ventricular failure, the right ventricular output (pulmonary blood flow) is decreased because of poor right ventricular ejection capability or increased pulmonary vascular resistance (afterload) or both. Under these adverse conditions, venoarterial bypass provides a means of optimizing preload and reducing right ventricular wall tension, while augmenting total systemic blood flow by rerouting a fraction of the systemic venous return extracorporeally around the lungs into the aorta. If an oxygenator is used in the bypass circuit, a system for supplementary gas exchange also is provided. Thus, systemic arterial desaturation is prevented even if there is coexisting respiratory dysfunction or high bypass flow rates are mandated by the need to maintain hemodynamic stability.

Employment of Venoarterial Bypass Support.
Acute right ventricular failure with life-threatening low cardiac output is the prime indication for mechanical circulatory assistance. The clinical picture of acute *right* ventricular power failure has many of the features of acute *left* ventricular failure. For instance, systemic hypotension (systolic arterial pressure <80 mm Hg) and many of the signs of reduced systemic blood flow (disorientation, oliguria, metabolic acidosis, cardiac index ≤1.8 liters/min/m^2) are present. The main distinguishing feature is that in acute right heart failure, right ventricular filling pressures are significantly elevated. Right atrial pressures are increased (≥20 mm Hg), while left atrial pressures are usually normal

or only mildly elevated. Pulmonary vascular resistance is frequently increased. If left ventricular failure also is present, *both* right and left atrial pressures will be elevated and the resultant hemodynamic picture may be difficult to distinguish from that of cardiac tamponade.

Conventional therapy for acute right ventricular failure normally includes administration of positive inotropic agents, optimization of preload and heart rate, and control of arrhythmias. The ability to control impedance to right ventricular ejection is limited because of the unpredictable response of the pulmonary vasculature to currently available vasodilators. Failure of these measures to achieve stabilization is taken to indicate that life-threatening cardiac dysfunction is present and mechanical circulatory assistance (venoarterial bypass support) is deployed.

PATIENT AND EQUIPMENT PREPARATION. To establish circulatory support, the femoral vessels are adequate access points. The groin and genitals are prepared; in the postcardiotomy patient this will have been done beforehand. Cannulation and initiation of support can easily be carried out in an ICU setting provided conditions of strict sterility are maintained. Adequate anesthesia usually can be achieved with local infiltration techniques, although light sedation may be required in patients who are wide awake. A urethral catheter is inserted, if this has not been done before.

The basic equipment required for establishment of right ventricular support includes two roller pumps (one arterial and one venous or recirculating pump), disposable membrane oxygenator with arterial and venous reservoirs, and a heat exchanger (Fig. 21-11). The ICU bed is elevated on shock blocks to facilitate venous drainage during bypass support. An ample length of extracorporeal tubing loop (venous side tubing length of approximately 2.0 m) to permit ample bed elevation and patient turning.

TECHNICAL CONSIDERATIONS. A vertical groin incision is preferred because it provides a better lie for the cannulae. Perfect hemostasis is ensured by liberal use of electrocautery and ligatures; this is mandatory because heparin anticoagulation and the thrombocytopenia attendant to prolonged bypass support will cause bleeding from the wound. To prevent edema and gangrene, the artery and vein should be cannulated proximally and distally (Fig. 21-12). A transverse arteriotomy and venotomy are preferable. To facilitate cannulation, the incision is carried to encompass three fourths the circumference of the vessels. Cannula sizes are dictated largely by the caliber of the vessels; a useful rule of thumb is to insert the largest cannulae that the vessels will safely accommodate.

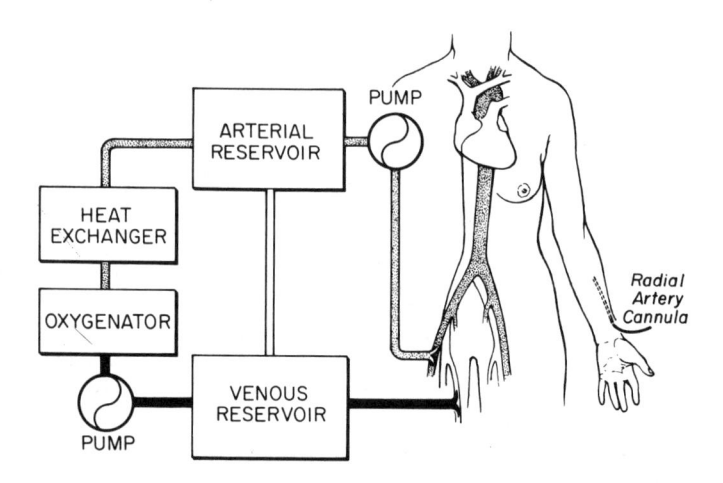

Figure 21-11. Schematic representation of a peripheral venoarterial bypass system used for postoperative support of a failing right ventricle.

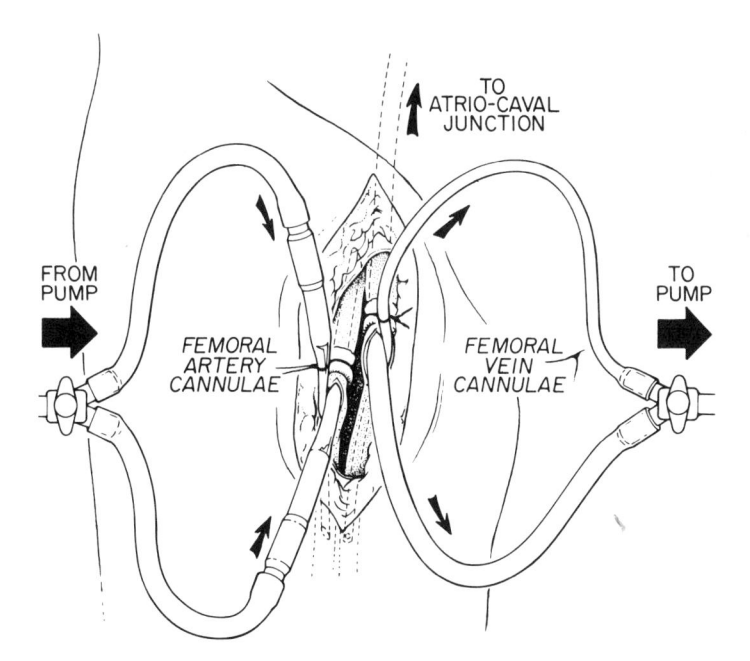

SPECIAL TECHNIQUES EMPLOYED IN THE INTENSIVE CARE UNIT

Figure 21-12. Technical details of venous and arterial cannulation. Note that both artery and vein are cannulated proximally and distally to maintain limb viability and prevent edema during prolonged support.

The cannulae are securely anchored and the wound is closed around the cannulae. Antibiotic ointment is applied at the points of cannula entry and exit and an occlusive dressing is used. Systemic antibiotics are mandatory.

The cannulae are now connected to the previously primed extracorporeal circuit.

INITIATION OF BYPASS SUPPORT. Circulatory assistance can be begun soon after the appropriate cannula connections are made. The bypass flow rate is gradually increased until satisfactory systemic arterial and right heart pressures are achieved. Further adjustments in flow rate are made after measurements of pulmonary blood flow are available (see Adjustment of Bypass Flow Rate).

ANTICOAGULATION. If heparin has not been given previously, systemic heparinization (200 IU/kg) is established before cannula insertion. During bypass support, heparin is administered continuously by infusion pump into a central vein or the extracorporeal circuit and titrated to maintain the ACT between 160 and 180 seconds. During weaning from support, as the bypass flow rate is reduced, additional heparin is administered (ACT between 180 and 200 seconds) to prevent clotting in the extracorporeal circuit from the reduced flow velocity and increased residence time within the extracorporeal circuit.

Hematologic function is carefully monitored with daily complete blood counts and assessment of the coagulation profile. It is helpful if frequent measurements of plasma hemoglobin and serum haptoglobins are taken, especially in patients requiring prolonged support.

ADJUSTMENT OF BYPASS FLOW RATE. Decisions about flow rate adjustments can be made from frequent measurements of pulmonary blood flow and right ventricular filling pressures. The object of therapy is to achieve levels of total systemic blood flow sufficient to maintain hemodynamic and metabolic stability at right ventricular filling pressures that are acceptable. Ideally, total systemic blood flow must be maintained at or above 2.5 liters/min/m^2 and right atrial pressures below 20 mm Hg. Absence of metabolic acidosis as well as a satisfactory urine output and hyperosmolality (relative to plasma) provide evidence of adequacy of total systemic blood flow.

Under conditions of femorofemoral venoarterial bypass, estimations of right ventricular output (pulmonary blood) may be made using one of two indicator-dilution methods. If the thermodilution method is employed, it is necessary to use a specially constructed thermodilution catheter that allows right ventricular injection of the thermal indicator so that none of it is lost into the bypass circuit during the measurement (Fig. 21-13). If the dye-dilution method is used, injection of the indocyanine green can be done through a pulmonary artery catheter with sampling via the radial artery. However, if the pulmonary blood flow (i.e., left ventricular output) is extremely low, mixing of central aortic blood with the returned pump-oxygenator blood will take place high up in the aorta at or above the takeoff of the brachiocephalic branches. Admixture of dye-containing with nondye-containing blood renders the measurement invalid. Thus, careful planning of the injection and sampling sites is necessary.

Total systemic blood flow is the *sum* of bypass and pulmonary blood flow. Pulmonary blood flow is equivalent to the right ventricular output, making the right ventricular contribution to total systemic blood flow easily calculated.

CRITERIA FOR DISCONTINUANCE OF SUPPORT. The criteria for weaning from venoarterial bypass support are similar to those followed for left ventricular assistance. Weaning is begun when there is clinical and hemodynamic evidence of a stable and adequate cardiac performance, with a steadily increasing right ventricular contribution to total systemic blood flow.

Bypass support is discontinued when right ventricular contribution to total systemic blood flow is 90 percent or more, provided total systemic blood flow is adequate (CI = 2.5 liters/min/m^2) and right atrial pressure is stable (<20 mm Hg).

DECANNULATION. This is generally done under local infiltration anesthesia. After removal of the proximal and distal cannulae,

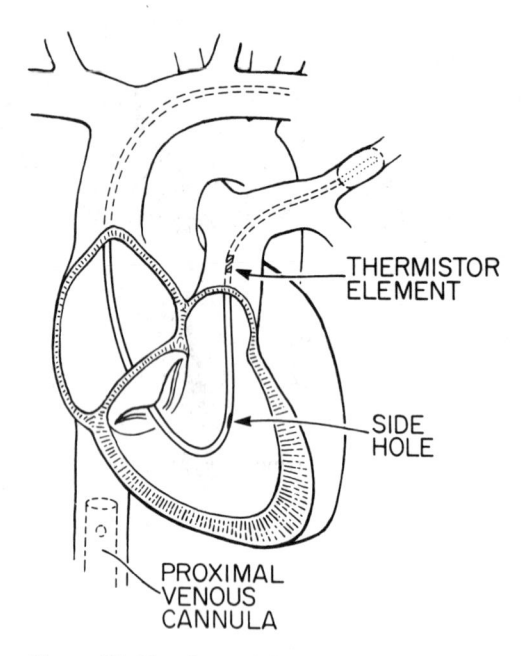

Figure 21–13. A specially configured thermistor-bearing, balloon-tipped, flow-directed catheter permits injection of thermal indicator into the right ventricle instead of the right atrium, and obviates loss of indicator into the bypass circuit during cardiac output measurements.

simple closure of the transverse vessel incisions accomplishes arterial and venous repair. Sometimes a vein patch graft repair of the femoral artery may be necessary. The wound is carefully debrided to provide clean and healthy tissue for primary closure.

REFERENCES

Abernathy WS: Complete heart block caused by the Swan-Ganz catheter. Chest 65:349, 1974.

Alpert JS, Dexter L: Blood flow measurement: the cardiac output. In Grossman W (ed): Cardiac Catheterization and Angiography. Philadelphia, Lea & Febiger, 1974.

Baird RJ, LaBrosse CJ, Lajos TZ, Thomas GW: Effects of a selective bypass of the left ventricle. Circulation 27:835, 1963.

Barratt-Boyes BG, Wood EH: Cardiac output and related measurements and pressure values in the right heart and associated vessels, together with an analysis of the hemodynamic response to the inhalation of high oxygen mixtures in healthy subjects. J Lab Clin Med 51:72, 1958.

Bartlett RH, Gazzanigia AB, Fong SW, Burns NE: Prolonged extracorporeal cardiopulmonary support in man. J Thorac Cardiovasc Surg 68:918, 1974.

Berger RL, Saini VK, Ryan TJ, Sokol DM, Keefe JF: Intra-aortic balloon assist for postcardiotomy cardiogenic shock. J Thorac Cardiovasc Surg 66:906, 1973.

——, Weisel RD, Vito L, Dennis RC, Hechtman HB: Cardiac output measurement by thermodilution during cardiac operations. Ann Thorac Surg 21:43, 1976.

Brandfonbrener M, Landowne M, Shock NW: Changes in cardiac output with age. Circulation 12:557, 1955.

Braunwald E, Covell JW, Maroke PR, Ross J: Effect of drugs and counterpulsation on myocardial oxygen consumption. Circulation 39, 40:IV-220, 1970.

Bregman D: Mechanical support of the failing circulation. Curr Prob Surg 13 (12): 1, 1976.

——, Bailin M, Bowman FO Jr, Parodi EN, Haubert SM, Edie RN, Spotnitz HM, Reemtsma K, Malm JR: A pulsatile assist device (PAD) for use during cardiopulmonary bypass. Ann Thorac Surg 24:574, 1977.

——, Goetz RH: Clinical experience with a new cardiac assist device—the dual-chambered intraaortic balloon assist. J Thorac Cardiovasc Surg 62:577, 1971.

——, Kripke DC, Cohen MN, Laniadu S, Goetz RH: Clinical experience with the uni-directional dual-chambered intra-aortic balloon assist. Circulation 43 (Suppl 1):82, 1971.

——, ——, Goetz RH: The effect of synchronous unidirectional intraaortic balloon pumping on hemodynamics and coronary blood flow in cardiogenic shock. Trans Am Soc Artif Intern Organs 16:439, 1970.

——, Parodi EN, Edie RN, Bowman FO Jr, Reemtsma K, Malm JR: Intraoperative unidirectional intra-aortic balloon pumping in the management of left ventricular power failure. J Thorac Cardiovasc Surg 70:1010, 1975.

Brown BG, Goldfarb D, Topaz SR, Gott VL: Diastolic augmentation by intra-aortic balloon. J Thorac Cardiovasc Surg 53:789, 1967.

Buckley MJ, Craver JM, Gold HK, Mundth ED, Daggett WM, Austen WG: Intraaortic balloon pump assist for cardiogenic shock after cardiopulmonary bypass. Circulation 48 (Suppl 3):90, 1973a.

——, Leinbach RC, Kastor JA, Laird JD, Kantrowitz AR, Madras PN, Sanders CA, Austen WG: Hemodynamic evaluation of intra-aortic balloon pumping in man. Circulation 41 (Suppl 2):130, 1970.

——, Mundth ED, Daggett WM, Gold HK, Leinbach RC, Austen WG: Surgical management of ventricular septal defects and mitral regurgitation complicating acute myocardial infarction. Ann Thorac Surg 16:598, 1973b.

Cappelletti RR, Reynolds BM: Left ventricular bypass support during surgical operations. Ann Surg 165:402, 1967.

Cerra F, Milch R, Lajos TZ: Pulmonary artery catheterization in critically ill surgical patients. Ann Surg 177:37, 1973.

Chun GMH, Ellestad MH: Perforation of the pulmonary artery by a Swan-Ganz catheter. N Engl J Med 284:1041, 1971.

Civetta JM, Gabel JC, Laver MB: Disparate ventricular function in surgical patients. Surg Forum 22:136, 1971.

Clauss RH, Birtwell WC, Albertal G, Lunzer S, Taylot WJ, Fosberg AM, Harken DE: Assisted circulation. I. The arterial counterpulsator. J Thorac Cardiovasc Surg 41:447, 1961.

Cohn JN, Tristane FE, Khatri IM: Studies in clinical shock and hypotension. VI. Relationship between right and left ventricular function. J Clin Invest 48:2008, 1969.

Connolly JE, Bacaner MB, Bruns EL, Lowenstein JM, Storli E: Mechanical support of the failing circulation in acute heart failure. Surgery 44:255, 1958.

Cross KW, Dawes GS, Mott JC: Cardiac output in the cat; a comparison between the Fick method and a radioactive indicator dilution method. J Physiol 136:240, 1957.

DeBakey ME: Left ventricular bypass pump for cardiac assistance: clinical experience. Am J Cardiol 27:3, 1971.

Dennis C, Carlens E, Senning A, Hall DP, Moreno JR, Cappelletti RR, Wesolowski SA: Clinical use of a cannula for left heart bypass without thoracotomy: experimental protection against fibrillation by left heart bypass. Ann Surg 156:623, 1962.

Dubois D, Dubois EF: A height-weight formula to estimate the surface area of man. Proc Soc Exp Biol NY 13:77, 1916.

Dunkman WB, Leinbach RC, Buckley MJ, Mundth ED, Kantrowitz AR, Austen NG, Sanders CA:

Clinical and hemodynamic results of intra-aortic balloon pumping and surgery for cardiogenic shock. Circulation 46:465, 1972.

Eliasch H, Lagerlöf H, Bucht H, Ek J, Eriksson K, Bergström J, Werkö L: Comparison of the dye-dilution and the direct Fick methods for the measurement of cardiac output in man. Scand J Clin Lab Invest 7 (Suppl 20):73, 1955.

Evonuk E, Imig CJ, Greenfield W, Eckstein JW: Cardiac output measured by thermaldilution of room temperature injectate. J Appl Physiol 16 (2):271, 1961.

Fegler G: Measurement of cardiac output in anaesthetized animals by a thermo-dilution method. J Exp Physiol 39:153, 1954.

Fitzpatrick GF, Hampson LG, Burgess JH: Bedside determination of left atrial pressure. Can Med Assoc J 106:1293, 1972.

Foote GA, Schabel SI, Hodges M: Pulmonary complications of the flow-directed balloon-tipped catheter. N Engl J Med 290:927, 1974.

Forrester JS, Diamond G, Ganz W, Danzig R, Swan HJC: Right and left heart pressures in the acutely ill patient. Clin Res 18:306, 1970.

———, ———, McHugh TJ, Swan HJC: Filling pressures in the right and left sides of the heart in acute myocardial infarction: a reappraisal of central-venous-pressure monitoring. N Engl J Med 285:190, 1971.

———, Ganz W, Diamond G, McHugh T, Chonette DE, Swan HJC: Thermodilution cardiac output determination with a single flow-directed catheter. Am Heart J 83:306, 1972.

Ganz W, Danoso R, Marcus HS, Forrester JS, Swan HJC: A new technique for measurement of cardiac output by thermodilution in man. Am J Cardiol 27:392, 1971.

———, Swan HJC: Measurement of blood flow by thermodilution. Am J Cardiol 29:241, 1972.

Geha DG, Davis NJ, Lappas DG: Persistent atrial arrhythmias associated with placement of a Swan-Ganz catheter. Anesthesiology 39:651, 1973.

Glassman E, Engelman RM, Boyd AD, Lipson D, Ackerman B, Spencer FC: A method of closed chest cannulation of the left atrium for left atrial-femoral artery bypass. J Thorac Cardiovasc Surg 69:283, 1975.

Gold HK, Leinbach RC, Sanders CA, Buckley MJ, Mundth ED, Austen WG: Intraaortic balloon pumping for control of recurrent myocardial ischemia. Circulation 47:1197, 1973.

Golden MS, Pinder T Jr, Anderson WT, Cheitlin MD: Fatal pulmonary hemorrhage complicating use of a flow-directed balloon-tipped catheter in a patient receiving anticoagulant therapy. Am J Cardiol 32:865, 1973.

Goodyer AVN, Huvos A, Eckhardt WF, Ostberg RH: Thermodilution curves in the intact animal. Circ Res 7:432, 1959.

Greene JF Jr, Cummings KC: Aseptic thrombotic endocardial vegetations: a complication of indwelling pulmonary artery catheter. JAMA 225:1525, 1973.

———, Fitzwater JE, Clemmer TP: Septic endocarditis and indwelling pulmonary artery catheters. JAMA 233:891, 1975.

Guyton AC, Jones CE, Coleman TG: Circulatory Physiology: Cardiac Output and Its Regulation. Philadelphia, Saunders, 1973, pp 21–134.

Hamilton WF, Moore JW, Kinsman JM, Spurling RG: Studies on the circulation. IV. Further analysis of the injection method, and of changes in hemodynamics under physiological and pathological conditions. Am J Physiol 99:534, 1932.

———, Riley RL, Attyah AM, Cournand A, Fowell CM, Himmelstein A, Noble RP, Remington JW, Richards DW Jr, Wheeler NC, Witham AC: Comparison of Fick and dye injection methods of measuring cardiac output in man. Am J Physiol 153:309, 1948.

Hattersley PG: Activated coagulation time of blood. JAMA 196:150, 1966.

Hill JD, de Leval MR, Fallat RJ, Branson ML, Eberhart RC, Schulte HD, Osborn JJ, Barber J, Gerbode F: Acute respiratory insufficiency. Treatment with prolonged extracorporeal oxygenation. J Thorac Cardiovasc Surg 64:551, 1972.

Hosie KF: Thermal-dilution technics. Circ Res 10:491, 1962.

Howell CD, Horvath SM: Reproducibility of cardiac output measurements in the dog. J Appl Physiol 14:421, 1959.

Huggins RA, Smith EL, Sinclair MA: Comparison between the cardiac output measured with a rotameter and output determined by the direct Fick method in open-chest dogs. Am J Physiol 160:183, 1950.

Jacobey JA, Taylor MJ, Smith GT, Gorlin R, Harken DE: A new therapeutic approach to acute coronary occlusion. II. Opening dormant coronary collaterals by counterpulsation. Am J Cardiol 11:218, 1963.

Jardin F, Gurdjian F, Blanchet F, Margairaz A: Massive pulmonary embolism with circulatory failure. Survival following sixty hours' support with a membrane lung. J Thorac Cardiovasc Surg 76:252, 1978.

Jurado RA, Estioko MR, Mindich BP, Benis AM, Kuhn LA, Mitchell BA, Litwak RS: Mechanical circulatory support of postcardiotomy low cardiac output accompanying severe resistive pulmonary hypertension. Presented at the New York Thoracic Society, Fall Session, 1979.

———, Matucha D, Osborn JJ: Cardiac output estimation by pulse contour methods: validity of their use for monitoring the critically ill patient. Surgery 74:358, 1973.

Kantrowitz A, Tjonneland S, Krakauer JS, Philips SJ, Freed PS, Butner AN: Mechanical intraaortic cardiac assistance in cardiogenic shock. Hemodynamic effects. Arch Surg 97:1000, 1968.

Kleiber M: Body size and metabolic rate. Physiol Rev 27:511, 1947.

Kolff WJ, Lawson J: Status of the artificial heart and cardiac assist devices in the United States. Trans Am Soc Artif Intern Organs 21:620, 1975.

Krause AH Jr, Bigelow JC, Page US: Transthoracic intraaortic balloon cannulation to avoid repeat sternotomy for removal. Ann Thor Surg 21:562, 1976.

Laird JD, Madras PN, Jones RT, Kantrowitz AR, Kothari ML, Buckley MJ, Austen WG: Theoretical and experimental analysis of the intraaortic balloon pump. Trans Am Soc Artif Intern Organs 14:338, 1968.

Lande AJ, Edwards L, Bloch JH, Carlson RG, Subramanian VS, Ascheim RS, Scheidt S, Fillmore S, Killip T, Lillelei CW: Prolonged cardiopulmonary support with a practical membrane oxygenator. Trans Am Soc Artif Intern Organs 16:352, 1970.

Lapin ES, Murray JA: Hemoptysis with flow-directed cardiac catheterization. JAMA 220:1246, 1972.

Lappas DG, Lell WA, Gabel JC, Civetta JM, Lowenstein E: Indirect measurement of left atrial pressure in surgical patients—pulmonary capillary wedge and pulmonary-artery diastolic pressures compared with left-atrial pressure. Anesthesiology 38:394, 1973.

Lefemine AA, Low HBC, Cohen NL, Lunzer S, Harken DE: Assisted circulation. III. The effect of synchronized arterial counterpulsation or myocardial oxygen consumption and coronary flow. Am Heart J 64:789, 1962.

Leighton RF, Czekajewski J: Use of a new cardiac output computer for human hemodynamic studies. J Appl Physiol 30:914, 1971.

Leinbach RC, Buckley MJ, Austen WG, Petschek HE, Kantrowitz AR, Sanders CA: Effects of intra-aortic balloon pumping on coronary flow and metabolism in man. Circulation 43, 44 (Suppl 1): I–77, 1971.

Lemen R, Jones JG, Cowan G: A mechanism of pulmonary artery perforation by Swan-Ganz catheter. N Engl J Med 292:211, 1975.

Lipp H, O'Donoghue K, Kesnekov L: Intracardiac knotting of a flow-directed balloon catheter. N Engl J Med 284:220, 1971.

Litwak RS, Koffsky RM, Jurado RA, Lukban SB, Ortiz AF Jr, Fischer AP, Sherman JJ, Silvay G, Lajam FA: Use of a left heart assist device after intracardiac surgery: technique and clinical experience. Ann Thorac Surg 21:191, 1976.

———, ———, Lukban SB, Jurado RA, Elster SK, Lajam FA, Brancato RW: Implanted heart assist device after intracardiac surgery. N Engl J Med 291:1341, 1974.

———, Lajam FA, Koffsky RM, Silvay G, Shiang H, Geller SA, Pederson FS: Obturated permanent left atrial and aortic cannulae for assisted circulation after cardiac surgery. Trans Am Soc Artif Intern Organs 19:243, 1973.

Lozman J, Powers SR Jr, Older T, Dutton RE, Roy RJ, English M, Marco D, Eckert C: Correlation of pulmonary wedge and left atrial pressures. A study in the patient receiving positive end expiratory pressure ventilation. Arch Surg 109:270, 1974.

Maroko PR, Bernstein EF, Libby P, DeLaria GA, Covell JW, Ross J Jr, Braunwald E: Effects of intraaortic balloon counterpulsation on the severity of myocardial ischemic injury following acute coronary occlusion: counterpulsation and myocardial injury. Circulation 45:1150, 1972.

Meisner H, Glanert S, Steckmeier B, Gams E, Hagl S, Heimisch W, Sebening F, Mesmer K: Indicator loss during injection in the thermodilution system. Res Exp Med 159:183, 1973.

Moulopoulos SD, Topaz S, Kolff WJ: Diastolic balloon pumping (with carbon dioxide) in the aorta: mechanical assistance of the failing circulation. Am Heart J 63:669, 1962.

Mueller H: Efficacy of intra-aortic balloon pumping and external counterpulsation in the treatment of cardiogenic shock. In Ledingham I McA (ed): Recent Advances in Intensive Therapy. Edinburgh, C. Livingstone, 1977, pp 191–202.

———, Ayres SM, Conklin EF, Giannelli S Jr,

Mazzara JT, Grace WJ, Nealson TF Jr: The effects of intra-aortic counterpulsation on cardiac performance and metabolism in shock associated with acute myocardial infarction. J Clin Invest 50:1885, 1971.

———, ———, Giannelli S, Conklin EF, Mazzara JT, Grace WJ: Effect of isoproterenol, 1-norepinephrine and intraaortic counterpulsation on hemodynamics and myocardial metabolism in shock following acute myocardial infarction. Circulation 45:335, 1972.

Mundth ED: Assisted circulation. In Sabiston DC, Spencer FC (eds):Surgery of the Chest. Philadelphia, Saunders, 1976, pp 1394–1415.

———, Buckley MJ, Daggett WM, McEnany MT, Gold HK, Leinbach RC, Austen WG: Surgical intervention for pre-infarction angina. Adv Cardiol 15:59, 1975.

———, Yurchak PM, Buckley MJ, Leinbach RC, Kantrowitz A, Austen WG: Circulatory assistance and emergency direct coronary artery surgery for shock complicating acute myocardial infarction. N Engl J Med 283:1382, 1970.

Nachlas MM, Siedband MP: The influence of diastolic augmentation on infarct size following coronary artery ligation. J Thorac Cardiovasc Surg 53:698, 1967.

Nahas GG, Visscher MB, Haddy FJ: Discrepancies in cardiac output measurement by two applications of the direct Fick principle. J Appl Physiol 6:292, 1953.

National Academy of Sciences—National Research Council: Mechanical Devices to Assist the Failing Heart. Pub No 1283. Washington, DC, National Academy of Sciences Printing Office, 1966.

Norman JC: An intracorporeal (abdominal) left ventricular assist device (ALVAD), XXX: clinical readiness and initial trials in man. Cardiovasc Dis Bull, Texas Heart Inst 3 (3):249, 1976.

O'Rourke MF, Shepherd KM: Protection of the aortic arch and subclavian artery during intraaortic balloon pumping. J Thorac Cardiovasc Surg 65:543, 1973.

Ortiz AF Jr, Lukban SB, Jurado RA, Litwak RS: The use of vein allografts as sidearms for intraaortic balloon insertion. Ann Thorac Surg 19:574, 1975.

Osborn JJ, Beaumont JO, Raison JCA, Russell J, Gerbode F: Measurement and monitoring of acutely ill patients by digital computer. Surgery 64:1057, 1968.

O'Toole JD, Wurtzbacher JJ, Wearner NE, Jain AC: Pulmonary-valve injury and insufficiency during pulmonary artery catheterization. N Engl J Med 301:1167, 1979.

Pace NL, Horton W: Indwelling pulmonary artery catheters: their relationship to aseptic thrombotic endocardial vegetations. JAMA, 233:893, 1975.

Pappas G: A smiple method of producing pulsatile flow during clinical cardiopulmonary bypass. Ann Thorac Surg 17:405, 1974.

Peters JP, Van Slyke DD: Quantitative Clinical Chemistry. Vol II. Methods. Baltimore, Williams & Wilkins, 1932, p 233.

Powell WJ Jr, Daggett WM, Magro AE, Bianco JA, Buckley MJ, Sanders CA, Kantrowitz AR, Austen WG: Effects of intraaortic balloon counterpulsation on cardiac performance, oxygen consumption, and coronary blood flow in dogs. Circulation Res 26:753, 1970.

Radvany P, Pine M, Weintraub R, Abelman WH, Bernhard WF: Mechanical circulatory support in postoperative cardiogenic shock. J Thorac Cardiovasc Surg 75:97, 1977.

Rahimtoola SH, Loeb HS, Ehsani A, Sinno MZ, Chuquimia R, Lal R, Rosen KM, Gunnar RM: Relationship of pulmonary artery to left ventricular diastolic pressures in acute myocardial infarction. Circulation 46:283, 1972.

Roe BB, Chatterjee K: Transaortic cannulation for balloon pumping: report of a patient undergoing closed chest decannulation. Ann Thorac Surg 21:568, 1976.

Rosensweig J, Chatterjee S: Restoration of normal cardiac metabolism and hemodynamics after acute coronary occlusion. Ann Thorac Surg 6:146, 1968.

Ross J Jr, Braunwald E: The study of left ventricular function in man by increasing resistance to ventricular ejection with angiotensin. Circulation 29:739, 1964.

———, Covell JW, Sonnenblick EH, Braunwald E: Contractile state of the heart characterized by force-velocity relations in variably afterloaded and isovolumic beats. Circ Res 18:149, 1966.

Rushmer RF: Cardiovascular Dynamics, 4th ed. Philadelphia, Saunders, 1976, pp 64–73.

Sanmarco ME, Philips, CE, Marquez LA, Hall C, Davila JC: Measurement of cardiac output by thermal dilution. Am J Cardiol 28:54, 1971.

Schenk WG Jr, Race D: Methods for measurement of blood flow. A current appraisal. J Surg Res 6:361, 1966.

Scott ML, Webre DR, Arens JF, Ochsner JL: Clinical application of a flow-directed balloon-tipped

cardiac catheter. Am Surg 38:690, 1972.
Seely RD, Nerlich WE, Gregg DE: Comparison of cardiac output determined by the Fick procedure and a direct method using the rotameter. Circulation 1:1261, 1950.
Sharp EH: Pulmonary embolectomy: successful removal of a massive pulmonary embolus with the support of cardiopulmonary bypass. A case report. Ann Surg 156:1, 1962.
Shore R, Holt JP, Knoefel PK: Determination of cardiac output in dog by the Fick procedure. Am J Physiol 143:709, 1945.
Sonnenblick EH: The mechanics of myocardial contraction. In Briller SA, Conn HL (eds): The Myocardial Cell: Structure, Function and Modification by Cardiac Drugs. Philadelphia, University of Pennsylvania Press, 1966, pp 173–250.
Soroff HS, Giron F, Ruiz U, Birtwell WC, Hirsch LJ, Deterling RA Jr: Physiologic support of heart action. N Engl Med 280:693, 1969.
———, Levine HJ, Sachs BF, Birtwell WC, Deterling RA: Assisted circulation. II. Effects of counterpulsation on left ventricular oxygen consumption and hemodynamics. Circulation 27:722, 1963.
Steingart RM, Meller J, Barovick J, Patterson R, Herman MV, Teichholz LE: Pulse doppler echocardiographic measurement of beat-to-beat changes in stroke volume in dogs. Circulation 62:542, 1980.
Stuckey JH, Newman MM, Dennis C, Berg EM, Goodman SE, Fries CC, Karlson KF, Blumenfeld M, Weitzner SW, Binder LS, Winston A: The use of the heart-lung machine in selected cases of acute myocardial infarction. Surg Forum 8:342, 1957.
Sugg WL, Rea MJ, Webb WR, Ecker RR: Cardiac assistance (counterpulsation in ten patients). Clinical and hemodynamic observations. Ann Thorac Surg 9:1, 1970.
———, Webb WR, Cook WA: Collective review. Assisted circulation. Ann Thorac Surg 3:247, 1967.
———, ———, Ecker RR: Reduction of extent of myocardial infarction by counterpulsation. Ann Thorac Surg 7:310, 1969.
Summers DN, Kaplitt M, Norris J, Rubin R, Nacht R, Arieff A, Lee M, Wechsler B, Sawyer DN: Intra-aortic balloon pumping: hemodynamic and metabolic effects during cardiogenic shock in patients with triple coronary artery obstructive disease. Arch Surg 99:733, 1969.

Swan HJC, Ganz W, Forrester J, Marcus H, Diamond G, Chonette D: Catheterization of the heart in man with use of a flow-directed balloon-tipped catheter. N Engl J Med 283:447, 1970.
Talpins NL, Kripke DC, Yellin E, Goetz RH: Hemodynamics and coronary blood flow during intra-aortic balloon pumping. Surg Forum 19:122, 1968.
Trinkle JK, Bryant LR: Mechanical support of the circulation: a new approach. Arch Surg 101:740, 1970.
Visscher MB, Johnson JA: The Fick principle: Analysis of potential errors in its conventional application. J Appl Physiol 5:635, 1953.
Warren JV: Determination of cardiac output in man by right heart catheterization. In Methods in Medical Research. Chicago, Year Book, 1948, p 224.
———, Stead EA Jr, Brannon ES: The cardiac output in man: a study of some of the errors in the method of right heart catheterization. Am J Physiol 145:458, 1946.
Weber KT, Janicki JS: Intra-aortic balloon counterpulsation. A review of phyiological principles, clinical results, and device safety. Ann Thorac Surg 17:602, 1974.
———, ———, Walker AA: Intra-aortic balloon pumping: an analysis of several variables affecting balloon performance. Trans Am Soc Artif Intern Organs 18:486, 1972.
Weikel AM, Jones RT, Dinsmore R, Petschek HE: Size limits and pumping effectiveness of intra-aortic balloons. Ann Thorac Surg 12:45, 1971.
Wessel HU, Paul MH, James GW, Grahn AR: Limitations of thermal dilution curves for cardiac output determinations. J Appl Physiol 30:643, 1971.
Williams BT, Sancho-Fornos S, Clarke DB, Abrams LD, Schenk WG Jr: Continuous, long-term management of cardiac output following open heart surgery. Ann Surg 174:357, 1971.
Wood EH, Bowers D, Shepherd JT, Fox IJ: O_2 content of mixed venous blood in man during various phases of the respiratory and cardiac output cycles in relation to possible errors in measurement of cardiac output by conventional application of the Fick method. J Appl Physiol 7:621, 1955.
Woods M, Scott RN, Harken A: Practical considerations for the use of a pulmonary artery thermistor catheter. Surgery 79:469, 1976.
Yahr WZ, Butner AN, Krakauer JS, Tomecek J, Tjonneland S, Kantrowitz A: Cardiogenic

shock: dynamics of coronary blood flow with intraaortic phase shift balloon pumping. Surg Forum 19:142, 1968.

Yu PN: Pulmonary arterial wedge pressure. In Pulmonary Blood Volume in Health and Disease. Philadelphia, Lea & Febiger, 1969, pp 31–32.

Zapol W, Pontoppidan H, McCullough N, Schmidt V, Blanc J, Kitz R: Clinical membrane lung support for acute respiratory insufficiency. Trans Am Soc Artif Intern Organs 18:553, 1972.

Zwart HHJ, Kralios A, Kwan-Gett CS, Backman DK, Foote JL, Andrade JD, Calton FM, Schoonmaker F, Kolff WJ: First clinical application of transarterial close-chest left ventricular (TaCLV) bypass. Trans Am Soc Artif Intern Organs, 16:386, 1970.

22. Cardiac Surgical Pharmacology

Roy A. Jurado

The rational use of drugs in the cardiac surgical patient is founded on a good working knowledge of basic pharmacology, a sound understanding of the pathophysiologic changes brought about by disease, and a clear insight into the physiologic alterations attendant on the perioperative state. Of particular importance are the numerous changes in organ system morphology and function associated with whole body perfusion (see Chapter 5). The electrolyte and acid-base changes, metabolic derangements, and ventilatory disturbances that occur during this period may modify the therapeutic action of certain pharmacologic agents and, not infrequently, lead to toxicity. In addition, either preexisting or coexisting organ system dysfunction (specifically hepatic or renal) may alter the bioavailability, metabolism, and pharmacokinetics of certain drugs. Moreover, the simultaneous use of several pharmacologic agents in the postoperative period increases the likelihood of adverse drug interactions. A clear understanding of these derangements and their relation to the therapeutic and toxic effects of drugs is essential to good patient care.

This chapter reviews the pharmacologic properties, physiologic actions, specific indications, and contraindications of six groups of drugs commonly used in cardiac surgery in the perioperative period. The pharmacologic agents included in this review are the following: (1) digitalis glycosides; (2) inotropic agents other than digitalis; (3) vasodilator drugs; (4) antiarrhythmic agents other than digitalis; (5) diuretics; and (6) drugs that alter blood coagulation. In the discussions that follow, only clinically important pharmacokinetic information will be included. Discussion of drug chemistry and structure-activity relationships likewise will be excluded.

DIGITALIS GLYCOSIDES

Digitalis has been the therapeutic keystone in the treatment of cardiac failure and other related disorders since Withering (1785) first described its use in dropsy and a variety of other conditions. In practice, the designation "digitalis glycosides" or simply "digitalis" has been used synonymously with the terms "cardiac glycosides" and "cardioactive glycosides." In this review, these terms will be used interchangeably.

There are now at least 300 known cardiac glycosides and congeners (Hoch, 1961). Despite their large number, cardiac glycosides exhibit and share a common and sometimes closely identical pattern of action. This pattern may be considered representative of the entire group and is commonly designated as "digitalis action." Individual differences in speed of onset, persistence of action, stability, absorption rates, and absolute doses exist. In the majority of instances, however, these are simply differences of degree and are frequently dose-related.

Although a great number of compounds possess digitalislike activity, only a few enjoy widespread acceptance for clinical use. For practical purposes, detailed knowledge of the properties of at most two or three preparations would be sufficient to cover most clinical needs. The choice of preparation in the individual patient is determined by: (1) speed of onset of action required; (2) desired route of administration; and (3) desired duration of action. In this review, discussion will be limited to the following preparations: ouabain, deslanoside, digoxin, digitoxin, and digitalis leaf. Ouabain typifies the rapid-onset and short-acting glycoside, while digitoxin and digitalis leaf are examples of long-acting compounds. Deslanoside and digoxin may be considered as intermediate-acting agents.

The two clinical effects of digitalis are improved myocardial contractility and slowing and control of the cardiac rate by increasing the refractory period of the atrioventricular node and bundle (His) and by increasing the vagal response of the sinoatrial node and conduction system.

Mechanism of Action

Inotropic Effects. The precise nature of the cellular action of digitalis glycosides is still controversial, although their positive inotropic effect was clearly established 44 years ago (Cattell and Gold, 1938). The bulk of scientific evidence, however, suggests that the inotropic effect of the digitalis glycosides is probably mediated through their effects on the transport systems that control the interrelated movements of sodium, potassium, and calcium across the cell (sarcolemma) membrane. Digitalis exerts a potent inhibitory effect on the transport enzyme known as Na^+, K^+-activated ATPase, which normally provides energy for the process by which sodium is removed from the cell, followed by a reciprocal influx of potassium (Albers et al., 1968).

While this highly specific interaction between cardiac glycosides and Na^+, K^+-activated ATPase has been clearly established, it is not entirely certain how this brings about an increase in the inotropic response of the cardiac myofiber. Recent studies employing highly sensitive isotopic techniques, however, have provided evidence that positive inotropic responses are accompanied by a net loss of potassium and a net uptake of sodium, accompanied by a net uptake of cellular calcium (Langer and Serena, 1970). Langer and Serena have postulated that inhibition of active cellular sodium transport may result in enhancement of calcium uptake, which in turn produces a positive inotropic response.

Moreover, more recent studies provide some evidence lending support to the interesting hypothesis that cardiac glycoside interaction with Na^+, K^+-activated ATPase inhibits outward movement of both sodium and calcium from the myocardial cell, resulting in an increase in the calcium pool available for excitation-contraction coupling (Schön et al., 1972). The presence of a calcium ATPase "pump" in the sarcoplasmic sacs has also been postulated (Entman et al., 1969). Digitalis interaction with Ca^{++} ATPase may promote reaccumulation and storage of additional calcium in the reticular sacs during the repolarization phase, with release of an increased amount of calcium during depolarization.

It appears that, whatever the underlying mechanism, cardiac glycosides increase the amount of calcium released to the contractile element at the time of excitation-contraction coupling; possibly this is related to interaction with the transport enzymes. It also seems that this increased calcium availability to the contractile element might be a crucial step in the chain of events leading to increased myocardial contractility (Lee and Klaus, 1971). Fig. 22–1 is a schematic representation of the proposed mechanisms by which digitalis glycosides produce their positive inotropic and electrophysiologic effects.

Electrophysiologic Effects. Despite major advances in the understanding of cardiac electrophysiology, many unanswered questions remain concerning therapeutic and toxic effects of digitalis on the electrical activity of the normal and diseased heart. There is, however, general agreement that interference of the transport of sodium, potassium, and calcium

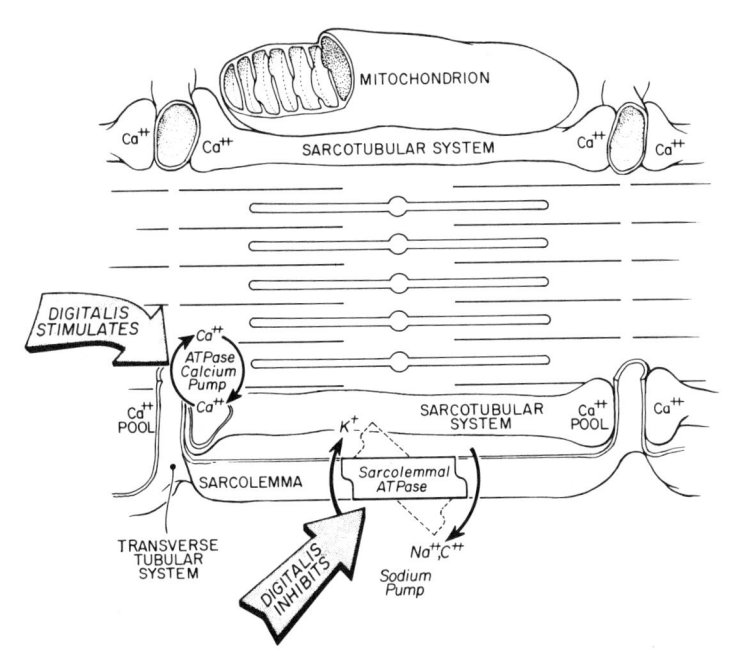

Figure 22-1. Schematic representation of the proposed mechanisms of digitalis action. It is believed that digitalis inhibits the "sodium-potassium pump" and stimulates the "calcium ATPase pump."

by inhibition of the cell membrane transport enzyme (Na$^+$, K$^+$-activated ATPase) underlies toxic effects on cardiac rhythm. The inhibition of this transport mechanism results in a net loss of potassium from the myocardial cell, presumably resulting in electrical instability.

For a clearer understanding of the electrophysiologic effects of digitalis, a brief review of the electrical attributes of the cardiac cell is in order. Cardiac cells are of two types: (1) those that initiate impulses and preferentially conduct them (specialized conducting cells); and (2) those that respond to stimuli by contracting (myocardial cells). They are histologically and histochemically different and behave differently under physiologic conditions, although myocardial cells may be able to generate stimuli under certain pathologic conditions.

In the resting state, the inside of the cell is electrically negative (from -80 and -90 mV) compared with the outside. The transmembrane resting potential is maintained by sodium and potassium gradients, which are in turn dependent on the integrity of the sodium-potassium transport system (Haas, 1972). If a depolarizing stimulus lowers the transmembrane potential of an adequate area of membrane rapidly enough from the resting or maximum diastolic potential to the threshold potential, excitation occurs (Weidmann, 1951). The occurrence of excitation is indicated by the development of an action potential.

On excitation of myocardial cells a transmembrane action potential can be recorded (Fig. 22-2, top panel). This consists of a rapid depolarization (phase O) resulting from a brisk intracellular movement of sodium into the cell—with reversal of the membrane potential, so that the inside becomes electropositive with respect to the outside by 20 to 30 mV. Repolarization (phases 1, 2, and 3), which is associated with extracellular migration of potassium, involves movement of current in the opposite direction and follows at a slower rate. An interval of electrical quiescence (the flat phase 4) follows each action potential with restoration of the transmembrane potential to the resting level. With each subsequent activation, the whole process is repeated.

The transmembrane potential recorded from specialized conduction tissue (that is, SA node, AV node, or His-Purkinje fibers) differs

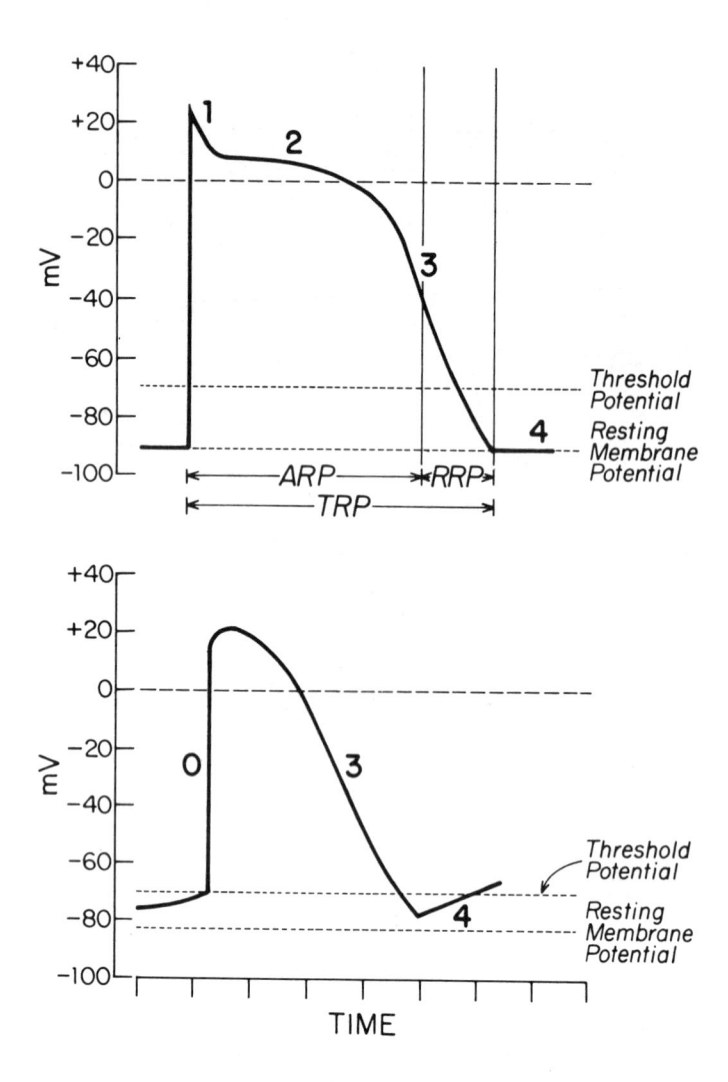

Figure 22-2. Transmembrane action potentials recorded from contracting myocardial cell (top panel) and from special conducting cells (bottom panel). ARP = absolute refractory period; RRP = relative refractory period; TRP = total refractory period.

from the above pattern in that after repolarization the membrane potential does not remain constant but exhibits a slow diastolic depolarization during phase 4 (Fig.22-2, bottom panel). If the threshold potential is reached during slow diastolic depolarization, spontaneous activation occurs—a process called automaticity. This property is common to all specialized cells, but the one that first attains the threshold potential usually acts as the dominant pacemaker, and the others, with slower diastolic depolarization during phase 4, are latent pacemakers.

In mammalian hearts, some part of the sinoatrial node usually acts as the pacemaker, because the rate of automatic firing is highest in this tissue. If a proximal pacemaker ceases to function, its impulse blocked, or if the automaticity of some other latent pacemaker is enhanced, specialized fibers other than the sinoatrial node may initiate ectopic impulses or may take over as the dominant pacemaker.

After depolarization, the cell becomes refractory to further stimuli until repolarization is complete. At first, there will be no response (absolute refractory period); this is followed by a phase (relative refractory period) during which depolarization can be produced if the stimulus is stronger than normal.

Within specialized conduction tissues of the heart, digitalis prolongs the refractory period and reduces conduction velocity, tending to slow the ventricular response to atrial fibrillation and atrial flutter, or to prolong the PR interval in the presence of normal sinus rhythm. In atrial and ventricular myocardium, on the other hand, the refractory period tends to be shortened, and the more rapid recovery time is reflected in a shortening of the QT interval of the electrocardiogram (Hoffman and Singer, 1964).

In the presence of toxic concentrations of digitalis, marked changes in transmembrane action potentials of specialized conduction cells occur (Hoffman, 1972). Purkinje cells develop diminished action potential amplitude and duration, with a shift in the resting potential toward less negative (i.e., closer to threshold potential) values. Decreased slope of the upstroke of the action potential (phase O) also occurs and is closely correlated with decreased conduction velocity. In addition, the slope of spontaneous diastolic depolarization toward threshold becomes steeper, resulting in increased automaticity of ectopic pacemaker foci.

Finally, there is increased heterogeneity of refractory periods in different cells, predisposing to reentrant rhythm disturbances. Whether ectopic beats and sustained tachyarrhythmias arising as a clinical manifestation of digitalis toxicity occur as a result of increased automaticity or reentry is not yet definitely known. It may well be that these and other mechanisms are operative at different times.

Autonomic Effects of Cardiac Glycosides. It is a well-established fact that digitalis increases the vagal response of the sinoatrial and atrioventricular nodes and the conduction system (Hoffman and Singer, 1964). Recent studies have shown that digitalis can influence preganglionic cardiac sympathetic nerve activity with substantial augmentation of the same at toxic doses, accompanied by the onset of ventricular tachyarrhythmias, including fatal ventricular fibrillation (Gillis et al., 1972). Additional neuroexcitatory effects observed included enhancement of vagal and phrenic nerve activity, the latter resulting in hyperventilation. Such neurally mediated effects are either prevented or reversed by spinal cord section (Gillis et al.) or sympathetic ablation by surgical and chemical methods (Wallace et al., 1967; Kelliher and Roberts, 1972). It is possible that these centrally mediated effects may play an important part in the genesis of digitalis toxic arrhythmias.

Effects of Digitalis on Organ Systems

Cardiac Effects. At therapeutic dose levels, digitalis acts primarily by increasing myocardial contractility. Both velocity and force of contraction are increased (Sonnenblick et al., 1966), whereas the duration of systole is slightly shortened (Weissler, 1964). This positive inotropic action of the drug is manifest in normal as well as failing heart muscle (Eddleman et al., 1951; Sanyal and Saunders, 1957; Braunwald et al., 1961). In the failing heart, this inotropic effect results in a recognized increase in cardiac output and usually a decrease in heart size. In the normal heart, however, the administration of cardiac glycosides results in no change or a slight decline in cardiac output (Burwell et al., 1927; Rodman et al., 1961), presumably because of reflex adjustments of the peripheral circulation.

The regulation and control of cardiac output is an exceedingly complex process, the inotropic state of the myocardium being only one of many important determinants. It has been clearly established that digitalis augments the contractile state of the normal myocardium in intact humans; however, reflex adjustments in the other determinants of cardiac output prevent a ready appreciation of this positive inotropic action.

In experimental studies using an isolated canine cardiac preparation, Covell et al. (1966) showed that digitalis administration increased myocardial oxygen consumption in the normal heart, whereas consumption was decreased in the failing heart. The increased energy expenditure in the normal heart is explained as a result of increased velocity of contraction and increased tension. In the failing heart, decreased oxygen consumption can be explained by an improvement in the mechanical efficiency that comes from a decrease in heart size typically brought about by digitalis action. A decrease in left ventricular end-diastolic volume results in a reduction in left ventricular end-diastolic pressure and, consequently, on the basis of simple physical principles (the Laplace relationship), a decline in myocardial wall tension.

In the light of the observations of Maroko et al. (1971) that a number of inotropic agents, including digitalis, increased the extent and severity of ischemic injury in experimental coronary occlusion in the nonfailing heart, a question of serious import arises concerning the use of digitalis and other inotropes in myocardial infarction. This is still an unsettled question in clinical practice.

The electrophysiologic effects of digitalis on the intact heart are complex, and are mediated by both autonomic and direct mechanisms. The initial effects on atrioventricular conduction are due to vagal stimulation, whereas direct effects become appreciable after full digitalization. Thus, within the atrioventricular node the refractory period is increased and conduction velocity is diminished, which may result in prolongation of the PR interval or overt toxicity in the form of second- or third-degree atrioventricular block. In ventricular muscle cells, on the other hand, the action potential tends to be shortened, and the more rapid recovery time is reflected in a shortening of the QT interval of the electrocardiogram (Hoffman and Singer, 1964). Digitalis exerts its salutary effects in certain types of supraventricular tachyarrhythmias, presumably through the above mechanisms.

Toxic dose levels of digitalis are characterized particularly by AV block and changes due to increased myocardial automaticity. Increased automaticity, on the other hand, is manifested by occasional premature systoles, ventricular ectopic tachycardia, or ventricular fibrillation.

Peripheral Vascular Effects. In normal subjects, digitalis tends to increase the tone of peripheral-resistance vessels, resulting in an increase in total peripheral resistance (Mason and Braunwald, 1964). Arteriolar and venous constriction likewise has been demonstrated in intact laboratory animals (Ross et al., 1960a, 1960b). Moreover, significant rises in peripheral vascular resistance have been observed in patients after rapid intravenous administration of digitalis (Kumar et al., 1973), and a marked peripheral vasoconstrictor effect that preceded the inotropic effect also has been reported (Cohn et al., 1969).

In normal canine preparations, digitalis produces generalized venoconstriction. This effect appears to be most marked in the hepatic veins, resulting in pooling of blood in the portal system and consequently diminished venous return to the heart (Ross et al., 1960a). It is believed that these venoconstrictive effects are probably of lesser magnitude in humans, although elevation of hepatic venous wedge pressure has been observed after digitalis administration in patients without heart failure (Baschieri et al., 1957).

Although other mechanisms may be operative, it is believed that the combined effect of some of these direct and neurally mediated peripheral actions contribute to the failure of digitalis to increase cardiac output in normal subjects. First, hepatic portal venous pooling tends to reduce venous return (preload) to the heart. Second, general arteriolar constriction results in an increase in systemic vascular resistance (afterload). Both actions would tend to counter the positive inotropic effect of the glycoside on the myocardium.

An increased level of sympathetic nervous activity accompanies congestive heart failure, producing systemic arteriolar and venous constriction (Mason and Braunwald, 1964). This may serve to maintain perfusion pressure in the face of a reduced cardiac output and to redistribute this lowered output among various regional circulatory beds with preferential perfusion of critical organs (Zelis and Mason, 1970). Moreover, sympathetic augmentation of myocardial contractility is essential in maintaining cardiac output. When digitalis is administered to patients in congestive heart failure, generalized vasodilation usually results instead of the vasoconstriction observed in normal subjects (Mason and Braunwald). The vasodilation is believed to be due to reflex withdrawal of sympathetic-induced vasoconstriction brought about by augmentation of cardiac output mediated by the positive inotropic action of the drug. This withdrawal of sympathetic activity also may account for the observation that venous pressure reduction often precedes diuresis after digitalis administration (Mason and Braunwald).

Effects on Kidney Function. Independent of its cardiovascular effects, digitalis exerts a direct renal action. It has been shown that digitalis inhibits tubular reabsorption of sodium (Hyman et al., 1956; Strickler and Kessler, 1961). Substantial inhibition of renal Na^+, K^+-ATPase and impairment of both tubular concentrating and diluting ability also have been demonstrated after direct infusion of large doses of ouabain into the renal artery (Torretti et al., 1972). While a direct renal action has been demonstrated, it is not clear what role this effect plays in the diuresis that is observed as a prominent manifestation of the therapeutic response to digitalis in edematous patients with congestive heart failure.

The prevailing view at present is that the diuresis is caused by the increase in cardiac output secondary to the inotropic drug action and reduction in ventricular afterload that accompanies generalized vasodilatation. The improved cardiac performance results in: (1) a reduction in capillary hydrostatic pressure (consequently promoting reabsorption of interstitial fluid); (2) an increase in renal blood flow and glomerular filtration rate (resulting in more complete reabsorption of sodium and water from the glomerular filtrate); and, presumably, (3) inhibition of the renin system with deactivation of certain edema-promoting hormonal mechanisms (i.e., secondary hyperaldosteronism) by virtue of improved renal perfusion (Davis, 1962).

Clinical Use

Indications. The two main indications for the clinical use of digitalis glycosides are congestive heart failure and certain types of supraventricular tachyarrhythmias.

CONGESTIVE HEART FAILURE. The chief clinical indication is myocardial failure, irrespective of the cause. Digitalis is most effective in patients with signs and symptoms of congestive heart failure due to valvular, hypertensive, ischemic, and congenital heart disease and certain cardiomyopathies. A consistent finding in this abnormal physiologic state is the presence of cardiac enlargement associated with diminished myocardial contractility, elevated ventricular filling pressures, and increased end-diastolic ventricular volumes. The administration of digitalis in this clinical setting generally results in an improvement of depressed myocardial contractility with a consequent increase in cardiac output and reduction of ventricular filling pressures and end-diastolic volumes. In turn, there is usually an accompanying diuresis with reduction in pulmonary or systemic venous hypertension.

However, when used in patients with mitral stenosis, where the main problem is mechanical obstruction to blood flow rather than impaired contractility, digitalis is of no demonstrable benefit unless atrial fibrillation or atrial flutter with a rapid ventricular response has replaced normal sinus conduction mechanisms or right ventricular failure has supervened (Beiser et al., 1968). Similarly, little benefit may result in patients with constrictive pericarditis or pericardial tamponade.

Idiopathic hypertrophic subaortic stenosis is another process in which digitalis is often of little value, and actually may be deleterious because it can increase left ventricular outlet obstruction by augmenting the contractility of the hypertrophied outflow tract segment. In the presence of associated congestive heart failure, however, as often happens in the late stages of the process, digitalis may be beneficial as in other cardiomyopathies.

Digitalis is relatively ineffective in "high-output" failure seen with thyrotoxicosis, anemia, arteriovenous fistulas, beriberi heart disease, and acute glomerulonephritis. In addition, patients with diffuse myocardial disease of any etiology often respond poorly to digitalis.

CARDIAC RHYTHM DISTURBANCES. Digitalis is of potential use in the management of some types of supraventricular tachyarrhythmias.

Paroxysmal atrial tachycardia, whether of atrial or atrioventricular functional (nodal) origin and when not caused by digitalis toxicity, frequently responds to adequate therapy with the glycosides. In practice, however, digitalis is used only after failure of simple measures, including vagal-stimulatory maneuvers (i.e., carotid sinus massage, physical stimulation of the pharynx) and cholinergic and fast-acting adrenergic pressor agents. Carotid sinus pressure should be repeated during the course of digitalization, since the combination of partial digitalization and this vagal stimulatory maneuver often will succeed when neither measure alone suffices. Maintenance digitalization usually abolishes or reduces the frequency of recurrent attacks.

Atrial fibrillation is one of the most common clinical indications for the use of digitalis. In this condition digitalis reduces the ventricular rate by increasing the refractory period of the conduction tissue; both vagal and direct mechanisms result in increased blockade of impulses at the atrioventricular junction. The fast, irregular atrial impulses being showered on the AV node are extinguished in greater number as the refractory interval is increased by digitalis, with consequent slowing of the ventricular rate. The refractory interval of the atrial mass, on the other hand, may be shortened; this favors perpetuation of atrial fibrillation with an increase in atrial rate, and, similarly, atrial flutter may be altered to reach the state of atrial fibrillation. The vagal effect of digitalis is responsible for the early shortened refractory period of the atrium. The general improvement in myocardial function, measured as increased contractile force, may have the later effect of converting the arrhythmias to a normal sinus rhythm.

In all instances of atrial fibrillation, it is best first to digitalize the patient and later, if regular sinus rhythm has not developed, to consider the additional use of quinidine or cardioversion. The cardiac glycosides prevent the tachycardia occasionally created by quinidine when it is given alone.

Atrial flutter, usually accompanied by 2:1 atrioventricular block in untreated cases, often can be managed with digitalis in doses sufficient to produce a degree of atrioventricular blockade resulting in a ventricular rate in the range of 70 to 100 per minute. This effect may require doses considerably in excess of the usual range. As in atrial fibrillation, when the arrhythmia is poorly tolerated by the patient it is often advisable to attempt direct current cardioversion before administration of doses of digitalis that would render the procedure hazardous. In the postoperative state, the ready availability of temporary pacemaker electrodes, prophylactically implanted at the termination of operative repair, provides an added measure of safety for electrical cardioversion even in the digitalized patient.

Wolf-Parkinson-White syndrome tachyarrhythmias may be terminated or prevented by digitalis in cases in which preferential effects on conduction or refractoriness in the normal or anomalous conduction pathways result in interruption of the reentrant circus movement. Quinidine or procainamide may be more effective in other cases, however, and an empirical approach is usually necessary.

Paroxysmal ventricular tachycardia presents a difficult problem because, if patients are left untreated, they usually develop heart failure or low cardiac output. At the same time, one hesitates to use a drug whose severe toxic effects closely resemble the condition being treated. In some cases, however, the resemblance is only superficial, and digitalis, though dangerous, may be critically helpful. Extrasystoles occurring in patients with heart failure may be based on anoxia and commonly disappear on digitalization and return of compensation.

Preparations. Table 22-1 lists some of the more commonly used cardiac glycoside preparations and summarizes the known pharmacokinetic data on these agents.

OUABAIN. This is the most rapidly acting of the glycosides currently available for clinical use. Therapeutic effects are discernible within 5 to 10 minutes and a positive inotropic action is noted within 20 minutes after intravenous administration, with the peak effect observed between 30 and 120 minutes. Ouabain is poorly and erratically absorbed from the gastrointestinal tract and is not meant to be administered orally; in fact, there is no oral preparation of the agent available. In practice, it is given intravenously. The plasma half-life in humans has been estimated to be 21 hours (Selden and Smith, 1972).

Ouabain, although predominantly excreted unchanged by the kidneys, has recently been found to have a substantial gastrointestinal excretion in both dogs and humans (Smith and Haber, 1973). The kidneys are the primary route of excretion, with 50 to 60 percent of an intravenous dose of H^3-ouabain found in the urine over a 24-hour period. Renal

TABLE 22-1 PHARMACOKINETICS OF COMMONLY USED GLYCOSIDE PREPARATIONS

Agent	Gastro-intestinal Absorption	Onset of Action (min)	Peak Effect (hr)	Average Half-Life in Normal Subjects	Primary	Secondary
Ouabain	Unreliable	5–10	½–2	21 hr	Renal	Gastro-intestinal excretion
Deslanoside	Unreliable	10–30	1–2	33 hr	Renal	--
Digoxin	55–75%*	15–30	1½–5	36 hr	Renal	Gastro-intestinal excretion
Digitoxin	90–100%	25–120	4–12	4–6 days	Hepatic (with entero-hepatic cycle)	Renal excretion of metabolites
Digitalis Leaf	Approximately 40%	NA†	NA†	4–6 days	Hepatic (with entero-hepatic cycle)	Renal excretion of metabolites

*Tablet form with good bioavailability; assumes normal small intestinal function.
†NA—Not available for intravenous use.
Adapted from Smith, T W and Haber, E (1973).

insufficiency promotes higher serum levels and prolongs the half-life of this agent. The pharmacokinetcs of ouabain are otherwise similar to those of digoxin, which will be discussed below.

DESLANOSIDE (CEDILANID-D; DESACETYL LANATOSIDE C). Except for the presence of an added glucose terminal residue, this agent is structurally identical to digoxin—an alteration that results in poor gastrointestinal absorption. Like ouabain, it is recommended only for parenteral use. After intravenous administration, the onset of action is 10 to 30 minutes, with the peak effect observed between 60 and 120 minutes. The half-life of 33 hours is essentially identical to that of digoxin. Its excretory pathway is primarily renal, and in the presence of renal dysfunction the half-life is prolonged. Although the onset of action is slightly more rapid, it is doubtful that it offers a distinct therapeutic advantage over parenteral use of digoxin.

DIGOXIN. This is the most widely used agent in clinical practice. This popularity stems chiefly from its intermediate duration of action, rapid onset, and flexibility of route of administration.

It has been estimated that about 85 percent of tritiated digoxin is absorbed when administered orally in alcoholic solution to normal human subjects. After intake of digoxin tablets approximately 75 percent is absorbed. There appears to be a large variation of bioavailability of various brands of digoxin and even within different lots of some manufacturers' products (Lindenbaum et al., 1971).

The small intestine is the primary site for absorption of digoxin, although a small amount may traverse the mucosa. Peak serum or plasma digoxin levels are reached about one to two hours after table ingestion in fasting subjects. Delayed gastric emptying for any reason will tend to delay this plasma peak, since only little absorption takes place before the small bowel is reached. Digoxin administration by the intramuscular route results in a slower and even more erratic absorption pattern than the oral or intravenous route, and also is attended in some patients by a considerable amount of pain. When a rapid onset of effect is required, it is certainly preferable to use the intravenous route; this avoids some of the uncertainty about the time when cardiac effects will peak and reduces the likelihood of giving an additional dose before the prior increment has had its full effect.

Approximately 20 to 25 percent of the circulating digoxin is bound to albumin, with the remainder existing in the unbound state. Digoxin is not metabolized in the body but is mainly cleared from the serum by the kidney by glomerular filtration and excretion of the unchanged molecule without significant tubular reabsorption or secretion of the drug. A small enterohepatic circulation also has been demonstrated. Its clearance is proportional to the renal creatinine clearance; thus the half-time for serum digoxin is prolonged in relation to decreased renal function. In anephric patients, approximately 5 percent of digoxin is excreted in the gastrointestinal tract per day. Diuresis, whether induced by water loading, drug administration, or diabetes insipidus, does not accelerate digoxin excretion.

Digoxin clearance from the body takes place in an exponential fashion. The half-life has been estimated to be 36 hours in subjects with normal renal function. Digoxin losses from the body are directly related to total body digoxin. Thus, approximately 37 percent of total body digoxin is excreted per day and must be replaced to maintain a steady state. For patients begun on maintenance digoxin without a prior loading dose, it takes about one week, the equivalent of four to five half-lives (Marcus et al., 1966), for the drug to accumulate, reach a plateau, and achieve a steady-state body concentration and kinetic equilibrium.

Studies of digoxin pharmacokinetics in infants and children indicate that tissue distribution of digoxin, half-life, and excretion are similar to those seen in adults (Dugan et al., 1972). Recommended doses of digoxin for children are two to three times greater than those for adults on a milligram per kilogram basis, and serum digoxin levels are significantly higher in children given therapeutic doses of digoxin. Children tolerate significantly higher serum concentrations than adults on usual maintenance digoxin therapy.

DIGITOXIN AND DIGITALIS LEAF. These two agents will be considered together since digitoxin is the principal active agent in digitalis leaf. Digitoxin is more completely absorbed from the gastrointestinal tract than digoxin, approaching 100 percent. Studies in dogs indicate that digitoxin is rapidly absorbed into the portal venous blood (Oliver et al., 1971). Peak concentrations are achieved within 15 minutes. Hepatic metabolism and biliary excretion of digitoxin delay its appearance in systemic veins, so that peak systemic concentrations are not achieved until 45 minutes after oral administration. Unlike digoxin, digitoxin is almost completely bound to serum albumin; that serum digitoxin levels are 20 times higher than those of serum digoxin for a comparable therapeutic effect may be explained by the large ratio of bound-to-free serum digitoxin.

Fifteen to 20 percent of total body stores of digitoxin are excreted per day, yielding a serum half-life of approximately four to six days. Because of the prolonged half-life, patients given maintenance doses of digitoxin require approximately one month (four to five half-lives) to reach kinetic equilibrium and steady-state body concentrations. It is apparent that loading doses are almost mandatory with digitoxin.

Unlike digoxin, digitoxin undergoes metabolism, primarily by the liver, and its metabolic products appear to have some pharmacologic effects (Doherty et al., 1971). Twenty-six percent of total body digitoxin undergoes enterohepatic circulation. Most of the digitoxin that is excreted in the bile is reabsorbed in the gastrointestinal tract, with only 2 percent excreted daily in the stool. This intestinal phase of the enterohepatic circulation has been used to remove digitoxin from the body with the aid of bile-sequestering agents. Digitoxin also is excreted by the kidneys to a lesser degree than digoxin. Because its metabolic products also are excreted by the kidneys, about 85 percent of the digitoxin leaving the body appears in the urine, primarily as inactive metabolites. However, because of digitoxin's hepatic metabolism, the presence of renal dysfunction only minimally affects the serum level and half-life of the active glycosides.

The relatively slow excretion of digitoxin results in only minor fluctuations in serum levels; however, this advantage is offset by the prolonged serum half-life, which has the negative feature of resulting in a longer duration of toxicity should overdosage occur. In general, it is safe to consider that a preparation with rapid onset of effects will exhibit rapid disappearance of effects. Digitoxin is undoubtedly the slowest in development of effects and slowest in disappearance of effects. Digoxin is more rapid in action. Ouabain has about the same rapidity of action as digoxin but has so often been used in relatively greater biologic potency that it has acquired a reputation of considerably faster action.

Compared to digitoxin, digitalis leaf is less completely absorbed from the gastrointestinal tract, approaching 40 percent. The average serum half-life has been estimated to be four to six days, essentially the same as that of digitoxin. The principal metabolic excretory pathway is similar to that of digitoxin. The agent is not available for parenteral administration.

Dosage Schedules. Dosage should be individualized and is largely empirical. Both the digitalization dosage and the maintenance dosage are determinted by numerous factors, such as absorption rate, excretion rate, degree of cardiac damage, and degree of other stresses (Jellife, 1968). Extensive clinical experience has produced some average dosages that can be used as rough guidelines (Table (22-2). The dosage schedules given in Table 22-2 are for adults; they usually are increased for infants and young children when calculated on a weight basis. A general estimate would place the dose per unit of the child's weight at about double. Premature infants, on the other hand, usually require relatively lower doses

TABLE 22-2 DOSES OF COMMONLY USED DIGITALIS PREPARATIONS*

	Average Digitalizing Dose		
Preparation	ORAL	INTRAVENOUS OR INTRAMUSCULAR	Daily Maintenance Dose, Oral
Ouabain	NA†	0.3–0.5 mg	NA†
Deslanoside	NA†	0.8–1.6 mg	NA†
Digoxin	1.25–1.5 mg	0.75–1.0 mg	0.25–0.5 mg
Digitoxin	0.70–1.2 mg	1.0 mg	0.10–0.20 mg
Digitalis Leaf	0.8–2.0 gm	NA†	0.1–0.2 gm

*Averages for adults without gastrointestinal, renal, or hepatic impairment.
†NA—Not available for use.

than the one-month to two-year-old group (Neill, 1964–65).

Digitalis Intoxication The clinical use of digitalis is accompanied by a high prevalence of toxic manifestations. Some estimates indicate that 10 percent of hospitalized patients receive digitalis and that 20 percent of them develop digitalis toxicity (Rodensky and Wasserman, 1961). Many factors contribute to the development of digitalis toxicity (see Table 22-3); some promote accumulation of digitalis in the body and the myocardium and others sensitize the myocardium to the toxic effects of digitalis. Perhaps the most important is the accumulation of excessive amounts of digitalis in the body and in the myocardium in particular.

Excessive digitalis accumulation is more commonly due to diminished excretion, although occasionally it reflects excessive dosage. Decreased renal and hepatic function with corresponding decreased excretion of the drug are important predisposing factors. Premature infants who are deficient in the usual excretory and metabolic processes as well as geriatric patients, who usually have decreased kidney function, are more likely to develop digitalis toxicity. In young people, large doses and high serum levels of the agent may be well-tolerated, whereas in the elderly lower doses lead to toxic manifestations. In the case of digoxin, this may relate to lower glomerular filtration rate, reduced creatinine clearance (Ewy et al., 1969), and decreased lean body mass with advancing age; in addition, the myocardium per se seems to be more sensitive with advancing age.

The rate of digoxin clearance from the serum has been found to be slowed in hypothyroidism and accelerated in hyperthyroidism (Doherty and Perkins, 1966). Hypothyroidism results in increased sensitivity to digitalis; both therapeutic and toxic effects are found at lower doses. Conversely, hyperthyroid patients are relatively resistant to digitalis and the dosage requirements are correspondingly higher.

Many factors modify the sensitivity of the myocardium to the therapeutic and toxic effects of digitalis (Fisch, 1971). The presence of associated myocardial ischemia, diffuse disease of the myocardium and conduction system, and sympathomimetic support of the myocardium all appear to increase myocardial sensitivity to digitalis and reduce the therapeutic-to-toxic ratio of the drug (Sodeman, 1965; Irons and Orgain, 1966; Morris et al., 1969).

Perhaps the most common predisposing influence is a decrease of intracellular potassium (Sodeman; Irons and Orgain), which may develop following the use of potassium-excreting diuretics, cardiopulmonary bypass (Ebert et al., 1965), prolonged use of corticosteroids, or any condition causing excessive

TABLE 22-3 FACTORS PREDISPOSING TO DEVELOPMENT OF DIGITALIS TOXICITY

A. Factors promoting excessive digitalis accumulation
  1. Excessive dosage
  2. Diminished excretion
     a. Renal disease
     b. Hepatic disease
     c. Prematurity
     d. Old age
     e. Hypothyroidism
B. Factors that lower myocardial toxic threshold for digitalis
  1. Local factors
     a. Myocardial ischemia
     b. Diffuse myocardial disease
  2. Systemic factors
     a. Old age
     b. Electrolyte abnormalities
        (1) Hypokalemia
        (2) Hypomagnesemia
        (3) Hypercalcemia
     c. Hypoxia
     d. Alkalosis
     e. Acidosis

Modified from Butler (1970).

potassium loss from the gastrointestinal tract. Potassium deficiency will potentiate those toxic effects of digitalis that appear as tachyarrhythmias or ventricular irritability. This may be seen even within usually nontoxic ranges of serum and myocardial digitalis. One also should remember that because serum potassium levels may not truly reflect intracellular potassium concentrations, toxic effects are frequently associated with normal serum potassium levels and also with levels of digitalis that may be within the therapeutic range. Hyperkalemia, on the other hand, potentiates the inhibition of atrioventricular conduction by digitalis.

Hypomagnesemia also predisposes to digitalis toxicity (Seller et al., 1970) and has been reported to result in increased binding of digoxin to the myocardium. This assumes significance because cardiopulmonary bypass has been associated with decreased serum magnesium levels (Scheinman et al., 1969). The loss of myocardial potassium induced by digitalis, which probably is partially responsible for arrhythmias, is inhibited by magnesium administration in experimental animals (Neff et al., 1972). Hypercalcemia potentiates the therapeutic and toxic effects of digitalis; in general, the administration of calcium in the digitalized patient should be avoided, if at all possible.

Hypoxia lowers the toxic threshold for digitalis (Irons and Orgain, 1966). There appears to be an additive effect in development of arrhythmias with both digitalis and hypoxia, both of which promote loss of potassium from the myocardium. Alkalosis does not appear to change the myocardial toxic threshold for digitalis as measured by the amount of digitalis necessary to produce ventricular arrhythmias in experimental animals; however, once toxicity occurs, alkalosis delays its reversal (Warren et al., 1968). Alkalosis is consistently associated with hypokalemia (Talso et al., 1962; Bliss et al., 1963; Warren et al., 1968) and may interfere with the transmyocardial transport of potassium and digitalis (Talso et al.; Warren et al.,). Although acidosis has been mentioned as a possible factor in digitalis toxicity, its role is unclear.

Treatment of Digitalis Toxicity. The therapeutic approach employed is determined by the severity of the arrhythmia observed. For instance, the more common and less severe manifestations, such as occasional ectopic beats, first-degree A-V block, or atrial fibrillation with a slow ventricular response, require only temporary withdrawal of the drug, close surveillance, and subsequent readjustment of the dosage schedule to prevent recurrence. On the other hand, active and vigorous therapy is indicated in the presence of more advanced arrhythmias that are either life-threatening or impair the efficiency of the heart as a pump.

When atrioventricular conduction is normal and renal function adequate, *potassium* administration is the standard and most effective method of treatment; this presupposes that digitalis had been discontinued. Ventricular irritability appears to relate to loss of intramyocardial potassium, which is not always accurately reflected in serum potassium levels. Therefore, even in the face of normal serum potassium levels, potassium administration is relatively innocuous and usually will be effective. When atrioventricular conduction is depressed, the use of potassium may be hazardous.

Diphenylhydantoin and lidocaine are extremely useful drugs in the treatment of digitalis toxic arrhythmias. These agents do not depress atrioventricular conduction and the effects on sinoatrial rate, atrial conduction, atrioventricular conduction, and conduction in the His-Purkinje system are minimal (Bigger et al., 1968; Bigger and Mandel, 1970).

Other agents that have been used effectively in digitalis-induced tachyarrhythmias include *propranolol, quinidine*, and *procainamide*. The latter agents have no specific antidigitalis action but rather act through their general antiarrhythmic mechanisms, which will be discussed in greater length in a later section of this chapter. While they are effective against digitalis-induced tachyarrhythmias, they tend to depress myocardial contractility while slowing sinoatrial and atrioventricular conduction rates; this negative inotropic action may be hazardous in patients who have markedly reduced cardiac performance and poor ventricular contractility.

Sinus bradycardia, sinoatrial arrest, and atrioventricular block of second or third degree may be treated effectively with *atropine;* occasionally *electrical pacing* will be required. When digitalis causes severe depression of atrioventricular conduction with slow ventricular rates, temporary ventricular pacing should be instituted. Similarly, in ventricular tachyarrhythmias when massive doses of antiarrhythmic agents must be administered that may suppress atrioventricular conduction, the combination of electrical pacing and drugs should be employed. Occasionally, where tachyarrhythmias fail to respond to antiarrhythmic agents, overdrive pacing may control the arrhythmia.

In the presence of digitalis intoxication, the use of *electrical cardioversion* is inadvisable because of the severe arrhythmias and conduction abnormalities that may ensue. Occasionally, however, direct current countershock must be employed because all other methods have failed to stop a life-threatening arrhythmia. In such a situation, the risks are reduced when lower energy levels are employed (Peleska, 1963).

A variety of other agents have been reported to be effective in the treatment of digitalis toxicity because of potent antiarrhythmic action. These include *potassium canrenoate* and *diphenidol*, but data on these agents are too meager for evaluation.

Immunologic reversal of digoxin toxicity, though still experimental, is a most promising approach to the problem. Schmidt and Butler (1971) have been able to show that sera from animals previously immunized with digoxin-albumin conjugates could reverse potentially lethal digoxin intoxication in dogs. In the presence of this antibody-rich serum, digoxin could be removed from the myocardium and digoxin toxicity reversed. The applicability of this technique in humans is still unknown.

The use of *steroid-binding resins (cholestyramine* and *colestipol)* may be helpful; these agents have been used to shorten the serum half-life of orally administered digitoxin in humans. Because digitoxin undergoes an enterohepatic circulation, agents that bind the drug within the gastrointestinal lumen should decrease half-life. Both cholestyramine (Caldwell et al., 1971) and colestipol (Bazzano and Bazzano, 1972) have been found effective in this regard. This therapeutic modality awaits further clinical trials.

Special Considerations

The Use of Digitalis in Patients Undergoing Cardiopulmonary Bypass. Special precautions must be taken in the administration of digitalis to patients undergoing corrective cardiac surgery requiring the use of cardiopulmonary bypass. Under these conditions, the stage is set for digitalis toxicity to occur in the postoperative period as a result of the interplay of multiple factors. First, many patients in or with a history of congestive heart failure will have been maintained on potassium-excreting diuretics preoperatively. Second, the marked kaliuresis that accompanies hemodilution perfusion (Ebert et al., 1965) increases the tendency for hypokalemia, especially if potassium supplementation has been less than optimal. Third, hypomagnesemia can occur postperfusion (Scheinman et al., 1969), further increasing the sensitivity of the myocardium to the toxic effects of digitalis (Seller et al., 1970). Fourth, certain postperfusion acid-base shifts may sensitize the myocardium to digitalis.

Moreover, factors promoting excessive accumulation of digitalis are operative in the postperfusion state. First, it has been observed that following a slight initial fall, attributed to dilutional factors, there is a rebound in serum digitalis concentration occurring some 13 to 16 hours after the onset of bypass, rising to or even surpassing the preoperative value (Coltart et al., 1971; Morrison and Killip, 1973). The explanation for this rebound phenomenon is still unclear. Second, a reduction in the urinary clearance rate of digoxin occurs in the early postbypass period (Coltart et al.). Third, although heretofore available experimental and clinical data on the effects of cardiopulmonary bypass on myocardial and serum digitalis concentrations have been conflicting (Kouchoukos et al., 1961; Austen et al., 1962; Beall et al., 1963; Ebert et al., 1963), more recent studies have demonstrated a constant myocardial digoxin concentration in the experimental canine model subjected to two hours of normothermic cardiopulmonary bypass (Molokhia et al., 1971).

Meanwhile, recent studies in man suggest that myocardial sensitivity to the toxic effects of digitalis may be increased during the first 24 hours after cardiopulmonary bypass. Morrison and Killip (1973) have shown that digitalis-induced toxic arrhythmias occurred at serum levels lower than those observed in patients toxic to the drug but who had not undergone cardiopulmonary bypass. The same investigators also demonstrated that the serum levels were higher in patients who had arrhythmia postbypass than in those who did not; moreover, a decline in serum level was associated with a prompt disappearance of the arrhythmia.

From the foregoing, it is apparent that the digitalized patient is at risk of developing glycoside toxicity in the postperfusion state. To minimize the possible occurrence of digitalis toxicity in the postperfusion period a number of measures are implemented and assiduously followed.

First, diuretics are stopped four to five days preoperatively, if at all feasible. Second, potassium supplementation is ensured preoperatively and carried into the postoperative period if renal function is adequate; potassium also is added to the perfusate during the conduct of cardiopulmonary bypass. Third, digitalis administration is stopped preoperatively. In the case of digoxin, the drug is discontinued the day before surgery. If long-acting glycosides such as digitoxin have been used, a switch to an intermediate-acting preparation (e.g., digoxin) is made seven to ten days preoperatively; henceforth, the digoxin protocol is followed. Fourth, the postoperative maintenance doses of digitalis must be carefully titrated to the clinical condition and the requirements of the individual patient, as his or her glycoside requirements may temporarily be less than the preoperative level owing to the increased sensitivity of the myocardium to digitalis. Digitalis requirements in the immediate postbypass period are best satisfied by the use of an intermediate-acting glycoside, such as digoxin, given intravenously in small incremental doses.

The Use of Digitalis in Renal Failure. In the presence of renal failure, the risks of digitalis toxicity are greater because of the altered pharmacokinetics of the glycosides and the electrolyte and acid-base changes frequently accompanying renal dysfunction and its treatment. The glycoside preparation of choice is the intermediate-acting digoxin, even though its main excretory pathway is primarily renal. The reason for this choice is the speedier return to normal body pool size after discontinuance of the drug if toxic levels are encountered. In the presence of end-stage renal failure it has been estimated that the biologic half-life of digoxin may be prolonged up to 4.4 days, while that of digitoxin may be twice as long.

It has been possible to successfully predict the appropriate dose of digoxin that can be used in patients with stable levels of renal insufficiency from the creatinine clearance and the known clearance rate of digoxin (Jellife, 1968). The application of this method combined with serial determinations of serum digoxin levels make safe use of the glycoside possible. A reduction in dosage is necessary to avoid toxicity. An average digitalizing dose in such patients is 1.0 to 1.5 mg of digoxin given over one to two days, with a daily maintenance dose of 0.125 mg for five to seven days per week. Naturally, there is considerable variation among patients.

For patients on hemodialysis, the risks are even greater, particularly during treatments. During dialysis, serum potassium drops, ionized serum calcium rises, and blood pH rises. All three changes increase the chance of an arrhythmia occurring. For this reason, careful attention to the dialysis flow rate, dialysate composition, and electrolyte balance are essential. The situation is even less predictable and therefore more risky with peritoneal dialysis.

Because of the high degree of tissue and serum protein binding of digoxin, only small amounts of the drug are recovered in the dialysate (Ackerman et al., 1967), preventing the drug from being effectively removed from the body by dialysis. The practical implication of this is that, if digitalis toxicity is even suspected, glycoside administration should be discontinued immediately—mere reduction in dosage would not suffice. It is far easier to replenish a depleted body pool of digitalis than the reverse.

INOTROPIC AGENTS OTHER THAN DIGITALIS

The Rationale for the Clinical Use of Inotropic Agents

A continuing cause of mortality after open intracardiac operations in patients coming to surgery with advanced myocardial dysfunction is low cardiac output, which manifests itself at the time of attempted discontinuance of perfusion and may persist for several days after operation. Similarly, acute pump failure associated with a low cardiac output—with or without the signs of congestive heart failure—remains a major cause of death after myocardial infarction. The low cardiac output syndrome—be it postoperative or postinfarctional—is characterized by a substantial reduction in total systemic blood flow, as provided by the heart, so that metabolic requirements are not satisfied; and underlying this, there is usually a significant reduction in the level of cardiac performance. In general, signs and symptoms attributable to a reduced cardiac output become clinically apparent when the cardiac index falls below 2.2 liters/min/m^2.

A discussion of the pathogenesis and clinical recognition of the low cardiac output syndrome is given in Chapter 9 and will not be repeated here. Suffice it to say that, whatever the underlying cause, the physiologic derangements that set the stage for a reduced level of cardiac performance usually can be categorized as one or more of the following: (1) abnormal ventricular pressure-volume relationships (preload); (2) diminished myocardial contractility; (3) increased outflow resistance to ventricular ejection (afterload); and (4) abnormal cardiac rate or rhythm.

The role of pharmacologic agents in the support of reduced cardiac performance is schematically outlined in Figure 22-3. In most instances, multiple factors are at play and dictate therapy; however, a persistently low level of cardiac performance almost always involves the element of poor myocardial contractility. In this setting, pharmacologic agents that increase the force of myocardial contraction (i.e., inotropes) are indicated (see Fig. 22-3).

In clinical practice, the mainstays of inotropic drug therapy are the adrenergic agents epinephrine, norepinephrine, isoproterenol, and dopamine. Other agents that have been used with varying degrees of success include dobutamine, a synthetic adrenergic drug, and glucagon. In this section, discussion will be confined to these drugs.

Adrenergic Drugs

Epinephrine, norepinephrine, and isoproterenol are the cardiac stiumlating agents that have found the most widespread application. Epinephrine and norepinephrine are endoge-

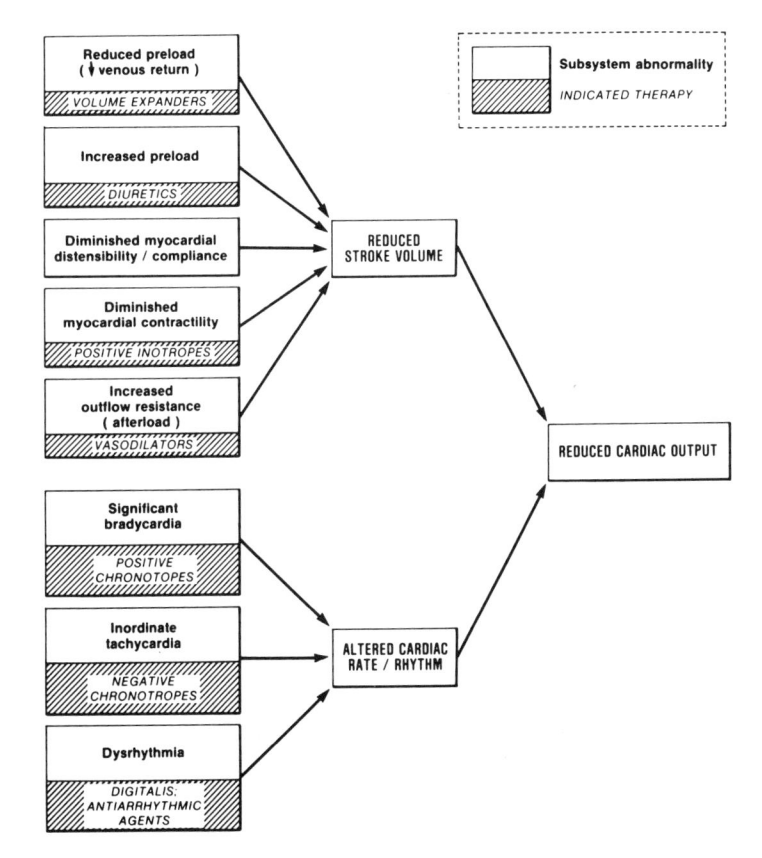

Figure 22-3. Schema showing the role of pharmacologic agents in the management of impaired cardiac performance.

nous catecholoamines, while isoproterenol is a synthetic amine. Dopamine, the immediate precursor of epinephrine, and dobutamine, another synthetic adrenergic drug, are now used with increasing frequency. This section will be devoted to discussions of the cardiovascular effects of these drugs.

Mechanism of Action. The concept of a dual adrenergic receptive mechanism, as origianlly proposed by Ahlquist (1948), is now widely accepted. Two distinct types of receptors, named *alpha* and *beta*, are distributed in varying patterns among the sympathetic effector cells situated in the different organs. Sympathetic effector cells may have alpha or beta receptors or both. In general, the cells of a sympathetically innervated organ have a preponderance of receptors of one type, although a small proportion of the second type also may be present. For example, the smooth muscles of blood vessels supplying skeletal muscles has a preponderance of beta receptors, by means of which epinephrine causes vasodilatation; at the same time, they also have a smaller number of alpha receptors, which, when selectively stimulated (for example, by a drug such as norepinephrine, which has specific alpha receptor-stimulating properties), produce vasoconstriction. Table 22–4 outlines the approximate distribution of the adrenergic receptors in the different cardiovascular effector organs where they have been determined.

Adrenergic drugs produce effects that are both excitatory and inhibitory. In general,

TABLE 22–4 RESPONSES OF CARDIOVASCULAR EFFECTOR CELLS TO ADRENERGIC STIMULATION

Cardiovascular Effectors	Adrenergic Receptor Type	Predominant Response
Heart		
S-A node	β	Increase in heart rate
Atria	β	Increased contractility; increase in conduction velocity
A-V node and conduction tissue	—	A-V node refractory period reduced
Ventricles	β	Increased contractility, conduction velocity; increase in rate of intrinsic pacemakers and automaticity
Blood Vessels		
Coronary	β, α	Vasodilatation
Skin and mucosa	α	Vasoconstriction
Skeletal muscle	α, β	Vasodilatation; vasoconstriction*
Cerebral	α	Vasoconstriction (mild)
Pulmonary	α	Vasoconstriction
Abdominal viscera	α, β	Vasoconstriction; vasodilatation*

*Usual response to circulating endogenous epinephrine: beta-receptor response (vasodilatation) predominates in blood vessels of skeletal muscles and liver; alpha-receptor response (vasoconstriction) in blood vessels of other abdominal viscera.

responses attributed to alpha-receptor activation are primarily excitatory, with the exception of intestinal relaxation. On the other hand, responses attributed to beta-receptor activation are primarily inhibitory, with the exception of myocardial stimulant effects (see Table 22–4). The responses to adrenergic drugs often can be clearly predicted on the basis of a knowledge of their selectivity in reacting with alpha or beta receptors. Epinephrine is, by far, the most potent activator of the alpha receptor; it is estimated to be two to ten times more active than norepinephrine and more than 100 times more potent than isoproterenol.

On the other hand, isoproterenol is perhaps the most active beta–receptor stimulator; it is two to ten times more potent than epinephrine and at least 100 times more active than norepinephrine. It appears that the chemical structure of the adrenergic agent predetermines which receptor or receptors will be activated and to what degree; in turn, the receptor and the natural function of the effector determines what the effector response will be. The foregoing concept provides a satisfactory explanation of the actions of the short-acting catecholamines, which produce their effects by a direct action.

Although the exact chemical nature of the adrenergic receptor remains largely unknown, there is now substantial evidence that —at least in the heart—the positive inotropic effects of catecholamines are largely mediated by the activation of the myocardial adenyl cyclase system, which, in turn, facilitates the conversion of adenosine triphosphate (ATP) to cyclic-3', 5'-adenosine monophosphate (cyclic AMP). A detailed review of the experimental evidence can be found in the publications of Sutherland and Robison (1966), Rasmussen (1970) and Epstein et al. (1970).

The present concept of the role of cyclic AMP as a mediator in the cardiac effects of catecholamines is illustrated in Figure 22–4. Briefly, this may be summarized as follows. In the myocardial cell, the catecholamine combines with a drug-specific beta receptor and, through some yet unknown mechanism, the myocardial adenyl cyclase system is activated. Adenyl cyclase, in turn, catalyzes the conversion of ATP to cyclic AMP. The latter

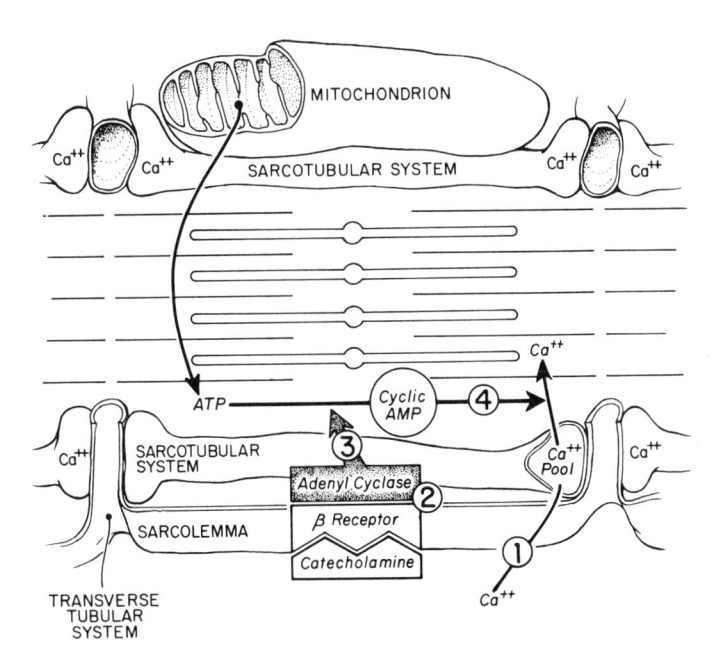

Figure 22–4. Proposed mechanisms of positive inotropic action of β-adrenergic drugs. Initial interaction between catecholamine and beta-receptor increases permeability of the cell membrane to calcium (1) and activates the myocardial adenyl cyclase system (2). Adenyl cyclase catalyzes the conversion of ATP to cyclic AMP (3). Cyclic AMP enhances mobilization of calcium from the sarcotubular stores, thereby increasing the amount of calcium released to the contractile myofilament during excitation-contraction coupling.

enhances the mobilization of calcium from the sarcotubular stores, thereby increasing the amount of calcium released to the contractile myofilament at the time of excitation-contraction coupling.

In addition, there is evidence that the initial interaction between catecholamine and beta receptor may, by itself, increase the permeability of the cell membrane to calcium (Rasmussen, 1970), causing extracellularly situated calcium to move intracellularly. The resultant increase in calcium concentration is thought to be ultimately responsible for augmenting myocardial contraction. Cyclic AMP is broken down to 5'-AMP and this reaction is catalyzed by a phosphodiesterase (Robison et al., 1967). Phosphodiesterase is inhibited by the methyl xanthines, particularly theophylline (Butcher and Sutherland, 1962). Theophylline is known to potentiate the positive inotropic action of norepinephrine (Rall and West, 1963), presumably by inhibiting the breakdown of cyclic AMP.

Epinephrine

Epinephrine is without doubt the most widely studied and best known of all the sympathomimetic amines.

Cardiac Effects. Epinephrine is a powerful cardiac stimulant. It acts directly on the beta receptors of the myocardium and of the cells of the intrinsic pacemakers and conduction tissues. It increases the force of myocardial (atrial and ventricular) contractility. It increases the heart rate through its effect on the sinoatrial node and by increasing the conduction velocity through the atria and ventricles. It also shortens the refractory period of atrial and ventricular muscle, although the refractory period of the human A-V node is slightly prolonged, presumably because of a reflex vagal discharge. The net result is that cardiac systole is shorter and more powerful and cardiac output is augmented (Table 22–5). Although cardiac work is increased, this is associated with a correspondingly greater increase in myocardial oxygen consumption resulting in a reduced cardiac efficiency.

Epinephrine also stimulates ventricular loci of pacemakers in humans. Ventricular extrasystoles may occur and may herald the onset of life-threatening ventricular arrhythmias if large doses are given. Although this is rarely seen with therapeutic doses in humans, ventricular premature beats, tachycardia, or fibrillation may be precipitated even by endogenously released epinephrine when the myocardium has been sensitized to this action of epinephrine by certain drugs, anesthetics, or disease (e.g., myocardial infarction).

Vascular Effects. Although large arteries and veins respond to epinephrine, its vascular action is exerted mainly on the smaller arterioles and precapillary sphincters. The response of a particular vascular bed to epinephrine action is determined in large measure by the presence and relative distribution of alpha and beta receptors (see Table 22–4). The blood vessels to *skin, mucosa,* and *kidney* are constricted by the action of alpha receptors; thus cutaneous, mucosal, and renal blood flow are usually reduced (see Table 22–4). On the other hand, blood flow to skeletal muscle is usually increased as a result of vasodilatation brought about by epinephrine action on the beta receptors situated in the smooth muscles of the supplying vessels. Although these vessels also contain alpha receptors, the beta receptors are sensitive to much lower concentrations of epinephrine; thus, at lower doses, vasodilatation is the predominant effect. At larger doses, both alpha and beta receptors are stimulated and the vasoconstrictor effect may become more pronounced, with a consequent increase in peripheral vascular resistance.

In experimental animals, epinephrine has been shown to produce a marked increase in coronary blood flow (Green and Kepchar, 1959). A similar effect has been demonstrated in humans, but whether the effective coronary blood flow, defined as the flow necessary to satisfy metabolic requirements, is actually increased is still an unsettled question. The net effect of epinephrine action on coronary

TABLE 22-5 COMPARATIVE EFFECTS OF CARDIOACTIVE SYMPATHOMIMETIC AMINES AFTER INTRAVENOUS INFUSION*

	Epinephrine	Norepinephrine	Isoproterenol	Dopamine	Dobutamine
Cardiac					
Heart rate	++,−†	+,−−†	+++	+,−†	0,+
Myocardial contractility	++	++	+++	++	++
Cardiac output	++	0,+,−	+++	++	++
Coronary blood flow	++	+++,−‡	++	+	
M$\dot{V}_{O_2}$	++	++	++	0,+	
Ectopics	++	++	+++	+	0
Blood Pressure					
Systolic	+++	+++	+	+	+
Diastolic	0,+,−	++	−	−	−
Mean	+	++	−	0,+	0
Peripheral Vascular Effects					
Cutaneous blood flow	−−	−	0,+	0,+	
Skeletal muscle blood flow	++	−	++	−	+
Renal blood flow	−	−	0,+	++	+§
Splanchnic blood flow	++	−	+	++	+§
Total peripheral resistance	−	+++	−−	−−	−

Key: 0=no change; +=increased; −=decreased: M$\dot{V}_{O_2}$=myocardial oxygen consumption.
*Half-lives (t½) of all amines short (measured in minutes).
†Reflex bradycardia.
‡Seen with larger doses of norepinephrine.
§Seen with larger doses of dobutamine.

blood flow is determined by the interaction of several factors.

The increase in cardiac output and aortic root pressure brought about by positive inotropism and chronotropism tend to augment coronary flow. On the other hand, the resultant increase in the vigor of contraction would tend to mechanically hinder flow by augmenting intramyocardial tension, with consequent reduction of effective coronary perfusion pressure (the difference between aortic diastolic pressure and intramyocardial compressive force or coronary sinus pressure, whichever is higher). Moreover, marked tachycardia will tend to further reduce coronary flow by shortening diastole, the time during which most of coronary flow occurs.

Both α- and β-adrenergic receptors have been demonstrated in the coronary arteries of humans and certain experimental animals (Zuberbuhler and Bohr, 1965); however, it is not yet clear whether epinephrine produces direct coronary vasodilatation through selective or preponderant beta-receptor stimulation. Some workers (Wegria, 1951; Gregg and Fisher, 1963) suggest that epinephrine may exert a metabolic dilator effect consequent on the increased force of contraction, and caused by locally produced metabolites and a relative myocardial hypoxia resulting from a discrepancy between the increased need for oxygen and the amount available. It is apparent that extremely complex mechanisms are involved. It is also possible that, in addition to the above, the hemodynamic state of the subject prior to epinephrine administration may play an equally important role in determining the net effect on coronary flow.

Whereas the effects of epinephrine on renal function are extremely variable, renal blood flow is consistently reduced while renal vascular resistance is increased (Gombos et al., 1962). On the other hand, hepatic blood is increased while splanchnic vascular resistance is reduced (Bearn et al., 1951).

Norepinephrine

Norepinephrine (levarterenol) is the chemical mediator liberated by postganglionic adrenergic nerves. In general, the responses to norepinephrine resemble the effects of stimulation of adrenergic nerves. It is a close chemical relative of epinephrine and shares numerous similarities in pharmacologic action with it (see Table 22–5). Both drugs act directly on effector cells, and their action differs mainly in the ratio of their effectiveness in stimulating α- and β-adrenergic receptors. While norepinephrine acts predominantly on alpha receptors, it has little effect on beta receptors, except those situated in the heart. Moreover, as an α-adrenergic stimulator it is weaker than epinephrine, though much more potent than isoproterenol (epinephrine, norepinephrine>isoproterenol). However, it is a much weaker beta receptor stimulator than isoproterenol and epinephrine (isoproterenol>epinephrine>norepinephrine).

Cardiovascular Effects. The nature of the cardiovascular effects are dose-related. In therapeutic doses, the systolic, diastolic, mean arterial, and pulse pressures all are increased. The cardiac output either is unchanged or decreased, while total peripheral resistance is increased—the latter representing a summation of its effect on the major vascular beds (Allwood et al., 1963). The blood flow is reduced through kidney, liver, skeletal muscle, and brain because of alpha receptor stimulation with resultant vasoconstriction. Adequate glomerular function is usually maintained unless the decrement in renal blood flow is substantial. The mesenteric vessels are constricted with reduction in splanchnic and hepatic blood flow.

Coronary blood flow is substantially increased, presumably because of both elevation of the aortic root pressure and coronary vasodilatation. Moreover, since it is a much weaker beta-receptor stimulator, less intramyocardial tension develops and the resultant effective head of coronary perfusion pressure is higher. Thus, the restrictive effect of enhanced myocardial contractility on coronary blood flow is lessened. The heart rate is usually decreased because of a compensatory reflex vagal activity that tends to overcome cardioacceleration and produces cardiac slowing.

Isoproterenol

Of all the sympathomimetic amines, isoproterenol is by far the most potent beta-receptor stimulator. Another characteristic of this amine is that it has almost no action on alpha receptors. The combination of these two unique properties is responsible for the prominence that isoproterenol enjoys in the clinical management of low cardiac output states, especially those that are primarily caused by diminished myocardial contractility and accompanied by significant vasoconstriction. Theoretically, isoproterenol would be the pharmacologic agent of choice in such situations, since it increases cardiac output by augmenting myocardial contractility and reduces peripheral vascular resistance (afterload) by producing vasodilation. Isoproterenol has been most effective in postcardiotomy low cardiac output states (Litwak et al., 1968; Mueller et al., 1968; Beregovich et al., 1971).

Cardiovascular Effects. The hemodynamic effects of isoproterenol are outlined in Table 22–5. After intravenous infusion of the drug, the systolic pressure increases slightly; however, since the diastolic pressure falls the mean arterial pressure may also drop. The heart rate is significantly increased, as is the force of myocardial contraction. Cardiac output is significantly augmented as a result of the positive inotropic and chronotropic effects of the drug. The improved circulatory dynamics may also help increase venous return.

Isoproterenol increases both coronary blood flow and myocardial oxygen consumption; measurements made in postoperative cardiac surgical patients have shown that the increase in coronary blood flow is of greater magnitude than the increase in myocardial oxygen consumption (Mueller et al., 1970). The significance of this observation will be discussed below. Vasodilatation is produced in the renal, mesenteric, cutaneous, and skeletal muscle vascular beds, mainly in the latter, resulting in a drop in peripheral vascular resistance (Allwood et al., 1963). Undesirable effects include tachycardia, palpitations, and ventricular premature contractions, which occur when large doses are employed.

Dopamine

Dopamine is a naturally occurring catecholamine (it is the immediate precursor of norepinephrine) that increases myocardial contractile force by a β-adrenergic action and produces mild vasoconstriction by an α-adrenergic action (McDonald and Goldberg, 1963). Dopamine also produces significant renal (McNay et al., 1965; McNay and Goldberg, 1966) and mesenteric vasodilatation (Eble, 1964) by a direct specific action that is not antagonized by either α- or β-adrenergic blocking agents. As with isoproterenol, this unique combination of properties provides the rational basis for the use of dopamine in certain forms of the shock syndrome associated with low cardiac output, diminished myocardial contractility, and elevated peripheral vascular resistance.

Cardiovascular Effects. The cardiovascular effects of dopamine (see Table 22–5) depend on the dose administered and the subject studied. When administered intravenously (1 to 10 μg/min), dopamine increases myocardial contractility (Whitsett and Goldberg, 1972; Velasco et al., 1974), cardiac output (Horwitz et al., 1962), renal blood flow (McDonald et al., 1964; McNay et al., 1965; McNay and Goldberg, 1966), and mesenteric blood flow (Eble, 1964) in normal subjects. These effects also have been observed in patients treated with dopamine for various types of circulatory shock and low cardiac output states (MacCannell et al., 1966; Talley et al., 1969; Loeb et al., 1971; Rosenbloom and Frieden, 1972; Holloway et al., 1973; Beregovich et al., 1974). Heart rate usually does not change, but may decrease at higher infusion rates (Doring et al., 1969). Mean arterial blood pressure is either slightly decreased or remains unchanged. Unlike isoproterenol, blood flow to the skeletal muscle vascular bed decreases (Ramdohr et al., 1972).

Coronary blood also is increased in dogs when the drug is given intravenously in doses that increase myocardial contractility or cardiac output (Cobb et al., 1972; Goldberg, 1972). Intravenous infusions of dopamine to patients with ischemic heart disease at rates that increase cardiac output and decrease peripheral vascular resistance do not seem to alter myocardial oxygen use (Goldberg, 1972; Crexells et al., 1973), although larger doses that increased heart rate and peripheral resistance could cause myocardial oxygen consumption to go up (Crexells et al.). Moreover, large doses of dopamine injected intravenously or into the coronary circulation can cause coronary vascular resistance to rise (Nayler et al., 1971).

A unique property of this amine not shared by other sympathomimetic amines is its ability to dilate the renal vascular bed and increase renal blood flow. The increase in renal blood in normal subjects is usually accompanied by increments in glomerular filtration rate and sodium excretion (McDonald et al., 1964).

Dopamine has been employed successfully in various clinical situations characterized by either hypotension, shock, congestive heart failure, or postoperative open heart myocardial dysfunction (MacCannell et al., 1966; Talley et al., 1969; Loeb et al., 1971; Rosenblum and Frieden, 1972; Beregovich et al., 1974). Available clinical evidence suggests that dopamine may possess, at least theoretically, certain advantages over the other sympathomimetic amines. In therapeutic doses, it augments cardiac output by increasing myocardial contractility and reducing afterload without altering arterial pressure, heart rate, and myocardial oxygen consumption. Afterload reduction is accomplished by a selective vasodilating action on critical vascular beds—namely, renal and mesenteric. Renal and mesenteric blood flow is augmented while vasodilatation of the relatively unimportant skeletal muscle vascular bed (a well-known β-adrenergic effect) is avoided; this highly desirable property is not shared with the other sympathomimetic amines.

Dobutamine

Dobutamine is a new synthetic catecholamine that is structurally related to epinephrine, norepinephrine, isoproterenol, and dopamine. It was synthesized in an attempt to produce a positive inotrope that lacked the heart rate-accelerating, arrhythmia-producing, and peripheral vascular effects of epinephrine, norepinephrine, and isoproterenol.

Cardiovascular Effects. Dobutamine has β-adrenergic effects on the heart with little action on the peripheral blood vessels. Its pharmacologic actions are very similar to those of dopamine, with the exception that dobutamine does not selectively dilate the renal vascular bed (Robie et al., 1974). Dobutamine exerts a positive inotropic action on the isolated heart muscle with little effect on spontaneous heart rate (Jewitt et al., 1974). In dogs, the positive inotropic effect may be seen without a significant increase in heart rate or diastolic arterial pressure and the tendency to produce ventricular arrhythmias is less (Kraft-Hunter and Hinds, 1973; Vatner et al., 1974).

There is accumulating clinical evidence that dobutamine augments cardiac output by increasing myocardial contractility and reducing peripheral vascular resistance with little or no effect on heart rate, ventricular irritability, and mean arterial pressure (Akhtar et al., 1973; Beregovich et al., 1973; Gunnar et al., 1973; Holloway et al., 1973). Dobutamine reduces the resistance in the coronary, mesenteric, and renal vascular beds, an indirect evidence that blood flow to these regional beds may be augmented (McRitchie et al., 1973). Moreover, in canine coronary artery ligation experiments, dobutamine was associated with smaller areas of myocardial necrosis and a lower incidence of ventricular arrhythmias than isoproterenol-treated animals (Tuttle et al., 1973).

The one property of this drug that is not desirable is its tendency to cause a redistribution of systemic blood flow favoring muscular beds at the expense of the kidneys and visceral beds. While it is true that it reduces the resistance in the renal and mesenteric vascular beds when given in smaller doses, this change is of small magnitude and larger doses are required before significant increases in blood flow to these regions become discernible (Vatner et al., 1974). Nevertheless, the drug holds some promise and is a potentially useful clinical agent; it certainly deserves further evaluation.

Glucagon

Although not a sympathomimetic amine, glucagon will be discussed here because it possesses certain desirable cardiovascular actions. Glucagon is a polypeptide hormone produced by the alpha cells of the pancreas. Although it acts primarily in the liver to increase cyclic AMP, thereby promoting glycogenolysis through activation of phospharylase (Sutherland et al., 1968), it also possesses positive inotropic and chronotropic effects on the heart (Farah and Tuttle, 1960; Regan et al., 1964; Whitehouse and James 1966; Parmley et al., 1968). The drug, as used clinically, is a purified extract of porcine pancreas.

Mechanism of Action. The positive inotropic action of glucagon is, like the catecholamines, believed to be mediated through the activation of the adenyl cyclase system, which results in the conversion of ATP to cyclic AMP with a consequent increase in intracellular calcium concentration during excitation (see Fig. 22–4). Glucagon is believed to combine with a specific receptor different from the β-adrenergic receptors, since glucagon action is not inhibited by β-adrenergic blockers (Glick et al., 1968). Glucagon also appears to stimulate catecholamine release, but the significance of this action is not yet fully understood (Glick et al.).

Cardiovascular Effects. Glucagon exerts a positive inotropic action. In the isolated cat papillary muscle preparation, it increases both the maximum velocity of muscle shortening and developed tension (Glick et al., 1968). In the intact anesthesized canine preparation, it produces a marked increase in myocardial contractility with a reduction in left ventricular end-diastolic pressure (Glick et al.). In patients studied at cardiac catheterization, glucagon increased arterial pressure, maximum left ventricular dp/dt, heart rate, cardiac index, and stroke work with no significant changes in left ventricular end-diastolic pressure, systolic ejection period, systolic ejection rate, and systemic vascular resistance (Parmley et al., 1968).

A modest chronotropic effect also has been demonstrated in the intact dog, an action substantially attenuated by β-adrenergic blockers without affecting the inotropism—suggesting the possibility that the chronotropic response is mediated by catecholamine receptors (Glick et al., 1968). In the human patient, the inotropic response was also manifest even in the fully digitalized state and was not accompanied by ventricular irritability or increased peripheral vascular resistance (Parmley et al., 1968).

A positive inotropic effect and an improvement in cardiac performance have been demonstrated in patients with low cardiac output after valvular replacement (Parmley et al., 1969) and in those with heart failure after acute myocardial infarction (Diamond et al., 1971). However, glucagon has been found to be relatively ineffective in ameliorating chronic congestive heart failure in the clinical (Nord et al., 1970) and experimental settings (Gold et al., 1970). Moreover, some evidence suggests that increasing duration and severity of the heart disease may adversely affect the response to glucagon (Nord et al.; Armstrong et al., 1971). Of interest is the experimental observation that, under conditions of chronic heart disease and failure, glucagon does not activate adenyl cyclase and fails to produce a positive inotropic effect (Gold et al.). As mentioned previously, activation of adenyl cyclase appears to be a critical step in the positive inotropic actions of both glucagon and catecholamines.

Despite its recognized limitations, glucagon may, under certain clinical conditions, prove to be useful both as the primary therapeutic agent or as an adjunct to more conventional measures. Obviously, this drug deserves further detailed study.

Clinical Use of Inotropic Agents

Cardioactive sympathomimetic amines frequently are administered in a variety of situations where there is "myocardial pump failure," particularly in postperfusion low cardiac output syndrome and in postinfarctional cardiogenic shock. However, it has become increasingly clear that the efficacy of these agents differs considerably, and often there is no unanimity of opinion about which is the "drug of choice" in any given clinical situation.

For instance, controversy surrounds the use of isoproterenol, a powerful β-adrenergic stimulator; yet it is frequently used in myocardial pump failure regardless of etiology (Kuhn et al., 1969; Talley et al., 1969) because of its potent inotropic action. However, its use is frequently attended by undesirable side effects, which include significant tachycardia, arrhythmias, and a reduced perfusion pressure (Gunnar et al., 1967; Smith et al., 1967). Isoproterenol also has been shown experimentally to extend infarct size after coronary occlusion (Maroko et al., 1971), to intensify myocardial ischemia after coronary narrowing resulting in acute cardiac failure (Vatner et al., 1974), and to impair left ventricular function when coronary blood flow is restricted (Maroko et al., 1973).

This undesirable effect does not appear to be an exclusive property of isoproterenol, however, as other conditions that increase myocardial oxygen requirements (including tachycardia and other inotropic agents such as glucagon and digitalis in the nonfailing heart) also produce extension of infarct size after experimental coronary artery ligation (Maroko et al., 1971; Maroko and Braunwald, 1973).

In contrast, it has been suggested that norepinephrine may be superior to isoproterenol in the treatment of postinfarctional shock (Kuhn, 1970). However, norepinephrine, while stimulating myocardial contractility, also causes a marked increase in peripheral resistance and a reduction in renal, splanchnic, and cerebral blood flow as a consequence of its potent α-adrenergic properties, further aggravating a situation already attended by marked arteriolar constriction due to sympathoadrenal discharge. Furthermore, norepinephrine may produce coronary vasoconstriction, especially when administered in large doses (Vatner et al., 1974). These actions are obviously undesirable.

The effects of epinephrine administration lie somewhere in between those of isoproterenol and norepinephrine. Dopamine is now used with increasing frequency because it increases myocardial contractility and cardiac output with less α-adrenergic vasoconstriction than norepinephrine and less cardiac acceleration than isoproterenol (Loeb et al., 1971; Goldberg, 1972). Nevertheless, dopamine exerts considerable α-adrenergic stimulation (Higgins et al., 1973; Vatner et al., 1973), which, in combination with its tendency to elicit arrhythmias, may limit its usefulness (Gunnar et al., 1972; Lipp et al., 1972).

The effects of dobutamine administration are similar to those of dopamine, except that dobutamine has very little or no effect on heart rate and ventricular irritability, a property that is obviously desirable. However, dobutamine does not possess the highly selective renal and mesenteric vasodilating actions of dopamine and, indeed, may favor redistribution of cardiac output to less important vascular beds, such as the skeletal muscle (Vatner et al., 1974). Glucagon has been used clinically with varying degrees of success, and its role is limited (Parmley et al., 1969; Diamond et al., 1971).

Ideally, an inotropic agent should have the following characteristics: (1) it must have a powerful and predictable cardiac stimulant action, increasing the force of myocardial contraction with minimal energy expenditure and oxygen consumption; (2) it must increase coronary blood flow substantially to more than offset the increased metabolic requirements brought about by positive inotropy so that, on balance, aerobiosis is maintained; (3) it must increase cardiac efficiency (more work performed for less expenditure of energy); (4) it should not produce tachycardia or elicit arrhythmias; (5) it should reduce ventricular afterload without producing a significant drop in perfusion pressure; (6) it must augment total systemic blood flow enough to satisfy total body metabolic requirements and favor redistribution of a reduced level of cardiac output to vital organs; and (7) it must have a short serum half-life (measured in seconds to a few minutes) to facilitate titration of dose to response. The foregoing discussion of the pharmacologic effects of currently available cardioactive agents makes it obvious that none of them fits the mold of the "ideal" inotrope.

In clinical practice, drug selection is based on careful consideration of the nature of the underlying cardiac disease, the patient's general condition and hemodynamic status, other therapy used, and the patient's response to such therapy. Needless to say, close surveillance of the patient and careful monitoring of moment-to-moment changes in his or her hemodynamic status are essential elements of the overall care plan. There are no hard-and-fast therapeutic rules, but the guidelines offered below may help the clinician formulate a therapeutic plan.

For instance, if the total peripheral vascular resistance is markedly elevated, use of a drug with a potent α-adrenergic action should be avoided except as part of an emergency resuscitative maneuver. Norepinephrine may be used temporarily to acutely elevate perfusion pressure in a patient with postinfarctional cardiogenic shock and profound hypotension before more appropriate therapeutic measures (including intraaortic balloon counterpulsation) could be initiated. On the other hand, if the total peripheral resistance is low or normal, the patient may benefit most from the use of a drug with combined α- and β-adrenergic stimulating action.

In the presence of significant tachycardia a strong β-adrenergic stimulator is contraindicated. Similarly, if significant coronary artery disease is present it is probably best to avoid use of a potent β-adrenergic stimulator (e.g., isoproterenol) because of the possibility of aggravating myocardial ischemia (Maroko et al., 1971) unless other measures designed to augment coronary blood flow (e.g., intraaortic balloon counterpulsation or coronary artery bypass) are employed concomitantly. A drug such as dobutamine may be superior to isoproterenol in such a situation (Tuttle et al., 1973) and may even be preferable over norepinephrine because of the latter's tendency to produce coronary vasoconstriction, when given in large doses (Vatner et al., 1974).

Extreme caution should always be exercised whenever a potent β-adrenergic stimulator such as isoproterenol is used because of its tendency to produce subendocardial ischemia even in subjects with normal coronary arteries (Buckberg et al., 1972). Although total coronary blood flow actually may be increased after isoproterenol administration (Mueller et al., 1970), the relative distribution of subepicardial to subendocardial blood flow may be the more important determinant in the genesis of isoproterenol-induced subendocardial ischemia (Buckberg et al.; Buckberg and Ross, 1973). Despite this undesirable effect, however, isoproterenol is still an important part of our therapeutic armamentarium; its margin of safety may be improved significantly if the dose administered can be titrated to both clinical response and measurements, albeit indirect, of available blood supply (e.g., diastolic pressure time index) in relation to oxygen demand (systolic pressure time index or tension time index), according to the concept advanced by Buckberg and his associates (1972, 1973).

As a matter of general principle, it is not sound pharmacologic practice to employ combined drug therapy (i.e., fixed-dose mixtures), especially if potent drugs are used. Perhaps an exception can be made when it is mandatory to use massive doses of a particular cardioactive sympathomimetic amine. In such situations, it may be safer to employ drug mixtures containing smaller amounts of each of two or more amines so that an optimal balance of α- and β-adrenergic action is rapidly achieved, while the toxic potential of each individual component of the mixture presumably is reduced. In practice, for instance, it is not uncommon to employ mixtures of isoproterenol and epinephrine, or of isoproterenol and dopamine; other drug combinations may be used as dictated by the hemodynamic status of the patient.

Dosage Schedule of Inotropic Agents

These potent agents preferably are administered by intravenous infusion to ensure rapid onset of action and easy titration of dose response. The recommended dosage ranges are given in Table 22–6. In general, smaller doses are used initially and are gradually increased until the desired therapeutic effects are achieved.

TABLE 22–6 USUAL CLINICAL DOSES OF INOTROPIC AGENTS

Drug	Infusion Rate
Epinephrine	0.5 to 1.5 μg/kg body weight/min
Isoproterenol	0.25 to 1.5 μg/kg body weight/min
Dopamine	10 to 50 μg/kg body weight/min
Dobutamine	2.5 to 10 μg/kg body weight/min
Glucagon	2 to 5 mg/min

VASODILATORS

Vasodilator drugs generally are employed to achieve one or both of the following therapeutic objectives: (1) to produce a prompt reduction of a markedly elevated blood pressure; and (2) to bring about a reduction in impedance to ventricular ejection and, therefore, of afterload. Acute reduction of the arterial pressure is the immediate therapeutic goal when hypertension is associated with acute aortic dissection, acute left ventricular failure, postoperative hemorrhage, or when the integirty of a tenuous vascular suture line is in jeopardy.

On the other hand, reduction in impedance to ventricular ejection has become an accepted adjunct to the therapy of low cardiac output syndromes, acute myocardial infarction, and chronic congestive heart failure not responsive to conventional therapy, as a means of either improving myocardial performance or protecting the myocardium from further ischemic injury or both (Franciosa et al., 1972; Chatterjee et al., 1973; Guiha et al., 1974; Parmley et al., 1974; Shell and Sobel, 1974; Walinsky et al., 1974). The probable mechanisms by which vasodilator drugs exert their salutary therapeutic effects are illustrated in Figure 22–5.

Pharmacologic vasodilatation may be achieved by a number of mechanisms: (1) ganglionic blockade; (2) adrenergic nerve terminal antagonism; (3) direct arteriolar dilatation; (4) α-adrenergic blockade; (5) β-adrenergic stimulation; (6) central nervous system action; or (7) a combination of some of these above actions. There is very little therapeutic advantage in the use of β-adrenergic drugs to produce vasodilatation because the powerful cardiac stimulant action of these agents tends to overshadow their peripheral vascular effects. α-adrenergic blockers have a similar drawback in that α-adrenergic blockade fre-

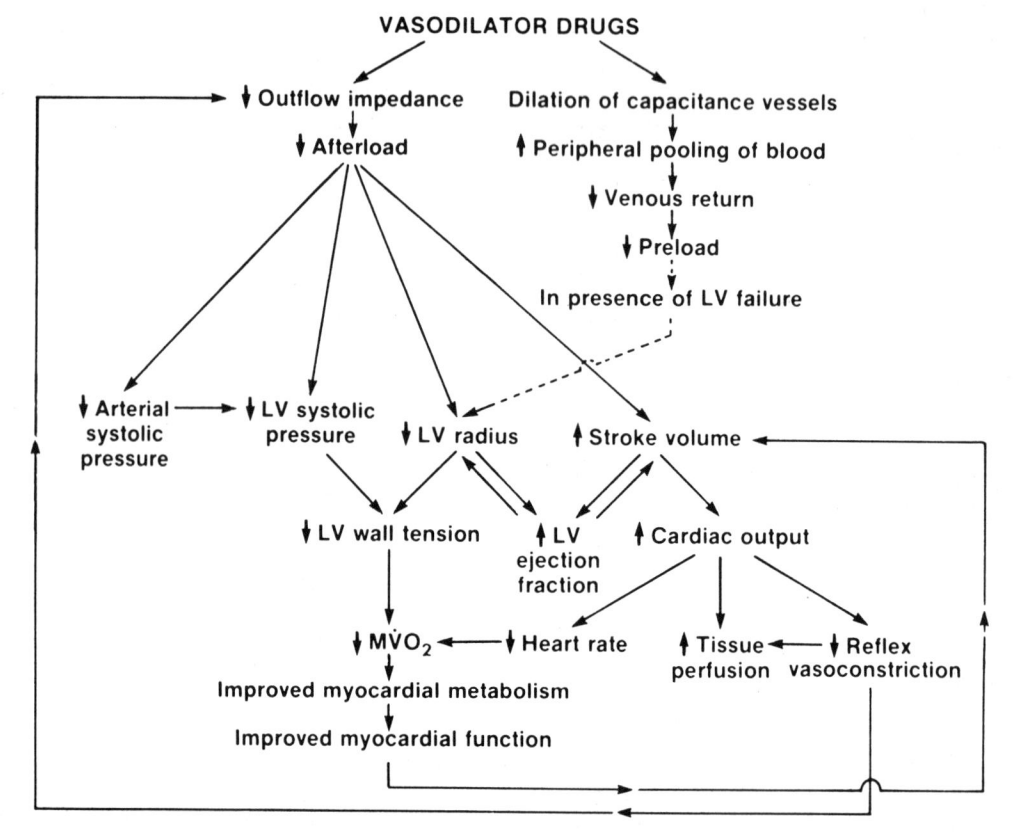

Figure 22–5. Usual hemodynamic changes brought about by vasodilator drug therapy.

quently is accompanied by a reflex increase in the heart rate and cardiac output resulting from the predominant action of unblocked β-adrenergic receptors. Therefore, for this discussion, consideration will be limited to those drugs listed in Table 22-7.

Trimethaphan

Trimethaphan is a ganglionic blocking agent. It produces arteriolar dilatation through blockade of sympathetic motor reflexes, a direct relaxing effect on the smooth muscles of blood vessels, and possibly through histamine release as well. It lowers arterial pressure and reduces total peripheral resistance (Bhatia and Frohlich, 1973). Heart rate is likewise lowered but the mechanism is not known. The effect on cardiac output is variable (Bhatia and Frohlich) and may depend largely on the hemodynamic state of the patient before treatment. In the absence of heart failure, cardiac output is often reduced, probably as a consequence of the dilatation of capacitance vessels, which results in peripheral pooling of blood and diminished venous return. In contrast, cardiac output is usually increased in patients in heart failure because of a decrease in venous return (preload) and a reduction in peripheral resistance (see Fig. 22-5).

Trimethaphan is used only for the production of controlled hypotension for short periods. Continuous intravenous administration is the only method of administration suitable for this purpose. It is generally administered with the aid of an easily regulated intravenous infusion pump through a central venous line to ensure predictable delivery of the desired amount of drug. Its advantages are that its hypotensive effects are extremely rapid in onset and the duration of action is extremely short, facilitating titration of dose to response. However, careful hemodynamic monitoring is mandatory for safe use of this potent drug.

The drug had been used extensively in the therapy of acute aortic dissections in combination with reserpine and guanethidine (Wheat and Palmer, 1968; Wheat et al., 1969). More recently, it has been successfully employed to reduce infarct size in hypertensive patients who developed acute myocardial infarction (Shell and Sobel, 1974). However, despite the clinical successes obtained with trimethaphan, the undesirable side effects that almost invariably accompany ganglionic blockade (postural hypotension, paralytic ileus, bladder distention, and sometimes myocardial depression) limit its usefulness. Furthermore, refractoriness is frequently observed after 24 to 48 hours of continuous therapy, necessitating the addition of other agents if therapeutic effects are desired beyond this period.

This drug is commercially available in a 10-ml vial containing 500 mg. The usual practice is to dilute the contents of the vial in 500 ml of intravenous solution for continuous infusion and to adjust the rate in accordance with the desired response. The recommended dosage range is 1 to 15 mg per minute.

Nitroprusside

Nitroprusside is a potent vasodilating agent that has been employed with increasing frequency within the last few years for a variety of clinical indications. Its clinical usefulness stems from its ability to rapidly lower arterial pressure and reduce peripheral vascular resistance.

Although the exact cellular mode of action is still unknown, it produces arteriolar and venodilatation by a direct relaxing effect on vascular smooth muscle (Johnson, 1929; Page et al., 1955; Palmer and Lasseter, 1975). Its pharmacologic action begins very quickly and is immediately reversible (see Table 22-7). Its effect on vascular smooth muscle appears to be highly specific and the drug is devoid of direct cardiac and central and autonomic nervous system effects. It is a highly potent vasodilator with a relatively low toxicity (Palmer and Lasseter).

In humans, it predictably lowers arterial pressure and total peripheral resistance (Schlant et al., 1962; Bhatia and Frohlich, 1973). Heart rate is usually increased, presumably as a reflex response to the hypoten-

TABLE 22-7 COMMONLY USED VASODILATOR DRUGS

Drugs	Onset of Action*	Peak Effect*	Duration of Action	Mechanism(s) of Action
Ganglionic Blocking Agent				
Trimethaphan	1–2 min	2–5 min	8–10 min	1. Blocks transmission in autonomic ganglia 2. Direct relaxing effect on vascular smooth muscle 3. Histamine release
Nonadrenergic Direct Vasodilators				
1. Nitroprusside	½–1 min	1–2 min	3–5 min	Direct arteriolar and venodilation
2. Hydralazine	10–20 min	20–40 min	3–8 hrs	Direct arteriolar dilatation
3. Diazoxide	1–2 min	2–3 min	4–12 hrs	Direct arteriolar dilatation
Adrenergic Nerve Terminal Antagonists				
1. Reserpine	1½–3 hrs	3–4 hrs	6–24 hrs	Depletes neurotransmitter (norepinephrine) and all other catecholamines from tissue stores
2. Methyldopa	2–3 hrs	3–5 hrs	6–12 hrs	Metabolized to alpha-methyl norepinephrine, a weak neurotransmitter that replaces norepinephrine at nerve terminals
3. Guanethidine	2–3 days‡	7–14 days‡	7–14 days‡	1. Interferes with transmission of sympathetic neuroeffector junctions 2. Depletes catecholamines from postganglionic nerve terminals in heart, blood vessels, and gastrointestinal tract
Mixed Action				
Chlorpromazine	1–3 min	3–5 min	8–10 min	1. Inhibition of centrally mediated pressor reflexes 2. Direct action of smooth muscle of blood vessels 3. ? α-adrenergic blockade

*After parenteral administration except where indicated othersise.
†Effect on cardiac output dependent on pretreatment hemodynamic state (see text).
‡After oral dose.
Abbreviations: AP-arterial pressure; TPR-total peripheral resistance; HR-heart rate; CO-cardiac output; CNS-central nervous system.
Key: 0=no change; (+)=increase; (−)=decrease.

Hemodynamic Effects				
AP	TPR	HR	CO	**Comments**
(−)	(−)	(+)	(−,+)†	1. Rapid onset and short duration of action 2. May depress myocardial contractility through adrenergic blockade 3. May lose effectiveness after 24 to 48 hours of continuous therapy
(−)	(−)	(+)	(−,+)†	1. Potential for thiocyanate toxicity 2. Unstable in stock solution
(−)	(−)	(+)	(+)	May increase cardiac work
(−)	(−)	(+)	(+)	1. May increase cardiac work 2. Rapid onset and prolonged duration of action 3. Produces sodium retention
(−)	(−)	(−)	(0,−)	1. Slow onset of action 2. Sedation and depression are common side effects 3. May depress myocardial contractility through direct action 4. Inconsistent effectiveness
(−)	(−)	(0,−)	(0)	1. Slow onset of action 2. Somnolence most common side effect but less marked than with reserpine 3. Inconsistent effectiveness
(−)	(−)	(−)	(−)	1. No CNS effect 2. Often causes orthostatic hypotension; may depress myocardial contractility and produce diarrhea 3. Fewer undesirable side effects than ganglionic blockers
(−)	(−)	(0)	(+,−)†	Short duration of action; not suitable for prolonged use

sion or reduction in cardiac output (Bhatia and Frohlich). The effect on cardiac output is variable, and the type of response is influenced by the hemodynamic state of the patient before drug administration (Schlant et al., 1962; Bhatia and Frohlich, 1973; Styles et al., 1973; Wildsmith et al., 1973). In the presence of left ventricular dysfunction, however, nitroprusside consistently produces an increase in cardiac output, presumably as a direct consequence of reductions in preload and afterload (see Fig. 22–5).

Nitroprusside has been used extensively and with greatest success in hypertensive crisis situations when prompt and effective lowering of arterial pressure is the immediate therapeutic objective (Gifford, 1961, 1962; Loggie, 1969). It also has been used in the therapy of acute aortic dissections and may soon largely replace trimethaphan as a first-line drug for this particular indication (Palmer and Lasseter, 1975). When used in the treatment of acute aortic dissections, nitroprusside always should be combined with a β-adrenergic blocker (e.g., propranolol), since it does not possess direct myocardial depressant effects and, indeed, may produce a reflex release of norepinephrine from cardiac nerve terminals.

More recently, nitroprusside has been employed to achieve a reduction of ventricular afterload—the ultimate objective being the enhancement of myocardial performance or the protection of a jeopardized myocardium from further ischemic injury or both. Franciosa et al. (1972) reported a significant reduction in ventricular filling pressure after nitroprusside therapy in patients with acute myocardial infarction and left ventricular dysfunction. This change in the state of ventricular dynamics was consistently associated with an increase in cardiac output and amelioration of the clinical signs of left ventricular failure.

It has also been suggested that the mortality rate in patients with postinfarctional cardiogenic shock could be reduced substantially with nitroprusside therapy (Chatterjee et al., 1973). In addition, it has been observed that the use of nitroprusside in combination with external counterpulsation produces significant hemodynamic improvement in patients with cardiogenic shock (Parmley et al., 1974). Moreover, Guiha et al. (1974) observed similar salutary effects in patients with chronic congestive heart failure that had been refractory to conventional therapy. It appears that the improvement in ventricular performance observed in these conditions after administration of nitroprusside is due to reductions in afterload and preload (see Fig. 22–5). This novel but promising approach deserves further detailed study.

Nitroprusside is administered by intravenous infusion, with careful monitoring of the patient's hemodynamic state. It is recommended that an infusion pump be used and that the drug be administered through a reliable and well-positioned central venous line to ensure predictable delivery of the desired amount of drug. The dose required to produce a given hypotensive effect is variable. The initial infusion rate is usually between 0.5 and 1.5 µg/kg/min, but doses as high as 50 µg/kg/min can be administered safely. Rarely, doses as high as 400 µg/kg/min given for short periods may be required (Palmer and Lasseter, 1975). When large doses are employed, plasma thiocyanate levels should be carefully monitored to avoid acute toxicity.

After intravenous administration, it is believed that nitroprusside combines directly with sulhydryl groups in the tissue and red blood cells and cyanide is released (Page et al., 1955). Circulating cyanide is then converted to thiocyanate in the liver. Thiocyanate is removed almost exclusively by renal excretory mechanisms, with a half-life of approximately seven days in people with normal renal function (Page et al.; Deichmann and Gerarde, 1969); the clinical implications are obvious. Symptoms of thiocyanate toxicity (fatigue, nausea, anorexia, disorientation, muscle spasms, and psychotic behavior) begin to appear at plasma levels of 5 to 10 mg/100ml. Hypothyroidism has been reported (Nourok et al., 1964) to occur during prolonged nitroprusside therapy, presumably as a result of thiocyanate interference with thyroid hormone synthesis.

Nitroprusside is photosensitive and must be protected from exposure to light during use to prevent degradation. In addition, it is recommended that a fresh solution be prepared and put up every four hours.

Hydralazine

Hydralazine has two distinct cardiovascular effects: a decrease in peripheral vascular resistance and an increase in cardiac output. It lowers arterial pressure by peripheral vasodilatation, with a marked reduction in total peripheral resistance. It acts directly on arteriolar smooth muscle, although it may also have some effect through the central nervous system (Schroeder, 1959; Reis and van Zweiten, 1967). It also produces an increase in cardiac output by increasing heart rate and stroke volume, probably by β-adrenergic stimulation (Brunner et al., 1967). This is probably responsible for its erratic effects in hypertensive emergencies and limits its usefulness as a hypotensive agent. Moreover, it has a relatively slow onset of action.

For these reasons, hydralazine is now only rarely, if ever, used in the therapy of hypertensive crises, and its use is generally limited to the treatment of moderate hypertension as an adjunct to other drugs. When used parenterally, it is usually given in doses of 10 to 50 mg at three- to six-hour intervals.

Diazoxide

Diazoxide is a nondiuretic thiazine (benzothiadiazine) derivative that reduces arterial pressure by direct arteriolar dilatation. Peripheral vascular resistance is reduced, accompanied by a reflex increase in heart rate and cardiac output. Its clinical use has been limited to the treatment of hypertensive crises. When given intravenously (5 mg/kg), it has a rapid onset of action (one to two minutes), with maximum effects achieved in two to three minutes; blood pressure then gradually returns to pretreatment levels over 4 to 12 hours.

Diazoxide produces a number of undesirable side effects, including sodium and water retention (Rubin et al., 1968), transient hyperglycemia and hyperuricemia. Natriuretic drugs are, therefore, administered concomitantly with diazoxide, but the effects on blood glucose and uric acid are not clinically important during the usually brief course of therapy.

Reserpine

Reserpine is believed to exert its antihypertensive effects by depleting the peripheral stores of catecholamines (Fawaz, 1963), probably by inhibition of an active transport system that maintains a normal concentration of norepinephrine at the storage site, with consequent impairment of the storage mechanism (Carlsson and Waldeck, 1967). In addition to its antihypertensive effect it may have a negative inotropic action as well (Nayler, 1963). Reserpine also exerts a central action, producing sinus bradycardia, sedation, a calming effect, and, in some cases, parkinsonian reaction, psychotic depression, and even suicide. It is possible that the central action is mediated through its effect on neurohumoral transmission in the central nervous system, perhaps involving norepinephrine or serotonin or both (Tomen, 1963). The CNS effect is apparently not essential to the antihypertensive effect of the drug.

Reserpine is most commonly employed in the treatment of mild hypertension and is usually used in conjunction with other agents. It is rarely used in the setting of a hypertensive crisis because of its erratic effect on arterial pressure and its slow onset of action (i.e., one hour after intravenous injection and two to three hours after intramuscular injection). It has been employed in the treatment of acute aortic dissections, mainly as an adjunct to other agents, for both its hypotensive and myocardial depressant effects (Wheat et al., 1969). The effective dose varies from one patient to another. It is usually recommended to start with a dose of 1 mg and to repeat the same or give double the initial dose every four hours, depending on the clinical response. When the required doses exceed 4 to 8 mg, it is best to switch to another drug.

Reserpine is relatively nontoxic, but a number of undesirable effects may occur if larger doses are used. For instance, there may be nasal stuffiness, increased gastrointestinal activity with stimulation of gastric secretion, activation of a peptic ulcer, severe depression, or extrapyramidal disturbances.

It appears that, by itself, its value as an antihypertensive agent is limited; maximum beneficial effects are obtained when the drug is used in combination with other agents in the therapy of mild hypertension.

Methyldopa

Alpha-methyldopa (or simply methyldopa) has an antihypertensive effect that is believed to be caused by the formation of a false neurotransmitter that replaces norepinephrine at the nerve terminals (Kopin, 1968). It has been shown that methyldopa can act as a substrate for dopa-decarboxylase (an enzyme necessary for the conversion of dopa to dopamine, the immediate precursor of norepinephrine) and leads to the formation of alpha-methylnorepinephrine. The latter replaces norepinephrine in the storage sites, thus depleting the sites of norepinephrine. The hypotensive effect is believed to be caused by the release at the nerve terminals of alpha-methylnorepinephrine, which is a weaker neurotransmitter than norepinephrine. In addition to its antihypertensive effect it exerts a central (sedative) action, presumably as a consequence of its ability to interfere with the biosynthesis of other important amines, including 5-hydroxytryptamine or serotonin (Clark, 1959).

Methyldopa, like reserpine, lowers arterial pressure by reducing peripheral vascular resistance. Usually the heart rate and cardiac output are not affected. In clinical practice, it is used mainly in the treatment of mild hypertension and usually in conjunction with other agents, such as reserpine and diuretics. Its value in the treatment of hypertensive emergencies is, like reserpine, limited both by its unpredictable effects and its slow onset of action (see Table 22-7). When used in hypertensive crises, the recommended dose is 500 to 1,000 mg intravenously. The response to this dose is extremely variable, however, and paradoxical hypertension has sometimes been observed. Accordingly, its clinical role has been limited to the treatment of mild hypertension and as an adjunct to more potent and predictable drugs in the management of hypertensive emergencies.

Methyldopa is relatively nontoxic, with undesirable effects generally developing with chronic use. Undesirable effects include mental depression, parkinsonism, hepatocellular damage, thrombocytopenia, and hemolytic anemia.

Guanethidine

Guanethidine exerts its hypotensive effect by producing selective sympathetic neuroeffector blockade. It not only blocks the release of norepinephrine (Fawaz, 1963), but it also brings about a depletion of norepinephrine at the storage sites by inhibiting the uptake of the amines (Shore and Giachetti, 1966). It produces a profound hypotensive effect by lowering peripheral vascular resistance. This is usually associated with bradycardia and a reduction in cardiac output (see Table 22-7). When guanethidine is given parenterally, an initial rise in arterial pressure may be observed, presumably because of release of norepinephrine and enhancement of the pressor effects of circulating norepinephrine from different storage sites (Athos et al., 1962).

Guanethidine has been reserved for use, usually in combination with other agents, in patients with severe diastolic hypertension. It also has been used in patients with milder forms of hypertension as an additional drug when less potent agents have not been effective. It has not been used as the primary drug in the treatment of hypertensive emergencies because of the paradoxical hypertension that it produces when given parenterally.

The main problems encountered with the acute use of guanethidine are orthostatic hypotension and diarrhea, the latter resulting from the predominance of unblocked parasympathetic impulses. Failure of ejaculation may occur after prolonged use.

Chlorpromazine

Chlorpromazine is a substituted phenothiazine that, although used primarily as an antipsychotic agent, possesses certain therapeutically useful actions on the cardiovascular system. It belongs to a large group of pharmacologically active compounds with actions on the central and peripheral nervous systems and important metabolic effects. For this section, discussion will be limited to the cardiovascular actions of chlorpromazine.

The substituted phenothiazines are known to act on the autonomic nervous system, producing α-adrenergic blockade, antiadrenergic uptake, and serotonergic and cholinergic blocking effects (Domino, 1971). The most consistent cardiovascular effect of chlorpromazine is a prompt reduction in arterial pressure, while the heart rate usually remains unchanged. The total peripheral resistance is decreased. The exact mechanism of the cardiovascular action is not entirely clear but could be caused by a combination of autonomic nervous system effects.

The effect on cardiac output is determined by the hemodynamic state of the subject. For instance, if the subject is normovolemic or hypovolemic the cardiac output will fall, presumably because of a peripheral pooling of blood and a reduction in venous return. The desirable clinical effect is an augmentation of cardiac output and a reduction in peripheral resistance. Both effects have been observed in postoperative patients after intravenous administration of chlorpromazine (Jurado et al., 1973).

Following intravenous injection, the onset of action is rapid and the maximum effect is achieved in three to five minutes (see Table 22-7). Although the dose required is dependent on the hemodynamic state of the individual patient, a dosage range of 2.5 to 50 mg has been found to be safe. It is recommended that the drug be administered intravenously in small incremental doses (i.e., 2.5 mg), at ten minute intervals, until the desired therapeutic effect has been achieved. Careful monitoring of the patient's hemodynamic state is, of course, mandatory.

Used in this fashion, chlorpromazine has been most effective in the management of postoperative open heart surgery hypertension in a previously normotensive patient whose cardiac performance is otherwise adequate. The mechanism of the arterial hypertension in this setting is not exactly known but may be related to postperfusion vasoconstriction. The rationale of therapy is the prompt reduction of ventricular afterload. The duration of chlorpromazine action is relatively short, and if larger doses (> 50 mg) of the drug are required consideration should be given to the use of other agents, such as nitroprusside or trimethaphan.

ANTIARRHYTHMIC AGENTS

For this section, readers are enjoined to reacquaint themselves with certain basic concepts in cardiac electrophysiology. To a certain degree, they have been reviewed in an earlier part of this chapter under *Digitalis Glycosides*. It will also be helpful to review some of the currently accepted concepts of the genesis of cardiac arrhythmias: to this end, the publications on the subject by Watanabe and Dreifus (1973), Hoffman and Cranefield (1964), Hoffman (1966), and Han (1969) will be extremely helpful.

Rational treatment of cardiac arrhythmias requires a precise understanding of the electrophysiologic basis for the arrhythmia and the mechanism of action of the therapeutic agent employed. However, the pathophysiology of cardiac arrhythmias is extremely complex and the actions of the drugs that are used in arresting or controlling them are equally so. Indeed, while the clinician might know the electrophysiologic effects of a particular drug, frequently he or she does not have a clear understanding of the underlying mechanism of action. It is therefore understandable that, in practice, therapy is not infrequently instituted on purely empirical grounds and based mainly on previous clinical experiences.

In this section, consideration will be limited to a group of primarily direct-acting agents that—although not chemically related to each other—share the common properties of diminishing automaticity and altering conduction velocity, refractory period, or membrane responsiveness. Included in this heterogeneous group are quinidine, procainamide, propranolol, lidocaine, and diphenylhydantoin. Other direct-acting agents that increase automaticity (e.g., isoproterenol) or decrease A-V conduction (e.g., digitalis) will not be discussed here. Similarly, agents that exert antiarrhythmic actions through indirect mechanisms will not be included. Examples of the latter group are certain adrenergic neuronal blockers (e.g., bretylium), cholinergic blockers (e.g., atropine), and cholinomimetic agents (e.g., edrophonium chloride and phenylephrine).

Edrophonium chloride, a quaternary ammonium compound that rapidly and reversibly inhibits acetylcholinesterase, is a potent cholinergic agent with a transient duration of action. Phenylephrine, a sympathomimetic agent with almost exclusive vasoconstrictor effects on the peripheral vascular system, produces an acute, transient elevation in blood pressure with reflex activation of the vagus nerves through the baroreceptor reflex. Both edrophonium and phenylephrine have been used effectively in the conversion of paroxysmal atrial tachycardia to normal sinus rhythm. Both agents exert their antiarrhythmic activity through their indirect cholinergic effects, with resultant slowing of the sinus rate, decrease in the effective refractory period and the action potential duration of the atrium, and slowing of atrioventricular conductivity.

The newer antiarrhythmic agents, such as disopyramide phosphate, a quinidine-like drug (Dreifus et al., 1973; Vismara et al., 1974), and verapamil (Schamroth et al., 1972) also will be excluded.

The genesis of cardiac arrhythmias involves exceedingly complex electrophysiologic mechanisms (Hoffman and Cranefield, 1964; Hoffman, 1966; Han, 1969; Watanabe and Dreifus, 1973), but the most important factors in the initiation and maintenance of cardiac arrhythmias appear to be the following: (1) altered automaticity; (2) decreased conductivity; (3) temporal dispersion of the refractory period; and (4) a combination of two or more of these mechanisms. Frequently, multiple mechanisms are operative in the genesis of a specific arrhythmia, and antiarrhythmic therapy should be directed toward the correction of the specific electrophysiologic abnormalities. Therapy should also include measures directed at the elimination of the predisposing and precipitating causes.

Classification of Antiarrhythmic Drugs

The comparative effects of the antiarrhythmic agents on the electrophysiologic properties of the heart are summarized in Table 22–8. In general, quinidine (Conn and Luchi, 1964), procainamide (Bigger and Heissenbuttel, 1969) and propranolol (Davis and Temte, 1968) reduce conduction velocity in cardiac tissues, whereas lidocaine (Bigger and Heissenbuttel; Bigger and Mandel, 1970) and diphenylhydantoin (Helfant et al., 1967; Rosati et al., 1967; Bigger et al., 1968) accelerate or do not influence this property. Quinidine (Conn and Luchi), procainamide (Bigger and Heissenbuttel), and propranolol indirectly (Wallace et al., 1966) prolong the refractory period; in contrast, lidocaine (Bigger and Heissenbuttel; Bigger and Mandel), diphenylhydantoin (Helfant et al., Rosati et al.; Bigger et al.), and propranolol directly (Davis and Temte; Singer and Ten Eick, 1969) shorten the refractory period.

All five agents depress automaticity of latent pacemakers and prolong the effective refractory period (measured by the ability of an early stimulus to evoke a propagated response) of the Purkinje fibers relative to the total action potential duration. By this latter effect, the rate of depolarization of the earliest premature beat will occur at a more negative membrane potential, thereby enhancing conduction in the Purkinje fibers and possibly

TABLE 22-8 COMPARATIVE ELECTROPHYSIOLOGIC EFFECTS OF COMMON ANTIARRHYTHMIC AGENTS*

Drugs	Automaticity S-A Node	Automaticity Latent Pacemakers	Excitability (Myocardium)	Conduction Velocity A-V Node	Conduction Velocity Purkinje System	Refractory Period	Refractoriness (ERP/APD)	Membrane Responsiveness
GROUP I								
Quinidine	Unchanged	Decreased	Decreased	Variable	Decreased	*Prolonged*	Increased	*Decreased*
Procain-amide	Unchanged	Decreased	Decreased	Decreased	Decreased	*Prolonged*	Increased	*Decreased*
Propranolol	Decreased	Decreased	Decreased	Decreased	Decreased	*Prolonged†* *Shortened‡*	Increased	*Decreased*
GROUP II								
Lidocaine	Unchanged	Decreased	Decreased	Unchanged	Increased	*Shortened*	Increased	*Increased*
Diphenyl-hydantoin	Unchanged	Decreased	Variable	Increased	Increased	*Shortened*	Increased	*Increased*

*Using therapeutic doses in intact subject.
†Indirect propranolol effect.
‡Direct propranolol effect.
Abbreviations: S-A=sinoatrial; A-V=atrioventricular; ERP=effective refractory period; APD=action potential duration.
N.B.: 1. Refractoriness is expressed as the ratio of the effective refractory period (ERP) relative to the action potential duration (APD).
2. Italics for emphasis only.
Table adapted from Hoffman and Bigger (1971).

eliminating reentrant beats generated by depressed conduction.

While all five agents decrease automaticity, there are important differences in their effects. Hoffman and Bigger (1971) have classified these drugs into two groups based on these differences. Thus, Group I, the quinidinelike group, includes quinidine, procainamide, and propranolol. These agents decrease automaticity and responsiveness and prolong the refractory period (see Table 22–8). Group II includes lidocaine and diphenylhydantoin; these drugs also decrease automaticity, but differ from those in the first group in that they increase responsiveness and shorten the refractory period (see Table 22–8).

Hemodynamic Effects

The hemodynamic effects of the five agents are summarized in Table 22–9. Quinidine depresses myocardial contractility and reduces arterial pressure and cardiac output; procainamide has similar effects (Hoffman and Bigger, 1971). The dose required to produce these effects depends on the route of administration and the status of the myocardium. Thus, doses in the recommended therapeutic ranges usually do not produce a significant negative inotropic effect in normal hearts but will readily produce depression in the presence of a damaged myocardium. β-adrenergic blocking agents have been reported to decrease cardiac rate, contractility, and output in humans (Hamer and Sowton, 1965; Epstein and Braunwald, 1966).

At therapeutic doses, lidocaine has minimal hemodynamic effects in normal subjects and in patients with heart disease. However, hypotension and depression of ventricular contractility have been reported with large doses of lidocaine both in experimental animals and humans (Frieden, 1965; Grossman et al., 1968; Jewitt et al., 1968; Lown and Vassaux, 1968). Diphenylhydantoin, when administered intravenously in therapeutic doses, is associated with some depression in myocardial contractility and a reduction in peripheral vascular resistance (Puri, 1971). An increase in left ventricular end-diastolic pressure (Leiberson et al., 1969) and a reduction in cardiac output (Mixter et al., 1966) also have been reported.

Clinical Use of Antiarrhythmic Agents

Whereas pharmacologic therapy is directed mainly at the correction of specific electrophysiologic abnormalities, a rational treatment plan should include measures designed to eradicate the inciting cause(s) of the arrhythmia and the deployment of other therapeutic modalities (e.g., electrical pacing and cardioversion) when indicated. The clinical role of the latter two measures is discussed in Chapter 10.

TABLE 22–9 HEMODYNAMIC EFFECTS OF THERAPEUTIC DOSES OF COMMON ANTIARRHYTHMIC DRUGS IN HUMANS

Drugs	Myocardial Contractility	Left Ventricular End-Diastolic Pressure	Arterial Pressure	Cardiac Output
Quinidine	Decreased	Increased	Decreased	Decreased
Procainamide	Decreased	Increased	Decreased	Decreased
Propranolol	Decreased	Increased	Decreased	Decreased
Lidocaine	No change or slight decrease	No change or slight decrease	Decreased	No change or slight decrease
Diphenylhydantoin	No change or slight decrease	No change or slight decrease	Decreased	No change or slight decrease

Quinidine and procainamide are useful in most types of supraventricular and ventricular tachyarrhythmias (Bigger and Heissenbuttel, 1969; Mason et al., 1970). Propranolol is particularly effective in suppressing supraventricular arrhythmias and in controlling ventricular rate (Gibson and Sowton, 1969; Mason et al.). Lidocaine (Bigger and Heissenbuttel; Mason et al.) and diphenylhydantoin (Conn, 1965; Damato, 1969) are most effective against ventricular tachyarrhythmias.

Diphenylhydantoin and lidocaine are the most effective agents in the management of rapid ectopic rhythms due to digitalis toxicity (Bigger et al., 1968; Bigger and Mandel, 1970). Propranolol is another agent that may be useful in the treatment of digitalis toxicity arrhythmias (Gibson and Sowton, 1969). The clinical applications of these agents are summarized in Table 22-10, and their relative effectiveness against the common arrhythmias are also shown. Table 22-11 shows the recommended dosage schedules, while known pharmacokinetic data on these agents are summarized in Table 22-12.

Lidocaine has the shortest half-life; this is a reflection of its weak tissue binding and its rapid inactivation by hepatic enzymes. The half-life of an intravenous bolus is about 10 minutes, and this rapid disappearance is thought to represent prompt volume distribution throughout the body (Thompson et al., 1971). On the other hand, the half-life of lidocaine after cessation of a sustained intravenous infusion is approximately 100 minutes (Thompson et al.), which presumably reflects degradation by the liver (Stenson et al., 1971). In the presence of liver disease or congestive heart failure, the lidocaine half-life is prolonged, in the range of 150 to 500 minutes (Thompson et al.).

Diphenylhydantoin has the most prolonged half-life (approximately 24 hours), a reflection of strong protein binding and hepatic degradation (Noach et al., 1958). Patients with liver disease and hepatic dysfunction have a prolonged diphenylhydantoin half-life. Of interest is the observation that the diphenylhydantoin half-life in patients with impaired renal function is shortened, presum-

TABLE 22-10 RELATIVE EFFECTIVENESS OF ANTIARRHYTHMIC AGENTS AGAINST COMMON ARRHYTHMIAS*

	Quinidine	Procainamide	Propranolol	Lidocaine	Diphenylhydantoin
I. Supraventricular Arrhythmias					
Atrial premature systoles	++++	+++	++	+	+
Paroxysmal atrial tachycardia	+++	+++	+++	+	++
Atrial flutter	+++	++	++	+	+
Atrial fibrillation	++++	+++	++	+	+
II. Ventricular Arrhythmias					
Ventricular premature systoles	+++	++++	++	++++	+++
Ventricular tachycardia	+++	++++	++	++++	+++
Ventricular fibrillation	+++	++++	++	++++	+++
III. Digitalis-induced arrhythmias	++	++	+++	++++	++++

*Scale of Effectiveness: ++++ = Excellent
+++ = Good
++ = Fair
+ = Poor

TABLE 22-11 RECOMMENDED DOSAGE SCHEDULE OF ANTIARRHYTHMIC AGENTS

Drugs	Intramuscular Route	Intravenous Route	Oral Route
Quinidine	Gluconate: 200–400 mg every 4–6 hours	Gluconate: 25 mg/min; total not to exceed 800 mg	Sulfate: 200–400 mg every 4–6 hours
Procainamide	250–500 mg every 4–6 hours	100 mg every 5 min; total not to exceed 1,000 mg	250–500 mg every 6 hours
Propranolol	—	1 mg/min; total not to exceed 0.1 mg/kg	10–30 mg every 6–8 hours
Lidocaine	—	Bolus: 25–50 mg every 5 min; total not to exceed 300 mg. Maintenance by drip: 1–4 mg/min	—
Diphenyl-hydantoin	—	100 mg every 5 min; total not to exceed 1,000 mg	100 mg every 6 hours

TABLE 22-12 COMPARATIVE PHARMACOKINETICS OF ANTIARRHYTHMIC AGENTS

Drugs	Protein Binding	Hepatic Metabolism	Renal Metabolism	Half-Life
Quinidine	++	90%	10%	5.0 hrs
Procainamide	+	10%	60%	3.0 hrs
Propranolol	+	90%	10%	2.3 hrs
Lidocaine	+	90%	10%	10 min*; 1.6 hrs†
Diphenylhydantoin	+++	90%	10%	24.0 hrs

Strength of binding interaction: ++++ > +++ > ++ > +
*Single bolus injection.
†Sustained intravenous infusion of therapeutic doses.

ably because of altered binding of the drug resulting in a greater unbound fraction (Letteri et al., 1971; Reidenberg et al., 1971).

Quinidine, procainamide, and propranolol have half-lives intermediate between those of lidocaine and diphenylhydantoin. Of the three agents, quinidine is most tightly bound to protein and has the longest half-life (five hours). Since quinidine (Conn, 1964) and propranolol (Bond, 1967) are primarily inactivated by hepatic metabolism, the half-life of these two agents are prolonged in the presence of hepatic dysfunction. In contrast, the half-life of procainamide will be prolonged in the presence of renal dysfunction (Koch-Weser, 1971).

All of the five agents are capable of producing undesirable cardiovascular, gastrointestinal, and central nervous system effects, which are more likely to occur in patients with myocardial damage than without it. Organic heart disease increases the sensitivity of the myocardium to toxic reactions, even at so-called therapeutic blood levels of the agents.

In addition, reduced cardiac output and the presence of organ system dysfunction will prolong the half-lives of the agents and contribute to toxicity. Perhaps, in the acutely ill patient, the most important side effects are those involving the cardiovascular system, since they are potentially life-threatening. All of the five agents are capable of producing serious conduction disturbances, profound hypotension, and significant reduction of cardiac output. These are especially prominent with propranolol, quinidine, and procainamide and less so with both lidocaine and diphenylhydantoin.

Because of their myocardial depressant action, the administration of antiarrhythmic drugs is generally discontinued in the preoperative period in patients undergoing corrective cardiac surgery, provided the patient's condition permits. The patient's condition, the presence or absence of hepatic or renal dysfunction, the clinical indication, and the specific drug used are factors to be considered in determining when to discontinue administration of antiarrhythmic agents. In general, diphenylhydantoin is discontinued three days before surgery. Quinidine, procainamide, and propranolol are stopped two days before, while lidocaine is discontinued one day before surgery.

Postoperatively, these drugs should be administered with extreme caution because of their hypotensive and negative inotropic effects. A thorough understanding of their electrophysiologic and hemodynamic effects and of their pharmacodynamic properties is essential to safe use of these drugs.

DIURETICS

Diuretics are useful in a wide variety of conditions that may be encountered in the care of the critically ill patient. However, they are primarily employed as adjuncts in the therapy of patients with acute ventricular failure and in those in chronic congestive heart failure, especially when edema, effusions, or anasarca are present. Frequently, the common denominator indicating diuretic therapy is the abnormal retention of water and salt. In some instances, however, diuretics are used in the clinical setting of the low cardiac output syndromes, even in the absence of overt signs of congestive failure, to improve ventricular performance by reducing preload and optimizing pressure-volume relationships in the ventricles (see Fig. 22–3). In addition, certain diuretics (particularly the benzothiadiazines) have been used in combination with other agents for the treatment of hypertension. Furosemide, specifically, has been advocated for use in the treatment of acute renal failure (Cantarovich et al., 1971), but the issue remains controversial.

In this section, only those drugs that augment urine flow by the mechanism of increasing renal solute excretion will be discussed. This includes those agents that inhibit renal transport of sodium (e.g., furosemide, ethacrynic acid, the benzothiadiazines, and organomercurials), the osmotic diuretics (e.g., mannitol), and the potassium-sparing diuretics (e.g., spironolactone, triamterene).

Table 22–13 lists the important pharmacologic actions of the more commonly used diuretic agents, while Table 22–14 summarizes pertinent pharmacodynamic information on these drugs.

Loop Diuretics

Furosemide and ethacrynic acid are two of the most potent diuretic agents available. These two agents, although chemically unrelated, share a similar mechanism of action and act on the same locus on the renal tubule (see Table 22–13). Both inhibit tubular reabsorption of sodium in the ascending limb of the loop of Henle (Hook and Williamson, 1965; Beyer et al., 1965), the locus of the countercurrent multiplier that is the basic mechanism responsible for urinary concentration and dilution.

Furosemide, by its effect on the countercurrent multiplier mechanism, abolishes the corticomedullary electrolyte concentration gradient and impairs the normal process of urinary concentration (Hook and Williamson,

TABLE 22-13   IMPORTANT PHARMACOLOGIC ACTIONS OF COMMONLY USED DIURETICS

Drugs	Mechanism of Action	Major Site(s) of Action	Other Actions
Furosemide	Inhibits tubular reabsorption of sodium	Ascending limb of the loop of Henle and distal diluting sites of renal tubule	1. May induce massive kaliuresis by presenting large sodium loads to the aldosterone-sensitive site of cation exchange 2. Reduces capacity of kidneys to regulate tonicity by interfering with countercurrent multiplier mechanism 3. Also promotes the excretion of chloride and hydrogen ions, hence tendency to produce metabolic alkalosis
Ethacrynic Acid	Same as furosemide	Same as furosemide	Same as furosemide
Benzothiadiazines (Thiazides)	Inhibit tubular reabsorption of sodium	Distal diluting sites (between diluting segment in ascending loop of Henle and portions of distal tubule where sodium reabsorption is modulated by aldosterone)	1. Also promote chloriuresis and kaliuresis 2. Increase osmolal clearance 3. Impair free-water clearance
Organomercurials	Reduce tubular reabsorption of sodium, presumably by inhibition of sulfhydryl-containing transport enzymes	Probably act mainly in proximal convoluted tubule*	1. Promote chloriuresis 2. Tend to produce metabolic alkalosis
Osmotic Diuretics	Increase obligatory water loss	Proximal and distal tubule	1. Expand extracellular fluid volume 2. May also interfere with tubular reabsorption of sodium by altering concentration gradients between tubular urine and tubular interstitium
Potassium-Sparing Diuretics Spironolactone	Competitively inhibits the binding of aldosterone to cellular receptors	Distal tubule	1. Reduces urinary loss of potassium 2. Most effective when secondary hyperaldosteronism a major factor in sodium retention
Triamterene	Inhibits sodium reabsorption and promotes potassium reabsorption	Distal tubule	Reduces urinary loss of potassium

*Controversial; drug action on other sites may be equally important.

TABLE 22-14 COMPARATIVE PHARMACODYNAMIC PROPERTIES OF COMMONLY USED DIURETICS

Drugs	Route of Administration	Dosage Range	Onset of Effect	Peak of Effect	Duration
Loop Diuretics					
Furosemide	IV; Oral	40–400 mg/day	IV: 5 min; Oral: 1 hr	IV: 30 min; Oral: 1–2 hrs	IV: 2 hrs; Oral: 6 hrs
Ethacrynic acid	IV; Oral	50–400 mg/day	IV: 15 min; Oral: 30 min	IV: 45 min; Oral: 2 hrs	IV: 3 hrs; Oral: 6–8 hrs
Benzothiadiazines					
Chlorothiazide	Oral	500–1,000 mg/day	1 hr	4 hrs	6–10 hrs
Hydrochlorothiazide	Oral	50–100 mg/day	2 hrs	4 hrs	12–18 hrs
Trichlormethiazide	Oral	4–8 mg/day	2 hrs	6 hrs	18–24 hrs
Chlorthalidone	Oral	100 mg/day	2 hrs	6 hrs	18–24 hrs
Organomercurials					
Meralluride	IM	0.5–2.0 ml IM; 3 times/week	2 hrs	6–8 hrs	12–24 hrs
Mercaptomerin	IM	0.5–2.0 ml IM; 3 times/week	2 hrs	6–8 hrs	12–24 hrs
Osmotic Diuretics					
Mannitol	IV	12.5–25 gm	15–30 min	45 min	2 hrs
Potassium-sparing Diuretics					
Spironolactone	Oral	25–100 mg/day	Gradual onset	48–72 after start of therapy	48–72 hrs after cessation of therapy
Triamterene	Oral	100–300 mg/day	2 hrs	6–8 hrs	12–18 hrs

1965). During solute diuresis, therefore, furosemide decreases tubular reabsorption of free water (Stason et al., 1966) and, like the thiazide diuretics, it inhibits free-water clearance during water diuresis. These observations support the view that the major site of action of furosemide is in the ascending limb of the loop of Henle and the distal diluting sites of the renal tubule.

Ethacrynic acid has a similar mode of action. It is capable of producing a significant reduction in the reabsorption of the filtered sodium load (Beyer et al., 1965). In the dog kidney, it abolishes the medullary hypertonicity and interferes with the ability to form a concentrated urine during hypovolemia (Goldberg, 1966) and also inhibits free-water clearance during water diuresis (Cannon et al., 1965).

Renal chloride excretion is greater than that of sodium after administration of both furosemide and ethacrynic acid. There is an accompanying increase in urinary titratable acidity and in potassium and ammonium excretion. Loss of potassium, hydrogen, and chloride ions may lead to hypokalemic or hypochloremic alkalosis (Larragh et al., 1966).

Furosemide and ethacrynic acid are effective orally and parenterally and both have a rapid onset of action with a relatively short duration of action, especially when administered intravenously (see Table 22-14). Because of rapid onset of action, they have become the diuretic agents of choice in the treatment of acute left ventricular failure and acute pulmonary edema. Moreover, patients in chronic congestive heart failure who have become refractory to less potent diuretics usually respond to furosemide and ethacrynic acid. Both agents remain effective in patients with low glomerular filtration rate, azotemia, and severe electrolyte disturbances. As mentioned previously, furosemide has been used in the treatment of acute renal failure (Cantarovich et al., 1971). Although its role in the latter condition remains controversial, furosemide has been shown to produce a decrease in renal vascular resistance and an increase in total renal blood flow (Hook et al., 1966), suggesting that it may be helpful in the treatment of acute ischemic renal failure. This potential application deserves further detailed study.

During use of these potent diuretics, careful observation and monitoring are necessary to guard against hyponatremia, hypochloremia, hypokalemia, and acute metabolic alkalosis. In practice, potassium chloride supplements are administered with the diuretics because of the tendency for hypokalemia and hypochloremic alkalosis to develop.

Benzothiadiazines (Thiazides)

The thiazides are believed to exert their diuretic effect primarily by inhibiting sodium reabsorption at the distal diluting sites (Larragh, 1962; Sullivan and Piroh, 1966). Osmolal clearance is increased and free-water clearance is impaired. Sodium reabsorption per se at the distal sites of sodium-for-potassium exchange is not altered; however, potassium secretion is increased by thiazide diuretics because of the increased load of sodium ions at the distal sites where potassium ions are secreted in exchange with sodium. The thiazides also possess a variable degree of inhibitory action on carbonic anhydrase. Inhibition of carbonic anhydrase and diminished hydrogen ion secretion also contribute to the kaliuretic action.

Because the thiazide diuretics also produce a significant kaliuresis, the serum potassium levels should be routinely monitored and supplemental potassium given as needed.

Organomercurials

Mercurials are believed to act primarily on the proximal convoluted tubules, although a distal site of action has been reported by several workers (Lambie and Robson, 1960; Sanabria, 1963; White and Rolf, 1963; Schmidt and Sullivan, 1966). They inhibit the sulfhydryl groups in transport enzymes, preventing the reabsorption of sodium and chloride, which are then excreted with an osmotically equivalent amount of water. The mercurials tend to produce a hypochloremic alkalosis. In the presence of metabolic alkalosis, the diuretic response to mercurials is markedly reduced; in this situation, acidifying salts such as ammonium chloride are administered to potentiate the diuretic effects of the mercurials. Although the use of the mercurial diuretics has declined in the past few years, these drugs remain among the most effective and useful diuretic agents available and may be employed when a more rapid onset of action is not required.

Mannitol

Mannitol is the reduced form of the sugar mannose and is an osmotic nonelectrolyte. Mannitol, unlike most sugars, is not metabolized. After intravenous infusion, its distribution is limited to the extracellular space, since it does not enter the cells. It is then freely filtered through the glomerulus and, since it is not reabsorbed, the amount of solute in the intratubular fluid is increased, which then preempts an equivalent volume of water within the tubular lumen. Even in the presence of antidiuretic hormone, the quantity of water reabsorbed from the tubular fluid is reduced during osmotic diuresis and a large volume of urine is presented to the distal tubules for excretion. It has also been reported that the reabsorption of sodium in the loop of Henle and the renal concentrating mechanism may be interfered with during mannitol diuresis (Goldberg and Ramirez, 1967).

Since mannitol can produce a sudden expansion of intravascular fluid volume, it must be used cautiously in patients with impaired cardiac performance.

Potassium-Sparing Diuretics

These are relatively weak diuretic agents that act mainly on the distal tubule. Spironolactone exerts its diuretic action by competing with aldosterone for specific receptor sites in the distal tubule, inhibiting the sodium-retaining action of aldosterone on the renal tubule (Liddle, 1958). Triamterene, on the other hand, is believed to exert its diuretic action by inhibiting sodium reabsorption and enhancing potassium reabsorption in the distal tubule (Liddle). These agents, therefore, cause a moderate increase in sodium and bicarbonate excretions in the urine and decreased urinary potassium and ammonia.

Spironolactone and triamterene are, by themselves, weak diuretic agents. These agents are most effective when used with the thiazides.

DRUGS THAT ALTER BLOOD COAGULATION

The rational use of drugs that influence the clotting mechanism of the blood is based on an understanding of the fundamental concepts of the mechanism of coagulation and lysis of a blood clot. These processes, which are not fully understood as yet, are reviewed in Chapter 15. For a more detailed discussion and review, the reader is encouraged to consult the reports of the International Committee on Blood Clotting Factors (1962). In this section, consideration will be limited to discussions of the pharmacologic properties of heparin and heparin antagonists, and the coumarin derivatives, warfarin and bishydroxycoumarin.

Heparin

Heparin is a naturally occurring mucoitin polysulfuric acid that has the property of prolonging the clotting of blood either in vivo or in vitro. The site of formation of heparin is not definitely established, but it is known that it is stored in mast cells, which are widely distributed in connective tissue. Heparin can be extracted from many organs particularly rich in mast cells. The liver and lungs of most species are rich in heparin. Commercial heparin is extracted from the lungs of domestic animals used for food by humans. Since heparin extracts obtained from different animals vary in potency, the final preparations are biologically standardized. Commercial preparations available in the United States generally contain not less than 100 U S P units per milligram.

Pharmacologic Properties. The major pharmacologic actions of heparin are almost entirely confined to the blood. While large doses of heparin given intravenously may affect blood lipid metabolism, the most significant effects are on blood coagulation.

Heparin inhibits the clotting of blood both in vivo and in vitro. When it is given in therapeutic doses, the *clotting time* is prolonged, while the *bleeding time* is generally unaffected. The *thrombin time* and one-stage *prothrombin time* are prolonged and thromboplastin generation is abnormal.

Heparin serves to prevent the formation of fibrin in the coagulation of blood through three closely related and interdependent mechanisms that affect the first three stages of coagulation. First, it retards the conversion of prothrombin to thrombin through its *antithromboplastin action* (Howell, 1925; Brinkhaus et al., 1939). Second, it exerts an *antithrombin action*, antagonizing the ability of thrombin to bring about the conversion of fibrinogen, by interacting with a plasma cofactor (Quick, 1938; Loomis, 1949). Third, heparin reduces platelet adhesiveness and inhibits the agglutination of platelets (Wright, 1951).

Clinical Use of Heparin. In clinical practice, heparin is used in a wide variety of conditions, primarily for the prevention and treatment of thrombosis and embolism. In cardiac surgery, heparin has a unique application; the use of extracorporeal circulation mandates the administration of heparin (see Chapter 5).

Heparin is not effective when given orally or rectally. Although it is well-absorbed after intramuscular and subcutaneous injections, the intravenous route is preferred. After intravenous administration, the onset of action is almost immediate, with the peak effect appearing in five to ten minutes. The clotting time will then gradually return to normal over the subsequent two to four hours. Although it is not appreciably destroyed by the blood itself, heparin disappears exponentially from the circulation. Since only 25 to 35 percent of a single dose of intravenously administered heparin can be recovered in the urine (Eiber et al., 1960), the rapid loss of heparin from the circulation must be due to extrarenal mechanisms. It is probable that heparin combines with plasma proteins and is, therefore, not readily available for passive renal excretion (Eiber and Danishefsky, 1957). It is also possible that exogenous heparin may be temporarily stored in the reticuloendothelial system. Olsson et al. (1963) reported that the rate of removal of heparin from the plasma is dependent on the dose. After intravenous injection, the half-lives of 100, 200, and 400 units per kilogram doses were estimated to be 56, 96, and 152 minutes, respectively.

For most clinical conditions requiring rapid and effective anticoagulation, a dose of 5,000 to 7,500 units of heparin given intravenously every six hours is generally adequate to prolong the clotting time to two to three times the control value. Since the metabolism of the drug can vary from patient to patient, appropriate checks of the clotting time should be made. When given by continuous drip infusion intravenously, a dose of 10 to 15 units per kilogram per hour is generally adequate for most conditions. For anticoagulation during the conduct of cardiopulmonary bypass, it has been our practice to administer an initial dose intravenously of 200 units per kilogram followed by additional doses of 100 units per kilogram for each hour of perfusion.

Toxicity of heparin is frequently due to overdosage, which is generally manifested as hemorrhagic phenomena from open wounds, skin puncture sites, and mucous membranes. Because of the short duration of action of aqueous heparin, treatment simply consists of a reduction in dosage. In the event of major hemorrhage, however, heparin administration must be discontinued and one of the heparin antagonists must be used to return the hemostatic mechanisms to safe levels.

Heparin Antagonists

Three compounds possess the property of reversing all the heparin actions on the coagulation mechanism. Hexadimethrene bromide, toluidine blue, and protamine sulfate are all capable of reacting directly with heparin to form inactive complexes. Of the three, only protamine sulfate is currently available for clinical use.

Protamine, a powerful heparin antagonist, is a low molecular weight protein found in the sperm of certain fish. The protamines are rich in arginine content, accounting for their strongly basic reaction, which is the basis for their antiheparin action. When the strongly basic protamine combines with the strongly acidic heparin, an inactive, stable salt complex devoid of anticoagulant action is formed.

The usual dose of protamine is 1.0 to 1.7 mg to antagonize each mg of heparin. Protamine should be given very slowly intravenously, no more than 5 mg per minute. In general, the quantity of protamine required decreases rapidly with the time elapsed after heparin injection.

To reverse the heparin effect after cardiopulmonary bypass, it has been our practice to adhere to the following dosage schedule. The initial dose is calculated on the basis of 3 mg of protamine per kilogram body weight (or 1.5 mg of protamine for every 100 units of initial dose heparin used), followed by three supplemental doses (each dose being one third the initial dose); the intravenous injections are given at half-hour intervals.

In general, this protamine regimen has been adequate. However, one should remember that the actual protamine requirement after cardiopulmonary bypass can vary widely, depending on the interplay of several factors, the most important of which are: (1) the decay of blood heparin levels as related to the duration of bypass and body temperature (Perkins et al., 1959); (2) additional heparin given in the form of heparinized blood (Tarhan et al., 1970); (3) supplemental doses to insure adequate heparin levels; (4) excessive heparin flush for arterial and venous monitoring lines; and (5) the amount of heparinized perfusate reinfused into the patient at the termination of bypass. Whenever the status of heparin reversal is uncertain, it is advisable to serially monitor the whole blood activated coagulation time (Hill et al., 1974) or, alternatively, to perform the "two-tube protamine titration" test described by Ellison et al. (1971) to determine more accurately the amount of protamine required.

To increase drug safety, certain precautions have to be taken when protamine is used to reverse the heparin effect after cardiopulmonary bypass. First, protamine must be administered very slowly because it can produce hypotension and bradycardia (Jacques, 1949; Egerton and Robinson, 1961) as well as depression of myocardial contractility (Fadali et al., 1974). It is now believed that protamine exerts a direct depressant effect on the myocardium and the peripheral vessels (Fadali et al.). Second, although protamine is thought to be nonantigenic, it can provoke an anaphylactoid type of reaction in the sensitive subject. For this reason, it is important to obtain a good history preoperatively. Specific emphasis should be given to eliciting a history of allergy to fish. When there is any doubt, a skin test for protamine should be performed.

Third, it is important to remember that protamine itself has anticoagulant properties (Shanberge et al., 1958; Andersen et al., 1959; Perkins et al., 1961; Hawskley, 1966; Berger et al., 1968). This anticoagulant action could in part be caused by interference with thromboplastin formation (Hougie, 1958), to its thrombocytopenic effects (Jacques, 1949; Hurt et al., 1956; Perkins et al.), or to other mechanisms. However, it appears that this anticoagulant effect is seen and becomes clinically significant only with larger doses of protamine (Ellison et al., 1971); these workers found that overdoses of as much as 800 mg/70 kg had minimal effects on the coagulation mechanisms of patients and volunteers.

COUMARIN DERIVATIVES

In this section, the pharmacologic properties of bishydroxycoumarin and warfarin will be discussed. The other oral anticoagulants (the indandione derivatives and other coumarin congeners) will not be considered because they are less frequently used in clinical practice. Moreover, one should remember that the coumarin and indandione derivatives all have essentially the same action in the body, their differences being mainly quantitative rather than qualitative. Therefore, for the sake of brevity, consideration will be limited to the two drugs in this group most commonly used clinically, namely, bishydroxycoumarin and warfarin.

Pharmacologic Properties

Bishydroxycoumarin and warfarin (hereinafter referred to as "the coumarin compounds" or "coumarins" for the sake of convenience) share one major pharmacologic action—the inhibition of blood clotting mechanisms. Like heparin, they are used for a wide variety of conditions for the prevention and treatment of thromboembolic disease. In cardiac surgery, the coumarins are the mainstays in the anticoagulant treatment of patients undergoing prosthetic cardiac valve replacement. Unlike heparin, however, the coumarin compounds have no effect in vitro and exert their effect in vivo only after a latent period of 12 to 24 hours.

The therapeutic action of the coumarin compounds depends on their ability to suppress the formation of prothrombin (factor II) and factors VII, IX, and X. The synthesis of these factors occurs in the liver and requires the presence of vitamin K. The exact mechanism underlying this action is still not completely known. However, because of the similarity in chemical structure of vitamin K and the coumarins, it is believed that these compounds may act as antimetabolites to block the utilization of vitamin K by the liver. This interference in the synthesis of factors II, VII, IX, and X results in a prolongation of both the prothrombin time and the coagulation time; the bleeding time is unaffected.

The coumarin drugs are all absorbed from the gastrointestinal tract, but at different rates. Warfarin is the only drug in the group that may be administered parenterally. After oral administration, warfarin is rapidly and completely absorbed by passive diffusion in the upper gastrointestinal tract and reaches its peak plasma concentration in three to nine hours (O'Reilly et al., 1963). In comparison, the absorption of bishydroxycoumarin is slow, imcomplete, and variable (O'Reilly et al., 1964). These differences in the rates and completeness in absorption partly account for the differences in the time required to produce the desired therapeutic effect.

The coumarins are highly bound (bishydroxycoumarin, 99 percent; warfarin, 97 percent) to the plasma proteins, predominantly to albumin (O'Reilly et al., 1963, 1964), but the binding is readily reversible. Coumarins bound to plasma proteins are pharmacologically inactive and are protected from biotransformation and excretion. Only the unbound (free) drug in the plasma is active; this fraction is in equilibrium with its sites of action and biotransformation and is susceptible to renal excretion. The bound fraction, on the other hand, constitutes a reservoir in the body and is gradually released as the concentration of the free (unbound) drug is reduced by biotransformation.

Metabolic breakdown of the coumarins is believed to take place in the hepatic microsomes by extensive hydroxylation through the action of mixed-function oxidase enzymes (Ikeda et al., 1968). While the high degree of binding of the coumarins to plasma proteins accounts for their long plasma half-life, individual variations in the half-life are mainly due to differences in the rates of biotransformation. In addition, the basic chemical structure of a specific compound appears to be an important determinant.

For example, it has been observed that the half-lives of compounds with a double coumarin ring system (examples: bishydroxycoumarin and ethylbiscoumacetate) increase with the plasma concentrations of the drugs (O'Reilly et al., 1964; Brodie et al., 1952). The plasma half-life of bishydroxycoumarin, after a single oral dose of 2 mg/kg, has been estimated to be 24 hours (Motulsky, 1964), whereas with a higher dose (e.g., 4 mg/kg) the half-life averaged approximately 48 hours (Vessel and Page, 1968). In contrast, the half-lives of the single coumarin ring compounds (examples: warfarin and acenocoumarin) are independent of their plasma concentrations.

Dosage Schedule

The dosage schedule for these compounds is determined by the desired therapeutic end point and must, therefore, be individualized. The prothrombin time must be monitored carefully and frequently until stability is attained. The oral route is preferable but may be contraindicated when gastrointestinal dysfunction is present. As pointed out before, warfarin may be administered parenterally. In practice, a loading dose is administered in the first day or two of therapy. Thereafter, much smaller daily maintenance doses are given and the exact amounts depend on the carefully monitored prothrombin time. The standard dosage schedule for bishydroxycoumarin is: 300 mg on the first day, 200 mg on the second day, and an average maintenance dose of 75 mg per day (range, 25 to 150 mg), depending on the therapeutic response. For warfarin, the standard schedule is an initial dose of 25 to 30 mg, and a maintenance dose of 2.5 to 25 mg per day.

It should be emphasized, however, that these dosage schedules have been designed for patients with normal liver function. In contrast, *patients with a history of congestive heart failure or hepatic dysfunction will require much smaller amounts (one fourth to one half the usual doses) of the anticoagulant drugs.* In this regard, one should remember that some patients may show significant elevation of the prothrombin time, in the absence of anticoagulant therapy, for the first 7 to 14 days after corrective cardiac surgery. These and other factors

TABLE 22–15 DRUGS THAT INCREASE THE ANTICOAGULANT EFFECTS OF THE COUMARINS IN HUMANS*

I. Drugs that inhibit hepatic microsomal enzyme activity:

    Allopurinol
    Chloramphenicol
    (with bishydroxycoumarin)

II. Drugs that interfere with prothrombin-complex synthesis:

    Antibiotics, oral (mainly chloramphenicol, chlortetracycline, and neomycin)

III. Drugs that reduce plasma prothrombin concentration:

    Salicylates

IV. Drugs that displace coumarins from protein-binding sites:

    Chloral hydrate
    Clofibrate
    Oxyphenbutazone
    Phenylbutazone
    Sulfonamides, long-acting

V. Drugs with unknown mechanism of action:

    Anabolic-androgenic steroids
    Quinidine
    Quinine
    Thyroid hormone

From: Adverse interactions of drugs. *The Medical Letter on Drugs and Therapeutics* (1973).

TABLE 22–16 DRUGS THAT DIMINISH THE ANTICOAGULANT EFFECTS OF THE COUMARINS IN HUMANS*

I. Drugs that induce increased activity of liver microsomal enzymes:

    Barbiturates
    Glutethimide
    Griseofulvin

II. Drugs that increase the action of some clotting factors:

    Contraceptives, oral

From: Adverse interactions of drugs. *The Medical Letter on Drugs and Therapeutics* (1973).

should be taken into consideration whenever anticoagulants are prescribed for the cardiac surgical patient (see below).

Toxicity

The principal toxicity of these compounds is the direct consequence of overdosage, resulting in marked depression of the synthesis of factors II, VII, IX, and X, which in turn leads to hemorrhagic complications. The coagulation defect produced by the coumarins can be directly combated by fresh whole blood transfusions, which supply the needed vitamin K-dependent coagulation factors to the patient. Large doses of vitamin K_1 oxide likewise will be effective by supplying the vitamin needed to enable the liver to synthesize the necessary coagulation factors; however, there is a latent period of three to four hours before the desired therapeutic effect is obtained.

Usually an overly prolonged prothrombin time or minor hemorrhage will respond satisfactorily to simple withdrawal of therapy. The need for vitamin K should be carefully assessed, since this complicates subsequent anticoagulant therapy. Moreover, because of the long half-life of the coumarins, the establishment of a new steady-state plasma concentration evolves rather slowly and the delay in reestablishing therapeutic levels may increase the likelihood of thromboembolism.

When significant hemorrhage occurs, the coumarin drug must be discontinued and fresh whole blood transfusions, along with vitamin K_1 oxide, should be administered.

Numerous factors influence the intensity and the duration of the anticoagulant activity of the coumarins. Among the more important ones are: the amount of vitamin K in the diet, the status of the hepatic function, the nature of the gastrointestinal flora, the presence or absence of gastrointestinal dysfunction, and the influence of drug interaction. The problem of drug interaction is discussed briefly below.

Drug Interaction

Perhaps no other group of therapeutic agents is more subject to drug interaction than the oral anticoagulants. For a comprehensive discussion of the problem of drug interaction involving anticoagulants the reader is referred to the review by Koch-Weser and Sellers (1971). In this section the interaction of drugs with coumarin will be discussed.

Pharmacologic agents can modify the anticoagulant action of coumarins through a number of possible mechanisms. They can: (1) alter the bioavailability of vitamin K; (2) interfere with coumarin absorption, protein binding, biotransformation, or excretion; (3) interfere with the synthesis and catabolism of factors II, VII, IX, and X without affecting the pharmokinetics of vitamin K or of the coumarins themselves; (4) alter the affinity for the coumarins at the hepatic receptor sites; or (5) interfere with other parts of the coagulation mechanism unrelated to prothrombin-complex activity. It is apparent that drug interaction may involve extremely complex mechanisms.

Some drugs in clinical use have definitely been shown to interact with the coumarins in humans. Those drugs known to increase the anticoagulant effect of the coumarins are listed in Table 22–15, while the drugs known to diminish their anticoagulant effect are listed in Table 22–16. The probable mechanism of drug interaction is indicated whenever the necessary information is available.

From the foregoing it is obvious that the clinician must exercise extreme caution in prescribing anticoagulant drugs. This is especially true for the cardiac patient who has had prosthetic valve replacement, since such a patient very frequently has secondary hepatic dysfunction. In addition, he or she usually receives several drugs simultaneously, including analgesics, antibiotics, sedatives, and hypnotics. The simultaneous use of several therapeutic agents undoubtedly increases the likelihood of adverse drug interactions.

REFERENCES

Ackerman G L, Doherty J E, Flanigan W J: Peritoneal dialysis and hemodialysis of tritiated digoxin. Ann Intern Med 67:718, 1967.

Adverse interactions of drugs. Med Lett Drugs Ther 15 (383): 77, 1973.

Ahlquist R P: A study of the adrenotropic receptors. Am J Physiol 153:586, 1948.

Akhtar N, Chaudhry M H, Cohn J N: Dobutamine: selective inotropic action in patients with heart failure. Circulation 48 (Suppl IV):136, 1973.

Albers A W, Kavat G J, Engel G J: Studies on the interaction of ouabain and other cardioactive steroids with sodium-potassium activated adenosine triphosphatase. Mol Pharmacol 4:324, 1968.

Allwood M J, Cobbold A F, Ginsburg J: Peripheral vascular effects of noradrenaline, isopropylnoradrenaline and dopamine. Br Med Bull 19:132, 1963.

Andersen M N, Mendelow M, Alfano C A: Experimental studies of heparin-protamine activity with reference to protamine inhibition of clotting. Surgery 46:1060, 1959.

Armstrong P W, Gold H K, Daggett W M, Austen W G, Sanders C A: Hemodynamic evaluation of glucagon in symptomatic heart disease. Circulation 44:67, 1971.

Athos W J, McHugh B P, Fineberg S E, Hilton J G: The effects of guanethidine on the adrenal medulla. J Pharmacol Exp Ther 137:229, 1962.

Austen W G, Ebert P A, Greenfield L J, Morrow A G: The effect of cardiopulmonary bypass on tissue digoxin concentrations in the dog. J Surg Res 2:85, 1962.

Baschieri L Ricci P D, Mazzuoli G F: Studi su la portata epatica nell' oumo: modificazioni del flusso epatico da digitale. Coure Circ 41:103, 1957.

Bazzano G, Bazzano G S: Digitalis intoxication: treatment with a new steroid-binding resin. JAMA 220:828, 1972.

Beall A C Jr, Johnson P C, Driscol T, Alexander J K, Dennis E W, McNamara D G, Cooley D A, DeBakey M E: Effect of total cardiopulmonary bypass on myocardial and blood digoxin concentration in man. Am J Cardiol 11:194, 1963.

Bearn A G, Billing B, Sherlock S: The effect of adrenaline and noradrenaline on hepatic blood flow and splanchnic carbohydrate metabolism in man. J Physiol (Lond) 115:430, 1951.

Beiser G D, Epstein S E, Stampfer M, Robinson B, Braunwald E: Studies on digitalis. XVII. Effects of ouabain on the hemodynamic response to exercise in patients with mitral stenosis in normal sinus rhythm. N Engl J Med 278:131, 1968.

Beregovich J, Bianchi C, D'Angelo R, Diaz R, Rubler S: Hemodynamic studies with dobutamine, a new inotropic agent. Circulation 48 (Suppl IV):144, 1973.

———, ———, Rubler S, Lomnitz E, Cagin N, Levitt B: Dose-related hemodynamic and renal effects of dopamine in congestive heart failure. Am Heart J 87:550, 1974.

———, Reicher-Reiss H, Kunstadt D, Grishman A: Hemodynamic effects of isoproterenol in cardiac surgery. J Thorac Cardiovasc Surg 62:957, 1971.

Berger R L, Ramasamy K, Ryan T J: Reduced protamine dosage for heparin neutralization in open-heart operations. Circulation 37, 38(Suppl II): II–154, II–157, 1968.

Beyer K H, Baer J E, Michaelson J K, Russo H F: Renotropic characteristics of ethacrynic acid: a phenoxyacetic saluretic-diuretic agent. J Pharmacol Exp Ther 147:1, 1965.

Bhatia S K, Frohlich E D: Hemodynamic comparison of agents useful in hypertensive emergencies. Am Heart J 85:367, 1973.

Bigger J T Jr, Bassett A L, Hoffman B F: Electrophysiological effects of diphenylhydantoin on canine Purkinje fibers. Circ Res 22:221, 1968.

———, Heissenbuttel R H: The use of procainamide and lidocaine in the treatment of cardiac arrhythmias. Prog Cardiovasc Dis 11:515, 1969.

———, Mandel W J: Effect of lidocaine on the electrophysiological properties of ventricular muscle and Purkinje fibers. J Clin Invest 49:63, 1970.

Bliss H A, Fishman W E, Smith P M: Effect of alterations of blood pH on digitalis toxicity. J Lab Clin Med 62:53, 1963.

Bond P A: Metabolism of propranolol, a potent specific beta adrenergic receptor blocking agent. Nature 213:721, 1967.

Braunwald E, Bloodwell R D, Goldberg L I, Morrow A G: Studies on digitalis. IV. Observations in man on the effects of digitalis preparations on the contractility of the nonfailing heart and on total vascular resistance. J Clin Invest 40:52, 1961.

Brinkhaus K M, Smith H P, Warner E D, Seegers W H: The inhibition of blood clotting: an unidentified substance which acts in conjunction with heparin to prevent the conversion of prothrombin to thrombin. Am J Physiol 125:683, 1939.

Brodie B B, Weiner M, Burns J J, Simson G, Yale E K: The physiologic disposition of ethylbiscoumacetate (Tromexan) in man and a method for its estimation in biological material. J Pharmacol Exp Ther 106:453, 1952.

Brunner H, Hedwall P R, Meier M: Influence of adrenergic beta-receptor blockade on the acute cardiovascular effects of hydralazine. Br J Pharmacol 19:182, 1967.

Buckberg G D, Luck J C, Payne D B, Hoffman J I E, Archie J P, Fixler D E: Experimental subendocardial ischemia in dogs with normal coronary arteries. Circ Res 30:67, 1972.

———, Ross G: Effects of isoprenaline on coronary blood flow: its distribution and myocardial performance. Cardiovasc Res 7:429, 1973.

Burwell C S, Neighbors DeW, Regen E M: The effect of digitalis upon the output of the heart in normal man. J Clin Invest 5:125, 1927.

Butcher R W, Sutherland E W: Adenosine 3', 5'-monophosphate in biological materials. II. The measurements of cyclic 3'-5'-AMP in tissues and the role of the cyclic nucleotide in the lipolytic response to epinephrine. J Biol Chem 237:1244, 1962.

Butler V P Jr: Digoxin: immunologic approaches to measurement and reversal of toxicity. N Engl J Med 283:1150, 1970.

Caldwell J H, Bush C A, Greenberger N J: Interruption of the enterohepatic circulation of digitoxin by cholestyramine. II. Effect on metabolic disposition of tritium-labelled digitoxin and cardiac systolic intervals in man. J Clin Invest 50:2638, 1971.

Cannon P J, Heinemann H O, Stason W B, Larragh J H: Ethacrynic acid: effectiveness and mode of diuretic action in man. Circulation 31:5, 1965.

Cantarovich F, Fernandez JC, Locatelli A, Perez Loredo J, Cristhot J: Furosemide in high doses in the treatment of acute renal failure. Postgrad Med J 47 (Suppl):13, 1971.

Carlsson A, Waldeck B: The accumulation of [^{3}H] noradrenaline in the adrenergic fibers of reserpine-treated mice. J Pharm Pharmacol 19:182, 1967.

Cattell M, Gold H: Influence of digitalis glycosides on the force of contraction of mammalian cardiac muscle. J Pharmacol Exp Ther 62:116, 1938.

Chaterjee K, Parmley W W, Ganz W, Forrester J, Walinsky P, Crexells C, Swan H J C: Hemodynamic and metabolic responses to vasodilator therapy in acute myocardial infarction. Circulation 48:1183, 1973.

Clark W G: Studies on inhibition of L-DOPA decar-

boxylase *in vitro* and *in vivo*. Pharmacol Rev 11:330, 1959.
Cobb F R, McHale P A, Bache R J, Greenfield J C Jr: Coronary and systemic hemodynamic effects of dopamine in the awake dog. Am J Physiol 222:1355, 1972.
Cohn J N, Tristani F E, Khatri I M: Cardiac and peripheral vascular effects of digitalis in clinical cardiogenic shock. Am Heart J 78:318, 1969.
Coltart DJ, Chamberlain DA, Howard MR, Kettlewell MG, Mercer JL, Smith TW: Effect of cardiopulmonary bypass on plasma digoxin concentrations. Br Heart J 33:334, 1971.
Conn H L: Quinidine as an antiarrhythmic agent. In Banyai A L, Gordon B L (eds): Advances in Cardiopulmonary Disease. Chicago, Yearbook, 1964, p 286.
———, Luchi R J: Some cellular and metabolic considerations relating to the action of quinidine as a prototype antiarrhythmic agent. Am J Med 37:685, 1964.
Conn R D: Diphenylhydantoin sodium in cardiac arrhythmias. N Engl J Med 272:277, 1965.
Covell J W, Braunwald E, Ross J Jr, Sonnenblick E H: Studies on digitalis. XVI. Effects on myocardial oxygen consumption. J Clin Invest 45:1535, 1966.
Crexells C, Bourassa M G, Biron P: Effects of dopamine on myocardial metabolism in patients with ischemic heart disease. Cardiovasc Res 7:438, 1973.
Damato A N: Diphenylhydantoin: pharmacological and clinical use. Prog Cardiovasc Dis 12:1, 1969.
Davis, J O: Adrenocortical and renal hormonal functions in experimental cardiac failure. Circulation 25:1002, 1962.
Davis L D, Temte J V: Effects of propranolol on the transmembrane potentials of ventricular muscle and Purkinje fibers of the dog. Circ Res 2:661, 1968.
Deichmann W B, Gerarde H W: Toxicology of Drugs and Chemicals. New York, Academic Press, 1969.
Diamond G, Forrester J, Danzig R, Parmley W W, Swan H J C: Acute myocardial infarction in man. Comparative hemodynamic effects of norepinephrine and glucagon. Am J Cardiol 27:612, 1971.
Doherty J E, Hall W H, Murphy M L, Beard O W: New information regarding digitalis metabolism. Chest 59:433, 1971.
———, Perkins W H: Digoxin metabolism in hypo- and hyperthyroidism: studies with tritiated digoxin in thyroid disease. Ann Intern Med 64:489, 1966.
Domino E F: Antipsychotics: phenothiazines, thioxanthenes, butyrophenones, and rauwolfia alkaloids. In DiPalma J R (ed): Drill's Pharmacology in Medicine. New York, McGraw-Hill, 1971, pp 464–474.
Doring D, Trenckmann H, Urbazek W: Die kardiovaskulären Wirkungen von Hydroxytyramin (Dopamin) und ihre Bedeutung für die Therapie des kardiogenen Schocks beim Herzinfarkt. Z Gesamte Inn Med 24:881, 1969.
Dreifus LS, Filip Z, Sexton DM, Watanabe Y: Electrophysiological and clinical effects of a new antiarrhythmic agent: Disopyramide. Am J Cardiol 31:129, 1973.
Dungan W T, Doherty J E, Harvey C, Char F, Dalrymple G V: Tritiated digoxin. XVIII. Studies in infants and children. Circulation 46:983, 1972.
Ebert P A, Jude J R, Gaertner R A: Persistent hypokalemia following open heart surgery. Circulation 31(Suppl):137, 1965.
———, Morrow A G, Austen W G: Clinical studies of the effect of extracorporeal circulation on myocardial digoxin concentrations. Am J Cardiol 11:201, 1963.
Eble J N: Proposed mechanism for the depressor effect of dopamine in the anesthetized dog. J Pharmacol Exp Ther 145:64, 1964.
Eddleman E E Jr, Willis K, Greve M J, Hayer H E: The effect of digitoxin on the apparent stroke volume, posteroanterior cardiac diameter, and the cardiac cycle in normal subjects as studied by the electrokymograph. Am Heart J 41:161, 1951.
Egerton W S, Robinson C L H: Anticoagulant and hypotensive properties of hexadimetrine and protamine. Lancet 2:635, 1961.
Eiber H B, Danishefsky I: Heparin in blood. Proc Soc Exp Biol Med 94:801, 1957.
———, ———, Borrelli FJ: Studies made with radioactive heparin in humans. Angiology 11:40, 1960.
Ellison N, Ominsky A J, Wollman H: Is protamine a clinically important anticoagulant: A negative answer. Anesthesiology 35:621, 1971.
Entman M L, Levey G S, Epstein S E: Mechanism of action of epinephrine and glucagon on the canine heart. Circ Res 25:429, 1969.
Epstein S E, Braunwald E: Beta-adrenergic receptor blocking drugs. N Engl J Med 275:1106, 1175, 1966.
———, Skelton C L, Levey G S, Entman M: Adenyl cyclase and myocardial contractility. Ann Intern Med 72:561, 1970.
Ewy G A, Kapadia G G, Yao L, Lullin M, Marcus F I: Digoxin metabolism in the elderly. Circulation 39:449, 1969.

Fadali M A, Ledbetter M, Papcostas C A, Duke L J, Lemole G M: Mechanism responsible for the cardiovascular depressant effect of protamine sulfate. Ann Surg 180:232, 1974.

Farah, A, Tuttle R: Studies on pharmacology of glucagon. J Pharmacol Exp Ther 129:49, 1960.

Fawaz G: Cardiovascular pharmacology. Ann Rev Pharmacol 3:57, 1963.

Fisch C: Digitalis intoxication. JAMA 26:1770, 1971.

Franciosa J A, Guiha N H, Limas C J, Rodriguera E, Cohn J N: Improved left ventricular function during nitroprusside infusion in acute myocardial infarction. Lancet 1:650, 1972.

Frieden J: Lidocaine as an antiarrhythmic agent. Am Heart J 70:713, 1965.

Gibson D, Sowton E: The use of beta-adrenergic receptor blocking drugs in dysrhythmias. Prog Cardiovasc Dis 12:16, 1969.

Gifford R W Jr: Hypertensive emergencies and their treatment. Med Clin North Am 45:441, 1961.

——: The treatment of hypertensive emergencies. Am J Cardiol 9:880, 1962.

Gillis R A, Raines A, Sohn Y J, Levitt B, Standaert F G: Neuroexcitatory effects of digitalis and their role in the development of cardiac arrhythmias. J Pharmacol Exp Ther 183:154, 1972.

Glick G, Parmley W W, Wechsler A S: Glucagon: its enhancement of cardiac performance in the cat and dog and persistence of its inotropic action despite beta receptor blockade with propranolol. Circ Res 22:789, 1968.

Gold H K, Prindle K H, Levey G S, Epstein S E: Effects of experimental heart failure on the capacity of glucagon to augment myocardial contractility and activate adenyl cyclase. J Clin Invest 49:999, 1970.

Goldberg L I: Cardiovascular and renal actions of dopamine: potential clinical applications. Pharmacol Rev 24:1, 1972.

Goldberg M: Ethacrynic acid: site and mode of action. Ann NY Acad Sci 139:443, 1966.

——, Ramirez M A: Effects of saline and mannitol diuresis on renal concentrating mechanism in dogs: alterations in renal tissue solutes and water. Clin Sci 32:475, 1967.

Gombos E A, Hulet W H, Bopp P, Goldring W, Baldwin D S, Chasis H: Reactivity of renal and systemic circulations to vasoconstrictor agents in normotensive and hypertensive subjects. J Clin Invest 41:203, 1962.

Green, H D, Kepchar J P: Control of peripheral resistance in major systemic vascular beds. Physiol Rev 39:617, 1959.

Gregg D E, Fisher L C: Blood supply of the heart. In Handbook of Physiology, Vol 2. American Physiological Society, 1963, pp 1551-1552.

Grossman J I, Lubow L A, Frieden J, Rubin I L: Lidocaine in cardiac arrhythmias. Arch Intern Med 121:396, 1968.

Guiha N H, Cohn J N, Mikulic E, Franciosa J A, Limas C J: Treatment of refractory heart failure with infusion of nitroprusside. N Engl J Med 291:587, 1974.

Gunnar R M, Loeb H S, Klodnycky M, Sinno M Z, Towne W: Hemodynamic effects of dobutamine in man. Circulation 48(Suppl IV):132, 1973.

——, ——, Pietras R J, Tobin J R: Ineffectiveness of isoproterenol in shock due to acute myocardial infarction. JAMA 202:1124, 1967.

Haas H F: Active ion transport in heart muscle. In DeMello W C (ed): Electrical Phenomena in the Heart. New York, Academic Press, 1972, p 163.

Hamer J, Sowton E: Cardiac output after beta-adrenergic blockade in ischaemic heart disease. Br Heart J 27:892, 1965.

Han J: Mechanisms of ventricular arrhythmias associated with acute myocardial infarction. Am J Cardiol 24:800, 1969.

Hawksley M: De-heparinization of blood after cardiopulmonary bypass. Lancet 1:563, 1966.

Helfant R H, Lau S H, Cohen S I, Damato A N: Effects of diphenylhydantoin on atrioventricular conduction in man. Circulation 36:686, 1967.

Hill J D, Dontigny L, de Leval M, Mielke C H Jr: A simple method of heparin management during prolonged extracorporeal circulation. Ann Thorac Surg 17:129, 1974.

Hoch J H: A Survey of Cardiac Glycosides and Genins. Columbia, University of South Carolina Press, 1961.

Hoffman B F: Effects of digitalis on electrical activity of cardiac membranes. In Marks B H, Weissler A M (eds): Basic and Clinical Pharmacology of Digitalis. Springfiled, Ill, Thomas, 1972, p 118.

——: The genesis of cardiac arrhythmias. Prog Cardiovasc Dis 8:319, 1966.

——, Bigger J T Jr: Antiarrhythmic drugs. In DiPalma JR (ed): Drill's Pharmacology in Medicine, 4th ed. New York, McGraw-Hill, 1971, pp 831-832.

——, Cranefield P F: The physiologic basis of cardiac arrhythmias. Am J Med 37:473, 1964.

——, Singer D H: Effects of digitalis on electrical activity of cardiac fibers. Prog Cardiovasc Dis 7:226, 1964.

Holloway E L, Schultz C S, Stinson E B, Harrison D C: Comparison of circulatory effects of dopamine and isoproterenol immediately following

cardiac surgery. Circulation 48(Suppl IV):177, 1973.
Hook J B, Williamson H: Effects of furosemide on renal medullary sodium gradient. Proc Soc Exp Biol Med 118:372, 1965.
———, Blatt AH, Brody MJ, Williamson HE: Effects of several saluretic-diuretic agents on renal hemodynamics. J Pharmacol Exp Ther 154:667, 1966.
Horwitz D, Fox S M, Goldberg L I: Effects of dopamine in man. Circ Res 10:237, 1962.
Hougie C: Anticoagulant action of protamine sulphate. Proc Soc Exp Biol Med 98:130, 1958.
Howell W H: The purification of heparin and its presence in blood. Am J Physiol 71:553, 1925.
Hurt R, Perkins H A, Osborn J J, Gerbode F: The neutralization of heparin by protamine in extracorporeal circulation. J Thorac Surg 32:612, 1956.
Hyman A L, Jacques W E, Abelmann W H: Observations on the direct effect of digoxin on renal excretion of sodium and water. Am Heart J 52:592, 1956.
Ikeda M, Ullrich V, Staudinger H: Metabolism *in vitro* of warfarin by enzymic and nonenzymic systems. Biochem Pharmacol 17:1663, 1968.
International Committee on Blood Clotting Factors: Thrombosis et hemorrhagica. Trans Weisbaden Conference 6(Suppl 1): 1962.
Irons G V Jr, Orgain E S: Digitalis-induced arrhythmias and their management. Prog Cardiovasc Dis 8:539, 1966.
Jacques L B: A study of the toxicity of the protamine salmine. Br J Pharmacol 4:135, 1949.
Jellife R W: An improved method of digoxin therapy. Ann Intern Med 69:703, 1968.
Jewitt D, Birkhead J, Mitchell A, Colin D: Clinical cardiovascular pharmacology of dobutamine; a selective inotropic catecholamine. Lancet 11:364, 1974.
Jewitt D E, Kishon Y, Thomas M: Lignocaine in the management of arrhythmias after acute myocardial infarction. Lancet 1:266, 1968.
Johnson C C: The actions and toxicity of sodium nitroprusside. Arch Int Pharmacodyn Ther 35:480, 1929.
Jurado R A, Matucha D, Osborn J J: Cardiac output estimation by pulse contour methods: validity of their use for monitoring the critically ill patient. Surgery 74:358, 1973.
Kelliher G J, Roberts J: Effect of 6-hydroxydopamine on ouabain-induced arrhythmia. Clin Res 20:857, 1972.
Koch-Weser J: Pharmacokinetics of procainamide in man. Ann NY Acad Sci 179:370, 1971.
———, Sellers E M: Drug interactions with coumarin anticoagulants. N Engl J Med 285:487, 547, 1971.
Kopin I J: False adrenergic transmitters. Ann Rev Pharmacol 8:377, 1968.
Kouchoukos N T, Goldring D, Burton R M: Effect of extracorporeal circulation upon the tissue digoxin concentration in the dog. Circulation 24:975, 1961.
Kraft-Hunter F, Hinds J E: Cardiac dynamic effects of increasing myocardial contractility without changing heart rate, mean aortic pressure in conscious instrumented dogs. Fed Proc 32:343, 1973.
Kuhn L A: Shock in myocardial infarction—medical treatment. Am J Cardiol 26:603, 1970.
———, Kline, H J, Goodman P, Johnson C D, Marano A J: Effects of isoproterenol on hemodynamic alterations, myocardial metabolism and coronary flow in experimental acute myocardial infarction with shock. Am Heart J 77:772, 1969.
Kumar R, Yankopoulos N A, Abelmann W H: Ouabain-induced hypertension in a patient with decompensated hypertensive heart disease. Chest 63:105, 1973.
Lambie A T, Robson J S: The effect of mersalyl on the renal tubular reabsorption of solute-free water. Clin Sci 20:123, 1960.
Langer G A, Serena S D: Effects of strophanthidin upon contraction and ionic exchange in rabbit ventricular myocardium: relation to control of active state. J Mol Cell Cardiol 1:65, 1970.
Larragh J H: The mode of action and use of chlorothiazides and related compounds. Circulation 26:121, 1962.
———, Cannon P J, Stason W B, Heinemann H O: Physiologic and clinical observations on furosemide and ethacrynic acid. Ann NY Acad Sci 139:453, 1966.
Lee K S, Klaus W: The subcellular basis for the mechanism of inotropic action of cardiac glycosides. Pharmacol Rev 23:193, 1971.
Leiberson A D, Schumacher R R, Childress R H, Boyd D B, Williams J F Jr: Effects of diphenylhydantoin on left ventricular function in patients with heart disease. Circulation 36:692, 1969.
Letteri J M, Melk H, Louis S, Kutt H, Durante P, Glazko A: Diphenylhydantoin metabolism in uremia. N Engl J Med 285:648, 1971.
Liddle G W: Aldosterone antagonists. Arch Intern Med 102:998, 1958.

Lindenbaum J, Mellow M H, Blackstone M O, Butler V P Jr: Variation in biologic availability of digoxin from four preparations. N Engl J Med 285:257, 1971.

Litwak R S, Kuhn L A, Gadboys H L, Lukban S B, Sakurai H: Support of myocardial performance after open cardiac operations by rate augmentation. J Thorac Cardiovasc Surg 56:484, 1968.

Loeb H S, Winslow E B J, Rahimtoola S H, Rosen K M, Gunnar R F: Acute hemodynamic effects of dopamine in patients with shock. Circulation 44:163, 1971.

Loggie J M H: Hypertension in children and adolescents. II. Drug therapy. J Pediatr 74:640, 1969.

Loomis T A: Antithrombin and heparin in human blood. J Lab Clin Med 34:631, 1949.

Lown B, Vassaux C: Lidocaine in acute myocardial infarction. Am Heart J 76:586, 1968.

MacCannell K L, McNay J L, Meyer M B, Goldberg L I: The use of dopamine in the treatment of hypotension and shock. N Engl J Med 275:1389, 1966.

Marcus F I, Burkhalter L, Cuccia C, Pavlovich J, Kapadia G G: Administration of tritiated digoxin with and without a loading dose: a metabolic study. Circulation 46:865, 1966.

Maroko P R, Braunwald E: Modification of myocardial infarction size after coronary occlusion. Ann Intern Med 79:720, 1973.

———, Kjekshus J K, Sobel B E, Watanabe T, Covell J W, Ross J R, Braunwald E: Factors influencing infarct size following experimental coronary occlusion. Circulation 43:67, 1971.

———, Libby P, Braunwald E: Effect of pharmacologic agents on the function of the ischemic heart. Am J Cardiol 32:930, 1973.

Mason D T, Braunwald E: Studies on digitalis. X. Effects of ouabain on forearm vascular resistance and venous tone in normal subjects and in patients with heart failure. J Clin Invest 43:532, 1964.

———, Spann J R Jr, Zelis R, Amsterdam E A: The clinical pharmacology and therapeutic applications of the antiarrhythmic drugs. Clin Pharmacol Ther 11:460, 1970.

McDonald R H Jr, Goldberg L I: Analysis of cardiovascular effects of dopamine in dog. J Pharmacol Exp Ther 140:60, 1963.

———, ———, McNay J L, Tuttle E P: Effects of dopamine in man: augmentation of sodium excretion, glomerular filtration rate, and renal plasma flow. J Clin Invest 43:1116, 1964.

McNay J L, Goldberg L I: Comparison of effect of dopamine, isoproterenol, norepinephrine on canine renal and femoral flow. J Pharmacol Exp Ther 151:23, 1966.

———, McDonald R H Jr, Goldberg L I: Direct renal vasodilatation produced by dopamine in dog. Circ Res 16:510, 1965.

McRitchie R J, Vatner S F, Tuttle R, Braunwald E: Cardiovascular effects of dobutamine, a cardiospecific β-adrenergic stimulant in conscious dogs. Circulation 48(Suppl IV):132, 1973.

Mixter C G, Moran J M, Austen W G: Cardiac and peripheral vascular effects of diphenylhydantoin sodium. Am J Cardiol 17:332, 1966.

Molokhia F A, Beller G A, Smith T W, Asimacopoulos P J, Hood W B Jr, Norman J C: Constancy of myocardial digoxin concentration during experimental cardiopulmonary bypass. Ann Thorac Surg 11:222, 1971.

Morris J J Jr, Taft C V, Whalen R E, McIntosh H D: Digitalis and experimental myocardial infarction. Am Heart J 77:342, 1969.

Morrison J, Killip T: Serum digitalis and arrhythmia in patients undergoing cardiopulmonary bypass. Circulation 47:341, 1973.

Motulsky A G: Pharmacogenetics. Prog Med Genet 3:49, 1964.

Mueller H S, Giannelli S Jr, Ayres S M, Conklin E F, Gregory J J: Effect of isoproterenol on ventricular work and myocardial metabolism in the postoperative heart. Circulation 37, 38(Suppl II):II-146, 1968.

———, Gregory J J, Giannelli S Jr, Ayres S: Systemic hemodynamic and myocardial metabolic effects of isoproterenol and angiotensin after open heart surgery. Circulation 42:491, 1970.

Nayler W G: A direct effect of reserpine on ventricular contractility. J Pharmacol Exp Ther 139:222, 1963.

———, McInnes I, Stone J, Carson V, Lowe T E: Effect of dopamine on coronary vascular resistance and myocardial function. Cardiovasc Res 5:161, 1971.

Neff M S, Mendelssohn S, Kim K E, Banach S, Swartz C, Seller R H: Magnesium sulfate in digitalis toxicity. Am J Cardiol 29:377, 1972.

Neill C W: The use of digitalis in infants and children. Prog Cardiovasc Dis 7:399, 1964–65.

Noach E L, Woodbury D M, Goodman L S: Studies on the absorption, distribution, fate and excretion of 4-C labelled diphenylhydantoin. J Pharmacol Exp Ther 122:301, 1958.

Nord H J, Fontanes A L, Williams J F Jr: Treatment of congestive heart failure with glucagon. Ann Intern Med 72:649, 1970.

Nourok D S, Glassock R J, Solomon D H, Maxwell M H: Hypothyroidism following prolonged sodium nitroprusside therapy. Am J Med Sci 248:129, 1964.

Oliver G C, Cooksey J, Witte C, Witte M: Absorption and transport of digitoxin in the dog. Circ Res 29:419, 1971.

Olsson P, Lagergren H, Ek S: The elimination from plasma of intravenous heparin: an experimental study on dogs and humans. Acta Med Scand 173:619, 1963.

O'Reilly R A, Aggeler P M, Leong L S: Studies on the coumarin anticoagulant drugs: the pharmacodynamics of warfarin in man. J Clin Invest 42:1542, 1963.

———, ———, ———: Studies on the coumarin anticoagulant drugs: a comparison of the pharmacodynamics of dicumarol and warfarin in man. Thromb Diath Haemorrh 11:1, 1964.

Page I H, Corcoran A C, Dustan H P, Koppanyi T: Cardiovascular actions of sodium nitroprusside in animals and hypertensive patients. Circulation 11:188, 1955.

Palmer R F, Lasseter K C: Drug therapy. Sodium nitroprusside. N Engl J Med 292:294, 1975.

Parmley W W, Chatterjee K, Charuzi Y, Swan H J C: Hemodynamic effects of noninvasive systolic unloading (nitroprusside) and diastolic augmentation (external counterpulsation) in patients with acute myocardial infarction. Am J Cardiol 33:819, 1974.

———, Glick G, Sonnenblick E H: Cardiovascular effects of glucagon in man. N Engl J Med 279:12, 1968.

———, Matloff J M, Sonnenblick E H: Hemodynamic effects of glucagon in patients following prosthetic valve replacement. Circulation 39(Suppl 1):163, 1969.

Peleska B: Cardiac arrhythmias following condenser discharges and their dependence upon strength of current and phase of cardiac cycle. Circ Res 13:21, 1963.

Perkins H A, Harkins G, Gerbode F, Rolfs M R, Acra J: Comparison of effects of protamine and polybrene with special emphasis on the factor VIII (AHG) deficiency induced. J Clin Invest 40:1421, 1961.

———, Osborn J J, Gerbode F: The management of abnormal bleeding following extracorporeal circulation. Ann Intern Med 51:650, 1959.

Puri P S: The effect of diphenylhydantoin sodium (Dilantin) on myocardial contractility and hemodynamics. Am Heart J 82:62, 1971.

Quick J A: The normal antithrombin of the blood and its relation to heparin. Am J Physiol 123:712, 1938.

Rall T W, West T C: The potentiation of cardiac inotropic responses to norepinephrine by theophylline. J Pharmacol 139:269, 1963.

Ramdohr B, Biamino G, Schröder R: Vergleichende Untersuchungen uber die Wirkung von Dopamin und Orciprenalin am gesunden Menschen: Muskeldurchblutung, Nierendurchublutung, Nierenfunktion. Klin Wocheschr 50:149, 1972.

Rasmussen H: Cell communication, calcium ion, and cyclic adenosinemonophosphate. Science 170:404, 1970.

Regan T J, Lehan P H, Henneman D H, Behar A, Hellems H K: Myocardial metabolic and contractile response to glucagon and epinephrine. J Clin Lab Clin Med 63:638, 1964.

Reidenberg M M, Odar-Cederloff I, von Bahr C, Borga O, Sjogvist F: Protein binding of diphenylhydantoin and desmethylimipromine in plasma from patients with poor renal function. N Engl J Med 285:264, 1971.

Reis H E, van Zweiten P A: Hypotensive effect of hydralazine, injected into the vertebral artery of the cat. Arch Int Pharmacodyn Ther 169:494, 1967.

Robie N W, Nutter D O, Moody C, McNay J L: *In vivo* analysis of adrenergic receptor activity of dobutamine. Circ Res 34:663, 1974.

Robison G A, Butcher R W, Sutherland E W: Adenyl cyclase as an adrenergic receptor. Ann NY Acad Sci 139:703, 1967.

Rodensky P, Wasserman F: Observations on digitalis intoxications. Arch Intern Med 108:171, 1961.

Rodman T, Gorczyca C A, Pastor B H: The effect of digitalis on the cardiac output of the normal heart at rest and during exercise. Ann Intern Med 55:620, 1961.

Rosati R, Alexander J A, Schaal S F, Wallace A G: Influence of diphenylhydantoin on electrophysiological properties of the canine heart. Circ Res 21:757, 1967.

Rosenblum R, Berkowitz W D, Lawson D: Effect of acute intravenous administration of isoproterenol on cardiorenal hemodynamics in man. Circulation 38:158, 1968.

———, Frieden J: Intravenous dopamine in the treatment of myocardial dysfunction after open-heart surgery. Am Heart J 83:743, 1972.

Ross J Jr, Braunwald E, Waldhausen J A: Studies on digitalis. II. Extracardiac effects on venous return and on the capacity of the peripheral vascular bed. J Clin Invest 39:937, 1960a.

———, Waldhausen J A, Braunwald E: Studies on digitalis. I. Direct effects on peripheral vascular resistance. J Clin Invest 39:930, 1960b.

Rubin A A, Taylor R M, Roth F E: A brief review of the development of diazoxide as an antihypertensive agent. Ann NY Acad Sci 150:457, 1968.

Sanabria A: Ultrastructural changes produced in the rat kidney by a mercurial diuretic (meralluride). Br J Pharmacol 20:352, 1963.

Sanyal P H, Saunders P R: Action of ouabain upon normal and hypodynamic myocardium. Proc Soc Exp Biol Med 95:156, 1957.

Schamroth L, Krikier D M, Garrett C: Immediate effects of intravenous verapamil in cardiac arrhythmias. Br Med J 1:660, 1972.

Scheinman M M, Sullivan R W, Hyatt K H: Magnesium metabolism in patients undergoing cardiopulmonary bypass. Circulation 39(Suppl I):235, 1969.

Schlant R C, Tsagaris T S, Robertson R J Jr: Studies on the acute cardiovascular effects of intravenous sodium nitroprusside. Amer J Cardiol 9:51, 1962.

Schmidt D H, Butler V P Jr: Immunological protection against digoxin toxicity. J Clin Invest 50:866, 1971.

Schmidt R W, Sullivan L P: Effect of meralluride on distal nephron transport of sodium, potassium, and chloride. J Pharmacol Exp Ther 151:180, 1966.

Schön R, Schönfeld W, Menke K-H: Mechanism and role of Na^+/Ca^{++} competition in (NaK)-ATPase. Acta Biol Med Ger 29:643, 1972.

Schroeder H A: The pharmacology of hydralazine. In Moyer J H (ed): Hypertension: The First Hahnemann Symposium on Hypertensive Disease. Philadelphia, Saunders, 1959, pp 332–344.

Selden R, Smith T W: Ouabain pharmacokinetics in dog and man: determination of radioimmunoassay. Circulation 45:1176, 1972.

Seller R H, Cangiano J, Kim K E, Mendelssohn S, Brest A N, Swartz C: Digitalis toxicity and hypomagnesemia. Am Heart J 79:57, 1970.

Shanberge J N, Barlas A, Regan E E: The effect of protamine on thromboplastin formation. J Lab Clin Med 52:744, 1958.

Shell W E, Sobel B E: Protection of jeopardized ischemic myocardium by reduction of ventricular afterload. N Engl J Med 291:481, 1974.

Shore P A, Giachetti A: Dual actions of guanethidine on amine uptake mechanisms in adrenergic neurons. Biochem Pharmacol 15:899, 1966.

Singer D H, Ten Eick R C: Pharmacology of cardiac arrhythmias. Prog Cardiovasc Dis 11:488, 1969.

Smith J H, Oriol A, Morch J, McGregor M: Hemodynamic studies in cardiogenic shock. Treatment with isoproterenol and metaraminol. Circulation 35:1084, 1967.

Smith T W, Haber E: Digitalis. N Engl J Med 289:945, 1973.

Sodeman W A: Diagnosis and treatment of digitalis toxicity. N Engl J Med 273:35, 93, 1965.

Sonnenblick E H, Williams J F Jr, Glick G, Mason D T, Braunwald E: Studies on digitalis. XV. Effects of cardiac glycosides on myocardial force-velocity relations in the nonfailing human heart. Circulation 34:532, 1966.

Stason W B, Cannon P J, Heinemann H O, Larragh J H: Furosemide: a clinical evaluation of its diuretic action. Circulation 34:910, 1966.

Stenson R E, Constantino R T, Harrison D C: Interrelationships of hepatic blood flow, cardiac output, and blood levels of lidocaine in man. Circulation 43:205, 1971.

Stickler J C, Kessler R H: Direct renal action of some digitalis steroids. J Clin Invest 40:311, 1961.

Styles M, Coleman A J, Leary W P: Some hemodynamic effects of sodium nitroprusside. Anesthesiology 38:173, 1973.

Sullivan L P, Pirch I H: Effect of bendroflumethiazine on distal nephron transport of sodium, potassium and chloride. J Pharmacol Exp Ther 151:168, 1966.

Sutherland E W, Robison G A: The role of cyclic-3-5'-AMP in responses to catecholamines and other hormones. Pharmacol Rev 18:145, 1966.

———, ———, Butcher R W: Some aspects of the biological role of adenosine 3', 5'-monophosphate (cyclic AMP). Circulation 37:279, 1968.

Talley R C, Goldberg L I, Johnson C E, McNay J L: A hemodynamic comparison of dopamine and isoproterenol in patients in shock. Circulation 39:361, 1969.

Talso P J, Remenchik A P, Cutilleta A: Altered myocardial potassium gradients in acute alkalosis and their relationship to acetystrophantidin sensitivity in the dog. Circulation 26:794, 1962.

Tarhan S, Moffitt E A, Lundborg R O, Wallace R B: Use of heparinized priming blood after whole body perfusion. Surgery 67:584, 1970.

Thompson P D, Rowland M, Melmon K L: The influence of heart failure, liver disease and renal failure on the disposition of lidocaine in man. Am Heart J 82:417, 1971.

Tomen J E P: Some aspects of central nervous system pharmacology. Ann Rev Pharmacol 3:153, 1963.

Torretti J, Hendler E, Weinstein E: Functional significance of Na-K-ATPase in the kidney: effects of ouabain inhibition. Am J Physiol 222:1398, 1972.

Tuttle R R, Pollock G D, Todd G, Tust R: Dobutamine: containment of myocardial infarction size by a new inotropic agent. Circulation 48 (Suppl IV):132, 1973.

Vatner S F, Higgins C B, Braunwald E: Effects of norepinephrine on coronary circulation and left ventricular dynamics in the conscious dog. Circ Res 34:812, 1974.

———, McRitchie R J, Braunwald E: Effect of dobutamine on left ventricular performance, coronary dynamics, and distribution of cardiac output in conscious dogs. J Clin Invest 53:1265, 1974.

———, ———, Maroko P R, Patrick T A, Braunwald E: Paradoxical effects of isoproterenol, nitroglycerin and exercise in conscious dogs with myocardial ischemia. Trans Assoc Am Physicians 86:201, 1973.

Velasco M, Tjandramaga T B, McNay J L: Differential dose-related effects of dopamine on systemic and renal hemodynamics in hypertensive patients. Clin Res 22:308A, 1974.

Vesell E S, Page J G: Genetic control of dicumarol levels in man. J Clin Invest 47:2657, 1968.

Vismara L A, Mason D T, Amsterdam E A: Disopyramide phosphate: Clinical efficacy of a new oral antiarrhythmic drug. Clin Pharmacol Ther 16:330, 1974.

Walinsky P, Chatterjee K, Forrester J, Parmley W W, Swan H J C: Enhanced left ventricular performance with phentolamine in acute myocardial infarction. Am J Cardiol 33:37, 1974.

Wallace A G, Schaal S F, Sugimoto T, Rozear M, Alexander J A: The electrophysiologic effects of beta-adrenergic blockade and cardiac denervation. Bull NY Acad Med 43:1119, 1967.

———, Troyer W H, Lesage M A, Zotti E F: Electrophysiologic effects of isoproterenol and beta-blocking agents in awake dogs. Circ Res 18:140, 1966.

Warren M C, Gianelly R E, Cutler S L, Harrison D C: Digitalis toxicity. II. The effect of metabolic alkalosis. Am Heart J 75:358, 1968.

Watanabe Y, Dreifus L S: Arrhythmias: mechanisms and pathogenesis. In Dreifus L S, Likoff W (eds): Cardiac Arrhythmias. New York, Grune & Stratton 1973, pp 35–54.

Wegria R: Pharmacology of coronary circulation. Pharmacol Rev 3:197, 1951.

Weidmann S: Effect of current flow on the membrane potential of cardiac muscle. J Physiol (Lond) 115:227, 1951.

Weissler A M, Gamel W G, Grode H E, Cohen S, Schoenfeld C D: The effects of digitalis on ventricular ejection in normal human subjects. Circulation 29:721, 1964.

Wheat M W Jr, Harris P D, Malm J R, Kaiser G, Bowman F O, Palmer R F: Acute dissecting aneurysms of the aorta. Treatment and results in 64 patients. J Thorac Cardiovasc Surg 58:344, 1969.

———, Palmer R F: Drug therapy for dissecting aneurysms. Dis Chest 54:344, 1968.

White H L, Rolf D: An analysis of the effects of meralluride and ouabain on sodium excretion by stop-flow and slow-flow techniques. J Pharmacol 141:326, 1963.

Whitehouse F W, James T N: Chronotropic action of glucagon on sinus node. Proc Soc Exp Biol Med 122:823, 1966.

Whitsett T L, Goldberg L I: Effects of levodopa on systolic pre-ejection period, blood pressure, and heart rate during acute and chronic treatment of Parkinson's disease. Circulation 45:97, 1972.

Wildsmith J A W, Marshall R L, Jenkinson J L, MacRae W R, Scott D B: Haemodynamic effects of sodium nitroprusside during nitrous oxide-halothane anaesthesia. Br J Aneasth 45:71, 1973.

Withering W: An Account of the Foxglove and Some of Its Medical Uses: With Practical Remarks on Dropsy and Other Diseases. Birmingham, M. Swinney, 1785.

Wright H P: Fourth Conference on Blood Clotting and Allied Problems. New York, Josiah Macy Jr Foundation 1951, pp 119–142.

Zelis R, Mason D T: Compensatory mechanisms in congestive heart failure: the role of the peripheral resistance vessels. N Engl J Med 282:962, 1970.

Zuberbuhler R C, Bohr D F: Responses of coronary smooth muscle to catecholamines. Circ Res 16:431, 1965.

Index

Abscess, annular, 410
Absolute refractory period, 544
Ac-globulin, 27
Acid-base abnormality, 165
Acid-base balance
    concepts of, 161-80
    nomenclature problems, 163-64
    notation system, 161-63
Acid-base compensation
    defined, 164, 166
    metabolic, 171
    neurosis, 399
    renal, 171-72
    respiratory, 170-71
Acid-base derangements
    mixed, 165, 166
    types, 164
Acid-base factors
    nonrespiratory, 166
    respiratory, 166
Acid-base imbalance, use of alkali, 175-77
Acid-base measurements, 139-40, 164
Acid-base states, description of, 166
Acidemia, 163, 356
Acidosis, 258, 450
    defined, 163
    and digitalis toxicity, 554
    dynamics of buffering and compensation for nonrespiratory, 167
Acidosis, nonrespiratory, drugs for treatment of,
    sodium bicarbonate, 177
    Tris buffer, 177
Acidosis, respiratory, 288
Acrylic plaques, 246
Actin, 189
Activated clotting time (ACT), 379. *See also* Activated coagulation time.
Activated coagulation time (ACT)
    during intra-aortic balloon counterpulsation, 524-25

Activated coagulation time (ACT) *continued*
    during left heart bypass support, 528-29
    during whole body perfusion, 98, 110
Adenosine triphosphate
    and adrenergic drugs, 559
    loss of regulatory effect of, 193
    and muscle contraction, role in, 186
    "plasticizing effect," 186
Adenovirus, 418
Adenylate cyclase, 189-90, 193, 559
β-Adrenergic agonists, positive inotropic actions of, 193-95
β-Adrenergic blocking drugs, 44
Adrenergic drugs, mechanism of action, 558-60
Adrenergic stimulation, responses of cardiovascular effector cells to, 558
Aerobic energy production, curtailment of, 185
Affinity hypoxia, 167, 169
Afterload. *See also* Arterial impedance; Vascular resistance; Ventricular afterload.
    defined, 508
    determinants of, 508
    elevation of, management, 221
    optimization of, 221
    and stroke volume, 134, 140-41, 204, 449
After-potentials, delayed, 244
Aging
    and acute renal failure, 355-56
    physiologic handicaps imposed by, 29
    and postsurgical infection rates, 406
    and pulmonary dysfunction, 340
    and sick sinus syndrome, 457
Agitation, postoperative, 390
Air embolism, 76, 258
    avoidance of, 109-10
    hyperbaria in, 391
Airway
    choice, 313
    patency, 317

599

INDEX

Airway *continued*
  positioning, 313-14
  pressure determination, 320
  total flow resistance, 338
  and tracheal damage, 314-17
Airway pressure, 320. *See also* Positive end-expiratory pressure; Ventilation patterns.
  determinants of, 319-21
  gas exchange, effects on, 318-20
  hemodynamic effects of, 291, 298-303, 319-21
  peak inflation pressure, 444
  zero end-expiratory pressure (ZEEP), 303, 321
Airway resistance, calculation of, 318
Alcoholism, 395
Aldosterone, 171
Alkalemia, 163
Alkalosis, 163, 258
  causes, 169
  defined, 164
  and digitalis toxicity, 554
Alveolo-capillary membrane, 144
Ambulation, postoperative, 150
Analgesia, postoperative, morphine sulfate, 132-33
Anatomic bleeding, 376
Anesthesia
  for cardiac surgery, 43-61
  local
    lidocaine, 46, 517
    local infiltration, 472, 490, 530, 532, 534
  maintenance of, 54-61
  and myocardial contractility, effect on, 210
  preanesthetic visit, 43-45
  propranolol discontinuation and, 44-45
  and renal function, effect on, 144-45
Anesthesiologist, in neonatal closed procedures, 435
Anesthetic management
  and diazepam, 48-49
  enflurane, 48
  halothane, 48, 50-51
  methoxyflurane, 48
  monitoring, 46-47
  morphine, 48-49
  neuroleptanalgesia, 48
  nitrous oxide, 48, 49-50
  principles for, choice of, 48
  and d-tubocurarine, 51
Anesthetics, drug interactions with, 43-44
Aneurysm, 390
Aneurysmectomy, 256
Angina pectoris, 455
Angiography, 254, 390, 411
Anicteric hepatitis, 422
Antiarrhythmic agents, 35, 575-80
  classification, 576-78

Antiarrhythmic agents *continued*
  clinical uses, 578-81
  dosage schedule, 580
  effectiveness, 579
  electrophysiology, 577
  hemodynamics, 578
  pharmacokinetics, 580
Antibodies
  antiheart, 418
  heart-reactive, 418
Antibiotic(s)
  bactericidal, 411
  dose in patients with normal renal function, 413-14
Antibiotic therapy
  in infants and children, 452
  postoperative
    cefazolin, 133
    cephalosporin, 133
    gentamicin, 133
    penicillin, 133
    vancomycin, 133
  preventive, 407-08
  prophylactic, 37
Anticoagulants, circulating, 376
Anticoagulation. *See* Activated coagulation time.
Anticoagulation therapy, postoperative
  oral warfarin sodium, 150
  prothrombin determination and, 150
Anticonvulsant therapy, 390
Antidiuretic hormone (ADH), 144, 171
Antigen(s)
  Australia, 422
  hepatitis B virus, 422
Antiheart antibodies, 418
Antihemophilic globulin, 89
Antiinflammatory-antipyretic-analgesic agents, 419
Antimicrobial therapy, optimal duration of, 413
Anoxia
  classification, 8
  tolerance, 8
Anxiety
  defined, 399
  strain factor in, 400
Aorta, juxtaductal coarctation of, 434
Aortic arch, interrupted, 434
Aortic crossclamping, 258
  and delineation of A-V conduction system, 247-48
Aortic regurgitation, 209
  hemodynamic data for valve replacement in, 208
Aortic valve disease, 208-9, 340
Aortic valve replacement, 104
  hemodynamic changes in patient recovering from, 136
Arrhythmias, 455
  atrial, 493

INDEX

Arrhythmias *continued*
  catheter-induced, 475-76
  causes, 243
  diagnosis and management of, 259-62
    postoperative, 262-71
  drug therapy
    digoxin, 272, 274-75
    disopyramide, 271, 274
    lidocaine, 271, 272-73
    procainamide, 271, 273
    propranolol, 271, 274
    quinidine, 271, 273-74
  epicardial electrodes
    for diagnosis of, 260-61
    for treatment of, 261-62
  genesis, 242, 250
  intraoperative
    diagnosis and treatment, 258
    electrode implantation, 258-59
    etiologic considerations, 258
  mapping of, 251-54
  nature of, 243-45
  postoperative, 250
  predisposing factors, 259
  triggered activity, 244
  ventricular, 493
Arrhythmogenic mechanism, 244
Arterial blood, three-variable system for acid-base studies with, 162
Arterial cannula, pressure gradient across, 99
"Arterial counterpulsator," 224
Arterial impedance, 204-05. *See also* Afterload; Ventricular afterload.
Arterial oxygenation, effect of body position
  during mechanical ventilation, 294
  site of airway collapse, 293
Arteriovenous oxygen content difference, determination of, 496-97
Arthralgia, 419
Aspergillus species, 411
Atelectasis, 423
  management of, 348-49
  in postperfusion lung, 128
  recognition of, 345
Atrial arrhythmias, 242
Atrial electrode implantation, 467-70
  coronary sinus approach, 468
  epicardial, 469
  in right atrial appendage, 468
Atrial fibrillation, 258, 265-66
  use of digitalis in, 548
Atrial flutter
  digitalis, 548
  type I, 263-65

Atrial flutter *continued*
  type II, 265
Atrial pacing, 245
Atrial quiescence incidence after heart surgery, 270
Atrioventricular block, partial, 455
Atropine, and digitalis toxicity, 554
Autologous blood prime, 77
Automaticity, abnormalities of, 244
Autoregulation, in kidney, 356
A-V bypass pathway, serial interruption of, 252
A-V conduction system, grid for mapping, 248
A-V junction, grid for mapping, 248
A-V node, 242
Avco-Roche IABP system, 515-16
Azotemia, 455

Bachmann's bundle, 242
Bacteremia, gram-negative, 410
Bacterial endocarditis, 462, 476
Bacteroides species, 424
Balloon. *See* Intra-aortic balloon.
Balloon counterpulsation. *See* Intra-aortic balloon counterpulsation.
Balloon pump. *See* Avco-Roche IABP system; Datascope IABP system.
Balloon-tipped, flow-directed catheters, 490. *See also* Catheters, pulmonary artery catheterization; Swan-Ganz catheters.
Benzothiadiazines (Thiazides), 584
  pharmacologic action, 582
Bernard, Claude, 14
Beta blockade, 35, 44-45
Beta receptor, 193
Biocompatibility, 88-89
Biologic feedback systems
  characteristics, 20
  negative loop, 20-22
  positive, 20-22
Bleeding
  laboratory diagnosis and treatment, 379-80
  postoperative, 125-26
  preoperative factors affecting, 373-76
  surgical, 380-81
Block
  artrioventricular, 455
  congenital, 456
  intraventricular, 455
  second-degree, 455
  sequential, 456
  third-degree, 455
  trifascicular, 456
Blood
  buffering, 176

Blood *continued*
  characteristics, 387
  coagulation
    drugs altering, 585-87
    mechanisms, 370-72
  hemoglobin content, 497
  loss, excessive, 126
  lysis, 373
  in pericardial space, inflammatory reaction to, 417-18
  syringe administration of, 434
  trauma, from cardiotomy suction systems, 72
  viscosity, 2, 3
  volume, acute postperfusion changes in, 90
Blood-compatible surfaces, nonthrombogenic, 65
Blood film oxygenators, 69-70
Blood flow
  and anesthesia in older patients, 388
  brain
    redistribution of, 8
    reduced, 387
  and heart disease, 19
  regional distribution of, 3, 387
Blood-gas exchange, monitoring of, 142, 143
Blood-gas measurements, 139-40
Bloodless prime, 78
Blood pool scan, gated cardiac, 304
Blood urea nitrogen (BUN), 146-47, 355
Body position, clinical significance in cardiac surgery, 204
Body weight, in acute respiratory failure, 261
Bohr effect, 83
Bradyarrhythmias, 217, 271
  from succinylcholine, 51
Bradycardia, 217, 250, 262, 455, 470
Brainstem dysfunction, 391
Brainstem syndromes, postoperative, 390
"Bridge proteins," 369
Bronchitis, recognition of, 345
Bronchopneumonia, 346
Bronchopulmonary disease, 33
Bronchopulmonary secretions, suction removal of, 327-28
Bronchoscopy, 349
Bubble oxygenators, 388, 436
Buffers, defined, 170
Bulk transport. *See* Blood flow.
Bundle branches, 243
"Butterfly" needles, 425

Calcium ATPase pump, digitalis inhibition of, 543
Calcium movements, 189
Calcium transport mechanism, of cardiac sarcoplasmic reticulum, 195

Caloric examination, 391
Candida species, 406, 409
Cannulation, 389
  aortic, 437
  arterial, 98
    pressure gradient across, 99
  of critically ill patient, 101-02
  malposition of, 389
  systemic venous, 99-101
  vena caval, 437
Carbon dioxide removal
  efficiency, 297
  factors influencing, 297-98
Cardiac cells, types, 543
Cardiac contraction, oxygen dependency of, 184
Cardiac death, acute, prediction of, 448
Cardiac dysfunction
  preoperative, 206-10
    aortic valve disease, 209-10
    congenital heart disease, 207-08
    coronary artery disease, 210
    mitral valve disease, 209-10
    myocardial disease, 210
    pressure and volume overload, 207
    renal failure, acute, 355
  severity of, 338
Cardiac failure. *See also* Congestive heart failure.
  and digitalis glycosides, 34
  management of patients in, 34-35
Cardiac function
  dependence on substrate delivery, 184
  postoperative maintenance and support of, 199-234
    afterload, 221-22
    left ventricular performance, 223-28
    myocardial contractility, 222
    postrepair management, 228-34
    rate and rhythm, 216-19
    ventricular filling pressures, 219-21
Cardiac index (CI)
  defined, 507
  effect of ventricular pacing on, 218
  influence of blood infusion on, 220
Cardiac management
  early postoperative analysis and management, 230-31
  operating room analysis and management, 229-30
Cardiac massage, resuscitative external, 416
Cardiac output (CO), 359
  and blood flow, 19
  and blood oxygen, 2-3
  calculation
    by dye-dilution, 500-502
    by thermodilution, 404-07
  cellular death and, 19
  defined, 494, 507

INDEX

Cardiac output (CO) *continued*
   and digital computers, 152
   digitalis and, 545-46, 547
   in diving animals, 9-10
   estimation of, 138-39
   hematocrit and, 3
   and hyperkalemia, 452
   low, 356
   measurement
      direct Fick method, 495-99
      hemodynamic parameters of, 507-09
      indicator-dilution methods, 499-504
      invasive methods, 495
      methods, 494-95
      noninvasive methods, 495
      pulse contour method, 217, 494-95
      rationale for, 494
      and postoperative pacing, 218
   and pancuronium, 53-54
   and postoperative pulmonary function, 344
   and urinary volume, 145
Cardiac pacing, and treatment of arrhythmias, 261-62. *See also* Pacing, postoperative.
Cardiac performance. *See also* Myocardial performance; Ventricular performance.
   impaired. *See also* Cardiac performance impairment; Intra-aortic balloon counterpulsation; Left heart assist device; Left heart bypass support; Ventricular performance.
      pharmacologic agents in management of, 557
      recognition of, 140-42
   maintenance and support of, 233
   postrepair pacing and, 217-19
Cardiac performance impairment, 230, 231-34
   adverse postoperative events, 213-14
   in infants and children, 449-50
   residual pathology, 213
   severe, mechanical support of, 223-30
   surgical trauma, 213
Cardiac rate. *See also* Heart rate.
   atropine-induced elevation of, 201
   autonomic nervous system and, 201
   and cardiac output, 201
   and digitalis, effects of, 542
   exercise and, 200, 201
   postoperative, optimization of, 216-18
   postoperative cardiac performance and, 233
   reserve capacity of, 200
Cardiac rhythm. *See also* Rhythms.
   disturbances, use of digitalis in, 548-49
   maintenance of stable, 524
Cardiac stimulating drugs, 557-58
   dobutamine, 58-59
   dopamine, 58

Cardiac stimulating drugs *continued*
   epinephrine, 58
   norepinephrine, 58
Cardiogenic shock, and IABC, 513
Cardioplegia, 470-71
   hypothermic, 106-09
   techniques for, 255
Cardiopulmonary bypass (CPBP), 66. *See also* Extracorporeal circulation; Whole body perfusion.
   and acute renal failure, 356
   cannulation, 98-102
   cardiac damage resulting from, 211
   cardiovascular operations without, 433-35
   digitalis in, use of, 555-56
   discontinuance measures, 110
   effects on pulmonary function, 341-43
   embolism avoidance, 109-10
   fibrinolysis in, excessive, 373
   heart-lung machine, 96
   heparin administration, 97-98
   infection, incidence of, 404-05
   intracardiac blood recovery, 102
   measures following, 96
   monitoring, 95-96
   myocardial preservation, 104-09
   perfusion techniques, 102-04
   priming perfusate, 96-97
   renal response to, 144-46
   vessel exposure, 97
Cardiovascular pathology, residual, 213
Cardiovascular subsystems
   in neonates and children, 447-50
      management concepts, 449
      impaired cardiac performance, 449-50
   performance. *See* Cardiovascular subsystem performance.
   postoperative examination of, 122-23
   and renal failure, acute, 360
Cardiovascular subsystem performance
   adequate, 138
   inadequate, 139
   postoperative assessment of, 133-42, 214-16
      acid-base measurements, 139-40
      blood-gas measurements, 139-40
      cardiac performance, 140-42
      clinical observations, 133-34
      electrocardiographic observations, 134
      hemodynamic measurements, 134-37
Cardioversion
   condenser discharge (DC), 271
   and digitalis toxicity, 554
Carotid endarterectomy, 388
Cascase systems, 372
Catecholamines, 193. *See also* Adrenergic drugs;

Catecholamines *continued*
  Dobutamine; Dopamine; Epinephrine; Inotropic agents; Isoproterenol; Norepinephrine.
Catheter(s). *See also* Pulmonary artery catheterization; Swanz-Ganz catheters.
  balloon-tipped, flow-directed, 490, 491, 497
  indwelling, 424
    intravascular, 493
  injection, 502
  intravascular, 444, 493
  lumen
    double, 491
    quadruple, 492
  sampling, 502
  Swan-Ganz, 490
  wedging, 492
    permanent, 494
Catheterization, 252
  and halothane, 53
Catheter-related infections
  clinical features, 425
  management, 425-26
  pathogenesis of, 425
Cedilanid-D, 550
Central depression, and postoperative pulmonary function, 344
Central nervous subsystem, postoperative examination, 123, 148-49
Cerebral arterial occlusive disease, 388
Cerebral blood flow
  CO_2 effect on, 5
  P_{CO_2}, 5
Cerebral dysfunction
  and blood pressure, low arterial, 388-89
  postoperative, factors contributing to, 387-89
  and preoperative neurologic damage, 388
Cerebral function, following CPBP, 91-92
Cerebral venous return, obstruction of, 389
Cervical node enlargement, 420
Chaenocephalus. See Icefish.
Chest massage, closed, 416
Chest physiotherapy, during mechanical ventilation, 329
Chest roentgenography, 26, 419
Chlorothiazide, pharmacodynamic properties of, 583
Chlorpromazine, 575
Chlorthalidone, pharmacodynamic properties of, 583
Cholestyramine, and digitalis toxicity, 555
Cinefluoroscopy, 411
Circulatory arrest
  cannulation and, 437
  combined surface and core cooling with, 438
  desirable, 438
  with perfusion cooling alone, 438

Circulatory arrest *continued*
  safe period of, 438
Circulatory assistance, mechanical, 223-30, 509-34
Circulatory failure, defined, 196
Circus movement, 244
Clark electrode, 497
Claudication, intermittent, 455
Closed procedures
  anesthesiologist, role of, 435
  in infants, management of, 434-35
"Closing capacity," defined, 295
"Closing volume," defined, 295
Coagulation
  cascade, 369
  defects, testing for, 27
  intrinsic mechanism of, 368
  proteins, activation of, 372
Coagulation disorders
  acquired
    circulating anticoagulants, 376
    cyanotic heart disease, 376
    drugs, 376
    liver disease, 375-76
    vitamin K deficiency, 375
  inherited
    hemophilia A, 373-74
    hemophilia B, 374-75
    von Willebrand's disease, 375
Coagulopathy, 376
Colestipol, and digitalis toxicity, 555
Colloids, misuse of, 344
Colorimetry, 497
Coma, postoperative, 390
Compensation
  defined, 164, 166
  metabolic, 171
  neurosis, 399
  renal, 171-72
  respiratory, 170-71
Complement fixation, 422
Complement systems, 373
Computer(s)
  analog, 503
  cardiac output, 503
  digital
    philosophy and objectives, 150-51
    potential, 152-54
    role in patient monitoring, 151-52
    schematic of physiologic variables in, 153
Computerized transaxial tomography, 390
Conduction system
  anatomy of, 241-43
  avoiding damage to, 243
  fibrosis of, 456

INDEX

Conduction system *continued*
   identification of, 245-50
Conduction tissue, 242
Confusional states, postoperative, 390
Congenital heart disease, 207-08
   management of patients with, 36
Congenital lesions, respiratory complications following surgery for, 337
Congestive heart failure, 435, 455
   and digitalis in, 547-58
   and postoperative pulmonary function, 344
Contact activation, 370
Continuous positive airway pressure (CPAP), in infants and children, 445
Continuous positive-pressure ventilation (CPPV), 330
Contractile proteins, impaired response to Ca^{2+}, 192
Convulsions, in ICU, 389-90
Coronary artery bypass grafting (CABG), 416
   hemodynamic response, 57
   resection of left ventricular aneurysms, 250-51
Coronary artery disease, 210
   and intravenous morphine, 49
   management, 35-36
   propranolol therapy, 35-36
   ventricular tachycardia associated with, 254
Coronary artery perfusion, gravity flow, 105
Coronary circulation
   and arterial P_{CO_2}, 6
   and collateral, anemia and, 12-13
   and hemodilution, 4
   and ischemia, 3
Coronary occlusion, effect on adequate body perfusion, 11-13
Coronary perfusion
   improper, 258
   pumps, 67
Coumarin derivatives. *See also* Anticoagulant therapy, postoperative.
   anticoagulant effects of, 589
   dosage schedule, 588-89
   drug interactions, 590
   pharmacologic properties, 587-88
   toxicity, 589
Counterpulsation principle, 509-10
Coxsackie B virus, 419
Creatine-kinase (CK), serum activity determination, 28
Cryosurgery, 253, 258
Crystalloids, 344
Cuvette densitometer, 502
Cyanosis, 347
Cyanotic congenital heart disease (CCHD), 377
Cyanotic heart disease (CHD), 376
Cyclic-3', 5'-adenosine monophosphate (cyclic AMP), 189-90

Cyclic-3', 5'-adenosine monophosphate *continued*
   catecholamine, cardiac effects of, 559
Cytomegalovirus, 418, 419

Datascope IABP system, 515-16
DC cardioversion, 271
Dead space, connector/adaptor-catheter, 503
Death, fear of, 400
Decannulation, 440
Delirium
   characteristics, 395
   postcardiotomy, 387
   treatment, 396
      chlordiazepoxide, 397
      chlorpromazine, 396-97
      diazepam, 397
      haloperidol, 397
Delta wave, 252
Denial, preoperative, 397-98
Depression
   etiology, 397-98
   during prolonged hospital care, 33
   treatment, 398
Densitometer, 503
Desacetyl lanatoside C, 550
Deslanoside, 550
Diabetes mellitus, in cardiac surgical patient, 32
Dialysis. *See also* Hemodialysis.
   indications for, 362
   peritoneal, 362
Dialysis-dependent patients, open heart surgery in, 364
Diaphragmatic stimulation, 474
Diazoxide, 573
Diffusion and cellular transport, 17-19
   characteristics of, 18
   circulation and, 18
   factors affecting rate of, 18-19
Digitalis glycosides, 541-56
   autonomic effects, 545
   cardiac effects, 545-46
   in cardiopulmonary bypass, 555-56
   clinical use, 547-49
   dosage schedules, 551-52
   electrophysiologic effects, 542-45, 546
   inotropic effects, 542
   intoxication, 552-54. *See also* Digitalis toxicity.
   and kidney function, 547
   peripheral vascular effects, 546-47
   pharmacokinetics of, commonly used, 549
   preparations, 549-51
      deslanoside, 550-51
      digitalis leaf, 551

Digitalis glycosides *continued*
  preparations *continued*
    digitoxin, 551
    oaubain, 549-50
  in renal failure, 556
Digitalis toxicity
  in cardiopulmonary bypass, 555
  electrical pacing in, 554
  electrophysiologic effects, 546
  factors predisposing to, development of, 553
  immunologic reversal of, 554-55
  transmembrane action potentials and, 545
  treatment, 554-55
Digitalization
  preoperative, 43-44
  prophylactic, 37-38
Digitoxin, 551
Digoxin, 550-51
  administration for arrhythmias, 274-75
Diphenidol, and digitalis toxicity, 554
Diphenylhydantoin
  and digitalis toxicity, 554
  dosage, 580
  effectiveness, 579
  electrophysiologic effects, 577
  hemodynamics, 578
  pharmacokinetics, 580
Diphtheroids, 409
Diseased sinus syndrome, 456
Disopyramide, administration for arrhythmias, 274
Disseminated intravascular coagulation (DIC), 379
  postoperative, 380
Diuretic(s), 581-85
  loop, 581-84
  osmotic, 582
  pharmacodynamics, 583
  pharmacology, 582
  potassium-sparing, 582, 585
Diuretic therapy, 34-35, 44
  and acute renal failure, 360
Diving animals
  master switch of, life in, 9-11
  self-induced ischemia in, 9
Dobutamine. *See also* Inotropic agents.
  cardiovascular effects, 564
  doses, usual clinical, 567
Dopamine. *See also* Inotropic agents.
  cardiovascular effects, 563-64
  doses, usual clinical, 567
Doppler echocardiography, 152
Double pH method, 140. *See also* Acid-base balance.
Douglas bag, 496
Drug intoxication, postoperative, 390

Drug therapy
  for arrhythmias, 271-75
    cardiac, 261-62
  for atrial flutter, 265
  and DC cardioversion, 271
  for ectopic atrial tachycardia, 268
  for extrasystoles, 270
  for paroxysmal atrial tachycardia, 263
  for ventricular tachycardia, 269
Ductal closure, induction of, 434
Ductal ligation, 434
Ductus arteriosus, closure, 10
Dye-dilution principle
  accuracy, 503-04
  and cardiac output calculation, 500-503
  limitations, 504
Dysrhythmias
  hemodynamic consequences of, 217
  postoperative occurrence, 216-17
Dysuria, 425

Echocardiography, 152, 411, 419
Echophonocardiography, 411
Ectopic rhythms, 242
Electrical pacing, and digitalis toxicity, 554
Electric razors, 477
Electrocardiogram, 419
Electrocardiography, 26-27
  postoperative, 134
Electrocautery, 470
Electrocoagulation current, 477
Electrode(s)
  atrial, 467-70
  bipolar, 258
  and cardiac arrhythmia
    diagnosis, 260-61
    treatment, 261-62
  displacement, 474, 475, 476
  endocardial screw, 469-70
  epicardial, 258-59
  fracture, 476-77
  implantation of, 258-59
  during intraoperative electrophysiologic studies, 246
  repositioning and replacement, 472-73
  stainless steel wire, 259
  temporary wire, 258
  transvenous, 468, 473
  unipolar, 258
Electroencephalography, 390-91
Electrograms
  abnormal, 251
  atrial, recording, 261

INDEX

Electrograms *continued*
   bipolar ventricular, types of, 256
   endocardial, 465
Electrolyte administration, postoperative, 127
Electromanometers, 490
Elema-Schonander servo-ventilator, 318
Embolism
   air, 391
   fat, 388
   gas, 388
   incidence of, 389
   micro-, 388
   pulmonary, 530
   silicone, 388
   systemic, 410
Emphysema, effect on ventilatory capacity and reserve, 340
Endocardial cushion defects, 245, 250
Endocardial mapping, 254
Endocardial resection, 257
Endocarditis
   fungal, 410
   prosthetic valve, 408-15
Endotracheal intubation, 347
   hemodynamic effect of, during anesthetic induction, 58
Endotracheal suction, effect of, 445
Endotracheal tube, 305
   immobilization of, 441
Epicardial mapping, 255
Epidemic hepatitis, 421
Epinephrine. *See also* Inotropic agents.
   cardiac effects, 560
   doses, 567
   vascular effects, 560-62
Epstein-Barr (EB) virus, 419
Erwinia species, 410
Escherichia coli, 405
Esophageal thermistor probe, 435
Ethacrynic acid
   alkalosis, 169
   pharmacodynamic properties of, 583
   pharmacologic actions of, 582
Excitability, phases, 457-58
Excitation-contraction coupling, calcium mobilization and coupling, 188-91
Exercise
   and cardiac output, oxygen consumption and work output during, 200
   and rate and stroke volume, 200, 201
   tolerance, in cardiac patient, 43
Exit block, 474
Extracorporeal circulation (ECC), 65-110. *See also* Car-

Extracorporeal circulation (ECC) *continued*
    diopulmonary bypass; Whole body perfusion.
   and acute cation changes, 91
   equipment
    filters, 72-73
    gas exchange devices, 67-72
    heat exchangers, 71-72
    pumps, 66-67
    suction systems, 72
    tubing for, 66
   host defense mechanisms impairment of, 405, 452
   leukocyte and platelet alterations, 91
   oxygen
    requirements, 80-81
    uptake, 81-82
   perfusate, 76-79
   perfusion rate, 81
   subsystem functional alterations associated with, 88-95
Extracorporeal membrane oxygenation (ECMO), 350
Extrasystoles, 270
Extubation
   criteria for early, 310
   management following, 310-11
   in infants and children, 447

Face tent, use with infants, 448
Factor VIII
   deficiency, 373-74
   inhibitors, 376
Fat emboli, 388
Fat globulinemia, 388
Feeding, postoperative, 149
Femorofemoral venoarterial bypass, 534. *See also* Venoarterial bypass support.
Fetus, human, in utero, 10-11
Fever, 420
Fiber shortening, maximum velocity of circumferential, 209
Fibrillation
   accidental induction of, 275
   atrial, 252
   ventricular, 252, 269-70
Fibrin, 372
   degradation, 89
   deposition, 367
Fibrinogen, 27, 89, 370, 372
   conversion, 367
Fibrinolysis, 368
   primary, 379
Fibrinolytic mechanism, 374
Fibrinolytic systems, 373

Fick principle, 495
Filters, for extracorporeal circulation, 72-73
Fleisch pneumotachograph, 496
Fluid and cation management in acute respiratory failure, 361-62
Fluid and electrolyte management, postoperative, 126-27
Fluid requirements, in infants and children, 241-52
Fluoroscopy
  and diagnosis of prosthetic valve malfunction, 411
  use during intra-aortic balloon insertion, 521
  use during pulmonary artery catheterization, 493
  use during transvenous pacemaker implantation, 463
Fossa ovalis, 242
Frank-Starling curves, 135
Frank-Starling mechanism, 449
Frank-Starling phenomenon, 140
Frank-Starling relationship, 201-03, 361
  ultrasound basis for, 202
Free water clearance, 147. *See also* Renal function.
Functional residual capacity (FRC), 295
Fungal infections, 425
Fungi, 409
Furosemide
  alkalosis, 169
  pharmacodynamic properties of, 583
  pharmacologic actions of, 582

Galvanometer deflection, negative, 504
Gas dispersion (bubble) oxygenators, 68
Gas emboli, 388
Gas exchange, abnormalities in, 338
Gas-hemoglobin affinity, 387
Gasoline engine distributors, 477
Gas tensions, 287
  and blood flow, 7
Gas transport, monitoring of, 142, 143
Gastrointestinal distention, 122
Gastrointestinal tract, postoperative distention of, 124
Giving up syndrome, 398
Glomerular filtration, reduced, 356
Glomerular filtration rate (GFR), 147, 357. *See also* Renal function.
Glucagon, 194. *See also* Inotropic agents.
  cardiovascular effects, 565
  mechanism of action, 564
  usual clinical doses, 567
Glutamic oxaloacetic transferase (SGOT), serum activity determination, 28
Glycosides, cardiac, positive inotropic actions of, 193-95
Gram-negative microorganisms, 409, 412
Great vessels, transposition of, 249
Gross pulmonary edema, 288

Guanethidine, 574-75

Hamilton equation, 503. *See also* Stewart-Hamilton equation.
Heart
  effects of digitalis, 545-46
  hypoxic, 184-86
  ischemic, 186-87
  as mechanochemical transducer, 183
  as obligatory aerobe, 184
Heart block, 245, 250
  causes, 456
  complete, 470
  congenital, 456
  sequential, 456
Heart failure, 195-97. *See also* Cardiac failure; Congestive heart failure.
  defined, 195-96
  myocardial catecholamine depletion in, 201
Heart-lung machine, 96
  factors influencing venous flow into, 100
Heart rate. *See also* Cardiac rate; Pacing; Pacing, postoperative.
  and cardiac output, 140, 200
Heat exchangers, 71-72
Hematocrit, 387
  cardiac output and, 2
  desired mixed, 436
  and oxygen delivery to tissues, 3
Hematologic function
  and left heart assist device, 529
  postoperative evaluation of, 149
Hematologic subsystem dysfunction, and acute renal failure, 359
Hematologic tests, 27
Hematomas, 382
Hemiplegia, 391
Hemoconcentration, 4
Hemodialysis, 362-63. *See also* Dialysis.
  and digitalis therapy, 556
  heparin and, 363
Hemodiluting prime, composition of, 79
Hemodilution, 436
  coronary circulation during, 4
  effect on buffers, 170
  induced, 3
  intravascular volume, 79
  methods, 78-79
  in myocardial infarction treatment, 13-14
  perfusion, 94
Hemodynamic effects
  during coronary artery bypass grafting, 57
  gallamine, 56

INDEX

Hemodynamic effects *continued*
   intravenous morphine, 50
   nitroglycerin, 60
   of nitrous oxide, 52, 54
   pancuronium, 55
   phentolamine, 60
   phenylephrine, 60
   d-tubocurarine, 55
Hemodynamic measurements
   arterial and atrial pressures, 134-38
   cardiac output, 138-39
Hemodynamic monitoring, 498
Hemodynamic performance
   effect of changes in airway pressure on, 298-304
   effects of mechanical ventilation on, 298
Hemoglobin saturation, 497
Hemolysis, 356
Hemophilia A (Factor VIII deficiency), 373-74
Hemophilia B (Factor IX deficiency), 374-75
Hemophilus species, 411
Hemorrhage
   and cardiac output, effect on, 21-22
   gastrointestinal, 363-64
   intercurrent, 391
Hemorrhagic complications, in open heart surgery, 367-84
   postoperative, cause of, 149
Hemostasis
   components of
      clotting, 370-73
      lysis, 373
      platelets, 368-70
      vasoconstriction, 367
   heparin and, 65-66
   mechanism, 367-68
Hemothoraces, and postoperative pulmonary function, 344
Heparin
   antagonists, 586-87
   clinical use, 585-86
   excess, 377-78
   pharmacologic properties, 585
Heparinization, 518
Hepatic damage, perfusion-related, 94-95
Hepatic dysfunction, and acute renal failure, 359
Hepatic enlargement, 420
Hepatic function, postoperative evaluation of, 148
Hepatitis
   anicteric, 422
   cholestatic, 422
   chronic active, 422
   epidemic, 421
   fulminant, 422
   homologous serum, 421

Hepatitis *continued*
   icteric, 422
   non-A-non B, 421
      virus, 420
   posttransfusion, 421
   recurrent, 422
   viral, 420-23
Hepatitis A, 421
Hepatitis A virus (HAV), 420
Hepatitis B, 421
Hepatitis B virus (HBV), 420
Hepatitis C, 421
Hepatitis C virus, 420
Hepatocellular necrosis, from halothane, 51
Hepatomegaly, 419
Hepatosplenomegaly, 419
Hibernation, blood flow during, 3-4
His bundle, 242-43
   mapping of, 246-47
   surgical interruption of, 253
Homeostasis, 20-22
   CO_2, 297-98
   hemodynamic, 48
   hydrogen ion, 164-75
   limits, 22
   renal, 144
Homologous blood transfusion, immunologic effects of, 77-78
Homologous blood prime, immunologic effects of, 77-78
Host defenses, after cardiopulmonary bypass
   impairment of, 405
   in infants and children, 452
Host resistance, supplementing, 407-08
Humidification, during mechanical ventilation, 327
Humidifier, cascade type of, 444
Hydralazine, 573
Hydrochlorothiazide, pharmacodynamic properties of, 583
Hydrogen ion
   activity, 163, 164
      abnormalities of, problems related to, 168
      and hemoglobin concentration and, effect to, 172
      and respiratory changes, 172-75
      temperature correction and, 172
   balance, 168
   deficit, treatment with acid, 177
   and homeostasis, 164-75
Hyperalimentation, 425
Hypercalcemia, and digitalis toxicity, 553
Hypercarbia, 4, 5, 12, 14
   during fetal life, 7-8
Hypergylcemia, 451
Hyperkalemia
   and digitalis toxicity, 553

Hyperkalemia *continued*
  drug therapy for, 361-62
Hypermetabolism, reduction of, 131-32
Hyperoxemia, 7
Hyperplasminemia, 379
Hypertension
  in cardiac surgical patient, 32
  chronic pulmonary venous, 281
  left ventricular failure associated with
    acute, 59
  pulmonary, 286-87, 303
    arteriolar, 339
    and phentolamine, 59
    venous, 338-39
Hyperthyroidism, and digitalis toxicity, 552
Hypertrophy, defined, 195
Hyperventilation, following acute myocardial infarction, 12
Hypoalbuminemia, 31
  and mechanical ventilation, 321-22
Hypocarbia, 347
  and mechanical ventilation, 321-22
Hypofibrinogenemia, 149
Hypoglycemia, 451-52
Hypokalemia, 91, 258
  and digitalis toxicity, 553-55
Hypomagnesemia, 555
  and digitalis toxicity, 553
Hyponatremia, 452
Hypoproteinemia, 31
Hypotension, 253, 388
  in cardiac surgical patient, 32-33
  and dialysis, 362-63
  and morphine, 49
  orthostatic, 397
  and d-tubocurarine, 53
Hypothermia, 258, 356
  global ischemic arrest, 105-06
  induced, 82-83
  induction of, 3
    during perfusion, 71
  in myocardial infarction treatment, 12, 13-14
  perfusion, 4, 436, 437
  temperature, 82-83
Hypothermic cardioplegia, 102, 440
"Hypothermic chamber," 438, 439
Hypothermic circulatory arrest, 436
Hypothermic ischemic arrest, 248-49
Hypothyroidism, and digitalis toxicity, 552
Hypoventilation, and mechanical ventilation, 313
Hypovolemia, 356
  and extracorporeal circulation, 90
Hypoxemia, 5, 14, 31, 347, 435
  during fetal life, 7-8

Hypoxemia *continued*
  and infarct size, 13
Hypoxia, 258
  affinity, 167, 169
  and digitalis toxicity, 553
  mechanism of negative inotropic action of, 191-93
Hypoxic pulmonary vasoconstriction (HPV), 290

Icefish (*Chaenocephalus*), 2, 3
Idiopathic hypertrophic subaortic stenosis, use of digitalis in, 547
Immunodiffusion, 422
Impulse conduction, abnormalities of, 244
Incisional pain, and postoperative pulmonary function, 343-44
Indicator-dilution principle, 499-500
Inductive coupling, 460
Indwelling nasotracheal tube, securing, 314, 315
Infarctectomy, 251
Infarction, right ventricular, 530
Infection(s)
  associated with open heart surgery, 403-26
  catheter-related, 424-26
  defined, 403
  fungal, 425
  incidence of, 403
  pathogenetic mechanisms in
    aging, 406
    anesthesia equipment, 406
    environmental, 404-05
    host defense impairment, 405
    use of prostheses, 405-06
  prosthetic valve, 408-15
  respiratory tract, 423-24
  urinary tract, 424-25
  viral, 418, 419-23
Infusate composition, in infants and children, 451-52
Infusion pumps, 434
Inorganic phosphate, accumulation of, 193
Inotropic agents. *See also* Catecholamines.
  clinical uses of, 565-67
  dobutamine, 564
  dopamine, 563-64
  dosage schedule, 467
  epinephrine, 560-62
  glucagon, 564-65
  isoproterenol, 562-63
  norepinephrine, 562
  rationale for, 556-57
Inotropic state, 449
Inotropism, 205
Inspiratory-expiratory ratio, 444
Instantaneous flow rate, defined, 318

INDEX

Intensive care area
  admission to, 122
  design, 120
  laboratory service for, 120-21
  maintenance, 121
  nursing staff, 121
Intensive care unit (ICU)
  left heart assist device monitoring in, 529-30
  neonate admission to
    laboratory studies, 443
    reception procedures, 442
    temperature control, 442-43
  and neurologic complications, diagnosis of, 389-90
  postoperative special techniques in, 489-534
  transfer of neonate to, 440-42
Intercellular transport system, digitalis effects on, 542-43
Intermittent mandatory ventilation (IMV), and weaning, 446
Intermittent positive-pressure ventilation (IPPV), 330
International Committee on Blood Clotting Factors (1962), 585
Internodal pathways
  anterior, 241
  middle, 242
  posterior, 242
Intra-aortic balloon (IAB), 510-13
  gases used for, 515-16
  insertion and removal, 514-15, 517-21, 526
  insertion sites, 521
  resistance to passage of, 519
  timing, 517, 522
  triggering, 516-17, 522
Intra-aortic balloon counterpulsation (IABC), 224-25, 509-26
  anticoagulation methods, 524-25
  clinical indications, 514
  contraindications, 514
  equipment and personnel requirements, 514-15
  hemodynamic and metabolic effects, 514
  initiation, 521-22
  local wound care, 525
  maintaining stable cardiac rhythm, 524
  monitoring limb viability, 525
  patient activity during, 524
  patient preparation for, 516-17
  physiologic considerations, 510-14
  removal of IAB, 526
  support, 36
  timing, 517, 522
  triggering, 516-22
  weaning from, 525
Intra-aortic balloon pump (IABP), commercial systems, 515-16

Intracellular water, 9, 10
Intraoperative electrical pacing, 59-61
Intrapericardial pressure, clinical significance in cardiac surgery, 204
Intrathoracic pressure, clinical significance in cardiac surgery, 204. *See also* Airway pressure.
Intraventricular block, 455
Ischemia
  anoxic tolerance in, 8
  cardiac pathology and, 211
  and coronary flow, 3, 4
  effect on electrolytes, 9
  and intracellular water, 9
  mechanism of negative inotropic action of, 191-93
  self-induced, 9
Isoenzymes, of creatine-kinase, 28
Isoproterenol. *See also* Inotropic agents.
  cardiovascular effects, 562-63
  usual clinical doses, 567

Janeway's lesion, 410

Kidney, effects of digitalis on, 547
Kinase, cyclic AMP-dependent protein, 194
Kinin systems, 373

Laboratory studies
  for cardiac patients, 26-28
  postoperative in infants, 443
Lactic acid, neonatal excretion of, 10-11
Lactic dehydrogenase (LDH), serum activity determination, 28
Laplace's law, 205
Left atrial pressure (LAP), 489, 490. *See also* Ventricular filling pressures; Left-heart filling pressures.
Left heart assist device (LHAD), 226, 227. *See also* Left heart bypass.
  cannula insertion, 527
  deployment of, 526
  discontinuance, 529-30
  extracorporeal circuit and connections, 527-28
  flow rate adjustment, 529
  heparin administration, 529
  intensive care unit management, 529-30
  operation room management of, 528-29
Left heart bypass
  direct left ventricular decompression and bypass, 226
  left atrial-systemic artery bypass, 226-28
  physiologic considerations, 225-26
Left heart distention, and pulmonary dysfunction, 341

Left heart dysfunction, and pulmonary function abnormalities, 32
Left heart filling pressure, estimation of, 489-90. *See also* Ventricular filling pressures.
Left heart vent system, 72
Leukocyte(s)
  effect of ECC on, 91
  morphologic changes in, 405
  phagocytic activity of, 91
Leukocytosis, 410, 416
Leukopenia, 405
Lidocaine
  and arrhythmias, 272-73
  and digitalis toxicity, 554
  dosage, 580
  effectiveness, 579
  electrophysiologic effects, 577
  hemodynamics, 578
  pharmacokinetics, 580
Limb viability, monitoring, 525
Lipid metabolism, and open heart surgery, 373
Lipids, accumulation of, 193
Lithium iodine cells, 460
Liver disease (hepatocellular damage), 375-76
Liver and kidney function tests, 27
Lobar collapse, recognition of, 345
Low cardiac output syndrome, 175-77. *See also* Cardiac performance, impaired.
Lumbar puncture, 391
Lung
  expansion, restriction by pleural fibrosis, 340
  function
    following open heart surgery, 281-306
    preoperative tests, 45
  mechanics
    monitoring of, 142, 143
    postoperative alterations in, 342-43
Lung compliance
  and anesthesia, effect on, 342-43
  defined, 318
  volume, 444
Lymphocytes, atypical, 420
Lymphocytosis, 419, 420

Macroemboli, platelet-fibrin, 356
Maculopapular eruption, 420
Magnetometers, 477
Malnutrition, and postsurgical infection rates, 406
Mannitol, 584
  pharmacodynamic properties of, 583
Master switch of life, 9, 11
Mechanical ventilation, 347, 416
  airway choice and care, 313-17

Mechanical ventilation *continued*
  care of patient requiring, 325-29
  controlled *vs* assist mode, 323
  criteria for reinstitution of, 311-12
  effects of, 291
  elective short-term, 312
  equipment choice, 318
  guidelines for proper conduct of, 317-25
  hypocarbia during, 321-22
  indications for prolonged, 312-13
  inspiratory-to-expiratory time ratio, 322
  in neonates and children, 443-44
  oxygen fraction in inspired gas, 322
  PEEP during, use of, 323-25
  physical principles, 317-18
  problems, 329-30
  respiratory rate, 322
  tidal volume, 321-22
  ventilation patterns, 318-21
  weaning from, 330-33
Mechanical work, generated by myocardium, 183
Mediastinitis, 415
Membrane oxygenators, 70, 436
Membrane pumps, 8-9
Meralluride, 583
Mercaptomerin, 583
Mercury-zinc cells, 460
Metabolic activity, obligatory increases in, 442
Metabolic compensation, 171
Methyldopa, 574
Microaggregates
  increased formation of, 344-45
  of leukocytes, platelets, and fibrin, 344
Microbiologic cleanliness, in operating room, 406-07
Microbubbles, 89
Microemboli, 89-90, 345, 388
  perfusion-related particulate, 258
Microorganisms, anaerobic, 424
Microwave ovens, 477
Minute volume, defined, 318
Mitral commissurotomy (postcommissurotomy syndrome), 417
Mitral stenosis
  and digitalis, 547
  pulmonary function in, 338
Mitral valve
  disease, 209-10, 281, 286, 340
  prosthetic, 250
  surgery, 243
Monitoring
  computer-based, 151-52
  intraoperative, 95-96
  postoperative, 120, 138-48, 214-16
Mosso, Antonio, 4

INDEX

Muscle relaxants
   gallamine, 53
   pancuronium, 53-54
   succinylcholine, 51-53
   d-tubocurarine, 53
Mustard procedure, 243, 250, 438
Mycobacterium chelonei, 405-06
Myocardial cell(s), 185, 543
   impaired calcium entry into, 192-93
Myocardial contractility
   control mechanisms
      phasic, 187-88
      tonic, 187
   and digitalis, 542
   drugs augmenting, 205
   factors reducing, 205
   maintenance of, 220
   measurement, 205-06
   pharmacologic support, 222-23
   regulation, 205
Myocardial damage
   enzyme markers of, 27-28
   identification of areas of, 250-51
Myocardial depression, 210
Myocardial disease, 210
Myocardial dysfunction, 259
   and postoperative pulmonary function, 344
Myocardial failure, 196
Myocardial hypoxia, 184
Myocardial infarction
   blood viscosity after, 12
   hypoxemia and, 13
   and reduced body temperature, 12
   and respiratory alkalosis, 12
   shock, 514
Myocardial injury, 470
   ischemia-induced, 211-12
Myocardial ischemia, 185
   and digitalis toxicity, 552
Myocardial oxygen consumption
   control of, 55-56
   during left-heart bypass, 225-26
   and morphine, 51
Myocardial perforation, 474-75
Myocardial performance, postsurgical factors affecting. *See also* Cardiac performance.
   adverse postoperative events, 213-14
   preoperative cardiac dysfunction and, 206-10
   surgical trauma, 210-13
   uncorrected cardiovascular pathology and, 213
Myocardial preservation
   coronary perfusion, 104-05
   hypothermia and global ischemic arrest, 105-06
   hypothermic cardioplegia, 106-09

Myocarditis, rheumatic, 210
Myosin, 187, 189

Narcotics
   addiction, 399
   disadvantages of, 49
   intravenous, 49
Nasal necrosis, prophylaxis against, 314
Nasotracheal aspiration, 349
National Academy of Sciences National Research Council, study on postoperative wound infections, 404
Nebulizer, ultrasonic, 327
Negative feedback system, 20-22
Negative heat, 506
Neonates
   cardiac surgical care of, 433-52
   digitalization, 449
   physiologic peculiarities in, 30-31
Neurologic abnormalities, and acute renal failure, 359
Neurologic complications, 387-92
   diagnosis, 389-91
   predisposing factors
      aging, 388
      cerebral arterial occlusive disease, 388
      reduced brain blood flow, 387
   psychiatric, 392, 395-400
Neurosis, compensation, 399
Neutrophilia, 419, 424
Nitroprusside, 569-73. *See also* Vasodilators; Vasodilator therapy.
Nonpulsatile pumps, 66
"No reflow phenomenon," 436
Norepinephrine, cardiovascular effects, 562. *See also* Inotropic agents.
Nursing care, during mechanical ventilation, 329
Nutritional status of cardiac surgical patient, 31

Obesity, 31-32
   and postsurgical infection rates, 406
   and pulmonary dysfunction, 340
Ohm's law, 83, 140, 318, 319, 494, 508-09
Oliguria, 146
Open-care bed, 440
Open heart surgery, 376-84
Open intracardiac surgery, in neonates and infants, 435-42
   completion, 440
   equipment and priming perfusate, 435-36
   perfusion conduct, 436-40
   preliminaries, 436
   transfer to ICU, 440-42

INDEX

Operating room
　analysis and management, 229-30
　left heart assist device monitoring in, 528-29
　and surgical infection control, 406
　transfer of patient from, 121-22
Operative trauma, renal response to, 144-46
Organ cooling, 437-38
Organic brain syndrome, 389
Organic mental syndrome, 455
　postoperative, 390
Organomercurials, 584
　pharmacologic actions of, 582
Osler's nodes, 410
Osmolality, ratio of urinary to plasma, 146
Ouabain, 549-50
Overdrive pacing, 244
Oximetric techniques, 498
Oxygen
　analyzer, 496
　and cardiac output, 2-3
　consumption
　　computer-assisted measurement of, 496
　　determination of, 495-96
　　reduction of, 131-32
　dissociation curve, 169
　requirements in ECC, 80-81
　tension, 86
　toxicity, 297
　uptake in CPBP, 81-82
　whole body consumption during surgery, 81
Oxygen-Fick method, 495-99
　clinical utility, 497-99
Oxygen-hemoglobin affinity, effects of pH on, 167
Oxygen-hemoglobin dissociation curve, temperature changes and, 172
Oxygenation, factors influencing
　cardiac output, 282-86, 325
　lung geometry, 281-82
　mechanical ventilation, 318-25
　oxygen consumption, 286-97
Oxygenator(s)
　basic concepts, 67-68
　blood film, 69-70
　bubble, 388, 436
　gas dispersion, 68
　membrane, 70-71, 436, 532
　pump, 388
　rotating disc, 70
　stationary vertical sheet, 70

Pacemaker(s), 262
　advanced function, 460
　classification, 458-60

Pacemaker(s) *continued*
　demand, 480-81
　electrical interference, 477
　electronic analysis, 481-84
　electronics, 461
　epinephrine stimulation of, 560
　failure due to exit block, 474
　generator replacement, 471-72
　"knock," 478-79
　lithium-powered, 472
　office analysis, 478-81
　patient education, 477-78
　patient follow-up, 478-81
　permanent cardiac, 455-84
　power sources, 460
　premature generator failure, 477
　programmable, 461-62, 470
　remote monitoring, 482-84
　special feature, 461-62
　wandering generator, 477
Pacemaker implantation
　epicardial, 466-67, 468
　　during open heart surgery, 470-71
　preoperative management, 462
　and respiratory depression, 462
　surgical techniques, 463-71
　transvenous, 463-66
　　veins used for, 464
Pacing
　atrial, 458
　　demand, 467
　　triggered, 467-68
　bifocal demand, 460
　bipolar, 459
　complications, 473-77
　electrophysiology, 457-58
　endocardial, 458
　epicardial, 458
　overdrive, 470
　permanent, indications for, 455-56
　sequential, 460
　unipolar, 458-59
　ventricular, 458-59
　　demand, 467
Pacing, postoperative
　cardiac arrhythmias, treatment of, 217, 261-62
　cardiac performance, support of, 215-16, 233
　cardiac rate augmentation with
　　atrial, 217
　　atrioventricular sequential, 219
　　ventricular, 217-18
　electrodes, temporary atrial and ventricular, placement of, 217, 259
　ventricular, hemodynamic effects of, 218

INDEX

Pacing modes
  asynchronous (fixed rate), 459
  atrial triggered, 459-60
  ventricular inhibited (demand), 459
  ventricular synchronous (standby), 459
Pain
  etiology, 398-99
  prolonged postoperative, 398-99
  treatment, 399
Palliation *vs* primary definitive repair, 434-35
Paradoxical aciduria, 169, 172
Paravalvular leak, 411
Paroxysmal atrial tachycardia, 548
Paroxysmal ventricular tachycardia, 548, 549
Partial thromboplastin time (PTT), 27
Patient care
  during mechanical ventilation
    chest physiotherapy, 329
    humidification, 327
    monitoring, 325-26
    nursing care, 329
    sedation, 326-27
    tracheobronchial toilette, 327-28
  goal, 17
  intraoperative, 23
  postoperative, 23
  preoperative
    diagnosis, 22-23
    management, 23
    scope, 22-23
Pectoral muscle stimulation, in pacing, 474
Pediatric patients, 433-52
Performance potential (reserve capability), 199
Perfusate. *See also* Cardiopulmonary bypass; Extracorporeal circulation.
  hemodilute, 436
  priming, 435-36
Perfusion. *See also* Cardiopulmonary bypass; Extracorporeal circulation; Open intracardiac surgery.
  equipment, 436
  hemodilution, 96
  hypothermia, 436, 437
  pathophysiology, 88-89
  pressure, 83-84
  pulsatile, 436
  rates, 81, 437
  resumption of, 438-40
  rewarming, 439
  techniques
    rate, 103
    systemic arterial pressure, 103-04
    temperature, 102-03
  temperature, 437-38
Pericardiocentesis, 475

Peripheral cooling, 4
Peripheral vascular system, effects of digitalis on, 546-47
Petecchiae, 410
Phlebotomy, 349
Phospholamban, 194
Physiologic dead space, potential sources of increased, 300
Physiologic dead space-to-tidal volume ratio (V_D/V_T), 338
Physiologic noise, 506
Plasma coagulation factors, 371
Plasma protein denaturation, during whole-body perfusion, 93, 405
Plasmin, 373
  excess, 378-79
Plasminogen, 373
Plasminogen activator liberation, 149
Plasminogen-plasmin system, 89
Platelet(s), 89, 368-70
  adequacy test for, 370
  effect of ECC on, 91
  and membrane alteration, 370
  release reaction, 369
  retention, 377
Platelet-biomaterial interaction, 370
Platelet-fibrin aggregates, 89
Platelet suppression, from drugs, 376
Pleural effusion, 346
  management of, 349
Pleuropericardial inflammation, 418
Pneumonia, bacterial, 423
Pneumonitis, 416
  management of, 348-49
  recognition of, 345-46
Pneumothoraces, and postoperative pulmonary function, 344
Pocket hematoma, in pacemaker implantation, 474
Polycythemia, 8, 440
Polyuria, 359
Positive end-expiratory pressure (PEEP), 295, 300, 302, 306, 319, 321, 340. *See also* Airway pressure.
  in infants and children, 444-45
  and mechanical ventilation, use during, 323-25
  and weaning, 446
Positive feedback system, 20-22
Postcardiotomy delirium, 392
Postextubation care, in infants and children, 447
Postextubation stridor, drug therapy for, 447
Postinfarction cardiogenic shock, 229
Postoperative fever, 344
Postoperative mediastinal infection
  clinical features, 416
  general considerations, 415
  pathogenesis, 415-16

INDEX

Postoperative mediastinal infection *continued*
   predisposition to, 415
   therapy, 416-17
Postperfusion period, 440
Postperfusion syndrome
   clinical features, 420
   incidence, 419
   management, 420
   pathogenesis, 419-20
Postpericardiotomy syndrome, 383
   autoimmune response, 418
   clinical features, 418-19
   defined, 417
   incidence, 417
   management, 419
   pathogenesis, 417-18
   viral illness and, 418
Potassium. *See also* Hyperkalemia; Hypokalemia.
   and digitalis toxicity, 553, 554
   intoxication, 359
   repletion, 452
Potassium canrenoate, and digitalis toxicity, 554
Preload. *See also* Ventricular filling pressure; Frank-Starling relationship.
   optimization of, 219-21
   and stroke volume, 140-41, 201-04, 449
Preoperative orders, for adult open heart surgery, 39
Priming solution. *See also* Cardiopulmonary bypass; Extracorporeal circulation.
   autologous, 77
   bloodless, 77, 78
   homologous, 77
   pump-oxygenator, 76
   volume, 76
Proaccelerin, 89, 371-72, 375-76
Procainamide
   and arrhythmias, 272-73
   and digitalis toxicity, 554
   dosage, 580
   effectiveness, 579
   electrophysiologic effects, 577
   hemodynamics, 578
   pharmacokinetics, 580
Prophylactic. *See* Antibiotic therapy, preventive.
Propranolol
   and arrhythmias, 274
   and digitalis toxicity, 554
   dosage, 580
   effectiveness, 579
   electrophysiologic effects, 577
   hemodynamics, 578
   pharmacokinetics, 580
Propranolol withdrawal syndrome, 35-36
Prostaglandin (PG) synthesis, 369-70

Prostaglandin synthetase inhibitor, 434
Prostheses, intracardiac or intravascular, 405-06
Prosthetic valve endocarditis
   clinical manifestations, 410-11
   general considerations, 408-09
   management, 411-15
   microbiology, 409-10
   operative intervention in, 414-15
   pathogenesis, 409
   pathology, 410
   prophylaxis, 415
Prosthetic valve obstruction, 410
Protamine, 586-87
   excess, 378
Protein denaturation, 388. *See also* Plasma protein denaturation.
Prothrombin, 27, 89, 371-72, 375
Pseudomonas aeruginosa, 406
Pseudomonas species, 425
Psychiatric complications
   anxiety, 399-400
   of cardiac surgery, 395-400
   depression, 397-98
   incidence, 395
   postoperative delirium, 395-97
   prolonged postoperative pain, 398-99
Psychosis, postoperative, 392
Pullup tourniquet, 518
Pulmonary artery catheterization. *See also* Catheters; Swan-Ganz catheters.
   complications, 493-94
   rationale for, 489
   technique, 490-93
Pulmonary artery end diastolic pressure (PAD), 489, 490
Pulmonary blood flow, calculation of, 499
Pulmonary capillary wedge (PCW) pressure, 489, 490
Pulmonary complications
   clinical recognition of, 345-47
      lobar collapse, 345
      pleural effusion, 346
      pneumonitis, 345-46
      respiratory failure, acute, 347
      segmental atelectasis, 345
      tracheobronchial secretion, increased, 345
      vascular overload, 346-47
   management of
      atelectasis, 348-49
      pleural effusion, 349
      pneumonitis, 348-49
      pulmonary edema, 349
      respiratory failure, acute, 349-50
      retained secretions, 348-49
   prevention of postoperative, 347-48

INDEX

Pulmonary dysfunction
  following CPBP, 92-94
  intraoperative factors
    cardiopulmonary bypass effects, 341-43
    left heart distention, 341
    surgical incision, 340-41
  postoperative, pathogenesis of, 309, 338-45
  preoperative factors
    anatomic, 340
    cardiac dysfunction severity, 338
    preexisting lung disease, 340
    pulmonary vascular disease, 339-40
    pulmonary venous hypertension, 338-39
  and renal failure, acute, 359
Pulmonary edema
  and respiratory failure, acute, 361
  management of, 349
Pulmonary embolism, 383, 530
Pulmonary extravascular water, measurements of, 339
Pulmonary function tests, 28
Pulmonary perfusion, monitoring of, 142, 143
Pulmonary subsystem, in neonates and children
  extubation, 447
  mechanical ventilation, 443-44
  positive end-expiratory pressure (PEEP), 444-45
  postextubation care, 447
  tracheal toilet, 445-46
  ventilator weaning, 446-47
  ventilatory control, 446
Pulmonary subsystem performance, analysis of. *See* Ventilation; Ventilatory and respiratory function, postoperative assessment of.
Pulmonary vascular disease, 287
Pulmonary vascular overload, 346-47
Pulmonic stenosis, 249
Pulsatile assist device, 514
Pulsatile flow, 104
Pulsatile pumps, 66-67
Pulse contour, during perfusion, 85-86
Pump lung, 293
Pump lung syndrome, 92-94, 347
Pump-oxygenator, 388. *See also* Cardiopulmonary bypass; Extracorporeal circulation.
  accidents associated with, 73-76
  perfusion, 405
Pumps. *See also* Cardiopulmonary bypass; Extracorporeal circulation.
  coronary perfusion, 67
  nonpulsatile, 66
  pulsatile, 66-67
  roller, 66
Purkinje cells, 545
Purkinje-like cells, 242
P wave, in arrhythmias, 260-61

QRS complex, in arrhythmias, 260-61
Quinidine
  administration for arrhythmias, 273-74
  and digitalis toxicity, 554
  dosage, 580
  effectiveness, 579
  electrophysiologic effects, 577
  hemodynamics, 578
  pharmacokinetics, 580

Radar, 477
Radioimmunoassay techniques, 422
Radioisotope brain scanning, 390
Radioisotopes, 460
Radio transmitters, 477
Rechargeable cells, 460
Recirculation curve, 500
Reentrant rhythms, 242
"Refined-clean" operations, 404
Refractory period
  absolute, 457
  effects of digitalis on, 542
  relative, 457
Regurgitation murmur, 410
Renal compensation, 171-72
Renal disease, intrinsic, and acute renal failure, 355
Renal failure
  body weight assessment, 361
  in cardiac surgery, 355-64
  cardiovascular manifestations, 359
  cardiovascular performance, 361
  complications in, 359
  dialysis, 362-63
  drug therapy, 363
  factors causing
    advanced age, 355-56
    advanced cardiac dysfunction, 355
    cardiopulmonary bypass, 356
    intrinsic renal disease, 355
    low cardiac output, 356
    surgical trauma, 356
  fluid and cation managment, 361-62
  gastrointestinal hemorrhage and, 363-64
  infection and, 363
  management of, 360
  nonoliguric, 358, 362
  nutritional support, 363
  oliguric, 358, 361
  pathophysiology and clinical patterns, 358-59
  patterns after cardiac surgery, 357
  pulmonary function, 361
  threatened acute, 357-58
  use of digitalis in, 556

Renal Failure Index, 357
Renal function
　changes in BUN and creatinine levels, 146
　evaluation of, 146-48
　postoperative assessment of, 144-48
Renal function tests, after cardiac surgery, 147
Renal performance, following CPBP, 94
Renal subsystem
　in infants and children, 450-52
　　fluid requirements, 451
　　infusate composition, 451-52
　postoperative examination of, 123
Reoperation, indications for, 126
Reperfusion injury, 106
Reserpine, 573-74
Reserve capacity, and homeostatic adjustments of rate and stroke volume, 200
Respiration, defined, 142
Respirator, weaning from, 131. *See also* Ventilators.
"Respirator lung," 296
Respiratory, acidosis, 288
Respiratory care
　essential elements of, 350
　preventive, 36-37
Respiratory changes
　acute steady-state, 172-73
　chronic, 173-75
Respiratory compensation, 170-71
Respiratory failure, 347
　management of, 349-50
　pathogenesis of postcardiotomy acute, 345
　pathogenetic mechanisms in, 346
Respiratory flow rate, calculation of, 318
Respiratory function values, after cardiac surgery, 143
Respiratory insufficiency, causes of, 286
Respiratory management, postoperative, 127-31
　preventive, 128-29
　ventilation, 129-30
　ventilators, 130-31
Respiratory rate, during mechanical ventilation, 322
Respiratory system
　postoperative examination of, 123
　preoperative assessment of, 45-46
Respiratory tract infections
　clinical features, 423-24
　management, 424
　pathogenesis, 423
Rest, for cardiac failure management, 34
Reticuloendothelial system, 405
Retrograde atrial activation, 252
Retrolental fibroplasia, in preterm infants, 444
Rewarming, neonatal, 439
Rheoencephalogram (REG), 5

Rhythm(s)
　automatic, 244, 261
　cardiac, factors affecting, 245
　ectopic, 242
　reentrant, 242, 244
　sinus, 245, 267
　supraventricular, 245
Roentgenogram, 416
　postoperative, 125
Roller pump, 66
Rotating disk oxygenator, 70
Roth's spots, 410

Safety devices, for extracorporeal circulation, 73-76
Sarcolemma depolarization, 185
Sarcoplasmic reticulum, 190
　impaired calcium release by, 192
Screen filtration pressure (SFP), 89
Second messengers, 369-70
Sedation, during mechanical ventilation, 326-27
Seizure activity
　drug therapy, 391
　postoperative, 389-90
Self-excitation, spontaneous, 244
Senning procedure, 438
Sensory impairment, postoperative, 390
Septicemia, 425, 476
Septic shock, 416
Serratia marcescens, 406
Serratia species, 411
Serum bactericidal activity, 411
Serum creatinine, 355
Serum hepatitis, 421
Serum prothrombin conversion accelerator, 27
Serum transaminase, 423
Short-wave diathermy, 477
Shunt(s), intracardiac, 503
　quantification of, 498
Shunt equation, 283, 285
Sick sinus syndrome, 456, 457
Sidearm graft, 519
Siggaard-Andersen nomogram, 162, 174, 450
Silicone emboli, 388
Sinus node
　electrophysiologic technique to identify, 246
　landmarks, 241
Sinus rhythm, 267
Skeletal muscle potentials, 477
Skin erosion, 476
Skin preparation, for cardiac surgery, 38
Sleep deprivation, 392
Slow flow syndrome, 145

INDEX

Sodium, fractional excretion of, 357
Sodium-potassium pump, digitalis inhibition of, 543
Sodium restriction, 34-35
Spectrophotometry, 497
Spike analysis, 459
Spironolactone
    pharmacodynamic properties of, 583
    pharmacologic actions of, 582
Splenic enlargement, 420
Splenomegaly, 410, 419
Spontaneous ventilation
    early extubation, criteria for, 310
    postextubation management, 310-11
    reinstitution of mechanical ventilation, criteria for, 311-12
Staphylococcus aureus, 405, 409, 410, 425-26
Staphylococcus epidermidis, 409
Stationary vertical sheet oxygenator, 70
Sternal dehiscence, 415
Sternotomy, 388, 415-17
Steroid-binding resins, and digitalis toxicity, 555
Steroid therapy, and postsurgical infection rates, 406
Stewart-Hamilton equation, 505. *See also* Hamilton equation.
Stokes-Adams attacks, 455, 462
"Stone heart" syndrome, 212
Streptococcus species, 409
Streptococcus viridans, 409, 410
Stroke index (SI)
    defined, 507
    influence of blood infusion on, 220
Stroke volume (SV)
    afterload, 204-05
    defined, 507
    factors determining, 140
    factors directly influencing, 449
    myocardial contractility
        measurement, 205-06
        regulation of, 205
    preload
        atrial contraction and, 204
        blood volume and, 204
        Frank-Starling relationship, 201-04
    reduced, guide to diagnosis of, 141
Stroke work index (SWI)
    calculation of, 507-08
    defined, 507
Stuart-Prower factor, 27, 371-72, 375
Suction systems
    for cardiac surgery, 72
    intracardiac, 102
    left heart vents in, 72

Supraventricular arrhythmia, hemodynamic changes associated with, 61
Surgery, cardiac
    anesthesia, 43-61, 95
    cardiovascular values conventionally monitored after, 134
    clinical response to, 119
    complications related to technical execution, 212
    daily fluid maintenance schedule, 127
    early general care
        antibiotic therapy, 133
        blood and fluid recording, 125-26
        fluid and electrolyte management, 126-27
        hypermetabolism reduction, 131-32
        oxygen consumption reduction, 131-32
        patient examination, 122-25
        postoperative bleeding, 125-26
        radiologic and laboratory examination, 125
        respiratory management, 127-31
        temperature, 125
    effects of
        anesthesia, 210
        cardiopulmonary bypass, 211
        myocardial injury during, 211-12
    intent of patient monitoring after, 119
    intraoperative monitoring, 95-96
    late bleeding complications in, 382
    muscle relaxants for, 51-54
    operative protocols, 95
    postoperative
        ambulation, 150
        anticoagulation therapy, 150
        feeding, 149
    premedication for
        diazepam, 46
        morphine, 46
        nitroglycerin, 46
        scopolamine, 46
    preoperative care, 33-39
    preparations for, 38-39
    psychologic preparation for, 33-34
    pulmonary complications after, 337
    renal failure in, 355-64
    surgical work-up, 25-28
Surgical incision, effect on pulmonary function, 340-41
Surgical risk
    factors affecting
        age, 29-31
        hypertension, 32-33
        metabolic disorders, 32
        nutritional status, 31-32
        secondary physiologic derangements, 32
    specific determinants of, 33

Swan-Ganz catheters, 382. *See also* Pulmonary artery catheterization.
  balloon inflation, 490-91
  balloon rupture, 493
  deflation protocol, 494
  pulmonary artery, 46
  thermistor-bearing, 96, 492
Sympathetic effector cells, 558
Sympathomimetic amines. *See also* Catecholamines.
  comparative effects after intravenous infusion, 561
  use in augmentation of myocardial contractility, 223
Syncopal episodes, 455
Systemic blood flow during perfusion
  distribution, 84-86
  pulse contour, 85-86
Systemic venous tone, clinical significance in cardiac surgery, 204

Tachyarrhythmias, 217, 244, 271
Tachycardia(s), 217, 244, 250, 347
  A-V junctional, 261
  ectopic atrial, 252, 261, 266-68
  and gallamine, 53
  identifying site of origin of, 256
  paroxysmal atrial, 252, 262-63
  reentrant, 253
  sinus, 261
  spontaneous automatic, 268-69
  supraventricular, 253, 262-69
  ventricular, 269
    associated with coronary artery disease, 254-57
    mapping of, 253-54
    techniques, 257-58
Tachypnea, 346, 347
Tamponade
  acute pericardial or mediastinal, 381-82
  cardiac, 220-21
  late mediastinal or pericardial, 382-84
Temperature, monitoring, 125
Temperature control, in infants, 442-43
Tetralogy of Fallot, 72, 83, 208, 249, 440, 450
  hemodynamic changes after total correction of, 137
Thermodilution cardiac output measurements, in infants, 439
  method, advantages of, 506-07
Thermodilution principle, 504-05
Thermodynamics, First law of, 183, 187
Thermoneutrality, 434
Thoracentesis, 349
Thoracic aortic aneurysm, 292
Thoracotomy, 435
Threshold potential, 544

Thrombin, excess (disseminated intravascular coagulation or DIC), 379
Thrombin generation, 372
Thrombocytopathias, 373
Thrombocytopenia, 149, 373, 376-77
Thrombopathy, 376
Thrombophlebitis, 426
Thrombosis, intracatheter, 493
Thrombosthenin, 368
Thrombus dissolution, 368
Tidal volume (TV), 321-22
  calculation, 444
Tissue perfusion, requirements of optimal, 2
Total flow resistance (TFR), 338
Total lung capacity (TLC), 295
Total static compliance (TSC), 338
Tracheal damage, prevention of, 314-17
Tracheal edema, drug therapy for, 447
Tracheal toilet, in infants and children, 445-46
Tracheobronchial infection, recognition, 345
Tracheobronchial suction, 445
Tracheobronchial toilette, 327-28
Tracheostomy, 330, 349, 415, 416
Transfusions, multiple, 344
Transmembrane action potentials, 544
Transmural pressure, right ventricular, 303
Transpulmonary pressures and compliance, distribution of, 228
Trauma
  anesthesia, 120
  of extracorporeal circulation, 119
  as source of fat emboli, 388
Triamterene
  pharmacodynamic properties of, 583
  pharmacologic actions of, 582
Trichlormethiazide, pharmacodynamic properties of, 583
Tricuspid regurgitation, 477
Trimethaphan, 569
Tropomyosin, 189, 190
Troponin, 188, 189, 190
Tubing. *See also* Extracorporeal circulation; Left-heart assist device; Venoarterial bypass support.
  polyvinylchloride (PVC), 66
  silicone elastomer, 66
Twiddler's syndrome, 477

Uhl's disease, 257
Ultrapore filtration, 345, 436
Urinary indices, 357
Urinary measurements, in acute respiratory failure, 361

INDEX

Urinary output
  adequate in infants, 451
  postoperative measurement of, 123-24
Urinary sodium concentration, measurements of, 147
Urinary tract infection(s)
  clinical features, 425
  incidence, 424
  management, 425
  pathogenesis, 424-25
Urinary urea nitrogen (UUN) measurements, 147
Urine
  characteristics in ARF, 358
  osmolality, 146
  quality, and renal function status, 146
  volume
    and cardiac output, 145
    inappropriate, 146

Vagal response, effects of digitalis on, 452
Van Slyke manometric apparatus, 497
Vascular disease, pulmonary, 339-40
Vascular lesions
  embolic cerebral, 388
  extracranial occlusive, 388
Vascular resistance, 508-09. *See also* Afterload.
Vasoactive effect, of oxygen, 5, 7
Vasoconstriction, 367
Vasodilating drugs
  chlorpromazine, 103
  halothane, 103
  sodium nitroprusside, 104
Vasodilator drug therapy, hemodynamic changes caused by, 568
Vasodilators
  chlorpromazine, 575
  diazoxide, 573
  guanethidine, 574-75
  hydralazine, 573
  mechanism of action, 568-69
  methyldopa, 574
  nitroprusside, 569-73
  pharmacokinetics, 570-71
  reserpine, 573-74
  therapeutic objectives, 567
  trimethaphan, 569
Vasodilator therapy
  nitroglycerin, 57
  sodium nitroprusside, 56-57
Vasodilator therapy in combination with
  methoxamine, 57
  phenylephrine, 57
Venoarterial bypass support, 531-34

Venoarterial bypass support *continued*
  anticoagulation, 533
  criteria for discontinuance, 534
  decannulation, 534
  flow rate adjustment, 533-34
  initiation, 533
Venoconstriction, and digitalis, 546
Venous cannulae, 100
Venous thrombosis, 476
Ventilation
  defined, 142
  efficiency of, 281
  manual, 310
  mechanical, 311-33
  monitoring of, 142, 143
  patterns, 318-21
  rate, in infants and children, 444
  spontaneous, 310-11
    vs mechanical, 129-30
  "triggered," 321, 323
Ventilation-perfusion (V/Q) imbalance, and mechanical ventilation, 313
Ventilator(s)
  Elma-Schonander servo-, 318
  "fighting," 329-30
  mechanical, 131
  pressure-cycled, 318
  pressure-limited, 130-31
  volume-controlled time-cycled, 443
  volume-cycled, 318
  volume-limited, 130-31
  weaning from, 446-47
Ventilator support, methodology of, 304-06
Ventilator therapy, effect on lung morphology, 297
Ventilatory and respiratory care
  in infants, 446
  postsurgical
    management techniques, 309-12
    mechanical, 312-33
Ventilatory and respiratory complications, management of, 337-50
Ventilatory and respiratory function, postoperative assessment of, 142-44
Ventricular afterload. *See also* Afterload; Vascular resistance.
  optimizing, 221-22, 449
  pharmacologic reduction, 221-22, 567
Ventricular contraction cycle, 457
Ventricular dysfunction
  left, hemodynamic changes in patient who succumbed from, 137
  right, postcardiotomy, 530
Ventricular dysplasia, right, 257

Ventricular failure. *See* Cardiac performance.
Ventricular failure, right, mechanical support for, 431-34
  discontinuance, 534
  flow rate adjustment, 533-34
  initiation, 533
  patient preparation, 532
  rationale, 531
  technical considerations, 532
Ventricular fibrillation, 470, 483
Ventricular filling pressures
  left, reliability of estimation methods, 490
  optimizing, 219-21
Ventricular pacing, hemodynamic changes associated with, 218
Ventricular performance, left, mechanical support
  intraaortic balloon counterpulsation, 224-25
  left heart bypass, 225-28
Ventricular power failure, 514
Ventricular septal defect, 249, 251, 448
Ventricular stroke work index, left (LVSWI), effect of morphine on, 52
Ventriculotomy, 449
Ventriculotomy of Guiraudon, 255
Vessel wall alteration, effect on blood flow, 368-69
Viral infection
  and postperfusion syndrome, 419
  and postpericardiotomy syndrome, 418
Viral hepatitis
  clinical features, 422-23
  drug therapy, 423
  immunologic methods, 421-22
  incidence, 421
  management, 423

Viral hepatitis *continued*
  pathogenesis, 421
Visual impairment, postoperative, 390
Vital sign monitor, 441
Vitamin K deficiency, 375
V_4 needle electrodes, placement of, 47
Von Willebrand's disease, 375
Vulnerable period, 458

Weaning
  from IABC support, 525
  infants and children from ventilator, 446-47
  from left heart assist device, 529-30
  from mechanical ventilation
    alternate methods, 332-33
    criteria for initiation of, 330-32
    extubation criteria, 332
  from ventilator support, 298-99
  from ventroarterial bypass support, 534
Whole body perfusion, 389. *See also* Cardiopulmonary bypass; Extracorporeal circulation.
  and acid-base balance, 87-88
  oxygen and carbon dioxide tensions, 86-87
  oxygen requirements, 80
  physiologic requirements and characteristics of, 80-88
  pressures, 83-84
  temperature, 82-83
Wolff-Parkinson-White (W-P-W) syndrome, 456
  A-V bypass pathways in, 253
  categories, 251-52
  digitalis in, 548
Wound infection, 475, 476